MOSBY'S

# Comprehensive
# Review
for
Veterinary Technicians

# MOSBY'S

# Comprehensive Review for Veterinary Technicians

## Third Edition

Edited by

**Monica M. Tighe, RVT, BA, MEd**
Professor, Veterinary Technician Program
St. Clair College of Applied Arts and Technology
Windsor, Ontario

**Marg Brown, RVT, BEd AD ED**
Professor, Veterinary Technician Program
Seneca College, King Campus
King City, Ontario

With 120 illustrations and 32 color plates

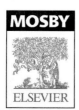

MOSBY

ELSEVIER

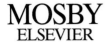

11830 Westline Industrial Drive
St. Louis, Missouri 63146

MOSBY'S COMPREHENSIVE REVIEW FOR VETERINARY
TECHNICIANS, EDITION 3

ISBN: 978-0-323-05214-6

---

**Notice**

Knowledge and best practice in this field are constantly changing. As new research and experience broaden our knowledge, changes in practice, treatment, and drug therapy may become necessary or appropriate. Readers are advised to check the most current information provided (i) on procedures featured or (ii) by the manufacturer of each product to be administered, to verify the recommended dose or formula, the method and duration of administration, and contraindications. It is the responsibility of the practitioner, relying on his or her own experience and knowledge of the patient, to make diagnoses, to determine dosages and the best treatment for each individual patient, and to take all appropriate safety precautions. To the fullest extent of the law, neither the Publisher nor the Editors assume any liability for any injury and/or damage to persons or property arising out or related to any use of the material contained in this book.

The Publisher

---

**Library of Congress Control Number 2007929331**

*Vice President and Publisher:* Linda Duncan
*Publisher:* Penny Rudolph
*Managing Editor:* Teri Merchant
*Publishing Services Manager:* Patricia Tannian
*Senior Project Manager:* Kristine Feeherty
*Design Direction:* Maggie Reid

Printed in the United States of America

Last digit is the print number: 9  8  7  6  5  4  3

To all past, present, and future veterinary technology students—
best wishes for a long, happy, and fulfilling career!

To all of our family, friends, and co-workers—we couldn't
do all that we do without you . . . thanks always!

# Contributors

**Patricia L. Bell, RVT, BSc**
Instructor, Veterinary Technology
    and Biotechnology Programs
Saskatchewan Institute of Applied Sciences
    and Technologies
Kelsey Campus
Saskatoon, Saskatchewan

**Emma K. Brown, RVT, MIAT**
Professor, Veterinary Technician
Seneca College of Applied Arts and Technology
King City, Ontario

**Marg Brown, RVT, BEd AD ED**
Professor, Veterinary Technician Program
Seneca College, King Campus
King City, Ontario

**Frances Cheslo, AHT, RVT**
Veterinary Partnership Specialist
Hill's Pet Nutrition Canada
Mississauga, Ontario

**Susan Cornwell, RVT**
Large Animal Technician
Ontario Veterinary College
University of Guelph
Guelph, Ontario

**Antoniette D'Amato-Scheck, LVT**
Licensed Veterinary Technician, Instructional Support
    Associate
Veterinary Science Technology
College of Technology at Delhi
State University of New York
Delhi, New York

**Barbara Donaldson, BA, BEd, MEd, RVT, VDT**
Canadian Veterinary Dental Technician Program
School of Health Sciences
St. Lawrence College
Kingston, Ontario

**Sheila R. Grosdidier, BS, RVT, MCP, HRP**
Consultant, Veterinary Management Consultation, Inc.
Evergreen, Colorado

**Joanne Hamel, RVT, BA**
Retired Professor
St. Lawrence College
Kingston, Ontario

**Kim Healey, RVT**
Large Animal Clinic
Ontario Veterinary College
University of Guelph
Guelph, Ontario

**Rachael J. Higdon, MBA, LVT**
Program Director, Veterinary Technology
Department of Health Sciences
Baker College
Clinton Township, Michigan

**Geraldine Higginson, BSc, MSc, RVT**
Avian and Exotics Department
Veterinary Teaching Hospital
Ontario Veterinary College
University of Guelph
Guelph, Ontario

**Mary E. Martini, RVT, RLAT**
Manager, Campus Animal Facilities
Ontario Veterinary College
University of Guelph
Guelph, Ontario

**Pierry McLean, AHT, RVT**
Linwood Veterinary Services
Linwood, Ontario

**Monica Dixon Perry, CVPM**
Consultant, Veterinary Management Consultation, Inc.
Evergreen, Colorado

**Elisa A. Petrollini, CVT, VTS (ECC)**
Nursing Student Small Animal Practicum Supervisor
Veterinary Technology Program
Harcum College;
Assistant Supervisor, Emergency Service Nursing
Matthew J. Ryan Veterinary Hospital
University of Pennsylvania
Philadelphia, Pennsylvania

**Sally R. Powell, CVT, VTS (ECC)**
Supervisor of Nursing, Emergency Service
Matthew J. Ryan Veterinary Hospital
University of Pennsylvania
Philadelphia, Pennsylvania

**Teri Raffel, AAS, CVT**
Instructional Assistant
Veterinary Technician/Laboratory Animal Technician
    Programs
Madison Area Technical College
Madison, Wisconsin

**Penny Rivait, RVT, BA, RLAT**
Professor, Veterinary Technician Program
St. Clair College of Applied Arts and Technology
Windsor, Ontario

**Ed Robinson, VT, AAS, BA**
Instructor, Veterinary Technology
Penn Foster Career Schools
Scranton, Pennsylvania;
Lab Technician Supervisor, VML Labs
Healthy Pen Corporation
Cranston, Rhode Island

**Shirley Sandoval, RVT, AAS**
Scientific Instructional Technician II, Large Animal
    Theriogenology
College of Veterinary Medicine
Washington State University
Pullman, Washington

**Pam Schendel, BS, RVT**
Clinical Pathology Teaching Technologist, Comparative
    Pathobiology Department
School of Veterinary Medicine
Purdue University
West Lafayette, Indiana

**Margi Sirois, EdD, MS, RVT**
Program Director
Penn Foster College
Scottsdale, Arizona

**Lucy Siydock, BSc(H), RVT, VTS(Anesthesia)**
Lead Hand, Anesthesiology
Veterinary Teaching Hospital
Ontario Veterinary College
University of Guelph
Guelph, Ontario

**Sandra Skeba, AHT**
Field Biologist
Songbird, Burrowing Owl, Prairie Dog
Hawks Aloft
Albuquerque, New Mexico

**Teresa Sonsthagen, BS, LVT**
Instructor, Animal and Range Sciences
North Dakota State University
Fargo, North Dakota

**Jane M. Sykes, AHT, Reg**
Imaging Coordinator, Imaging Division
Lawson Health Research Institute
London, Ontario

**Marianne Tear, BA, MS, LVT**
Manager II, Division of Laboratory Animal Resources
Wayne State University;
Program Coordinator, Veterinary Technology
Wayne County Community College District
Detroit, Michigan

**Monica M. Tighe, RVT, BA, MEd**
Professor, Veterinary Technician Program
St. Clair College of Applied Arts and Technology
Windsor, Ontario

**James A. Topel, CVT**
Instructor, Veterinary Technician and Laboratory Animal
    Technician Programs
Madison Area Technical College
Madison, Wisconsin

**William L. Wade, LVT, LATG**
Operations Manager, Division of Laboratory Animal
    Resources
Duke University
Durham, North Carolina

**Dan Walsh, RVT, MPS**
Instructional Technologist, Veterinary Technology
School of Veterinary Medicine
Purdue University
West Lafayette, Indiana

**Elizabeth Warren, RVT**
Instructor, Health Professions Institute
Austin Community College
Austin, Texas

**Kisha L. White-Farrar, BSc, RVT**
Fort Worth, Texas

# Preface

*Mosby's Comprehensive Review for Veterinary Technicians,* Third Edition, is a reference book written by and for veterinary technicians. It is a must read for those needing a concise overview of veterinary technology. This strategic manual is extremely practical for those studying for the national accreditation examinations, students wishing to review important components, and graduates reviewing essential information.

The content is presented in an easy-to-read outline format. Each chapter includes learning outcomes, a clear and concise description of the important components, extensive references, and updated multiple-choice questions. Each chapter has been rewritten and updated by the original author or new authors to reflect changes in the field. Substantial material has been added to some of the chapters, and practical components have been emphasized.

This text is not meant to cover all areas of veterinary technology extensively; however, it is an excellent primary review guide that highly complements every veterinary technology textbook.

Appendixes include abbreviations, a metric system overview, medical terminology, species information, normal values, and veterinary technician resources. An important feature is the comprehensive test with an answer key, which includes 300 multiple-choice questions that cover each of the chapters equally. The makeup of this comprehensive test in no way reflects the percentage of topics on any credentialing examination.

A further essential addition is the inclusion of updated figures and color plates that will assist with the understanding of the content.

Once again, this textbook should prove to be an important asset to the veterinary technology profession.

## ACKNOWLEDGMENTS

We would like to extend our thanks and appreciation to Teri Merchant and Elsevier for their continued support of the Veterinary Technician profession. For many years Elsevier has assisted veterinary technicians by providing resources to increase their knowledge and understanding of veterinary science and ultimately benefit their ongoing learning experience. It is companies such as Elsevier that facilitate learning and teaching for veterinary technician students and their instructors.

**Monica M. Tighe and Marg Brown**

# Contents

## PART I  BASIC AND CLINICAL SCIENCES

1. **Animal Anatomy and Physiology, 2**
   Penny Rivait
2. **Urinalysis and Hematology, 24**
   Dan Walsh, William L. Wade,
   Antoniette D'Amato-Scheck, and Pam Schendel
3. **Cytology, 54**
   Margi Sirois
4. **Parasitology, 73**
   Ed Robinson
5. **Diagnostic Microbiology and Mycology, 98**
   Sandra Skeba
6. **Clinical Chemistry, 112**
   Joanne Hamel
7. **Virology, 126**
   Patricia L. Bell
8. **Immunology, 134**
   Patricia L. Bell

## PART II  CLINICAL APPLICATIONS

9. **Restraint and Handling, 144**
   Teresa Sonsthagen
10. **Sanitation, Sterilization, and Disinfection, 164**
    Teri Raffel
11. **Radiography, 173**
    Marg Brown
12. **Alternative Imaging Technology, 194**
    Jane M. Sykes and Pierry McLean

## PART III  PATIENT MANAGEMENT AND NUTRITION

13. **Genetics, Theriogenology, and Neonatal Care, 206**
    Marianne Tear and Margi Sirois
14. **Companion Animal Behavior, 231**
    Emma K. Brown
15. **Small Animal Nutrition, 243**
    Frances Cheslo
16. **Large Animal Nutrition and Feeding, 263**
    James A. Topel
17. **Laboratory Animal Medicine, 287**
    Mary E. Martini
18. **Exotic Animal Medicine, 311**
    Geraldine Higginson

## PART IV  ANESTHESIA AND PHARMACOLOGY

19. **Anesthesia, 334**
    Lucy Siydock
20. **Pharmacology, 367**
    Elizabeth Warren
21. **Pharmaceutical Calculations, 393**
    Monica M. Tighe

## PART V  MEDICAL AND SURGICAL NURSING

22. **Surgical Preparation and Instrument Care, 400**
    Rachael J. Higdon
23. **Small Animal Nursing, 414**
    Monica M. Tighe
24. **Equine Nursing and Surgery, 453**
    Susan Cornwell and Kim Healey
25. **Ruminant, South American Camelid, and Pig Nursing, Surgery, and Anesthesia, 471**
    Shirley Sandoval
26. **Veterinary Dentistry, 490**
    Barbara Donaldson
27. **Emergency Medicine, 507**
    Sally R. Powell and Elisa A. Petrollini
28. **Zoonoses, 523**
    Kisha L. White-Farrar

## PART VI  PRACTICE MANAGEMENT AND SELF-MANAGEMENT

29. **Personal, Practice, and Professional Management Skills and Ethics, 541**
    Monica Dixon Perry, Sheila R. Grosdidier, and Marg Brown

## APPENDIXES

A  Abbreviations and Symbols, 562
B  The Metric System and Equivalents, 568
C  Medical Terminology, 569
D  Species Names, 573
E  Normal Values, 574
F  Additional Veterinary Technician Resources, 575
G  Comprehensive Test with Answer Key, 576
H  Answer Key to Chapter Review Questions, 594

Color plates follow page 52

# PART I

# Basic and Clinical Sciences

## CHAPTER 1

# Animal Anatomy and Physiology

*Penny Rivait*

## OUTLINE

Definitions
Cell Structure and Physiology
   Prokaryote: "Before Nucleus"
   Eukaryote: "True Nucleus"
Movement In and Out of Cells
Tissues
   Epithelial Tissue
   Connective Tissue
   Muscle Tissue
   Nervous Tissue

Membranes
Directional Terminology
Body Systems
   Skeletal System
   Muscular System
   Nervous System
   Cardiovascular System
   Central Vascular System
   Digestive System
   Lymphatic System

Respiratory System
Excretory System
Reproductive System: Male
Reproductive System: Female
Endocrine System
Integumentary System
Senses

## LEARNING OUTCOMES

After reading this chapter you should be able to:

1. Explain the various processes that enable substances to move in and out of cells.
2. List the structural and functional characteristics of the four primary body tissues and their subtypes.
3. Define and be able to use all directional terms.
4. Classify and identify basic bones and joints.
5. List the three types of muscle and state the distinct characteristics of each.
6. Describe the divisions of the nervous system and state how they relate to each other.
7. List the parts of the brain and state their functions.
8. List the parts of the cardiovascular system and state their functions.
9. Explain the cardiac cycle and identify its components on a typical electrocardiogram.
10. Compare and contrast the structure and function of arteries and veins.
11. Explain the process of digestion.
12. Name the parts of the ruminant stomach and state their functions.
13. Describe the structure and function of lymph vessels, lymph nodes, and lymphatic organs.
14. Name the parts of the respiratory system and state their functions.

15. Describe the three basic processes of respiration.
16. Define *tidal volume, residual volume, dead space, apnea, eupnea,* and *dyspnea.*
17. Explain the anatomy and functions of the excretory system.
18. Explain the anatomy and physiology of the male and female reproductive systems.
19. Explain the estrous cycle.
20. Describe the processes of parturition and lactation.
21. List the endocrine glands; state the hormones they release and their functions.
22. Describe the structure and function of all sense organs.

Anatomy and physiology are the essential foundations of veterinary technology. Many clinical procedures, such as positioning of a patient for a radiograph, preparing for a surgical procedure, or simply placing a catheter, involve a working knowledge of anatomy and physiology. Understanding the unique interrelationships of the animal's body systems is critical in assisting with the management of disease.

## DEFINITIONS ▰▰▰▰▰▰▰▰

I. Anatomy: the science of the structure of the body and the relation of its parts
II. Physiology: the science of how the body functions

## CELL STRUCTURE AND PHYSIOLOGY ▰▰▰▰

Cells are the basic unit of life. Cells are either prokaryotes or eukaryotes.

### Prokaryote: "Before Nucleus"

I. A cell that lacks a true membrane-bound nucleus
II. All bacteria are prokaryotes

### Eukaryote: "True Nucleus"

I. A cell that has a membrane-bound nucleus and contains many different membrane-bound organelles
II. All multicellular organisms are composed of eukaryotic cells
III. Composition of eukaryotic cells
Three major parts: cell membrane, cytoplasm, and nucleus
  A. Cell membrane (plasma membrane)
    Separates the cell from its external environment
    1. Consists of a double phospholipid layer with interspersed proteins (fluid-mosaic model); also contains carbohydrate chains and cholesterol
    2. Semipermeable; therefore allows various substances to move in and out of the cell
    3. Some cells have surface modifications, such as hairlike projections (cilia) that are used for surface movement, a single longer projection (flagellum) that is used for cellular movement, or microvilli that increase surface area (especially in absorptive cells)
  B. Cytoplasm
    Encompasses everything within the cell except the nucleus. Organelles within the cytoplasm have very specialized functions
    1. Ribosomes
      a. Float freely or are attached to the endoplasmic reticulum
      b. Composed of protein and ribosomal ribonucleic acid (RNA)
      c. Site of protein synthesis
    2. Mitochondria
      a. "Powerhouse" of the cell
      b. Contains mitochondrial deoxyribonucleic acid (DNA) and protein
      c. Double membrane with the inner membrane extending into folds called cristae
      d. Cristae increase surface area for production of adenosine triphosphate (ATP)
      e. ATP is produced through the process of cellular respiration (Krebs cycle, citric acid cycle, tricarboxylic acid cycle)
      f. Cells that use large amounts of energy (e.g., skeletal muscle) have large numbers of mitochondria
    3. Endoplasmic reticulum (ER)
      a. Rough endoplasmic reticulum (RER)
        (1) Hollow system of flattened membranous channels with attached ribosomes
        (2) Acts as transportation network for proteins
      b. Smooth endoplasmic reticulum (SER)
        (1) Hollow system of flattened membranous channels without attached ribosomes
        (2) Not involved in protein synthesis
        (3) Important in synthesizing cholesterol, steroid-based hormones, and lipids; also important in detoxification of drugs, breakdown of glycogen, and transportation of fats
        (4) Liver cells, intestinal cells, and interstitial cells of the testes have large amounts of SER
    4. Golgi complex (Golgi apparatus)
      a. Stacked, saucer-shaped membranes that function as a receiving, packaging, and distribution center
      b. Modifies and packages substances received from the ER and then exports them from the cell or releases them into the cytoplasm for internal use
      c. Produces lysosomes
    5. Lysosomes
      a. Contain digestive enzymes that digest intracellular bacteria and break down nonfunctional organelles
      b. Are the principal organelles in digestion of nutrients
      c. Autolysis (i.e., self-digestion of the cell) occurs if the lysosome enzymes are released into cytoplasm
      d. Large numbers found in phagocytic cells
    6. Peroxisomes
      a. Membrane-bound organelles that contain strong oxidase and catalase enzymes
      b. Use oxygen to detoxify toxic substances, especially alcohol and formaldehyde
      c. Very important in converting free radicals (normal byproducts of cellular metabolism but harmful to biological molecules if left to accumulate) into hydrogen peroxide, which is converted to water by catalase enzymes

d. Large numbers found in liver and kidney cells

7. Cytoskeleton
   a. Consists of microtubules, microfilaments, and intermediate filaments, which are all made of proteins
   b. Provides an elaborate internal framework that gives the cell form, structure, and support; anchors organelles; and enables movement

8. Centrioles
   a. Microtubules arranged to form a hollow tube
   b. Important in organizing the mitotic spindle
   c. Form the base of cilia and flagella

C. Nucleus
   1. Control center of the cell
   2. Contains DNA, which governs heredity and protein synthesis
   3. DNA is in the form of chromatin in the nondividing cell and in the form of chromosomes in the dividing cell
   4. Has a double, semipermeable nuclear membrane or envelope
   5. Contains one or more nucleoli, which manufacture the ribosomal units

## MOVEMENT IN AND OUT OF CELLS

I. Definitions
   A. Solute: a substance that can be dissolved
   B. Solvent: a substance that does the dissolving
   C. Solution: when the solute has dissolved and is no longer distinguishable from the solvent (a uniform mixture)
   D. Intracellular: within a cell
   E. Extracellular: outside of a cell
   F. Intercellular: between cells (interstitial)

II. Passive processes: no energy is expended by the cell
   A. Diffusion
      1. Movement of molecules (e.g., water and ions) from a high concentration to a low concentration
      2. Oxygen enters a cell and carbon dioxide exits a cell by simple diffusion through the lipid layer of the cell membrane
   B. Facilitated diffusion
      1. Diffusion with the aid of carrier proteins
      2. Glucose enters the cell by this method
   C. Osmosis
      1. Movement of water through a semipermeable membrane from a region of low solute (high solvent) to a region of high solute (low solvent)
      2. Water constantly moves in and out of the cell by osmosis

3. Osmotic pressure is the amount of pressure necessary to stop the flow of water across the membrane

D. Filtration
   1. Substances are forced through a membrane by hydrostatic pressure; small solutes will pass through; larger molecules will not
   2. Important in kidney function

III. Active processes: energy is expended by the cell
   A. Endocytosis: materials are taken into the cell
      1. Phagocytosis ("cell eating"): cell membrane extends around solid particles
         a. Some white blood cells and macrophages are phagocytic
      2. Pinocytosis (bulk-phase) ("cell drinking"): cell membrane extends around fluid droplets
         a. Important in absorptive cells in small intestine
      3. Receptor mediated: specialized membrane receptors bind to substances entering the cell
         a. Enzymes, insulin, hormones, iron, and cholesterol enter the cell by this method
   B. Exocytosis: materials are expelled by a cell
      1. Waste products are excreted and useful products are secreted into the extracellular space
      2. Hormones, neurotransmitters, and mucus are released from the cell by this method
   C. Active transport
      1. Movement of molecules from a low concentration to a high concentration with the aid of carrier proteins
      2. Sodium-potassium pump is an active transport pump within cell membranes; most ions and amino acids move into cells by this method

IV. Hypotonic, hypertonic, and isotonic
   A. Hypotonic: extracellular fluid is less concentrated than the intracellular fluid
      1. Red blood cells placed in a hypotonic solution will gain water through osmosis and burst (hemolysis)
   B. Hypertonic: extracellular fluid is more concentrated than the intracellular fluid
      1. Red blood cells placed in a hypertonic solution will lose water through osmosis and *crenate* (shrivel)
   C. Isotonic: concentrations of the extracellular and intracellular fluids are equal
      1. Red blood cells placed in an isotonic solution will remain unchanged, because osmotic pressures are equal

## TISSUES

I. Tissue: groups of similar cells with related functions
II. Histology or microanatomy: the study of tissues
III. Four primary types of tissue

A. Epithelial
B. Connective
C. Muscle
D. Nervous

## Epithelial Tissue

I. Covers body surface, lines body cavities, and forms the active part of glands
   A. Functions are protection, secretion, excretion, filtration, absorption of nutrients, and receipt of sensory information
II. May form simple (one cell layer) or stratified (more than one cell layer) tissue
III. Subtypes
   A. Squamous epithelium
      1. Flat, thin, platelike cells
      2. Simple squamous epithelial tissue lines blood vessels (endothelium), alveoli of lungs, and thoracic and abdominal cavities
      3. Stratified squamous epithelial tissue is found in areas of wear: nonkeratinized tissue lines the mouth, esophagus, vagina, and rectum; keratinized tissue makes up the epidermis
   B. Cuboidal epithelium
      1. Cube-shaped cells
      2. Simple cuboidal epithelial tissue is important in absorption and secretion; forms the active part of glands and small ducts, ovary surface, and kidney tubules
      3. Stratified cuboidal epithelial tissue is fairly rare but lines the ducts of sweat, salivary, and mammary glands
   C. Columnar epithelium
      1. Tall, rectangular-shaped cells
         a. Simple columnar epithelial tissue lines the digestive tract from stomach to rectum and is important for absorption and secretion; these cells also have a surface modification known as microvilli and are associated with mucus-secreting cells known as goblet cells
         b. Simple columnar epithelial tissue with cilia lines bronchi, uterine tubes, and uterus
         c. Stratified columnar epithelial tissue is relatively rare but is found in mammary ducts and portions of the male's urethra
   D. Pseudostratified columnar epithelium
      1. Appears to be more than one layer, but all cells touch the basal membrane
      2. Usually ciliated and often associated with goblet cells; found in the respiratory tract
   E. Transitional epithelium
      1. May resemble both cuboidal and squamous shapes depending on the thickness of the organ but is found in areas where a great degree of distention is needed, such as the urinary bladder, ureters, and part of the urethra (cuboidal when bladder is empty and squamous when bladder is full)
   F. Glandular epithelium
      1. Highly specialized epithelial cells with the ability to secrete various products
      2. Classified as endocrine or exocrine
         a. Endocrine: ductless and secrete hormones directly into the bloodstream (e.g., estrogen secreted by ovaries)
         b. Exocrine: have ducts and secrete onto an epithelial surface (e.g., sweat glands)
            (1) Exocrine glands are numerous and classified in many different ways, especially by their structure, method of secretion, and type of secretion

## Connective Tissue

I. Widely distributed throughout the body and composed of three elements: cells, fibers, and matrix (ground substance)
II. Has a variety of functions depending on tissue type (connects and supports, protects, insulates, transports fluids, and stores energy)
III. Fiber types
   A. Collagen fibers (white fibers): long, straight, very strong white fibers composed of collagen
   B. Elastic fibers (yellow fibers): long, thin, branching, stretchable yellow fibers composed of elastin
   C. Reticular fibers: fine, collagen fibers in a complex network
IV. Cell types
   A. Many different cell types depending on the tissue; immature and active cells have the suffix -*blast*, and mature cells have the suffix -*cyte*
V. Connective tissue types are divided into two categories: connective tissue proper and specialized connective tissue and their subtypes (Table 1-1)

## Muscle Tissue

I. Skeletal (striated)
   A. Voluntary control
   B. Long, parallel striated fibers with multiple nuclei located at their periphery
   C. Attach to and move bones
II. Smooth
   A. Involuntary control
   B. Spindle-shaped, smooth cells with a centrally located nucleus
   C. Found in walls of hollow organs (e.g., digestive tract, blood vessels)
III. Cardiac
   A. Involuntary control

**Table 1-1** Connective tissue categories

| Type/subtype | Examples and composition |
|---|---|
| **CONNECTIVE TISSUE PROPER** | |
| *Loose* | |
| Areolar | Most widely distributed; supports organs; protects and provides flexibility for all three fiber types |
| | Fibroblasts, macrophages, mast cells, white blood cells |
| Adipose | Insulates, protects, cushions |
| | Reserve energy composed of fat cells (adipocytes) |
| Reticular | Supportive tissue |
| | Found in spleen, liver, lymph nodes, and bone marrow |
| | Network of fine reticular fibers, macrophages, and fibroblasts |
| *Dense* | |
| Regular | Tendons (bone to muscle), ligaments (bone to bone), and aponeuroses (muscle to muscle) |
| | Collagen fibers arranged in a parallel pattern and fibroblasts provide strong attachments |
| Irregular | Dermis of the skin, organ capsules, joint capsules |
| | Collagen fibers arranged in an irregular pattern, elastic fibers, fibroblasts |
| | Provide strength and support to areas experiencing tension from all directions |
| Elastic | Ligaments that contain more elastic fibers than collagen; nuchal ligament in horse's neck |
| **SPECIALIZED** | |
| *Cartilage* | |
| Hyaline | Nose, trachea, larynx, embryonic skeleton, costal cartilage, articular cartilage |
| | Collagen fibers and chondrocytes support with some flexibility |
| Elastic | Pinna, auditory canal, epiglottis, elastic fibers |
| | Provides shape and great flexibility |
| Fibrocartilage | Intervertebral discs, pubic symphysis, disk in stifle thick collagen fibers, and chondrocytes |
| | Provide strong support |
| *Bone (Osseous)* | |
| Compact (dense) | Bones, collagen fibers, osteocytes, and calcified matrix |
| | Supports, protects, houses blood-producing tissue, stores calcium and other minerals |
| *Blood* | |
| Spongy (cancellous) | Latticelike bone structure |
| | Erythrocytes, leukocytes, thrombocytes, plasma |

B. Long, striated cells that are joined at points known as intercalated discs; have a single, centrally located nucleus

C. Found only in the heart (myocardium)

## Nervous Tissue

I. Specialized for conducting electrical impulses

II. Major locations are brain, spinal cord, and nerves

III. Two major cell types: neurons, which conduct impulses; and neuroglial (glial) cells, which are supporting cells and do not conduct impulses

## MEMBRANES

I. Membranes are made up of more than one tissue, which is usually a type of epithelial tissue attached to a type of connective tissue.

II. There are three types of membranes
  A. Mucous membranes (mucosae)
    1. Membranes that line hollow organs and connect to the exterior
    2. Usually stratified, squamous, or simple columnar epithelium attached to loose connective tissue known as lamina propria

3. Mucous membranes are adapted to absorb and secrete; normally secrete mucus, which lubricates both the respiratory and digestive pathways
4. The color of mucous membranes is used to evaluate many conditions in animals (e.g., blue mucous membranes indicate hypoxia)

B. Serous membranes (serosa)
1. Membranes that line body cavities but do not connect to the exterior
2. Simple squamous epithelium connected to a layer of loose connective (areolar) tissue
3. Secretes a thin, watery fluid (i.e., serous fluid), which reduces friction between parietal and visceral surfaces
4. Serous membranes are named according to their location and organ (e.g., parietal peritoneum and visceral peritoneum, parietal pericardium and visceral pericardium, parietal pleura and visceral pleura)

C. Cutaneous membranes (integument or skin)
1. Consist of keratinized, stratified squamous epithelium (epidermis) attached to a layer of dense irregular connective tissue (dermis)
2. Because it is exposed to the environment, it provides durability, protection, and waterproofing

## DIRECTIONAL TERMINOLOGY

I. Cranial: toward the head (e.g., the thoracic vertebrae are cranial to the sacral vertebrae)
II. Caudal: toward the tail (e.g., the lumbar vertebrae are caudal to the cervical vertebrae)
III. Dorsal: toward the backbone (e.g., the thoracic vertebrae are dorsal to the sternum)
IV. Ventral: away from the backbone (e.g., the umbilicus is on the ventral surface of the cat)
V. Medial: closest to the median plane (e.g., the tibia is medial to the fibula)
VI. Lateral: farthest from the medial plane (e.g., the ribs are lateral to the sternum)
VII. Proximal: the point closest to the backbone; used especially in reference to limbs (e.g., the greater trochanter is on the proximal end of the femur)
VIII. Distal: the point farthest from the backbone; used especially in reference to limbs (e.g., the fabella is located at the distal end of the femur)
IX. Anterior: toward the head; used especially in reference to limbs (e.g., the patella is on the anterior aspect of the rear leg)
X. Posterior: toward the tail; used especially in reference to limbs (e.g., the Achilles tendon is on the posterior aspect of the rear leg)
XI. Palmar: bottom of the front foot
XII. Plantar: bottom of the rear foot

## BODY SYSTEMS
### Skeletal System

I. Osteology: study of bones
II. Skeletal divisions
A. Axial skeleton
1. Bones found on the midline or attached to it (excludes the limbs)
2. Examples include the ribs, skull, vertebral column, and sternum
B. Appendicular skeleton
1. All bones that are present in the limbs (e.g., femur, humerus)
III. Function of bones
A. Support soft tissues of the body
B. Protect vital organs (e.g., heart)
C. Act as levers for muscle attachment
D. Store minerals
E. Produce blood cells
IV. Types of bone
A. Compact (dense) bone
1. Has very few spaces, appears solid, and provides strength and support
2. Made of haversian systems (osteons); each system is composed of the following:
a. Central haversian canal: houses blood vessels and nerves
b. Canaliculi: very small canals that radiate out, connecting all lacunae to each other and to the central haversian canal
c. Lamellae: concentric rings of bone
d. Lacunae: small spaces that house osteocytes (mature bone cells)
B. Spongy (cancellous) bone
1. No haversian systems
2. Has large spaces between latticelike pieces of bone known as trabeculae
3. Spaces are filled with marrow
V. Types of bone cells
A. Osteoblast: immature bone cell that produces the bone matrix known as osteoid
B. Osteocyte: mature bone cell; each cell occupies a lacunae in bone
C. Osteoclast: very large multinucleated cells that are capable of dissolving bone matrix and releasing minerals, which is a process known as osteolysis, or resorption
1. It is important for the body to maintain a balance between osteoblast and osteoclast activity
VI. Classification of bones
A. Long bones
1. Consist of a long cylindrical shaft (diaphysis), two ends (epiphyses), and a marrow cavity (e.g., radius, femur)

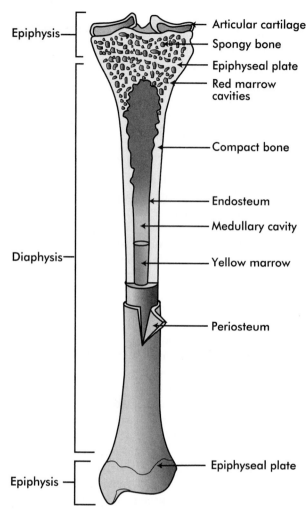

Epiphysis

Diaphysis

Epiphysis

Articular cartilage
Spongy bone
Epiphyseal plate
Red marrow cavities

Compact bone

Endosteum
Medullary cavity

Yellow marrow

Periosteum

Epiphyseal plate

**Figure 1-1** Parts of a long bone. (From Colville T, Bassert JM: *Clinical anatomy and physiology for veterinary technicians,* St Louis, 2002, Mosby.)

2. Main supporting bones of the body
3. Parts of a long bone (Figure 1-1)
   a. Diaphysis: shaft
   b. Epiphysis: proximal or distal end of the bone
   c. Articular cartilage: hyaline cartilage that covers the ends of the bones
   d. Periosteum: fibrous membrane covering outside of bone; rich in blood, nerves, and lymphatic vessels
   e. Endosteum: lines the marrow cavity
   f. Medullary (marrow) cavity: space within the bone center that contains marrow (red or yellow); red marrow is hematopoietic tissue that produces blood cells; yellow marrow is primarily fat
   g. Epiphyseal cartilage: region between diaphysis and epiphysis where bone grows in length; often referred to as the *growth plate*; becomes the epiphyseal line in mature animals

B. Short bones
   1. Small, cube-shaped bones
   2. Two thin layers of compact bone with spongy bone between the layers
   3. Function as shock absorbers (e.g., carpus, tarsus)
C. Flat bones
   1. Thin, flat bones
   2. Two layers of compact bone with spongy bone between the layers; resembles a sandwich
   3. Have a protective function (e.g., pelvis, scapula, ribs, and many bones of the skull)
D. Pneumatic bones
   1. Contain sinuses (e.g., frontal)
E. Irregular bones
   1. Unpaired bones with complicated shapes that do not fit any other category (e.g., vertebra, some skull bones) (Table 1-2)
F. Sesamoid bones
   1. Small short bones attached to tendons
   2. Reduce friction along a joint (e.g., patella)
VII. Osteogenesis (ossification): formation of bone (Figure 1-2)
   A. Endochondral
      1. Bones formed from cartilage bars laid down in the embryo
      2. Majority of bones in the body are formed by this method
   B. Intramembranous
      1. Bones formed from fibrous membranes laid down in the embryo
      2. Most flat bones are formed by this method
      3. Osteoblasts produce new bone and become mature osteocytes
VIII. Skeletal species differences (see Table 1-2 for species variations)
   A. Cat has a clavicle; dog does not
   B. Male dogs have a nonarticulating bone (os penis) in the penis
IX. Articulations (joints)
   A. Formed when two or more bones are united by fibrous, elastic, or cartilaginous tissue
   B. Classification by function
      1. Synarthrosis: immovable joint (e.g., skull sutures)
      2. Amphiarthrosis: slightly movable joint (e.g., pubic symphysis)
      3. Diarthrosis: freely movable joint (e.g., stifle)
   C. Classification by structure
      1. Fibrous: united by fibrous tissue; no joint cavity; synarthroses (e.g., skull sutures)
      2. Cartilaginous: united by cartilage; no joint cavity; amphiarthroses (e.g., intervertebral discs, pubic symphysis)

**Table 1-2**  Vertebral formulas

| Species | No. of cervical vertebrae | No. of thoracic vertebrae | No. of lumbar vertebrae | No. of sacral vertebrae | No. of caudal or coccygeal vertebrae |
|---|---|---|---|---|---|
| Dog, cat | 7 | 13 | 7 | 3 | 21-23 |
| Horse | 7 | 18 | 6 | 5 | 15-20 |
| Cow | 7 | 13 | 6 | 5 | 18-20 |
| Pig | 7 | 14-15 | 6-7 | 4 | 20-23 |
| Sheep | 7 | 13 | 6-7 | 4 | 16-18 |
| Human | 7 | 12 | 5 | 5 | 4 |

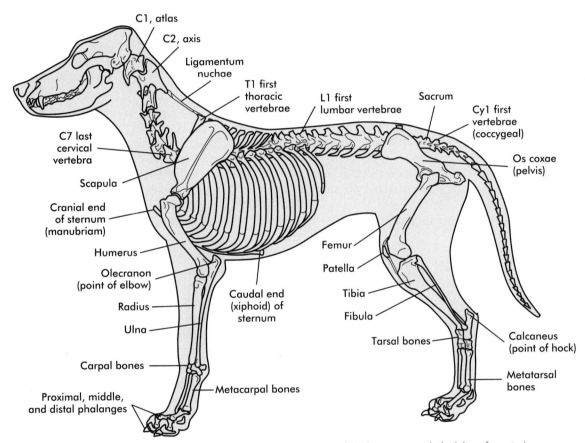

**Figure 1-2**  Canine skeleton. (From Colville T, Bassert JM: *Clinical anatomy and physiology for veterinary technicians*, St Louis, 2002, Mosby.)

3. Synovial: joint cavity filled with synovial fluid; synovial membrane and joint capsule; diarthroses (e.g., all joints of the limbs)
   a. Majority of the joints in the body are synovial
   b. They are classified into several types (Table 1-3)

## Muscular System

I. Function
   A. Produces movement of entire body or parts
   B. Maintains posture
   C. Produces heat

II. Types
There are three types of muscle: skeletal, smooth, and cardiac
   A. Skeletal muscle (striated, voluntary)
      1. Skeletal muscle cells are long, striated fibers that run parallel to each other
      2. Cells are multinucleated with the nuclei on the periphery
      3. Functional unit is a sarcomere
      4. Each muscle fiber is a muscle cell consisting of many myofibrils
      5. Myofibrils are composed of myofilaments (i.e., actin and myosin)

**Table 1-3**  Types of synovial joints

| Synovial joint | Structure | Location | Movement |
|---|---|---|---|
| Ball and socket (spheroid) | Ball-shaped head articulates with cup-shaped depression | Shoulder, hip | Flexion, extension, abduction, adduction, rotation, circumduction |
| Arthrodial (condyloid) | Oval articulating surfaces | Radiocarpal joints | Flexion, extension |
| Trochoid (pivot) | Rounded end of one bone articulates with a ring of bone | Atlantoaxial | Rotation |
| Hinge (ginglymus) | Cylindrical bone fits into depression | Stifle, elbow | Flexion, extension |
| Gliding | Flat, articulating surfaces | Radioulnar, intervertebral | Flexion, extension |
| Saddle | Concave surface articulates with a convex bone | Carpometacarpal, in primates only | Flexion, extension, abduction, adduction, rotation, circumduction |

B. Smooth muscle (visceral, nonstriated, involuntary)
1. Smooth muscle cells are spindle shaped with one centrally located nucleus and no striations
2. Responsible for involuntary movement (e.g., digestion)
3. Two types of smooth muscle: single unit or visceral smooth muscle and multiunit smooth muscle
4. Single-unit smooth muscle is found in sheets and forms the walls of many hollow organs (e.g., intestines); contraction occurs in waves
5. Multiunit smooth muscle is found as individual fibers, and the fibers are activated by the autonomic nervous system (e.g., arrector muscle of hair, eye muscles)

C. Cardiac muscle (myocardium)
1. Involuntary, striated cells that branch to form a network
2. Cells are joined by intercalated discs, which aid in conduction of the nervous impulse to coordinate contraction

D. Contraction of skeletal muscle by mechanism described in the sliding-filament theory
1. A nerve impulse travels down a motor nerve axon
2. Acetylcholine is released into the synaptic cleft, transmitting the impulse to the sarcolemma
3. Impulse is conducted into the T tubules and to the sarcoplasmic reticulum
4. Calcium is released from the sarcoplasmic reticulum
5. Calcium binds to troponin, which causes a change in the conformation of tropomyosin

6. This change exposes the myosin binding sites on the actin
7. ATP is hydrolyzed, providing the energy required for contraction
8. Myosin binds to actin, forming cross-bridges during this active phase of muscle contraction
9. Myosin continues to attach, pull, and detach, which moves the actin toward the center of the sarcomere
10. When the nerve impulse stops, calcium is actively transported back into the sarcoplasmic reticulum and muscle relaxes; energy is also required for relaxation
11. All-or-none principle states that muscle fibers either contract to their fullest or not at all

E. Skeletal muscle actions
1. Flexor: usually decreases the angle of a joint
2. Extensor: usually increases the angle of a joint
3. Abductor: moves a bone away from the midline
4. Adductor: moves a bone toward the midline
5. Levator: produces a dorsally directed movement
6. Depressor: produces a ventrally directed movement
7. Sphincter: decreases the size of an opening

## Nervous System

The central nervous system (CNS) consists of the brain and spinal cord.

I. Brain
A. Cerebrum
1. Site of motor control, interpretation of sensory impulses, and areas of association

Nervous System

## ORGANIZATION

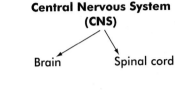

**Central Nervous System (CNS)**

Brain       Spinal cord

**Peripheral Nervous System (PNS)**

Afferent division (receptors to CNS)       Efferent division (CNS to body)

Somatic NS (CNS to skeletal muscles)       Autonomic NS (CNS to smooth muscle and glands)

Sympathetic NS       Parasympathetic NS

2. Basic arrangement consists of outer gray matter, which contains neuron cell bodies, and inner white matter, which consists mainly of axons
3. Surface area increased by gyri (elevations) and sulci (fissures)

B. Diencephalon
1. Region of thalamus and hypothalamus
2. Thalamus acts as a relay station for sensory impulses and interprets some sensations, such as temperature and pain
3. Hypothalamus regulates many homeostatic functions (e.g., body temperature, fluid balance, thirst, urine output, food intake, emotion, and behavioral patterns) and has an important connection with the endocrine system

C. Brain stem
1. Consists of midbrain, pons, and medulla oblongata
2. Midbrain serves as a connecting link
3. Pons contains important respiratory centers
4. In the medulla oblongata, nerve fibers cross from left to right, and vice versa
5. Medulla also influences respiratory rate, heart rate, vomiting, coughing, and sneezing
6. Throughout the brain stem is the reticular activating system (RAS), which is responsible for sleep/wake cycles

D. Cerebellum
1. Responsible for coordination and balance

II. Spinal cord
A. Runs through the vertebral foramen
B. Basic arrangement consists of outer white matter, which contains nerve fibers, and a butterfly-shaped inner region of gray matter composed of neuron cell bodies
C. Contains ascending and descending nerve tracts
D. Major function is to convey sensory (afferent) nerve impulses from the periphery to the brain and to conduct motor (efferent) nerve impulses from the brain to the periphery
E. Brain and spinal cord are protected by bone and meninges

III. Meninges
A. Dura mater: outer layer composed of dense, fibrous connective tissue
B. Arachnoid (arachnoidea) mater: middle layer consisting of very delicate and elastic connective tissue
C. Pia mater: transparent, delicate connective tissue that contains tiny blood vessels and adheres to the surface of the brain and spinal cord
D. Epidural space: between bone and dura mater; contains loose connective tissue, blood vessels, and fat; injection of anesthetic agents into this region causes temporary nerve paralysis
E. Subarachnoid space: contains cerebrospinal fluid and large blood vessels

IV. Cerebrospinal fluid (CSF)
A. Colorless, watery fluid; contains protein, glucose, ions, and other substances
B. pH and pressure are particularly important
C. Cushions and nourishes the brain
D. A lumbar or CSF tap is used for CSF sampling

V. Blood-brain barrier
A. The blood-brain barrier protects the brain from fluctuations in chemical levels that are present within the bloodstream
B. Endothelial cells of the capillaries in the brain are joined by tight junctions, thereby forming an impermeable barrier (i.e., the blood-brain barrier)
C. Lipid-soluble substances, such as oxygen, carbon dioxide, and steroid hormones, enter the brain by dissolving through the capillary cell walls
D. Essential substances (e.g., glucose and amino acids) are transported into the brain by facilitated diffusion
E. Many other substances (e.g., waste products and drugs) are blocked by the blood-brain barrier

VI. Peripheral nervous system (PNS)
A. Consists of all nerve processes connecting to the CNS; includes all cranial and spinal nerves

B. Divided into two major divisions: afferent (sensory) and efferent (motor)

C. Afferent or sensory nerves carry impulses from sensory receptors to the CNS for interpretation

D. Efferent or motor nerves carry impulses from the CNS to skeletal muscle as part of the somatic division and to smooth muscle, glands, and heart as part of the autonomic system

E. All voluntary movements are part of the somatic division

F. The autonomic division serves all the involuntary functions and is further divided into sympathetic and parasympathetic nervous systems

  1. Sympathetic nerve fibers elicit the fight-or-flight response in emergencies or stressful situations (e.g., increased heart rate, respiratory rate, and blood flow)

  2. Parasympathetic nerve fibers are responsible for quiet activities (e.g., digestion, heart rate) and return the body to normal levels after the sympathetic response

VII. Principal cells of the nervous system

A. Neuron (nerve cell)

  1. Composed of dendrites, cell body, and axon

  2. Dendrites receive the impulse and conduct it to the cell body, which in turn conducts it to the axon, which leads the impulse away to a synapse

  3. Nerve impulses are generated by action potentials

  4. An action potential is depolarization followed by repolarization; the electrical charge of the cell is reversed and then returned to normal

  5. Impulses travel in one direction

  6. Nerve cell bodies cannot regenerate if damaged

  7. Some nerve cells have an insulative covering known as myelin; myelin is interrupted at the nodes of Ranvier—impulses jump from node to node, making transmission along myelinated nerve fibers faster than along nonmyelinated nerve fibers. This mode of conduction is known as saltatory conduction.

B. Neuroglial cells (glial)

  1. Connective tissue cells within the CNS and PNS; are supportive and protective only and do not transmit impulses

  2. There are six types: four are found in the CNS and two in the PNS

  3. Glial cells in the CNS

    a. Astrocytes: star shaped, most abundant, support nervous tissue, stimulate formation of blood-brain barrier

    b. Oligodendrocyte: smaller, wrap around axons to form myelin in CNS

    c. Microglia: phagocytic cells

    d. Ependymal: ciliated, which helps circulate CSF

  4. Glial cells in the PNS

    a. Schwann cells: wrap around axons to form myelin in peripheral nerves; comparable to oligodendrocytes in the CNS

    b. Satellite cells: surround cell bodies but function is unknown

VIII. Reflexes

A. Automatic response to a stimulus

  1. Reflex arc involves a stimulus that is picked up by sensory receptors

  2. The impulse is transmitted along a sensory neuron to the spinal cord, where it synapses with an interneuron (three-head neuron reflex) or directly with a motor neuron (two-head neuron reflex)

  3. Impulse hits the effector organ, causing a response

  4. Some typical reflexes are the stretch reflex (knee-jerk reflex), withdrawal reflex, corneal reflex, and papillary light reflex

## Cardiovascular System

The cardiovascular system includes the heart *(cardio)* and blood vessels *(vascular)*.

I. Function

A. Heart provides the force to circulate blood to all parts of the body

II. Structure (Figure 1-3)

A. Myocardium is the heart (cardiac) muscle

B. Cardiac muscle cells are striated and are connected by intercalated discs

C. Intercalated discs have a low electrical resistance; therefore the impulse spreads very quickly and all cells seem to function as one

III. Protective layers

A. Pericardium: a double-walled membranous sac covering the myocardium

  1. The outer layer, enveloping the heart, is a tough fibrous connective tissue known as fibrous pericardium; deep to this layer is a more delicate layer known as serous pericardium

  2. Serous pericardium has two layers: the parietal layer adheres to the fibrous pericardium, and the visceral layer adheres to the myocardium

  3. Space between the two layers of serous pericardium is the pericardial cavity, filled with pericardial fluid, which reduces friction when the heart beats

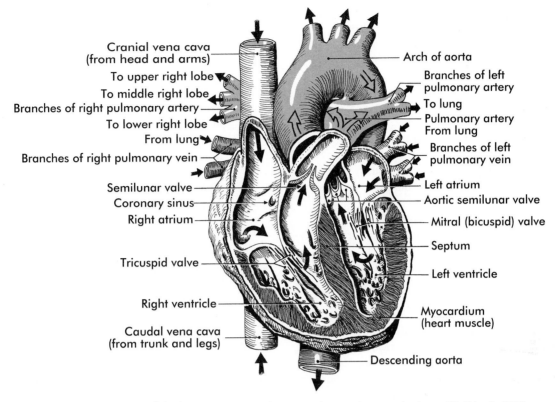

**Figure 1-3** Anatomy of the heart. (From McBride DF: *Learning veterinary terminology*, ed 2, St Louis, 2002, Mosby.)

B. Endocardium: a serous membrane lining the inner chambers of the heart

IV. Pulmonary circulation
  A. Consists of the precava (cranial vena cava or superior vena cava) and postcava (caudal vena cava or inferior vena cava)
  B. Precava and postcava empty into the right atrium; blood then passes through the tricuspid valve into the right ventricle and through the pulmonary artery (passes pulmonary semilunar valve) to the lungs, where the blood is oxygenated and returned to the heart via pulmonary veins

V. Systemic circulation (somatic circulation)
  A. Oxygenated blood in the left atrium flows through the bicuspid (mitral) valve to the left ventricle and out of the aorta (passes aortic semilunar valve) to all parts of the body
  B. Two branches come off of the aortic arch in dogs and cats
    1. Innominate artery (brachiocephalic), which branches into the right subclavian artery and right and left common carotid arteries
    2. Left subclavian artery

VI. Coronary circulation
  A. Coronary arteries provide nutrients and oxygen to the myocardium; coronary veins drain waste and carbon dioxide from the myocardium

VII. Cardiac cycle
  A. One complete cycle: as atria contract (systole), the ventricles relax (diastole); and as ventricles contract, the atria relax
  B. Atrial diastole: atria are at rest
    1. Right atrium is receiving blood from the precava and postcava while the left atrium is receiving blood from the pulmonary veins
  C. Atrial systole: atria are contracting
    1. Sinoatrial (SA) node fires, causing contraction of the atria; blood is pushed through the tricuspid and bicuspid valves into the right and left ventricles
  D. Ventricular diastole
    1. Ventricles receive blood from the atria
  E. Ventricular systole
    1. Impulse from the SA node has been conducted to the atrioventricular (AV) node, which conducts the impulse down the bundle of His (AV bundle) to the Purkinje fibers
    2. Ventricles are now stimulated to contract; blood is forced through the semilunar valves into the pulmonary artery to the lungs, and out of the aorta to all parts of the body

VIII. Heart sounds
  A. Auscultation (listening to heart sounds)
    1. Lubb, dupp, pause

a. *Lubb* is the first sound; it is a long sound made when the AV valves close

b. *Dupp* is the second sound; it is a short, sharp sound made when the semilunar valves close

IX. Heart rate

A. Animal heart rates vary with age, size, breed, health, and fitness

B. Dog: 70 to 160 beats per minute

C. Cat: 150 to 210 beats per minute

D. Heart rate may also be affected by chemicals, hormones, temperature, behavior, and respiratory rate

X. Electrocardiography (ECG [or EKG])

A. Electrocardiogram records the electrical activity of the heart

B. First wave is the P wave, which represents the electrical events during atrial systole (depolarization)

C. Large QRS complex represents the electrical events of ventricular systole (depolarization)

D. T wave represents the electrical events during ventricular diastole (repolarization)

E. Atrial diastole occurs during ventricular systole; therefore, it is masked by the QRS complex

## Central Vascular System

I. Blood vessels

A. Arteries

1. Carry blood away from the heart

2. Carry oxygenated blood (except for pulmonary artery)

3. Are thicker and stronger than veins

4. Pressure within is greater than in veins

B. Arterioles

1. Small arteries

2. Lead to capillaries and regulate the blood flow into them

C. Capillaries

1. Consist of one layer of endothelium

2. Microscopic diameter

3. Exchange of oxygen and carbon dioxide takes place here

D. Venules

1. Emerge from capillaries and enlarge into veins

E. Veins

1. Are larger than arteries and have thinner walls

2. Venous blood pressure is low; therefore they have valves to prevent the backflow of blood

3. Carry blood back to the heart

II. Fetal circulation

A. Lungs, kidneys, and digestive tract are nonfunctional in fetus but must be nourished with oxygen

B. Exchange of nutrients and waste takes place within the placenta

C. Oxygenated blood enters the fetus via one umbilical vein

D. Vein ascends toward the fetal liver and divides into two; one branch joins the hepatic portal vein and enters the liver, while the majority of blood flows into the ductus venosus, which connects to the postcava

E. Postcava enters the right atrium; precava from the head also enters the right atrium

F. Most of the blood goes directly through the foramen ovale to the left atrium, into the left ventricle, and out of the aorta to all parts of the fetus

G. Blood that goes into the right ventricle passes into the pulmonary artery; most blood is diverted through the ductus arteriosus into the aorta (a small amount goes to the lungs)

H. Blood in the descending aorta branches into the iliac arteries; the two umbilical arteries branch off and return deoxygenated blood to the placenta

## Digestive System

The digestive system breaks down foodstuff into absorbable nutrients to fuel the body. There are anatomical variations among different species depending on their diet.

I. Process

A. Digestive system uses five basic processes to prepare the food for utilization by the body

1. Ingestion of food

2. Peristalsis: moving food through the digestive tract

3. Mechanical and chemical digestion

4. Absorption

5. Defecation

II. Types of diets

A. Herbivore: plant-eating animal (e.g., rabbit, cow, horse, sheep)

B. Carnivore: meat-eating animal (e.g., cat, dog, tiger)

C. Omnivore: plant- and meat-eating animal (e.g., rats, pigs, humans)

III. Histological layers

A. Walls of gastrointestinal tract or alimentary canal can be divided into four layers

1. Mucosa, closest to the lumen: three sublayers

a. Epithelium: stratified squamous and simple columnar

b. Lamina propria: connective tissue

c. Muscularis mucosae: smooth muscle

2. Submucosa: loose connective tissue

3. Muscularis externa: two or three layers of smooth muscle depending on location

a. Oblique muscle: stomach has all three layers

b. Circular muscle

c. Longitudinal muscle

4. Serosa: loose connective tissue

IV. Structures
  A. Mouth
    1. Receives food and mixes it with saliva during mastication
    2. Bolus is formed
  B. Pharynx
    1. Common passageway for digestive and respiratory systems
  C. Esophagus
    1. Muscular tube running from the pharynx to the cardia (opening to stomach)
    2. Food moves through the esophagus via peristalsis
  D. Stomach
    1. Simple stomach: monogastric animals
      a. Found in humans, pigs, horses, and dogs
      b. Four regions: esophageal, cardiac, fundic, pyloric
        (1) Esophageal region is nonglandular
        (2) Cardiac region produces mucus
        (3) Fundic region is the true body of the stomach and contains true gastric glands, which have four distinct cell types
          (a) Mucous neck cells, which secrete mucus
          (b) Chief cells, which produce the enzyme pepsinogen
          (c) Parietal cells, which produce hydrochloric acid
          (d) Endocrine cells, which produce the hormone gastrin
        (4) Pyloric region produces mucus
      c. Has inner folds known as rugae
      d. Food is mixed in the stomach with secretions from the digestive glands until it is reduced to a liquid known as chyme
      e. pH of stomach is acidic
    2. Ruminant stomach
      a. Found in cattle, sheep, goats, and llamas
      b. All ruminants are herbivores, but not all herbivores are ruminants
      c. Animal regurgitates food (bolus), remasticates (rechews), and swallows it again (deglutition)
      d. Composed of four compartments: rumen, reticulum, omasum, and abomasum
        (1) Rumen: called "fermentation vat"
          (a) Largest compartment
          (b) Food is mixed and churned in a favorable environment (i.e., proper pH, temperature, bacteria, and anaerobic conditions)
        (2) Reticulum: called "hardware compartment"

          (a) Most cranial compartment that is not completely separate from the rumen
          (b) Also called the "honeycomb"
          (c) Acts as a passageway for food, paces the contraction of the rumen, and is the usual site for ingested foreign objects
        (3) Omasum
          (a) Grinds up the food and absorbs water and bicarbonate
          (b) Composed of many layers of laminae, which resemble leaves
        (4) Abomasum
          (a) True glandular stomach
          (b) Mixes the food with enzymes, initiating chemical digestion
  E. Small intestine
    1. Divided into three regions: duodenum, jejunum, ileum
    2. Major site of digestion and absorption
    3. Three specialized structures increase the surface area of the small intestine
      a. Circular folds: deep, mucosal folds
      b. Intestinal villi: long, slender projections
      c. Microvilli: columnar epithelial cells have microvilli
    4. Produces digestive enzymes (proteases, amylases, and lipase)
  F. Large intestine
    1. Cecum found at the ileocecocolic junction
    2. Colon (ascending, transverse, descending)
    3. Has no villi, circular folds, or secreted enzymes; large number of goblet cells secrete mucus
    4. Absorbs water, produces vitamins B and K, and propels waste toward the rectum
  G. Rectum
    1. End portion of the large intestine that secretes mucus
  H. Anus
    1. Terminal ending of gastrointestinal tract
    2. Has two sphincters: one internal involuntary sphincter and one external voluntary sphincter
  I. Other organs that are involved
    1. Pancreas: releases sodium bicarbonate, which neutralizes acidic chyme and digestive enzymes into the duodenum
      a. Trypsin: to digest proteins
      b. Lipase: to digest fat
      c. Amylase: to digest starch
    2. Liver: produces bile, which emulsifies fats
    3. Gallbladder: stores bile and releases it into the duodenum when fats are present

a. Under the influence of cholecystokinin (CCK)

b. Rats and horses do not have a gallbladder

V. Digestive process (simple stomach)

A. Food enters the mouth and is mixed with salivary amylase (from salivary glands: parotid, sublingual, mandibular, and zygomatic)

B. Amylase begins to break down starch

C. Food entering the stomach is mixed with gastric juice composed of protein-digesting enzymes, hydrochloric acid, and mucus

D. Rennin (chymosin) is also present in the young to coagulate milk

E. In the small intestine, the chyme is acted on by pancreatic enzymes

1. Pancreatic amylase: to act on starch

2. Trypsin: to act on proteins

3. Chymotrypsin: to act on proteins

4. Elastase: to act on elastin

5. Peptidases: to act on large peptides (proteins)

6. Lipase: to act on fats

7. Nucleases: to act on nucleic acids

F. Pancreatic enzymes are delivered in an alkaline fluid to help neutralize the acidic chyme

G. Small intestine also secretes enzymes

1. Trypsin: to act on dipeptides

2. Maltase, sucrase, and lactase: to act on disaccharides

3. Nuclease: to act on nucleic acids

4. Chyme is mixed with enzymes through segmentation and moves via peristalsis

5. Monosaccharides and amino acids are absorbed through the intestinal capillaries, and fats are absorbed through the lacteals of the intestinal villi

H. Large intestine absorbs water, produces vitamins B and K, and moves solid waste to the rectum for defecation

I. Defecation of undigested waste occurs through the anus

## Lymphatic System

I. Function

A. Absorbs protein-containing fluid that escapes from capillaries in tissues and returns it to the venous system

B. Transports fats from digestive tract to blood

C. Produces lymphocytes

D. Develops immunity

II. Structure

A. Lymph vessels

1. Blind end tubes, running parallel to venous system, that eventually empty into pre-cava

2. Resemble veins but have thinner walls and more valves; lymph is filtered through the lymph nodes

B. Lymph nodes (glands)

1. Oval-shaped structures

2. Filter lymph

3. Produce lymphocytes

C. Lymph organs

1. Tonsils

a. Mass of lymphoid tissue embedded in mucous membrane

b. Supplied with reticuloendothelial cells

2. Spleen

a. Largest mass of lymphoid tissue

b. Phagocytic function

c. Produces lymphocytes

d. Stores and releases blood as needed

3. Thymus

a. Important in developing immune response in the young

b. Eventually replaced by fat in the adult, depending on the species

## Respiratory System

I. Structures

A. Nostrils (nares)

1. External openings

B. Nasal cavity

1. Lined with mucous membrane

2. Houses turbinate bones

3. Air is warmed by capillaries, moistened, and filtered

C. Pharynx

1. Nasopharynx: from posterior nares to soft palate

2. Oropharynx: from soft palate to hyoid bone

3. Laryngopharynx: from hyoid bone to larynx

4. Eustachian tube: from middle ear to nasopharynx

D. Larynx (voice box)

1. Consists of cartilage (e.g., thyroid, cricoid, arytenoid, and epiglottis)

2. Epiglottis covers the glottis during swallowing

3. Vocal folds attach to arytenoid cartilage

E. Trachea

1. Consists of noncollapsible, C-shaped, cartilaginous rings

2. Lined with ciliated columnar cells

3. Divides into bronchi at the tracheal bifurcation

F. Bronchi

1. Right and left cartilaginous bronchi enter the lungs

2. Passageways become progressively smaller, and the amount of cartilage diminishes

G. Bronchiole
1. Consists of smooth muscle, no cartilage
2. Lead to the alveoli
H. Lungs
1. Varying number of lobes, depending on species
2. Covered with visceral pleura
3. House microscopic air sacs known as alveoli, where exchange of oxygen and carbon dioxide takes place

II. Physiology
A. Respiration of mammals: three basic processes
1. Ventilation: movement of air between the atmosphere and the lungs
2. External respiration: exchange of gases between the alveoli and the blood
3. Internal respiration: exchange of gases between the blood and the cells
B. Ventilation
1. Inspiration (inhalation)
a. Nervous impulse from the brain causes the diaphragm and external intercostal muscles to contract
b. Diaphragm moves caudally and the chest moves ventrally; therefore the size of the thoracic cavity is increased, which decreases intrathoracic pressure and intraalveolar pressure
c. Because intraalveolar pressure is now less than atmospheric pressure, air moves into the lungs
2. Expiration (exhalation)
a. Diaphragm and external intercostal muscles relax
b. Diaphragm moves cranially and the chest moves dorsally; this decreases the size of the thoracic cavity, which increases intrathoracic pressure and intraalveolar pressure
c. Because intraalveolar pressure is now greater than atmospheric pressure, air moves out of the lungs
d. Expiration is a passive process

III. Lung volumes
A. Tidal volume: the volume of air exchanged during normal breathing
B. Inspiratory reserve volume: the amount of air inspired over the tidal volume
C. Expiratory reserve volume: the amount of air expired over the tidal volume
D. Residual volume: air remaining in the lungs after a forced expiration
E. Dead space: air in the pathways of the respiratory system

IV. Respiratory rate
A. Dog: 10 to 30 breaths per minute
B. Cat: 24 to 42 breaths per minute
C. Horse: 8 to 16 breaths per minute

V. Control of respiration
A. Medullary rhythmicity center in the medulla oblongata, a region that has inspiratory and expiratory neurons
B. Apneustic area in the pons, which prolongs inspiration
C. Pneumotaxic area in the pons, which inhibits the apneustic area and causes expiration
D. Hering-Breuer reflex: stretch receptors in the lungs that prevent the lungs from overinflating
E. Carbon dioxide: an increase in carbon dioxide causes an increase in respiratory rate
F. Other factors may affect the rate of respiration (e.g., pain, cold, blood pressure, pH, oxygen, stress)

VI. Terminology
A. Pneumothorax: air in the thoracic cavity
B. Atelectasis: collapsed lungs
C. Pleuritis (pleurisy): inflammation of the pleural membranes
D. Pneumonia: inflammation of the lungs caused primarily by bacteria, viruses, or chemical irritants
E. Eupnea: normal, quiet respiration
F. Dyspnea: difficult breathing
G. Apnea: no breathing

## Excretory System

I. Anatomy
A. Kidneys
1. Extract and remove metabolic waste from the blood; blood pressure provides the force
2. Size and shape vary according to the species; majority are bean shaped
3. Right kidney is more firmly attached and cranial to the left kidney
4. Microscopic unit is the nephron
5. Outer cortex: contains the glomerulus, Bowman's capsule, proximal convoluted tubules (PCTs), and distal convoluted tubules (DCTs)
6. Medulla: contains the loop of Henle and most of collecting tubules
7. Medulla is arranged into various numbers of pyramids
8. Apex of the pyramid is the papilla, which opens into the minor calyx, major calyx, and renal pelvis
B. Ureters
1. Consist of smooth muscle
2. Capable of peristalsis to move urine to the urinary bladder
C. Urinary bladder
1. Consists of smooth muscle
2. Lined with transitional cell epithelium

D. Urethra
1. Tube of smooth muscle to transport urine from the urinary bladder to the exterior

II. Physiology: three phases to urine production
A. Filtration
1. Blood enters glomerulus by the afferent arteriole
2. Various pressures cause water, salt, and small molecules to move out of the glomerulus into Bowman's capsule
a. The filtrate is now called the glomerular filtrate; rate at which it is formed is called the glomerular filtration rate (GFR)
B. Reabsorption
1. Occurs in the PCTs and loop of Henle; substances needed by the body are reabsorbed from the glomerular filtrate into the peritubular capillaries
C. Secretion
1. Substances are selectively secreted from the peritubular capillaries into the DCT

III. Urination (micturition)
A. The voiding of urine
B. Filtrate flows into collecting ducts, renal pelvis, ureter, urinary bladder, and urethra and is voided as urine
C. Urine is water plus waste products (e.g., urea, excess ions)

IV. Hormonal influence
A. Antidiuretic hormone (ADH [vasopressin])
1. Increase in ADH release increases the reabsorption of water within the kidney
B. Aldosterone
1. Stimulates sodium reabsorption in the kidney

## Reproductive System: Male

I. Male anatomy
A. Testicles
1. Two oval glands in a skin-covered scrotum
2. Seminiferous tubules produce sperm
3. Interstitial cells of Leydig produce testosterone
4. Epididymis adheres to the side of the testicle; it connects the seminiferous tubules to the vas deferens and provides storage for sperm and a place for maturation
5. Testicles develop inside the abdomen but descend into the scrotum (after birth in dogs and cats), where the body temperature is more favorable for sperm development
B. Vas deferens (ductus deferens)
1. Connects the epididymis to the urethra
2. Is a part of the spermatic cord, along with blood vessels and nerves
3. Spermatic cord passes through the inguinal ring; at this point, the vas deferens separates and joins the urethra

C. Accessory sex glands
1. These glands produce semen
2. Semen provides a transport medium for sperm, protects the sperm against the acidity in the female genital tract, and provides a source of nutrition
3. Glands vary with the species
4. Dogs have a prostate only
5. Cats have a prostate and bulbourethral (or Cowper's) glands
6. Stallions have seminal vesicles (vesicular glands), prostate, bulbourethral glands, and ampulla
D. Penis
1. Houses the urethra, which transports sperm into the female genital tract
2. Consists of a shaft and the tip, known as the glans penis
3. Erectile tissue surrounds the urethra; with sexual excitement the tissue becomes engorged with blood, leading to an erection, followed by the release of sperm during ejaculation
a. Penis of the dog and stallion is composed of mostly erectile tissue and a small amount of connective tissue
b. Penis of the bull, ram, and boar is composed of mostly connective tissue and very little erectile tissue
(1) These animals achieve erection by the straightening of the sigmoid flexure (S shaped)
4. Dog penis is unique in that it has a very long glans penis and a nonarticulating bone (os penis)
5. Cat penis is retracted and covered with spiny epithelial projections

II. Male physiology
A. Follicle-stimulating hormone (FSH) is secreted from the pituitary, causing spermatogenesis to begin
B. Spermatogonia in the testicle undergo meiosis; each cell will give rise to four mature sperm, each containing the haploid number of chromosomes
C. Interstitial cell–stimulating hormone (ICSH) is secreted from the pituitary, causing the interstitial cells of Leydig to produce testosterone

## Reproductive System: Female

I. Female anatomy
A. Ovaries
1. Paired oval organs found in the abdomen
2. Produce ova and hormones
B. Oviduct
1. Conducts ova from ovary to uterine horn or uterus (depending on the species)

C. Uterine horns and/or uterus
1. Presence or absence of uterine horns varies with the species
2. In dogs and cats, young develop within the uterine horns
3. In monotocous or uniparous (giving birth to one offspring at a time) animals, young develop in the body of the uterus
4. In polytocous or multiparous (giving birth to more than one offspring at a time) animals, young develop in uterine horns

D. Cervix
1. Cervix is the opening to the uterus; some species have a double cervix (e.g., rabbits)
2. Female reproductive system consists of the following histological layers:
   a. Endometrium: epithelial cells, mucous membrane, and glands
     (1) Varies in thickness during the reproductive cycle
     (2) Is reabsorbed in animals with an estrous cycle and sloughed in animals with a menstrual cycle (primates)
   b. Myometrium: smooth muscle
   c. Perimetrium: serous covering, which is continuous with peritoneum

D. Vagina (birth canal)
1. Muscular tube from the cervix to the urethral orifice

E. Vulva
1. The external genital organ
2. Many female animals have a common urogenital pathway

II. Female physiology
A. Types of estrous cycles
1. Monestrous: usually one cycle per year, and usually in seasonal breeders (e.g., mink)
2. Diestrous: cycle in spring and fall (e.g., dog)
3. Polyestrous: more than one cycle per year (continuous) (e.g., swine)
4. Seasonally polyestrous: cycle continuously in specific seasons (e.g., cat, horse, sheep)
5. Reflex or induced ovulators: ovulate after being bred (e.g., cat, rabbit, mink, ferret)
6. Spontaneous ovulator: ovulation occurs naturally regardless of coitus (e.g., humans)

III. Estrous cycle
A. Proestrus
1. Period of preparation
2. Under influence of FSH from the pituitary
3. New ovarian follicles grow and release estrogen, which builds up the uterus and uterine horns

B. Estrus ("standing heat"): period of sexual receptivity
1. Female is sexually receptive to the male
2. Uterus and uterine horns are ready to receive an embryo
3. Release of luteinizing hormone (LH) from the pituitary causes ovulation in dogs
4. Cats and rabbits are nonspontaneous, or induced, ovulators and ovulate when bred; they have a longer estrus if not bred
5. Dogs may have a bloody discharge; cats exhibit behavioral changes (e.g., rubbing, lordosis, vocalization)

C. Metestrus
1. Short postovulatory phase
2. Each ruptured follicle develops into a corpus luteum
3. Corpus luteum produces progesterone, which causes final maturation of uterine horns and/or uterus and inhibits development of new follicles

D. Diestrus
1. Corpus luteum continues to secrete hormones
2. If pregnancy does not occur, the corpus luteum degenerates
3. If pregnancy occurs, the corpus luteum is maintained and continues to secrete hormones; in some species secretion occurs for the entire pregnancy, and in others only until the placenta is developed
4. Some animals remain in this stage and appear pregnant; this is known as pseudopregnancy

E. Anestrus
1. Long period of inactivity in seasonally polyestrous animals

IV. Fertilization and pregnancy
A. Copulation or coitus is the act of mating or sexual intercourse
B. Male will mount the female and insert the penis; ejaculation deposits semen into the vagina
C. Fertilization begins with the union of sperm and egg within the oviduct
D. Zygote undergoes mitotic divisions as it is propelled through the uterine tubes and then implants in the uterine horns or uterus, depending on the species
E. Placenta forms to allow the exchange of nutrients and waste products between mother and fetus (fetal and maternal blood do not mix)
F. Fetal membranes form around the developing embryo for protection
G. As the embryo grows, it develops a placenta and attaches to the endometrial lining of the uterus

**Table 1-4**  Endocrine glands

| Gland | Hormone/steroid hormone | Action |
|---|---|---|
| Thyroid | Thyroxin | Accelerates metabolism |
| | Calcitonin | Regulates calcium levels |
| Parathyroid | Parathormone | Regulates calcium and phosphorus levels |
| Adrenal cortex | Glucocorticoids, mineralocorticoids, gonadocorticoids | Protein and carbohydrate metabolism, stress resistance, antiinflammatory effects, regulates sodium and potassium levels, male and female sex hormones |
| Adrenal medulla | Epinephrine, norepinephrine | Stimulate sympathetic nervous system; "fight or flight" |
| Pituitary (master gland) | Growth hormone | Stimulates growth |
| | Thyroid-stimulating hormone (thyrotropic) | Stimulates thyroid gland |
| | Adrenocorticotropic hormone (corticotropin) | Stimulates adrenal cortex |
| | Follicle-stimulating hormone | Growth of ovarian follicle |
| | Luteinizing hormone (interstitial cell–stimulating) | Causes ovulation; stimulates testosterone production |
| | Prolactin | Stimulates lactation |
| | Oxytocin | Causes uterine contractions |
| | Antidiuretic hormone (vasopressin) | Causes water reabsorption |
| Pancreas | Insulin | Decreases blood glucose |
| | Glucagon | Increases blood glucose |
| Ovary | Estrogen | Female sex characteristics |
| | Progesterone | Prepares uterus and uterine horns |
| Testes | Testosterone | Male sex characteristics |

H. Between implantation and parturition, the developing organism is called a fetus

I. Protective fetal membranes
   1. Amnion: forms a fluid-filled sac closest to the fetus; this is filled with amniotic fluid
   2. Allantois: a two-layered membrane; one layer adheres to the amnion, the other layer to the chorion; fluid fills this cavity
   3. Chorion: outermost layer, which attaches to the endometrium
      a. Type of fetal attachment varies with species

V. Parturition: act of giving birth
   A. Labor
      1. Under the influence of oxytocin from the pituitary, the uterus and/or uterine horns begin to contract
      2. Delivery of fetus: fetus is pushed through the cervix and vagina
      3. Delivery of placenta: placenta (afterbirth) is delivered after the birth of each fetus

VI. Gestation period: length of time from fertilization to birth
   A. Cat and dog: average 63 days
   B. Horse: average 336 days
   C. Cow: average 285 days

VII. Dystocia: difficult birth
   A. May result in the need for a cesarean section

VIII. Lactation: milk production
   A. First milk is colostrum; contains antibodies, proteins, and vitamins and is important for the neonate
   B. Milk production is under the influence of prolactin from the pituitary

## Endocrine System

Endocrine glands (Table 1-4) are ductless and produce chemical substances (hormones) that have a specific effect on a target area. The hormones are secreted directly into the bloodstream.

I. Characteristics
   A. Hormones may
      1. Change the permeability of a cell
      2. Change the permeability of an organelle
      3. Activate or inactivate an enzyme system
      4. Change the rate of enzyme production

II. Control
   A. Hormone secretion is regulated through a feedback system; as the hormone levels rise, their secretion is inhibited
   B. Only the adrenal medulla is under neural control

## Integumentary System

### Anatomy

I. Skin consists of two layers of skin and one underlying layer of subcutaneous tissue
  A. Epidermis
    1. Superficial layer is the stratum corneum; this is a nonvascular, cornified layer
    2. Constantly being shed and replaced
    3. Deep to this is the actively growing stratum germinativum
    4. Melanocytes (pigment cells) produce melanin, giving skin its color, and are found in this region
  B. Dermis (corium)
    1. Deep to the epidermis
    2. Contains arteries, veins, capillaries, lymphatics, and nerve fibers
  C. Hypodermis
    1. Deep to the dermis is the subcutaneous layer consisting of connective and adipose tissue

### Function

I. Protective barrier, sense organ, and site for vitamin D synthesis
II. Contains many glands and nerve receptors (e.g., Meissner's corpuscle [touch receptor], sweat glands, Ruffini's endings [heat receptor], Pacini's corpuscles [pressure receptor], sebaceous glands)

### Hair

I. Hair contains an inner medulla covered by the thicker cortex, which in turn is covered by a keratinized layer called the cuticle
II. Hair is produced within a follicle, with growth originating in the bulb region
III. The portion of a hair that is below the skin is known as the root; the region above the skin is the shaft
IV. Number of hairs per follicle varies
V. Each hair follicle is supplied with sebaceous glands and an arrector muscle of hair
VI. Contraction of this muscle is responsible for the raised hairs seen in frightened cats
VII. Types
  A. Normal guard or cover hair; usually accompanied by shorter wool hair in the same follicle
  B. Wool hair: shorter, wavy, no medulla (e.g., sheep)
  C. Tactile hairs (sinus hairs) (e.g., whiskers): used as feelers; very sensitive to movement

### Specialized Integument

I. Horns, claws, and hooves grow from a specialized dermis and consist of cornified epidermal cells

## Senses

### Vision

I. Anatomy: eye
  A. Sclera: outermost fibrous coat (white of the eye)
  B. Choroid: vascular coat between the sclera and retina
  C. Retina: nervous coat housing photoreceptors (e.g., rods and cones)
  D. Vitreous humor: clear, watery fluid filling the vitreous body
  E. Lens: focuses light onto the retina
  F. Iris: colored, contractile membrane between the lens and the cornea; regulates amount of light passing through the pupil
  G. Pupil: opening in the center of the iris
  H. Aqueous humor: clear, watery fluid filling the anterior and posterior chambers
  I. Cornea: transparent covering on the eye
  J. Conjunctiva: mucous membrane that lines the eyelids
  K. Nictitating membrane: third eyelid
II. Lacrimal apparatus
  A. Tears from the lacrimal gland located in the upper eyelids flow onto the eyeball to flush debris from the eye and moisten and lubricate it
  B. Tears drain from a lacrimal duct in the medial canthi of the upper and lower lids into the nasal cavity via the nasolacrimal duct
III. Physiology
  A. Light passes through the pupil, is refracted by the lens, and hits the photoreceptors (i.e., rods and cones of the retina)
  B. Rods respond to dim light; more are present in nocturnal animals
  C. Cones respond to bright light and color
  D. Nervous impulses from rods and cones are passed via the optic nerve to the brain

### Hearing

I. Anatomy: ear; consists of three regions
  A. Outer ear
    1. From the pinna up to and including the tympanic membrane
    2. Air filled
  B. Middle ear
    1. Houses three ossicles: malleus (hammer), incus (anvil), and stapes (stirrup)
    2. Air filled; communicates with the nasopharynx by way of the eustachian tube
  C. Inner ear
    1. Houses the cochlea and semicircular canals
    2. Fluid filled

3. Cochlea houses the organ of Corti (hearing receptors)
4. Semicircular canals contain nerve receptors for perception of balance

II. Physiology
  A. Sound waves are transmitted through the outer ear and strike the tympanic membrane
  B. Sound is concentrated and conducted through the three ossicles to the round window of the cochlea
  C. Cochlea houses the organ of Corti, which when stimulated conducts a nervous impulse along the auditory nerve to the brain

III. Deafness
  A. Nerve deafness
    1. Results from malfunction of receptors or auditory nerve
    2. Most common in blue-eyed cats with white coats, Sealyham terriers, Scotch terriers, border collies, and fox terriers
  B. Transmission deafness
    1. Results from malfunction in transmission of sound waves from outer to inner ear

## Smell

I. Associated with the olfactory bulb
II. Receptors lie in the mucous membranes of the nasal cavity
III. Odor is dissolved in receptors and transmitted to the brain

## Taste

I. Taste receptors are enclosed in gustatory papillae on the tongue
II. Three types of gustatory papillae: fungiform, foliate, and vallate
  A. Fungiform papillae: mushroom shaped; scattered among filiform papillae on the surface of the tongue
  B. Foliate papillae: leaf shaped and found on the lateral borders of tongue (really parallel folds of lingual mucosa)
  C. Vallate (circumvallate) papillae: large, circular projections surrounded by a cleft
    1. Contain taste buds and serous glands in all domestic animals
    2. Contain mucous glands in the horse
III. Two other types of papillae are mechanical: filiform and conical
  A. Filiform: thorn shaped; help direct food toward pharynx and are used for lapping and grooming
    1. These papillae are shorter and softer in the horse, hence the velvetlike tongue
  B. Conical (also lenticular papillae in ruminants): cone shaped; larger than filiform papillae

# Glossary

**anatomy** The study of the form and structure of the body

**apnea** No breathing

**articulation** Where two or more bones meet; also called a joint

**canthi (singular, canthus)** The junction of the upper and lower eyelids at either corner of the eyes

**carnivore** Meat-eating animal

**conjunctiva** Mucous membrane that lines the eyelids

**cornea** Transparent covering on the eye

**coronary circulation** Blood circulation that nourishes the myocardium

**dead space** Air in the respiratory passageways

**dyspnea** Difficult breathing

**dystocia** Difficult birth

**endocrine glands** Secrete hormones directly into the bloodstream

**estrous cycle** Interval from the beginning of one period of sexual receptivity to the beginning of the next

**estrus** Time of the female's cycle when she is receptive to a male

**eupnea** Normal respiration

**exocrine glands** Secrete substances through ducts, usually onto an epithelial surface

**extracellular** Outside of a cell

**herbivore** Plant-eating animal

**hormone** Chemical substance that has a specific effect on target area

**hypertonic** Having a higher osmotic pressure than another solution

**hypotonic** Having a lower osmotic pressure than another solution

**intercellular** Between the cells

**intracellular** Within a cell

**isotonic** Having equal osmotic pressures

**lacrimal apparatus** Lacrimal duct conducts tears from the medial corners to the nasal cavity

**lactation** Milk production

**laminae (singular, lamina)** Thin, flat layer or membrane

**meninges** Protective coverings of the brain and spinal cord

**monestrous** Having one estrous cycle per year

**monotocous** Producing one offspring at birth

**myocardium** Heart muscle

**nonspontaneous ovulator** Ovulation occurs only when bred

**omnivore** Animal that eats meat and plants

**osmotic pressure** Amount of pressure necessary to stop the flow of water across a membrane

**osteology** Study of bones

**parturition** Act of giving birth

**physiology** Study of body functions

**polyestrous** Having more than one estrous cycle per year

**polytocous** Giving birth to several offspring at one time

**residual volume** Air remaining in the lungs after a forced expiration

**ruminant** Animal with a four-chambered stomach; animal that commonly chews its cud

**spontaneous ovulator** Ovulation occurs naturally within the cycle

**tidal volume** Volume of air exchanged during eupnea

# Review Questions

1 The process by which bone is formed from cartilage bars is known as
   a. Intramembranous ossification
   b. Endochondral ossification
   c. Heteroplastic osteogenesis
   d. Chondrabar osteogenesis

2 Skeletal muscle is composed of
   a. Parallel, multinucleated fibers
   b. Interconnected, uninucleated fibers
   c. Spindle-shaped, uninucleated fibers
   d. Parallel, uninucleated fibers

3 The scientific discipline that studies the functions of living things is
   a. Anatomy
   b. Systemic anatomy
   c. Physomy
   d. Physiology

4 The canine foreleg is composed of the following bones
   a. Tibia, radius, ulna
   b. Humerus, radius, ulna
   c. Humerus, radius, fibula
   d. Femur, tibia, fibula

5 A dog that has had a major hemorrhage accidentally receives a large transfusion of distilled water into the cephalic vein. This would probably have
   a. No result as long as the water was sterile
   b. Serious, perhaps fatal, results, because the red blood cells would shrink
   c. No effect, because the dog was dehydrated
   d. Serious, perhaps fatal, results, because the red blood cells would burst

6 In the digestive tract, the three histological layers of the mucosa are
   a. Stratified squamous, simple columnar, stratified squamous
   b. Epithelium, lamina propria, muscularis mucosae
   c. Submucosa, muscularis externa, serosa
   d. Muscularis mucosae, lamina propria, columnar epithelium

7 In the dog, the SA node is located in the
   a. Left auricle
   b. Right atrium
   c. Left ventricle
   d. Right ventricle

8 Which one of the following hormones is not secreted by the pituitary?
   a. FSH
   b. ACTH
   c. Cortisone
   d. Growth hormone

9 All of the following are major sites of lymphatic tissue except
   a. Tonsils
   b. Thymus
   c. Spleen
   d. Kidneys

10 Which of the following statements about the middle ear is false?
   a. It contains three ossicles
   b. Infection in the middle ear is called otitis media
   c. It communicates with the nasopharynx by means of the eustachian tube
   d. The cochlea is located here

**BIBLIOGRAPHY**

Colville T, Bassert J: *Clinical anatomy and physiology for veterinary technicians*, St Louis, 2002, Mosby.

Frandson RD, Wilke W, Fails AD: *Anatomy and physiology of farm animals*, ed 6, Philadelphia, 2003, Lippincott Williams & Wilkins.

Marieb E, Hoehn K: *Human anatomy and physiology*, ed 7, San Francisco, 2007, Pearson Benjamin Cummings.

Martini F: *Fundamentals of anatomy and physiology*, ed 7, San Francisco, 2006, Pearson Benjamin Cummings.

McBride DF: *Learning veterinary terminology*, ed 2, St Louis, 2002, Mosby.

Romich JA: *An illustrated guide to veterinary terminology*, ed 2, Clifton Park, NY, 2006, Thomson Delmar Learning.

Ruckebusch Y, Phaneuf L-P, Dunlop R: *Physiology of small and large animals*, St Louis, 1991, Mosby.

Sherwood L, Klandorf H, Yancey P: *Animal physiology from genes to organisms*, Belmont, Calif, 2005, Thomson Brooks/Cole.

## CHAPTER 2

# Urinalysis and Hematology

*Dan Walsh*    *William L. Wade*    *Antoniette D'Amato-Scheck*    *Pam Schendel*

## OUTLINE

Urinalysis
   Specimen Collection and
     Handling
   Chemical Components
   Microscopic Evaluation
   Uroliths

Hematology
   Blood Collection and Sampling
   Erythrocyte (Red Blood Cell)
     Evaluation
   Leukocyte (White Blood Cell)
     Evaluation

Thrombocyte (Platelet)
   Evaluation
Total Protein
Instrumentation

## LEARNING OUTCOMES

After reading this chapter you should be able to:

1. Describe, compare, and evaluate the various collection methods for urine and blood sample.
2. Describe the various procedures for the evaluation of urine and blood sample.
3. Explain the various components of the test results as they relate to the "normal" physiological and pathophysiological patient.
4. Identify and limit preanalytical patient variables and care influences, and specimen collection, handling, and timing influences that affect results.

**V**eterinarians and researchers depend on clinical laboratory test results to complement the presenting complaint, history, and examination, thus offering the patient the best possible care. Consistent and accurate results provided by the veterinary technician are an essential component of this care. Regardless, if the tests are performed in-house or forwarded to a reference laboratory, preanalytical patient variables and care, specimen collection, handling, and timing influence the results.

## URINALYSIS

A complete urinalysis includes the evaluation of the physical, chemical, solute, and microscopic components of the urine, and may include microbiological cultures, identification and sensitivity testing, and identification of urinary calculi.

  I. The information gained from these evaluations is used to assess the urinary system and aid diagnosis of nonurinary tract disorders
    A. Whether we are looking for or confirming a diagnosis, screening for an asymptomatic disease during an annual health or presurgical exam, monitoring the progress of a disease, or assessing the efficacy and safety of a treatment, urinalysis helps in patient evaluation
    B. The tests are usually easily performed, using a minimum of supplies, diagnostic instrumentation, and veterinary technician time

### Specimen Collection and Handling

  I. Containers
    A. Collect the specimen in a clean (preferably sterile and disposable), dry, opaque container to prevent contamination and degradation of the light-sensitive components (e.g., bilirubin and urobilinogen)
      1. The container should be nonbreakable and fitted with a tight lid after collection, to prevent contamination, spillage, or evaporation

2. Sterile containers should be used for urine samples collected by cystocentesis or catheterization for bacterial culture
3. The sterile aspiration syringe used for these procedures makes an acceptable container

B. Timing of urine formation vs. collection vs. analysis
   1. Formation
      a. Because urine is stored in the bladder after formation, the urine is not necessarily "fresh" upon collection
      b. Deterioration of components may have occurred from the natural breakdown of formed elements, and may be influenced by the presence of bacteria and change in pH
   2. Collection
      a. Fasted, postprandial, postrest, random vs. timed, singular vs. serial
      b. A singular sample gives a "snapshot" in time, whereas a series of samples allows for changes due to variation in activity
      c. A postrest sample will likely be more concentrated then a sample collected after activity and water consumption
      d. A 3 to 6 hour postprandial sample may be more reflective of the diet
   3. Analysis
      a. Degradation occurs from the instant of formation and subsequent collection
      b. To be reliable and best reflect the patient's condition, a urinalysis should be performed within 20 to 30 minutes of collection

C. Methods of collection
   1. Free flow (clean catch, spontaneous micturition or voiding)
      a. Simple, noninvasive procedure but unsatisfactory for bacterial culture
      b. Preferably, a midstream sample is collected, avoiding initial or end portion of the voided urine
      c. Vulva or prepuce should be cleansed before collection
      d. Variations
         (1) Commercially available absorbable urine sponges
             (a) For chemistry and physical evaluation only
             (b) Not for microscopic urinalysis
         (2) Litter pan
             (a) Replace regular absorbable litter with inert nonabsorbable litter
         (3) Manual expression
             (a) Must be performed with care and patience; avoid excessive pressure to the bladder

         (b) Should never be attempted on an animal with a suspected urethral obstruction
      (4) Metabolism cage
          (a) Usually of value to determine urine volume only
          (b) Extended time between collection and testing may increase the possibility of contamination and sample degradation
          (c) To assist in maintaining sample quality, cold pack collection reservoirs are available, as are alarm-sensitive cages, which alert personnel of the presence of a sample
      (5) Tabletop, cage, floor
          (a) May be adequate for screening if the surface is clean and free of disinfectant residues, and the sample is analyzed in an expedient manner
          (b) These samples are usually contaminated, not suitable for bacterial culture, and offer limited diagnostic information
      (6) Client-collected samples
          (a) Usually, client-collected samples are not satisfactory because of improper collection procedures, the extended time between collection and testing, and the use of improper containers and storage
          (b) Although not always practical, it is best to have the client bring the patient to the clinic
          (c) Under these circumstances, the client should be asked to discourage the pet from voiding urine for 2 to 3 hours before the appointment to facilitate collection at the clinic
   2. Cystocentesis
      a. Performed by inserting a needle through the ventral abdominal wall and into the urinary bladder
      b. Perform the procedure using aseptic technique on a patient with a full bladder, thus providing a better anatomical reference and minimizing possible damage to other abdominal organs
      c. Collection through cystocentesis avoids contaminants from the lower portions of the urinary tract, making the sample suitable for bacterial culture
   3. Transurethral catheterization
      a. Performed by passing a rubber, plastic, or metal catheter through the urethra and into the urinary bladder

b. Type and size of catheter depends on size, gender, and species of animal

c. Catheterize as aseptically and atraumatically as possible to avoid complications for the patient and catheter-induced cell and bacterial contamination of the sample

d. Sample is aspirated into a syringe attached to the exposed end of the catheter

D. Preservation

1. For microscopic evaluation, centrifuge immediately

2. Refrigerate (~35° to 46° F [~2° to 8° C]) for an additional 2 to 12 hours if necessary, but bring sample to room temperature (~68° to 77° F [~20° to 25° C]) before evaluation, especially if evaluating specific gravity (SG) and crystals

   a. Cold urine may also interfere with enzymatic reactions on the urine chemistry dipsticks

3. Freezing (≤ 32° F [≤ 0° C]) is satisfactory for common urine chemical analytes, but will most likely destroy the cellular elements

4. Chemicals

   a. The sample can be preserved by the addition of acidifiers (e.g., boric acid, hydrochloric acid), formaldehyde, toluene, thymol, phenol, chloroform, sodium fluoride, and commercial chemical urinary preservatives

   b. Although one or more urine elements may be preserved by the chemical, it may be at the expense of other elements in the urine

E. Sample variables

1. Samples should be analyzed within 20 to 30 minutes of collection to maximize validity of information and to minimize postcollection analytical variables

2. One, more, or all results may be directly or indirectly influenced by nonpathological internal and external influences (e.g., exercise, water intake, diet, medication, collection method, degree of restraint, environmental factors [e.g., temperature, humidity])

   a. The veterinarian interprets individual test results in light of these variables, the results of other urine and clinical evaluation procedures, and in concert with the physical examination and history

3. Precollection and postcollection (preanalytical), "artifactual" or iatrogenic variables may increase or decrease values, resulting in false positive or negative results.

| Component | Variation to deterioration of sample and/or influences on test methods |
|---|---|
| Ammonia | Increase from proliferation of urease-producing bacteria |
| Bacteria | Increase from the in vitro proliferation of bacteria that normally inhabit the vagina, labia, urethra, or prepuce; or arise from urinary tract infections or contamination from external sources |
| | Bacterial concentration approximately doubles every hour at room temperature (~68°-77° F [~20°-25° C]) |
| Bilirubin | Decrease from exposure to light and oxidation at room temperature |
| Casts | Decrease due to alkalinization (pH > 7.0) or dilution of urine (SG ~ < 1.008-1.010) |
| Color | Darkens with exposure to light and urochrome degradation |
| | Brown-black discoloration with blood substitutes |
| Crystals | Types and numbers increase or decrease with pH and temperature changes (colder temperature causes increase) |
| Erythrocytes | Hemolysis caused by dilute and/or alkaline urine, or freezing |
| Glucose | Decrease from metabolism by cells or bacteria and/or from the inhibition of the enzymatic reaction on the chemistry strip if the urine is cold |
| Hemolysis | Increases due to the deterioration of the erythrocytes in alkaline or dilute urine blood |
| Ketones | May decrease with the presence of bacterial metabolism and volatilization of acetone |
| Leukocytes | Decrease with alkalinization and/or dilution of urine, or freezing |
| Nitrites | Increase when bacteria convert nitrate to nitrite |
| | Decrease when nitrite is converted to nitrogen and evaporates |
| Odor | Becomes stronger from the ammonia produced from bacterial metabolism |
| pH | Usually increases (alkaline) with the presence of urease-producing bacteria and/or the loss of $CO_2$ |
| | Decreases (acidic) with the proliferation of non–urease-producing bacteria and yeasts converting glucose to acids |
| Proteins | Increase from bacteria proliferation, alkalinization, contamination with chemicals (e.g., disinfectants: quaternary ammonium or chlorhexidine), some medications (check package insert), blood substitutes, anesthetics, or elevated body temperature |
| | Decrease with acidic urine |
| Turbidity | Develops from presence of bacteria, proliferation of crystals, or precipitation of amorphous material |
| Somatic cells | Deteriorate with rise in pH or freezing |
| Urobilinogen | Decreases upon exposure to light |
| Yeasts/fungi | Increase from external contamination or resistant urinary tract infection |

II Physical evaluation

A. Volume: influenced by several factors, including water intake, environmental temperature, physical activity, size, species, diet, and medications

1. Ideally, various sequential samples should be evaluated over 24 hours to determine the various internal and external influences on urine volume and the other physical, chemical, and microscopic analytes

B. Terms related to urine volume and output

1. Pollakiuria: refers to frequent urination; often confused with polyuria by clients

2. Polyuria
   a. Increase in urine output or production
   b. Associated with nephritis, diabetes mellitus, and polydipsia

3. Oliguria
   a. Decrease in the formation or elimination of urine
   b. Occurs with shock, dehydration, water conservation, or renal failure

4. Anuria
   a. Complete absence of urine formation or elimination
   b. Can occur from renal shutdown; usually associated with obstruction

5. Continence: storage of urine in the bladder as it fills

6. Incontinence: dribbling of urine at frequent intervals

7. Micturition: physiological term for emptying the bladder

8. Dysuria: difficulty or pain upon urination

C. Color

1. In most species, urine is light-yellow to dark
   a. Yellow is normally due to urochrome pigments
   b. Urobilin may also influence the color

2. Color generally correlates with specific gravity (SG [concentration]), volume, and pigments from internal or external sources
   a. Light-colored urine tends to have a lower SG; darker urine generally has a higher SG
   b. Bile pigments are likely contained in yellow-brown to greenish urine that foams when shaken
   c. Red or reddish-brown urine indicates hematuria (red blood cells [RBCs]) or hemoglobinuria (hemoglobin [Hb])
   d. Brown urine may contain myoglobin from muscle cell breakdown (myoglobinuria)
   e. Medications and diet may influence color
   f. Increase in urine volume results in urine dilution and lighter color
   g. Urine collected after a period of rest tends to be darker in color due to increased concentration

D. Some species have variable color of urine

1. Rabbit urine commonly varies from yellow to cloudy-white to orange-red-brown from porphyrin pigments

2. Horse urine is browner upon standing from oxidation

III. Transparency (turbidity, cloudiness): presence of particulate matter

A. Transparency is described as clear, hazy, cloudy, turbid, opaque, or flocculent (large particulate matter that readily settles out)

B. Cloudy urine can be associated with the presence of cellular debris, such as RBCs, white blood cells (WBCs), epithelial cells, crystals, bacteria, casts, mucus, semen, and lipids

1. Bacterial proliferation or crystal formation can cause urine to become cloudy upon standing

C. Normal freshly voided urine in many species is clear; exceptions include

1. Horse, because of the presence of calcium carbonate crystals and mucus secreted by glands in the renal pelvis

2. Rabbit, hamster, and guinea pig, because of the presence of calcium salts

3. Feline urine commonly is slightly cloudy, because of the presence of fat

4. On standing, urine typically becomes more cloudy with the increased number of bacteria and possible formation of crystals (e.g., calcium carbonate crystals form in cattle urine)

D. Microscopic evaluation is necessary to distinguish possible causes of turbidity

IV. Odor

A. Not highly diagnostic; varies with species and gender of the patient

1. Odors are commonly described as
   a. "Normal" (characteristic for the species and gender)
   b. Ammoniacal (urease-producing bacteria)
   c. Putrid (bacterial degradation of protein)
   d. Fruity/sweet (e.g., ketones, glucose)
   e. "Disagreeable"

2. Strong urine odor is typical in mice and uncastrated male cats, goats, and pigs

3. In some cases, a sweet or fruity odor can indicate the presence of ketones (ketonuria) and is commonly associated with diabetes mellitus, pregnancy toxemia in sheep, or acetonemia (ketosis) in cows

4. Ammonia is due to bacterial proliferation, which may be from infectious or contaminating

organisms, and will result in increased odor upon standing

It may be indicative of improper storage rather than the health of the patient

    5. Odor may be influenced by diet and medications

V. Specific gravity (SG, Sp. Gr., urine specific gravity [USG])

  A. Density of a liquid compared with that of distilled water

    1. In practical applications, it is used to assess the ability of the renal tubule to concentrate or dilute filtrates from the glomerulus, indicating how well the kidney can maintain water and osmotic balance

    2. The urine SG is interpreted by the veterinarian in concert with the patient's hydration status, and blood urea nitrogen and serum creatinine levels

  B. Terms related to SG

    1. *-sthen* (strength), *iso-* (the same as), *hypo-* (less than), *hyper-* (greater than)

    2. Isosthenuria ("fixed SG" [SG ~1.008 to 1.012])

      a. The glomerular filtrate has the same SG as the plasma. The urine has neither been diluted nor concentrated in the kidney tubules

    3. Hyposthenuria (SG < ~1.008)

      a. Tubules are diluting the urine below the SG of plasma

    4. Hypersthenuria (baruria [SG > ~1.012])

      a. Tubules are concentrating the urine above the SG of plasma

    5. Maximum urine concentration (SG) values

      a. Species-specific maximum concentration capacity (SG) of the tubules

    6. Functionally adequate urine concentration (SG) values

      a. Species-specific sufficient concentrating (SG) ability, suggesting a sufficient number of "normally" functioning nephrons to prevent azotemia (presence of nitrogen wastes [e.g., urea, creatinine] in the blood) assuming renal blood flow is sufficient and there are no other influencing factors to impair the function of the nephrons

    7. Inappropriate urine concentration (SG) values

      a. Values below the questionable range

    8. Questionable SG values

      a. Values marginally below the functionally adequate range

  C. Normal (reference) SG values vary and fluctuate widely from day to day and within the same day, and are related to the individual, species, diet, activity, water and electrolyte balance of the body, as well as possible pathologies

    1. A single value within the normal or outside the normal range for an individual or the species does not necessarily reflect renal function or dysfunction

  D. Methods of SG evaluation

    1. Refractometer (total solids [TS] meter)

      a. Solute in the urine bends light passing through the urine to a degree that is proportional to the concentration of the solute

      b. Approximately measures SG or total solids of urine

      c. Refractometers are calibrated within a specific temperature range; operating outside of this range may cause erroneous results; check manufacturer's instructions

      d. Ensure that results are read from the SG scale, which differs by species, and from the total protein and refractive index scales

      e. To approximate the SG if the reading is off the scale, dilute the urine 1:1 with distilled water and adjust results accordingly by multiplying the last two digits of the reading by 2

        (1) For example, a urine sample diluted 1:1 with distilled water with a reading of 1.030 will have an SG of 1.060 (2 × 30) when adjusted for the 1:1 dilution

        (2) Do not attempt to make the dilution on the refractometer, because of the difficulty of obtaining an even mixture of urine and distilled water

      f. The relative specific refractivity of the urine of cats, rabbits, and guinea pigs differs from that of dogs, large animals, and humans

        (1) Therefore the use of the commonly used human-based urine SG scale will give falsely elevated SG results for cats, and falsely low SG results for guinea pigs and rabbits

        (2) Preferably, use refractometers with scales calibrated for the specific species

      g. Glucose, protein (albumin), radiopaque dyes, urea, sodium chloride, and some antibiotics will raise the SG value (e.g., ~0.004 for each gram of glucose per deciliter of urine, and ~0.003 for each gram of protein per deciliter of urine)

| Species | Approximate possible maximum range | Common (daily variable-functional) range | Questionable (marginal) to adequate values* |
|---------|-----------------------------------|------------------------------------------|--------------------------------------------|
| Canine | ~1.001-1.075 | ~≥ 1.015-1.045 | ~1.030>1.040+ |
| Feline | ~1.001-1.085 | ~≥ 1.035-1.060 | ~1.035>1.045+ |
| Large animals | ~1.001-1.040 | ~≥ 1.015-1.030 | ~>1.025+ |

*Consistent successive results at the low end of or below these values from samples collected at various times throughout the day may indicate a disorder and would most likely be considered an "inappropriate" value.

(1) To correct the SG, subtract the relevant increase for each gram of analyte (e.g., protein or glucose) per deciliter of urine

h. Quality control (QC): check the zero setting/calibration of the refractometer daily with distilled water (1.000 SG [± 0.05%]), and with a known control (5% NaCl solution = 1.022 SG [± 0.001])

(1) Adjust refractometer according to manufacture's instructions

2. Urinometer
   a. A "hydrometer" calibrated for urine
   b. When the urinometer is placed in a cylinder filled with urine, it will displace a volume equal to its weight
      (1) Therefore the more solute present in the urine, the less volume will be displaced and the higher the urinometer will float, denoting a higher specific gravity
   c. Requires a large volume of urine (~5 to 15+ mL), whereas the refractometer requires only a drop or two
   d. Read results at bottom of the meniscus on the urinometer float
   e. Urinometers are calibrated to read samples at room temperature; correct the specific gravity reading for the urine, if the temperature of the urine is not at the calibrated temperature of the urinometer. Check manufacturer's instructions
   f. Quality control
      (1) Check the accuracy of the urinometer with distilled water (SG 1.000) at the calibrated temperature

3. SG reagent test strips
   a. An indirect colorimetric method, where an increased color change is correlated with increased concentration of ionic solutes
   b. Developed for use with human urine samples
   c. Least reliable method of determining SG in animals, especially if SG is greater than 1.030, the upper limit of the test strips
      (1) High concentrations of protein and/or ketones may give falsely elevated

values, whereas alkaline and/or dilute urine (low SG) may give false low values, and high urine lipid content may either raise or lower values

d. Not influenced by the presence of glucose or urea
e. Read results by comparing color changes with color scale on container
f. See specific manufacturer's instructions

4. Osmometry
   a. Unit: milliosmol/kg [L] = mOsm/kg [L]
   b. Likely the most representative method of analyzing urine solute concentration
   c. Measures number of dissolved particles in the urine
      (1) Costly instrumentation (osmometers) and time-consuming method, therefore more likely used in research and reference laboratories
   d. Urine osmolality can be roughly "guesstimated" from the USG by multiplying the last two digits of the USG by 36 (e.g., USG: 1.030 ≅ 1080 [30 × 36] mOsm/kg [L])

E. Urine SG values
   1. Commonly reported SG values
   2. Increased SG occurs with dehydration, decreased water intake, acute renal disease, and shock
      a. In these situations, it would be expected that SG would be consistently higher than ~1.035 in the feline, 1.030 in the canine, and 1.025 in large animals
      b. Decreased SG occurs with increased fluid intake and in renal and other diseases

## Chemical Components

I. Urine pH
   A. Used to generally assess the body's acid-base balance
      1. pH number expresses the hydrogen ion ($H^+$) concentration or the acidity
         a. pH < 7 is decreased pH, or acid urine
         b. pH > 7 is increased pH, or basic or alkaline urine
   B. Reagent strips are most commonly used to determine pH; after being dipped into urine

sample, the color change is compared with the color on a scale on the container

1. Common findings are between pH 5.5 and 8.5 across species

C. pH is often affected by diet

1. Herbivores commonly have an alkaline pH (~7 to 8.5); nursing herbivores commonly have more acid urine
2. Carnivores have an acidic pH (e.g., feline ~6 to 7)
3. Urine of omnivores may be either acid or basic
4. Urine tends to become less acid after meals, because of the "alkaline tide" (postprandial gastric secretion of hydrochloric acid)

D. Loss of $CO_2$ occurs when samples are left open and standing at room temperature, resulting in higher pH readings

E. Standing urine, containing urease-producing bacteria, also increases the reading

F. In highly acidic urine, a false reduction of the pH reading may result because of dripping from the protein pad onto the pH pad. Therefore technique and timing are critical. See package insert

II. Protein

A. Proteinuria usually describes an abnormal level of proteins or protein metabolites in the urine

B. Small amounts of protein pass through the glomerulus, but most are resorbed by the renal tubules

C. Detection of protein levels is commonly made with a reagent test strip

1. Lower limits of detection: ~30 to 50 mg/dL, which are specific for relatively large amounts of albumin

D. Color comparison is made and results are recorded in mg/dL

1. The results for the healthy patient are none or trace (10 mg/dL), and the veterinarian will interpret the protein results in concert with the USG

E. Results are considered semiquantitative because of variables in chemical reaction and color chart comparison

F. Errors can occur

1. False-positive or falsely elevated values may result when the urine is alkaline and highly concentrated, or if the test strip is left in contact with the urine for an extended period or not read at the appropriate time; check the package insert
   a. If proteinuria is caused by globulins, or Bence-Jones protein (indicative of multiple myeloma) rather than albumin, or if

protein is present in dilute or acidic urine, false-negative results can occur

2. Depending on the reader and individuality in color determination, different values may be obtained
3. Proteinuria in diluted urine indicates greater protein loss than in concentrated urine
4. Small amounts of albumin may go undetected with routine chemistry dipstick tests

G. Proteinuria results from several prerenal and postrenal causes

H. Values must be taken in context with hematology and chemistry results, other urinalysis results, or other methods of evaluating protein levels

1. Urine protein–to–creatinine (UPC) ratio (lower limits of detection: ~$\geq$5 mg/dL) reflects the amount of protein excreted over 24 hours based on a single urine sample
2. Sulfosalicylic acid (SSA) turbidometric test (lower limits of detection: ~$\geq$ 5 to 10 mg/dL)
   a. Detects globulins and Bence-Jones protein in addition to albumins
   b. Used as a confirmatory test for chemistry test strip positive results, especially samples with an alkaline pH
3. Microalbumin (MA) test (lower limits of detection: ~$\geq$1 mg/dL); detects small quantities of albumin in the urine
   a. Microalbumin level has been associated with a variety of nonrenal and renal diseases, including being an indicator of early renal disease
   b. The full extent of the usefulness of this test is still under study
   c. Currently, the available efficacious tests in veterinary medicine are species-specific immunologic (enzyme linked immunosorbent assay [ELISA]) tests
      (1) Human MA test strips do not completely match the results of the species specific veterinary tests

III. Glucose

A. Detectable levels of sugar are referred to as glucosuria or glycosuria and depend on glucose levels in the blood

1. Glucose is not commonly detected in healthy animals; it passes through the glomerulus and is resorbed in the proximal tubules
   a. Unless the renal threshold is reached (e.g., ~170 to 180 mg/dL [>6.8 mmol/L] in dogs), glucosuria does not usually occur
   b. Therefore, unless there is excess of glucose reaching the tubules that cannot be resorbed or there is a functional deficit

of the tubules, glucose will not be detectable

B. Testing is usually performed with reagent test strips to detect glucose, and/or reagent tablets to detect sugars (glucose and other reducing sugars) in the urine
   1. If the proteinaceous labile enzymes found in the glucose test pads become inactive, a false-negative result occurs
      a. Check with the manufacturer for details on prolonging the life of unopened, in-date packages by freezing

C. Hyperglycemia along with glucosuria can be attributed to diabetes mellitus created by insulin deficiency or function
   1. For confirmation of diabetes mellitus, blood glucose level should be evaluated

D. Other factors, such as fear, stress, excitement, intravenous infusion of glucose, and other diseases also cause glucosuria
   1. Fasting is recommended before glucose testing to avoid higher levels after a high-carbohydrate meal
      a. False-positive results can occur after the use of various drugs, such as salicylates, ascorbic acid, and penicillin

IV. Ketones

A. Ketones include acetone, and acetoacetic and β-hydroxybutyric acids
   1. Acetone and β-hydroxybutyric acid are derived from acetoacetic acid and result from the catabolism of fatty acids
      a. Usually, ketones are filtered by the glomerulus and resorbed by the tubules
   2. Ketones are produced during fat metabolism and are important sources of energy
   3. Excessive ketones are toxic, producing central nervous system depression and acidosis

B. In normal animals, very small amounts are found in the blood
   1. If there is increased fat metabolism, excess ketones spill into the urine, causing ketonuria
      a. Ketonemia (excess ketones in circulation [ketosis, acetonemia]) results in ketonuria

C. Commonly, in large animals, ketosis (pregnancy toxemia) is associated with hypoglycemia consequential to high glucose demands, resulting in increased fat metabolism
   1. Typically occurs in early lactation or late pregnancy, whereas in small animals, ketosis occurs with diabetes mellitus; lack of insulin prevents carbohydrate utilization

D. Several reagent test strips or separate reagent tablets can be used to measure ketone levels
   1. Color intensity is proportional to ketone concentration
   2. These tests are most sensitive to acetoacetic acid and acetone

V. Bile pigments

A. Commonly detected bile pigments include bilirubin and urobilinogen
   1. Only conjugated bilirubin is found in the urine
   2. A small amount of urobilinogen, from the breakdown of bilirubin by bacteria in the intestines, is excreted into the urine

B. Determination of bile pigments is made with reagent test strips and tablet tests, with the tablet tests being more accurate
   1. A rough determination of the presence of bilirubinuria can be determined if urine is shaken and a yellow foam forms
   2. Positive bilirubin test pads in cats are usually reliable, whereas in dogs there can be a significant number of false-negative and false-positive results
      a. Urobilinogen is not easily detected; therefore urobilinogen test pads in both dogs and cats have not been always reliable

C. Bilirubinuria can be seen in several diseases, including biliary obstruction, hepatic infections, toxicity, and hemolytic anemia
   1. Light will oxidize bilirubin if urine is left standing, resulting in a false-negative result
   2. Because the liver and kidneys of dogs and cattle have an enzyme that can conjugate bilirubin, slight bilirubinuria may be present in these species

VI. Blood

A. Presence of intact RBCs in the urine is referred to as hematuria, whereas the presence of free hemoglobin is hemoglobinuria, and presence of myoglobin is myoglobinuria
   1. Hematuria, hemoglobinuria, and myoglobinuria change the color of urine to pink to red to brown
      a. A crude method to distinguish between myoglobinuria and hemoglobinuria is to evaluate the plasma/serum for the presence of hemolysis
         (1) If the urine and plasma/serum are fresh and both are reddish, hematuria is most likely present
         (2) Colorless plasma is indicative of myoglobinuria, because myoglobin does not emit a color in the plasma
         (3) Myoglobinuria is accompanied by intact red blood cells; an elevated plasma/serum creatine kinase (CK)

may also suggest the possibility of myoglobin in the urine, because an increase in both may indicate insult to muscle tissue

   b. To distinguish hematuria from hemoglobinuria and myoglobinuria

     (1) Precentrifugation: with hematuria, urine is cloudy because of the presence of intact erythrocytes

     (2) Postcentrifugation of the urine

       (a) The supernatant will remain colorless in the case of hematuria

       (b) If hemoglobinuria and myoglobinuria are present, the urine supernatant will still be reddish

  B. Occult blood may also be present, with no visible changes to the urine

  C. Hematuria is associated with disease of the urogenital tract

    1. Hemoglobinuria indicates some intravascular hemolysis

     a. Caution: postcollection hemolysis occurs with improperly handled or stored urine

    2. Myoglobinuria generally indicates a muscle pathology or overexertion

  D. Besides color interpretation, blood or blood components in the urine are detected with reagent strips as well as tablets

    1. Because these do not differentiate the cause of blood in urine, microscopic evaluation to determine RBC number, animal history and examination, and other tests should be included in the evaluation process

VII. Nitrite level in urine in humans is used as an indirect indication of bacteriuria

  A. It is believed that ascorbic acid normally present in canine and feline urine usually gives false-negative results

  B. Bacterial cultures and microscopic evaluation of fresh urine samples are the best methods for detecting the presence of bacteriuria

VIII. Leukocyte tests are designed to detect the presence of leukocyte esterase, found in all types of white blood cells, except lymphocytes

  A. False-positive results for cats and false-negative results for dogs are common; therefore it is best to evaluate fresh urine samples microscopically for the presence of leukocytes

  B. In addition, false-negative results may occur in patients with glucosuria and elevated USG, and in those treated with certain antibiotics (e.g., tetracycline)

  C. Falsely elevated results have been observed in old samples and those contaminated with feces

  D. Check package insert

IX. Urobilinogen is formed in the gastrointestinal (GI) tract by anaerobic bacteria breaking down conjugated bilirubin, with small amounts eliminated in the urine and the majority in the feces

  A. When elevated, the test may be indicative of liver or GI tract dysfunction or intravascular hemolysis

    1. Because of the instability of urobilinogen, false negatives have been observed in acidic urine, old samples, and those exposed to light and air

    2. False positives have been observed when the reagent strips have been stored close to a heat source

    3. Unlike in humans, a significantly increased urobilinogen level with the chemistry dipstick has not been observed in most patients; therefore the usefulness of the test in animals is questionable

## Microscopic Evaluation

Examination of the urine sediment is highly valuable when used with the urine physical and chemistry tests, and hematology and serum/plasma chemistries. Microscopic evaluation may be considered a form of exfoliate cytology.

I. Sample preparation

  A. Best sample is obtained after a period of extended rest, because it is more likely to be highly concentrated

  B. Refrigerate the sample if it cannot be examined within 20 to 30 minutes. Room temperature storage can result in bacterial growth, natural chemical breakdown, and cell lysis

  C. Thoroughly mix the specimen, transfer to a conical-tip centrifuge tube, and centrifuge sample at the speed and time specified by the centrifuge manufacturer

    1. At least 5 mL fresh urine is ideal, but "micro" methods and containers are available for smaller samples

  D. Note the volume of sediment; leave a small amount of the supernatant and resuspend the sediment by gently tapping the bottom of the tube with your finger

    1. Using a pipette, transfer a small drop of urine to a clean microscope slide and examine (Note: Do not use a wooden stick, because cells and other constituents commonly adhere to the stick)

     a. Cover-slipping is optional, based on experience and personal preference

     b. Viewing of stained (e.g., wet: Sternheimer-Malbin, 0.5% new methylene blue [NMB]) or unstained urine is based on experience and personal preference

(1) If you do stain, do not attempt to mix the stain on the slide with the urine. Mix in the tube for the best suspension of stain and urine

(2) The type of stain will specifically influence the appearance of the microscopic elements. Use an unstained sample to distinguish between stain artifacts and urine constituents

(3) Diff-Quik can also be used for stained urine preparation, with films prepared in methods similar to blood and other cytology films. Because urine is a fluid with typically low protein content, it may be washed off the slide in the staining process. Use of serum-coated slides may limit the loss of supernatant

E. Reduce illumination (lower condenser), view entire area under the coverslip through a 10× (low power field [LPF]) objective, and then through a 40× (high power field [HPF]) objective

F. Crystals and cast numbers are typically estimated as the average number per LPF

  1. Epithelial cells and blood cells are estimated as the average number per HPF

  2. Bacteria and sperm are noted as few, moderate, or many under HPF

G. Contaminated or unrefrigerated "stale" samples should be avoided

  1. Samples that have not been thoroughly resuspended after centrifugation may yield a non-representative sediment

  2. Sediments that were allowed to dry on the microscope slide may make cells unrecognizable

  3. Stain precipitate may mimic cells and crystals

II. Components of sediment (Figure 2-1)

A. Normally, very few WBCs (leukocytes) are found (Color Plates 1 and 2)

  1. Most cells in urine are neutrophils, which appear spherical, granular, and larger than RBCs, but smaller than epithelial cells

  2. Excessive number of WBCs is referred to as pyuria or leukocyturia

  3. An increased number indicates active inflammatory disease along the urinary tract, but can also be contaminants from the genital tract

  4. More than a few (5 to 8 per HPF) should be regarded as abnormal and further investigated

  5. Note any evidence of bacteria

B. The number of RBCs (erythrocytes) is also normally small (Color Plates 1 and 3)

  1. Excessive number of RBCs is referred to as hematuria

  2. Hematuria is associated with trauma, calculi, infection, and benign or malignant neoplasia

3. RBCs appear as pale yellow refractive disks, usually uniform in shape and smaller than WBCs

  a. Sample manipulation can create distortion, crenation, and hemolysis, and confusion with fat or yeast

    (1) Fat droplets (Color Plate 5) will float in and out of planes of focus; RBCs do not. Additionally, fat drops usually vary more in size, do not take on a crenated appearance, and will stain shades of iridescent orange with Sudan III or IV stain

    (2) If a small amount of 2% acetic acid is added to the slide and the structures disappear, they were RBCs

4. In concentrated urine, RBCs may lose fluid and become crenated (shrunken and spiked)

  a. In dilute urine they may swell or lyse, becoming ghost cells

5. More than a few (5 per HPF) should be noted as abnormal and further investigated

6. RBCs may be a contaminant of the female genital tract in void samples or poorly collected catheterized samples

C. Epithelial cells (Color Plate 2)

  1. Three types usually found in urine sediment: squamous, transitional, and renal

  2. Squamous cells are derived from the urethra, vagina, and vulva, and are the largest cells found in urine sediment

    a. These are partially or fully cornified, appearing as flat, irregularly shaped cells with angular borders, and if present, have small round nuclei

    b. Usually not seen in samples obtained by cystocentesis or catheterization

    c. Their presence is not considered significant

  3. Transitional cells come from the bladder, ureters, renal pelvis, and part of the urethra

    a. Wide variation in size; may be round, pear shaped, or caudate, typically with granular cytoplasm

    b. Increased numbers are associated with inflammation, such as cystitis

  4. Renal cells originate from the renal tubules, are found in small numbers, are slightly larger than WBCs, and are sometimes difficult to differentiate from WBCs

    a. Usually round with a large nucleus

    b. Increased numbers indicate renal tubular disease

D. Casts (cylinduria) (see Figure 2-1)

  1. Formed in and taking the cylindrical shape of the distal and collecting tubules of the kidneys

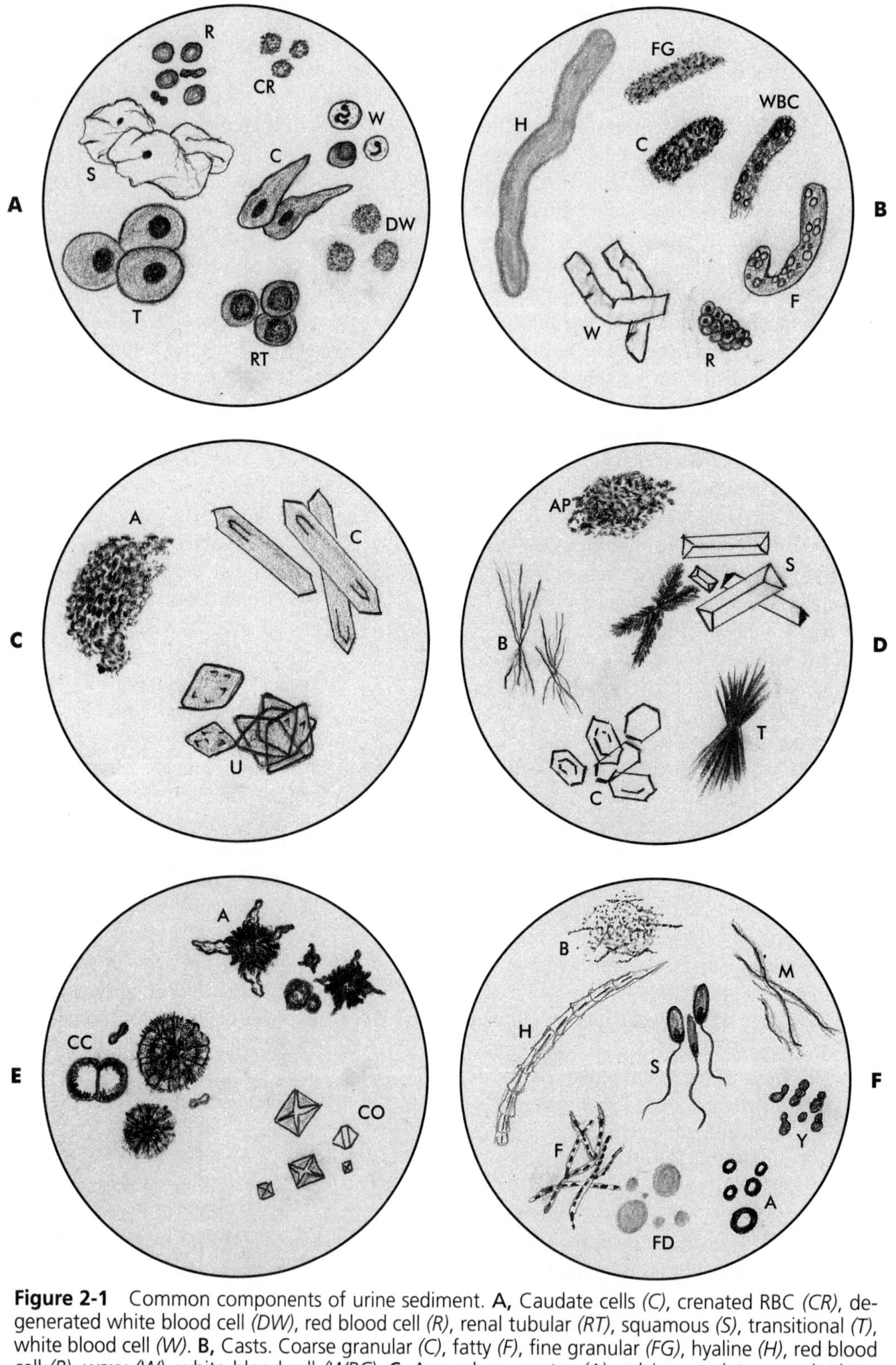

**Figure 2-1** Common components of urine sediment. **A,** Caudate cells (C), crenated RBC (CR), degenerated white blood cell (DW), red blood cell (R), renal tubular (RT), squamous (S), transitional (T), white blood cell (W). **B,** Casts. Coarse granular (C), fatty (F), fine granular (FG), hyaline (H), red blood cell (R), waxy (W), white blood cell (WBC). **C,** Amorphous urates (A), calcium oxalate monohydrate (C), uric acid (U). **D,** Amorphous phosphate (AP), bilirubin (B), cystine (C), struvite/triple phosphate (S), tyrosine (T). **E,** Ammonium biurate/"thorn apple" (A), calcium carbonate (CC), calcium oxalate dihydrate/"envelope" (CO). **F,** Air bubbles (A), bacteria (B), fat droplets (FD), fungi (F), hair (H), mucus (M), sperm (S), yeast (Y). (Drawings by Toni D'Amato-Scheck, AAS, LVT, from Walsh D, D'Amato-Scheck T, editors: *Clinical technician lab manual,* State University of New York at Delhi, 2001.)

a. Common to all cast formation is an acid environment, presence of mucoproteins, increased time of flow through the tubules, and increased salt concentration
2. Dissolve in alkaline urine; so analyze fresh samples immediately
3. Any structures that are in the tubules at the time the casts are formed may embed themselves in the cast
4. Casts are commonly indicative of renal tubular irritation, inflammation, and degeneration, and larger numbers of casts may help localize pathology to the renal tubules, but numbers and types of casts do not always indicate the prognosis or severity of the disease
   a. May be only a few casts in severe chronic nephritis
   b. Types of casts may be more indicative of the time span the cast has been present in the tubule and the "aging process" of the cast
      (1) For example, casts degrade in the following order: degenerating tubule > hyaline cast > renal tubular cells adhere to hyaline cast > renal tubular cell cast > coarse granular cast > fine granular > waxy
   c. Usually no casts are found, but it is not unusual to find one or two hyaline casts or granular casts per LPF in moderately concentrated urine in the apparently healthy patient
      (1) The presence of renal tubular cell casts and increased number of granular casts are commonly indicative of tubular degeneration, whereas white cell casts suggest inflammation of the tubules, and RBC casts indicate bleeding into the tubules
      (2) Cell casts are usually always significant
   d. The conditions may be acute, minor and reversible, or chronic and permanent
5. Hyaline casts
   a. A few may be seen in normal urine
   b. Clear, colorless, refractile, and composed of mucoprotein
   c. Cylindrical with relatively symmetrical sides and rounded ends
   d. Indicates mildest form of renal irritation
   e. Seen with low light and may be mimicked by mucus strands
6. Cellular casts (tubular epithelial, red and white blood cell)
   a. Epithelial casts contain cells from renal epithelium

(1) Seen in acute nephritis and renal tubule degeneration
   b. RBC casts occur when RBCs adhere to the hyaline cast during hemorrhage into the tubules
      (1) RBC casts are fragile, but in fresh urine, they appear similar to the "free" RBCs, being yellow to orange-red in unstained urine
   c. WBC casts occur in an inflammatory process
      (1) Composed primarily of neutrophils
      (2) Easily visually confused with renal tubular cell casts, especially if the tubular cells are degenerated
      (3) Look for free WBCs. They may be more commonly found in the presence of WBC casts
      (4) Form granular casts as the WBCs degenerate
7. Granular casts (Color Plates 5 and 6)
   a. Most common type seen in animals
   b. Commonly, contain pieces (granules) of degenerate epithelial cells and WBCs or precipitated plasma proteins or by-products of protein metabolism
   c. The "cellular" granules may deteriorate from larger pieces of cellular material, coarse granular casts, to small cellular fragments, fine granular casts
   d. Seen in greater numbers with acute nephritis; may indicate severe kidney disease
8. Fatty (lipid) casts
   a. Fatty casts contain small to variable-size, refractile fat droplets
      (1) The lipids come from degenerated cells where the lipid had accumulated
      (2) Not unusual in cats with renal disease and dogs with diabetes mellitus, as well as other tubular diseases
9. Waxy casts are wide, square ended, colorless to dull gray, with comparatively refractile edges, and commonly have a "brittle" appearance
   a. More opaque than hyaline casts and indicate chronic to severe tubular degeneration, with conditions of extremely low passage rates
   b. Can be seen with more light than hyaline casts
E. Crystals (see Figure 2-1)
   1. May be normal or abnormal
      a. Term *crystalline* may or may not be of clinical significance
   2. Crystal formation is influenced by pH, temperature, concentration, diet, and medication

3. Struvite (magnesium ammonium phosphate, triple phosphate) (Color Plates 3 and 4)
   a. Appear as classic "coffin lids"—three- to six-sided colorless prisms normally found in alkaline urine
   b. May be associated with urease-producing bacteria of lower urinary tract disease, often in association with uroliths
   c. Can be found in slightly acidic urine
4. Amorphous phosphate/urates (Color Plate 7)
   a. Phosphates found in alkaline urine appear as granular precipitate
   b. Urates are similar but are found in acidic urine
   c. Ammonium biurate crystals are round and brownish, with long spicules, sometimes having a "thorn-apple" or "mange mite" appearance
      (1) Seen in liver disease or portal caval shunts
      (2) Commonly found in Dalmatians
5. Calcium carbonate (Color Plate 7)
   a. Often found in normal horses
   b. Resemble dumbbells, oval, wheel-like in shape
6. Calcium oxalate (Color Plate 7)
   a. Small, colorless envelopes, sometimes dumbbell or ring formed, usually with a characteristic X form in the center
   b. Generally in acidic urine, but can be seen in neutral or alkaline urine
   c. Dihydrate calcium oxalate crystals are found in normal urine
      (1) Monohydrate calcium oxalate crystals seen in animals with ethylene glycol toxicity, or in large animals that ingested oxalates
      (2) Also associated with calcium oxalate urolithiasis
7. Leucine/cystine/tyrosine (Color Plate 6)
   a. May indicate hepatic disease
   b. Leucine crystals are small and round, with sectioned centers
   c. Tyrosine crystals appear spiculated and spindle shaped
   d. Cystine crystals are flat and hexagon shaped (six sided)
      (1) Their presence may indicate metabolic defect of cystine metabolism
      (2) Possible association with uroliths
   e. All three are found in acidic urine
8. Uric acid
   a. Acid urine and associated with metabolic defect
9. Bilirubin crystals (Color Plate 4) often found if there is bilirubinuria

10. Some drugs, such as sulfonamides, may precipitate and form crystals
11. Crystals may form in standing urine, especially if the urine is refrigerated or if the sample is left open to the air and moisture is lost
    a. Warming of the urine may cause crystals to dissolve
F. Other cells may be found in urine sediment
   1. Spermatozoa (Color Plates 4 and 6) can be seen in the urine of an intact male, but they are clinically insignificant
   2. Parasite ova in the urine sediment may indicate fecal contamination or urine parasites
   3. Fat droplets are highly refractile, spherical, and of various shapes and sizes; thus they are often difficult to differentiate from other cells, especially RBCs; however, they can be stained with Sudan stain, and are in focus just on the underside of the coverslip
   4. Bacteria (Color Plate 2) may not be detected in the sediment until their numbers approach more than 10,000 per mL
      a. When stains are used, be careful to avoid precipitated or bacteria contaminated stains, because both may be falsely identified as sediment bacteria
      b. Cultures, Gram staining, and antimicrobial sensitivity testing should be used for identification of bacteria and selection of the antimicrobial agent

## Uroliths

I. The Minnesota Urolith Center reports the most common type of feline uroliths (urinary stones, concretions) to be calcium oxalate, followed by struvite, whereas historically in the dog, struvite is more common than calcium oxalate
II. The canine numbers seem to be gradually reversing with more recent submissions
   A. Although there are in-house chemical methods for the determination of the composition of the stones, quantitative mineral analysis at reference laboratories tends to provide the most accurate determinations
III. Reference laboratories use such techniques as polarizing light microscopy, infrared spectroscopy, and energy dispersive x-ray spectroscopy (EDAX)

## HEMATOLOGY

The most commonly performed hematology procedure is the complete blood count (CBC). It commonly includes determination of total erythrocyte counts, relative and absolute leukocyte counts, packed cell volume (PCV), total plasma protein, Hb level, RBC indices, and blood film evaluation.

I. Blood profiles (hemograms) can be expanded to include such parameters as platelet and reticulocyte values, and red cell mean diameters

II. It should be understood that actual values vary with the methodology, laboratory performing the tests and population of patients tested
   A. Abnormal patients may fall within the reference value range, whereas normal patients may be outside of the range
   B. Reference value ranges for the species tend to be wide, whereas individual patient normal ranges are narrower

## Blood Collection and Sampling

I. General rules
   A. Collect the smallest amount of blood necessary to perform all tests plus an adequate amount for retest or errors
      1. This will usually be approximately two times the initial amount necessary to accomplish the tests
      2. Use syringes and vacuum collection devices proportional to the size of the patient and volume needed
   B. Ethylenediaminetetraacetic acid (EDTA) is the best anticoagulant for hematology in most mammals
      1. When used in the proper ratio of anticoagulant to blood, it will cause the least changes in cell morphology
         a. For birds and reptiles, heparin is a better anticoagulant
      2. When using anticoagulants, fill the tube to at least 90% of its capacity to maintain the proper anticoagulant-to-blood ratio
         a. Do not put in more than the volume that a vacuum tube will collect
         b. Inadequate sample amount will cause crenation of the erythrocytes and changes in the leukocytes
   C. Be cautious when aspirating with a syringe, or a vacuum collection device that is too large
      1. Excessive vacuum may cause cell destruction and injury to the patient
   D. When transferring blood from a syringe to a vacuum container, either
      1. Remove the stopper from the tube and the needle from the syringe
         a. Gently push on the plunger to evacuate the blood from the syringe
         b. Better for preserving cell morphology
      2. Carefully pass the needle through the stopper and allow the vacuum to pull the blood from the syringe
         a. Simultaneously pushing the plunger on the syringe along with the vacuum from the tube will cause excessive pressure and damage cells

E. Avoid frequent collection from the same site
   1. May cause localized increases in the numbers of leukocytes and platelets, trauma, pain, and increased chance for hematoma formation
F. Samples collected immediately postprandial may be lipemic
G. Fear, excitement, struggling, stress, treatment, and restraint may cause relative changes in the patient's values, because of redistribution of cells from and to the marginal (storage) and circulating pools of blood
   1. Stress (glucocorticoid-induced) leukogram: mature neutrophilia, monocytosis, lymphopenia, eosinopenia
   2. Develops over several hours and persists for several days
      a. Physiological (epinephrine, excitement, "fight or flight") leukogram: lymphocytosis, mature neutrophilia
   3. Develops immediately and can resolve in as short as 30 minutes; more common in cats
   4. Relative polycythemia (transient increase in RBC mass): lacks total plasma protein increases, resulting from splenic contraction in
      a. Exercise, epinephrine release from fear, excitement or pain
      b. Manual compression of the spleen while restraining or lifting the patient
      c. Dehydration
      d. Relative anemia
         (1) Usually resulting from a dilution effect due to fluid administration
   5. Physiological thrombosis due to
      a. Splenic contraction sequential to epinephrine release, resulting from excitement and exercise
      b. Manual compression of the spleen while restraining and lifting the patient
H. Medications and fluids may have biological or dilution effects on the sample or may influence the test procedure
I. Patient history, such as recent vaccinations, surgery, and geographical origin, may influence results
J. Time of collection to time of testing is critical
   1. Sample degradation starts immediately after collection
   2. EDTA prevents coagulation but does not preserve the sample

## Erythrocyte (Red Blood Cell) Evaluation
(Figure 2-2, Table 2-1)

I. Erythrocyte PCV (measured value)
   A. Also termed hematocrit (HCT) (calculated value)
   B. Determines percentage of RBCs in the circulating blood volume

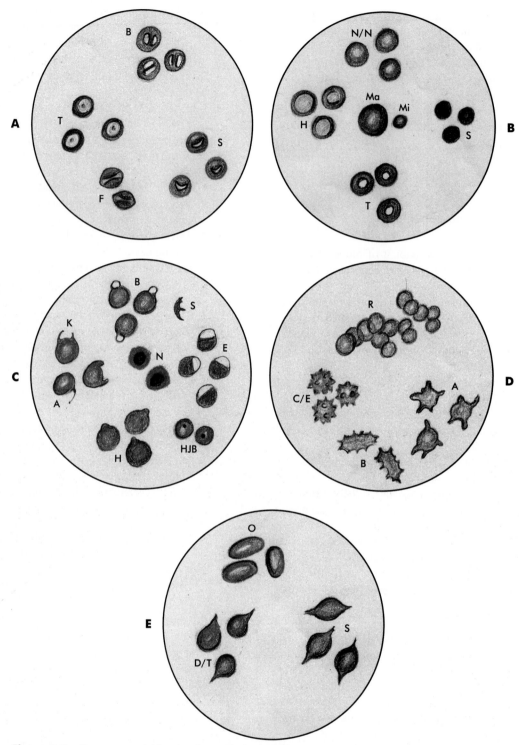

**Figure 2-2** Common red blood cell morphological changes and inclusions. **A,** Stomatocytes *(S)* and leptocytes: bar cell *(B)*, folded *(F)*, target cell *(T)*. **B,** Hypochromic *(H)*, macrocyte *(Ma)*, microcyte *(Mi)*, normocyte/normochromic *(N/N)*, spherocyte *(S)*. **C,** Apple stem cell *(A)*, blister cell *(B)*, eccentrocyte *(E)*, Heinz body *(H)*, Howell-Jolly body *(HJB)*, nucleated red blood cell *(N)*, schistocyte *(S)*. **D,** Acanthocyte *(A)*, burr cell *(B)*, echinocyte *(C/E)*, rouleaux *(R)*. **E,** Dacrocyte/teardrop *(D/T)*, ovalocyte *(O)*, spindle/fusiform cell *(S)*. (Drawings by Toni D'Amato-Scheck, AAS, LVT, from Walsh D, D'Amato-Scheck T, editors: *Clinical technician lab manual*, State University of New York at Delhi, 2001.)

**Table 2-1** Erythrocyte variations

| Erythrocyte variations | Description | Notes |
| --- | --- | --- |
| • Variations may be in vivo due to species, breed, environmental influences on the patient, and pathologies or in vitro due to problems in analytical methods, and preanalytical and postanalytical patient, collection, sample, and processing variables<br>• There may be multiple variations in or on a given cell or blood film<br>• Colors are as visualized with Romanowsky-Wright's-type stains, unless otherwise noted. Variations may occur with age, brand, and lot number of stain and staining techniques | | |
| **ANISOCYTOSIS** (Color Plates 13 to 16) (A general term denoting variation in erythrocyte size (only microcytic or macrocytic or combinations of sizes); combinations of sizes are not unusual in normal cattle and cats) | | |
| Normocyte | Commonly used to describe typical size of erythrocyte for a species | In some texts used to describe the typical shape, size, and color for species. For various species: Normocytes in mammals with discoid cells range from ~1.5 μm D in the Malay Chevrotain (Lesser Mouse Deer) to 7 μm D in the dog to ~10.8 μm D in the Northern Elephant Seal. The normocytes of the various species of reptiles, fish, birds, and amphibians have similar variations in size. Shape also varies and influences size. Camelids and nonmammals have elliptical cells |
| Macrocyte | Larger than typical erythrocytes for the species | Increased MCV, typically polychromatic, with the exception of equines. Usually immature cell. Sign of regeneration. When macrocytic and polychromatic they may be termed "macrocytic polychromatic erythrocytes" |
| Microcyte | Smaller than typical erythrocytes for the species | Decreased MCV |
| **ARRANGEMENT—CELLULAR ORGANIZATION—"BEHAVIOR" VARIATIONS** | | |
| Rouleaux (pronounced "ruu low") formation | RBCs appearing like elongated, tumbled stacks of coins | Common on the blood films of healthy equines, and to a lesser extent in cats, pigs, and dogs. Increases in any species may be indicative of an inflammatory or neoplastic condition. When present, rouleaux formations are observed throughout the film |
| Agglutination (autoagglutination) | Indiscriminate three-dimensional clumping of erythrocytes | Caused by immunoglobins bound to the erythrocytes. Although indicative of immune-mediated hemolytic anemia (IMHA [AIHA]), the Coombs test is more sensitive in identifying this condition. These clumps will be observed throughout the blood film. The erythrocytes are "immunologically" bound and will not disperse with the addition of normal saline to a drop of the patient's blood. These are not microclots caused by difficulty in collection of the sample or clotting pathologies |
| **COLOR VARIATIONS** | | |
| Normochromasia | Typical color erythrocyte for the species. Usually pinkish-red and influenced by the amount of central pallor. Mammals such as camels and llamas, which have elliptical, more or less flat erythrocytes, lack central pallor | Suggests an adequate amount of hemoglobin in the cell and typical MCHC for the species. Varying degrees of central pallor and complementary biconcavity may be present in those species having a discoid-shaped erythrocyte, with the dog having the most central pallor, and horse and goat the least in the common species |

Continued

**Table 2-1** Erythrocyte variations—cont'd

| Erythrocyte variations | Description | Notes |
|---|---|---|
| Hypochromasia | Lacking typical color of the erythrocyte for the species. Having an increased central pallor | Resulting from an inadequate amount of hemoglobin. Having a decreased MCHC. Common with an iron deficiency anemia. |
| Hyperchromasia (although mentioned in textbooks, the term is not commonly used—see Notes) | Appears as an increase in color intensity | Suggests an absolute increase in the amount of hemoglobin within the cell and increase in MCHC. True hyperchromasia most likely does not exist, but the presence of hemolysis, Heinz bodies, and lipemia may produce interferences in the tests and result in an artifactual "calculated" increase in MCHC. Spherocytes have the appearance (illusion) of being hyperchromic and smaller due to the change in shape, from discoid to spherical (ball-like), resulting in the lack of concavity and visible central pallor |
| Polychromasia (polychromatophilic, diffuse basophilia, polychromatophil) (Color Plates 13 to 15) | Varying degrees of bluish-staining of the erythrocyte cytoplasm. These cells are usually also macrocytic | This is indicative of varying aged-younger cells and is due to the presence of ribosomes in the cell. If stained with a vital stain (e.g., NMB), the reticular structure would be seen and the cell would be noted as a reticulocyte. This sign of regeneration is indicative of an active bone marrow. Polychromatic cells are not unusual in normal dogs and pigs, are fairly common in young pigs and rats, and are extremely rare in horses of any age. When macrocytic and polychromatic, they may be termed "macrocytic polychromatic erythrocytes" |
| **INCLUSIONS** (Because these are within the cell, they stay in focus when focusing up and down) | | |
| Basophilic stippling (Color Plate 16) | Variable size and number of blue granules distributed throughout the RBC; stay in focus with the RBC when focusing up and down | May be found in lead poisoning; regenerative response |
| Heinz bodies | Usually a singular, ~1-4 μm in diameter, "roundish," "noselike" protrusion from the surface of the erythrocyte, giving the RBC a "lightbulb" appearance. Most easily observed on the edge of the RBC | An oxidative injury resulting in denaturing of the hemoglobin. Heinz bodies will not stain with Wright's-type stains but will with vital stains, such as NMB. They are not uncommon in low numbers in healthy cats and may be associated with hemolytic anemia in all species. Seen in cats ingesting acetaminophen and dogs ingesting onions, acetaminophen, and other oxidative substances and drugs. |
| Howell-Jolly body (Color Plate 15) | Usually a singular, relatively round, nonprotruding, dark-purple inclusion approximately ~1 μm in diameter observed on the surface of the RBC | Remnants of nuclear chromatin. Sign of regeneration. Also found in splenectomized patients |
| Nucleated red blood cell (NRBC), metarubricyte (Color Plate 13) | Macrocytic cell with a polychromatic cytoplasm and nuclear appearance commensurate with the age of the RBC. Immature nonmammalian RBCs will be rounder and larger than their mature oval counterpart | Immature red cell, usually rubricytes and metarubricytes. The mature nonmammalian species cytoplasm will be pinkish-red |
| Siderotic granules/inclusions (siderocytes, Pappenheimer bodies, focal basophilic stippling) | Bluish, varying sized and shaped granules, usually distributed toward the periphery of the RBC | Contain iron. Found in such conditions as lead toxicity and hemolytic anemia |

**INFECTIOUS AGENTS** (Intracellular and extracellular parasites, bacteria, protozoa, and viral) (these are the more common agents)

| | | |
|---|---|---|
| *Aegyptianella* spp. | Very small organisms lacking pigmented granules and varying in appearance with the species and stage of development | Intracytoplasmic (within the cytoplasm), *Pirohemocyton*-like (*piro-* = "pear-shaped") virus of birds |
| *Anaplasma* spp. (Color Plate 16) *A. marginale* | Commonly numerous, small, ~1 μm in diameter, coccoid (round to oval) shaped, usually purple bodies typically on the margin of the RBC. Commonly smaller than Howell Jolly bodies and not as round | Worldwide occurrence *A. centrale*: endemic in Middle East, South America, southern Africa |
| *Babesia* spp. *B. bigemina* (bovine) *B. bovis* (bovine) *B. caballi* (equine) *B. canis* (canine) *B. equi* (equine) *B. gibsoni* (canine) | Common characteristics: colorless to light-blue cytoplasm and purple-to-red nuclei. More common in the RBCs at the feathered edge of the film *B. canis*: teardrop-pear-shaped structures, commonly in pairs *B. gibsoni*: round to oval and elongated | Intracellular (within the cell) piroplasmid protozoan of mammals, fish, reptiles (turtles, snakes, lizards) *B. felis* and *B. cati* are not believed to be currently present in North America |
| *Cytauxzoon felis* | Oval-ring-like, ~1(± 0.5) μm in diameter with clear center; small, blue nucleus; commonly at one end of the ring | Intracellular protozoan |
| Distemper viral inclusion body | If present, found on immature erythrocyte, variable in shape: round to oblong to irregular, ~1-2 μm in diameter, blue-gray to pale blue to dark violet-reddish-pink in color; smooth-glassy to granular in texture | Not commonly found. Usually larger than Howell Jolly bodies. Present in the viremic stage. Can be also found in all types of white blood cells |
| *Mycoplasma* spp. (formerly *Eperythrozoon* spp.) *Candidatus M. ovis* (formerly *E. ovis* [ovine]) *M. wenyonii* (formerly *E. wenyoni* [bovine]) *M. haemosuis* (formerly *E. suis* [porcine]) | Small (~0.5 μm), blue, singular or multiple pleomorphic (coccoid, rod, or ring shaped) organisms. May be on or off the RBC. Ring form common | *Mycoplasma* bacteria. Also present in llamas |
| *Mycoplasma* spp. (formerly *Haemobartonella* spp.) *M. haemofelis* (Ohio strain, large strain [formerly *H. felis*]) | Pleomorphic, small. On or off cell  Small, dark blue rods on the edge of the cell or ring form on the surface of the cell; RBC agglutination is not uncommon. Ring forms are uncommon | *Mycoplasma* bacteria. Epicellular (immediately beneath the membrane of the cell). Serological testing is more sensitive than a blood film for diagnosis. Most pathological strain. Common with FeLV-positive cats. *Candidatus M. haemominutum* (small strain, California strain): Pathological significance to cats is unclear |
| *M. haemocanis* (formerly *H. canis*) | Small, individual blue cocci to rods, more commonly in chains that are branching and "Y" shaped and go across the RBC | Found more commonly in splenectomized dogs or those that have splenic pathologies |

*Continued*

**Table 2-1** Erythrocyte variations—cont'd

| Erythrocyte variations | Description | Notes |
|---|---|---|
| *Haemoproteus (Hemoproteus)* spp. | Appearance varies with stage of development of the gametocyte but commonly does not distort the cell, despite occupying ~50% of the cellular area; may semiencircle the nucleus; stains dark purple to pale blue to pink. Granular purplish-pink pigmented material present | Intracellular, protozoa of birds |
| *Hemogregarina* spp. *Hematozoon* (snakes) *Hemogregarina* (semiaquatic freshwater turtles) *Karyolus* (Old World lizard) | Individual genera are difficult to differentiate in the erythrocytes. Common characteristics: 1-2 "sausage-shaped" intracytoplasmic gametocytes, which cause a distortion of the host erythrocyte and lack refractile pigment granules | Affects reptiles, fish, amphibians |
| *Leucocytozoon* spp. | Fills and distorts cell with a light- to dark-staining gametocyte; commonly elongated and spindle-shaped cell; commonly has a two-nuclei appearance: darker purplish-staining host erythrocyte nucleus and lighter purplish-pinkish staining parasite nucleus; no granular pigmented material | Intracellular, protozoa of birds |
| Microfilaria *Dirofilaria immitis* (heartworm [dogs, cats, ferrets]) | Vary with species. Earthwormlike with a blunt and pointed end. Stain blue | Microfilaria are extracelluar nematodes seen in amphibians, birds, reptiles, fish, and mammals. Microfilaria may be "sheathed" (e.g., *Folayella furcata* found in reptiles). *D. immitis* must be distinguished from the non-disease producing *Acanthocheilonema (Dipetalonema) reconditum* |
| *Plasmodium* spp. | Highly variable in appearance depending on species of *Plasmodium* and stage of development, but commonly erythrocytes are not distorted and have refractile, granular, pigmented material | Intracellular, flagellate protozoa of birds, reptiles (especially lizards and snakes); avian malaria |
| *Trypanosoma* spp. | Slender and wormlike in appearance, with undulating membrane, narrowed posterior, and single flagellum | Extracellular protozoan of amphibians, birds, reptiles, fish, amphibians, and mammals. Usually an incidental finding in birds. Transmitted by blood-sucking insects |
| **POIKILOCYTOSIS** (Color Plates 9 and 12) (true [nonartifactual], pathological) (a general term denoting nondescript variations in *shapes* of erythrocytes that are scattered throughout the blood film. *Note:* There is apparently not a total agreement on the definitions and causes for all terms used to describe the shapes of erythrocytes. Poikilocytosis is common in clinically healthy swine of all ages, young goats, and cattle. Normal shapes may vary from virtually flat [e.g., goat] to biconcave [e.g., dogs and primates] discs to elliptical [e.g., camelids and nonmammals]) | | |
| Acanthocytes (spur cell) | Varying number of unevenly sized and spaced "fingerlike" blunt projections | Commonly seen in hepatic associated diseases. May be seen in apparently healthy young cattle and goats. Metabolic/membrane disorder |

| | | |
|---|---|---|
| Blister cell | Blister or vesicle on side of RBC formed by a thin cell membrane, forming an area devoid of hemoglobin; giving the RBC a "padlock-like" appearance | An oxidative injury found with iron deficiency. Metabolic/membrane disorder |
| Keratocytes (horn cells) | Ruptured blister with two upright cattle "horn-like" projections | Keratocytes and apple-stem cell will most likely become schistocytes (see later) |
| Apple-stem cell | Ruptured blister forming a single projection | |
| Crystallized hemoglobin | Rod to cubical, usually dark red appearance | Not unusual in cats, llamas, and young puppies. No known pathological significance |
| Dacryocytes (dacrocyte, teardrop cells) | Teardrop-shaped erythrocytes with a single elongated or pointed end | May be found in bone marrow disorders of dogs and cats, iron deficiency in ruminants and modified ruminants, and kidney and splenic disorders of dogs. Result of mechanical fragmentation |
| Drepanocyte (sickle cell) | Change to a spindle shape (fusiform), being elongated and coming to a more or less sharp-to-round point on both ends | This in vitro phenomenon may occur in the blood of deer, Angora goat, and some British-breed sheep as a result of an alteration of the hemoglobin due to temperature, oxygen and pH changes |
| Eccentrocyte (hemighosts) | Red at one end of the RBC and colorless at the other, giving a "half moon" appearance to each side | Hemoglobin accumulated at one end of the cell. Found in hemolytic diseases. Seen in dogs ingesting onions, acetaminophen. Oxidative of hemoglobin. May be found with Heinz bodies |
| Elliptocyte (ovalocyte) | Oval or elliptical erythrocyte, being more flat than concave | Normal shape for camelids and nonmammalian species. They have been found in a variety of bone marrow disorders in dogs and cats, hepatic conditions in cats, and hereditary disorders in dogs. Metabolic/membrane disorder in mammals other than camelids |
| Echinocyte | Round-to-elongated cell with relatively evenly sized, shaped, and spaced blunt or pointed projections | Erythrocytes with ruptured cell membranes. Appearance may vary on the blood film depending on the thickness of the area. Metabolic/membrane disorder |
| Burr cell (echino elliptocytes) | Appear as elongated ruffled, with relatively evenly sized and spaced, short, blunt projections | An in vivo change; May be indicative of renal disease |
| Crenation (type I echinocyte) | Relatively round ruffled erythrocyte with sharp, evenly spaced spicules, which are commonly seen on the edge of the RBC | An in vitro artifactual change affecting all the erythrocytes on the entire film or in a given area of the film; indicative of excessive anticoagulant, alteration in pH from slow drying of blood films caused by thick films and environmental factors |
| Type III echinocytes | Very short, evenly spaced, fine spicules found on the surface the mature erythrocyte | An in vivo change, more common in animals bitten by rattle snakes |
| Ghost cells | Extremely pale to colorless, appearing round to smudgelike; may be more visible with decreased light | Virtually devoid of hemoglobin in the cytoplasm; in vivo resulting from very recent intravascular hemolysis or in vitro in the blood tube or in the preparation of the blood film. If a result of blood film preparation, they will usually appear as red smudges |
| Leptocytes | Thin, folded RBC. Commonly larger and polychromatic | Increased cell membrane compared with the total cell volume and internal contents. Found when there is increased production of erythrocytes, and hepatic conditions. Metabolic/membrane disorder |
| Target cells (codocytes) | "Targetlike" or "bullseye" appearance with red center and alternating red and white rings | Increased surface area of the cell membrane or decreased cytoplasmic volume; may be found in such conditions as hepatic disorders, iron deficiency anemia, and immune mediated hemolytic anemia |
| Bar cells (knizocyte) | Red "barlike" outfolding across the center of the cell appearing similar to the international "no" symbol (⊘) | See Target Cell for causes |

Continued

**Table 2-1** Erythrocyte variations—cont'd

| Erythrocyte variations | Description | Notes |
|---|---|---|
| Schistocytes (schizocytes) | Varying size and shaped fragments of erythrocyte; common irregular shapes include triangles, helmet, crescents; nondescript | Usually formed from intravascular shearing of the cell. Diseases may include disseminated intravascular coagulopathy (DIC), iron deficiency, and vascular neoplasms. Result of mechanical fragmentation |
| Spherocyte (Color Plates 13 to 15) | Dark red staining, appearing smaller than average size, round, lacks central pallor | Common in hemolytic anemias |
| Stomatocytes | Cup-shaped erythrocytes with an oval, elongated "smiley face" appearance to the central pallor | There may be an in vitro artifact in a thick blood film or in vivo artifact resulting from a hereditary condition in dogs or drug induced. Metabolic/membrane disorder |
| **ARTIFACTS** (Because they are on the surface of the cell, they will not stay in focus with the cell when focusing up and down) | | |
| Cellular overlap | Crowded cells with uneven distribution of all types of cells | Thick area of blood film |
| Crenation | See Echinocyte | |
| Ghost cells | See Ghost Cells | |
| Overstaining (pseudopolychromasia) | General bluish or greenish staining of cells regardless of age | Greenish staining may be due to the exposure of sample to formalin; bluish staining may be due to prolonged exposure to the basophilic component of the stain |
| Stain precipitate | Varying shape and size, usually purple granules on and around the cell to do not stay in focus with the cell when focusing up and down | Check film, staining and drying technique, and condition of stain. Do not shake stain container to attempt to resuspend precipitate |
| Stomatocyte | See Stomatocyte | |
| Refractile artifacts (water droplets/ residue, refractory bubbles) | Varying shape and size "bubbles" that refract when focusing up and down | Check blood film staining, rinsing and drying technique. Blood on slide may not have been before staining. May be water residue or gas trapped as it escapes the cell |
| Torocytes (punched-out cells) | Abrupt change from dense red to white area giving a "punched-out" appearance, as contrasted to a gradual change with a normal central pallor; may appear smaller than normal RBCs | Must be distinguished from hypochromic RBCs. Artifact of improper spreading of blood on slide |

*FeLV*, Feline leukemia virus; *MCHC*, mean corpuscular hemoglobin concentration; *MCV*, mean corpuscular volume; *NMB*, new methylene blue; *RBC*, red blood cell.

C. Most easily measured by filling a microcapillary or hematocrit tube with fresh, anticoagulated blood

D. Tubes are sealed and centrifuged at high speed

1. Actual time depends on the speed and centrifugation angle

2. Hematocrit centrifuges are often preset for speed

3. Goat and sheep blood should be centrifuged for twice the time of dog blood

a. The mean size of small RBCs (< 4 to 5 μm) in goat and sheep blood increases cell numbers and subsequent packing time

E. Results are determined by use of a scale on the centrifuge, hand-held card, or mechanical reader

F. Results are reported as percentage (%) in conventional units (or as liter per liter [L/L] in SI units)

G. Color (e.g., hemolysis, icterus) and clarity (e.g., lipemia) of plasma, presence of microfilaria, and total plasma protein (TPP) can be evaluated from the plasma fraction of the PCV (hematocrit) tube

H. The hydration status of the patient will relatively influence the values; dehydration relatively increases the value and overhydration relatively decreases values

I. A calculated HCT may vary from an actual PCV, because of influences of methodology

II. Erythrocyte total numbers

A. Determined by using an automated (e.g., impedance counter, flow cytometry, etc.) or a manual cell counting device (*Note*: As of the printing of this text, manual methods are limited to the use of Thoma erythrocyte-diluting pipettes, due to the elimination of availability of commerically prepared disposable erythrocyte-diluting pipette-reservoir counting systems)

B. Automated counters require calibration for cell size, depending on species

C. Manual counts are made with a hemocytometer and are usually not as accurate

D. Both methods require that the sample be diluted before counting

E. Total erythrocyte count usually has no advantage over the PCV except to determine the RBC indices

F. Total RBC numbers are reported as millions per microliter ($n \times 10^6/\mu L$, or $n \times 10^{12}/L$ in SI units)

III. Hemoglobin

A. Part of the RBCs responsible for carrying oxygen and carbon dioxide

B. Assists in acid-base regulation by eliminating carbon dioxide

C. Can be measured by photometric methods, or directly or indirectly measured on automated cell counters

D. Used for determining erythrocytic indices

E. Measured in g/dL (g/L)

F. For a quick guesstimation, the normal animal Hb content is about one third of the PCV

1. This ratio is based on a typically healthy patient with an average RBC size of 7 μm

IV. Erythrocyte indices

A. Determined by use of the total RBC numbers, Hb content, and PCV; many electronic instruments automatically include these values

1. Used in classifying some anemias

B. Mean corpuscular volume (MCV)

1. Mean volume of a group of erythrocytes

2. Terminology with regard to their size

a. Macrocytosis = increased MCV

b. Microcytosis = decreased MCV

c. Normocytosis = size appropriate for the species

d. Anisocytosis = varying cell size (not used as a descriptor for MCV)

3. MCV is calculated by multiplying PCV (%) by 10 and dividing the product by the total RBC count (number of millions)

a. As an example, for a PCV of 45% (use as a whole number) and an RBC count of 5,000,000/μL (5 million):

(1) $(45 \times 10) \div 5.0 = 450 \div 5.0 = 90$ fL

4. MCV is recorded in femtoliters (fL); normal ranges vary among species

5. For SI units, divide the PCV (L/L) by the RBC count and multiply by 1000

C. Mean corpuscular hemoglobin (MCH)

1. Mean weight of Hb contained in the average RBC

a. MCH is calculated by multiplying the Hb concentration by 10 and dividing the product by the total RBC count (number of millions); for example, for an Hb level of 15 g/dL and RBC count of 5,000,000/μL:

$(15 \times 10) \div 5.0 = 150 \div 5.0 = 30$ pg

b. Results are recorded in picograms (pg)

2. Considered the least accurate of the indices, because Hb level and RBC count are less accurate than PCV

D. Mean corpuscular hemoglobin concentration (MCHC) is the concentration (proportion) of Hb in the average RBC

1. Terminology regarding hemoglobin concentration

a. Hypochromasia = decreased MCHC/increased level of central pallor

b. Hyperchromasia = increased MCHC (usually artifactual)

(1) No true hyperchromic state is thought to exist

c. Normochromasia = MCHC appropriate level of central pallor for the species

2. MCHC is calculated by multiplying the Hb concentration by 100 and dividing the product by the PCV (%)
   a. For Hb of 15 g/dL, and PCV of 45% (use as a whole number):
      (1) $(15 \times 100) \div 45 = 1500 \div 45 = 33$ g/dL or 33%
   b. Results are reported in g/dL (g/L)
      (1) For SI units, divide the Hb concentration (g/L) by the PCV (L/L)
      (2) Considered the most accurate of the RBC indices because it does not require the RBC count
E. Red cell distribution (RDW) is an electronic measurement of width of the RBCs
   1. Higher RDWs indicate increased anisocytosis, whereas normal values indicate normal cell size variations

V. Reticulocyte count
A. Expression of the percentage of RBCs that are reticulocytes, or immature erythrocytes still containing the ribosomes
B. Wright's stain causes a polychromatophilic staining, or diffuse, blue-gray color
C. Cats possess two forms: aggregate and punctate
   1. Only the aggregate form should be counted
   2. Similar to other species, this contains large clumps that appear polychromatophilic
D. A few drops of blood are mixed with an equal amount of NMB stain
   1. This mixture is used to prepare a conventional blood film that shows up as deep blue granular material in the young RBCs
E. Percentage of reticulocytes per 1000 RBCs or an absolute count in reticulocytes per milliliter is reported
   1. Absolute reticulocyte count/$\mu$L = reticulocyte % $\times$ total RBC count/$\mu$L
F. Useful in assessing the bone marrow response to anemia in all domestic animals, except for horses, because they do not release reticulocytes from the bone marrow

## Leukocyte (White Blood Cell) Evaluation

I. Total leukocyte counts may be made manually or with automated cell counters
A. For a manual count, a Neubauer hemocytometer and Unopette (Becton, Dickinson and Co., Franklin Lakes, NJ) dilution system is used for sample preparation
   1. Erythrocytes are lysed with this system to limit interference with the count
B. Automated counters use a variety of methods including impedance, quantitative buffy coat, and flow cytometry

C. Nucleated red blood cells (NRBCs) may interfere with the leukocyte counts, because they mimic the leukocyte and inflate the count
   1. Manual counting methods and those automated systems that lack the sophistication to address correcting for the presence of NRBCs must be manually corrected using the values gained in the WBC count and an enumeration of the number of NRBCs observed in the counting and identification of 100 WBCs on the differential film
      a. Example: total WBC is 9000/$\mu$L ($n \times 10^9$/L) 10% NRBCs or 900 absolute NRBCs
         (1) $9000 - 900 = 8100$/$\mu$L as the corrected total WBC
D. Avian and reptilian leukocyte count
   1. Birds and reptiles have NRBCs, which makes determining a WBC count difficult with the mammalian methods
      a. With the advent of laser flow technology, the possibility of an automated counting method of nonmammailian blood cells exists. Manual methods are crude and include the use of various reagents to highlight the cells (0.1% Phloxine B Diluent in propylene glycol or Natt and Herrick's solution)
E. Increased WBC count is leukocytosis
F. Decreased WBC count is leukopenia

II. Leukocyte evaluation and differentiation
A. WBC evaluation and differentiation is performed by examining the stained blood film
   1. Traditional stains include Wright's, Wright-Giemsa, and Diff-Quik (American Scientific Products, McGaw Park, Ill)
   2. Techniques vary
      a. Follow manufacturer's directions
B. Cells should be examined and counted in an area of the blood film where distribution and staining properties are best
   1. Monolayer of cells is preferable; examination is completed under 100 $\times$ oil immersion magnification
   2. Avoid "feathered edge counting" because of increased number of artifacts, but scan this area because it is not uncommon for blood parasites and basophils to be located here
   3. If a coverslip is put on immersion oil, there is more definition of cells
C. Leukocyte differential numbers should always be reported as absolutes
   1. Percentage of each cell type is multiplied by the total WBC count/$\mu$L
      a. Example: 60% neutrophils $\times$ 10,000 WBC/$\mu$L total = 6000 (absolute) neutrophils/$\mu$L
D. Leukocyte morphology (Table 2-2)

**Table 2-2** Leukocyte morphology

| WBC variations | Description | Notes |
|---|---|---|
| | | **NEUTROPHILS*** |
| Neutrophils (Color Plates 8 to 12, 15, and 16) | Irregular, segmented nucleus with coarse clumped chromatin staining dark purple<br>Cytoplasm is pale blue with faint granulation | Granulocyte; also classed as an acidophil in reptiles; most common peripheral WBCs in companion animals<br>Species variations: second most common WBC in cattle; horse neutrophils show more segmentation than dog neutrophils; granules in canine neutrophils are commonly not distinctive; avian and other nonmammalian neutrophils are commonly called heterophils and have rectangular granules vs. rounder granules in mammalian species<br>Average life span of 10 hours<br>Phagocytic and bactericidal properties<br>*Neutropenia* may be due to decreased survival of cells, reduced or ineffective production, or sequestration; will likely produce a *degenerative left shift* (more immature than mature neutrophils)<br>Immature neutrophil stage; inflammation is usually indicated by increased bands; increase may also be due to stress, exercise, glucocorticoid use, or leukemia |
| | | Increased numbers of immature neutrophils=*left shift*<br>*Degenerative left shift*=number of immature exceeds the number of mature cells and decreasing total WBC count<br>*Regenerative left shift*=number of mature neutrophils exceeds the number of immature, but total WBC is at a typical to increasing number of WBCs<br>*Orderly left shift*=number of each immature cell stage decreases with the degree of immaturity of the cell stages |
| Neutrophilic bands (Color Plate 15) | Sausage to horseshoe shaped; symmetrical nuclear borders with rounded ends | |
| Pelger-Huët anomaly | Hyposegmented bilobed nucleus that appears like a "peanuts in a shell" or "eye glasses," with cytoplasm appearing mature and chromatin condensed | Congenital, nonpathological disorder in dogs and cats<br>"False left shift"<br>A transient pseudo–Pelgar-Huët anomaly may occur with some severe inflammatory diseases in cattle, horses, and pigs<br>Also may be present in eosinophils and basophils |
| Neutrophilic metamyelocyte | Compared to the band: nucleus more kidney bean–shaped, chromatin less condensed, cytoplasm deeper blue | One stage younger than bands; rarely found in circulating blood |
| Toxic neutrophils (reactive neutrophils) | | Changes with toxicity and functioning of the cell=reactivity (cell performing its typical defensive function); often indicative of bacterial disease; many times more evident in the feline |
| Döhle bodies | Appear as small, gray-blue cytoplasmic inclusions | Indicative of mild toxemia |
| Basophilia | Blue cytoplasm, usually with vacuoles | Slightly more severe signs of toxicity and reactivity |
| Hypersegmentation (Color Plate 11) | Nuclear segmentation increased for what is typical for the species<br>Increased segmentation beyond what is typical for the species | Implies older neutrophils; *right shift*=an increased number of hypersegmented neutrophils |
| Barr body (sex bud or lobe) | Appendage on the nucleus shaped like a drum stick or tennis racket | Found typically on the neutrophils of females and occasionally hermaphrodites; may also be found on other granulocytes |

*Polymorphonuclear (PMN); synonyms: heterophil in avian, reptile, and fish; and pseudoeosinophil in rabbits, and some rodents. It is an older term but still may be seen in laboratory animal and European literature.
*RBC*, Red blood cell; *WBC*, white blood cell.

*Continued*

**Table 2-2** Leukocyte morphology—cont'd

| WBC variations | Description | Notes |
|---|---|---|
| **LYMPHOCYTES** (Color Plates 8, 11, and 13) | | |
| Lymphocyte | Typically round, larger than RBC; vary in size from small to large; large nucleus, staining deep purple with dense chromatin, usually eccentrically placed and occupying most of the cytoplasmic area; cytoplasm typically darker at the periphery of the cell and becomes lighter as it approaches the nucleus (perinuclear clear zone, "ballerina skirting" effect), and may have small purple-pinkish granules (azurophilic) | Agranulocyte Function in immunologic defense Cattle tend to have more lymphocytes than neutrophils |
| Reactive (activated) lymphocytes | Possibly more pronounced: perinuclear zone, basophilic cytoplasm, azurophilic granules, or cytoplasmic vacuolization; possible nuclear variations including indentation | A sign of antigenic stimulation |
| Kurloff body | Large, single, granular inclusion in the cytoplasm | Guinea pig |
| Plasma cell | Eccentric, round nucleus with condensed/clumped chromatin; deep blue staining cytoplasm; perinuclear to juxtanuclear (next to) clear zone (Golgi apparatus); smaller nucleus in relation to cytoplasm compared to typical lymphocyte | End stage of B lymphocyte differentiation; rarely seen in circulating blood |
| **MONOCYTES** (Color Plates 9 and 14) | | |
| | Variable nuclear shape (kidney bean shape, elongated, lobulated) with diffuse chromatin, not as intensely stained; blue-gray cytoplasm, possibly with vacuoles and fine pink granules; may be difficult to distinguish from band neutrophils or metamyelocytes | Largest of the peripheral WBCs; circulate briefly in blood before entering tissues as macrophages |
| **EOSINOPHILS** (Color Plates 10 and 12) | | |
| | Nuclear structure similar to neutrophils but chromatin not as coarsely clumped; distinctive red- to pink-staining cytoplasmic granules that vary in size and shape among species | Granulocyte; also classed as an acidophil in reptiles Dog: varying size, round red granule, similar in color to RBCs on the film Cat: eosinophil granules tend to be rod shaped, small, and numerous Horse: intense orange-red, large, round, granules (strawberry-like in appearance) Cattle, sheep, and pig: stain intense pink and are round Increase is noted in the presence of parasites and allergic or hypersensitive reactions Increase tends to parallel increases in basophils and mast cells |
| **BASOPHILS** (Color Plate 10) | | |
| | Cytoplasmic granules stain blue to blue-black (lavender in cat) and vary in number, with a few commonly indistinct granules in dog, and more numerous and distinct granules in horse and cow; gray-blue cytoplasm often with small vacuoles; when present, it is not unusual to find basophils more to the periphery of the film | Basophils: a rare finding in peripheral blood Involved with hypersensitivity reactions |

## LEUKOCYTE INFECTIOUS INCLUSIONS

| | | |
|---|---|---|
| Bacteria Ehrlichia (E.) | Clinically significant if neutrophils contain phagocytized bacteria. Morula containing several, small, blue to purple coccoid shaped bodies | E. canis: dog monocytes and lymphocytes<br>E. ewingii: dog neutrophils and eosinophils (granulocytic ehrlichiosis)<br>E. phagocytophila: cattle<br>Equine: causes Potomac horse fever, can also infect dogs and cats |
| Neorickettsia (Ehrlichia) risticii | Similar appearance to canine Ehrlichia | Equine neutrophils and eosinophils |
| Anaplasma phagocytophila (Ehrlichia equi) | Similar appearance to canine Ehrlichia | |
| Histoplasma capsulatum | Varying number of ~3-μm diameter, round to oval in shape, light blue cytoplasm; pink to purple, granular, eccentrically located nucleus | Yeasts |
| Hepatozoon canis | Elliptical, light blue staining | Dogs: neutrophils, eosinophils and monocytes |
| Canine distemper viral inclusions | Varying size and shape with pinkish-reddish to light purple inclusion, granular to smooth texture organism, with or without a halo effect | Dogs: neutrophils and monocytes |
| Lysosomal storage disease | Varying appearances: pinpoint purple granules in the cytoplasm of WBCs similar to toxic granulation but without other toxic signs; multiple vacuoles in lymphocytes, possibly with granules in the vacuole | Dogs: any WBC<br>Example of lysosomal storage diseases include: gangliosidosis, mannosidosis, mucopolysaccharidosis, and Niemann-Pick disease |

## OTHER LEUKOCYTE VARIATIONS

| | | |
|---|---|---|
| Basket (smudge) cells | Lacy, netlike, or with crisscross "basket weave" pattern; nuclear remnant, lacking intact cytoplasm | May be in vivo from an overwhelming pathology or in vitro from excess anticoagulation, rough handling of the sample, or extended period of time from collection to processing |

## Thrombocyte (Platelet) Evaluation

I. General information
 A. Anuclear cytoplasmic fragments from bone marrow megakaryocytes in mammal; nucleated in nonmammalian species
 B. Vary in size, shape, and color
  1. In mammals, usually pale blue cytoplasm, varying in shape, with filamentous projections when activated. Most species may have more or less obvious granules, which are usually reddish-purple
   a. Platelets from equines have a tendency not to stain as brilliantly as those of other species
  2. Platelets from nonmammalian species usually are more oval than round; commonly smaller than RBCs; with virtually clear, colorless cytoplasm; and possibly have cytoplasmic vacuoles and granules
 C. May be found in clumps (especially in cat)
 D. Thrombocytes (platelets) are an important component of hemostasis
 E. "Adequate" number is a subjective term, which varies with the laboratory and is meaningful only if the patient does not have occult or obvious bleeding
  1. Commonly, estimates of ~6 to 10+ platelets per oil immersion field in most mammalian species, and ~12+ per 1000 RBCs in birds have been considered adequate. Average number of platelets in 10 oil immersion fields, in an area where RBCs are evenly distributed, is multiplied by 20,000 for a rough estimate per μL
  2. With decreased estimates, platelet aggregation on the blood film or tube of blood must be ruled out before thrombocytopenia (decreased platelet numbers) is confirmed
   a. Look for platelet clumps, commonly located around the feathered edge and in the thicker areas of the film
 F. Actual counts can be done manually with the hemocytometer or an automated cell counter and is the preferred method of evaluating the number of platelets
  1. Thrombocytopenia
   a. Decreased platelet number, due to a variety of primary and secondary causes with possible common clinical manifestations
    (1) Examples: trauma and associated hemorrhage, rodenticide poisonings, immune-mediated, medication side effects, neoplasms, and infectious agents
     (a) Examples include *Babesia, Ehrlichia, Haemobartonella, Rickettsia,*

*Toxoplasma,* feline leukemia virus (FeLV), feline infectious peritonitis (FIP), and feline immunodeficiency virus (FIV)
    b. In mammals, commonly a platelet number <100,000/μL is a red flag, and when <20,000 to 50,000/μL, spontaneous bleeding may occur
 C. Thrombocytosis: increased platelet number, usually exceeding 1,000,000/μL
  1. Essential (idiopathic, primary hemorrhage)
  2. Thrombocythemia: chronic and extremely elevated platelet count caused by a bone marrow disorder
   a. Reactive (secondary) thrombocytosis: transient sequela to trauma, splenectomies, specific medications, and various diseases not originating in the bone marrow
   b. Physiological thrombocytosis
    (1) Commonly caused by movement of platelets from the storage pools (e.g., spleen) as a result of stress and exercise
IV. Mean platelet volume (MPV) provides an average size of platelets
 A. An increased value suggests the presence of younger or reactive giant (macro-, mega-) platelets (Color Plate 8), a regenerative response
 B. A decreased value implies the presence of microplatelets (small), possibly caused by immune-mediated platelet destruction
 C. Healthy patients in some species (e.g., cats) have highly variable platelet size

## Total Protein

I. Combination of various proteins produced mostly by the liver
II. Abnormalities indicate diseases in tissues responsible for protein synthesis, catabolism, and loss
III. Total plasma or serum protein measured in g/dL (g/L)
IV. Commonly measured with a refractometer or automated chemistry analyzer
V. Influenced by the hydration status of the patient

## Instrumentation

I. Quantitative buffy coat analysis (QBC), flow cytometry, impedance counter
II. Each of these methodologies has their place in the clinical laboratory. General principles must be recognized when using any of these instruments
 A. The results will be only as good as the sample that is provided
 B. Each instrument has its limitations, which may include

Precursor blood cells in order of least immature to most mature cells

| Erythrocyte | Granulocyte | | Agranulocyte | Thrombocyte |
|---|---|---|---|---|
| Rubriblast | Myeloblast | Monoblast | Lymphoblast | Megakaryoblast |
| Prorubricyte | Progranulocyte | Promonocyte | Prolymphocyte | Promegakaryocyte |
| Rubricyte | Myelocyte | Monocyte | B and T lymphocytes | Megakaryocyte |
| Metarubricyte | Metamyelocyte | | | Platelet |
| Polychromatic | Band | | | |
| erythrocyte | Mature | | | |

1. Species specificity due to cell size variations (especially RBCs) and presence of NRBCs and platelets, and cell behavior (e.g., rouleaux)
   a. Some instruments require modifications and validation when the blood of a different species is "counted" to accommodate these differences
2. Limitations on the number of cells (high and low) that may be accurately counted
3. Limitations on the ability of the instrument to discriminate between cell types when the cells are similar in appearance (e.g., size, weight, nuclear components, cytoplasmic inclusions)
4. Susceptibility to common inferences (e.g., microfilaria, platelet and WBC aggregates, microclots)
5. Select an instrument based on the species to be tested, parameters (e.g., WBC, RBC, MCH, MCHC, RDW, MPV, platelet, HCT, Hb, differential, "mini-differential")
6. When working properly the results will generally be more accurate and more rapid than those from manual methods
7. All instruments and methods must have a quality control program that includes actual counts on known control samples for the species routinely tested, calibration confirmation, and recalibration of instruments when necessary
   a. Despite recommendations from some manufacturers that these procedures be performed on a weekly or monthly basis, these tasks should be performed at least daily, whenever the instrument is shut down and reactivated, and when a problem occurs and is resolved
8. All cell identification must be confirmed on a stained blood film

# Glossary

**absolute** Actual change in number of cells
**absolute count** Calculation of absolute cell numbers based on percentage of type multiplied by the total cell count

**acanthocyte** Erythrocyte with irregularly shaped margins
**agglutination** Process in which particles aggregate or clump together
**agranulocyte** WBCs, such as monocytes and lymphocytes, that do not have obvious cytoplasmic granules when viewed under a light microscope
**an-** Without, not, lacking (prefix)
**anemia** Below normal values in PCV, RBC count, or Hb level
**anisocytosis** Variation in RBC size; without even cell size
**anuria** Complete absence of urine formation or elimination
**azurophilic granules** Large homogeneous and dense granules that stain blue with Romanowsky stain
**basophilia** Increased number of basophils
**basophilic stippling** Presence of small, blue-staining granules in the erythrocyte
**bilirubinuria** Detectable conjugated bile pigments in the urine
**buffy coat** Layer of WBCs, platelets, and NRBCs above the packed RBCs in centrifuged blood
**codocyte** Form of leptocyte or target cell
**continence** Storage of urine in the bladder as the urine is produced
**crenation** Erythrocytes with spiny projections on the margin of the cell
**-cytosis** Increased number of cells (suffix)
**dysuria** Difficult or painful urination
**eosinopenia** Decreased number of eosinophils
**eosinophilia** Increased number of eosinophils
**erythrophagocytosis** Engulfing, or phagocytosis, of the erythrocyte
**erythropoiesis** Production of RBCs
**exfoliative cytology** Study of cells shed from body surfaces, such as tissues, lesions, and fluids
**extreme (marked)** Greatly increased
**exudates** Fluid escaped from blood vessels with a high content of protein and cellular debris
**glucosuria** Detectable levels of glucose in the urine (glycosuria)
**granulocyte** WBC containing granules
**granulomatous** Composed of a tumorlike mass or nodule of granulation tissue
**hematuria** Presence of intact erythrocytes in the urine
**hemoglobinuria** Free Hb in the urine
**hemolysis** Destruction of RBCs
**heterophil** Avian neutrophil
**hyper-** Increased (prefix)
**hypersegmented** Neutrophil with more than five lobes in the nucleus

**hypertonic**  Greater than isotonic concentration

**hypo-**  Decreased (prefix)

**hypochromic**  Erythrocyte with lack of or decrease in staining intensity, low cellular Hb, increased amount of central pallor

**hypotonic**  Less than isotonic concentration

**incontinence**  Dribbling of urine at frequent intervals

**iso-**  Similar, the same (prefix)

**isotonic**  Similar osmolality to normal plasma

**ketonuria**  Excessive ketones (e.g., acetone) in the urine

**left shift**  Presence of an increased number of immature (non-segmented) neutrophils in the circulation

**leptocyte**  Thin, flattened, hypochromic erythrocyte that has a normal diameter and a decreased mean corpuscular volume

**leukemia**  Neoplastic disease in which a significant number of immature blast cells are found in the bone marrow and blood

**leukemoid response (reaction)**  Leukocytosis with a neutrophilia, marked left shift with bands and earlier precursors, and reactive lymphocytes

**leukocytosis**  Increase in circulating WBC numbers

**leukopenia**  Decrease in circulating WBC numbers

**lymphocytosis**  Increased number of circulating lymphocytes

**macro-**  Larger (prefix)

**macrocyte**  RBC with a diameter that is larger than normal

**macrocytic**  Increased number of large RBCs, increased MCV

**marked (extreme)**  Greatly increased

**mast cell**  Tissue cell having granules that contain histamine and heparin

**meta-**  After (prefix)

**micturition**  Physiological term for empting the bladder

**micro-**  Smaller (prefix)

**microcyte**  RBC with a diameter that is smaller than normal

**microcytic**  Increased number of small RBCs

**monocytopenia**  Decreased number of monocytes

**monocytosis**  Increased number of monocytes

**neutropenia**  Decreased number of neutrophils

**neutrophilia**  Increased number of neutrophils

**NMB**  New methylene blue, a basic dye used to stain cell nuclei and granules

**normo-**  Typical for a species (prefix)

**normochromic**  Normal, pink-staining erythrocyte

**normocyte**  Most commonly used to describe an erythrocyte of the typical size for a given species; occasionally in older texts it is used to describe an erythrocyte with the typical shape, size, and/or color for a particular species

**NRBC (nRBC)**  Nucleated RBC; an immature erythrocyte

**oliguria**  Decrease in urine formation

**pan-**  Overall (prefix)

**pancytopenia**  Decrease in the RBC, WBC, and platelet lines

**PCV**  Packed cell volume, or hematocrit

**-penia**  Decreased number of cells (suffix)

**-philia**  Increased number of cells (suffix)

**plasma**  Fluid portion of the blood in which cells are suspended

**poikilocytosis**  Variation in general RBC shape

**pollakiuria**  Frequent urination

**polychromasia**  Erythrocytes that have a bluish tint when stained with regular blood stains and are reticulocytes (granular precipitates) with NMB

**polyuria**  Increased urine production (volume)

**postprandial**  Immediately after eating

**pro-**  Before (prefix)

**proteinuria**  Abnormal level of proteins in the urine

**RBC**  Red blood cell or erythrocyte

**relative**  Proportional (percentage) change in number

**right shift**  Presence of an increased number of hypersegmented neutrophils in circulation

**rouleaux**  Erythrocytes formed in stacks or columns

**schistocyte**  Fragmented erythrocyte; "helmet cell"

**sedimentation rate**  Rate at which RBCs settle in their own plasma in a given amount of time

**smudge cell**  Nucleated cell that has ruptured during smearing because of mechanical damage or increased fragility of the cell

**spherocyte**  Small, dense, dark-staining erythrocyte

**supravital staining**  Use of a stain that has a low toxicity so that vital and functional processes can be studied in live cells

**thrombocytopenia**  Decreased number of platelets (thrombocytes)

**thrombocytosis**  Increased number of platelets (thrombocytes)

**toxic neutrophils**  Neutrophil showing certain morphological changes, such as vacuolation, toxic granules, increased basophilia, or nuclear changes

**WBC**  White blood cell, or leukocyte

# Review Questions

1 Of the following collection methods, which is primarily of use for urine volume only?
   a. Cystocentesis
   b. Metabolism cage
   c. Client-collected samples
   d. Catheterization

2 Urine samples should be analyzed within _____ for maximum valid information
   a. 1 hour
   b. 2 minutes
   c. 30 minutes
   d. 12 hours

3 Normal freshly voided urine of many species is clear. Exceptions include which of the following species?
   a. Rabbit
   b. Horse
   c. Hamster
   d. All of the above

4 It is recommended that urine sample size be standardized. An adequate sample of fresh urine is considered to be
   a. 1 mL
   b. 5 mL
   c. 10 mL
   d. 20 mL

5 The fluid portion of the blood from which fibrinogen has been removed is termed
   a. Serum
   b. Plasma
   c. Buffy coat
   d. Packed cells

**6** If used in the proper ratio to blood, which anticoagulant is most recommended to cause the least changes in cell morphology?
 a. Heparin
 b. EDTA
 c. Potassium chloride
 d. Acid-citrate-dextrose (ACD)

**7** To maintain proper anticoagulant to blood ratio, sample tubes should be filled to at least what capacity?
 a. 90%
 b. 50%
 c. 75%
 d. 60%

**8** Blood samples collected immediately postprandial may be
 a. Icteric
 b. High in TPP
 c. Lipemic
 d. Low in RBCs

**9** Which urine collection method is optimal for bacterial culture?
 a. Manual expression
 b. Cystocentesis
 c. Midstream
 d. Litter pan pour off

**10** Pollakiuria is defined as
 a. Complete absence of urine formation
 b. Increased urine production
 c. Frequent urination
 d. Decreased urine formation

## BIBLIOGRAPHY

Baker P: Lecture notes, Seneca College, King City, Ontario, 2005.

Bush BM: *Interpretation of laboratory results for small animal clinicians*, London, 1991, Blackwell.

Campbell TW: *Avian hematology and cytology*, Ames, 1995, Iowa State University Press.

Chew DJ, DiBartola SP: *Interpretation of canine and feline urinalysis*, St Louis, 1998, Ralston Purina.

Cowell RL: *Veterinary clinical pathology secrets*, St Louis, 2004, Hanley & Belfus.

Cowell RL, Tyler RD: *Diagnostic cytology and hematology of the horse*, ed 2, St Louis, 2002, Mosby.

Cowell RL, Tyler RD, Meinkoth JH: *Diagnostic cytology and hematology of the dog and cat*, St Louis, 1999, Mosby.

Free HM, editor: *Modern urine chemistry*, Elkhart, Ind, 1991, Miles Diagnostic Division.

Fudge AM: *Laboratory medicine: avian and exotic pets*, Philadelphia, 2000, Saunders.

George JW: The usefulness and limitations of hand-held refractometers in veterinary laboratory medicine: a historical and technical review, *Vet Clin Pathol* 30:201, 2001.

Harvey JW: *Atlas of veterinary hematology: blood and bone marrow of domestic animals*, Philadelphia, 2001, Saunders.

Hendrix CM: *Laboratory procedures for veterinary technicians*, ed 4, St Louis, 2002, Mosby.

McCurnin DM, Bassert JM, editors: *Clinical textbook for veterinary technicians*, ed 6, St Louis, 2006, Saunders.

Osborne CA, Stevens JB: *Urinalysis: a clinical guide to compassionate patient care*, Shawnee Mission, Kan, 1999, Bayer.

Raskin RE, Meyer DJ: *Atlas of canine and feline cytology*, Philadelphia, 2001, Saunders.

Rebar AH et al: *A guide to hematology in dogs and cats*, Jackson, Wyo, 2002, Teton New Media.

Sink CA, Feldman BF: *Laboratory urinalysis and hematology for the small animal practitioner*, Jackson, Wyo, 2004, Teton New Media.

Thrall MA et al: *Veterinary hematology and clinical chemistry*, Baltimore, 2004, Lippincott Williams & Wilkins.

Walsh DJ, Wade WL: The differential film: errors and normal variations, *Vet Tech* 17:7, 1996.

Wernery U et al: *A color atlas of camelid hematology*, Ames, 1999, Iowa State University Press.

## CHAPTER 3

# Cytology

*Margi Sirois*

## OUTLINE

Indications
Specimen Collection
Concentration Techniques
Characteristics of Fluid Samples
Slide Preparation

Fixation and Staining
  Techniques
Evaluation and Interpretation
Cytology of Inflammation
Neoplastic Lesions

Noninflammatory, Nonneoplastic
  Lesions
Collection and Evaluation of
  Common Lesions

## LEARNING OUTCOMES

After reading this chapter, you should be able to:

1. Describe a variety of sample collection and processing techniques for cytology samples.
2. Identify common normal cells found in cytology samples.
3. Identify common abnormal cells in cytology samples.
4. Describe methods for differentiation of inflammatory and neoplastic cytology samples.

**M**icroscopic examination of cells, primarily those exfoliated from tissues, lesions, and internal organs, has become an increasingly valuable tool in veterinary diagnostics. Fluid aspirates also provide valuable diagnostic information to the clinician. Sample collection can be easily performed, and in most cases no special equipment is required.

## INDICATIONS

I. Purpose
  A. Differentiation between inflammatory processes and neoplastic diseases
  B. Identification of cell types present to aid in diagnosis and treatment

II. Advantages
  A. Can be collected quickly and easily
  B. No specialized equipment is required
  C. Inexpensive
III. Disadvantages
  A. Quality control concerns
    1. Improper specimen collection can damage cells
    2. Staining techniques are variable and subject to greater error than standard staining methods
    3. Formalin fumes near specimen collection or processing areas cause cells to become partially fixed and therefore unusable for cytological evaluation

## SPECIMEN COLLECTION

I. Fine needle biopsy
  A. Used to collect samples from the skin, lymph nodes, and internal organs
  B. Samples may be collected with the aspiration or nonaspiration technique
  C. Samples should be collected from several areas and depths within the tissue by redirecting the needle into other locations
    1. Aspiration method requires a needle and syringe
      a. Recommended needle sizes range from 22 to 25 gauge, attached to a 3- to 12-mL syringe
    2. Softer masses require smaller syringes and smaller-gauge needles; firmer masses require larger-bore syringes and larger-gauge needles

a. Negative pressure pulls cells into the hub of the needle

b. Pressure must be released each time the needle is redirected into the mass

3. The nonaspiration method, also referred to as the capillary technique or stab technique, uses a needle or a syringe without the plunger attached to a needle

a. Cells are forced into the hub of the needle from the pressure of the puncture

D. Samples are collected and pushed onto clean microscope slides for staining

II. Centesis

A. Includes thoracocentesis, cystocentesis, arthrocentesis, cerebrospinal fluid (CSF) taps, and abdominocentesis

B. Collection site should be aseptically prepared

1. If samples are being submitted for microbiology testing, a surgical scrub should be performed

2. Surgical preparation should also be done for CSF and joint taps

C. Usually performed with animal in standing position

1. For cystocentesis, dorsal or lateral recumbency may be used

2. CSF is usually completed in lateral recumbency

D. Fluids may be centrifuged for sediment examination or submitted for bacterial culture

III. Solid mass imprinting

A. For collection and preparation of cytologic specimens from external lesions or samples removed during surgical procedures

B. Samples of external lesions can be collected with a single imprint or the Tzanck method

1. Remove gross debris before imprinting

2. For Tzanck preparations, make multiple imprints from the lesion before cleaning, after cleaning, after debridement, and after removal of any scabs

a. Also imprint the underside of scabs removed

C. Can also be performed on surgically removed tissues

1. Fresh edge is cut to expose the center of the mass

2. The specimen is blotted to remove excess fluid and blood

D. Multiple small imprints are made onto a clean slide

IV. Scraping

A. Prepared from tissues collected during necropsy or surgery or from external lesions on the living animal

B. Scrapings are made using a clean scalpel blade on a freshly cut surface of tissue or on a surface external lesion that has been cleaned and blotted

V. Swab technique

A. Used as an aid in determining stage of estrous cycle, evaluating uterine and vaginal disease, and in collecting samples from ears

B. Also useful for evaluation of fistulated lesions

C. Rayon swabs should be used for collection of samples to be cultured, because cotton may inhibit growth of some bacteria

1. Ear swabs samples may contain excess wax that may interfere with sample evaluation

a. Pass the slide briefly through a flame or expose it to gentle heat from a warm hair dryer to dissolve the wax before staining the smear

D. For vaginal cytology, vulva and surrounding area are cleaned, and a vaginal speculum is carefully introduced

1. Sample of the vaginal mucosa is taken with a sterile swab moistened with sterile saline

a. Swabs of fistulated lesions should be taken before and immediately after cleaning the site

b. Samples are rolled onto clean slides for staining

VI. Tissue biopsy

A. Involves sampling of a piece of tissue for cytological and/or histopathological examination

B. Hair at skin biopsy sites should be carefully clipped to avoid inflammatory artifact from skin irritation

C. Skin lesions are sampled without removal or disturbance of or any scales, crusts, or surface debris, because they may offer valuable diagnostic information

D. Wedge biopsy usually involves excision of an entire lesion and then removal of a wedge of tissue through a transition zone to normal tissue

E. Punch biopsy most commonly done with Keyes cutaneous biopsy punches

1. Two or three punch biopsy specimens of various lesions are collected

2. The punch is gently rotated in one direction until the punch blade has sectioned the tissue

F. Specimens collected by the wedge or punch method should be removed gently by grasping the margin of the tissue with a pair of fine forceps

1. The specimen is blotted gently on a paper towel to remove excess blood and placed on a splint (small piece of wooden tongue depressor or cardboard)

2. The tissue is allowed to dry onto the splint
3. The splint is immersed or floated specimen-side down in the fixative
G. Specimens collected by endoscopy can be gently flushed from the tip of the endoscope using sterile saline
H. Tissue samples for histopathological examination are fixed in 10% formalin
   1. To allow for proper infiltration of the tissue with formalin, samples should be no more than 1 cm wide
   2. Large tissues should be prepared by slicing into the tissue at 1-cm increments while leaving the sections attached
   3. Formalin volume should be 10 times the specimen volume
   4. With large tissues, the sample can be removed to a smaller jar with less formalin once it has been fixed for 24 hours

VII. Transtracheal and bronchial washes
   A. Evaluation of mucous secretions from the trachea, bronchi, and bronchioles, and in differential diagnosis of inflammation, neoplasia, mycosis, and bacterial and protozoal diseases
   B. Two techniques
      1. Percutaneous technique provides samples with the least contamination
         a. Requires placement of a jugular catheter within the tracheal lumen through the cricothyroid ligament
         b. Saline is infused through the catheter at a maximum dose of 1 to 2 mL/10 lb (4.5 kg)
         c. When the animal coughs or the entire dose has been given, a small amount of fluid is aspirated and the catheter is removed
      2. Orotracheal technique
         a. Requires that the patient be lightly anesthetized
         b. Sterile endotracheal tube is inserted
         c. Large-bore indwelling catheter is then placed down the endotracheal tube so that the catheter extends just beyond the end of the endotracheal tube
         d. Saline is infused at a dose of 1 to 2 mL/10 lb (4.5 kg), and then a small amount of aspirate is collected
         e. Bronchoalveolar lavage (BAL) is an orotracheal technique used to collect samples specifically from the lower respiratory tract
            (1) Bronchoscopy is the preferred method for performing a BAL, but specialized equipment (e.g., bronchoscope) is required

VIII. Nasal flush
   A. Aids in diagnosis of diseases affecting the upper airway
   B. Fluid (normal saline) is infused into the nasal cavity through the nares using a syringe and tubing, and then aspirated
   C. Specimens are processed as for a tracheal wash

## CONCENTRATION TECHNIQUES

I. May be needed if cellularity of sample is low
II. Place anticoagulated fluid in a standard clinical centrifuge
III. Spin for 5 minutes at 1000 to 2000 rpm (165 to 400 $g$)
IV. Pour off supernatant. Leave a few drops in the tube and then gently resuspend sediment
V. Prepare multiple smears using several different smearing techniques
VI. Gravitational sedimentation and membrane filtration are specialized concentration techniques used with CSF

## CHARACTERISTICS OF FLUID SAMPLES

I. The total volume collected must be recorded at the time of collection
II. Before preparation of any fluid sample, the gross characteristics of the sample, such as color, turbidity, and odor, should be determined
   A. Color and turbidity: influenced by protein concentration and cell numbers
      1. Gross discoloration, with increased turbidity, may be due to iatrogenic contamination with peripheral blood, recent or old hemorrhage, inflammation, or a combination of these
         a. Recent hemolysis imparts a reddish discoloration to the supernatant
         b. Hemorrhage that occurred at least 2 days previously generally causes a yellowish supernatant, usually with little erythrocytic sediment
         c. Clumps of platelets may be observed in recent, often iatrogenic hemorrhage; these clumps are not obvious after approximately 1 hour
   B. Inflammation also may discolor body fluids, with the degree of turbidity reflecting leukocyte numbers
   C. Color may vary from an off-white or cream to a red-cream or dirty brown, depending on the number of erythrocytes also involved and the integrity of the cells present
   D. Total nucleated cell count (TNCC) and total protein should also be determined
      1. Usually the sample can then be characterized as a transudate, exudate, or modified transudate (Figure 3-1)

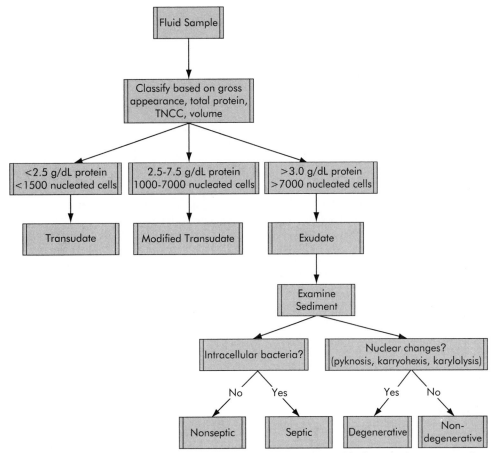

**Figure 3-1** An algorithm to classify effusions as transudates, modified transudates, or exudates, based on total protein content and total nucleated cell count *(TNCC)*.

2. Transudate samples are clear or colorless, with TNCC less than 500/mL and total protein less than 3 g/dL
   a. Transudates are more commonly found in ascites and are usually colorless
3. Modified transudates are moderately cellular and have total protein concentrations between 2.5 and 7.5 g/dL
   a. They are often amber or pink and turbid
4. Exudates are characterized by increased cellularity and total protein greater than 3.0 g/dL
   a. This higher cell count and protein value are usually indicative of inflammation

## SLIDE PREPARATION

I. Preparation of smears from solid masses
   A. Compression prep method (Figure 3-2)
      1. Also referred to as a squash preparation
      2. Small amount of aspirate is placed in the center of a clean slide
      3. Second slide is placed over the sample at a 90-degree angle and is carefully slid apart from the bottom slide

4. Excessive pressure can distort and rupture cells
   B. Modified compression preparation (Figure 3-3)
      1. Combination method especially useful when cells are unusually fragile or the sample is thin
      2. Small amount of aspirate is placed in the center of a clean slide
      3. Second slide is placed on top at a 90-degree angle
      4. Second slide is rotated 45 degrees and then lifted straight off
   C. Starfish method (Figure 3-4)
      1. Most useful for highly viscous samples
      2. Small amount of aspirate is placed in the center of a clean slide
      3. Tip of the needle is then used to pull the sample out into several projections, forming a starfish pattern
II. Preparation of smears from fluid samples
   A. Line smear (Figure 3-5)
      1. Used when fluid samples cannot be concentrated or when the amount of sediment is very small

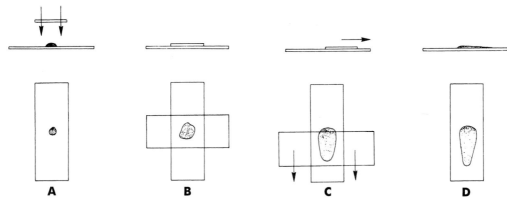

**Figure 3-2** Squash preparation. **A,** A portion of the aspirate is expelled onto a glass microscope slide, and another slide is placed over the sample. **B,** This spreads the sample. If the sample does not spread well, gentle digital pressure can be applied to the top slide. Care must be taken not to place excessive pressure on the slide, causing the cells to rupture. **C,** The slides are smoothly slid apart. **D,** This usually produces well-spread smears but may result in excessive cell rupture. (From Cowell RL, Tyler RD, Meinkoth JH: *Diagnostic cytology and hematology of the dog and cat*, ed 2, St Louis, 1999, Mosby.)

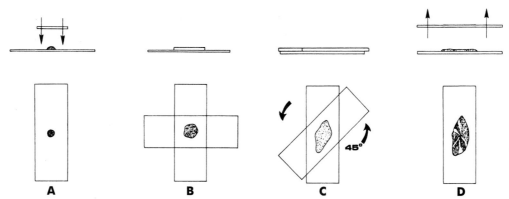

**Figure 3-3** A modification of the squash preparation. **A,** A portion of the aspirate is expelled onto a glass microscope slide, and another slide is placed over the sample. **B,** This causes the sample to spread. If necessary, gentle digital pressure can be applied to the top slide to spread the sample more. Care must be taken not to use excessive pressure and cause cell rupture. **C,** The top slide is rotated about 45 degrees and lifted directly upward, producing a spread preparation with subtle ridges and valleys of cells (**D**). (From Cowell RL, Tyler RD, Meinkoth JH: *Diagnostic cytology and hematology of the dog and cat*, ed 2, St Louis, 1999, Mosby.)

2. Small drop of the sample is placed near the end of a clean glass slide, and a second slide is used to spread the specimen in a manner similar to that used for preparation of a peripheral blood film
3. When the smear covers approximately three fourths of the slide, the second slide is abruptly lifted off the first
4. This produces a smear with a thick edge that contains a line of concentrated sediment from the sample
5. Smear should be dried quickly with a hairdryer or some other method
  B. Wedge smear
    1. Small amount of aspirate is placed on one end of a clean slide

2. Second slide is then used to smoothly pull the sample toward the other end
3. This technique produces a film similar to that used for a whole blood differential count

## FIXATION AND STAINING TECHNIQUES ▬▬▬

I. Fixation of cytology slides
  A. Slides must be thoroughly air-dried and fixed before stain is applied
  B. The preferred fixative for cytology specimens is 95% methanol
    1. The methanol must be fresh and not contaminated with stain or cellular debris
    2. The prepared cytology slides should remain in the fixative for 2 to 5 minutes

3. Greater fixative times will improve the quality of the staining procedure and will not harm the samples

II. Stain

  A. Stains should be applied according to the recommendations of the manufacturer

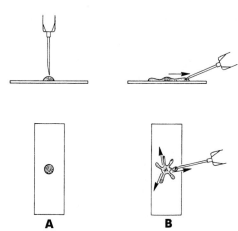

**Figure 3-4** Needle spread, or "starfish" preparation. **A,** A portion of the aspirate is expelled onto a glass microscope slide. **B,** The tip of a needle is placed in the aspirate and moved peripherally, pulling a trail of the sample with it. This procedure is repeated in several directions, resulting in a preparation with multiple projections. (From Cowell RL, Tyler RD, Meinkoth JH: *Diagnostic cytology and hematology of the dog and cat*, ed 2, St Louis, 1999, Mosby.)

    1. Denser, thicker preparations tend to require a longer time to stain structures correctly

  B. Types of stains

    1. Romanowsky stains

      a. Include Wright's, Giemsa, and Diff-Quik

      b. Provide satisfactory staining of cytological specimens

      c. Some variation in staining quality is evident: consistent use of one type is recommended

    2. New methylene blue

      a. Will stain nuclei, mast cell granules, and most infectious agents

      b. Can be applied directly to an air-dried slide

      c. Selected uses include determining the presence of nucleated cells, bacteria, fungi, and mast cells

    3. Gram staining

      a. For classification of bacterial agents

      b. Gram-negative bacteria and cells stain pink; gram-positive organisms stain purple

    4. Other stains

      a. Hematoxylin and eosin stain: normally used for histological evaluations

      b. Papanicolaou's stains

        (1) Commonly used in human gynecological examinations

        (2) Multiple steps required in staining technique

        (3) Excellent for accentuating nuclear detail

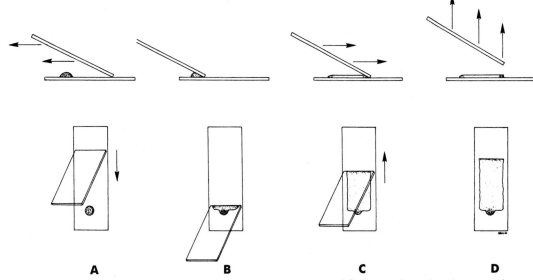

**Figure 3-5** Line smear concentration technique. **A,** A drop of fluid sample is placed onto a glass microscope slide close to one end, and another slide is slid backward to contact the front of the drop. **B,** When the drop is contacted, it rapidly spreads along the juncture between the two slides. **C,** The spreader slide is then smoothly and rapidly slid forward. **D,** After the spreader slide has been advanced about two thirds to three fourths the distance required to make a smear with a feathered edge, the spreader slide is raised directly upward. This produces a smear with a line of concentrated cells at its end, instead of a feathered edge. (From Cowell RL, Tyler RD, Meinkoth JH: *Diagnostic cytology and hematology of the dog and cat*, ed 2, St Louis, 1999, Mosby.)

## EVALUATION AND INTERPRETATION

I. Initial examination
   A. Low power (×100) to evaluate overall cellularity, quality of preparation
      1. Scan for large objects, such as cell clusters, parasites, fungal hyphae, and crystals
   B. High power (×430) to determine predominant cell types
   C. Oil immersion (×1000) to describe cellular characteristics
   D. Algorithms, such as the one in Figure 3-6, should be used to assist with differentiation
   E. The cytology report should indicate the cell types present, their appearance, and relative proportions
II. Cells commonly found in exfoliative cytology
   A. Neutrophils
      1. May resemble those in blood, be degenerative, or have undergone morphological changes
         a. Hypersegmentation: more than five lobes
         b. Pyknosis: condensed nucleus
         c. Karyolysis: loss of nuclear membrane
         d. Karyorrhexis: fragmented nucleus (Color Plate 17)
   B. Lymphocytes: usually appear the same as in peripheral blood
   C. Plasma cells
      1. Represent activated lymphocytes
         a. Appear as oval cell with eccentric nucleus, basophilic cytoplasm, and a perinuclear clear zone (Color Plate 18)
   D. Eosinophils: usually appear the same as in peripheral blood
   E. Macrophages (Color Plate 19): large cells derived from the monocyte found in peripheral blood
      1. Oval to pleomorphic nucleus with lacy to condensed chromatin
      2. Abundant blue cytoplasm with vacuoles
      3. May be multinucleated or giant cells (nuclei uniform in size and shape)
      4. May contain phagocytized material
   F. Mesothelial cells (Color Plate 20)
      1. Cells that line the pleural, peritoneal, and visceral surfaces
      2. Round, usually with one round to oval nucleus, but may be multinucleated
      3. May have nucleoli, corona (a fringe border), be seen singularly or in clusters
      4. Nuclear chromatin is finely reticulated
      5. May react to the presence of excess fluid by developing abnormal morphologies that should not be confused with malignant changes
      6. Cytoplasm is slightly basophilic and may contain phagocytic debris
         a. Difficult to distinguish from macrophages once they are activated
   G. Mast cells
      1. Round to oval with round to oval nuclei
      2. Numerous blue to purple cytoplasmic granules
   H. Erythrocytes: may be free in sample or seen inside phagocytic cells, particularly macrophages

## CYTOLOGY OF INFLAMMATION

I. Inflammation is a normal physiological response
   A. Chemotactic factors released from damaged tissue attract neutrophils and macrophages to the inflamed site
   B. Eosinophils and basophils may also be evident
II. Classifications: inflammation can be classified as purulent, pyogranulomatous, granulomatous, or eosinophilic, based on the relative percentages of cells present
   A. Purulent inflammation (Color Plate 17)
      1. May also be referred to as suppurative or acute inflammation
      2. Most common type of inflammation, with the majority being caused by bacteria
      3. Samples usually characterized by greater than 85% neutrophils
      4. Small numbers of macrophages and lymphocytes may also be present
   B. Pyogranulomatous inflammation (Color Plate 21)
      1. May also be referred to as chronic/active
      2. Consists of macrophages and 50% to 75% neutrophils
   C. Granulomatous inflammation
      1. May also be referred to as chronic inflammation
      2. Greater than 70% of cells mononuclear (monocytes, macrophages, giant cells) with few neutrophils
   D. Eosinophilic
      1. Consists of greater than 10% eosinophils
      2. Often a few mast cells, plasma cells, and lymphocytes

## NEOPLASTIC LESIONS

I. Best indication is presence of homogeneous population of cells, which may or may not be pleomorphic
II. May be benign or malignant and may have associated inflammation
III. Benign neoplasia (hyperplasia) is characterized by homogeneous populations of the same cell type with no evidence of malignant characteristics within cells
IV. Malignant neoplasia is characterized by morphological changes in cytoplasm and nuclei

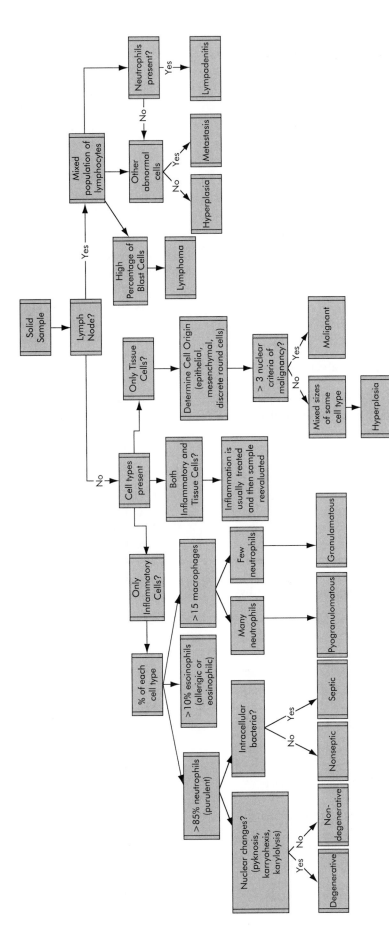

**Figure 3-6** An algorithm to help evaluate cytologic preparations.

V. A minimum of three criteria should be met before determining malignancy in a cytological sample
  A. Five criteria are more diagnostic
     1. Not as indicative of neoplasia if inflammation is also present or changes are only in cytoplasm
VI. Criteria of malignancy (Table 3-1)
  A. General criteria of malignancy
     1. Anisocytosis and macrocytosis
     2. Hypercellularity
     3. Pleomorphism (except lymphoid tissue)
  B. Cellular changes
     1. Anisocytosis: abnormal variation in size of cells of same type
     2. Pleomorphism: variability in the size, shape, and appearance of same cell type
     3. Hypercellularity: increased cell exfoliation
  C. Nuclear changes: most important criteria for determining malignancy
     1. Anisokaryosis: any unusual variation in overall nuclear size
     2. High or variable "N:C ratio": specifically, an increased ratio of the size of the nucleus to that of the cytoplasm
     3. Increased mitotic activity: mitosis is rare in normal tissue, and cells usually divide evenly in two. Any increase in the presence of mitotic figures or cells that are not dividing equally is considered a criterion for malignancy
     4. Coarse chromatin pattern: chromatin pattern is coarser than normal and may appear ropy or cordlike
     5. Nuclear molding: deformation of nuclei by other nuclei within the same cell or adjacent cells
     6. Multinucleation: multiple nuclei within a cell
     7. Nucleoli that vary in size, shape, and number
        a. Anisonucleoliosis
        b. Angular nucleoli
        c. Multiple nucleoli
  D. Cytoplasmic changes
     1. Extreme basophilia of cytoplasm
     2. Vacuolation
  E. Boundaries may be irregular and indistinct
VII. Tissue origin
  A. Malignant neoplasia should be characterized by origin of tissue cells present
  B. Common neoplastic tissue cells include epithelial, mesenchymal, and discrete round cell
     1. Epithelial cell tumors
        a. Also referred to as carcinoma or adenocarcinoma
        b. Samples tend to be highly cellular, and often exfoliate in clusters
        c. Cells tend to be large to very large
           (1) Show marked variation
           (2) Nuclei are round with smooth to slightly coarse chromatin pattern that increases with increased malignancy
           (3) Nuclei contains one or more notable nucleoli
           (4) Cytoplasm is moderate to abundant
        d. Increased N:C ratio with nuclear molding evident
     2. Mesenchymal cell tumors or spindle cell tumors (Color Plate 22)
        a. Also referred to as sarcoma and are usually less cellular
        b. Tend to exfoliate singly or as wispy spindles
           (1) Cytoplasm tails away from nucleus: fusiform shape
           (2) Generally small to medium sized
           (3) Moderate degree of light to medium blue cytoplasm
           (4) Round to oval nucleus with smooth fine chromatin that is lacy
           (5) Nucleoli more evident as malignancy increases
              (a) Also change in shape, chromatin pattern, and N:C ratio
     3. Discrete round cell tumors
        a. Exfoliate very well but are usually not in clumps or clusters
        b. Individual round cells that are small to medium sized
        c. Round cell tumors include histiocytoma, lymphoma, mast cell tumors, plasma cell tumors, transmissible venereal tumors, and melanoma
           (1) Histiocytoma and transmissible venereal tumor appear similar, except that histiocytoma is not usually highly cellular
              (a) Histiocytoma cells have poorly defined boundaries, contain a few vacuoles, and have a moderate amount of pale blue cytoplasm
              (b) Boundaries of transmissible venereal tumors appear distinct; there are usually many definite vacuoles with a light smoky to medium blue cytoplasm
           (2) Lymphosarcomas can be recognized by the presence of large numbers of cells with prominent nucleoli
              (a) Cells are round; size and characteristics depend on the type of lymphosarcoma

**Table 3-1** Easily recognized general and nuclear criteria of malignancy

| Criteria | Description | Schematic representation |
|---|---|---|
| **GENERAL CRITERIA** | | |
| Anisocytosis and macrocytosis | Variation in cell size, with some cells ≥1.5 times larger than normal | |
| Hypercellularity | Increased cell exfoliation due to decreased cell adherence | Not depicted |
| Pleomorphism (except in lymphoid tissue) | Variable size and shape in cells of the same type | |
| **NUCLEAR CRITERIA** | | |
| Macrokaryosis | Increased nuclear size. Cells with nuclei larger than 10 μm in diameter suggest malignancy | |
| Increased nucleus-to-cytoplasm (N:C) ratio | Normal nonlymphoid cells usually have an N:C ratio of 1:3 to 1:8, depending on the tissue. Increased ratios (1:2, 1:1, etc.) suggest malignancy | RBC. See Macrokaryosis |
| Anisokaryosis | Variation in nuclear size. This is especially important if the nuclei of multinucleated cells vary in size | |
| Multinucleation | Multiple nucleation in a cell. This is especially important if the nuclei vary in size | |
| Increased mitotic figures | Mitosis is rare in normal tissue | normal abnormal |
| Abnormal mitosis | Improper alignment of chromosomes | See Increased Mitotic Figures |
| Coarse chromatin pattern | The chromatin pattern is coarser than normal; it may appear ropy or cordlike | |
| Nuclear molding | Deformation of nuclei by other nuclei within the same cell or adjacent cells | |
| Macronucleoli | Nucleoli are increased in size. Nucleoli ≥5 μm strongly suggest malignancy. For reference, RBCs are 5-6 μm in the cat and 7-8 μm in the dog | RBC |
| Angular nucleoli | Nucleoli are fusiform or have other angular shapes, instead of their normal round to slightly oval shape | |
| Anisonucleoliosis | Variation in nucleolar shape or size (especially important if the variation is within the same nucleus) | See Angular Nucleoli |

*RBC,* Red blood cell.

(b) Plasma cell tumors can be recognized by large numbers of cells with an eccentrically located nucleus, trailing basophilic cytoplasm, and a prominent perinuclear zone

(3) Mast cells can be recognized by their prominent purple/black granules (Color Plate 23)

(a) Granules not as dark in cats

(b) Few to many cells with moderate amount of cytoplasm

(c) Round nuclei stain pale

(4) Melanoma is generally characterized by cells with prominent dark black granules

(a) Cells from poorly differentiated tumors may contain few or no granules (amelanotic melanoma)

## NONINFLAMMATORY, NONNEOPLASTIC LESIONS

These include cysts, such as epidermal inclusion cysts (sebaceous cysts), hyperplasia, dysplasia, hematoma, seroma, adipocytes, and salivary mucocele.

## COLLECTION AND EVALUATION OF COMMON LESIONS

I. Cutaneous and subcutaneous tissues

A. Collection is usually made by swabbing, scraping, imprint, or fine needle aspiration

B. Collect sample before and after cleaning the lesion

C. If scabs are present, remove them before sample collection

D. Scraping should be performed at several levels within the lesion (Tzanck prep)

E. Common inflammatory lesions include bacterial, fungal, and parasitic infections

1. Infectious agents are often visible within phagocytic cells

a. Gram-positive cocci (*Staphylococcus* sp., *Streptococcus* sp.)

b. Gram-negative bacilli (*Nocardia* sp., *Actinomycetes* sp., *Pseudomonas* sp.)

c. Fungi (*Microsporum* sp.)

d. Parasites (*Leishmania* sp.)

2. Noninfectious inflammation may result from injection site reactions, trauma, insect bites, snakebites, etc.

F. Common neoplastic lesions are numerous and include lipomas, mast cell tumors, histiocytomas, squamous cell carcinomas, fibromas, and hemangiosarcomas

1. Skin is the most common site for neoplasia in dogs and cats

II. Respiratory system

A. Tracheal and bronchial samples

1. Usually collected with transtracheal wash or by endoscopy

2. Aids in determining cause of chronic coughing

3. Presence of mucus makes actual cell counts difficult

a. Estimate of increased or normal numbers on stained sediment smears may be useful

(1) Inflammatory conditions will increase mucus production

b. Mucus will appear as twisted or whorled blue to pink amorphous sheets

c. Eosinophilic, spiral mucus casts from small bronchioles (Curschmann's spirals) suggest a chronic bronchiolar problem (Color Plate 24)

(1) Increased cellularity often accompanies a granular appearance

4. Normal cell types

a. Columnar and cuboidal epithelia can be ciliated or nonciliated

(1) Columnar cells are elongated or cone shaped, with a generally round to oval nucleus showing a finely granular chromatin pattern at one end of the cell

(2) Cuboidal cells are similar except they are more square in shape

b. Neutrophils are similar to those found in peripheral blood with greater toxic changes

(1) Increase in neutrophils indicates inflammation

c. Alveolar macrophages will generally have an eccentrically placed, round to bean-shaped nucleus

(1) Cytoplasm is abundant, blue-gray, and granular

d. If oral contamination occurs, superficial squamous cells may be common

(1) Large epithelial cells with small nucleus and abundant angular cytoplasm

5. Increase in macrophages and neutrophils is not normal

6. Eosinophils are commonly seen in allergic disease

7. Mast cells may also be present and have little diagnostic significance unless found in high numbers

a. Red-purple intracytoplasmic granules are characteristic

8. Bacterial and fungal diseases are routinely identified by transtracheal wash

B. Lung tissue
  1. Fine needle aspiration is used to collect samples from masses identified radiographically
     a. Complications include pneumothorax and hemorrhage
  2. Tissues removed during biopsy are prepared by scraping and/or impression
  3. Normal cell types found are similar to those obtained from transtracheal wash
  4. Common neoplasms of lung tissue include carcinoma and adenocarcinoma
     a. Inflammation may be the result of bacterial (*Mycobacterium* sp.), fungal (*Cryptococcus* sp., *Blastomyces* sp.), parasitic (*Toxoplasma* sp., *Pneumocystis* sp.), and viral diseases
  5. Nasal exudates and masses
     a. Usually collected by aspiration or nasal flushing
     b. Bacterial and fungal organisms may be present
     c. Trauma or foreign body inflammation is common
     d. Neoplasia of nasal cavities is uncommon but usually malignant

III. Oral cavity
  A. Usually collected by swabbing, imprint, or scraping
  B. Normal flora includes the bacterium *Simonsiella* sp.
  C. Neoplasia may occur on lips, cheeks, palate, gingiva, tonsils, or tongue
     1. Watch carefully for oral melanomas
     2. Epuli are commonly seen

IV. Sensory organs
  A. Specimens are usually collected from eyelids using scraping or fine needle aspiration
     1. Sebaceous gland tumors are common
  B. Samples for evaluation of the conjunctiva are usually collected by scraping with a flat round-tip spatula
     1. May help identify the cause of chronic conjunctivitis
  C. Samples for evaluation of corneal lesions are collected by applying topical anesthetic and scraping the lesion
  D. Secretions from ear canals are collected with cotton swabs
     1. Bacterial and fungal (*Malassezia* spp.) infections are common (Color Plate 25)
     2. Parasites (*Otobius* sp., *Otodectes* sp.) may also be present
     3. Neoplasia is uncommon and usually benign

V. Glandular tissues
  A. Samples from mammary, parathyroid, thyroid, and salivary glands are usually collected by fine needle aspiration
  B. Common inflammatory and benign neoplastic conditions include mastitis, cysts, sialoceles, and lymphocytic thyroiditis
  C. Mammary tumors are common in female dogs and cats and are usually malignant. These are often histologically mixed (contain a variety of cell types)
  D. Malignant neoplastic conditions of salivary, thyroid, and parathyroid tissues are extremely rare

VI. Lymph nodes
  A. Lymph node tissue: complex cytology evaluations
     1. Normal lymph nodes
        a. Consist of 75% to 95% small lymphocytes
           (1) Smaller than a neutrophil and has scant, pale blue cytoplasm
           (2) Round nuclei is about the size of a red blood cell (RBC) with dense aggregated chromatin
        b. Only a few plasma cells, medium and large lymphocytes, and macrophages
        c. Reticular and endothelial cells are common, but because of aspiration techniques, the large swollen nuclei often appear without any cytoplasm
        d. Small numbers of neutrophils, eosinophils, and mast cells are occasionally present
        e. Cytoplasmic fragments referred to as lymphoglandular bodies are round, homogeneous, basophilic structures about the size of platelets
        f. Free nuclei that are pink and amorphous result from the aspiration pressure forcing fragile lymphocytes to rupture and release the nuclei
     2. Wide variety of diseases can manifest with changes in lymph node cytology
     3. Inflammation (lymphadenitis)
        a. Will have an increase in inflammatory cells: neutrophils, eosinophils, and macrophages (Color Plate 26)
           (1) Likely have more than 5% neutrophils or 3% eosinophils
     4. Hyperplasia (benign neoplasia)
        a. Cytologically similar to a normal lymph node
     5. Mixed (both inflammatory and neoplastic cells present)

6. Neoplasia (lymph node cells with abnormal nuclear features or presence of large number of blast cells)
7. Metastasis (neoplastic cells from other body tissues that spread to lymph nodes) (Color Plate 27)

VII. Bone marrow
A. Used when the differential blood cell count demonstrates ambiguous or unexplained abnormal results
B. Samples may be collected by aspiration or by removing a bone marrow core
C. Use different sites for each collection when collecting both an aspirate and a core sample
D. Proper restraint is crucial; sedation or local anesthesia may be needed; aseptic technique is required
E. Aspiration biopsy collection sites: head of the femur, head of the humerus, iliac crest, or femoral canal
F. Core biopsy
1. Core samples allow the architecture of the cells to remain intact
2. Overall cellularity of the marrow is most accurately determined with a core sample
3. The core sample is collected using a 16- to 18-gauge Jamshidi needle
4. The most commonly used site for collection is the iliac crest
G. Preparing marrow smears
1. Line smears, starfish smears, wedge films, and compression smears can also be used for bone marrow samples
2. Smears must be prepared and stained immediately, or the sample mixed with 0.5 mL of 2% to 3% ethylenediaminetetraacetic acid (EDTA) in saline
3. Staining time must be increased depending on the cellularity and thickness of the sample
4. One slide is usually stained to detect the presence of hemosiderin
5. Romanowsky's stain can be used for aspiration samples; hematoxylin and eosin stain is preferred for core biopsy samples
H. Evaluation of bone marrow films
1. Evaluated with results of a differential count from a concurrent peripheral blood film
2. The sample is described as acellular (aplasia), hypercellular (hyperplasia) or hypocellular (hypoplasia), based on the proportion of nucleated cells versus fat present
   a. Samples from adult animals are usually about 50% nucleated cells and 50% fat
   b. Samples from juvenile mammals are usually 25% fat
   c. Samples from geriatric animals usually have marrow consisting of approximately 75% fat
   d. Samples are then further characterized by describing the type of cells present (e.g., hypoplasia/myeloid).

I. Cells in bone marrow
1. Myeloid cells are relatively large and pale-staining cells
   a. Myeloblast, promyelocyte, myelocyte, and metamyelocyte
   b. Metamyelocytes, bands, and segmented myeloid cells make up 80% to 90% of myeloid cells
2. Erythroid cells are smaller and have clumped basophilic nuclei
   a. Rubriblast, prorubricyte, rubricyte, and metarubricyte
   b. Rubricytes and metarubricytes usually account for 80% to 90% of the erythroid cells
3. The ratio of myeloid cells to erythroid cells (M:E ratio) is determined by counting 500 nucleated cells and classifying them as erythroid or myeloid
   a. Alternative systems for evaluation of bone marrow include erythroid maturation index, myeloid maturation index, and left shift index for both myeloid and erythroid cell lines
4. Megakaryocytes: not evenly distributed in a bone marrow aspirate; very large cells with multiple fused nuclei; often seen in clusters (Color Plate 28)
5. More than 10 per low-power field would indicate an increase in this cell line
6. Other components of bone marrow
   a. Osteoblasts: much larger than plasma cells and nuclear material is paler
   b. Plasma cells: may contain inclusions representing immunoglobulin (Russell bodies) (Color Plate 29)
   c. Osteoclasts: contain multiple nuclei and may appear somewhat fused and similar in appearance to megakaryocytes
      (1) Seen most often in samples from young, actively growing animals
      (2) Blue cytoplasm that may contain granular material of variable sizes that stains a deep red
   d. Macrophages and mast cells
   e. Lymphocytes: usually present in low numbers

(1) Lymphoblasts and prolymphocytes: difficult to distinguish from rubriblasts and prorubricytes

(2) Reactive lymphocytes and normal, mature lymphocytes may also be present

f. Hemosiderin: found in macrophages in bone marrow and free of cells

(1) Small gray to black granules when traditional blood film stains are used

(2) Almost always absent in bone marrow preparations from cats

(3) Decrease or absence of hemosiderin is significant in most other species

I. Reporting of results

1. Results include overall cellularity and either M:E ratio, maturation index, or left shift index.

2. Sample is described in narrative form; unique patterns and morphological abnormalities described

3. Hemosiderin, increased presence of mitotic figures, increased presence of osteoblasts, osteoclasts, mast cells, phagocytized material, and metastatic cells from other organs are recorded when present

4. The data are reported along with the concurrent differential count from a peripheral blood film

5. Inflammatory conditions are classified according to the primary cell type(s) present as fibrinous, chronic, chronic granulomatous, or chronic pyogranulomatous

6. Neoplastic disorders of hematopoiesis are classified as either lymphoproliferative or myeloproliferative

VIII. Hepatobiliary tissues

A. Samples for cytological evaluation of the hepatobiliary system may be collected by fine needle aspiration or biopsy

B. Normal findings in hepatobiliary cytology include hepatocytes and blood cells

C. Hepatocytes commonly contain bile pigments and hemosiderin

D. Abnormal findings usually involve changes in the morphology of the hepatocytes (vacuoles, excessive or unusual granulation, or unstained areas within the cytoplasm)

E. Common nonneoplastic disorders include feline hepatic lipidosis

F. Inflammatory disorders include amyloidosis, hepatitis, and cholangiohepatitis

G. Often blood chemistry and physical examination assist in identifying the cause of any inflammatory or nonneoplastic condition

H. Common neoplastic disorders include epithelial cell tumors, lymphosarcoma, and hemangiosarcoma

I. Metastasis from other body tissues is a common finding

IX. Fluid aspirates: may involve removal and evaluation of abnormal fluid accumulation (e.g., abdominocentesis, thoracocentesis) or removal and evaluation of body fluids normally found (e.g., arthrocentesis, spinal tap)

A. Abdominal and thoracic fluid

1. Accumulations of thoracic or abdominal fluid indicate pathology in other body systems

2. Sample is collected by fine needle aspiration into a sterile EDTA collection tube

a. If cultures or biochemical testing are required, additional samples should be collected in a transport media container and a plain sterile blood collection tube

3. Samples are initially evaluated for volume, total nucleated cell count, total protein, color, and clarity

4. Abdominal and thoracic fluids should be classified as to type of effusion (transudate, exudate, modified transudate) using the classification system described previously

5. Techniques for preparation of slides depend on the character of the sample

a. Samples with low cellularity should be concentrated before preparation or prepared as line smears

b. Turbid samples usually have high cellularity and can be prepared with direct smears

6. Cells seen in most thoracic effusions include neutrophils, mesothelial cells, macrophages, lymphocytes, and other peripheral blood cells

a. Predominance of neutrophils indicates an inflammatory process

(1) Neutrophils should be evaluated for degenerative characteristics, toxic granulation, presence of phagocytized material, etc.

b. Common inflammatory conditions include infectious peritonitis, infectious pleuritis, and feline infectious peritonitis

c. Macrophages and mesothelial cells look similar in effusions

(1) They may appear atypical, but this is an expected response to the presence of abnormal fluid around the cells and should not be confused with neoplasia

d. Increased number of lymphocytes usually indicates neoplasia, particularly lymphosarcoma

e. Chylous effusions often have a predominance of mature lymphocytes (Color Plate 30)

f. Reactive lymphocytes are present in inflammatory conditions and can be differentiated from neoplastic cells by evaluating the cytoplasm

(1) Reactive lymphocytes are larger than small lymphocytes and usually have scant to moderate deep blue cytoplasm

(2) Neoplastic lymphocytes usually have moderate clear to light blue cytoplasm

(a) Nucleus shape is variable, and nuclei contain finely stippled nuclear chromatin and nucleoli

(b) They are larger than neutrophils

g. Increased number of mast cells indicates a mast cell tumor

h. Other neoplastic conditions that may be identified cytologically include carcinoma, sarcoma, and mesothelioma

i. Some tumors do not exfoliate well into effusions. The absence of neoplastic cells does not rule out neoplasia

B. Synovial fluid

1. Evaluation of synovial fluid may aid in differential diagnosis of lameness

2. Collection method: arthrocentesis usually involves fine needle aspiration from the flexed joint space, but techniques vary depending on the joint of interest

3. Normal synovial fluid contains a variety of proteins, electrolytes, and other substances (e.g., glucose) similar to blood plasma

4. Synovial fluid does not clot unless the sample is contaminated with blood or intraarticular hemorrhage is present

a. If needed, heparin is the anticoagulant of choice

5. Samples should be evaluated for volume, total nucleated cell counts, color, turbidity, viscosity, total protein, and mucin concentration

6. Abnormal cytological findings include increased RBCs, vacuolization of large mononuclear cells (macrophages and/or clasmatocytes), and other degenerative characteristics (karyorrhexis, pyknosis)

7. Infectious disorders are uncommon but usually bacterial in origin

a. Phagocytized bacteria normally would be evident

8. A variety of degenerative joint diseases can occur (e.g., arthritis, systemic lupus erythematosus) and are usually immune mediated

a. Radiography is often used for confirmation

C. Cerebrospinal fluid

1. Evaluation of cerebrospinal fluid (CSF) can aid in diagnosis of neurological disorders

2. Sample collection is by needle and syringe on the anesthetized patient

a. Ultrasound guidance is common

3. Site of collection depends on suspected neuropathy; lumbar puncture and atlantooccipital space are the most common collection sites

4. CSF should be examined for total cellularity, color, turbidity, total protein, and total RBC count. Biochemical testing may also be needed

5. CSF fluid generally needs to be concentrated before performing cytological evaluation

6. In normal CSF tap, most cells are small lymphocytes, with a few monocytes and macrophages (look like monocytes with phagocytic vacuoles)

a. Neutrophils are not normally found unless the tap was traumatic

7. Increases in total nucleated cells or alterations in the relative proportions of the various cell types indicate a pathological condition

8. A variety of inflammatory disorders can occur, including bacterial meningitis, feline infectious peritonitis, and toxoplasmosis

9. Neoplastic cells are a rare finding in CSF

X. Urogenital system

A. Kidney tissue

1. Samples are usually collected by fine needle aspiration or biopsy

2. Renal tubular epithelial cells and peripheral blood cells are common findings

3. Large polygonal to round, found singly or in clusters

4. Abundant light-blue cytoplasm with round, centrally located nucleus

5. Abnormal findings include lymphoid cells, lymphoblasts, and plasma cells

6. Inflammation is a common finding and may be septic (pyelonephritis) or nonseptic

a. Benign cysts also occur

7. Renal lymphosarcoma is common in cat; carcinoma is common in dog

8. Majority of renal tumors in dog and cat are malignant

B. Urinary tract
1. Cytological evaluation of the urinary tract may aid in differentiation of urinary tract masses
2. Samples can be collected with routine urine collection methods or by fine needle aspiration of radiographically identified masses
3. Infectious cystitis is characterized by the presence of large numbers of neutrophils. Infectious agents may also be present, either free or within phagocytic cells
4. Neoplasia of the urinary tract usually involves bladder epithelial cells
5. Prostatic enlargement usually requires cytological evaluation
   a. Samples are collected by fine needle aspiration
   b. Prostatitis is common and characterized by large numbers of neutrophils that may also be septic
   c. Benign hyperplasia is common in older animals
   d. Prostatic carcinoma may also occur
C. Vaginal cytology
1. Indicated to assist in timing mating programs, such as artificial insemination in small animals, or to evaluate infectious or neoplastic processes
2. History and clinical signs are important for proper interpretation of cytology specimen
3. Samples with very large numbers of degenerate neutrophils may indicate vaginitis, pyometra, or metritis
4. Transitional cell carcinoma or squamous cell carcinoma may also be identified cytologically
5. Cells commonly found vary depending on the stage during the estrous cycle
   a. Basal cells are small with small amount of cytoplasm
   b. Parabasal cells are generally uniform in shape and are small and round with a small amount of cytoplasm (Color Plate 31)
   c. Intermediate cells are twice the size of parabasal cells
      (1) As they increase, the cytoplasm becomes more irregular, folded, and angular
      (2) Superficial cells are the largest cells seen
         (a) With age the nuclei become pyknotic, fade, and occasionally disappear
         (b) Cytoplasm is abundant, angular, and folded

         (c) Commonly referred to as cornified cells
6. Identification of cell populations during the estrous cycle is easily accomplished through cytologic examination
   a. Anestrus
      (1) Predominantly noncornified squamous epithelial cells
      (2) Smaller cells, basophilic cytoplasm, and large, round nucleus
         (a) Cells are intermediate or parabasal
      (3) Some neutrophils but no RBCs
   b. Proestrus (Color Plate 32)
      (1) In early to mid-proestrus, there is a mixture of parabasal, intermediate, and superficial cells
         (a) Neutrophils and RBCs are present
      (2) By late proestrus, there is a decrease in neutrophil numbers
         (a) Mostly large intermediate and superficial cells
         (b) RBCs may or may not be present
         (c) Bacteria often present
   c. Estrus
      (1) All superficial cells
      (2) Many appear to be anuclear or have small pyknotic nuclei
      (3) RBCs may be present, but no neutrophils
      (4) Bacteria often present
   d. Metestrus
      (1) Parabasal and intermediate cells replace superficial cells
      (2) Neutrophil numbers increase
      (3) RBCs generally absent but may be present
      (4) Cytologically, late estrus to early metestrus resembles early or mid-proestrus
   e. Testes
      (1) Sample collection by fine needle aspiration can aid in differentiation of testicular enlargement
      (2) Inflammatory conditions (orchitis and epididymitis) appear similar to other inflammatory processes
      (3) Common neoplastic conditions include Sertoli cell tumors and interstitial cell tumors
      (4) Transmissible venereal tumor may be present on external genitalia
         (a) May also be found in the oral and nasal cavities

f. Semen evaluation
   (1) Avoid exposing semen samples to marked changes in temperature (especially cold), water, disinfectants, or variations in pH
   (2) Laboratory equipment and supplies used in semen collection and examination should be clean and dry and warmed to about 37° C (98.6° F)
   (3) Semen evaluation includes measurement of ejaculate volume, evaluation of gross appearance, sperm motility, sperm concentration, sperm morphology, and live:dead sperm ratio
      (a) The opacity and color of the sample should be recorded as thick, creamy, opaque; milky opaque; opalescent milky; or watery
      (b) Sperm motility: subjective assessment; two methods of assessment
      (c) Wave motion: classified as very good, good, fair, and poor, based on the amount of "swirling" activity observed in a drop of semen on a microscope slide at low-power (×40) magnification
      (d) Motility: progressive motility of individual spermatozoa is determined on a relatively dilute drop of cover-slipped semen, examined at ×100 magnification
   (4) Sperm concentration: semen samples are diluted and counted with a hemocytometer
   (5) Live:dead sperm ratio: staining with a vital dye permits discrimination between live and dead spermatozoa
   (6) Sperm morphology: assess a nigrosin and eosin stained smear; the percentage of abnormal spermatozoa and their types are recorded after observing 100 to 500 cells
      (a) Abnormalities are divided into head, midpiece, and tail problems
      (b) Abnormalities often are categorized as primary or secondary

XI. Miscellaneous
   A. Musculoskeletal system
      1. Muscle tissue samples can be collected in a manner similar to that used for cutaneous and subcutaneous lesions
         a. Bone tissue samples are collected by fine needle aspiration or biopsy
      2. Primary muscle tissue tumors are extremely rare
      3. Inflammatory disorders of bone tissue (osteomyelitis) can be caused by a variety of infectious agents, such as fungi and bacteria
      4. Neoplastic disorders of bone are common
         a. Osteosarcoma is characterized by highly cellular samples and pleomorphic cell types
         b. Chondrosarcoma is characterized by the presence of a diffuse cartilaginous matrix with embedded cells
         c. Fibrosarcoma and hemangiosarcoma may also occur in bone tissue
   B. Spleen
      1. Samples for analysis of the spleen can be collected by fine needle aspiration or biopsy
      2. Care must be taken when collecting samples by fine needle aspiration to avoid fracturing delicate splenic tissues
      3. Cytology evaluation is combined with clinical signs (e.g., degree of splenic enlargement) when determining diagnosis
      4. Hyperplasia can result from a variety of infectious or immune-mediated conditions, including parasites and fungi
      5. Splenic enlargement can also occur as a result of extramedullary hematopoiesis involving the spleen
      6. Neoplastic disorders of the spleen include hemangiosarcoma, fibrosarcoma, and several other tumor types
   C. Rectal mucosa
      1. Presence of mucus or blood in fecal samples may indicate the need for rectal mucosal scraping
      2. Normal cells in rectal scrapings include columnar epithelial cells and bacteria
      3. Infections with *Histoplasma* or *Balantidium* organisms may be identified with rectal scraping
      4. Lymphosarcoma may be identified with rectal scraping
         a. Most other intestinal masses require fine needle aspiration for evaluation

## ACKNOWLEDGMENT ▬

The author recognizes and appreciates the original work of Marg Brown and Bill Wade, on which this chapter is based.

# Glossary

**abdominocentesis** Removal of fluid from the abdominal cavity
**adenocarcinoma** Tumors of epithelial cell origin that tend to be highly cellular and often exfoliate in clumps or sheets
**adenoma** Benign epithelial tumor
**adipocytes** Fat storage cell

**amyloidosis** Deposition of an almost insoluble protein in various tissues

**anisocytosis** Abnormal variation in size of cell

**anisokaryosis** Abnormal variation in size of nucleus

**anisonucleoliosis** Abnormal variation in size of nucleoli

**arthrocentesis** Removal of fluid from a joint

**benign** Neoplasia that is characterized by homogeneous populations of cells that are not malignant, including lipoma, fibroma, papilloma, and adenoma

**biopsy** Removal of cells or tissues for microscopic or chemical examination

**carcinoma** Tumors of epithelial cell origin that tend to be highly cellular and often exfoliate in clumps or sheets

**centesis** Act of puncturing a body cavity or organ with a hollow needle to draw out fluid

**chemotactic** Molecules that attract and guide the movement of cells, such as phagocytes

**cholangiohepatitis** Inflammation of the biliary and liver parenchyma

**chondrosarcoma** Malignant tumor of the cartilage cells or their precursors

**chylous effusion** A milky liquid that contains a high concentration of lymph fluid

**clasmatocyte** Synovial fluid monocytic leukocytes other than lymphocytes, monocytes, and macrophages

**cystocentesis** Aspiration of fluid from the urinary bladder

**effusion** Fluid in a body cavity that is abnormally increased in volume

**epulis** Benign tumor of mixed cells found in the oral cavity

**erythrocytophagia** Phagocytosis of erythrocytes

**exfoliative cytology** Study of cells from body surfaces

**exudate** Effusion characterized by greater than 3.0 g/dL of protein and greater than 7000 nucleated cells/mL

**fibroma** A tumor of the fibrous or well-developed connective tissue

**fibrosarcoma** Sarcoma found in fibrous connective tissue

**fistula** Abnormal passage between two internal organs or from an internal organ to the body surface

**granulomatous** Inflammatory condition characterized by greater than 70% of mononuclear cells (monocytes, macrophages, giant cells) with few neutrophils

**hemangiosarcoma** Malignant neoplasia consisting of epithelial cells and fibroblasts

**hemosiderin** Insoluble form of intracellular iron storage

**hepatocytes** Liver cells

**histiocytoma** Tumor of discrete round cell origin that tends to exfoliate singly and have high cellularity

**histopathology** Microscopic study of diseased tissues

**hypercellularity** Abnormal increase in number of cells present

**hyperplasia** Abnormal increase in overall cell numbers as a result of an external stimulus

**hypersegmentation** Excessive division into segments or lobes

**in situ** Within the body

**karyolysis** Loss of nuclear membrane

**karyorrhexis** Fragmentation of the cell nucleus

**lymphadenitis** Inflammation of the lymph nodes

**lymphoblast** Immature, nucleated precursor of the mature lymphocyte; also called large lymphocyte

**macrocytosis** Increase in number of abnormally large cells

**macrophage** Tissue phagocyte derived from the peripheral blood monocyte

**malignant** Neoplasia that displays multiple abnormal nuclear criteria

**mast cell** Tissue cell containing granules of histamine and heparin that stain dark purple

**melanoma** Tumor arising from cells that contain melanin

**mesenchymal** Muscular, connective tissue and vessels that are derived from the embryonic connective tissue in the mesoderm

**mesoderm** Middle of the three primary germ layers of the embryo

**mesothelial** Cells that line pleural, peritoneal, and visceral surfaces

**mesothelioma** Rare malignant tumor derived from mesothelial cells

**metastasis** Neoplasia that is present in an area other than where it initially developed

**modified transudate** Effusion characterized by moderate cellularity and increased total protein

**mucocele** Accumulated mucous secretion in a cavity

**neoplasia** Any new or abnormal growth, especially if it is uncontrolled and progressive; a tumor

**osteomyelitis** Inflammation of the bone

**osteosarcoma** Malignant tumor of the bone

**papilloma** Common wart

**percutaneous** Performed through the skin

**perinuclear** Space between the inner and outer nuclear membranes

**plasma cell** Activated lymphocyte characterized by eccentrically located nucleus, basophilic cytoplasm and a perinuclear clear zone

**pleomorphic** Abnormal variation in size and/or shape of cells of the same type

**pleuritis** Inflammation of the pleura

**pneumothorax** Air in the pleural cavity that causes lung collapse

**purulent** Inflamed area containing greater than 85% neutrophils

**pyknosis** Condensed nucleus

**pyogranulomatous** Inflammatory process consisting of macrophages and 50% to 75% neutrophils

**sarcoma** Malignant tumor derived from connective tissue cells

**sialocele** Common nonneoplastic condition of salivary gland characterized by fluid-filled cavities composed primarily of epithelial cells

**suppurative** Purulent inflammation containing greater than 85% neutrophils

**thoracocentesis** Removal of fluid from the thoracic cavity

**transudate** Effusion with less than 2.5 g/dL protein and fewer than 1500 cells/mL

# Review Questions

**1** The preferred sample preparation technique when cellularity is low is
  a. Wedge smear
  b. Starfish smear
  c. Line smear
  d. Squash prep

**2** The presence of yellowish supernatant after centrifugation of an effusion usually indicates
   a. Iatrogenic contamination with peripheral blood
   b. Recent hemorrhage
   c. Inflammation
   d. Hemorrhage that occurred at least 2 days previously

**3** A chylous effusion typically appears
   a. Milky
   b. Pink
   c. Amber
   d. Colorless

**4** The presence of predominantly anuclear cornified epithelial cells indicates
   a. Proestrus
   b. Anestrus
   c. Diestrus
   d. Estrus

**5** Cells that line the pleural, peritoneal, and visceral surfaces are
   a. Plasma cells
   b. Mast cells
   c. Mesothelial cells
   d. Macrophages

**6** Cells that contain a perinuclear clear zone are
   a. Plasma cells
   b. Mast cells
   c. Mesothelial cells
   d. Macrophages

**7** A cytology sample containing 90% neutrophils is described as
   a. Chronic inflammation
   b. Granulomatous inflammation
   c. Purulent inflammation
   d. Pyogranulomatous inflammation

**8** A criterion of malignancy that involves variability in the size and shape of same cell type is referred to as
   a. Anisocytosis
   b. Anisokaryosis
   c. Pleomorphism
   d. Nuclear molding

**9** A bone marrow sample from a juvenile animal that contains 50% fat is described as
   a. Hypoplastic
   b. Hyperplastic
   c. Inflammatory
   d. Neoplastic

**10** A deformation of nuclei by other nuclei within the same cell or adjacent cells is referred to as
   a. Nuclear molding
   b. Angular nuclei
   c. Anisonucleosis
   d. Multinucleation

## BIBLIOGRAPHY

Baker R, Lumsden J: *Color atlas of cytology of the dog and cat*, St Louis, 2000, Mosby.

Cowell R, Tyler R, Meinkoth J: *Diagnostic cytology and hematology of the dog and cat*, ed 2, St Louis, 1999, Mosby.

Meyer DJ: The management of cytology specimens, *Comp Cont Educ Pract Vet* 9:1, 1987.

Perman V: *Cytology of the dog and cat*, South Bend, Ind, 1979, American Animal Hospital Association.

Raskin R, Meyer D: *Atlas of canine and feline cytology*, Philadelphia, 2001, Saunders.

Rebar A: *Handbook of veterinary cytology*, St Louis, 1980, Ralston Purina.

## CHAPTER 4

# Parasitology

*Ed Robinson*

## OUTLINE

Feces Examination
   Gross Examination of Feces
   Standard Vial Gravitation
      Flotation Technique
   Quantitative Fecal Examination
   Commercial Flotation Kits
   Direct Smear
   Centrifugal Flotation Technique
   OVC Puddle Technique

Preservation of Parasitic Samples
Blood Parasite Examination
   Modified Knott's Technique
   Commercial Filter Technique
   Buffy Coat Method
Enzyme-Linked Immunosorbent
   Assay
External Parasite Identification
   Skin Scraping

Skin Digestion Technique
Cellophane Tape Method
Baermann Technique
External and Internal Parasite
   Identification

## LEARNING OUTCOMES

After reading this chapter, you should be able to:

1. List the scientific and common names of parasites.
2. Define and describe the life cycles of various parasites.
3. Describe clinical signs associated with each parasite.
4. Describe how to identify a parasite infestation.
5. Define treatment and control of parasite infestations.
6. Define various basic laboratory techniques for the identification of parasites.

The parasite/host relationship is unique. A parasite is an organism that in its natural habitat feeds and lives on or in another organism. The parasite may cause clinical signs in the host, but its goal is to use the host to live and reproduce without causing death. However, a parasite infection of sufficient numbers can overwhelm the host and cause death. Familiarity with life cycles helps us to control parasites. For example, heartworm in dogs can be controlled with preventives. In other cases, such as flea infestation, the environment and the host need to be treated. Proper identification of parasites or ova allows the veterinarian to determine which treatment regimen is appropriate. This chapter describes common parasites by host, beginning with the domestic dog and cat and moving on to horses, food animals, and some common laboratory animals. See parasite tables at the end of the chapter.

## FECES EXAMINATION
### Gross Examination of Feces

I. Gross characteristics of feces should be recorded and reported to the veterinarian
II. Characteristics noted include consistency, color, and presence of blood, mucus, or adult parasites, including tapeworm segments

### Standard Vial Gravitation Flotation Technique

I. Based on specific gravity of parasitic material and fecal debris
  A. Specific gravity of most parasite eggs is between 1.100 and 1.200
  B. Specific gravity of water is 1.000
  C. Flotation solution must have a higher specific gravity than that of the parasitic material to facilitate flotation of parasite eggs, oocysts, etc.
II. A simple, inexpensive technique but of poor efficiency
  A. Materials
    1. Vial (approximately 2 inches deep by 1 inch in diameter)

2. Two paper cups
3. Wire strainer
4. Tongue depressor
5. Glass slide and coverslip
6. Solution of sodium nitrate with specific gravity of 1.200 to 1.250 when mixed manually and 1.200 with commercial preparations.
   a. Other common flotation solutions
      (1) Sugar solution: inexpensive, does not crystallize or distort eggs, specific gravity of 1.330
      (2) Zinc sulfate solution: for *Giardia* cysts, specific gravity of 1.180
      (3) Saturated sodium chloride solution: specific gravity up to 1.200
B. Fill a paper cup with approximately 60 mL of sodium nitrate solution
C. Using a tongue depressor, add approximately 2 to 4 g (0.5 to 1 teaspoon) of feces
D. Mix feces well with sodium nitrate solution
E. Strain, using wire strainer, into a second cup. Remove as much fluid as possible from the fecal material in the strainer
F. Discard feces on the strainer and wash strainer with hot water for reuse
G. Swirl strained fecal suspension in the cup to randomly disperse eggs and pour mixture into vial until fluid projects above rim of the vial, creating a positive meniscus
H. Place a coverslip on top of the fluid and allow eggs to float upward
I. After a minimum of 10 to 15 minutes, remove coverslip (straight up), trying not to tilt fluid back into vial, and place it on a glass slide
J. Using ×10 objective, systematically examine entire area under the coverslip, noting type and number of parasites seen
   1. Sample should also be examined using ×40 objective for small protozoa
K. Although the procedure cannot be classified as quantitative, results are reported as follows:
   1. 1 to 100 eggs seen: graded as one plus (+)
   2. 101 to 300 eggs seen: graded as two plus (++)
   3. 301 or more eggs seen: graded as three plus (+++)

## Quantitative Fecal Examination

I. Quantitative procedures are used to determine the number of eggs present per gram of feces
   A. Examples include the Wisconsin double centrifugation technique and the McMaster technique
   B. Other quantitative procedures can be found in the reference books listed at the end of this chapter

## Commercial Flotation Kits

I. Common examples
   A. Ovassay (Synbiotics, San Diego, Calif)
   B. Fecalyzer (EVSCO Pharmaceuticals, Buena, NJ)
   C. Ovatector (BGS Medical Products, Venice, Fla)
II. Kits are easy to use but moderately expensive and have low sensitivity; are commonly used in clinics.
III. A kit generally comes with a vial, which may or may not have a cap; an insert (or funnel or filter), to collect or pick up feces; and possibly flotation solution
IV. Follow insert instructions

## Direct Smear

I. Direct smear is used to
   A. Detect protozoa in feces
   B. Quickly estimate the number of parasites
II. Materials
   A. Microscope slides and coverslips
   B. Applicator sticks or tongue depressors
   C. Lugol's iodine (especially for *Giardia*) or new methylene blue stain (optional)
III. Procedure
   A. Place a drop of saline or water on a slide with an equal amount of feces. A drop of stain may be added at this time
   B. Mix feces and saline with applicator stick
   C. Make a very thin smear on the slide
   D. Remove large pieces of feces on slide for easier viewing
   E. Examine smear using ×10 objective for parasite eggs and larvae, and ×40 objective for protozoal organisms

## Centrifugal Flotation Technique

I. Centrifugal flotation technique used to
   A. Concentrate ova in feces
   B. Detect *Giardia* oocysts more efficiently than regular flotation technique
II. Materials
   A. Paper cups
   B. Tongue depressor
   C. Cheesecloth or tea strainer
   D. 15-mL centrifuge tube
   E. Water
   F. Fecal solution
   G. Centrifuge
   H. Microscope slide and coverslip
   I. Wire loop, transfer pipette, or glass rod
   J. Lugol's iodine for *Giardia* oocysts (optional)
III. Procedure
   A. Place approximately 1 teaspoon of feces in a paper cup and mix with enough water to make a semisolid solution

B. Place tea strainer or cheesecloth over second paper cup and empty the fecal mixture into it. Wash strainer (if used)

C. Pour contents of second cup into 15-mL centrifuge tube

D. Centrifuge for 3 minutes at 450 to 650 *g* (about 1500 rpm)

E. Pour supernatant off and add fecal flotation solution to about the 10-mL mark on the centrifuge tube (or ¾ full). Place a stopper or other cover over the tube and mix by inverting 4 to 5 times

F. Recentrifuge for 5 minutes

G. Without removing the tube from the centrifuge, use the wire loop, glass rod, or transfer pipette to transfer the surface film to a glass slide (touch transfer pipette to surface, don't aspirate solution)

H. Examine under microscope at ×10 for parasite eggs and ×40 for protozoan organisms

## OVC Puddle Technique (for *Cryptosporidium* Oocysts)

I. Materials
A. Microscope slide and coverslip
B. Applicator stick
C. Saturated sugar solution (e.g., corn syrup)
II. Procedure
A. Place a drop of sugar solution on a glass slide
B. Add a small amount of feces to slide and mix
C. Add a coverslip and examine under ×40 objective
1. Oocysts of *Cryptosporidium* are up to 5 μm in diameter and are slightly pink
2. There may be fungal spores present that are similar in size and shape to an oocyst; however, spores usually will bud if observed for a period of time

## PRESERVATION OF PARASITIC SAMPLES

I. Fresh specimens should be packaged in leak-proof containers, sealed, and labeled
A. Label should include the following information: date, location where specimen was obtained, owner's name, animal's species, animal's name or identification number, referring veterinarian, clinic address, and telephone number
II. Feces can be sent fresh or mixed at a ratio of 1:3 with 10% formalin
III. Whole parasites or segments can be preserved in alcohol or formalin

Examples of ova are illustrated at the end of the chapter.

## BLOOD PARASITE EXAMINATION (*Dirofilaria immitis* AND *Acanthocheilonema* [FORMERLY *Dipetalonema*] *reconditum*)
### Modified Knott's Technique

I. Materials
A. 15-mL centrifuge tube and centrifuge
B. 2% formalin
C. Methylene blue stain
D. Pasteur pipettes and bulbs
E. Slides and coverslips
II. Procedure
A. Place 1 mL of EDTA blood in a 15-mL conical centrifuge tube
B. Add 9 mL of 2% formalin (or water)
C. Mix by inversion and shake to lyse the red blood cells
D. Spin in centrifuge for 5 minutes at 1000 rpm or let stand for 1 hour
E. Decant supernatant by inverting tube once and letting it drain
F. Add 2 drops of methylene blue stain to the sediment and mix with a pipette by gently aspirating the mixture
G. Place a drop of the mixture on a slide, add coverslip, and examine under ×10 objective
H. Examine entire slide for microfilariae

## Commercial Filter Technique

I. Common example of a commercial kit
A. Difil-Test (EVSCO, Buena, NJ)
II. These kits come with filters, lysing solution, stain, and directions
III. Most kits require 1 mL of whole blood to test for heartworms
IV. Mix blood with 10 to 12 mL of lysing solution
V. Place a new filter in the filter holder, inject the fluid into the filter holder, and rinse with 10 mL of water
VI. Place the filter on a slide, and add a drop of stain
VII. Add a coverslip to the slide, and examine slide

## Buffy Coat Method

I. A concentration method using a small amount of blood
II. Is quick and can be performed after evaluation of a packed cell volume (PCV) and before total protein evaluation
III. Materials
A. Microhematocrit tubes and sealer
B. Centrifuge
C. Microscope slides and coverslips
D. Saline
E. Methylene blue stain
F. Small file or glass cutter

IV. Procedure
    A. Centrifuge blood-filled microhematocrit tube for 3 minutes
    B. Read PCV
    C. Examine surface of buffy coat (white blood cells) layer of the blood under microscope
       1. When a blood-filled microhematocrit tube is spun in the centrifuge, the blood separates into three layers
          a. Plasma
          b. White blood cell layer (buffy coat)
          c. Red blood cell layer
    D. Use a file to scratch tube at level of the buffy coat. Snap tube and gently tap tube to place buffy coat on slide
    E. Add a drop of saline and a drop of methylene blue stain to the buffy coat. Add coverslip, and examine for microfilariae
    F. Use remaining plasma from the hematocrit tube to evaluate total protein

## ENZYME-LINKED IMMUNOSORBENT ASSAY ▬

I. Enzyme-linked immunosorbent assay (ELISA) kits do not detect microfilariae. They detect only the host's response to parasites or antigens present in the blood
II. This test can be used to identify
    A. Occult heartworm
    B. *Dirofilaria immitis*
III. Common examples
    A. DiroCHEK (Synbiotics, San Diego, Calif)
    B. PetChek/Snap (Idexx, Westbrook Me)
    C. Witness (Binax, Scarborough, Me)
IV. ELISA antigen detection system
    A. Monoclonal antibody is bound to the walls of a well in a test tray, to a membrane, or to a plastic wand
    B. If the specific antigen is present in the sample, it will bind to this antibody and to the second enzyme-labeled antibody that is added
    C. When a color-producing agent is added to the mixture, the agent reacts to develop a specific color that indicates presence of the antigen in the sample
    D. If the sample contains no antigen, the second antibody is washed away during a rinsing process and no other color reactions take place
V. ELISA tests are easy to perform when following manufacturer directions and take approximately 10 to 15 minutes to complete

## EXTERNAL PARASITE IDENTIFICATION ▬
### Skin Scraping

I. Materials
    A. No. 10 scalpel blade
    B. Mineral oil in a dropper bottle
    C. Microscope slides
    D. Microscope

II. Procedure
    A. Add mineral oil to a slide and dip scalpel blade into it
    B. Begin scraping by holding skin between thumb and index finger of one hand and scalpel blade in the other hand
    C. While scraping, the blade must be held perpendicular to the skin
       1. Holding the blade at any other angle could result in an incision into the skin
    D. Depth of scraping depends on the suspected parasite
       1. *Sarc*optes (burrowing mite) and Demodex (hair follicle mite): scrape until blood begins to seep from the abrasion
       2. Chorioptes (nonburrowing mite) and Cheyletiel*la* (walking dandruff): skin is scraped superficially to collect loose scales and crusts
    E. All of the harvest (material scraped from the skin) is placed on a slide with mineral oil
    F. After adding a coverslip, examine entire slide under the ×10 objective
    G. For thorough evaluation, examine at least 10 slides

### Skin Digestion Technique

I. Used for scraping samples where there is a large amount of scurf and skin debris
II. Materials
    A. Conical centrifuge tube
    B. 4% NaOH
    C. Hot plate, beaker
    D. Centrifuge
III. Procedure
    A. Place the skin scraping (with scalpel blade if desired) in a 15-mL conical centrifuge tube
    B. Add about 10 mL of 4% NaOH solution
    C. Place the tube in the water bath (glass beaker with water) on the hot plate. Allow the water to boil gently for 5 to 10 minutes
    D. Remove the centrifuge tube, and centrifuge at 1000 rpm (×264 $g$) for 5 minutes
    E. Decant supernatant, mix sediment with a pipette, place a drop on a slide, add a coverslip, and examine under the microscope (×10)

### Cellophane Tape Method

I. Used for mites and pinworms that are primarily on the skin surface and the hair (e.g., *Cheyletiella* sp., *Oxyuris equi*)
II. Materials
    A. Cellophane tape
    B. Mineral oil
    C. Microscope slides

III. Procedure
    A. Using cellophane tape, lift off dermis from skin surface
    B. Place a drop of mineral oil on a slide and stick tape on top of the slide
    C. Examine slide using ×10 objective

## Baermann Technique

I. This is used for removing lungworm larvae from small amounts of feces
II. Materials
    A. Paper cup
    B. Disposable cellulose tissue (Kimwipe)
    C. Elastic band
    D. Sedimentation jar
    E. Long Pasteur pipette with bulb
    F. Dissecting microscope

III. Procedure
    A. Place the fecal sample in a paper cup
    B. Cover the opening of the cup with a disposable cellulose tissue and secure with an elastic band
    C. Fill a sedimentation jar halfway with warm water
    D. Invert the paper cup with the feces, and punch a small hole in the bottom of the cup
    E. Immerse the tissue end of the cup into the water in the sedimentation jar
    F. Tuck the overhanging tissue into the jar
    G. After 12 to 18 hours, withdraw a sample from the bottom of the sedimentation jar
        1. Gently tilt the paper cup, and insert a long Pasteur pipette down to the bottom of the jar
        2. Refill the pipette three or four times, and place the fluid collected into a small Petri dish
    H. Examine with a dissecting microscope
        1. The larvae should be alive and motile

# EXTERNAL AND INTERNAL PARASITE IDENTIFICATION (Tables 4-1 to 4-5)

**Table 4-1**    Diagnostic characteristics of internal parasites of domestic animals

| Parasite | Location | Prepatent period | Diagnostic stage | Test | Method of infection | Clinical signs | Control |
|---|---|---|---|---|---|---|---|
| | | | | **DOG** | | | |
| Toxocara canis | Small intestines | 3-5 wk | Dark brown, thick-walled egg, with a pitted eggshell; single-celled zygote, 75-90 μm | Fecal flotation or centrifugal flotation | Ingestion of infective egg Paratenic host Transplacentally Transmammary Ingestion of larvae in bitch's feces | Poor growth, emaciation, intestinal blockage, vomiting, diarrhea, death | Remove feces from environment |
| Ancylostoma caninum | Small intestines | 2-3 wk | Clear, smooth, thin-walled hookworm egg; zygote 8- to 16-cell morula; 55-65 × 27-43 μm | Fecal flotation or centrifugal flotation | Skin penetration Ingestion of infective larvae Transmammary Paratenic host Larval "leak" Transplacentally | Anemia, weakness, melena | Remove feces from environment |
| Uncinaria stenocephala | Small intestines | 2 wk | Hookworm egg; 63-93 × 32-55 μm | Fecal flotation or centrifugal flotation | Ingestion of infective larvae Skin penetration (not likely) | Usually no obvious clinical signs In heavy infection in dogs, hypoproteinemia, dehydration, weakness | Remove feces from environment |
| Trichuris vulpis | Large intestines | 3 mo | Smooth, amber, thick-walled, barrel-shaped egg with bipolar plugs; single-celled zygote, 72-90 × 2-40 μm | Fecal flotation or centrifugal flotation | Ingestion of infective larvae | In heavy infection, severe watery diarrhea, hematochezia (frank blood in feces) leading to rapid dehydration and death | Remove from environment |
| Eucoleus bohmi | Nasal sinuses | Unknown | Smooth, yellow-brown, thick-walled egg with a striated shell and asymmetric bipolar plugs; single-celled zygote | Fecal flotation or centrifugal flotation | Ingestion of infective egg | Upper respiratory signs, sneezing and nasal discharge | |
| Filaroides spp. | Lungs | 5-10 wk | L1 with S-shaped tail lacking a dorsal spine; esophagus third of length of body; 265-330 μm long | Fecal flotation or centrifugal flotation Baermann | Paratenic host Ingestion of infective egg | Chronic coughing | |

| | | | | | | | |
|---|---|---|---|---|---|---|---|
| Crenosoma spp. | Lungs | 19-21 days | L1 with a straight, pointed tail; esophagus third of length of body; 265-330 μm | Baermann | Ingestion of infected snails | Coughing | |
| Spirocerca lupi | Esophagus | 5-6 mo | Clear, smooth, thick-walled, paperclip-shaped, larvated egg; 30-37 × 11-15 μm | Flotation or centrifugal flotation | Ingestion of intermediate host (dung beetle); Ingestion of paratenic host | Vomit, dysphagia, weight loss, sudden death; Most infections not diagnosed until necropsy | In endemic areas, dogs should be prevented from eating dung beetles, frogs, mice, and lizards, and they should not be fed raw chicken scraps |
| Dirofilaria immitis | Heart | 6-8 mo | Microfilaria (L1) lacks an esophagus | Modified Knott's millipore filtration; ELISA antigen test | Transmission from infective mosquito bites; Transplacental infection of microfilariae only | Lethargy, exercise intolerance, signs referable to right-sided cardiac enlargement | Use of preventives, reduce exposure to mosquitoes in endemic areas |
| Dipetalonema reconditum | Subcutaneous tissue | 9 wk | Microfilaria | Modified Knott's tissue millipore filtration | Transmission from infective flea bites; Ingestion of fleas | Considered to be nonpathogenic, microfilariae may cause problems in kidney tubules | Control flea population |
| Dioctophyma renale | Kidney | 5 mo | Dark brown, thick-walled, barrel-shaped egg with a pitted shell and an operculum at each pole; single-celled zygote; 71-84 × 46-52 μm | Sedimentation of urine | Ingestion of intermediate host (annelid worm); Ingestion of paratenic host (i.e., fish and green frogs) | May be none. Vague abdominal pain after kidney rupture; Adult worms often found in abdominal cavity at surgery | Surgical removal—nephrectomy if in the kidney |
| Dracunculus insignis | Subcutaneous tissue | 309-410 days | Comma-shaped larva with an esophagus and a straight tail; 500-750 μm long | Direct smear of fluid in blister | Ingestion of crustaceans in infected water | Pea-sized blisters on legs, elbow, and axillary area, break open; Adult worms coiled in subcutaneous tissue | Surgical removal |

*Continued*

**Table 4-1** Diagnostic characteristics of internal parasites of domestic animals—cont'd

| Parasite | Location | Prepatent period | Diagnostic stage | Test | Method of infection | Clinical signs | Control |
|---|---|---|---|---|---|---|---|
| | | | | **CAT** | | | |
| Toxocara cati | Small intestines | 8 wk | Dark brown, thick-walled, pitted egg; single-celled zygote; 65-75 μm | Fecal flotation or centrifugal flotation | Ingestion of infective eggs; Transmammary; Ingestion of paratenic host | Usually none, cat may vomit worm or two | Clean up environment |
| Ancylostoma | Small intestines | 3 wk | Hookworm egg; 55-76 × 34-45 μm | Fecal flotation or centrifugal flotation | Skin penetration; Ingestion of infective larvae; Transmammary infection | Anemia, emaciation, weakness, melena, death | |
| Dirofilaria immitis | Heart | 6-8 mo | Microfilaria (L1) lacks an esophagus | ELISA antigen or ELISA antibody | Transmission from infective mosquito bite | Acute: diarrhea/vomiting, tachycardia, syncope, sudden death. Chronic: coughing, vomiting, weight loss, anorexia, dyspnea, lethargy | Use of preventives, reduce exposure to mosquitoes in endemic areas |
| Aelurostrongylus abstrusus | Bronchioles, alveoli | 4-6 wk | L1 with S-shaped tail and a dorsal spine; 360 μm long; esophagus one fourth the length of body | Baermann | Ingestion of infected snail; Ingestion of paratenic host | Usually asymptomatic, may see chronic coughing | |
| Platynosomum fastosum | Liver | 8-12 wk | Dark amber, oval, operculated egg containing a miracidium; 34-50 × 20-35 μm | Sedimentation of feces | Ingestion of intermediate host (snail) | Severe infections characterized by anorexia, persistent vomiting, diarrhea, jaundice, death | |
| Toxoplasma gondii | Small intestines | 1-3 wk | Clear, smooth, thin-walled spherical oocyst; single-celled zygote; 8-10 μm | Fecal flotation or centrifugal flotation | Ingestion of cysts in meat; Ingestion of sporulated oocysts | Most infections are latent or asymptomatic. Young animal's signs may include fever, anorexia, cough, dyspnea, diarrhea, jaundice, and central nervous system dysfunction | Cats should not be fed raw meat; remove litter daily before sporulation can occur |

**DOG AND CAT**

| Parasite | Location | Prepatent period | Egg/Larval description | Diagnosis | Transmission | Clinical signs | Control |
|---|---|---|---|---|---|---|---|
| *Toxascaris leonina* | Small intestines | 11 wk | Clear, smooth, thick-walled eggshell with wavy internal membrane; single-celled zygote and does not completely fill the eggshell; 75 × 85 μm | Fecal flotation or centrifugal flotation | Ingestion of infective eggs; Ingestion of paratenic host | Heavy worm burdens may cause weakness, dehydration, poor condition | Clean environment |
| *Ancylostoma braziliense* | Small intestines | 3 wk | Hookworm egg; 75-95 × 41-45 μm | Fecal flotation or centrifugal flotation | Ingestion of infective larvae; Skin penetration | Anemia, diarrhea, melena, emaciation, weakness | Clean environment |
| *Capillaria aerophilus* | Trachea, bronchi | 6 wk | Rough, granular, thick-walled, barrel-shaped, straw-colored egg with asymmetric bipolar plugs; single-celled zygote; 58-79 × 29-40 μm | Fecal flotation or centrifugal flotation | Ingestion of infective eggs | Light infection—none; Heavy infection—signs of bronchitis; bronchi and bronchioles may fill with blood and mucus | |
| *Capillaria plica* (dog) *Capillaria felis-cati* (cat) | Urinary bladder | 60 days | Rough, striated, thick-walled, barrel-shaped, amber-colored egg with asymmetric bipolar plugs; single-celled zygote; 60-68 × 24-30 μm | Sedimentation of urine | Ingestion of intermediate host (earthworm) | Usually none, may be signs of chronic cystitis, frequent urination, painful urination, hematuria | |
| *Strongyloides stercoralis* | Small intestines | 8-14 days | L1 with a rhabditiform esophagus and a straight pointed tail; L3 with a filariform esophagus and a bipartite tail | Baermann; Fecal culture | Skin penetration; Ingestion of infective larvae; Transmammary | Heavy infection—mucoid diarrhea in young animals; Emaciation and reduced growth rate | |
| *Physaloptera* spp. | Stomach | 56-83 days | Smooth, clear, thick-walled, larvated egg; 45-53 × 29-42 μm | Fecal flotation or centrifugal flotation | Ingestion of intermediate host (beetles) | Cause gastritis and duodenitis, often resulting in vomiting, anorexia, and dark feces | |
| *Dipylidium caninum* | Small intestines | 3 wk | Proglottid with bilateral genital pores; eggs containing 6-hooked hexacanth embryos in packets; 35-60 μm | ID proglottids; Fecal flotation or centrifugal flotation | Ingestion of a cysticercoid in intermediate host, (i.e., flea, lice) | Usually none, may see segments in feces; May see "scooting" | Control of intermediate hosts |

*Continued*

**Table 4-1** Diagnostic characteristics of internal parasites of domestic animals—cont'd

| Parasite | Location | Prepatent period | Diagnostic stage | Test | Method of infection | Clinical signs | Control |
|---|---|---|---|---|---|---|---|
| *Taenia* spp. | Small intestines | 2 mo | Dark brown, thick, radially striated eggshell; 6-hooked hexacanth embryo; 32-37 µm; rectangular proglottids with unilateral genital pore | ID proglottid | Ingestion of cysticercus in intermediate host (i.e., rabbit, rodent) | Usually none, may see segments in feces | Restrict pets from eating wildlife |
| *Echinococcus* spp. | Small intestines | 47 days | Similar to *Taenia* eggs | Fecal flotation or centrifugal flotation | Ingestion of hydatid or alveolar hydatid cysts in intermediate host (i.e., moose, sheep, goats, cattle, horse, deer [*E. granulosus*] or rodents [*E. multilocularis*] | Usually none | Restrict pets from eating raw meat, viscera, and wildlife |
| *Mesocestoides* spp. | Small intestines | 16-20 days | Smooth, thin egg capsule containing 6-hooked hexacanth embryo, 20-25 µm; globular proglottid with parauterine body | Fecal flotation or centrifugal flotation ID proglottid | Complete life cycle is unknown, arthropods/mammals/reptiles/birds are suspected intermediate hosts | Usually none | Control environment |
| *Spirometra mansonoides* | Small intestines | 10-30 days | Unembryonated, thin-walled, smooth, amber-colored egg; operculated; 70×45 µm | Fecal flotation or centrifugal flotation | Ingestion of intermediate host (crustaceans, water snake) | Vague/none | Control environment |
| *Paragonimus kellicotti* | Lung | 1 mo | Smooth, golden brown, urn-shaped, operculated egg; 75-118×42-67 µm | Sedimentation of urine | Ingestion of metacercariae in crayfish | Often none, may be intermittent chronic coughing | Control environment |
| *Nanophyetus salmincola* | Small intestines | 1 wk | Rough, brown, operculated egg; 52-82 × 32-56 µm | Sedimentation of feces | Ingestion of metacercariae in various tissues in fish | None; clinical signs due to salmon poisoning complex caused by rickettsial organism | Control environment |
| *Isospora* spp. | Small intestines | 4-12 days | Clear, spherical to ellipsoid thin-walled oocyst; size varies with species | Fecal flotation or centrifugal flotation | Ingestion of sporulated oocyst | Persistent diarrhea, may lead to dehydration and death | Clean environment to prevent accumulation and sporulation of oocysts |

| Organism | Location | Prepatent period | Egg/oocyst description | Diagnosis | Transmission | Clinical signs | Prevention/Control |
|---|---|---|---|---|---|---|---|
| *Sarcocystis* spp. | Small intestines | 7-33 days | Thin-walled oocyst with 2 sporocysts containing 4 sporozoites each or sporocyst; size varies with species | | Ingestion of cysts in muscle tissue—various intermediate hosts | None | Restrict pets from eating raw meat, offal |
| **HORSE** | | | | | | | |
| *Parascaris equorum* | Small intestines | 10 wk | Rough, brown, thick-walled, spherical egg; single-celled zygote; 90-100 µm | Fecal flotation or centrifugal flotation | Ingestion of infective egg | Adult horses—none Foals—may retard growth, may cause colic (e.g., intussusception, or volvulus of gut) | |
| *Eimeria leukarti* | Small intestines | 15-33 days | Dark brown, piriform, thick-walled oocyst; 70-90 × 49-69 µm | Fecal flotation or centrifugal flotation | Ingestion of sporulated oocysts | Not pathogenic, no clinical signs | |
| Cyathostomes (small strongyles) | Large intestines | 2-3 mo | Smooth, thin-walled, clear strongyle egg; zygote 8- to 16-cell morula; size varies with species | Fecal flotation | Ingestion of infective larvae | Poor growth, decreased performance, profuse diarrhea In acute conditions, large number of worms seen grossly in feces | |
| *Strongylus* spp. (large strongyles) *Strongylus vulgaris S. ledentatus S. equinus* | Large intestines | 6-12 mo | Strongyle egg | Fecal flotation or centrifugal flotation | Ingestion of infective larvae Larvae not too pathogenic, adults may cause anemia, loss of condition | Colic, fever, diarrhea, weight loss, death | Strategic deworming |
| *Oxyuris equi* | Large intestines | 5 mo | Clear, smooth, thin-walled egg with 1 side flattened; operculated; 90 × 42 µm | Cellophane tape preparation | Ingestion of infective eggs | Pruritus ani, fraying of hairs on tail head May see female worms passed in feces, white egg masses on perianal skin | Removal of egg masses on perianal skin with soap and water; clean stalls and woodwork |

*Continued*

**Table 4-1**  Diagnostic characteristics of internal parasites of domestic animals—cont'd

| Parasite | Location | Prepatent period | Diagnostic stage | Test | Method of infection | Clinical signs | Control |
|---|---|---|---|---|---|---|---|
| *Anoplocephala* spp. | Small and large intestines | 1-2 mo | Clear, thick-walled, square eggs with a pear-shaped (piriform) apparatus containing a hexacanth embryo | Fecal flotation or centrifugal flotation | Ingestion of cysticercoid in pasture mite | Most asymptom-atic, but *A. perfo-liata* causes colic and death due to intestinal accident | |
| *Strongyloides westeri* | Small intestines | 8-14 days | Smooth, thin-walled, larvated egg; 40-50 × 32-40 μm | Fecal flotation or centrifugal flotation | Transmammary Skin penetration Ingestion of infective larvae | No obvious signs in adult horses Diarrhea in foals | |
| *Gasterophilus* spp. | Stomach | | 2.5-cm, robust grub with rows of spines and straight spiracular slits (breathing tubes) | Identification of third stage larva | Ingestion of larvae | Bots in tongue and gums may cause ulcers on surface of tongue and tooth problems Bots in stomach occasionally cause perforation of stomach wall with fatal peritonitis | Remove bot eggs from horse's legs and shoulder area |
| **CATTLE, SHEEP, GOAT** | | | | | | | |
| Trichostron-gyles: *Haemonchus, Ostertagia, Cooperia, Trichostron-gylus* | Abomasum, small intestines | 15-28 days | Strongyle egg | Fecal flotation or centrifugal flotation | Ingestion of infective larvae while grazing | Clinical signs depend on age, host resis-tance, and number of worms Acute signs; seen mainly in younger animals, diarrhea, anorexia, and loss of condition Chronic signs are more subtle—may see poor weight gain and general poorly doing animal | Try to prevent pasture con-tamination by strategic worming of animals |
| *Dictyocaulus* spp. | Lungs | 3-4 wk | L1 with dark granular intestines; esophagus one third the length of larva; straight pointed tail; 550-580 μm long | Baermann | Ingestion of infective larvae | Coughing, dyspnea | |

| | | | | | |
|---|---|---|---|---|---|
| *Strongyloides* spp. | Small intestines | 3-4 wk | Thin-walled egg with parallel sides; 40-60 × 20-25 µm | Ingestion of infective larvae | Rarely a clinical problem |
| *Oesophagostomum* spp. | Large intestines | 45 days | Strongyle egg | Ingestion of infective larvae | Usually not a clinical problem in cattle and goats in moderate numbers<br>In sheep, large numbers can cause diarrhea and weight loss |
| *Skrjabinema* spp. | Large intestines | 25 days | Clear, smooth, thin-walled egg with one side flattened, single-celled zygote | Ingestion of infective egg | Typical of pinworms Eggs deposited on perianal skin—possibly pruritus ani<br>Seen in goats, rarely in sheep |
| *Eimeria* spp. | Small and large intestines | 10-30 days | Smooth or rough, thin-walled, clear to yellowish brown oocysts; single-celled zygote; size varies with species | Ingestion of infective egg | Light infections, usually no clinical signs<br>Heavy infections, diarrhea, sometimes bloody, and tenesmus<br>Note: clinical signs are possible before oocysts pass in the feces; repeat fecal examination will eventually reveal oocysts |
| *Moniezia* spp. | Small intestines | 6 wk | Thick-walled, clear, triangular to square egg with a piriform apparatus containing a hexacanth embryo | Ingestion of cysticercoid in a free-living pasture mite | Not considered very pathogenic. Heavy burdens may affect weight gain |
| *Thysanosoma actinoides* | Bile ducts | | Thin-walled egg with hexacanth embryos in packets; 21-45 µm | | |

*Continued*

**Table 4-1** Diagnostic characteristics of internal parasites of domestic animals—cont'd

| Parasite | Location | Prepatent period | Diagnostic stage | Test | Method of infection | Clinical signs | Control |
|---|---|---|---|---|---|---|---|
| *Fasciola* spp. | Liver | 10-12 wk | Dark amber, oval, operculated egg; 130-150 × 63-90 µm | Sedimentation of feces | Ingestion of metacercariae | Devastating disease in sheep, is dependent on the number of metacercariae eaten over a short period of time Produces a distended, painful abdomen, anemia, and sudden death Chronic disease may show signs of anemia, unthrifti-ness, submandibular edema, and reduced milk secretion | |
| *Bunostomum* spp. | Small intestines | 2-3 wk | Strongyle egg | Fecal flotation or centrifugal flotation | Ingestion of infective larvae Skin penetration | Ruminant hookworms Occasionally low worm burdens Heavy infections can cause anemia | Strategic deworming |
| *Chabertia ovina* | Large intestines | 47-63 days | Strongyle egg | Fecal flotation or centrifugal flotation | Ingestion of infective larvae | Larvae and adults can cause small hemorrhages with edema in the colon: the feces may be coated with mucus when passed | Deworming |
| *Trichuris* spp. | Large intestines | 2-3 mo | Dark, brownish, thick walled, symmetric bipolar plugs; smooth egg with single-celled varies with species zygote; 50-60 × 21-25 µm | Fecal flotation or centrifugal flotation | Ingestion of infective larvae Skin penetration | Clinical signs are unlikely, heavy worm burdens seldom seen In occasional heavy infections may see dark feces, anemia, and anorexia *Trichuris* is not transmissible between ruminants and dogs | Deworming |

| Organism | Site | Prepatent period | Egg/Oocyst description | Diagnosis | Transmission | Clinical signs | Treatment |
|---|---|---|---|---|---|---|---|
| *Capillaria* spp. | Small intestines | | Brownish, thick-walled striated egg with asymmetric bipolar plugs; single-celled zygote; 45-52 × 21-30 µm | Fecal flotation or centrifugal flotation | Ingestion of infective eggs | None | No treatment |
| **CATTLE** | | | | | | | |
| *Cryptosporidium muris* | Abomasum | 4-10 days | Clear, smooth, thin-walled oocyst containing 4 sporozoites; 5 × 7 µm | Fecal flotation or centrifugal flotation | Transmission by the fecal-oral route Oocysts shed in the feces are immediately infective | Usually seen in calves 1-3 wk old Diarrhea, tenesmus, weight loss, anorexia are usually seen | Disease is usually self-limiting Supportive therapy is recommended (i.e., fluids) |
| **SHEEP** | | | | | | | |
| *Protostrongylus rufescens* | Lungs | 30-37 days | L1 with a straight, pointed tail 48-56 µm long without a dorsal spine; 340-400 ×19-20 µm | Baermann | Ingestion of intermediate host (slug or snail) | Chronic eosinophilic granulomatous pneumonia | |
| *Mullerius* spp. | Lungs | 6 wk | L1 are 300-320 × 14-15 µm with S-shaped tail bearing a dorsal spine | Baermann | Ingestion of infective larvae in slugs on pasture | More common in goats Coughing | |
| **PIG** | | | | | | | |
| *Eimeria* spp. | Small intestines | 4-10 days | Smooth or rough, thin-walled oocyst; single-celled zygote; size varies with species | Fecal flotation or centrifugal flotation | Ingestion of sporulated oocysts | Essentially nonpathogenic May see diarrhea Adult pigs usually do not show clinical signs but contaminate the environment Nursing piglets: diarrhea, dehydration, emaciation | |
| *Isospora* spp. | Small intestines | 5 days | Smooth, clear, thin-walled oocyst; single-celled zygote; 17-25 × 16-21 µm | Fecal flotation or centrifugal flotation | Ingestion of sporulated oocysts | | |

*Continued*

**Table 4-1**    Diagnostic characteristics of internal parasites of domestic animals—cont'd

| Parasite | Location | Prepatent period | Diagnostic stage | Test | Method of infection | Clinical signs | Control |
|---|---|---|---|---|---|---|---|
| *Balantidium coli* | Large intestines | | Thin-walled, greenish cyst with hyaline cytoplasm; 40-60 µm; 30-150 × 25-120 µm trophozoite with rows of cilia | Fecal flotation or centrifugal flotation  Direct smear | Ingestion of cysts | Found commonly in the feces of swine, not considered pathogenic | Not usually treated |
| *Ascaris suum* | Small intestines | 7-9 wk | Brownish yellow, thick-walled, mammilated egg; single-celled zygote; 50-80 × 40-60 µm | Fecal flotation or centrifugal flotation | Ingestion of infective egg | Nursing pigs may show dyspnea  Growing pigs—reduced weight gains  Adult pigs—usually none | |
| *Strongyloides ransomi* | Small intestines | 3-7 days | Smooth, thin-walled, larvated egg with parallel sides; 45-55 × 26-35 µm | Fecal flotation or centrifugal flotation | Larvae can be transmitted via colostrums  Ingestion of larvae | Heavy infections in piglets produce severe diarrhea when 10-14 days of age, with high mortality | |
| *Oesophagostomum* spp. | Large intestines | 32-42 days | Strongyle egg | Fecal flotation or centrifugal flotation | Ingestion of infective larvae | Reduced weight of gain in grower pigs | |
| *Hyostrongylus rubidus* | Stomach | 15-21 days | Strongyle egg | Fecal flotation or centrifugal flotation | | | |
| *Metastrongylus* spp. | Lungs | 24 days | Rough, clear, thick-walled, larvated egg with a corrugated surface; 45-57 × 38-41 µm | Fecal flotation or centrifugal flotation | Ingestion of infective larvae | Diarrhea, anorexia, decreased weight gain | |
| *Trichuris suis* | Large intestines | 2-3 mo | Brownish yellow, smooth, thick-walled egg with symmetric bipolar plugs; single-celled zygote 50-56 × 21-25 µm | Fecal flotation or centrifugal flotation | Ingestion of the intermediate host (earthworm) | Coughing and predisposition to bacterial and viral respiratory infections | |
| *Trichinella spiralis* | Small intestines | 2-6 days | L3 encysted in striated muscles; esophagus composed of stichocytes (single cells stacked on top of one another); cysts are 400-600 × 250 µm | Squash preparation of muscle | Ingestion of larvae in muscle, (i.e., carnivorism) | Usually no clinical signs. Economic loss at slaughter | |

## DOG, CAT, CATTLE, HORSE, SHEEP, GOAT, PIG

| Parasite | Location | Prepatent period | Morphology | ID adult | Method of infection | Clinical signs | Zoonotic |
|---|---|---|---|---|---|---|---|
| *Thelazia californiensis* | Eye | 3-6 wk | Adult worm in conjunctival sac and tear duct | | Flies (*Musca* spp., *Fannia* spp.) deposit infective larvae on the eye while feeding on ocular secretions | Excessive tearing, conjunctivitis, corneal opacity and ulceration | Not commonly seen |
| *Giardia duodenalis* | Small intestines | 7-10 days | Smooth, clear, thin-walled cyst with 2-4 nuclei; 4-10×8-16 μm Piriform, bilaterally symmetric greenish trophozoite with 2 nuclei and 4 pair of flagella; 9-20×5-15 μm | Fecal flotation or centrifugal flotation; Fecal ELISA antigen; Direct smear | Ingestion of cyst stage | Predominantly diarrhea | |
| Trichomonads | Digestive tract | | Spindle-shaped to piriform trophozoite with 3-5 anterior flagella, an undulating membrane, and 1 posterior flagellum | Direct smear | Ingestion of trophozoite | Diarrhea | |
| *Cryptosporidium* spp. | Small and large intestines | 4-10 days | Clear, thin-walled, spherical oocyst containing 4 sporozoites; 5×5 μm | Fecal flotation or centrifugal flotation | Ingestion of oocysts | Diarrhea, dehydration, anorexia | |

**Table 4-2** Diagnostic characteristics of blood parasites of domestic animals

| Parasite | Definitive host | Location | Prepatent period | Diagnostic stage | Diagnostic test |
|---|---|---|---|---|---|
| *Babesia* spp. | Humans, dogs, cattle, horses | Blood (erythrocytes) | 10-21 days | Paired piriform (tear-shaped) merozoites in erythrocytes | Romanowsky-stained blood film, indirect fluorescent antibody test |
| *Trypanosoma* spp. | Humans, dogs, cats, cattle, sheep, horses | Blood and lymph, heart, striated muscle, reticuloendothelial muscle | Acute and chronic disease | Trypanosome form, spindle-shaped flagellate with undulating membrane, central nucleus and kinetoplast, found in blood Amastigote form, intracellular spherical bodies with single nucleus and rod-shaped kinetoplast, found in myocardium, striated muscle cells, and macrophages | Blood smears; xenodiagnosis (clean vector allowed to feed on suspect patient and organism isolated from the vector), biopsy, animal inoculation, serology |
| *Leishmania donovani* | Humans, dogs | Intracellular in cytoplasm of macrophages of reticuloendothelial system | Several mo up to 1 yr | Amastigote form, oval, single nucleus, with a rod-shaped kinetoplast, in clusters within the cytoplasm of macrophages | Impression smears and biopsy of skin, lymph nodes, and bone marrow |

From Johnson EM: Diagnostic parasitology. In Pratt PW: *Principles and practice of veterinary technology*, St Louis, 1998, Mosby.

**Table 4-3** Zoonotic internal parasites

| Parasite | Host | Reservoir | Infective stage | Condition |
|---|---|---|---|---|
| Toxocara spp. | Dogs, cats | Dogs, cats | Egg with L2 | Visceral larva migrans |
| Ancylostoma spp. | Dogs, cats | Dogs, cats | L3 | Cutaneous larva migrans |
| Uncinaria stenocephala | Dogs, cats | Dogs, cats | L3 | Cutaneous larva migrans |
| Toxoplasma gondii | Cats | Cats, raw meat | Sporulated oocyst, bradyzoite, tachyzoite | Toxoplasmosis |
| Strongyloides stercoralis | Dogs, cats, humans | Humans, dogs, cats | L3 | Strongyloidiasis |
| Dipylidium caninum | Dogs, cats, humans | Flea | Cysticercoid | Cestodiasis |
| Taenia saginata | Humans | Bovine muscle | Cysticercus | Cestodiasis |
| Taenia solium | Humans | Porcine muscle | Cysticercus | Cestodiasis |
| | Humans | Humans | Egg | Cysticercosis |
| Echinococcus granulosus | Dogs | Dogs | Egg | Hydatidosis |
| Echinococcus multilocularis | Dogs, cats | Dogs, cats | Egg | Hydatidosis |
| Spirometra mansonoides | Dogs, cats | Unknown | Procercoid in arthropod | Sparganosis |
| Sarcocystis spp. | Humans | Cattle, pigs | Sarcocyst in muscle | Sarcocystiasis |
| | Dogs, cats | Dogs, cats | Oocyst | Sarcosporidiosis |
| Cryptosporidium parvum | Mammals | Mammals | Oocyst | Cryptosporidiosis |
| Balantidium coli | Humans, pigs | Humans, pigs | Cyst, trophozoite | Balantidiasis |
| Ascaris suum | Pigs | Pigs | Egg with L2 | Visceral larva migrans |
| Trichinella spiralis | Mammals | Porcine and bear | Encysted L3 muscle | Trichinellosis |
| Thelazia spp. | Mammals | Fly | L3 | Verminous conjunctivitis |
| Giardia duodenalis | Mammals | Mammals | Cyst | Giardiasis |
| Babesia microti | Rodents, humans | Hard tick | Sporozoite | Babesiosis |
| Trypanosoma | Mammals | Reduviids | Trypanosomal form in kissing bug | Chagas' disease |
| Leishmania donovani | Mammals | Phlebotomine fly | Leptomonad form in sand fly | Leishmaniasis |

From Johnson EM: Diagnostic parasitology. In Pratt PW: *Principles and practice of veterinary technology*, St Louis, 1998, Mosby.

**Table 4-4** Common parasites in laboratory animals

| Parasite/hosts | Transmission | Clinical signs | Diagnosis |
|---|---|---|---|
| **Pinworms** | | | |
| *Syphacia obvelata*, mice, hamsters | Ingestion of infective egg Retroinfection | Usually none Heavy infections: impaction, intussusception, rectal prolapse | Eggs are thin walled Flattened along one side measuring 100-142 × 30-40 μm |
| *Syphacia muris*, rats | Eggs hatch in perianal region, and larvae migrate back into the colon | Poor growth rate | Eggs larvate within 6-24 hr. *S. muris*: eggs measure 72-82 × 25-36 μm |
| *Aspiculuris tetraptera*, mouse | Ingestion of infective egg | Often none | Eggs on fecal float are elliptical, thin shelled 89-93 × 36-42 μm |
| *Passalurus ambiguous*, rabbit | Ingestion of infective egg | Usually none Large numbers in young animals may cause gastric disturbance | Eggs are slightly flattened, 95-103 × 43 μm |
| **Tapeworms (dwarf)** | | | |
| *Hymenolepis nana*, mouse, rat, hamster | Ingestion of egg | Heavy infection in mice can cause weight loss, poor growth, intestinal occulsion and impaction | Eggs are oval with a hexacanth larvae 40-45 × 34-37 μm |
| *Hymenolepis diminuta*, mouse/rat/hamster | Ingestion of cysticercoid in paratenic host Autoinfection | Heavy infection in hamsters can cause intestinal occlusion and impaction | |
| *Cysticercus pisiformis*, rabbit | Ingestion of cysticercoid | Usually none | Eggs semispherical 60-66 μm with dark outer capsule, hexacanth larvae |
| | Larval stage of *Taenia pisiformis* | Cysts in peritoneal cavity Heavy infection: abdominal distention | Cysticercus with opaque body at one end with an inverted scolex |
| *Multiceps serialis*, rabbit | Larval stage of *Taenia multiceps* | Swelling, puffy skin | Cyst in subcutaneous tissue (may be palpable) |
| **Coccidia** | | | |
| *Eimeria* spp., *E. separata*, rat | Ingestion of sporulated oocysts | Nonpathogenic | Smooth-walled ellipsoidal oocysts 10-19 × 10-17 μm |
| *Eimeria* spp., mouse | Ingestion of sporulated oocysts | Nonpathogenic—moderate infections causing diarrhea | Typical oocyst |
| *Eimeria caviae*, guinea pig | Ingestion of sporulated oocysts | Usually none Heavy infections: diarrhea, anorexia, lethargy, death | Smooth, oval, light brown oocyst measuring 13-26 × 12-23 μm |
| *Eimeria* spp., rabbits | Ingestion of sporulated oocysts | Mild to severe Heavy infection: anorexia, severe diarrhea, distended abdomen, death | Characteristic oocysts |
| *Cryptosporidium* sp. *Klossiella muris*, mouse *K. cobayae* *K. caviae*, guinea pig | Ingestion of oocyst Ingestion of sporocyst | Diarrhea None—mild nephritis | Smooth walled oocyst 7 × 5 μm Sporocyst passed in the urine |

Continued

**Table 4-4** Common parasites in laboratory animals—cont'd

| Parasite/hosts | Transmission | Clinical signs | Diagnosis |
|---|---|---|---|
| **Fleas** | | | |
| *Leptopsylla segnis*, mouse | | None | Very small flea<br>1-3 mm in length |
| *Spilopsyllus cuniculi*, rabbit | | Intermediate host for *H. diminuta* and *H. nana*<br>Adults feed in clumps inside pinna<br>Vector of myxoma virus | 1.2-1.5 mm in length<br>Head long and slender |
| **Lice** | | | |
| *Polyplax spinulosa*, rat<br>*Polyplax serrata*, mice | Direct contact | Large numbers cause irritation and anemia<br>Vector for *Haemobartonella muris* (rat)<br>Vector for *Eperythrozoon coccoides* (mice) | Three pairs of legs end in clasping claws<br>Eggs laid on host cemented firmly to the base of the hair |
| *Gliricola porcelli*, guinea pig | | General body surface | Broad head, elongated body<br>Eggs have distinctive operculum |
| *Gryopus ovalis*, guinea pig | | Preference for head and face | Broad head<br>Eggs with operculum |
| **Mites** | | | |
| **Fur dwelling** | | | |
| *Myobia musculi* | Direct contact | Mange, head and face | First pair of legs modified for gripping hair<br>One claw on second pair of legs |
| *Radffordia*<br>*Mycoptes musculinus*, rat/mouse | | Mange, shoulders and back<br>Mange, shoulders and back | Two claws on the second pair of legs |
| *Cheyletiella parasitivorax* | Direct contact | Occasional mange, shoulders and back<br>None | Medium-sized mite, very active, yellowish white body<br>Short palpi with claw curving inward |
| *Listorphorus gibbus*, rabbit | | | *Listorphorus* spp., smaller mite, body laterally compressed, broad head |
| *Chirodiscoides caviae*, guinea pig | Direct contact | None | Small mite, twice as long as broad |
| **Surface dwelling** | | | |
| *Psoroptes cuniculi*, rabbit | Direct contact | Ear cankers | Macroscopic, moving rapidly inside ear pinnae |
| *Sarcoptes* spp.<br>*Notoedres* spp., mice/rats/rabbit | Transfer of larvae and nymphs | Located in epidermal tunnels<br>Causes generalized mange and alopecia | Round, fat mites<br>Short, stubby legs<br>Nonjointed pedicles |
| **Follicle dwelling** | | | |
| *Demodex* spp., hamster/gerbil/rat | Mite found in hair follicles | Dry, scaly skin with scabby lesions | Cigar-shaped mite with stumpy limbs placed evenly along the body |

**Table 4-5** Ectoparasites: general

| Parasite/host | Transmission and life cycle | Clinical signs and location | Diagnosis |
|---|---|---|---|
| *Melophagus ovinus* (sheep ked) | Obligatory parasite; spends entire life on host | Rubbing and scratching causes damage to wool and skin | Macroscopic Large numbers can cause anemia |
| *Hypoderma* spp. (cattle grub) | Fly → egg → larva (migrate through host) → pupate on ground | Irritation to cattle, reduced weight gain, milk production, economic loss at slaughter | Macroscopic |
| *Oestrus ovis* nasal bot (sheep, goat) | Fly (L1-L3 in host) → pupate on ground | Nasal discharge, sneezing, rubbing nose | Macroscopic |
| *Cuterebra* spp. (lagomorph, dog, cat) | Fly → egg on ground, L1 on host migrate to L3 → pupate on ground | Fibrotic cyst in subcutaneous tissue Secondary infection with abcessation | Macroscopic |
| **LICE** | | | |
| *Anoplura* (sucking) | | Lice on skin usually in areas that can be protected from being rubbed off | Adult, dorsoventrally flattened, head narrower than thorax; nymph, small adult; egg (nit) elongate, operculate, glued to hairs |
| *Haematopinus* spp. | Cattle, pig, horse | Pruritic | |
| *Linognathus* spp. | Dog, cattle, sheep | | |
| *Solenopotes* spp. | Cattle | | |
| *Pediculus* spp. | Humans | | |
| *Mallophaga* (biting) | | Lice on skin and hair; cause rubbing and scratching | Adult, dorsoventrally flattened, head wider than thorax; nymph, small adult; egg elongated, operculated, whitish |
| *Damalinia* spp. | Horse, cattle, sheep | | |
| *Felicola subrostratus* | Cat | | |
| *Trichodectes canis* | Dog | | |
| **FLEAS** | | | |
| *Ctenocephalides* spp. | Dog, cat | Adult on skin of host; larvae and pupae in the bedding/living area of host; can cause flea allergy dermatitis | Adults seen grossly Flea "dirt" (feces) on host |
| **TICKS** | | | |
| Hard | | | |
| *Dermacentor* spp. | Dog, cat three-host tick | Vectors for Rocky Mountain spotted fever, tularemia, Q fever | Scutum ornate; basis capitulum parallel sided, palps short with festoons |
| *Ixodes scapularis* | Animals, humans three-host tick | Vector for Lyme disease (*Borrelia burgdorferi*) | Scutum ornate; basis capitulum parallel sided, palps long, without festoons |
| *Rhipicephalus sanguineus* | Primarily dog three-host tick | Vector for *Babesia canis* and *Ehrlichia canis* | Scutum ornate; basis capitulum angular, palps short, with festoons |

*Continued*

**Table 4-5** Ectoparasites: general—cont'd

| Parasite/host | Transmission and life cycle | Clinical signs and location | Diagnosis |
|---|---|---|---|
| Soft<br>*Argasid* | Birds | Not routinely seen | Soft ticks have a leathery dorsal surface that lacks a hard plate (scutum) |
| **MITES** | | | |
| *Sarcoptes* spp., pig, dog, cat, horse, cattle, humans | Egg → larvae → nymph → adult all takes place on the host<br>Transmission by direct contact | Scratching, chewing, self-excoriation causing crust and scab formation<br>Secondary infections can occur | Round mite with short stubby legs; posterior two pairs not extending beyond margins of the body; long unsegmented pedicles; dorsal spines |
| *Demodex* spp., dog, cat, cattle, goat, humans | Adults in hair follicles lay eggs, larvae and nymphs at mouth of follicles<br>Transmission by direct contact | More common in dogs<br>Lesions consist of varying degrees of scaling, alopecia, erythema, hyperpigmentation | Adult, anterior half of mite; eggs elongate; stubbly legs on adults may be seen on fecal float |
| *Cheyletiella* spp., dog, cat, rabbit (also called "walking dandruff") | All stages on host, mites feed on epidermal debris<br>Transmission by direct contact | Dorsal seborrhea, generally nonpruritic | Adult, oval, long legs that extend beyond the margins of the body; terminal appendage on each leg is a fine comblike structure |
| *Chorioptes* spp., cattle, sheep, goat, horse | Mites live on surface of the skin<br>Transmission by direct contact | Tail mange: cattle<br>Scrotal mange: sheep<br>Leg mange: horse | Adult, oval, long legs that extend beyond the margins of the body; pedicles are short and unsegmented with large suckers |
| *Psoroptes* spp., cattle, sheep, goat, horse | Transmission by direct contact or with infested material | Pruritus, alopecia<br>Skin becomes thick and wrinkled<br>Animals may become emaciated and die<br>Not commonly seen | Adults, oval, long legs that extend beyond the margins of the body; pedicles are long and segmented |
| *Otodectes cynotis*, dogs, cats | Transmission by direct contact with infected host | Shaking head, scratching ears<br>Severe infestations: head tilt, otitis media circling, convulsions | Adults, white motile with otoscope<br>Adults, large, short unjointed pedicles with suckers on some legs |

## ACKNOWLEDGMENT ■■■■■■■■■■

The editors and author recognize and appreciate the original work of Mary Lake, on which this chapter is based.

# Glossary

**acariasis** Infestation by mites

**alopecia** Deficiency of hair or loss of coat

**anthelmintic** "Against worms"; therefore a drug used to remove worms

**arthropod** Invertebrate animals having segmented external coverings and jointed legs (e.g., ticks and mites)

**Baermann technique** Generally used for removing lungworm larvae from small amounts of feces

**cestode** Commonly called tapeworms; flat, segmented worms

**efficacy** Effectiveness of a drug

**ELISA** Enzyme-linked immunosorbent assay

**erythema** Redness of the skin

**final host** Normal host or definitive host; type of animal in which the adult worm is found

**flagellum** A long, whiplike, mobile appendage arising from the surface of a cell used for locomotion

**hexacanth** Infective stage of development in a cestode egg after fertilization takes place

**infective** Developed to a stage capable of causing infection

**intermediate host** Any organism in which a parasite lives during its larval or nonreproductive stage

**intussusception** A prolapse of one or more parts of the small intestine or colon into the lumen of the intestine immediately adjacent to it. This condition usually causes an intestinal obstruction

**kinetoplast** An accessory body found in many protozoa; it contains DNA and replicates independently

**mange** Infestation by mites

**melena** Dark, tarry stool

**meniscus** Curved upper surface of a liquid on the top of a container

**metacercaria** The encysted resting or maturing stage of a trematode parasite in the tissues of a second intermediate host or on vegetation

**morula, morulated** Solid mass of cells clustered together

**myiasis** Invasion of living tissue by fly maggots

**nematode** Free-living or parasitic unsegmented worms, usually cylindrical and elongated in shape and tapering at the extremities

**noninfective** Not yet developed to a stage capable of causing infection

**oocysts** A stage of the life cycle of coccidial parasites. It contains a zygote and under specific conditions sporulates to become a mature infective oocyst. It can remain infective for long periods in dry conditions

**operculum** A lid or covering; the plug of a trophoblast that helps close the gap in the endometrium made by the implanting blastocyst

**OVC** Ontario Veterinary College

**paratenic host** One in which the parasite does not develop to adult, remains alive for long periods, and does not rely on host exclusively to complete its life cycle

**PCV** Packed cell volume

**pediculosis** Infestation by lice

**piriform** Pear-shaped

**prepatent infection** Occurs when worms have not yet developed to mature adults; therefore no eggs are being shed and a diagnosis is not possible by fecal examination or other laboratory testing

**prepatent period (ppp)** Period of time between infection of the host and when eggs or larvae can be recovered by laboratory methods

**protozoa** Unicellular organisms

**rpm** Revolutions per minute

**sporocyst** A cyst that contains oocysts of coccidia in which sporozoites develop

**sporozoite** A spore formed after fertilization

**trophozoite** The active, motile, feeding stage of flagellate protozoa (e.g., *Giardia* spp.)

**trematode** Group of parasites that are hermaphroditic, have two suckers (oral and ventral), and require an intermediate host; commonly called flukes

**volvulus** Torsion of a loop of intestine causing an obstruction

**zoonosis** Disease of animals that can be transmitted to humans

**zygote** The cell resulting from a union of a female and male gamete. A fertilized ovum

# Review Questions

1 ELISA tests can detect
   a. *Dirofilaria immitis*
   b. *Dirofilaria* antigen
   c. Microfilaria
   d. Only occult heartworm

2 *Eimeria steidae* is associated with
   a. Hepatic coccidiosis in rabbits
   b. Cecal coccidiosis in chickens
   c. Renal coccidiosis in geese
   d. Intestinal coccidiosis in dogs

3 Biting lice have which characteristic?
   a. Head wider than thorax
   b. Feed on blood
   c. Narrower head than thorax
   d. Barely move

4 Cutaneous larva migrans is caused by
   a. *Toxocara cati*
   b. *Trichuris vulpis*
   c. *Ancylostoma caninum*
   d. *Aelurostrongylus* sp.

5 Visceral larva migrans is caused by ingestion of
   a. *Echinococcus* sp.
   b. *Toxocara* sp.
   c. *Uncinaria* sp.
   d. *Dioctophyma renale*

6 The intermediate host for the bovine tapeworm, *Moniezia* sp., is a
   a. Bird
   b. Pasture mite
   c. Snail
   d. Mudworm

**7** *Eimeria* spp. when sporulated contain
   a. Four sporocysts with two sporozoites
   b. Two sporocysts with four sporozoites
   c. One sporocyst with three sporozoites
   d. None of the above
**8** The term *pediculosis* means
   a. Infestation by mites
   b. Invasion of living tissue by fly maggots
   c. Intense itching and hair loss
   d. Infestation by lice

**9** Which of the following is not true about ticks?
   a. Often carry disease-causing organisms
   b. Are generally picked up from wooded areas
   c. Feed on blood
   d. Adult ticks have six legs
**10** The prepatent period for *Dirofilaria immitis* is
   a. 6.5 weeks
   b. 3 months
   c. 8 months
   d. 6.5 months

## APPENDIX

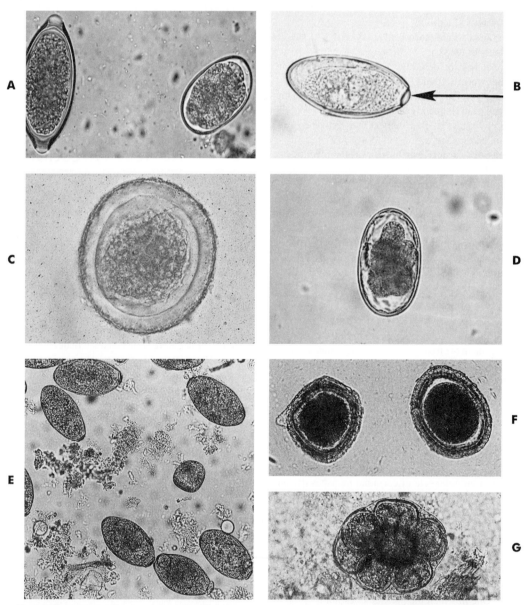

**Figure A-1**   A, *Trichuris vulpis* and *Ancylostoma caninum*. B, *Oxyuris equi*. C, *Parascaris equorum*. D, Strongyle type of ovum. E, *Fasciola hepatica/Moniezia* sp. F, *Toxocara canis*. G, *Dipylidium caninum*.

## BIBLIOGRAPHY

Arkness JE, Wagner JE: *The biology and medicine of rabbits and rodents*, ed 4, Philadelphia, 1995, Lippincott Williams & Wilkins.

Barta JR: *Principles of disease*, lecture notes from Veterinary Parasitology, Ontario Veterinary College, 2001, Guelph, Ontario, Canada.

Coles EH: *Veterinary clinical pathology*, ed 4, Philadelphia, 1986, Saunders.

Hendrix CM, Robinson E: *Diagnostic parasitology for veterinary technicians*, ed 3, St Louis, 2006, Mosby.

Hendrix CM, Sirois M: *Laboratory procedures for veterinary technicians*, ed 5, St Louis, 2007, Mosby.

Ivens VR et al: *Principal parasites of domestic animals in the U.S*, Urbana, Ill, 1989, University of Illinois.

Lautenslager P: *Notes from veterinary parasitology for animal health technicians*, Centralia, Ontario, Canada, 1982, Centralia College.

Owen DG: *Parasites of laboratory animals, Handbook #12*, London, 1992, Royal Society of Medicine Services.

Peregrine A: *Anthelmintics registered in Canada, principles of disease in veterinary medicine*, lecture notes from Veterinary Parasitology, Guelph, Ontario, Canada, 2001, Ontario Veterinary College.

Sirois M, editor: *Principles and practice of veterinary technology*, St Louis, 2003, Mosby.

Sloss MW, Kemp RL: *Veterinary clinical parasitology*, Ames, 1978, Iowa State University Press.

## CHAPTER 5

# Diagnostic Microbiology and Mycology

*Sandra Skeba*

## OUTLINE

Purpose
Equipment
  Light Microscope
  Incubator
  Sterilizing Heat Sources
  Media
  Miscellaneous Equipment
Bacteriological and Fungal Media
  Basic Media
  Specific Types of Media: Plates
  Basic Media: Tubes
Types of Specimens
  Sterile Areas
  Nonsterile Areas
  Abscessed Areas
Collection and Culture of Specimens
  Swab Specimen
  Liquid Specimen

Solid Specimen
Urine Specimen
Blood Specimen
Fecal Cultures
Fungal Cultures
Transport and Shipping of
  Specimens
Basic Diagnostic Tests
  Acid-Fast Stain
  Bile Esculin
  Catalase Test
  Coagulase Test
  Gram Stain
  Kirby-Bauer Sensitivity
  Miniature Biochemical
    Test Kits
  Optochin Susceptibility
  Oxidase Test

Bacterial Identification
  Gram-Positive Cocci
  Gram-Negative Cocci
  Gram-Negative Rods
  Gram-Negative Spirochetes
  Gram-Negative Coccobacilli
  Gram-Positive Rods
  Mycoplasma
  Obligate Intracellular Bacteria
Fungal Identification
  Dermatophytes
  Saprophytes
  Yeast
  Dimorphic Fungi

## LEARNING OUTCOMES

After reading this chapter you should be able to:

1. List and describe equipment needed to perform diagnostic microbiology.
2. Describe and list the purposes of various bacterial and fungal media.
3. Describe the types of samples that may be obtained from the body for microbiological culture.
4. Describe the collection and transport of specimens.
5. Explain bacterial identification procedures for gram-positive and gram-negative bacteria.
6. Explain fungal identification.
7. Describe how to perform various diagnostic tests to identify specific bacteria and fungi.

**M**icrobiology is the study of microscopic organisms. Clinical microbiology is the identification of these organisms, including bacteria, fungi, parasites, and viruses, that cause clinical illness. In this chapter we will explore the fundamental components of a working clinical microbiology laboratory, the most common causes of bacterial and fungal diseases of domestic animals, and how to use this information to assist the veterinarian in the diagnosis and treatment of these diseases.

## PURPOSE

The purpose of a veterinary clinical microbiology laboratory is to

I. Assist the veterinarian in the diagnosis and treatment of bacteriological and fungal disease
II. Provide accurate identification of the causes of infections

III. Provide useful information about the organisms cultured (e.g., antibiotic sensitivity)
IV. Maintain cost- and time-effectiveness while presenting all of the above
    A. Many practices send out cultures to commercial laboratories because their low volume of samples makes keeping media impractical
    B. Competent staff must be available to perform microbiological procedures
    C. Not every bacterium or fungus can be identified in the small veterinary lab, but patients may benefit from the quick turnaround time when common pathogens are identified in-house

## EQUIPMENT

### Light Microscope

I. Probably the most expensive piece of equipment needed
II. Parts of a light microscope
    A. Eyepiece(s): one in a monocular microscope; two in a binocular microscope. The eyepiece(s) magnify the viewed field 5, 10, or 15 times ($\times 5$, $\times 10$, or $\times 15$; most are $\times 10$). A binocular microscope is more expensive but is preferred because of the ease in viewing and increased clarity
    B. Light source: an attached, internal light bulb with a variable intensity best illuminates the viewed slide
    C. Light condenser: another means of increasing or decreasing the amount of light on the slide; most good microscopes have two: one directly above the light source and one under the stage
    D. Stage: the platform on which the slide is placed for viewing; most stages are movable with two knobs on the side of the microscope: one for horizontal movement and one for vertical movement
    E. Objectives: magnify the specimen
    F. Focus: most microscopes have two types of focus-adjusting knobs: a coarse focus for initially viewing the specimen and a fine focus for sharpening the image
III. There are many different models available; for use in a clinical microbiology laboratory, must have at least three objectives
    A. $\times 10$ (dry): used to scan the slide
    B. $\times 40$ (dry): used to identify fungal elements
    C. $\times 100$ (oil immersion): used to differentiate stained bacteria

### Incubator

An incubator allows an organism to be grown under controlled conditions. There are many different types of incubators available, but for most clinical microbiology laboratories, all that is needed is an incubator that keeps the specimens at 37° C (98.6° F), which is human body temperature, and room air oxygen concentration.

I. Most cultures are grown overnight and held at least 48 hours
II. Most veterinary cultures are grown at 37° C (98.6° F), including reptile and amphibian cultures
    A. Even though reptiles and amphibians are poikilothermic (i.e., their bodies stay at ambient temperature), most organisms present will grow at 37° C (98.6° F)
    B. This temperature is especially critical when performing such standardized tests as the Kirby-Bauer sensitivity

### Sterilizing Heat Sources

I. Bunsen burner
    A. Attaches to gas wall outlets
    B. Allows flame to be ignited with a spark striker
    C. Quickly sterilizes the metal loop used for transferring microorganisms to be inoculated into growing media
    D. Also used to heat-fix slides for staining procedures
II. Electric heating element
    A. Usually ceramic, an enclosed heater that sterilizes metal loops
    B. Eliminates the need for a natural gas source
    C. Provides more even heating of loop
III. Alcohol lamps
    A. Usually a small glass lamp with a wick that extends into alcohol in the base
    B. Wick must be ignited with another flame source (e.g., matches)
    C. Does not sterilize metal loops as quickly or thoroughly as a Bunsen burner
    D. Less expensive than previously mentioned options

### Media

I. Must choose appropriate type of media for isolation needs
    A. Nutritive media grow all types of bacteria (and some fungi)
    B. Selective media grow only certain types of bacteria (e.g., gram-negative or gram-positive types) or fungi
    C. Differential media contain elements that differentiate between certain types of bacteria (e.g., lactose fermenters [LFs] or hydrogen sulfide [$H_2S$] producers)
II. All media must be examined for accidental bacterial/fungal contaminants before use
III. All media plates are incubated upside down (media side up) to prevent condensation from dripping onto cultures

## Miscellaneous Equipment

I. Metal loop: for transferring bacterial or fungal specimens onto media or slides; many sizes are available

II. Glass microscope slides and coverslips: for placing a specimen to be examined under the microscope

III. Wooden applicator sticks: disposable; used when performing quick identification tests

IV. Sterile cotton-tipped applicators: many uses, including applying specimens to media or microscope slide

V. Wax or permanent markers: to identify specimens on media or slides

VI. Filter paper: used to perform some identification tests

## BACTERIOLOGICAL AND FUNGAL MEDIA
### Basic Media

I. Agar: a semisolid media
II. Broth: a liquid media
III. Plate: a flat, round container of agar
IV. Tube: a screw-top container; can contain broth or agar
V. Slant: a tube of agar that has been allowed to gel at an angle
VI. Selective media: contain compounds that inhibit growth of certain types of organisms
VII. Differential media: contain compounds that identify certain characteristics of organisms grown on the media

### Specific Types of Media: Plates

I. Columbia colistin–nalidixic acid agar (CNA) with 5% sheep's blood
A. Selects for gram-positive organisms using colistin and nalidixic acid
B. Phenylethyl alcohol (PEA) agar is another media used for gram-positive bacteria selection

II. MacConkey II agar (MAC)
A. Selects for gram-negative organisms using crystal violet as a gram-positive bacterial inhibitor
B. Differentiates between lactose fermenters (LFs) and non–lactose fermenters (NLFs) using a neutral red indicator that colors LF colonies purple
C. Designed to inhibit the swarming of *Proteus* spp. bacteria

III. Mueller-Hinton agar (MH)
A. General-use medium specially formulated to give standardized results during antibiotic sensitivity testing
B. Can be enriched with blood for more fastidious organisms

IV. *Salmonella-Shigella* agar (SS)
A. Selects for pathogenic enteric gram-negative bacteria
B. Differentiates colonies on the basis of lactose fermentation [see MacConkey II Agar (MAC)]
C. Differentiates $H_2S$-producing bacteria by use of ferric citrate in the formula, which produces black pigment in hydrogen sulfide–producing colonies
D. Other gram negative selective/differential media include Hektoen enteric agar and Levine eosin methylene blue agar

V. Trypticase soy agar with 5% sheep's blood (TSA); also referred to as blood agar plate (BAP)
A. General, nutritive medium for cultivation of fastidious microorganisms
B. Used for the observation of bacterial hemolytic reactions

### Basic Media: Tubes

I. Bile esculin agar (BE)
A. Slanted medium used to identify bacteria that hydrolyze esculin, especially enterococci
B. Positive reaction is indicated by ferric citrate, which reacts by producing a dark brown color

II. Brain heart infusion (BHI)
A. Enriched broth used to bring bacteria to a certain turbidity level when performing diffusion antibiotic sensitivity testing (Kirby-Bauer)

III. Dermatophyte test medium (DTM)
A. Solid-tubed medium, supplemented with gentamicin and chlortetracycline; used to isolate pathogenic fungi
B. Differentiation is provided by phenol red, which causes a color change in the presence of acid-producing, rapidly growing pathogenic fungi

IV. Gram-negative broth (GN)
A. Selective enrichment medium for *Salmonella* and *Shigella* spp. used in fecal culturing

V. Motility test medium
A. Semisolid medium used to demonstrate motility of bacteria

VI. Mycosel agar
A. Selective fungal medium that contains cycloheximide and chloramphenicol to inhibit bacterial growth. Sabouraud dextrose agar with chloramphenicol is used in a similar way

VII. Nutrient agar slant (NA)
A. Media used for the cultivation and transport of nonfastidious organisms

VIII. Oxidation fermentation medium with dextrose (OF)
A. Semisolid medium used to determine dextrose use in gram-negative bacteria

IX. Sodium chloride 0.85% (NaCl 0.85%)

A. Sterile solution used for diluting gram-negative bacteria for API testing

X. Thioglycollate broth (THIO) without indicator –135C

A. General-use broth that grows most bacterial organisms, including anaerobes and some fungi

XI. Trypticase soy broth (TSB)

A. General-use broth that grows most bacteria, particularly fastidious organisms

B. Used primarily in blood cultures and sterility testing

XII. Urea agar slant (UREA)

A. Used to determine urease production of bacteria

B. Positive result is indicated by the presence of a phenol red indicator

## TYPES OF SPECIMENS

There are three types of areas of the body to consider when obtaining a specimen for microbiological culture.

### Sterile Areas

I. Body areas or cavities that do not normally contain bacteria or fungi; any bacteria encountered in these specimens should be considered abnormal. The samples most commonly cultured include

A. Blood

B. Urine

C. Spinal fluid

D. Joint fluid

E. Solid organs

F. Milk

G. Lower respiratory tract

### Nonsterile Areas

I. Body areas that, when healthy, contain resident bacteria and fungi (normal flora) that must be distinguished from disease-causing organisms; these areas include

A. Hair/fur

B. Skin

C. Sputum or saliva

D. Intestinal tract/feces

E. Ears

F. Upper respiratory tract, including nares and trachea

### Abscessed Areas

I. Areas that the body has filled with exudative material in response to inflammation or irritation

A. Sterile abscesses have no bacterial etiology and their culture will result in no growth

B. Primary infection abscesses usually contain only one type of pathogen (the cause of the original infection)

C. Secondary infection abscesses contain multiple opportunistic pathogens, bacterial or fungal, that invaded after the original infection

## COLLECTION AND CULTURE OF SPECIMENS

### Swab Specimen

I. Culturette or sterile cotton-tipped swab

A. Commonly used when culturing ears, nares, and abscesses

B. Liquid specimen may be squirted onto a swab, then submitted

C. Prepackaged sterile swabs may contain a small amount of liquid or gel used as a transport medium, which keeps the organisms viable while in transit (usually for up to 48 hours)

D. Use swab to inoculate one third of each plate: BAP, CNA, MAC

E. Place remaining swab into THIO broth. If swab is plastic or wood, break off cleanly against side of tube so that specimen end of swab is immersed in the medium (break off at a low enough height so that swab end does not protrude from tube). If swab is metal, use clean utility scissors to cut swab off at a good site and flame the cut end of the swab and cool before allowing to rest in broth

F. Streak inoculated plates for isolation (Figure 5-1)

G. Gram stain can be made from the swab if a flamed, sterile microscope slide is used. Smear sample onto the slide after inoculating the plates but before the swab is placed in the broth. It is best to get a second swab for gram staining

H. Incubate overnight

### Liquid Specimen

I. Aspirate in syringe, sterile tube, etc.

A. Typically, liquid specimens presented are abscess material, tracheal wash, bronchial wash, nasal discharge, joint fluid, or spinal fluid

B. Inoculate each of the plates (usually BAP, MAC, and CNA) with a small drop of specimen

C. Inoculate thioglycollate broth with a few drops of specimen

D. Use flamed, cooled loop to spread inoculant on one third of each plate; then streak each plate for isolation (see Figure 5-1)

E. Gram stain specimen from syringe/tube

### Solid Specimen

I. Solid specimens include hard abscess material and tissue samples, including organs, skin, and scales

II. Usually the best way to culture these materials is to place a small amount in nutritive broth (THIO or TSB) overnight, then subculture the broth onto the plated media

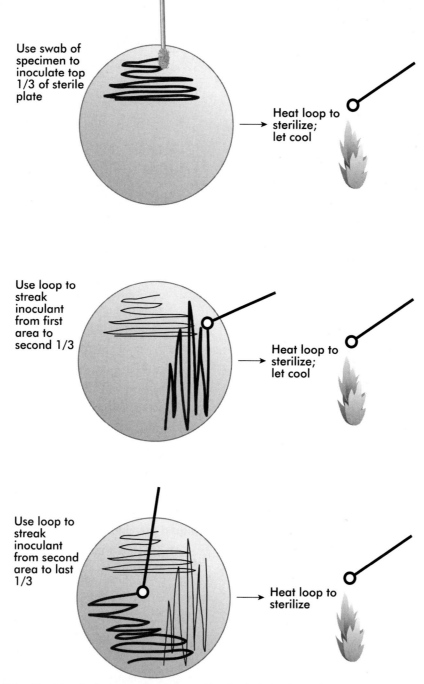

Use swab of specimen to inoculate top 1/3 of sterile plate

Heat loop to sterilize; let cool

Use loop to streak inoculant from first area to second 1/3

Heat loop to sterilize; let cool

Use loop to streak inoculant from second area to last 1/3

Heat loop to sterilize

**Figure 5-1** Streaking for isolation. Goal of streaking for isolation is to obtain individual bacterial colonies that are far enough away from other colonies that they can be tested separately and identified.

III. Use aseptic technique when collecting tissue samples, especially at necropsy

## Urine Specimen

I. Best urine specimen for culture is obtained by cystocentesis; sterile catheterization may also be used. A specimen obtained by free catch may contain normal flora from the skin and genital area

II. Use a sterile, calibrated, nonreusable loop to inoculate 10 μL of urine on a BAP

III. Spread inoculant evenly over entire surface of plate. Any colonies that grow will be counted; the results multiplied by 100 will give bacteria per mL of urine. Numbers below 1000 colonies/mL are usually not considered clinically significant

IV. Inoculate MAC and CNA plates as for liquid specimens

V. A urine sample is generally not placed in THIO because of the high incidence of false-positive readings from contamination (even cystocentesis)

## Blood Specimen

I. Mammal
  A. Disinfect rubber tops of two TSB tubes and venipuncture site with a surgical preparation solution
  B. Collect blood directly into TSB tube from venipuncture (i.e., with Vacutainer). One tube is vented to allow aerobic growth; one is left sealed for anaerobic growth
  C. If patient/vein size does not allow direct venipuncture, place noncoagulated blood into broth via syringe (use clean needle if possible or remove needle from syringe before inoculating)
  D. If two tubes are inoculated, one is vented using aseptic technique with a Vacutainer needle (leave needle in place with cover on loosely)
  E. Tubes should be observed every day for hemolysis or cloudiness. Anaerobic activity may be indicated if lid pops off tube
  F. If signs of growth are observed, treat tubes as liquid specimens and subculture/gram stain
  G. Keep tubes at least 8 days, after which subculture to TSA plate and gram stain to confirm negative result

II. Avian, reptile, amphibian, and fish blood
  A. If patient is large enough, follow mammal protocol
  B. For small patients, place at least five drops of aseptically drawn blood into THIO broth. Avoid use of anticoagulants, which may interfere with bacterial growth
  C. Observe tube daily. Treat as liquid specimen if signs of growth occur
  D. These specimens tend to look positive because of the presence of red blood cell nuclei; subculture is required to verify negative
  E. Confirm negatives at 8 days, as for mammals

## Fecal Cultures

I. All fecal cultures are inoculated onto MAC and SS plates and into GN broth
II. GN broth, regardless of plate findings, is subcultured onto an SS plate at 24 and/or 48 hours
III. Be aware of species-specific pathogens when looking for possible pathogenic colonies: in most carnivores and hoofstock, *Salmonella* spp. are a main concern. In primates, one must also look for *Shigella* spp. Both are NLFs, but *Salmonella* spp. are $H_2S$ producers and *Shigella* spp. are not
IV. Pathogenic $H_2S$-positive *Salmonella* can be distinguished from the common nonpathogenic $H_2S$-positive *Proteus* spp. by a simple urea test (*Proteus* spp. are urea positive)
V. Of concern in some primates and hoofstock is *Yersinia pseudotuberculosis*. This is a NLF that does not produce $H_2S$. This bacterium is urea positive, however, and could be overlooked if urea tests are performed to rule out pathogens. For this reason, any NLF colonies encountered in a primate or hoofstock fecal sample should be fully identified
VI. Gram stain all fecal specimens
  A. *Campylobacter* spp., curved gram-negative rods that can appear as "seagull" or W shapes, may be presumptively identified by their pathognomonic shape. They are difficult to culture because of fastidious oxygen requirements
  B. Large quantities of large, spore-forming, gram-positive rods may indicate a clostridial problem
  C. Yeast may also be detected on gram stains. They are especially significant in avian patients

## Fungal Cultures

I. Examine specimen for fungal elements (yeast, hyphal segments) under the microscope, if possible
II. If the specimen is to be incubated for dermatophytes (hair and/or skin samples, most often) place into a small slant tube of DTM
III. All other fungal cultures are placed in Mycosel slants
  A. If the sample is liquid, as in tracheal or bronchial wash, a clean needle on the syringe is used to scratch a few lines in the fungal medium; then a couple of drops of the specimen are placed on the medium
  B. If the sample is on a swab, aseptically break the end of the swab off so it fits in the tube of medium; then gently embed the swab into the agar using flamed, cooled forceps
  C. Pieces of hair or skin can be aseptically placed on top of the medium
IV. If unsure of the organism, place in both DTM and Mycosel media (as in severe skin infections)
V. Cultures are placed at room temperature in a dark area and examined daily for fungal growth
  A. Dermatophyte fungi (which invade the hair and skin) will often grow within 3 or 4 days and turn DTM red
  B. Saprophytic fungi (which are opportunistic environmental fungi) can take up to 3 weeks to grow
VI. Cultures should be held for 1 month to confirm negative results

## TRANSPORT AND SHIPPING OF SPECIMENS ■

I. Samples to be sent to an outside lab should be shipped as quickly as possible
  A. Refrigeration helps organisms stay viable. Do not freeze samples

B. Commercially available swab transport systems, such as Culturettes, have a small amount of liquid or gel at the swab end that helps the organisms survive transport. Screw top containers must be taped closed

C. All specimens must be labeled with full identification of the owner, animal, sample type, and test(s) to be performed

D. If the sample is to be picked up by a local lab, their transport system is usually sufficient

E. Samples shipped through commercial carriers (FedEx, for example) need to be placed in a secure, waterproof, primary container with absorbent material. This primary container (or several primary containers) is then placed in a secondary container that is also durable and watertight

   1. The outer shipping container is usually a box or envelope that protects the contents from damage

   2. Wet or dry ice, if needed, is placed between the secondary container and the shipping container

F. It is the law to properly prepare and identify biological specimens for transport. Contact the shipping agency for detailed regulations

## BASIC DIAGNOSTIC TESTS
### Acid-Fast Stain

I. Make a saline or water suspension of sample on slide (not too thick); allow to air dry

II. Heat-fix slide by passing through a flame, specimen side up, three or four times. Let slide cool to touch

III. Flood slide with carbol fuchsin stain; allow to sit for 5 minutes. Rinse with tap water until water runs clear

IV. Rinse the slide briefly (15 to 20 seconds) with an acid alcohol solution to decolorize, then rinse again with tap water

V. Flood slide with malachite green counterstain; let sit for 50 to 60 seconds. Rinse under tap water and blot dry

   A. Mycobacteria will stain as thin red or pink rods against a green or bluish background. A few yeasts will also stain pink; they are clearer and smaller

### Bile Esculin

I. Inoculate a bile esculin agar slant with a *Streptococcus* colony to be tested

II. Place in incubator

III. Examine within a few hours. If agar turns black, test is positive (enterococcal streptococci are positive)

IV. Incubate negative result overnight to confirm

### Catalase Test

I. Using a wooden applicator stick, smear a small amount of the colony to be tested on a clean glass slide

II. Place a drop of 3% hydrogen peroxide on the specimen

III. Observe for bubbling, which indicates a positive reaction. *Staphylococcus* are catalase positive, *Streptococcus* are catalase negative

### Coagulase Test

I. Place a sample of the *Staphylococcus* colony to be tested into a small amount of liquid rabbit plasma with ethylenediaminetetraacetic acid (EDTA)

II. Incubate overnight

III. Coagulase-positive staphylococci will cause the plasma to gel

IV. Coagulase-negative staphylococci will not affect the plasma's liquid state

### Gram Stain

Follow directions from the gram stain kit. Usual staining procedure is

I. Specimen is placed on a microscope slide

II. Colony from a plate is suspended in water, or a flamed, cooled loop is used to transfer a drop of thioglycollate broth

III. Allow to air dry

IV. Heat-fix by passing slide quickly through a flame, specimen slide up, about four times, and cool

V. Flood slide with crystal violet stain; let sit 1 minute

VI. Rinse with tap water until water runs clear

VII. Flood slide with Gram's iodine; let sit 1 minute

VIII. Rinse with tap water until water runs clear

IX. Flood slide with decolorizer, rock back and forth about 10 seconds, and then rinse slide with tap water. Repeat if specimen is very dark, but try not to overdecolorize

X. Flood slide with safranin counterstain, allow to sit for 30 to 50 seconds, and then rinse with tap water until water runs clear

XI. Dry on blotting (bibulous) paper or allow to air dry

XII. Observations under oil immersion (×100) objective: gram-positive bacteria stain purple or dark blue. Gram-negative bacteria stain pink

   A. Overdecolorizing or using an old colony can cause false gram-negative reactions

   B. Forgetting to decolorize or not decolorizing a heavy specimen sufficiently may yield a false-positive result

### Kirby-Bauer Sensitivity

I. Bacteria to be tested are diluted in 5 mL BHI broth (or 5 mL 0.85% saline if an API strip is being set up) to match a 0.5 McFarland standard of cloudiness (which is available commercially)

II. Using a sterile cotton-tipped applicator, the sample is inoculated onto a Mueller-Hinton plate in a sweeping, overlapping fashion to cover the entire surface evenly (the opposite goal of streaking for isolation)

III. Antibiotic sensitivity disks are placed on the agar surface with the antibiotic disk dispenser. Disks must be taped lightly onto the agar surface so they adhere to the media while the plate is being incubated (upside down)

IV. Inhibition zones are read with a millimeter ruler after incubation overnight at 37° C. Measure the complete clear zone across the antibiotic disk, where bacteria did not grow. Several readings can be taken if the zones are unclear or irregular. Refer to an antibiotic sensitivity chart, because not all inhibition zones mean the same for each antibiotic or bacteria type

## Miniature Biochemical Test Kits (for Gram-Negative Identification)

I. Examples include Micro ID, Enterotube, Minitek, and API 20E
II. API 20E can be used to illustrate the basic concept
  A. Each little cup of the API strip is a separate test (each test used to be performed separately, but now the results can be assessed quickly and easily)
  B. The 0.85% saline suspension of bacteria used for setting up the API 20E is also used to inoculate the Mueller-Hinton plate for Kirby-Bauer sensitivity testing
  C. When the API 20E instruction sheet is followed correctly, the main causes for improper readouts are using mixed colonies of bacteria; using too few colonies; trying to identify a gram-positive colony; or using old, nonviable colonies
  D. Other tests for identification of enteric bacteria exist; follow manufacturer's instructions

## Optochin Susceptibility

I. A small paper disk impregnated with 5 µg optochin is placed on a BAP inoculated heavily with the streptococcus colony to be tested, which is then incubated.
  A. *Streptococcus pneumoniae* are sensitive to optochin and will show a marked zone of inhibition (no growth) around the disk, while other α-hemolytic streptococci are unaffected

## Oxidase Test

I. Using a wooden applicator stick, smear a small to moderate amount of colony to be tested on a piece of white filter paper
II. Place a drop of oxidase reagent on the paper

III. Smeared sample will turn dark blue if positive (some colonies appear blue when initially placed on the filter paper: watch closely for color change)
IV. Many colonies will turn dark after 5 or more minutes, so record only immediate color change

## BACTERIAL IDENTIFICATION*

Examine bacteriological plates after overnight incubation. Observe the morphology of the colonies. Each colony of the same type of bacteria will look the same. Growth on the TSA and CNA plate indicates the bacteria are gram positive. Growth on the TSA and MAC plate indicates the bacteria are gram negative. Growth only on the TSA plate indicates a fastidious organism; gram stain a representative colony.

### Gram-Positive Cocci (Figure 5-2)

Gram-positive cocci are composed mainly of three groups: staphylococci (staph), streptococci (strep), and micrococci. The micrococci are not often encountered in the veterinary laboratory.

I. *Staphylococcus* spp.
  A. Note if colony causes any hemolysis on the blood agar plate. Staphylococci are either hemolytic or nonhemolytic
  B. First test performed on any gram-positive colony is the catalase test (staphylococci are catalase positive)
  C. Coagulase test is performed on the colony (generally, the coagulase-positive staphylococci are more pathogenic)
  D. Mueller-Hinton sensitivity test is performed using BHI broth as a colony diluent
  E. Some samples (such as skin swabs) can be expected to have staph growth. It may be wise to ask the requesting veterinarian if a sensitivity test should be performed
  F. Often staph colonies growing in a broth tube will resemble comets or shooting stars
  G. Staph, especially those that are coagulase positive, can cause skin or other infections, such as bumblefoot in birds
II. *Streptococcus* spp.
  A. Streptococci are catalase negative
  B. Note any hemolysis surrounding the colonies on the BAP. Streptococci hemolysis is graded into
    1. α-Hemolysis (incomplete hemolysis): agar surrounding the colony is greenish
    2. β-Hemolysis (complete hemolysis): agar surrounding the colony is clear
    3. γ-Hemolysis (no hemolysis): agar surrounding the colony is unaffected

*Note that these procedures are basic. They are described in greater detail in a clinical microbiology book, which is the final reference when identifying organisms.

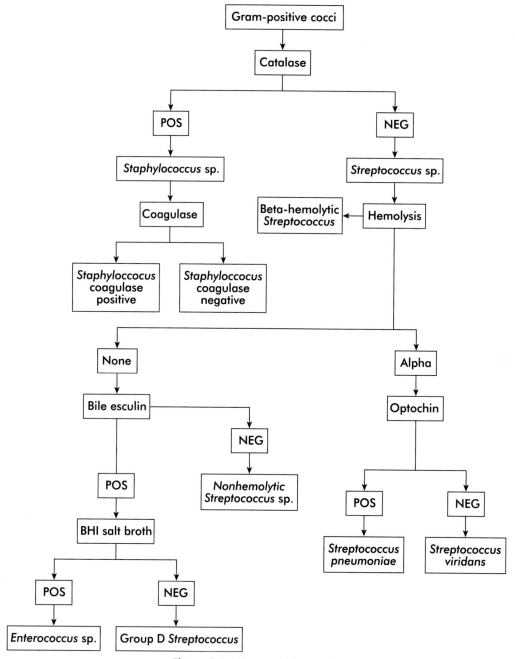

**Figure 5-2**   Gram-positive cocci.

C. Sensitivity is performed using BHI broth. (An MH plate with 5% sheep's blood can be used to promote the growth of the streptococci)

D. *Streptococcus* spp. that do not grow well on the MH plate, especially β-hemolytic *Streptococcus*, will be sensitive to most antibiotics

E. Enterococci or enterococcal streptococci (e.g., *Streptococcus faecalis*) are found in the alimentary tract but are opportunistic pathogens elsewhere in the body. To determine if a colony is an *Enterococcus*, a bile esculin test is performed; enterococci are bile esculin positive

F. Many *Streptococcus* spp. will grow like stars suspended in the broth

G. Streptococci can be responsible for many illnesses in animals, including pneumonia, mastitis, and septicemia

H. The optochin disk test distinguishes *S. pneumoniae* from other α-hemolytic streptococci

## Gram-Negative Cocci

I. *Neisseria* spp. are often found as normal flora in the respiratory tract of many animals; as pathogens, they mainly cause concern in humans

A. *N. gonorrhoeae* is the cause of human gonorrhea
B. *N. meningitidis* causes human meningitis
C. *N. weaveri*, found in the canine mouth, can cause infections in dog bites
D. *N. iguanae* can cause abscesses in iguanid lizards

## Gram-Negative Rods (Figure 5-3)

I. Enterobacteriaceae, or enteric (gut) bacteria, are gram-negative rods that are commonly isolated in veterinary medicine
II. Gram-negative rods grow on the BAP and MAC plate (they will often overgrow gram-positive cocci on the BAP, which makes the CNA plate essential for recovering these)
III. Note the lactose reaction of the colony on MAC agar
   A. If the colony is a NLF, it will be clear. Perform an oxidase test
   B. LFs are dark pink or purple. All LFs are oxidase negative

IV. Colony is prepared for API 20E and sensitivity testing using sterile 0.85% saline. Other commercial tests can be used; follow the instructions
V. If searching for fecal pathogens, all NLFs must be identified and/or ruled out
   A. For example: *Proteus* spp. and *Salmonella* spp. are both NLFs and H$_2$S positive. *Proteus*, however, is urea positive; a urea test can distinguish these bacteria within a few hours
   B. *Shigella* and *Pseudomonas* look similar on an MAC plate. To rule out suspicious colonies, perform an oxidase test: *Shigella* will be oxidase negative
   C. *Aeromonas* spp. are a light LF, appearing creamy pink on an MAC plate. They are oxidase positive
   D. These organisms are readily identified by most commercial gram negative test kits
VI. Anaerobic gram negative rods
   A. *Bacteroides* spp. are common pathogens in veterinary medicine. *B. fragilis* causes diarrhea in a

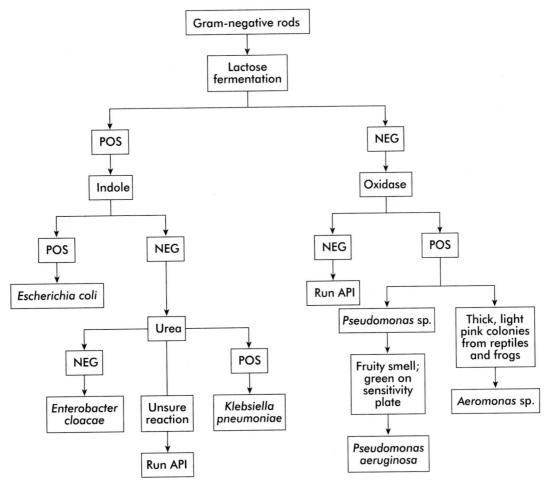

**Figure 5-3** Gram-negative rods.

wide variety of species and is seen in soft tissue abscesses, mastitis, and periodontitis

B. *Fusobacterium* spp. are normal inhabitants of the oral cavity and intestinal tract but can cause infections in dog and cat bites. They also are a cause of thrush in horses and bovine foot rot

C. Because these anaerobes do not form spores, they need proper handling and prompt transport for successful culture

VII. Some of the nonenteral gram-negative rods, such as *Pseudomonas* and *Aeromonas* spp., can be serious primary pathogens, especially in birds, reptiles, fish, and amphibians

## Gram-Negative Spirochetes

I. *Campylobacter* spp. are bacteria found in the digestive tracts of many mammals. In hoofed mammals they can be normal flora; in others (especially primates and carnivores) they can cause a chronic debilitating diarrhea

A. Shape of *Campylobacter* is often characteristic: two small, curved, gram-negative rods join end-to-end to form a seagull or W shape. These can be difficult to see on a gram stain, and other forms may be present (spiraled), so a negative gram stain is not diagnostic

B. *Campylobacter* requires a microaerophilic environment to grow and often are overgrown by more vigorous organisms. Special media and growing conditions are required for culture

II. *Yersinia* spp. may be encountered in reptile/amphibian cultures and primate or ruminant fecal cultures. These bacteria are halophilic (requiring salt to grow). Most media have sufficient salt to enable the bacteria to grow and be identifiable by API

III. Other spirochetes include *Leptospira* spp., *Borrelia* spp., and *Helicobacter* spp.

## Gram-Negative Coccobacilli

I. *Moraxella bovis* are large gram-negative cocci that sometimes resemble fat rods; they cause pinkeye in cattle

II. Gram-negative coccobacilli include *Bordetella* spp. and *Pasteurella* spp. These organisms are of concern to the veterinary microbiology laboratory because they can cause respiratory disease in dogs *(Bordetella bronchisepticum)* and in cats and rabbits *(Pasteurella multocida)*. *Brucella abortus* is a serious pathogen in cattle, causing abortions

III. These organisms can be identified in the API system

IV. Care must be taken not to misidentify these as streptococci, because they may not grow on MAC. Any flat, shiny, gray colony (especially if it has no look-alike on the CNA plate) should be gram stained

V. It can be difficult to tell coccobacilli from cocci, so it is best to work with young colonies. Older colonies

of streptococci may lose their ability to hold a positive gram reaction

## Gram-Positive Rods

I. Most small microbiology laboratories do not attempt to identify *anaerobic* gram-positive rods, such as *Clostridium* spp.

II. Note their presence and whether they have spores on gram stain

III. They will grow anaerobically in THIO, toward the bottom, but not on regular plates. For this reason it is important to gram stain the broth

IV. Most common *aerobic* gram-positive rods encountered are *Bacillus* spp.

A. These are large, parallel-sided rods that grow on the blood agar plate only

B. Colonies often have a "grainy" or "mucoid" appearance and can be hemolytic and spore forming

C. They grow at the top of the broth in the THIO tube

D. Sensitivities can be performed but often are not necessary because *Bacillus* spp. are mostly found in culture as normal flora or environmental contaminants

E. Prominent exception is *B. anthracis*, which causes sudden death in cattle and sheep, and skin and lung lesions in humans

F. *B. piliformis* causes acute fatal enteritis in rodents and foals

V. *Corynebacterium* spp. are small gram-positive rods that are often curved and pleomorphic, giving them a "Chinese letters" look on gram stain

A. In people and animals, they are often found as normal flora of the alimentary tract, especially the mouth and skin

B. Pathogenic *Corynebacterium* include

1. *C. equi* (foal pneumonia), *C. pseudotuberculosis* (caseous lymphadenitis in sheep and goats), and *C. renale* (urinary tract infections in cattle, pigs, and male sheep)

VI. *Listeria monocytogenes* and *Erysipelothrix rhusiopathiae* are also small rods

A. *Listeria* spp. are small, non–spore-forming rods that are catalase positive; *Erysipelothrix* spp. are pleomorphic rods that are catalase negative

B. *Listeria* spp. can infect the brainstem

C. *Erysipelothrix* spp. are most commonly found in cases of septicemia and occasionally are a cause of endocarditis in dogs

VII. *Mycobacterium* spp. are long, thin, gram-positive rods that sometimes branch. These can be serious pathogens. They do not grow on typical bacteriological media

A. *M. tuberculosis* causes pneumonia in humans and other primates

B. *M. avium* causes a fatal, untreatable gastrointestinal and respiratory infection in birds
   1. These bacteria are difficult to culture: it takes months and specialized media
   2. Their presence in sputum or tissue can be demonstrated by their ability to retain an acid-fast stain, which is a test that can be performed in most veterinary laboratories

## Mycoplasma

I. *Mycoplasma* spp. are small bacteria that lack a cell wall and therefore are not easily stained and observed in exudates

II. Pneumonia and arthritis are the most common diseases associated with *Mycoplasma* spp.

III. Identification of *Mycoplasma* spp. can be made only at a reference laboratory

## Obligate Intracellular Bacteria

I. *Chlamydia*, *Ehrlichia*, and *Rickettsia* are examples of obligate intracellular bacteria

II. These are gram-negative rods that are often host specific. Because they must be grown in cell cultures, diagnosis is made clinically by serology, or by special staining to highlight the organisms within the host's cells
   A. *Chlamydia* spp. cause genital and upper respiratory infections in humans, cats, pigs, and birds
   B. *Ehrlichia canis* causes canine hemorrhagic fever, a tick-borne disease
   C. *Rickettsia rickettsii* is the cause of Rocky Mountain spotted fever, also tick-borne, in humans and dogs

## FUNGAL IDENTIFICATION

Fungi are identified by their characteristic microscopic morphology.

I. A small piece of clear cellophane tape is pressed gently but firmly onto the fungal colony, sticky side down. The tape is placed, sticky side down, on a microscope slide to which a drop of saline or lactophenol cotton blue has been added. The slide is examined under the microscope for hyphal identification

II. Other specialized techniques and media can be used to identify fungi, but these are generally more time consuming and not commonly done in small laboratories

III. TSA plate will often grow yeast, if present in a sample. Therefore any colonies that are not easily recognized should be gram stained (or make a wet mount with saline) and examined microscopically

IV. In very heavy fungal infections (e.g., avian aspergillosis) the fungus will often grow on top of the THIO and/or the surface of the TSA plate. These colonies are usually readily identified as fungi by their dry, fuzzy appearance

## Dermatophytes

I. Found in hair, skin, nails, and claws, they are the cause of ringworm in humans and animals

II. Main dermatophytes affecting animals are *Microsporum* spp. and *Trichophyton* spp.

III. Most dermatophytes cause a color change in dermatophyte test medium (from orange to red)

IV. These fungi are distinguished by their large macroconidia, visible microscopically. The shape of the macroconidia identifies the organism

## Saprophytes

I. Saprophytic fungi are found in the environment and are opportunistic pathogens

II. The saprophytes include
   A. *Aspergillus* spp., which can cause pneumonia, especially in birds
      1. Some species can also cause disease by their presence in feed and hay
      2. They create a toxin known as aflatoxin, which can cause a severe immunosuppressive effect in animals ingesting affected feed
   B. *Mucor* spp. and *Rhizopus* spp. can cause lymph node, lung, and liver lesions in immunosuppressed animals

## Yeast

A cream-colored colony growing only on the TSA plate could be yeast.

I. *Candida* spp. can be found infecting mucous membranes, especially in the gastrointestinal tract (including the mouth), genital tract, respiratory tract, and ears

II. *Candida albicans* causes many diseases, especially when predisposing conditions exist, such as
   A. Immunosuppression
   B. Primary bacterial infection
   C. Prolonged antibiotic use
   D. *Candida albicans* can be identified by means of the germ tube test
      1. An isolate of yeast is incubated in rabbit plasma with EDTA for 2 to 3 hours, and then examined microscopically
      2. *C. albicans* produces germ tubes, which grow from the side of the yeast like tiny hyphae
      3. True germ tubes do not "pinch in" at the point of attachment to the parent yeast cell
   E. Commercial agglutination tests also exist for identification of *C. albicans* and many other yeasts

III. *Cryptococcus neoformans* is an encapsulated yeast that can cause severe nasal infections in dogs and cats and meningitis in people (this is a very zoonotic organism)
   A. Cultures or nasal exudates can be examined under the microscope with a drop of India ink to highlight the thick capsule

IV. *Malassezia pachydermatis* is found in the external ear and is emerging as the cause of seborrheic dermatitis and hypersensitivity reactions

  A. It can be identified by its appearance on a gram stain as an oval, bottle-shaped, budding yeast

V. Yeast can be normal flora in the ears, genitals, and oral cavity

## Dimorphic Fungi

I. Dimorphic fungi exhibit yeastlike growth when in animal tissue and saprophytic fungus–type growth in the environment

II. These fungi are highly zoonotic and must be handled using protective measures

  A. They are identified by their characteristic microscopic appearance

  B. Infections can also be diagnosed by serology testing

III. Dimorphic fungi of special clinical concern

  A. *Histoplasma capsulatum:* causes respiratory tract infections in dogs, cats, and humans

  B. *Blastomyces dermatitidis:* causes blastomycosis, a respiratory and/or skin infection in dogs and humans

  C. *Coccidioides immitis:* causes respiratory disease in dogs and humans; can also affect bones and internal organs

  D. All of these organisms can be presumptively identified by cytological examination of the clinical specimen

# Glossary

**aerobic** Requiring oxygen to live

**agar** Semisolid medium

**anaerobic** Requiring the absence of oxygen to live

**aseptic technique** Performed with as little opportunity for contamination as possible

**broth** Liquid medium

**coccobacillus** An oval-shaped bacterium that is between the coccus and bacillus forms of bacteria

**culture** Deliberate growing of an organism under controlled conditions

**differential medium** Microbiological medium that contains compounds that identify certain characteristics of organisms grown on the medium

**dimorphic fungus** A fungal organism with two growth forms: moldlike and yeastlike

**enteral bacteria** Bacteria found in the gastrointestinal tract

**halophilic** Bacteria that require a high concentration of salt for optimal growth

**microaerophilic** Bacteria that require oxygen for growth but at a lower concentration than what is present in the atmosphere

**nlf** Non–lactose fermenters

**normal flora** Organisms found in a healthy animal

**opportunistic pathogen** Organism able to infect an area already compromised by injury or infection

**optochin susceptibility test** A test to distinguish between *Streptococcus pneumoniae* and other α-hemolytic streptococci

**plate** Flat, round container of agar

**pleomorphic** Having many shapes

**selective medium** Microbiological medium that contains compounds that inhibit growth of certain types of organisms

**slant** Tube of agar that has been allowed to gel at an angle

**tube** Screw-top container that can contain broth or agar

**zoonotic** Capable of causing disease in animals and humans

# Review Questions

**1** An in-house microbiology laboratory must be
  a. Run without the veterinarian's input
  b. Completely automated
  c. Have the ability to identify every possible organism
  d. Cost effective, staffed by proficient personnel, and aware of clients' needs

**2** The oculars (or eyepieces) of a microscope
  a. Have no magnification abilities
  b. Multiply the magnification of the objectives by 5, 10, or 15
  c. Add 10 to the magnification of the objectives
  d. Control the amount of light entering the microscope

**3** Nutritive media
  a. Select for different types of bacteria
  b. Differentiate types of bacteria
  c. Grow most bacteria
  d. Are not used for most microbiological procedures

**4** MacConkey agar is an example of
  a. A differential and selective medium
  b. A general nutritive and differential medium
  c. A general nutritive medium
  d. A selective medium

**5** Sterile abscesses
  a. Do not need to be cleaned with a disinfectant before sampling
  b. Contain only one type of organism
  c. Contain many types of organisms
  d. Contain no bacterial or fungal organisms

**6** Bacterial cultures are incubated
  a. At room temperature
  b. At the patient's body temperature
  c. At human body temperature
  d. In the refrigerator

**7** The very best specimen for urine culture is obtained
  a. Via aseptic catheterization
  b. Via free catch
  c. Via cystocentesis
  d. Off of the cage floor

**8** Fungal cultures are incubated
  a. At room temperature
  b. At the patient's body temperature
  c. At human body temperature
  d. In the refrigerator

**9** A streptococcal colony on a blood agar plate with a greenish zone around it is said to be
 a. Hemolytic
 b. α-Hemolytic
 c. β-Hemolytic
 d. Nonhemolytic

**10** Dermatophyte fungi are found
 a. Infecting skin hair and nails
 b. To commonly cause pneumonia
 c. As normal flora on most animals
 d. As free-living fungi in the environment

## BIBLIOGRAPHY

Forbes BA et al: *Bailey and Scott's diagnostic microbiology*, ed 12, St Louis, 2007, Mosby.

Hendrix CM, Sirois M: *Laboratory procedures for veterinary technicians*, ed 5, St Louis, 2007, Mosby.

Mahon CR, Manuselis G: *Textbook of diagnostic microbiology*, ed 2, Philadelphia, 2000, Saunders.

McCurnin DM, Bassert JM, editors: *Clinical textbook for veterinary technicians*, ed 6, St Louis, 2006, Saunders.

Power D, editor: *Manual of BBL products and laboratory procedures*, Cockeysville, Md, 1988, Becton-Dickinson.

Quinn PJ et al: *Clinical veterinary microbiology*, St Louis, 1994, Mosby.

Sirois M, editor: *Principles and practice of veterinary technology*, ed 2, St Louis, 2004, Mosby.

Songer JG, Post KW: *Veterinary microbiology: bacterial and fungal agents of disease*, St Louis, 2005, Saunders.

## CHAPTER 6

# Clinical Chemistry

*Joanne Hamel*

## OUTLINE

General Information
Kidney Function
   Creatinine
   Urea (Urea Nitrogen)
   Water Deprivation/Urine
      Concentration Tests
Pancreatic Function
   Urine Glucose
   Serum/Plasma Glucose
   Serum Amylase
   Serum Lipase
   Trypsinlike
      Immunoreactivity

Liver Function
   Bilirubin
   Urine Urobilinogen
   Total Serum/Plasma Proteins
   Albumin
   Globulins
   Albumin-Globulin Ratio (A:G)
   Enzymes
   Bile Acids
Electrolytes and Minerals
   General Information
   Serum Sodium
   Serum Potassium

   Serum Chloride
   Serum Calcium
   Serum Phosphorus
   Serum Magnesium
   Measurement of Electrolytes
Thyroid Function
   Thyroid Hormone: $T_4$
   Free Thyroid Hormone ($FT_4$) by
      Dialysis
   Canine Thyroid Stimulating
      Hormone
   Serum Cholesterol

## LEARNING OUTCOMES

**After reading this chapter you should be able to:**

1. Identify common laboratory tests used to evaluate kidney, pancreatic, and liver function, as well as electrolytes and minerals, and some miscellaneous tests, in small and large animals.
2. Understand the significance of abnormal results of these tests.
3. Provide samples required and proper conditions under which the tests are performed.
4. Identify common tests that appear in various chemistry profiles.

It is essential that all blood samples destined for biochemical analysis be collected with care, using the correct anticoagulants or no anticoagulants. One must pay close attention to any special requirements when collecting blood samples. The results are only as good as the samples tested.

Evaluation of the chemical constituents of whole blood, plasma, and serum has become increasingly realistic in the practice setting. Instrumentation, equipment, and procedures have been greatly modified to allow relatively rapid and reliable diagnostics. Chemical components are routinely assayed by use of chemical reagent test strips or automated dry chemical analysis machines. Box 6-1 and Tables 6-1 to 6-3 at the end of the chapter provide the commonly requested tests, biochemistry reference values, a summary of function tests, and a conversion chart for SI and conventional units.

## GENERAL INFORMATION

I. Components of whole blood
   A. Whole blood: composed of fluid and cellular components
      1. Plasma is the fluid portion
      2. Erythrocytes, leukocytes, and thrombocytes compose the cells
   B. Plasma: fluid portion of the blood in which cells are suspended; 90% water and 10% dissolved

proteins, hormones, lipids, enzymes, salts, carbohydrates, vitamins, and waste materials

C. Serum: fluid portion with fibrinogen protein removed; derived when whole blood is allowed to clot

II. Sample handling

A. The following should be kept in mind when handling samples

1. Samples should be collected from calm, fasted patients when possible

2. Avoid hemolysis by selecting needles of the correct size and dry syringes or new evacuated tubes

3. To avoid chemical interaction with the specimen, serum is the sample of choice for all tests

    a. Blood samples taken for serum separation are allowed to clot, centrifuged, and separated, or use SST (serum separator tubes) if possible

      (1) This eliminates the use of sodium fluoride for collection of serum glucose

    b. Samples are allowed to clot at room temperature for 20 to 30 minutes

    c. Separate the clot by "rimming" with a wooden applicator stick around the inside of the tube

    d. Blood tubes are counterbalanced and centrifuged for 10 minutes at 2000 to 3000 rpm

      (1) Centrifuge as soon as possible and transfer the serum or plasma to chemically clean and properly labeled test tubes

    e. Several types of blood tubes and devices are designed to facilitate serum separation

    f. Serum is carefully pipetted or poured off into a suitable container and labeled

    g. Serum may be refrigerated or frozen; freezing may affect some test results

    h. Quality of serum

      (1) Lipemic serum: cloudy, excessive lipids, often due to diet, metabolic disease

      (2) Hemolytic serum: pink to reddish tint; caused by damage to red blood cells, either physiological or iatrogenic

      (3) Icteric serum: yellow tinge; indicative of liver disease

    i. Samples for whole blood or plasma should be collected with an anticoagulant. If plasma is used, be sure that the anticoagulant chosen does not interfere with the tests requested

    j. Types of anticoagulants include

      (1) Heparin: available in sodium, potassium, lithium, and ammonium salts

        (a) Good choice for plasma samples because there is little interference with chemical assays; use at 20 units/mL of blood

    k. Ethylenediaminetetraacetic acid (EDTA): anticoagulant of choice for hematological tests because it has little effect on morphology

      (1) Should not be used for chemical assays of plasma

    l. Sodium fluoride: a glucose preservative with some anticoagulant properties

    m. Samples should be analyzed immediately

      (1) When this is not possible, samples should be refrigerated until tests can be performed (return to room temperature before testing)

      (2) Collect sufficient sample for the tests requested

    n. Each laboratory should establish a set of normal values that will reflect test procedures and conditions used

## KIDNEY FUNCTION ▰▰▰▰▰▰▰

More than 75% of the glomeruli of both kidneys must be nonfunctional before serum chemistry changes occur. The nephron parts are so closely related that malfunction in one area will eventually affect another.

### Creatinine

I. A byproduct of muscle metabolism that is produced at a constant rate and filtered out almost entirely by the glomeruli

A. A constant small amount is produced daily

II. Increased serum creatinine levels are seen when there is a lack of functional glomeruli

III. Serum creatinine concentrations are influenced by

A. Fluid and hydration levels

B. Prerenal factors, such as shock

C. Postrenal factors, such as bladder and urethral obstructions

IV. Used to evaluate glomerular function

V. Sample required

A. Serum or plasma may be used

B. Hemolysis does not influence the results

C. Bilirubinemia will cause false increases

### Urea (Urea Nitrogen)

I. Urea is an end product of protein metabolism and is excreted primarily by the kidneys

A. Up to 40% is reabsorbed by the tubules for reexcretion

B. Rate of reabsorption is inversely proportional to the amount of urine output

II. Evaluates glomerular filtration and function

III. Nonrenal causes of increased serum urea nitrogen include
   A. The amount of protein ingested and absorbed
   B. Fever
   C. Corticosteroids

IV. Levels are increased in renal insufficiency

V. Etiology of increased levels include
   A. Prerenal factors, such as shock and dehydration
   B. Postrenal factors, such as obstruction in the ureters, bladder, or urethra

VI. May be decreased in anorexia, liver disease, tubular injury

VII. Sample required
   A. Serum preferred
   B. Plasma should not be collected with ammonium oxalate
      1. False increases will be produced
   C. Plasma should not be collected with fluoride
      1. Decreases will be produced
   D. Samples should be nonlipemic
   E. It is recommended to fast the animal for 18 hours before testing
   F. Serum or plasma should be tested as soon as possible because bacterial contamination will reduce the amount of urea in the sample

### Water Deprivation/Urine Concentration Tests

I. The patient is gradually deprived of water over 3 to 5 days until there is a stimulus for endogenous antidiuretic hormone (ADH) release
   A. This usually occurs at about 5% weight loss

II. If sufficient ADH, specific gravity of normal urine concentration is 1.025

III. Failure to concentrate urine over the duration of the test is indicative of insufficient ADH or tubular dysfunction

IV. This test should never be performed on animals that are dehydrated or have increased serum urea

## PANCREATIC FUNCTION ▬▬▬▬▬

The pancreas has endocrine and exocrine functions. Pancreatic endocrine function involves the production of glucagon and insulin. Diabetes mellitus, or a deficiency of insulin resulting in hyperglycemia, is the most common endocrine disorder of the pancreas. Pancreatic exocrine function involves the production of lipase, amylase, and trypsin. Most pancreatic disturbances occur in the exocrine function of the pancreas. Dogs seem to have a greater incidence than cats.

### Urine Glucose

I. Glycosuria (glucosuria) exists when blood glucose levels exceed the renal threshold for absorption of glucose in the proximal convoluted tubules

II. A diagnosis of diabetes mellitus is not made unless glycosuria accompanies hyperglycemia

III. Clinitest tablets (Ames) are not specific for glucose and will give a positive reaction with any reducing sugars
   A. This is considered a screening test only

IV. Reagent sticks such as Clinistix, Chemstrip, and others are specific for measuring glucose
   A. These sticks use glucose oxidase, peroxidase, and a color indicator

V. False-positive test outcomes in urine may result from
   A. Ascorbic acid
   B. Morphine
   C. Salicylates
   D. Penicillin
   E. Tetracycline
   F. Intravenous fluids containing glucose
   G. General anesthetics, etc.

VI. Sample required
   A. Freshly voided, morning sample

### Serum/Plasma Glucose

I. Most test procedures use glucose oxidase, which is specific for measuring glucose in samples

II. Hyperglycemia may result from
   A. Diabetes mellitus
   B. Several nonpancreatic causes such as stress and hyperadrenocorticism (Cushing's disease)

III. Hypoglycemia may result from
   A. Malabsorption
   B. Severe liver disease
   C. Prolonged contact of the serum or plasma with the cellular component of the blood

IV. Glucose tolerance tests may be used to determine how well an animal is able to utilize carbohydrates

V. Sample required
   A. Serum is preferable
      1. Sodium fluoride may be used if the plasma cannot be removed from the cells immediately
      2. It is essential to collect and treat the sample properly to obtain meaningful results
   B. Centrifuge sample immediately
      1. Remove plasma or serum and transfer to another test tube

VI. Blood cells will continue to use glucose at a rate of 7% to 10% per hour if allowed to remain in contact with the serum or plasma

VII. A fasting sample is preferred, 16 to 24 hours in dogs and cats

VIII. Ruminants should not be fasted

### Serum Amylase

I. Amylase acts to break down starches and glycogen

II. Increased serum amylase levels are seen in
  A. Acute, chronic, and obstructive pancreatitis
  B. Hyperadrenocorticism
  C. Liver disease
  D. Upper gastrointestinal inflammation or obstruction
    1. Renal failure
III. Animals have a greater serum amylase activity level than humans (10 times greater in the dog and cat) so it is recommended to dilute the serum with normal saline before testing if using tests designed for human samples
IV. Amyloclastic test: should be used for dogs because maltose does not influence the results
V. Amylase concentrations are not considered useful in cats
VI. Sample required
  A. Nonlipemic serum or heparinized plasma
  B. Hemolysis may elevate the values

## Serum Lipase

I. Lipase breaks down the long-chain fatty acids of lipids into fatty acids and alcohols
II. Lipase is usually in low levels in serum but serum levels increase in cases of pancreatitis (chronic and acute)
III. Increased serum lipase is also seen in
  A. Renal failure
  B. Hyperadrenocorticism
  C. Dexamethasone treatment
  D. Bile tract disease
IV. Manual methods for measuring lipase are cumbersome, but with the newer colorimetric and new dry chemistry kits, it is easier to evaluate serum lipase levels
V. It is recommended to perform serum amylase and lipase tests on patients suspected of having acute pancreatitis
VI. Some cats with pancreatitis do not have elevated serum lipase levels
VII. Sample required
  A. Nonhemolyzed, nonlipemic serum or heparinized plasma

## Trypsinlike Immunoreactivity

I. Trypsinlike immunoreactivity (TLI) on serum
  A. Considered the test of choice
    1. A highly specific and sensitive assay for exocrine pancreatic insufficiency in dogs
  B. Trypsinogen, a trypsinlike substance, is synthesized in the pancreas and normally released in trace amounts into the circulation
    1. The amount of this hormone detected by ligand assay techniques can be used to determine if the animal has exocrine pancreatic insufficiency (EPI)
  C. Suspect animals are fasted for 12 hours; serum is collected and sent away for analysis
    1. Normal TLI for the dog is 5.2 to 35 µg/L

    2. Dogs with EPI have levels less than 2.5 µg/L
  D. EPI may result from chronic pancreatitis, juvenile atrophy, and pancreatic hypoplasia
    1. Lack of functional tissue leads to maldigestion of food because inadequate amounts of lipase, trypsin, and amylase can be produced
  E. This condition is a common cause of malabsorption in dogs but rarely occurs in cats

## LIVER FUNCTION

No one test is totally satisfactory for determining the presence or absence of liver disease. A liver profile is usually ordered, and other special tests can be done as well. Seventy percent of the liver is nonfunctional before serum chemistry changes are noted.

## Bilirubin

I. Bilirubin is produced by the metabolism of heme by the mononuclear phagocytic system (formerly called the reticuloendothelial system)
II. Hyperbilirubinemia refers to increased serum bilirubin levels
  A. Hyperbilirubinemia can cause jaundice
III. Conjugated and unconjugated forms of bilirubin are found normally in serum or plasma
  A. The unconjugated or initial form of bilirubin is lipid soluble, bound to serum proteins, and carried to the liver to be conjugated
  B. The conjugated form is found mainly as glucuronic acid, which is water soluble and more readily excreted from the body via the biliary system to the intestines and kidney
    1. Some is "regurgitated" back into the liver and circulatory system
    2. The bile secretes the remainder in conjugated form to the intestines
  C. The conjugated form is unbound to serum proteins, so it can pass into the urine through the glomerulus
IV. Increases in the total amount of bilirubin are significant
V. Total bilirubin and conjugated (direct form) bilirubin are measured
  A. The amount of unconjugated bilirubin is determined by subtraction
VI. Bilirubin measured in urine is always the conjugated form, unless there is renal damage
VII. Increased unconjugated serum bilirubin levels indicate prehepatic jaundice, an inability of the liver cells to take up unconjugated bilirubin, or an inability to conjugate the bilirubin within the liver cells
VIII. Prehepatic jaundice is due to moderate to severe intravascular hemolysis and will be accompanied by a decreased hematocrit

A. In cattle, most hyperbilirubinemia is caused by hemolysis
   1. Unfortunately, serum bilirubin levels rarely increase sufficiently to aid in diagnosis
IX. Increased serum conjugated bilirubin levels are seen with hepatic jaundice or cholestasis (posthepatic jaundice)
X. A more marked rise in conjugated bilirubin is noted with posthepatic jaundice
XI. Some dogs have a lower renal threshold for bilirubin
   A. Bilirubin in the urine is considered a sensitive indicator of liver disease in dogs
   B. Cat, pig, sheep, and horse do not normally have bilirubin in their urine
   C. Occasionally, normal cattle will exhibit biliuria
XII. Horses will have increased unconjugated serum bilirubin in prehepatic and hepatic conditions
   A. Increased unconjugated levels also will be seen in many nonhepatic diseases (cardiac insufficiency, constipation, colic)
   B. Unconjugated and conjugated serum bilirubin levels increase after fasting
XIII. In cattle, sheep, goat, and pig
   A. Even in severe liver diseases, only slight increases in total bilirubin will be noted
   B. Most increased total bilirubin levels are due to hemolytic disorders; thus serum bilirubin measurements are not useful indicators of liver disease
XIV. Most testing methods for serum contain diazo reagent, which reacts specifically with bilirubin
   A. Ictotest tablets contain diazo reagent and measure bilirubin in urine. This test
      1. Is highly specific
      2. Is sensitive to small amounts of bilirubin
      3. Rarely produces false-positive results
      4. May be semiquantitative with serial dilutions of the urine
   B. Reagent strips
      1. Examples: Ictostix, Multistix use diazo reagent
      2. Considered less sensitive to bilirubin in urine than Ictotest
XV. False-positive results are caused by some medications
XVI. Samples required
   A. Nonlipemic, nonhemolyzed serum or plasma
   B. Remove serum or plasma from the clot or cells within 3 hours
   C. Store samples in the dark, because up to 50% bilirubin will be lost in the first hour of collection if left in light
   D. Samples can be refrigerated or frozen
   E. Freshly collected urine must be tested immediately for bilirubin

## Urine Urobilinogen

I. In small animals other than cats and dogs, the results are not as useful in pinpointing liver problems; testing is not routine
II. In humans and dogs, the amount of urine urobilinogen will increase in hepatocellular disease and decrease with obstructive problems
III. No urobilinogen or a decreased amount is a common finding in normal dogs
IV. Sample required
   A. Freshly voided urine sample
   B. In urine left sitting out, urobilinogen is converted to urobilin, which cannot be detected with tests used for urobilinogen

## Total Serum/Plasma Proteins

I. Proteins in serum samples are easily subjected to denaturation from heat, exposure to strong acids or bases, enzymatic action, exposure to urea and other substances, and ultraviolet (UV) light
II. Total serum proteins (TSPs) and serum albumin are measured, and the serum globulins are determined by subtraction
III. Levels are affected by
   A. Altered rates of protein synthesis in the liver
   B. Altered breakdown or excretion of proteins
   C. Dehydration or overhydration
   D. Altered distribution of proteins in the body
IV. Serum protein indicates the hydration level in the animal
   A. Animals that are in shock or overhydrated will have decreased serum protein
   B. Dehydrated animal will have increased serum protein
V. TSP also can be used as a guide to the nutritional status of an animal
VI. Goldberg refractometer (American Optical Company, Greenwich, Conn) is most commonly used to measure TSP in clinics
   A. Refractometer is considered a good screening method
   B. Results obtained are affected by electrolytes, lipids, hemolysis products, urea, and glucose in the sample
   C. It is essential to have a clear sample
VII. Wet and dry chemistry methods for measuring protein use the biuret method for measuring serum proteins
VIII. Total dye binding is used in an automated serum analyzer to also measure total serum proteins
IX. Sample required
   A. Nonhemolyzed, nonlipemic serum or plasma collected with EDTA or heparin
   B. Serum gives slightly lower values

C. Avoid contact with detergents and UV light, which will denature the proteins

## Albumin

I. Serum albumin and globulin levels change in response to several diseases
II. As a general rule, when changes occur, the albumin level decreases, whereas the globulin level increases to maintain a constant TSP level
III. Globulin fraction can be divided into subfractions
IV. TSP and albumin are measured, and the globulin fraction can be obtained by subtracting the smaller from the larger value
V. Albumin dye binding is used to measure serum albumin levels
VI. Increases in this fraction are rare; seen sometimes in shock
VII. Decreased albumin may occur in
  A. Chronic liver disease
  B. Starvation/malnutrition
  D. Malabsorption
  E. Enteritis, colitis, parasites
  F. Pregnancy and lactation
  G. Prolonged fever
  H. Uncontrolled diabetes
  I. Trauma
  J. Nephritis, nephrosis
  K. Ascites, protein losing enteropathy
  L. Blood loss

## Globulins

I. Globulin fractions, along with albumin, can be separated by electrophoresis
  A. The globulin fraction of serum proteins is quite complex and can be subdivided into α-globulins, β-globulins, and γ-globulins
II. Fibrinogen is one of the coagulation factors and is used in the clotting process
  A. Fibrinogen is part of the globulin fraction and is sometimes measured separately
    1. Plasma must be used
    2. This protein makes up about 4 g/L of the total plasma protein fraction
III. Electrophoresis shows relative increases and decreases in the different fractions
  A. These can be related to specific diseases
IV. Different species show different normal electrophoretic patterns
V. In general, increases in globulins may be seen with
  A. Inflammation/infections
  B. Antigenic stimulation
  C. Neoplasia or abnormal immunoglobulin production
VI. Globulin fraction usually increases when albumin decreases

## Albumin-Globulin Ratio (A:G)

I. Is calculated by dividing the serum albumin results by the globulin results
II. Should be evaluated along with the protein profile
III. May provide early indication of abnormal protein profile
IV. In dogs, horses, and sheep the A:G is > 1; in cattle, pigs, and cats the A:G ratio is ≤1

## Enzymes

Biological enzymes are classified as plasma/serum specific (normally present in plasma/serum) and non–plasma/serum specific
I. Non–plasma specific enzymes
  A. Assayed during clinical diagnosis, because these enzymes increase in concentration in serum if
    1. Tissue cells are destroyed
    2. There is an increase in their production
    3. There is obstruction of their excretory route
    4. There is a decrease in circulation
  B. Test kits should contain all required substrates, coenzymes, and cofactors
  C. It is important to perform tests at the temperature indicated in the instructions
    1. This is usually 30° C
  D. It is important to handle samples carefully, paying careful consideration to any special requirements for anticoagulants and separation
  E. Historically there have been many units of measurement used for measuring the same enzymes (e.g., serum alkaline phosphatase has been measured in Bodansky units, Bessey-Lowry-Brock units, King-Armstrong units, and others)
    1. The international unit (IU) of measurement for enzyme assays replaces the old units
      a. IU is the amount of enzyme that will catalyze the conversion of one micromole of substrate per minute
    2. It is advisable for labs to establish their own normal values
II. ALT
  A. Also known as alanine aminotransferase or alanine transaminase
    1. Formerly called SGPT (serum glutamic pyruvic transaminase)
  B. Found in large amounts in the hepatocytes of dog, cat, and primate
    1. Considered a useful and specific test for liver function in these species
  C. This enzyme is not present in large enough amounts in liver cells of horse, ruminant, or pig to be of diagnostic significance
  D. Serum ALT increases if hepatocytes are damaged, but the damage may not necessarily be irreversible

1. The increase is due to an isolated incident if the initial ALT is increased but declines on subsequent serial tests
2. If ALT remains elevated or increases, the cause is chronic

E. Some drugs can increase ALT in dog but not in cat

F. Sample required
   1. Nonhemolyzed, nonlipemic serum, or plasma collected with EDTA or sodium citrate
   2. Do not freeze

III. AST
   A. Also known as aspartate aminotransferase or aspartate transaminase
      1. Formerly called SGOT (serum glutamic-oxaloacetic transaminase)
   B. Present in all tissues of the body, especially in cardiac muscle, skeletal muscle, and the liver
      1. Not an organ-specific enzyme
   C. AST assays should be run with other enzyme assays, especially ALT, when evaluating liver function
   D. For species in which ALT is not useful, AST is sometimes used as an alternative to ALT in diagnosing liver disease
      1. In this case other causes of increased AST should be ruled out before focusing on the liver
   E. Horse has higher normal AST values than other species
      1. Test method used should be specific for this species
      2. Samples should be diluted before assaying
   F. AST should be evaluated with ALT for dog and cat
      1. Increased ALT with normal to mildly elevated AST may indicate reversible liver damage
      2. Marked elevations in ALT and AST indicate hepatocellular necrosis
      3. Increased AST with normal ALT may indicate that the source of AST is not liver
   G. Samples required
      1. Nonhemolyzed, nonlipemic serum or plasma
      2. Specimen should be centrifuged and removed from the cells immediately, because AST will leak out of the red blood cells into the serum or plasma

IV. AP
   A. Alkaline phosphatase
   B. Present in almost all tissues of the body, especially in liver and bone
      1. Used as an indication of intrahepatic or posthepatic cholestasis
   C. Increases in AP are due to increased production of the enzyme rather than reduced excretion of the enzyme through the bile system
      1. This enzyme is normally present in serum in small amounts
   D. Increased AP is common in young animals, because of the increased rate of bone growth
   E. Increased AP in adult animals may be seen with bone injury or in obstructive liver disease
   F. Glucocorticoids and some anticonvulsant drugs will markedly increase AP for up to 2 weeks after administration
   G. Samples required
      1. Serum or heparinized plasma

V. LDH
   A. Lactate dehydrogenase
   B. Found in most tissues of the body, including liver, muscle, and red blood cells
   C. Elevations in serum are considered nonspecific because they may be due to damage or necrosis of any tissues containing this enzyme
   D. Samples required
      1. Serum or plasma collected with any anticoagulant other than EDTA or the oxalates

VI. GGT
   A. γ-Glutamyltransferase
   B. Found in liver, pancreas, and kidney
   C. Elevations in serum usually caused by liver source
      1. GGT is elevated primarily in cholestasis but will be increased in all liver diseases
      2. In small animals, increased GGT will usually be accompanied by increased ALT
      3. GGT increase is a good indicator for small animal fatty liver disease
      4. Some medications also will cause an increase in GGT

VII. SD
   A. Sorbitol dehydrogenase
   B. Found primarily in liver cells; will be elevated in serum in cases of hepatocellular damage or necrosis
   C. Sometimes used in large animals to replace ALT when diagnosing liver disease
   D. Very unstable
      1. Much of the activity is lost within 8 hours of sample collection
      2. This is a limiting factor if samples are being processed by out-of-clinic laboratories

## Bile Acids

I. Formed in the liver, secreted into the bile, and stored in the gallbladder between meals
II. Secreted into the intestinal tract where they aid in fat absorption and digestion
III. Most reabsorbed in the ileum, filtered from the blood by the liver, and recycled
   A. Mechanism is so efficient that normally serum values are very low
      1. Normal resting values: cat, 5 μmol/L; dog, 9 μmol/L

2. Two-hour postprandial values: cat, 10 µmol/L; dog, 30 µmol/L
IV. Increased serum bile acid levels are noted in all forms of liver disease, because the liver cannot clear the acids from the blood
V. Decreased serum bile acid levels are noted in delayed gastric emptying and ileal disease
VI. Sample required
  A. Serum

## ELECTROLYTES AND MINERALS ▬▬▬
### General Information

I. Sodium, potassium, chloride, and bicarbonate are the four electrolytes in plasma
II. Minerals of importance are calcium, phosphate, and magnesium
  A. These two groups are often simply called electrolytes
  B. These are the anions (negatively charged ions) and cations (positively charged ions) found in the fluids of all animals
III. Electrolytes help to maintain water balance, osmotic pressure, and normal muscular and nervous functions; act as activators for enzyme reactions; and function in acid-base balance

### Serum Sodium

I. Most abundant extracellular cation that plays a major role in the distribution of water and the maintenance of osmotic pressure of fluids in the body
  A. If sodium is retained, water is retained
II. Hypernatremia, or increased serum sodium, is rare unless the animal is deprived of water
III. Hyponatremia, or decreased serum sodium, is quite common and is seen in such conditions as renal failure, vomiting, or diarrhea; use of diuretics; excessive ADH; congestive heart failure; water toxicity; or excessive administration of fluids
IV. Sample required
  A. Nonhemolyzed serum is preferred
  B. Plasma collected with lithium or ammonium heparin is also acceptable
  C. Remove from cells as soon as possible

### Serum Potassium

I. Cation that is 90% intracellular
  A. Serum levels are so low that measurement of serum potassium does not give much information about the body's potassium levels
II. Hyperkalemia, or increased serum potassium, will be seen in adrenal cortical hypofunction, acidosis, or late-stage renal failure
III. Hypokalemia, or decreased serum potassium, will be seen in alkalosis, insulin therapy, or excess fluid loss due to diuretics, vomiting, and diarrhea

IV. Samples required
  A. Nonhemolyzed serum or heparinized plasma (plasma preferred)
  B. Remove from the cells as soon as possible
    1. Especially important in cattle and horse, which have sufficient potassium in their red blood cells to alter serum chemistry results

### Serum Chloride

I. It is the most abundant extracellular anion
  A. Chloride plays an important role in water and electrolyte balance and osmotic pressure
    1. Concentration is regulated by the kidneys
  B. There is a close relationship between sodium and chloride levels
    1. Hyperchloremia is increased serum chloride
      a. May be due to metabolic acidosis or renal tubular acidosis
    2. Hypochloremia is decreased serum chloride
      a. May be due to excessive vomiting, anorexia, malnutrition, or diabetes insipidus, or may accompany hypokalemia
II. Samples required
  A. Nonhemolyzed serum preferred
  B. Also heparinized plasma
  C. Remove serum from cells as soon as possible

### Serum Calcium

I. About 99% of the body's calcium is in bone
II. Remaining calcium
  A. Maintains neuromuscular excitability and tone
  B. Acts as an enzyme activator
  C. Is important in coagulation
  D. Helps in transport of inorganic ions across cell membranes
III. Calcium and phosphorous levels are closely related and have an inverse relationship
  A. Both are regulated by parathyroid hormone (PTH), calcitonin, and vitamin D
IV. Serum calcium levels vary with serum protein and serum albumin levels
  A. These should be evaluated with serum calcium
V. Hypercalcemia, or increased serum calcium, seen in
  A. Pseudohyperparathyroidism
  B. Hyperparathyroidism
  C. Excessive vitamin D intake
  D. Bony metastases
VI. Hypocalcemia or decreased serum calcium may be seen in
  A. Malabsorption
  B. Eclampsia
  C. Pancreatic necrosis
  D. Hypoalbuminemia
  E. Gastrointestinal stasis or blockage in ruminants

F. Postparturient lactation in cow, bitch, ewe, and mare

G. Hypoparathyroidism

VII. Sample required

    A. Nonhemolyzed serum or heparinized plasma

## Serum Phosphorus

I. Most of the body's phosphorus (80%) is found in bone

    A. Remaining 20% functions in the body in carbohydrate metabolism and energy storage, release, and transfer; phosphorus is also incorporated into nucleic acids

II. Serum calcium and serum phosphorous levels are closely related and have an inverse relationship

III. PTH regulates serum phosphorus

IV. Hyperphosphatemia, or increased serum inorganic phosphorus, may be seen in renal failure, anuria, excessive vitamin D intake, ethylene glycol poisoning, and hypoparathyroidism

V. Hypophosphatemia, or decreased serum inorganic phosphorus, may occur in

    A. Primary hyperparathyroidism

    B. Malabsorption

    C. Inadequate intake

    D. Hyperinsulinism

    E. Diabetes mellitus

    F. Lymphosarcoma

    G. Hyperadrenocorticism

VI. Sample required

    A. Nonhemolyzed serum or heparinized plasma

    B. Remove serum or plasma from the cells as soon as possible

## Serum Magnesium

I. Magnesium (cation) is found in all body tissues, and its level is closely related to calcium and phosphorus levels

II. Imbalance in the calcium-magnesium ratio can lead to muscle tetany in cattle and sheep

III. Sometimes calcium and magnesium have a reciprocal relationship; other times they have a direct relationship

IV. Sample required

    A. Nonhemolyzed serum or plasma

## MEASUREMENT OF ELECTROLYTES

I. Flame photometry: serum sodium and serum potassium

II. Ion-selective electrodes: all of the electrolytes

III. Coulometric methods: serum chloride

IV. Atomic absorption: serum calcium, serum magnesium

V. Colorimetric methods: serum calcium, serum phosphorus

## THYROID FUNCTION

### Thyroid Hormone: $T_4$

I. Thyroxine ($T_4$)

    A. Total $T_4$ measurement provides a baseline measure of resting thyroid hormone concentration

        1. Assessment for hyperthyroidism or hypothyroidism

        2. $T_4$ levels may be low because of diseases not of thyroid origin; a single low result does not necessarily indicate hypothyroidism

        3. $T_4$ levels in cats fluctuate from day to day; a single low test result should not be used to rule out hyperthyroidism

II. Sample required

    A. Serum collected in SST

### Free Thyroid Hormone ($FT_4$) by Dialysis

I. Measures the portion of $T_4$ that is not bound to protein

    A. Useful in diagnosis of hyperthyroidism in cats where $T_4$ levels are normal or only slightly elevated

    B. $FT_4$ level not as influenced as $T_4$ level by medications and diseases that might cause false low $T_4$ results

II. Sample required

    A. Serum collected in SST

### Canine Thyroid Stimulating Hormone

I. Thyroid stimulating hormone is responsible for stimulating the synthesis of thyroid hormones in the thyroid gland

    A. Canine thyroid stimulating hormone (cTSH), when measured along with $FT_4$ level, can provide diagnostic accuracy for hypothyroidism. cTSH will be elevated and $FT_4$ will be decreased

II. Sample required

    A. Serum

### Serum Cholesterol

I. Mostly derived from liver synthesis; also from the adrenal cortex, ovaries, testes, and intestinal epithelium

II. Increases usually associated with hypothyroidism

    A. Will also occur with lipemia

    B. Associated with diabetes mellitus, hyperadrenocorticism, nephrotic syndrome, some liver diseases, bile duct obstruction, and pregnancy

III. Not a liver-specific test

IV. Sample required

    A. Nonhemolyzed; 12-hour fast is recommended; fluoride and oxalate anticoagulants may cause false increases in enzymatic test results

**Box 6-1** Summary of Function Tests

**LIVER FUNCTION TESTS**
AST (aspartate aminotransferase)
ALT (alanine aminotransferase)
AP (alkaline phosphatase)
Total serum bilirubin
Direct/conjugated bilirubin
Bile acids
Glucose
Cholesterol
Urine bilirubin
Urine urobilinogen
Total serum protein
Serum albumin
Electrophoresis: protein fractionation
Plasma fibrinogen
Hematology

**KIDNEY FUNCTION TESTS**
Serum creatinine
Blood urea nitrogen
Urine concentration/water deprivation tests
Endogenous creatinine clearance tests
Serum electrolytes and minerals: sodium, potassium,
    calcium, phosphorus, magnesium, chloride
Hematology

**PANCREATIC FUNCTION TESTS**

*Endocrine Function*
Serum glucose
Urinalysis; urine glucose
Glucose tolerance tests

*Exocrine Function*
Serum amylase
Serum lipase
Trypsinlike immunoreactivity assay

**TESTS FOR MUSCLE DISEASE**
Creatine kinase
AST
LDH

**DIGESTIVE TRACT TESTS**
Serum amylase
Serum lipase
Fecal trypsin
Examine feces for parasites, fat, starch, muscle fibers
Plasma turbidity test
Glucose tolerance test
Total serum protein
Hematology
Xylose absorption test
Serum folate
Serum $B_{12}$

**ENDOCRINE FUNCTION TESTS**

*Parathyroid Gland*
Parathormone (PTH)
Serum and urine calcium
Serum and urine phosphorus
Serum alkaline phosphatase

*Thyroid Gland*
Thyroxine: total serum $T_4$
Free $T_4$ by equilibrium dialysis
Canine thyroid stimulating hormone
Serum cholesterol
Serum protein

**ADRENAL CORTEX FUNCTION TESTS**
Serum glucose
Serum cholesterol
Alkaline phosphatase
Serum sodium
Serum potassium
Leukogram

**ELECTROLYTES**
Serum sodium
Serum potassium
Serum chloride

**MINERALS**
Serum calcium
Serum phosphorus
Serum magnesium

**Table 6-1**   Biochemistry reference intervals

|  | Unit | Canine | Feline | Bovine | Equine | Porcine |
|---|---|---|---|---|---|---|
| Albumin | g/L | 29-43 | 30-44 | 34-43 | 30-37 | 27-39 |
| Alkaline phosphatase | U/L | 22-143 | 16-113 | 33-114 | 119-329 | 0-500 |
| Alkaline transaminase | U/L | 19-107 | 31-105 | — | — | — |
| Amylase | U/L | 299-947 | 482-1145 | — | — | — |
| AST | U/L | — | — | 56-176 | 259-595 | — |
| Total bilirubin | μmol/L | 0-4 | 0-3 | 0-5 | 21-57 | 0-4 |
| Calcium | mmol/L | 2.30-2.80 | 2.22-2.78 | 2.10-2.70 | 2.75-3.25 | 1.80-2.90 |
| Chloride | mmol/L | 104-119 | 114-123 | 91-103 | 95-104 | 99-105 |
| Cholesterol | mmol/L | 3.60-10.20 | 2.00-12.00 | 2.90-8.00 | 1.70-2.70 | 2.0-5.0 |
| Creatinine | μmol/L | 20-150 | 50-190 | 40-80 | 80-130 | 90-240 |
| Glucose | mmol/L | 3.3-7.3 | 4.4-7.7 | 2.1-3.8 | 3.7-6.7 | 3.6-5.3 |
| Lipase | U/L | 60-848 | 29-77 | — | — | — |
| Magnesium | mmol/L | 0.70-1.00 | 0.80-1.10 | 0.85-1.20 | 0.6-1.00 | 0.8-1.6 |
| Phosphorus | mmol/L | 0.90-1.85 | 0.80-2.29 | 1.46-2.83 | 0.73-1.71 | 1.6-3.4 |
| Protein | g/L | 55-74 | 66-84 | 70-94 | 58-75 | 61-81 |
| Potassium | mmol/L | 3.8-5.4 | 3.6-5.2 | 3.7-5.4 | 3.1-4.3 | 4.7-7.1 |
| Sodium | mmol/L | 140-154 | 147-157 | 134-149 | 136-144 | 140-150 |
| Urea | mmol/L | 3.5-9.0 | 6.0-12.0 | 3.0-8.3 | 4.2-8.9 | 3.0-8.5 |

Courtesy the Animal Health Laboratory, Laboratory Services Division, University of Guelph, Guelph, Ontario, Canada.
Results vary from laboratory to laboratory and depend on the method used, as well as the animal's breed, sex, age, and environment.

**Table 6-2**   Biochemical reference values: conventional units

|  | Cattle | Sheep | Goat | Swine | Horse | Dog | Cat |
|---|---|---|---|---|---|---|---|
| Alanine aminotransferase (ALT; SGPT) (U/L) | — | — | — | — | — | 17-69 | 34-55 |
| Alkaline phosphatase (AP; SAP) (U/L) | 41-94 | 0-140 | 42-775 | — | 83-283 | 5-73 | 14-25 |
| Amylase (U/L) | — | — | — | — | 9-34 | 700-1700 | 1000-1700 |
| Aspartate aminotransferase (AST; SGOT) (U/L) | 42-98 | 31-111 | 67-117 | — | 153-411 | 12-37 | 11-29 |
| Bile acids (μg/mL) | — | — | — | — | 0-5 | 0-5 | 0-5 |
| Bilirubin |  |  |  |  |  |  |  |
|   Total (mg/dL) | 0-1.9 | 0-0.4 | 0-0.1 | 0-0.2 | 0.2-6.0 | 0-0.4 | 0-0.5 |
|   Direct (mg/dL) | 0-0.4 | 0-0.3 | — | — | 0-0.4 | 0-0.1 | 0-0.1 |
| Calcium (mg/dL) | 8.0-10.5 | 11.5-13.0 | 8.5-10.2 | 11.0-11.3 | 11.2-13.8 | 8.7-11.8 | 9.2-11.9 |
| Chloride (mEq/L) | 95-110 | 98-110 | 99-110 | 100-105 | 98-110 | 99-110 | 117-123 |
| Cholesterol (mg/dL) | 39-177 | 40-58 | 80-130 | 117-119 | 46-177 | 117-345 | 100-165 |
| Creatine phosphokinase (CPK; CK) (U/L) | 66-220 | 0-330 | 108-211 | — | 92-307 | 12-292 | 0-540 |
| Creatinine (mg/dL) | 1.0-2.7 | 1.2-1.9 | — | 1.0-2.7 | 1.2-1.9 | 0.7-1.6 | 1.2-2.1 |
| Gamma glutamyltransferase (GGT) (U/L) | 13-32 | 35-67 | 43-71 | — | 11-44 | 0-11 | 0-1 |
| Glucose (mg/dL) | 35-55 | 30-65 | 58-76 | 65-95 | 60-100 | 55-102 | 55-114 |
| Iron (μg/dL) | 57-162 | 166-222 | — | 91-199 | 73-140 | 94-122 | 68-215 |
| Lipase (U/L) | — | — | — | — | 40-78 | 52-305 | — |
| Magnesium (mg/dL) | 1.2-3.5 | 1.9-2.5 | 2.8-3.6 | 1.9-3.9 | 1.8-2.5 | 1.5-2.4 | 1.9-2.7 |
| Phosphorus (mg/dL) | 4.0-7.0 | 4.0-7.0 | 7.5-12.3 | 4.0-11.0 | 3.1-5.6 | 2.8-7.6 | 4.6-7.1 |
| Potassium (mEq/L) | 3.9-5.8 | 4.8-5.9 | 3.5-6.7 | 4.7-7.1 | 3.0-5.0 | 3.7-5.6 | 4.0-4.5 |
| Sodium (mEq/L) | 132-152 | 145-160 | 142-155 | 140-150 | 132-150 | 137-149 | 147-156 |
| Sorbitol dehydrogenase (SDH) (U/L) | 18-46 | 14-41 | 35-80 | — | 0-15 | — | — |
| Triglycerides (mg/dL) | — | — | — | — | 5-55 | 10-140 | 30-100 |
| Urea nitrogen (mg/dL) | 6-27 | 8-20 | 15-33 | 8-24 | 10-20 | 7-21 | 18-34 |

**Table 6-2** Biochemical reference values: conventional units—cont'd

| | Cattle | Sheep | Goat | Swine | Horse | Dog | Cat |
|---|---|---|---|---|---|---|---|
| **Acid-base** | | | | | | | |
| Bicarbonate (mmol/L) | 20-30 | 21-28 | 26-30 | 18-27 | 23-32 | 17-24 | 17-24 |
| pH | 7.35-7.50 | 7.32-7.50 | — | — | 7.32-7.55 | 7.31-7.42 | 7.24-7.40 |
| $Pco_2$ (mm Hg) | 34-45 | — | — | — | 38-46 | — | — |
| **Proteins** | | | | | | | |
| Total protein (g/dL) | 5.7-8.1 | 6.0-7.9 | 5.9-7.4 | 7.9-8.9 | 6.0-7.7 | 5.4-7.1 | 5.4-7.8 |
| Albumin (g/dL) | 2.1-3.6 | 2.4-3.0 | 2.7-3.9 | 1.8-3.3 | 2.9-3.8 | 2.6-3.3 | 2.1-3.3 |
| $\alpha_1$-Globulin (g/dL) | 0.7-1.2 | 0.3-0.6 | 0.5-0.7 | 0.3-0.4 | 0.7-1.3 | 0.2-0.5 | 0.2-1.1 |
| $\alpha_2$-Globulin (g/dL) | — | 0.3-0.6 | — | 1.3-1.5 | 0.7-1.3 | 0.3-1.1 | 0.4-0.9 |
| $\beta_1$-Globulin (g/dL) | 0.6-1.2 | 1.1-2.6 | 0.7-1.2 | 0.1-0.3 | 0.4-1.2 | 0.7-1.3 | 0.3-0.9 |
| $\beta_2$-Globulin (g/dL) | — | — | 0.3-0.6 | 1.3-1.7 | — | 0.6-1.4 | 0.6-1.0 |
| $\gamma_1$-Globulin (g/dL) | 1.6-3.2 | 0.9-3.3 | 0.9-3.0 | 2.2-2.5 | 0.9-1.5 | 0.5-1.3 | 0.3-2.5 |
| $\gamma_2$-Globulin (g/dL) | — | — | — | — | — | 0.4-0.9 | 1.4-1.9 |

Updated from first edition by B.W. Parry, University of Melbourne, Werribee, Victoria, Australia.
Reproduced from Blood DC, Studdert VP: *Saunders comprehensive veterinary dictionary*, ed 2, Philadelphia, 1999, Saunders.
All enzymes measured at 37° C. Reference values may be influenced by the method of measurement and by the animal's breed, sex, age, and environment. Hence these values are guidelines only.

**Table 6-3** Conversion factors for biochemistry data

| Analyte | Conventional unit | Multiplication factor | SI unit | Multiplication factor | Conventional unit |
|---|---|---|---|---|---|
| Alanine aminotransferase | U/L | 1 | U/L | 1 | U/L |
| Albumin | g/dL | 10 | g/L | 0.10 | g/dL |
| Alkaline phosphatase | U/L | 1 | U/L | 1 | U/L |
| Amylase | U/L | 1 | U/L | 1 | U/L |
| Aspartate aminotransferase | U/L | 1 | U/L | 1 | U/L |
| Bicarbonate | mEq/L | 1 | mmol/L | 1 | mEq/L |
| Bile acids | µg/mL | 2.547 | µmol/L | 0.3926 | µg/mL |
| Bilirubin | mg/dL | 17.10 | µmol/L | 0.058 | mg/dL |
| Calcium | mg/dL | 0.2495 | mmol/L | 4.008 | mg/dL |
| Chloride | mEq/L | 1 | mmol/L | 1 | mEq/L |
| Cholesterol | mg/dL | 0.02586 | mmol/L | 38.67 | mg/dL |
| Creatine (phospho)kinase | U/L | 1 | U/L | 1 | U/L |
| Creatinine | mg/dL | 88.4 | µmol/L | 0.011 | mg/dL |
| Gamma glutamyltransferase | U/L | 1 | U/L | 1 | U/L |
| Glucose | mg/dL | 0.0555 | mmol/L | 18.0 | mg/dL |
| Iron | µg/dL | 0.1791 | µmol/L | 5.583 | µg/dL |
| Lipase | U/L | 1 | U/L | 1 | U/L |
| Magnesium | mg/dL | 0.4114 | mmol/L | 2.431 | mg/dL |
| $Pco_2$ | mm Hg | 0.1333 | kPa | 7.502 | mm Hg |
| Phosphorus | mg/dL | 0.3229 | mmol/L | 3.097 | mg/dL |
| Potassium | mEq/L | 1 | mmol/L | 1 | mEq/L |
| Proteins | g/dL | 10 | g/L | 0.10 | g/dL |
| Sodium | mEq/L | 1 | mmol/L | 1 | mEq/L |
| Sorbitol dehydrogenase | U/L | 1 | U/L | 1 | U/L |
| Triglycerides | mg/dL | 0.01129 | mmol/L | 88.6 | mg/dL |
| Urea (nitrogen) | mg/dL | 0.3570 | mmol/L | 2.80 | mg/dL |

From Blood DC, Studdert VP: *Saunders comprehensive veterinary dictionary*, ed 2, Philadelphia, 1999, Saunders.

# Glossary

**amyloclastic test** Method of measuring serum amylase by measuring the disappearance of a starch substrate

**anion** Negatively charged ion

**anticoagulant** Chemical used to inhibit clotting of whole blood. The liquid portion of the sample harvested is plasma

**azotemia** Increased level of urea in blood samples

**bile** A fluid produced by the liver and stored in the gallbladder that aids in digestion. This substance is primarily composed of bile acids or salts, bile pigments, and cholesterol

**cation** Positively charged ion

**Cushing's syndrome** Hyperactivity of adrenal cortices secondary to excessive pituitary excretion of adrenocorticotropic hormone

**dry chemistry** Method of chemical analysis. All the reagents needed for a particular test are incorporated into a multilayered film slide. These special slides are used in automated analyzers

**electrolytes** Ions capable of carrying an electric charge

**electrophoresis** Separation of ionic solutes, such as serum proteins, based on their rates of migration in an applied electric field

**endogenous** Something produced within an organism or caused by something within an organism

**hemolysis** Destruction of red blood cells, causing release of hemoglobin

**hypercalcemia** Excess calcium in the blood

**hyperchloremia** Excess chloride in the blood

**hyperglycemia** Increased blood glucose level

**hyperkalemia** Excess potassium in the blood

**hypernatremia** Excess sodium in the blood

**hyperparathyroidism** Excessive activity of the parathyroid glands

**hyperphosphatemia** Excess phosphates in the blood

**hypocalcemia** Blood calcium level below normal

**hypochloremia** Abnormally low level of chloride in the blood

**hypoglycemia** Decreased blood glucose level

**hypokalemia** Abnormally low potassium level in the blood

**hyponatremia** Salt depletion or abnormally low level of sodium in the blood

**hypoparathyroidism** Underactive parathyroid glands

**hypophosphatemia** Blood phosphate levels below normal

**icterus** Jaundice; result of excess bilirubin in the blood

**lipemia** Excess lipids in the blood

**malabsorption** Impaired intestinal absorption of nutrients

**malassimilation** Gastrointestinal tract is unable to take up nutrients because of faulty digestion or impairment of the transport mechanisms across the intestinal mucosa

**metastasis** Growth of pathogenic organisms or abnormal cells distant from the primary site of development

**osmotic pressure** Hydrostatic pressure required to stop osmosis, which is the diffusion of molecules of a dilute solution passing through the walls of a semipermeable membrane into a more concentrated solution

**plasma** Liquid portion of blood in which proteins, cells, electrolytes, nutrients, and products of metabolism are suspended

**prehepatic** Before the liver

**radioimmunoassay** Technique that measures the rate of immune complex formation using radiolabeled isotopes

**saccharogenic test** Method for measuring serum amylase by measuring reducing sugars that are produced by amylase action

**serum** Liquid portion of blood that has been allowed to clot; contains all the same constituents as plasma except fibrinogen, which is consumed in the clotting process

**SST** Serum separator tubes

**steatorrhea** Large amounts of fat in the stool

# Review Questions

1 Serum creatinine levels can be influenced by
   a. Amount of protein in an animal's diet
   b. Lipemia
   c. Hemolysis
   d. How well the glomeruli are filtering

2 Serum samples collected for measurement of blood glucose levels
   a. Should ideally be collected right after an animal has eaten
   b. Should be collected using EDTA
   c. May be collected in SST (serum separator tubes) and used for other tests as well
   d. Are preferred over plasma samples because they are easier to collect

3 Which of the following is considered to be the best test for evaluating pancreatic function in dogs?
   a. Serum lipase levels
   b. Trypsinlike immunoreactivity
   c. Serum protease levels
   d. Bile acids

4 Serum or plasma samples destined for tests including total bilirubin levels should be
   a. Stored in a dark place
   b. Removed from the cells within three hours of collection
   c. Nonlipemic and nonhemolyzed
   d. All of the above

5 Calculation of the A:G ratio
   a. Is accomplished by dividing the serum albumin fraction by the globulin fraction
   b. Often assists with early detection of serum protein abnormalities
   c. Should be evaluated with the protein profile
   d. All of the above

6 Which of the following liver enzyme tests is considered a specific test for liver disease in dogs, cats, and primates only?
   a. AST
   b. ALT
   c. AP
   d. SD

**7** Which of the following statements regarding liver enzyme tests is not true?
   a. Most of these tests can be determined at room temperature
   b. Nonhemolyzed, nonlipemic samples are preferred
   c. Samples should be separated as soon as possible, because the levels of some of the chemicals will be altered if the serum or plasma remains with the cells
   d. Specific instructions for each test must be followed to ensure reliable results

**8** Which of the serum protein fractions rarely increases in a disease state?
   a. Albumin
   b. α-Globulins
   c. β-Globulins
   d. γ-Globulins

**9** Bile acids
   a. Are usually found in low levels in the bloodstream
   b. Will be increased in all forms of liver disease
   c. Are removed from circulating blood by the liver
   d. All of the above

**10** Accurate diagnosis of hypothyroidism in dogs is best achieved with measurements of
   a. cTSH and $T_4$ measurements
   b. $T_4$ and total $T_4$ measurements
   c. Serum cholesterol
   d. cTSH and serum cholesterol

**BIBLIOGRAPHY**

Bishop ML, Duben-Engelkirk JL, Fody EP, editors: *Clinical chemistry: principles, procedures, correlations*, ed 5, Philadelphia, 2004, Lippincott Williams & Wilkins.

Bistner S, Ford R, Raffe MR: *Kirk and Bistner's handbook of veterinary procedures and emergency treatment*, ed 7, Philadelphia, 2000, Saunders.

Burtis CA, Ashwood ER, editors: *Tietz fundamentals of clinical chemistry*, ed 5, Philadelphia, 2001, Saunders.

Fenner WR: *Quick reference to veterinary medicine*, ed 3, Ames, Iowa, 2000, Blackwell.

Hendrix CM, Sirois M, editors: *Laboratory procedures for veterinary technicians*, ed 5, St Louis, 2007, Mosby.

Kaneko JJ, Harvey JW, Bruss ML, editors: *Clinical biochemistry of domestic animals*, ed 5, New York, 1997, Academic Press.

Kaplan A, Szabo LL: *Clinical chemistry: interpretation and techniques*, ed 4, Philadelphia, 1994, Lippincott Williams & Wilkins.

Latimer KS, Mahaffey EA, Prasse KW: *Duncan and Prasse's veterinary laboratory medicine: clinical pathology*, ed 4, Ames, Iowa, 2003, Blackwell.

McCurnin DM, Bassert JM, editors: *Clinical textbook for veterinary technicians*, ed 6, St Louis, 2006, Saunders.

Simpson JW, Else RW: *Digestive disease in the dog and cat*, ed 2, London, 1996, Blackwell Scientific.

Sirois M, editor: *Principles and practice of veterinary technology*, ed 2, St Louis, 2004, Mosby.

Sirois M, editor: *Veterinary clinical laboratory procedures*, St Louis, 1995, Mosby.

## CHAPTER 7

# Virology

*Patricia L. Bell*

---

## OUTLINE

Composition and Control
Viral Infections
Nomenclature

Sampling Techniques
Collection of Specimens
Submission of Samples

In-Clinic Laboratory Testing of
Samples
Prevention

## LEARNING OUTCOMES

**After reading this chapter you should be able to:**

1. Describe the composition of a virus.
2. Describe the process of virus replication.
3. Describe, in general, different types of viral infections.
4. Describe sampling techniques, including the collection of specimens and submission of samples.
5. Describe various diagnostic testing procedures commonly performed in the clinic.
6. Explain common techniques for the prevention of contracting a virus or reducing the effects of viral diseases.

This chapter begins by reviewing the basic features of viruses, including their composition, control, and replication. The chapter also contains a brief summary that defines common methods of studying the collection, culturing, and submission of clinical specimens for diagnostic laboratory analysis and laboratory diagnostic techniques. A list of a few of the most common viral diseases for different species and their vaccine availability are provided at the end of the chapter.

## COMPOSITION AND CONTROL

I. Viruses are not cellular
   A. Viruses consist of protein and nucleic acid; some have lipids and carbohydrates

II. Viruses do not possess a nucleus, cytoplasm, cell membrane, or cell wall
III. Viruses are obligate intracellular parasites
   A. Viruses depend on host cell metabolism for their reproduction
   B. Animal viruses are most commonly cultured in mice, embryonated chicken eggs, or tissue culture
IV. Virus sizes vary
   A. Largest is poxvirus ($300 \times 240 \times 200$ nm)
   B. Smallest is parvovirus (22 nm diameter)
   C. Prions are considered to be smaller life forms
V. Classification
   A. Viruses are classified on the basis of
      1. Their shape as seen on electron microscopy
      2. Composition of their nucleic acid core (genome)
      3. Whether the virus possesses an envelope
VI. Envelope
   A. Lipid membrane that surrounds the virus is termed the envelope
      1. Enveloped viruses are easily killed
         a. Hypochlorite (common household bleach) dissolves fats
         b. Freezing and thawing process will render the virus inert because of the breakdown of the envelope by frozen water molecule
   B. "Naked virus" does not possess an envelope
      1. Naked viruses are more refractory
      2. It is more difficult to disinfect an area where these viruses have been located

a. Steam sterilization is recommended to kill all viruses at the temperature of 121° C (250° F) at 15 pounds per square inch (psi) for 30 minutes

b. Many commercial viricidal compounds, designed to be used in a clinical setting, are available to destroy different types of viruses

VII. Genomes

A. Mammalian genomes are composed of double-stranded DNA (deoxyribonucleic acid), from which various RNAs (ribonucleic acids) are transcribed

B. Viral nucleic acid can be DNA or RNA; can also be double or single stranded

1. Viruses with a nucleic acid core composed of RNA also possess a reverse transcriptase enzyme to create DNA from their RNA when they infect a mammalian host cell

2. Oncogenic viruses are common in the group, which have an RNA nucleic core; they are potentially cancer-causing agents

C. Some double-stranded DNA viruses can incorporate their DNA sequences into host cell DNA and be replicated during mitosis

1. This does not cause cellular damage and therefore no clinical signs: these are termed latent infections

2. Virus may lie dormant for years until the host is stressed because of age, malnutrition, water deprivation, shipping, surgery, or trauma, when the virus reemerges to produce intact virions and disease

VIII. Replication—there are four basic stages of replication for most viruses: attachment, penetration-uncoating, replication, and assembly-release

A. Attachment

1. Virus must gain access to the host cell to which it can bind

2. This is done via the virus portal entry

3. Portal entry is usually the mucosal surface to the respiratory, urogenital, or gastrointestinal tract

4. Breaks in the integument are a rare method of entry except when insect vectors are involved

5. Cell membrane is bound in a complementary fashion by the viral binding proteins

6. Viral binding proteins determine the species affected and the type of pathology caused

B. Penetration-uncoating

1. Most viruses produce enzymes that degrade the host cell membrane sufficiently to permit the nucleic acid core to enter

2. As it does so, the core exits the capsid (the outer shell of the virus), which remains on the host cell exterior

3. Exiting of the capsid is the uncoating process and occurs simultaneously with penetration

C. Replication

1. Aim is for the virus to produce thousands of copies of itself to ensure survival, but it lacks the ability to do so on its own

2. Thus the virus's nucleic acid redirects the host cell DNA to ignore its own needs and to instead produce viral components, such as capsid fragments and viral nucleic acid

3. This results in the breakdown of the host cell membrane, and this change initiates the immune response (see Chapter 8)

4. Because the virus is hidden in the host cell, the immune system is not able to respond to the virus specifically

5. Virus has already reproduced many copies of itself, which readily invade other cells and begin replication before the immune system is activated

D. Assembly-release

1. After all the various components of the virus structure have attained a critical concentration, assembly occurs spontaneously

2. Viral components come together to produce virions

a. Virions can be visualized on electron microscopy

b. They are cytoplasmic, nuclear, or both, depending on where they occur within the host cell

3. Virions almost immediately leave the cell

4. Most viruses exit the cell by causing it to rupture, termed the lysogenic cycle

5. Cell is destroyed; this causes the overall signs of disease

6. Most viruses that undergo replication are released from the host cell, spread to neighboring cells, and begin again the process of replication

7. Some viruses will be shed in secretions of the host body

8. Other viruses enter the systemic circulation and spread throughout the body; this is called a viremia—such infections can cause overall bodily signs, such as rashes

IX. Limitation of viruses

A. Some viruses are restricted to certain body temperatures

1. Nasal passages of mammalian respiratory tract average 2° C (35° F), which is lower than that of the lower respiratory tract and therefore remain susceptible to upper respiratory tract infections

B. Some viruses are limited by the surface proteins found on certain cell types (these form localized infections)

C. Other viruses enter the systemic circulation and spread throughout the body

## VIRAL INFECTIONS

I. Viral infections of any type can affect the host with regard to clinical signs in one of two ways
   A. Apparent infection: causes clinical disease
      1. This disease may be peracute to chronic
   B. Silent, nonapparent, or subclinical infection: does not result in overt signs
      1. This may result in a transient carrier state
      2. Such carriers (also known as persistently infected) are difficult to identify
         a. They therefore can sometimes infect a herd despite quarantine precautions
II. Examples
   A. Neurons in rabies victims or the T lymphocytes in cats infected with the feline immunodeficiency virus (FIV)
      1. These are cells that have become inactive or malfunction because of a virus
   B. Equine infectious anemia virus causes an immunological reaction within the host in which the immune system does more harm than the virus
      1. Immune system attacks the red blood cells, resulting in the anemia
III. Viral infections predispose an affected animal to secondary diseases (usually bacterial in nature) that can be worse than the primary viral disease
   A. Oncogenesis occurs with some viruses
      1. Infected cells transform, resulting in neoplasm with potential for malignancy, such as Marek's disease in chickens

## NOMENCLATURE

I. Viral family names end in the suffix *-viridae*
II. Viral genus names end in suffix *-virus*
III. Names are not underlined or italicized

## SAMPLING TECHNIQUES

I. Analysis of samples is not usually done within a veterinary practice but instead at a commercial, regional, or state diagnostic laboratory
II. Analysis of samples is not usually completed in time to treat the sick animal, but it is used to confirm a diagnosis and for epidemiological reasons
III. Laboratory test results are only as reliable as the quality of the samples submitted and the history provided
IV. Virus is most easily cultured from specimens just before the onset of signs and for a short time afterward

V. Animals that have been showing clinical signs for a few days generally are not sampled for viruses

## COLLECTION OF SPECIMENS

I. Representative animal from a herd should be sent for full examination (i.e., necropsy)
II. Examine ill and contact animals and sample from both, because the virus titer (concentration) is highest before signs
III. To identify a disease via an antibody titer
   A. Bleed at least six readily identifiable animals with early clinical signs
   B. Bleed the same animals 2 to 4 weeks later
   C. Change in titer means a positive diagnosis of a current disease and not immunity from previous recovery from the disease
IV. If unsure what samples to collect, take a wide range for the virologist to choose from, or call the laboratory and discuss sample collection with the personnel
V. Use one of the following transport media
   A. Sterile Hanks' balanced salt solution plus 10% bovine serum albumin
   B. Sterile skim milk
   C. Sterile charcoal transport medium, which is available commercially
VI. Note: A virus will survive 3 weeks without refrigeration and therefore will survive shipping
VII. Antibiotics may be added to control bacterial contamination
VIII. Keep specimens cool, 1° to 4° C (34° to 39° F), but do not freeze
IX. Postmortem tissues collected aseptically from several areas of the body can be used for histopathology
   A. Sections should be no larger than 3 to 5 mm ($\frac{3}{16}$ inch) thick
   B. Sections should be fixed in 10% formalin
   C. Less than 1 g of tissue in transport medium
   D. Do not freeze these samples
X. Collection from a live animal
   A. Heparinized plasma for immediate submission
   B. Serum may also be collected, which may be frozen

## SUBMISSION OF SAMPLES

Most laboratories will provide submission forms. The following pertinent information is needed for diagnosis.
   I. Sampling information
   II. Animal species
   III. Age and sex of the patient(s)
   IV. Size of the herd, flock, and kennel involved where applicable
   V. Number of animals affected
   VI. Duration of the illness to date
   VII. Clinical signs

VIII. Losses, if any

IX. Similar cases in the area

X. Vaccination history (if not available, note on form)

XI. Treatment given up to the time of sampling

XII. Disease suspected

XIII. Specimens submitted and labeled appropriately

## IN-CLINIC LABORATORY TESTING OF SAMPLES

I. Viruses are identified initially on the basis of

A. Clinical history

B. Specimen sample submitted

C. Immunoreactivity

D. One or a combination of histopathology, advanced laboratory tests, and electron microscopy

II. In some instances the most commonly used techniques have been adapted to kit form, so they may be used in a clinical setting or out in the field

A. Fluorescent antibody (FA) test

1. This test uses antibodies of known specificity that bind viral antigens

2. Binding can then be visualized through conjugation (labeled) with a fluorescent dye

3. Such a procedure can be performed using frozen tissue sections, tissue imprints, tissue scrapings, and blood smears

4. Selection depends on the viral life cycle within the host

5. Often such results are available rapidly (in less than 1 hour)

a. Accuracy depends on the application to appropriate specimens that are in good condition (fresh with little to no autolysis)

6. This may not be an applicable test method if the required samples cannot be obtained from live animals

B. Enzyme-linked immunosorbent assay (ELISA) test

1. Popular test kit method in which a known specific antibody is adsorbed, usually in a small plastic well in a well plate or a specially designed membrane (kit dependent)

2. These antibodies will have patient sample applied

3. Common diseases that are screened in this manner are feline leukemia virus (FeLV), parvovirus, and heartworm

a. Viral antigen, if present in the animal's serum, is tightly and specifically bound by the adsorbed antibodies

b. Another antibody of the same specificity, which is labeled (most frequently with an enzyme), is applied to produce a sandwich formation

c. Another alternative to the enzymatic label is a fluorescent label

d. Very important wash step is then performed to remove any unbound labeled antibody (which would be the case if the animal does not possess the viral antigen in its serum and therefore is negative for FeLV)

e. If the viral antigen is present, the labeled antibody will not be removed because the binding is very strong

f. Substrate is then added; it must be one that reacts with the enzyme with which the second antibody is labeled

g. Reaction produces a visible color change to permit the technician to recognize the unhealthy animal's state

h. In some cases in which no vaccine is available, the viral antigen can be bound to the well or membrane to detect antibody in the patient's serum as an indicator of the disease; this technique is the one of choice in such cases and where the viral titer remains low in the body

C. Latex agglutination (LA) test

1. Another popular test kit; it uses the same principles as the ELISA test

2. Antiviral antibodies are adsorbed to microscopic latex beads. If the applied sample contains the antigen (virus), it will be bound by these antibodies and produce agglutination

3. Because of the granular appearance of the latex beads in solution, it is very important to run positive and negative controls simultaneously

4. Such a method can be used to detect parvovirus from fecal samples of ill dogs or rotavirus in the feces of various species with rotaviral diarrhea

## PREVENTION

There are three major factors involved in preventing occurrence or reducing the effects of viral diseases.

I. Health measures

A. Good hygiene

B. Prompt disposal of dead animals

C. Proper nutrition

D. Clean and adequate water supply

E. Reasonable population density to reduce stress

F. Screening and quarantine of new animals before their entry into the household or herd

II. Immunization if possible and maintenance of current vaccinations

III. Treatment of viral disease (Table 7-1)

**Table 7-1**  Common diseases and vaccine availability

| Disease | Etiology | Vaccine available |
|---|---|---|
| **BOVINE** | | |
| Leukemia | Retrovirus | No |
| Spongiform encephalopathy | Prion | No |
| Viral diarrhea | Pestivirus | Yes, killed and modified live virus (MLV) (caution when using in pregnant cows and those incubating the disease) |
| Calf scours complex | Rotavirus and coronavirus | Yes, but best when given to the dam and passed through colostrums |
| Foot and mouth | Picornavirus | Yes, killed, resulting in short-term immunity; not always effective |
| Infectious rhinotracheitis | Herpesvirus | Yes, MLV and killed |
| Parainfluenza-3 | Paramyxovirus | Yes, killed and attenuated-live |
| Respiratory syncytial virus | Paramyxovirus | No |
| Vesicular stomatitis | Vesiculovirus | No, not in North America |
| **PORCINE** | | |
| Encephalomyocarditis | Picornavirus | No |
| Hemagglutinating encephalomyelitis | Coronavirus | No |
| Hog cholera | Pestivirus | Yes, MLV |
| Porcine parvovirus infection | Parvovirus | Yes, killed and MLV |
| Pseudorabies | Herpesvirus | Yes, attenuated (effectiveness is low) or recombinant (subunit) |
| Reproductive and respiratory syndrome | Arteriviridae | Yes |
| Rotavirus infection | Rotavirus | Yes, MLV and killed |
| Swine influenza | Orthomyxovirus | Yes, inactivated |
| Swine pox | Poxvirus | No |
| Transmissible gastroenteritis | Coronavirus | Yes, attenuated-live and killed Planned infections are done in epidemic areas only |
| Vesicular exanthema of swine | Calicivirus | No |
| **OVINE AND CAPRINE** | | |
| Border disease | Pestivirus | No |
| Bluetongue | Orbivirus | Yes, MLV and killed (used in some countries—not in the United States, where import restrictions are used for control) |
| Caprine arthritis-encephalitis | Lentivirus | No |
| Contagious ecthyma | Poxvirus | Yes |
| Progressive pneumonia of sheep | Lentivirus | No |
| Scrapie | Prion | No |
| **EQUINE** | | |
| Coital exanthema | Herpesvirus | No |
| Encephalomyelitis | Arbovirus | Yes, MLV |
| Influenza | Orthomyxovirus | Yes, killed |
| Infectious anemia | Nononcogenic retrovirus | No |
| Viral arteritis | Togavirus | Yes, MLV |
| West Nile encephalomyelitis | Flavivirus | Yes, killed (adjuvanted) or recombinant |
| Rhinopneumonitis | Varicella virus | Yes, killed and MLV; caution—high abortion risk |
| **CANINE** | | |
| Coronavirus infections | Coronavirus | Yes, killed |
| Distemper | Morbillivirus | Yes, MLV; can use measles followed by distemper or a combination in very young pups |
| Herpesvirus infection | Herpesvirus | No |
| Infectious hepatitis | Adenovirus | Yes, MLV and killed |

**Table 7-1**  Common diseases and vaccine availability—cont'd

| Disease | Etiology | Vaccine available |
|---|---|---|
| Infectious tracheobronchitis | Parainfluenza virus, adenovirus-2, morbillivirus; possibly reovirus, herpesvirus, adenovirus-1 | Yes, polyvalent vaccines due to simultaneous morbillivirus, and bacterial infections |
| Parvoviral enteritis | Parvovirus | Yes, MLV; possibly not effective owing to viral mutation |
| Rabies | Rhabdovirus | Yes, MLV and killed<br>*Note:* is potential in *all* warm-blooded animals |
| Leptospirosis (bacteria) | *Leptospira* spp. | Yes |
| Lyme disease (bacteria) | *Borrelia burgdorferi* | Yes, killed vaccine and recombinant |
| **FELINE** | | |
| Feline respiratory complex: calicivirus (FCV) | Calicivirus | Yes, polyvalent MLV |
| Feline respiratory complex: rhinotracheitis (FRV) | Herpesvirus | Yes, polyvalent MLV (in combination with FCV) |
| Infectious peritonitis | Coronavirus | Yes, MLV (not entirely effective) |
| Immunodeficiency virus | Lentivirus | No |
| Leukemia | Oncogenic retrovirus | Yes killed, effectiveness varies, recombinant (subunit or gene-deleted) |
| Panleukopenia | Parvovirus | Yes, inactivated and MLV |
| Rabies | Rhabdovirus | Yes, MLV and killed<br>*Note:* is potential in *all* warm-blooded animals |
| **AVIAN** | | |
| Encephalomyelitis | Enterovirus | Yes, killed and MLV |
| Infectious laryngotracheitis | Herpesvirus | Yes, MLV |
| Influenza | Orthomyxovirus | No |
| Leukosis | Retrovirus | No |
| Coronal enteritis of turkeys | Coronavirus | No |
| Duck plague | Herpesvirus | No |
| Fowl pox | Poxvirus | Yes, attenuated-live or recombinant (vectored) |
| Infectious bronchitis | Coronavirus | Yes, killed and MLV polyvalent; full immunity may not occur |
| Marek's disease | Herpesvirus | Yes |
| Psittacine beak and feather | Circovirus | No |
| Newcastle disease | Paramyxovirus | Yes, inactivated (adjuvanted), MLV or recombinant (vectored) |
| Infectious bursal disease | Birnavirus | Yes, inactivated and MLV |

See Chapter 8 for an in-depth explanation about types of vaccines.

# Glossary

**adjuvant** Substances added to a vaccine (commonly mineral oil, alum, bacterial fractions, some sugars, or combinations of these) that increase the antigenicity and therefore the degree of the immune response

**adsorb** To attract and retain other material on the surface

**altered self** Any change in the molecular configuration of one's cells that may result in attack by the immune system. This state may be a result of viral invasion of cells, cancer, radiation, or poisoning

**autoclave** Instrument with a chamber in which materials are rendered sterile via a treatment with the necessary steam heat and pressure for a specific period of time

**autolysis** Rupture and death of a cell

**capsid** Shell of protein that protects the nucleic acid of a virus

**DNA** Standard short form for deoxyribonucleic acid, the physical basis for the genetic code. It forms a double-stranded helix in animals. Under strict and specific physiological regulations, it codes for the production of RNA. In viruses it may be single- or double-stranded

**genome** Entire genetic complement of an organism. In animals it involves DNA and RNA, but in viruses it is one or the other

**inactivated** Rendered inert or nonfunctional by exposure to heat of sufficient temperature and duration

**latent** Quiescent state awaiting later reactivation, which may occur years later. In the case of latent viruses, they insert their DNA into the host cell DNA to be replicated together. Frequently stress is implicated in the viruses' resurgence and resultant disease state

**lysin** Agent that ruptures (bursts) and therefore kills host cells

**lysogenic cycle** Ability to cause lysis or produce lysins; ability to exit a host cell by rupturing that cell causing its death

**naked virus** A virus that does not have a lipid membrane

**nucleic acid core** Molecule of DNA or RNA, either of which can be double or single stranded. The term is used synonymously with "viral genome"

**obligate intracellular parasite** A parasite that lives within a host cell. The host cell is its only means of survival

**oncogenesis** Production of tumors

**parasite** One organism that survives at the detriment of another

**portal of entry** Pathway by which a pathogenic agent gains entry to the body

**prion** Proteinaceous infectious particle, the smallest known microorganism. Laboratory tests indicate that although this microorganism does not possess any nucleic acid, it consists of protein and is capable of producing disease

**psi** Old, standard unit of pressure that is still widely in use; denotes pounds per square inch

**recombinant** Produced through DNA technology using the pathogen's genome to create the antigenicity and immune response. Because the virus is not intact there is no risk of disease to the patient

**refractory** Resistant, capable of withstanding adverse conditions and surviving

**reverse transcriptase RNA** Enzyme of RNA viruses that catalyzes the transcription of RNA to DNA, which is then incorporated into a genome of the host cell self-recognized by the immune system as one's own molecular configuration and therefore tolerated

**RNA** One form of nucleic acid, of which there are three forms: ribosomal, messenger, and transfer. It codes for the assembly of proteins. Some viruses, such as the retroviruses, possess only RNA in their genome, but because they possess a reverse transcriptase enzyme, they can "reverse code" for DNA

**subclinical** Used to describe the early stages or a very mild form of a disease

**titer** Strength per volume of a volumetric test solution

**T lymphocyte** Lymphocytes that do not produce antibody; rather they primarily act to destroy altered self in the body due to viral infection or neoplastic transformation

**tolerance** State of being tolerated by the immune system and therefore not attacked. In health this occurs in one's own body only; if it is conveyed to microorganisms, it will result in an immunodeficiency

**viremia** Stage of some infections where the virus enters the blood and spreads throughout the body

**viricidal** Term meaning virus killer; frequently used to describe disinfectant chemicals with this capacity

**virion** Intact, functional virus particle, capable of infecting a host cell

# Review Questions

1 Which of the following statements is true about viruses?
   a. They are microscopic, cellular, parasitic organisms
   b. They are all readily destroyed by ordinary household soaps and other disinfectants
   c. They are obligate intracellular parasites
   d. All of the above

2 Which of the following is not a major factor in reducing the effects of or preventing viral disease?
   a. Treatment
   b. Immunization
   c. Replication cycle of the virus
   d. Health measures

3 Envelope viruses are rendered inert with
   a. Freezing and thawing
   b. Heat
   c. Soap and water
   d. None of the above

4 Which of the following is used to classify a virus?
   a. Their shape, as seen via electron microscopy
   b. Type of genome it possesses
   c. Presence or lack of an envelope
   d. All of the above

5 Autoclaving to sterilize a virally contaminated material requires the following same parameters as for a bacterially contaminated material
   a. 121° C, 15 psi for 30 minutes
   b. 250° F, 150 psi for 15 minutes
   c. 121° C, 10 psi for 15 minutes
   d. 250° F, 100 psi for 30 minutes

6 Complete the following statement: "Viruses are spread between contacts most effectively"
   a. During the acute stage of the disease
   b. Before the onset of clinical signs and for a very short time afterward
   c. At the beginning of convalescence
   d. None of the above

7 When submitting samples to a diagnostic laboratory virology department, it is important to
   a. Include a thorough case history
   b. Use an approved shipping medium
   c. Take serum samples from readily identifiable animals, now and up to 4 weeks later
   d. All of the above

8 Viral diseases are treated by administering antibiotics
   a. True
   b. Only during the viremic stage
   c. Only as a supportive measure to control opportunistic infections
   d. Only if the disease is due to an enveloped virus

9 Viral diagnostic tests include
   a. Fluorescent antibody test
   b. Electron microscopic visualization
   c. Enzyme-linked immunosorbent assay
   d. All of the above

**10** The following is an acceptable transport media for viruses
   a. Skim milk medium
   b. Sterile William's solution
   c. Sterile carbon transport medium
   d. Formaldehyde

## BIBLIOGRAPHY

Black JG: *Microbiology principles and applications*, ed 3, Englewood Cliffs, NJ, 1996, Prentice Hall.

Blood DC et al: *Saunders comprehensive veterinary dictionary*, ed 3, Oxford, 2007, Saunders.

Gershwin LJ et al: *Immunology and immunopathology of domestic animals*, ed 2, St Louis, 1995, Mosby.

Quinn PJ et al: *Clinical veterinary microbiology*, St Louis, 1994, Mosby.

Roberts AW, Carter GR, Chengappa MM: *Essentials of veterinary microbiology*, ed 5, Philadelphia, 1995, Lippincott Williams & Wilkins.

*The Merck veterinary manual*, ed 9, Whitehouse Station, NJ, 2005, Merck.

Turgeon ML: *Immunology and serology in laboratory medicine*, ed 3, St Louis, 2003, Mosby.

Tizard I: *Veterinary immunology: an introduction*, ed 7, St Louis, 2004, Saunders.

## CHAPTER 8

# Immunology

*Patricia L. Bell*

## OUTLINE

Innate or Nonspecific Immunity
Adaptive or Specific Immunity
Antibodies
  IgM
  IgG
  IgA
  IgE
  IgD

Primary vs. Secondary Immune
  Responses
Types of Acquired Immunities
Transfer of Maternal Immunity to
  the Offspring Including the Role
  of Vaccines
Immunopathological
  Mechanisms

Types of Vaccines
  Vaccine Difficulties
  Vaccine Precautions
  Adverse Vaccine Reactions

## LEARNING OUTCOMES

After reading this chapter you should be able to:

1. Briefly describe in general terms how the immune system defends the body from an infection.
2. Describe innate and adaptive immunity.
3. Compare and contrast primary versus secondary immune responses and how they relate to vaccine protocols.
4. List and describe antibody classes, their roles in the immune response, and how they are used in diagnoses.
5. Describe different types of acquired responses.
6. Describe hypersensitivities and cell-mediated and humoral immunodeficiencies.
7. Describe the types of vaccines and give advantages and disadvantages of each.
8. Explain the transfer of maternal immunity to the offspring, and explain the differences between the species.
9. Describe various components that can cause the immune system to not respond to a vaccine.
10. Recognize clinical signs of an immune response, including the response to a vaccine.
11. Recognize life-threatening reactions (anaphylaxis) to a vaccination.

This chapter deals with the general physiological mechanisms involved in an innate and adaptive immune response, as well as primary versus secondary immune responses. This is done so that the manipulations of the immune system by vaccines, which are discussed later, can be better understood. In the adaptive system, the section on antibodies is expanded so that the sections on maternal transfer of immunity to offspring, types of acquired immunity, and vaccines themselves are clear. Other sections included are immunopathological mechanisms and vaccine difficulties and precautions. Each section provides some background information and stresses clinical and diagnostic considerations.

### INNATE OR NONSPECIFIC IMMUNITY ▬▬

I. Definition: the immunity with which we are born
II. Includes physical and chemical barriers to an antigen, such as
   A. Intact skin, stomach acids, commensal organisms, mucus production, cilia, lysozyme in tears, and body temperature
III. Also involves the humoral and cell mediated systems
   A. They include reactions involved in the inflammatory responses, particularly the functions of the phagocytes, which are the body's first line of defense for containing and halting the spread of the pathogen

B. Wound healing also occurs because of this process
IV. If the innate system is successful, the adaptive immune response will not be activated and antibody production will not occur
V. Especially important features of innate immunity
   A. Occurs immediately after an antigen's entry (which is important because antibody production takes days)
   B. Treats all antigens the same (no specificity involved)
   C. Strength and speed of the response do not increase with subsequent encounters with the same antigen (no memory involved)
   D. Common clinical signs of an innate system response are primarily due to histamine release
      1. Clinically seen as swelling or edema, because plasma moves from the circulation into the tissues
      2. Redness and excess heat from vasodilation and increased blood flow
      3. Release of extra mucus occurs in some areas

## ADAPTIVE OR SPECIFIC IMMUNITY

I. Definition: the response of the defenses of the body to a specific substance (antigen)
II. Individuals produce antibodies
III. Response is highly specific
IV. Adaptive immunity possesses a memory, so the body's response becomes more rapid and stronger with each encounter with the same antigen
V. During the adaptive response, immunity is created
   A. Cell-mediated immune response involves T lymphocytes and the phagocytes (neutrophils, monocytes, and macrophages)
      1. Macrophage engulfs the pathogen, digests and kills it, and presents a piece of it (epitope) on its surface
      2. T-helper lymphocytes bind to the epitope presented on the macrophage surface
      3. T-helper lymphocyte then presents the epitope to a B lymphocyte
         a. Macrophage and T-helper cell then produce specific cytokines (also called lymphokines)
         b. Examples of lymphokines are
            (1) Interleukin-1: produced by the macrophage and causes the T-helper cell to release more interleukins
            (2) Interleukin-2: causes more T cells to be produced
            (3) Also releases interleukin-4 and interleukin-6 (they cause the B-lymphocyte to clone and produce memory cells and antibodies)

B. Strength that the immune system attains and therefore the individual's level of immunity reached depends on
   1. Genetics, general state of health, the dosage of antigen, the antigen's portal of entry and persistence (rate of clearance) in the body, and the number of times it has been encountered previously
VI. Antibody will bind and neutralize the antigen by providing a physical barrier between the antigen and the host cells

## ANTIBODIES

I. Definition: noncellular components (they are glycoproteins) of the adaptive immune response that bind specifically to parts of the antigen called antigenic determinants or epitopes
II. By binding to the antigen, antibodies prevent the antigen from doing further harm (neutralizing) and they enhance other immune responses
III. Five classes of antibodies (also called immunoglobulins [Ig])

### IgM

I. During the primary immune response to a particular antigen, stimulated (antigen-bound) B cells (also known as B lymphocytes, plasma- or antibody-forming cells) secrete IgM antibody
   A. Because of its large size, this antibody class is confined to the vascular system
   B. It comprises about 10% of the antibody pool in most mammals

### IgG

I. Most plasma cells produce IgG antibody molecules during secondary and subsequent immune responses (to the same antigen)
   A. IgG can cross the placental barrier (transplacental immunity) in species with a lower number of placental membranes (dog, cat, rodent, and primate) to convey short-term immunity to the newborn

### IgA

I. If a plasma cell resides in a lymph node that drains portals of entry such as the gastrointestinal tract, urogenital tract, or the conjunctiva of the eyes, it will produce IgA antibodies
   A. Here it binds the potential invader, blocking its ability to bind to the host tissue, and making it too large to pass through the mucosal membrane
   B. This class of antibody is found in body secretions, including tears, mucus, and colostrum
      1. After about 18 hours of life, the neonate will begin to produce stomach acids, and the antibodies

of the colostrum will be digested, rendering them useless for immune purposes. So ingestion of the colostrum must occur very early in life or the neonate may not be protected

## IgE

I. It is found in minute levels in the plasma of healthy animals
  A. IgE boosts local inflammatory reactions
  B. It also helps protect animals against helminths by attracting eosinophils to the site of infestation
  C. If an individual produces excess IgE, such a response may become damaging to self
     1. If the reaction is localized, it is termed an allergy
     2. When it acts systemically, it is a hypersensitivity reaction called anaphylaxis; it may induce anaphylactic shock, which can be fatal

## IgD

I. It is found on lymphocyte membranes and in negligible amounts in body fluids
  A. Primary role is as an antigen receptor for B cells

## Primary vs. Secondary Immune Responses

I. There are two stages to the adaptive immune response
II. It is these stages that are manipulated by modern vaccine therapy
  A. Primary immune response occurs the very first time the adaptive response engages a particular substance (antigen) and only then; this could be due to disease or the first vaccination
     1. Response is slow and takes several days to become clinically detectable
     2. IgM antibody is produced
     3. Response is weak because the antibody titer remains relatively low
     4. IgM antibody does not last long in the body
     5. Clinical signs are longer lasting with a disease situation
  B. Secondary immune response occurs with the second or subsequent encounter with the same antigen; this could be due to disease or a booster vaccine
     1. Response is rapid, taking only 1 or 2 days to become clinically detectable
     2. IgG antibody is produced
     3. Response is strong; the antibody titer can be up to 105 times higher than for the primary response
     4. IgG persists in the system up to months or even years after the response has occurred
     5. Clinical signs are usually less severe and of shorter duration than those of the primary response with a disease situation

III. Physiology of these stages must be taken into account when using antibody titers to determine an animal's health status
  A. Blood samples are drawn to obtain data regarding a patient's antibody type and titer
     1. IgM antibody titer to a particular antigen infers either a recent initial vaccination for that disease (check the vaccination history) or a current disease state
     2. IgG antibody titer to a particular antigen infers either that booster vaccines have been administered at some time previously (check the vaccination history), that the animal has recovered from this disease at some time in the past (check the clinical history if available), or a current disease state. Retest in 2 to 4 weeks
     3. If the retesting of the titer shows the IgG antibody level to be close to the previous test level, then the animal has antibodies from a previous disease recovery (convalescent state) or a vaccine. If the titer is increasing the animal is currently ill (actively infected state)

## TYPES OF ACQUIRED IMMUNITIES ▬▬▬

I. Definitions
  A. Acquired immunities: occur after birth
  B. Natural immunity: without medical (human) intervention
  C. Artificial immunity: medically induced immunity
  D. Active immunity: the individual's own immune system produced the antibodies (and therefore long-term immunity occurs)
     1. This is known as a seroconversion
  E. Passive immunity: antibodies were "donated" and therefore the individual's immune system was not stimulated to produce the antibodies (nor any memory cells)
     1. This involves short-term immunity because these antibodies will be quickly catabolized and cleared from the body, and no replacements will be synthesized
  F. Acquired natural active immunity
     1. Usually induced by disease recovery
  G. Acquired natural passive immunity
     1. Antibodies are passed to the fetus or neonate
        a. From the mother across the placental barrier (species dependent)
        b. Or via ingestion of colostrum by the neonate
  H. Acquired artificial active immunity
     1. Via vaccination
  I. Acquired artificial passive immunity
     1. Antibodies produced in one animal are infused into another animal

2. Initial animal is administered a pathogen, vaccination series, or a bacterial toxin repeatedly until that animal is "hyperimmune" (possesses a very high antibody titer)
3. During the hyperimmune state a portion or all of the animal serum is removed, and the antibodies are harvested and can be used for the following
   a. To produce an antiserum, which can then be given to other animals, to convey short-term immunity
      (1) Common example is in the treatment of people after exposure to the rabies virus
   b. To produce a toxoid (in the case of the use of a bacterial toxin on the initial animal), which can be administered to other animals
      (1) Common example is the anti–tetanus toxoid for potential *Clostridium tetani* exposure
      (2) It is also available for the treatment of other clostridial pathogens

## TRANSFER OF MATERNAL IMMUNITY TO THE OFFSPRING INCLUDING THE ROLE OF VACCINES

I. Dam can pass on only the antibodies that she possesses
   A. Vaccines are important to neonatal health
      1. It is critical that the breeder female be fully vaccinated and that those vaccines be up to date. If not, her progeny may not have the needed immunity to survive until their own immune systems are finished developing
      2. Check the vaccine protocol carefully to determine when the mother should be vaccinated to provide maximum immunity to the young. Some cannot be administered during pregnancy; others must be given close to parturition
   B. Check the vaccine protocol with regard to immunizing young animals and follow them carefully
      1. If vaccines are given too soon, the maternal antibodies may block the neonate's immune system from responding, so no immunity occurs
      2. Neonate's immune system may not be ready to react to the vaccine, so no immunity occurs
      3. If given too late, the maternal antibodies may be gone and the disease can occur during the time the infant is left unprotected, without any antibodies of its own
II. Route by which immunity (antibody) is transferred from mother to offspring is determined by the placental barrier as well as the type of antibody involved
   A. It is the number of membranes, which comprise the placenta, that determines how much IgG

antibody can cross from the maternal into the fetal circulation
   1. Three membranes allow 100% of the maternal IgG antibody to cross
   2. This type of placentation occurs in humans and other primates and protects them from systemic infections
   3. These neonates still require IgA antibody, which cannot cross the placental barrier but is obtained via the ingestion of colostrum. Such ingestion conveys immunity to the gastrointestinal tract to help prevent neonatal diarrhea
   4. Dog and cat possess four membranes in their placentas, and therefore most of their maternal immunity is conveyed through the ingestion of colostrum
   5. Ruminants have five membranes, whereas pig, horse, and donkey have six membranes in their placentas. These numbers block all antibodies from crossing. As a result, colostrum is the only source of immune transfer in these species, and its ingestion is crucial

## IMMUNOPATHOLOGICAL MECHANISMS

I. Disorders result from inappropriate or inadequate immune responses and are labeled as hypersensitivities, autoimmune reactions, or immunodeficiencies
II. Immunoproliferative disorders can also occur, in which the proliferation of the leukocytes becomes aberrant, excessive, and/or nonfunctional
   A. Example: lymphosarcoma, for which the theory of an oncogenic viral etiological agent has been proposed
      1. This type of pathology is usually studied as a hematological disorder even though it severely compromises the immune system's ability to function
III. Four types of hypersensitivity reactions (some of which occur in isolation, but more often more than one type occurs simultaneously)
   A. Type 1 involves the animal producing an excess of IgE antibody
      1. If this is a genetically based condition, it is known as an atopy
      2. It can produce very problematic, even fatal, conditions
         a. Too much IgE antibody means too many mast cells degranulate, and in turn too much histamine is released
         b. This results in allergies of various forms dependent on the allergen's (an antigen that induces an allergic response) portal of entry, such as
            (1) Inhalation, ingestion, or movement through the skin

(2) It may result in allergy development or anaphylactic shock and death

3. Unfortunately allergies are relatively common in animals and can occur to almost any compound from feedstuffs and pharmaceuticals to environmental items, and POTENTIALLY EVEN VACCINES!

   a. Common examples: canine atopic dermatitis and contact dermatitis (classic flea bite hypersensitivity and sweet itch fit here) but the latter does not involve atopy

B. Type 2 occurs when an animal produces antibodies against its own cells that are then lysed by complement

   1. Results in an autoimmune disorder
   2. Examples: autoimmune hemolytic anemia, equine infectious anemia, immune-mediated thrombocytopenia, pemphigus, and systemic lupus erythematosus

C. Type 3 occurs when antibodies bind to an antigen and form large complexes that become deposited in body tissues; often joints and vessel walls or kidneys are involved

   1. It produces inflammation and tissue necrosis at these sites
   2. A common example: rheumatoid arthritis

D. Type 4 is the result of the actions of the cell-mediated immunity (CMI)

   1. They infiltrate the area in which the allergen occurs. Then redness, hard lump formation, and necrosis occur
   2. These create a granuloma
   3. Example: flea collar sensitivities

IV. Immunodeficiency

A. Definition: lack of a particular immune system component and/or a malfunction

B. Types

   1. Congenital, cell-mediated immunodeficiency
      a. Example: cyclic neutropenia in gray collies and their crosses
      b. They experience a cyclic decrease of all cellular elements (most notably the neutrophils), during which time they have a very low resistance to infection
   2. Congenital, humoral immunodeficiencies include the inability to produce certain classes of antibody
      a. IgG deficiency in cattle; IgM deficiency in horse, Doberman pinscher, and basset hound; and IgA deficiency in other dogs
   3. Combined immunodeficiency can be seen in some Arabian horses and basset hounds that do not possess a thymus, no lymphoid organs, and a very low number of lymphocytes

   a. Such animals survive their first few months primarily because of the antibodies received from their mothers
   b. Usually they succumb to adenoviral pneumonia (horse) or the distemper vaccine (dog)
   4. Deficiencies due to cell-mediated immunity alone are rare
   5. Acquired deficiencies (occurring after birth)
      a. These are common especially in the cat owing to feline leukemia and feline AIDS viruses
      b. They occur in animals that do not receive colostrum or that nurse from mothers with poor immunity and therefore produce low-quality colostrum
      c. They also develop in old age as the immune system weakens and deficiencies begin to develop

C. Other general causes of inappropriate immune reactions

   1. Breakdown of tolerance to usually "ignored" material, such as dust (i.e., chronic alveolar emphysema in horses) or autoimmune disease occurs

## TYPES OF VACCINES

I. Vaccines are important in the preventive health care program, because they reduce the chances of a particular disease occurring

II. Ideal vaccine would be safe and effective and have no undesirable side effects

III. There are many types of vaccines

A. Killed or inactivated vaccines

   1. Organisms (bacteria or virus) used to produce these vaccines are killed, often by chemical treatment
   2. These are safe, stable (store well) vaccines
   3. They require repeated dosages to maintain protective immunity, and this increases their cost
   4. Immunity conveyed may be weak owing to the effects of killing the organism
   5. Adjuvants (compounds to boost the immune response) are often added, which can cause severe reactions at the site of administration

B. Attenuated-live/modified-live vaccines (MLVs)

   1. These use live but attenuated or otherwise avirulent organisms
   2. They convey strong, long-lasting immunity
   3. They can cause abortions; mild immunosuppression or residual virulence can cause mild disease (rare) and have been implicated in some autoimmune diseases

C. Recombinant vaccines

   1. These are produced through DNA technology
   2. They possess a high degree of efficacy and safety

3. Not many are available, and they are expensive
4. Types include subunit, gene deleted, and vectored

D. Monoclonal/polyvalent vaccines
   1. Monoclonal vaccines produce immunity directed against a specific pathogen only
   2. Polyclonal vaccines produce immunity directed against more than one pathogen simultaneously
      a. These are also termed "-way" vaccines, such as three-way or four-way, depending on the number of diseases they protect against
      b. They contain a mix of antigens

E. Other similar therapies include
   1. Use of bacterial toxins; such vaccines are termed toxoids
      a. Animal still produces its own antibodies; therefore the immunity is long-lived
   2. Use of antitoxins that contain antibodies directed against the toxins produced by the pathogen
   3. Use of antisera that contain antibodies directed against the pathogen itself
      a. In the above two situations, the animal is given antibodies from another already immune animal, and therefore this type of immunity is short-lived

## Vaccine Difficulties

I. Vaccines are not guaranteed to work, because an individual may react to proteins carried over from the culture environment of the virus, chemicals used to kill the virus, or even the adjuvant itself
   A. Adjuvant may not perform adequately, the epitopes may be altered during processing, or they may not be very immunogenic in the first place

II. Usually vaccines are sold as a lyophilized powder to which a particular amount of sterile distilled water is added
   A. Amount of water must be correct because the concentration is important in inducing a good response
   B. Do not mix vaccines in the same syringe unless the protocol states it is safe to do so, because the resultant combination could inactivate the vaccines
   C. It must be handled gently after reconstitution so that no mechanical damage occurs, and it must be delivered to the appropriate area in the body for which it was designed to work
      1. Some are to be injected subcutaneously; others are for intramuscular injection

2. If administered incorrectly, there may not be sufficient inflammation or the vaccine may be cleared so rapidly that it does not stimulate the immune system
3. Nonstimulation can occur with accidental intravenous administration; but it could also result in anaphylaxis
4. Use of excessive alcohol at the injection site using any type of vaccine has also been implicated

III. Vaccine must be stored properly during shipping, because temperature extremes can cause a loss of antigenicity

IV. After all proper precautions are taken, there is still no guarantee the vaccinated animal will respond appropriately
   A. Young animal that is immunologically compromised may succumb to illness from a live vaccine, or may not develop immunity to killed or other vaccines
   B. Even if an animal does not become ill from the administration of a vaccine, there is no way of knowing what the animal's immune status is unless an antibody titer is done
   C. Vaccines may not be effective when administered to certain populations of animals, such as animals that are
      1. Immunosuppressed
      2. Heavily infested with parasites
      3. Very stressed
      4. Malnourished
      5. Incubating disease
      6. Showing signs of an abscess at the site of inoculation

V. Viruses are capable of a process called antigenic drift
   A. Example: canine parvovirus
   B. Such a virus mutates its genome and its epitopes so that preexisting antibodies from previous vaccines are now unable to bind and therefore are useless
   C. As a result, a previously ill and recovered animal or a previously vaccinated animal is no longer immune

## Vaccine Precautions

I. Following the recommended vaccination schedule increases an animal's chances of developing a protective immunity

II. If a vaccine is given too early in life, the maternal antibodies in the circulation may prevent the young animal's immune system from properly responding to the vaccine, lessening its efficacy
   A. Neonate's immune system may not be sufficiently developed to respond

III. Boosters must be administered at correct times to maintain the necessarily high level of immunity to prevent disease

## ADVERSE VACCINE REACTIONS

I. Adverse reactions are rare; when they do occur, they are usually mild and/or localized
  A. Common clinical signs include
    1. Slight fever, lethargy, soreness at the injection site, and possibly anorexia
    2. These clinical signs usually subside in a day
    3. Client must be warned of the possibility of such an occurrence, but also educated to not be alarmed
  B. Common causes include
    1. Cell culture (that the viruses are grown in) proteins carried over into the vaccine
    2. Adjuvants added

C. Severe reactions involving anaphylaxis are rare; common clinical signs include
  1. Vomiting
  2. Salivation
  3. Incoordination
  4. Urticaria
  5. Dyspnea
    a. Epinephrine may be used to treat these potentially life-threatening cases
D. Vaccines have been implicated in cases of fibrosarcoma in cat and immune-mediated hemolytic anemia and thrombocytopenia in dog
  1. These situations are currently under investigation
  2. Occurrence is rare
  3. Benefits of vaccines still greatly outweigh the risks involved
  4. Protocols may be altered to less frequent administrations to help prevent these problems from occurring (Table 8-1)

**Table 8-1**  Examples of vaccine protocols

| Species | Age/time of year | Vaccine |
|---|---|---|
| Canine | 8-10 wk | Distemper, adenovirus II, parainfluenza, and parvovirus |
| | 10 -12 wk | Distemper, adenovirus II, parainfluenza, and parvovirus |
| | 16 wk | Distemper, adenovirus II, parainfluenza, parvovirus, and rabies |
| | 1 yr | Distemper, adenovirus II, parainfluenza, parvovirus, and rabies |
| Vaccines boosters should be administered 3-4 wk apart<br>Annual boosters for distemper, adenovirus II, parainfluenza, parvovirus<br>Rabies should be boosted every year or every 3 yr depending on animal's location and type of vaccine used<br>Additional vaccines—leptospirosis, corona virus, *Bordetella* spp., and Lyme disease—may be required depending on location and client requests | | |
| Feline | 8-10 wk | Feline viral rhinotracheitis, calicivirus, and panleukopenia |
| | 10 -12 wk | Feline viral rhinotracheitis, calicivirus, panleukopenia, and rabies |
| | 10 wk or older | FeLV booster in 3-4 wk (recommend test first) |
| | 1 yr | Feline viral rhinotracheitis, calicivirus, panleukopenia and rabies |
| Vaccine boosters should be administered 3-4 wk apart<br>*Note:* Administration of rabies vaccine should be over the right hind leg. All other vaccines near left hind leg. This is due to the concern over injection site sarcomas documented in 1:10 000 cases, believed to be linked to the rabies vaccine<br>Rabies should be boosted every year or every 3 yr depending on animal's location and type of vaccine used | | |
| Horses<br>  Foals | Spring of yearling year | Western and eastern equine encephalitis, tetanus, West Nile, twice 4-6 wk apart |
|   Adults | Spring (spring and fall if traveling) | Western and eastern equine encephalitis, tetanus<br>Rabies if in endemic area<br>Anthrax if in endemic area |
| | Spring and fall | Equine influenza and strangles (specifically the intranasal variety of both) |
| *Note:* See Chapter 24 for further information | | |
| Cattle | Spring | Blackleg |
| Additional vaccines for cattle include bovine viral diarrhea, infectious bovine rhinotracheitis, parainfluenza 3, calf scours, and anthrax if in endemic area and/or client requests them | | |

*Note:* This is an example from the Western College of Veterinary Medicine, Saskatoon, Saskatchewan, Canada. Every municipality, province, state or veterinary practice may have their own vaccine protocols, which must be followed.
*Note:* In Canada, animals must be over 12 weeks of age to be vaccinated for rabies.

# Glossary

**adjuvant** Substance added to vaccines to enhance their antigenicity

**allergen** Material that invokes an allergic response, usually localized, in an individual

**antigen** Material capable of eliciting an antibody response in an animal

**antigenic drift** Process of mutation whereby an antigen changes its epitopes, thereby rendering previous immunity (and vaccines) useless or clinically reduced. A common occurrence in influenza viruses; occurred recently in the canine parvovirus

**antiserum** Serum containing antibodies directed against the various epitopes of an antigen that elicited their production

**atopy** A hereditary condition involving immunoglobulin E hypersensitivity

**autoimmune reaction** Occurs when tolerance to self breaks down and the immune system attacks self; it is usually an unhealthy state

**avirulent** Without disease-causing properties; this may be induced by multiple subculturing of some pathogens

**cell-mediated immunity** Branch of the immune system where cells, rather than antibody, play the predominant role. It occurs in both the innate and adaptive branches of the immune system

**colostrum** "First milk" secreted by a mother. In many species it is high in proteins, including antibodies, and therefore is a form of passive natural immunity

**commensal** Living on or within another organism and deriving benefit while befitting or not harming the host

**congenital** Born with; possibly but not necessarily hereditary

**epitope** Structural component of an antigen against which immune responses are made and to which an antibody binds; also called antigenic determinant

**etiological agent** Cause of the disease

**fibrosarcoma** Tumor from collagen-producing fibroblasts

**gene-deleted** Specific genes are removed from the pathogen so it becomes harmless and can produce a safe vaccine that elicits strong immunity. These are also known as genetically attenuated. This attenuation cannot be reversed

**genome** Genetic inventory

**granuloma** Dysfunctional tissue filled with eosinophils, fibroblasts that produce a scar, and large macrophages

**hypersensitivity** Normal reaction of the immune system, which for one reason or another becomes exaggerated and does damage to self

**immunodeficiency** Lack of all or part of the immune system's function with varying degrees of compromise to the animal's health; may be fatal

**immunoproliferative disorder** Characterized by the rapid production of lymphoid cells producing immunoglobulins

**lyophilized** Freeze-dried

**memory** One of the unique components of the immune system; it permits the recognition of an antigen that has been encountered before; because of the production of a greater number of B-cells (memory cells), the response is therefore faster and stronger. It goes hand-in-hand with specificity

**necrosis** Breakdown and death of cells, usually a result of inflammation

**pemphigus** A group of immune-mediated diseases of skin and mucous membranes

**phagocyte** White blood cell of the innate immune response that recognizes material as foreign to the body and engulfs it for digestion to render it harmless to the body

**polyclonal** Pertaining to several clones; derived from different cells

**self** One's own cells and molecules that the immune system, in health, does not attack but tolerates

**seroconversion** Changeover from a nonexistent or low antibody titer to one that is elevated; it usually implies an immune level

**specificity** Increased speed and strength of the immune system when encountering the same antigen for a second or subsequent time

**sub-unit** Genes from a pathogen are placed in another microbe so as to clone pathogen products. These gene products are then extracted, isolated, and purified for use in vaccine production; may also fall under the heading of antigens generated by genetic engineering

**sweet itch** Dermatitis of horses caused by hypersensitivity to the bites of *Culicoides* spp.; characterized by intense itching along the middle of the back

**tolerance** Lack of responsiveness by the immune system. Tolerance is healthy when it occurs to self, but is immunosuppressive when it occurs to antigens; can be induced by drugs, such as steroids

**toxoid** A toxin treated to destroy its toxicity without destroying antigenicity

**vectored** Specific pathogenic material is inserted into a nonpathogenic organism as a carrier for vaccine production. The antigenic proteins are not purified, and the recombinant organism itself may be used as a vaccine. Also known as live recombinant organisms

# Review Questions

**1** Innate immunity
   a. Is recognized by the clinical signs of fever and chills
   b. Is solely created by the actions of the neutrophils
   c. Occurs after the adaptive immune response
   d. Type of immunity with which one is born and does not develop after birth

**2** Which are clinical signs of anaphylaxis?
   a. Vomiting
   b. Dyspnea
   c. Incoordination
   d. All of the above

**3** Booster vaccines are given to
   a. Elicit a primary immune response
   b. Cause the production of IgM antibodies
   c. Stimulate the innate immune system
   d. Elicit a secondary immune response and a higher antibody titer

**4** Which of the following is false with regard to vaccine therapy?

  a. Vaccines may not be effective when given to a patient that is currently not showing clinical signs but is incubating a disease

  b. Vaccines may be responsible for certain types of anemia in dogs

  c. Vaccines are an example of acquired natural active immunity

  d. Recombinant vaccines are very effective and safe

**5** When administering a vaccine, to ensure the maximum immunity possible in the patient, it is important that you

  a. Follow the timing given by the manufacturer in the written protocol

  b. Use the correct route of administration

  c. Store the vaccines correctly and reconstitute them according to the manufacturer's instructions

  d. All of the above

**6** Which of the following species receive no maternal antibody during gestation?

  a. Cat

  b. Cow

  c. Dog

  d. Primate

**7** It is important that all neonates receive colostrum within what time period?

  a. The first 18 hours of life

  b. The first 24 hours of life

  c. The first 2 days of life

  d. The first week of life

**8** An example of acquired natural active immunity is

  a. Ingestion of colostrum

  b. Recovery from disease

  c. Vaccination

  d. Maternal antibodies crossing the placental barrier in cats

**9** The following statement describes an allergy

  a. It involves the excess production of IgE antibody and release of histamine

  b. It is rare in all species of animals, but when it occurs it is always hereditary

  c. It is a localized reaction to an allergen in animals that produce too much IgA antibody to that compound

  d. It is a type 2 hypersensitivity reaction

**10** The only antibody that can enter tissue spaces and cross the placental barrier in some species is

  a. IgG

  b. IgA

  c. IgD

  d. IgM

## BIBLIOGRAPHY

Alberts B et al: *Molecular biology of the cell*, ed 4, New York, 2002, Garland.

Facts on File Conference Highlights Agricultural Biotechnology International Conference, June 11–14, 1996, Saskatoon, Canada.

Gershwin L et al: *Immunology and immunopathology of domestic animals*, ed 2, St Louis, 1995, Mosby.

Janeway CA, Travers P: *Immunobiology, the immune system in health and disease*, London, 1994, Garland.

Roitt I, Brostoff J, Male D: *Immunology*, ed 6, London, 2001, Mosby.

Steinberg M, Cosloy S: *The Facts on File dictionary of biotechnology and genetic engineering*, ed 3, New York, 2006, Facts on File.

Tizard I: *Veterinary immunology: an introduction*, ed 7, St Louis, 2004, Saunders.

# PART II

# Clinical Applications

## CHAPTER 9

# Restraint and Handling

*Teresa Sonsthagen*

## OUTLINE

Dog Restraint
  Danger Potential
  Behavioral Characteristics
  Considerations for Restraint
  Restraint Equipment
Cat Restraint
  Danger Potential
  Behavioral Characteristics
  Considerations for Restraint
  Restraint Equipment
Horse Restraint
  Danger Potential
  Behavioral Characteristics
  Approaching a Horse
  Capturing a Horse
  Leading a Horse

Tying
  Restraint for General
    Examinations
  Restraint for Dental Procedures
  Distraction Techniques
  Tail Tie
  Picking Up Feet
  Foals
  Casting
Cattle Restraint
  Danger Potential
  Behavioral Characteristics
  Restraint
Sheep Restraint
  Danger Potential
  Behavioral Characteristics

Anatomy and Physiology
  Restraint
Goat Restraint
  Danger Potential
  Behavioral Characteristics
  Anatomy
  Restraint
Pig Restraint
  Danger Potential
  Behavioral Characteristics
  Anatomy and Physiology
  Restraint
Knots

## LEARNING OUTCOMES

After reading this chapter you should be able to:

1. Know the danger potential of each species so that your safety is kept in mind when restraining successfully.
2. Predict the common behavioral characteristics so that the most successful method of restraint will be used.
3. Keep in mind the considerations of restraint so that the animal is handled safely and will recover as soon as possible after the restraint procedure.
4. Be comfortable with the restraint equipment available for the species and use the proper tool for the procedure.

This chapter will reacquaint you with some of the basic restraint techniques taught in most veterinary technology programs. Without good basic knowledge of behavior, safety measures, and proper restraint techniques, the patient could injure the veterinary technician, veterinarian, and the owner, or injury could result to the patient. Restraint should be safe and firm, yet gentle. Restraint should be safe for the animal, safe for the person performing the restraint, and safe for the person performing the procedure.

This chapter will cover the restraint of cats, dogs, horses, cattle, sheep, goats, and pigs and is designed to refresh your memory on how the basic restraint techniques are performed, how most animals behave, and which safety measures should be used to ensure no one is injured. Restraint of rabbits and rodents will be covered in Chapter 17.

## DOG RESTRAINT ■■■■■■■■■

### Danger Potential

I. Canine teeth are a main means of defense

II. Toenail scratches are painful but not usually serious

### Behavioral Characteristics

I. Determined by breed, training, previous experiences, and human association

  A. The normal dog is a well-cared-for, sociable animal

    1. The pet or working dog is recognized by a happy attitude—wags tail, comes to greet you

    2. It has been taught definite social behaviors—sit, stay, down, and off

    3. Clients with new puppies should be advised on how to teach social behavior

    4. Dogs are usually docile but can be pushed into biting by painful procedures, harsh treatment, injury, or pain

  B. Nervous, frightened dogs

    1. Recognized by anxious expression, rapid head movement, sclera evident, grimacing, trembling lips, avoidance of eye contact, and shivering. They may cower or they may be boisterous

    2. Some nervous dogs nip out of excitement

    3. Expect these dogs to bite

      a. Approach them slowly, let them come to you, don't back them into a corner

      b. After they allow you to touch them, quickly but gently restrain their heads and snuggle them close to your body

  C. Vicious or aggressive dogs

    1. Recognized by head held low, hackles raised, tail straight out

    2. Dogs will bite, especially if challenged

    3. These dogs will try to make eye contact with you. This is a challenge

      a. Challenge definition: looking the dog in the eye, body faced forward

      b. The best action on your part is to slowly back away and avoid eye contact. Keep body sideways to the dog, look out the corner of your eye, and do not crouch

      c. If they look away it usually means they have backed off

    4. Both small and large dogs are capable of inflicting serious damage

      a. Small dogs can be more aggressive than large dogs, but keep in mind that a large dog can cause more damage

    5. Dogs do not always exhibit obvious characteristics of aggressiveness; some will attack without much warning

### Considerations for Restraint

Look at the type of animal, behavior, and past treatment received from humans to determine what type of restraint will be needed. Keep in mind the following seven points while restraining.

I. Rough handling will usually provoke retaliation; if the animal is pushed too far you will cause it to defend itself

  A. Minimal restraint is often the best way to start, moving up to more restrictive forms as necessary.

  B. A good grip around the muzzle or neck (Figure 9-1) secures the head.

  C. Two fingers between the legs secures them from slipping through your hands

II. If injured and in pain, a dog can be confused and disoriented, which makes determining its behavior unpredictable

  A. Always muzzle these dogs; the only exception is a dog with head injuries

    1. Apply the muzzle tightly or not at all

    2. The muzzle should not be left on longer than 20 minutes without a break

  B. When manipulating a dog, avoid putting pressure on the injured area; pressure can cause more damage or more pain, which in turn can cause the animal to go into shock or retaliate

III. Aggression and hostility

  A. Do not take chances with aggressive and hostile dogs; use the restraint tools necessary to keep yourself safe. These tools include

    1. Capture poles or rabies stick

    2. Gloves

    3. Blanket if the dog is small

    4. Cage or run doors, used as a shield

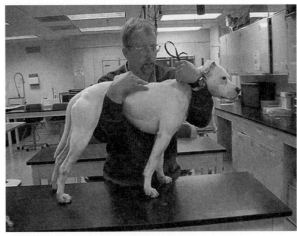

**Figure 9-1** Restraining a dog's head and body. (From Sheldon CC, Sonsthagen T, Topel JA: *Animal restraint for veterinary professionals,* St Louis, 2006, Mosby.)

IV. Fear and/or nervousness
  A. Attempt to reason and soothe the dog but exercise caution
    1. Use muzzles or rope leashes to remove them from cages or runs
    2. Sometimes you have to sedate animals before they are brought into the clinic
V. Old/young
  A. Special care is required when dealing with the very old and the very young
    1. Geriatric animals have to be handled with care and consideration
      a. If hospitalized, they will miss human contact; visits by the owners should be encouraged
      b. They are sensitive to stress
      c. They are most likely arthritic, so manipulation and pressure placed on joints can be very painful
      d. Comfort measures, such as a soothing voice, blankets or pads, and treats, are a must
    2. Puppies are difficult to hold onto because they are full of boundless energy and curiosity
      a. You must always maintain contact with them
      b. Examination table can cause fractures or dislocations
      c. When carrying them, keep a secure hold
VI. Pregnant animals should be treated the same as a geriatric patient
  A. Pregnant animals are prone to injury from increased weight, which puts pressure on hips, spine, and shoulders
  B. Pressure to the abdomen can be traumatic and should be avoided
  C. Stress and physiological changes may cause the bitch to abort
VII. Pets that are dominant are usually difficult to handle if their owners are present, because the pets have not learned to be submissive to people
  A. Owners may be asked to leave the room
    1. Most dogs calm down because they do not know what to expect from strangers
    2. If the owner refuses to leave, explain that the dog will have to be muzzled to protect the staff and the owner, and that a muzzle will also calm the dog
  B. When the owner is not present and the dog is still misbehaving
    1. Speak to the dog in a commanding voice
    2. It may be necessary to rap it under the chin or use a choker collar
    3. Be firm, consistent, and very persistent in getting the dog to behave
    4. If the dog wins the first battle, you will lose the war

**Restraint Equipment**

I. Choker collars are used only as a discipline tool
  A. The correct use is to sharply snap the collar closed and then release; this correction should be done immediately after bad behavior
  B. If not placed on the neck correctly, pressure will not be released
    1. Hold the collar so that it makes a "D" and slip it over the dog's neck
    2. Check for proper release. When pulling up on the collar and letting it loose, the loop around the neck should loosen up immediately
  C. Do not pull and tug continuously on the choker collar, because the dog will get used to the stimulus and not react
  D. Never use a choker collar as an everyday collar. Many animals have been caught on fences and have hung themselves because the loops can get caught in chain link and other nooks and crannies
II. Gentle Leaders/Promise/Halti collars
  A. These collars are used for training and for behavior modifications
  B. They work on the premise of a bitch making corrections to a puppy with pressure behind the ears and over the muzzle
  C. These collars must be fitted properly to each individual to work properly
III. Two types of leashes
  A. Leather leashes should be at least 6 feet (2 m) long and are ideal for training with choker collars, because they do not give and seldom break or tear
  B. Nylon, flat or round, rope leashes are usually 4 to 5 feet (1.5 to 2 m) in length, with a loop like a choker collar that will loosen when the standing part is released. They are used in several ways
    1. A nervous or vicious dog can be removed from a cage by using the rope leash
      a. A large noose is flipped over the dog's head; the dog can be pulled to the edge of the cage, keep the leash taut, grab a back leg, and quickly lower the dog to the floor
      b. Never just drag the dog out of the cage and let it drop to the floor; this can cause injury to the neck, back, and legs
    2. For vicious dogs, rope leashes can be used to cross-tie them
      a. Two leashes are placed around the dog's neck and held taut in opposite directions. This allows you to approach the rear to give an injection or to place a muzzle
  C. Chain or hard rope leashes should be avoided because they can injure the hands

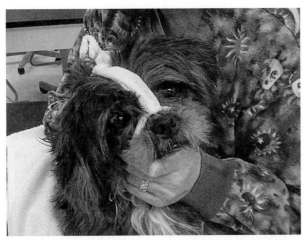

**Figure 9-2** Proper fit of gauze muzzle. (From Sheldon CC, Sonsthagen T, Topel JA: *Animal restraint for veterinary professionals,* St Louis, 2006, Mosby.)

IV. Capture pole or rabies pole is a long pole with a rope or covered wire protruding from the end to form an adjustable noose. The noose is slipped over the head of an aggressive animal
  A. Slide the noose in and out several times before using to make sure it is working correctly and can be quickly released in an emergency
  B. Once the animal is captured, the head can be controlled well enough to apply a muzzle or give an injection in the rear leg
V. Muzzles; two types
  A. The commercially prepared muzzle should be fitted to the dog at the store
    1. If it does not fit properly, the dog may bite with its incisors
  B. The gauze muzzle is a temporary muzzle constructed of roll gauze
    1. Tear off enough gauze to go around the nose of the dog twice and up behind the ears
    2. Make the first loop by tying a large open, loose overhand knot centered in the gauze; quickly slip this loop over the dog's nose
    3. Crisscross the gauze under the muzzle
    4. Bring the ends up behind the ears and tie with a bow
    5. If the dog is a brachycephalic breed, like a boxer, tie the ends behind the ears with an overhand knot. Bring one end of the gauze between the eyes, then under the loop around the nose, and tie to the other end in a bow, which will end up on top of the head. This prevents the loops from slipping off (Figure 9-2)
      a. This same method is used to muzzle cats
VI. A harness works extremely well for small dogs
  A. They cannot slip out of them
  B. If necessary you can lift them out of harm's way

VII. Voice commands. Fortunately, of all the animals we have to deal with, the dog will respond readily to the human voice
  A. A soft crooning voice comforts and calms and should be used throughout a restraint procedure
  B. The tone of voice should not be high pitched
    1. A high-pitched tone simulates the yelps and barks of littermates, which can make the dog think it is dominant over you
  C. A sharp, low, commanding tone often gets the dog's attention; this is similar to the low barks or growls of a dominant bitch or dog
    1. Avoid a yelling tone, which can frighten or cause aggression
  D. Always be consistent with your vocal tones so you do not confuse the dog
    1. If you sound like a littermate at one time (high-pitched voice) and then later yell at the dog, it may become very confused and act out

## CAT RESTRAINT
### Danger Potential

Of all domestic animals, the cat is one of the most difficult to handle because of its agility and formidable weaponry.
  I. Teeth are capable of inflicting serious wounds that often become infected
  II. Claws are razor sharp; all four feet can be used simultaneously and are the main means of defense

### Behavioral Characteristics

  I. Normal behavior
  A. Cats are aloof, independent creatures; they are not pack animals and do not have the pack instinct like a dog
  B. They are, however, social animals and will live peacefully with an established pecking order in a group of cats
  C. They are highly intelligent and curious creatures, often getting into serious situations because of it
  D. Cats are extremely territorial and mark their territory by spraying urine and rubbing scent glands (found by the commissure of the lips and at the base of the tail) on furniture, the boundaries of their yard, and their owner
    1. New places are thoroughly investigated; cats will explore everything and mark it as their territory
    2. When confined to a small space like a cage or small room, a cat's first instinct is to escape
      a. If escape is impossible the cat will defend the area as its own territory
      b. This often explains why a placid cat turns aggressive when that territory is "invaded"
  E. Most cats are placid and friendly in general, especially if well treated

II. Depressed behavior
   A. A depressed cat may stop eating and drinking
   B. The cat may be depressed as a result of boarding or removal from a familiar environment
      1. Depression results from lack of freedom and interaction with people
   C. It may sit in the litter box or huddle in the corner under newspapers or a towel
   D. If depression continues, the cat can become weak and could turn hostile if pushed
   E. These cats can/should be handled gently and often
III. If hostile, pound for pound, cats are among the most fearsome animals alive
   A. Hostile cats are difficult to handle
      1. They do not respond or submit to restraint, and if they escape they are very difficult to capture
   B. They will fight until they are too weak to fight anymore. You should handle these cats with restraint tools, such as gloves, towels, nets, or capture poles
   C. You can recognize them by observing their body language
      1. Ears pinned back or flat
      2. Vocalizing from hissing, low growls to screams
      3. Fur on tail and hackles raised
      4. Pawing at you

## Considerations for Restraint

Cats in general are not difficult to handle if you understand their actions. Observe each cat to determine the best method to use.

   I. Make sure all doors and windows are locked. Cats can squeeze through very small openings and are extremely difficult to catch when they are on the floor and running
   II. With a calm cat, begin with the least amount of restraint and become firmer as the situation demands. Make your adjustments in small increments—too firm too fast will often anger the cat
   III. Do not begin restraint until all participants are ready to start, because cats tolerate manipulation for only a very short period
   IV. Stay calm but firm, and be consistent with your voice and the restraint techniques chosen
   V. Few cats attack without warning, so angry cats should be covered with a large towel or blanket and scooped up. Wear protective gloves when doing this, because the blanket will not prevent bites or scratches
   VI. If you are aware of the cat's instinctive territorial trait, many problems can be avoided
      A. Cornered cats will attempt to escape and if unable to do so will fight
      B. Allow the cat to leave its territory by walking out of the cage, or quickly reach in with rope leash, capture pole, or gloved hands and remove it

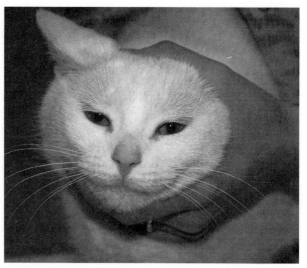

**Figure 9-3** Cat head restraint. (From Sheldon CC, Sonsthagen T, Topel JA: *Animal restraint for veterinary professionals,* St Louis, 2006, Mosby.)

   VII. Distraction techniques work very well on the cat; this involves inflicting mild pain to a certain area so the cat does not pay attention to what is going on elsewhere. Do not start the techniques too early, because they can backfire and make them angry fast
      A. "Caveman" pets: vigorous pats on the head or body
      B. Tapping or blowing on the nose
      C. Vigorous rubbing on top of the head
   VIII. Head and leg restraint is very important with cats for the safety of the people doing the procedure. There are several methods of securing the head
      A. Wrap your hand completely around the cat's head with thumb ending up on top of head (Figure 9-3)
      B. Scruff the cat and hang onto the back legs with a finger in between (Figure 9-4)

## Restraint Equipment

   I. A rope leash described in canine restraint is used in the same manner
      A. You occasionally capture one or both front legs, along with the neck. If you are gentle it still works well
   II. A towel, pillowcase, or small blanket can be used to surround a hostile cat
      A. One method is to center the towel over the cat and then sweep the flaps of the towel under the cat, wrapping its legs in the folds of the towel similar to the way a taco is wrapped
      B. A second method is to place the towel on the table, depositing the cat in the first third of the towel, wrapping the other two thirds tightly around the

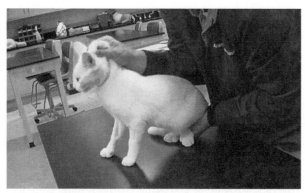

**Figure 9-4** Scruffing cat neck and securing back legs. (From Sheldon CC, Sonsthagen T, Topel JA: *Animal restraint for veterinary professionals,* St Louis, 2006, Mosby.)

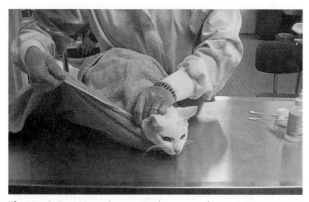

**Figure 9-5** Wrapping a cat in a towel. (From Sheldon CC, Sonsthagen T, Topel JA: *Animal restraint for veterinary professionals,* St Louis, 2006, Mosby.)

cat, and tucking in the end closest to the tail, much like a burrito is wrapped (Figure 9-5)

III. Gloves are made of thick leather that should cover your arms up to the elbow
   A. Disadvantages of gloves
      1. Tactile sense is lost, which may result in applying too much pressure
      2. They will not protect you from bites but do reduce the number of scratches you receive
   B. Use of gloves
      1. Place your hand partially in one gauntlet
      2. Offer that hand to the cat while it is trying to bite or scratch
      3. Reach in with your other hand, fully encased in a gauntlet, and grab the animal by the scruff of the neck. This same technique can be used on small to medium-sized dogs

IV. Feline restraint bag (cat bag) is usually made of canvas or thick nylon. This bag completely encloses the body of the cat. The head is held in place and there are access zippers or Velcro strips to allow the legs

to be brought out. Never leave the cat unattended, because it can roll off the table
   A. Advantages to using a cat bag
      1. It usually has a calming effect; after a cat realizes it cannot escape, it will calm down
      2. The feet can no longer be used against you
   B. Disadvantages
      1. The cat can still bite
      2. You must be careful not to get the fur and skin caught in the zipper
      3. Large and/or angry cats are difficult to place into the bag
      4. The jugular vein is not easily accessible
      5. To prevent spread of disease and ectoparasites, the bag should be disinfected after each use

V. If you are alone and need to perform a simple and painless procedure, floral tape or Vet wrap works well to bind the legs together
   A. First tape front legs together and then tape rear legs together
      1. A towel over the head may also prove beneficial
   B. Remove the tape from the back legs first and then the front legs
   C. Never leave cat with legs bound like this alone on top of a table because it could roll off and severely injure itself
   D. The use of adhesive tape could pull and remove hair

VI. Leather/nylon or gauze muzzles work well and protect the handler from bites
   A. Most commercial muzzles also cover a cat's eyes
   B. Reusable muzzles should be disinfected to prevent spread of respiratory diseases

VII. An Elizabethan collar can also protect the handler from bites

## HORSE RESTRAINT
### Danger Potential

I. Rear feet
   A. The kicking range of the hind feet is 6 to 8 feet (2 to 2.5 m) straight out, with the furthest extension of the foot the most dangerous for handlers
   B. The aim is usually very accurate
   C. To pass safely behind a horse, you can either
      1. Stay at least 10 to 12 feet (3.5 to 4 m) behind or to the side
      2. Stay in direct physical contact with the horse by placing a hand on the rump

II. Front feet
   A. If a horse rears it can knock a person to the ground
   B. It can strike a handler's head and arms with or without rearing

III. Teeth
  A. Front incisors can cause major injuries, because the horse can lock its jaws, which will cause further damage as the bitten area is pulled from the horse's mouth
  B. Discipline is a must if a horse bites
    1. This may include a sharp jerk on the halter or a firm pop on the nose

## Behavioral Characteristics

I. The horse is nervous and suspicious by nature. It is quick to detect threats and react to them in a manner that may be dangerous to humans
  A. As part of its flight instinct, if suddenly frightened or hurt, reactions may include rearing, biting, kicking, or running away, all without obvious warning
  B. Keep alert and never treat a horse complacently
  C. Always move slowly and deliberately. Quick motions and loud noises will almost always frighten a horse into evasive action
II. Horses often show some warning signals that should be heeded to prevent possible injuries. The most expressive parts of a horse are the ears; however, the tail, eyes, and mouth are also useful indicators of behavior
  A. Ears
    1. If the horse is alert, the ears are pricked forward
      a. The horse sees what is coming and usually will not become startled
    2. If the horse is nervous or uncertain, the ears are constantly moving back and forth
      a. Offer comforting words and be ready for a flight response
    3. If the horse is angry or fearful, the ears are pinned back
      a. Expect these horses to strike, kick, or rear up
    4. If the horse is concentrating, the ears are pinned back (out to the sides)
      a. It is usually busy performing what it is meant to do
  B. Tail
    1. Nervousness is indicated by wringing or circling. Comfort measures are also appropriate: gentle pats and quieting talk
    2. When the horse is in pain or sleeping, the tail is straight down. If in pain, a harsh stimulus may cause a fight-or-flight response. If sleeping and startled, expect the same
    3. Fear is shown by the tail being clamped tight between the gluteal muscles. Comfort measures are a must with this horse. Be ready for the fight-or-flight response

## Approaching a Horse

I. Approach from the front and slightly to the left side
  A. Horses are accustomed to being handled from this near (left) side
  B. The right side is referred to as the far side
II. Move slowly without sudden movements or loud noise
  A. If the horse moves away, stop. If you do not stop, the horse will think it is being chased and will flee
III. Talk to the horse and perhaps offer it some grain so it will approach you; a quick hand can get a rope around its neck while its head is in the bucket
IV. Some horses will need to be put in a smaller pen to catch them
  A. Luring them into the pen with grain is a much better method than chasing them
V. When approaching a horse from the rear
  A. Begin talking to it before you get close. A startled horse may kick or jump forward and injure itself or you

## Capturing a Horse

I. Check the halter and lead rope for splits or fraying
II. A horse can easily break a defective lead rope and/or halter
III. Slip the lead rope around the horse's neck and tie a single overhand knot to keep the rope from slipping off. Proceed to put the halter on the horse
IV. Hold the neck strap of the halter in the left hand, reach under the horse's neck, and hold the head still so the right hand can bring the halter over the horse's neck
V. Slide the nose band of the halter onto the nose and buckle the neck strap behind the ears
  A. Keep your movements slow and deliberate
VI. Check to make sure the halter is settled correctly on the horse's face
VII. Attach the lead rope to the center ring of the halter under the chin. Untie the end of the lead rope from around the neck. The left hand should hold the loose end of the rope in neat loops with the entire rope held in front of you
  A. Never wrap the loose end of the lead rope around your hand
  B. Never have the rope loose behind you

## Leading a Horse

I. Gather the lead rope in your left hand. Do not wrap it around your hand. If the horse bolts, it could snag, causing a severe injury
II. Always walk on the left side of the horse with your right hand on the lead rope approximately 5 to 6 inches (12 to 15 cm) from the halter ring

III. Stay close to the shoulder
- A. Do not get too far in front of the horse because it can rear up and strike with a front foot or it can accidentally step on the back of your heels as it walks. It can also bite you on the shoulder or back
- B. When stopping, stand facing the same direction as the horse

## Tying

I. A horse should always be tied to a sturdy, vertical object with a well-fitting halter and suitable lead rope

II. The knot used to tie the lead rope should be a quick release knot, such as the halter tie
- A. The horse can be released quickly if it gets into trouble

III. Allow about 2 to 3 feet (0.75 to 1 m) of lead rope so the horse can adjust the angle of its neck and shift its position as it desires
- A. The horse may tangle its front feet in the rope if a longer rope is left
- B. A shorter rope may frustrate the horse enough to cause it to attempt to free itself

IV. Check the area around your tied horse for possible hazards that could cause serious injuries

V. Never pass under the neck of a tied horse to get to the other side. This is a very dangerous practice that could result in serious injuries if the horse is startled

## Restraint for General Examinations

I. Stand on same side of horse as the person who is working on the animal
- A. By standing on the same side, the horse has the option of moving away from both of you to escape
  1. If there are people on both sides, the animal will pick the smallest of the barriers and try to move over that. Unfortunately, that may be a person bending or kneeling

II. Never stand directly in front of the horse
- A. It can rear up and come down on top of you
- B. It can strike out with its front feet
- C. It can run you over in an effort to escape

III. Hold head level with the withers; if the head is held higher, the horse has an advantage and can easily escape

IV. Cross tying
- A. Used to prevent a horse from rearing and from moving its forequarters from side to side
- B. The horse can still strike with its front feet and move its rear quarters
  1. Snap a lead rope onto the cheek piece ring on each side of the halter. Tie each lead rope to the side of the stanchion, to stocks, or to beams
  2. Tie the ropes high enough to prevent the horse from rearing and entangling its feet in the ropes

3. Use a quick release knot, such as the halter tie, or use a quick release buckle
4. Cross tying allows you access to the horse's entire body but does not prevent it from swinging its rear end

V. Stocks
- A. A narrow stall with removable or semiopen sides and a gate at both ends
  1. Lead the horse through the back gate and close the front after it is in the stocks
  2. Do not go into the stocks with the horse; pass the rope around the bars as needed to keep the horse moving
  3. Stocks are used usually for rectal and uterine examination or procedures on the head

VI. Blindfolds
- A. Can be used to control an obstinate or a fearful horse
- B. The horse will usually calm down and depend on you to guide it wherever you want it to go
- C. Work slowly and talk constantly to reassure the horse

## Restraint for Dental Procedures

I. Place your left hand on the bridge of the horse's nose with your thumb under the noseband of the halter, and place your right hand on the nape of the neck; push the head down

II. To hold the tongue, reach in at the commissure of the lips, grasp the tongue, and slowly pull it out to the side through the diastema of the lower jaw

## Distraction Techniques

I. Twitches are used on obstinate horses that will not allow procedures to be performed
- A. Through the release of endorphins, which mask the pain, twitches distract the horse's attention from other procedures by applying a mild pain to the upper muzzle
- B. Of the three types (chain, humane, and rope), the chain is most common (Figure 9-6)
  1. Place the loop of chain over your left hand, catching one side of the loop between your little finger and ring finger
  2. Grasp as much of the horse's upper lip with your left hand as possible, press the bottom edges together to protect the delicate inner surface, and quickly slide the handle up so the chain loop rests high up around the lip
  3. Tighten the chain by twisting the handle until the twitch is fitted snugly on the lip so lip curls upward
  4. Tighten and loosen the chain on the muzzle to keep the twitch effective. If steady pressure is applied the muzzle would lose circulation,

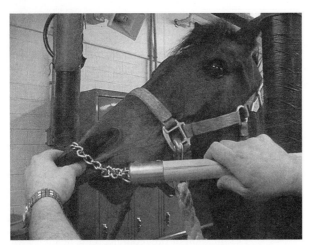

**Figure 9-6** Application of a twitch. (From Sheldon CC, Sonsthagen T, Topel JA: *Animal restraint for veterinary professionals,* St Louis, 2006, Mosby.)

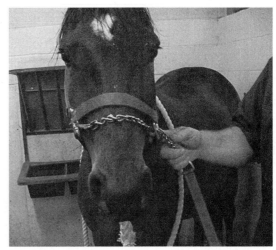

**Figure 9-7** Chain shank on a horse. (From Sheldon CC, Sonsthagen T, Topel JA: *Animal restraint for veterinary professionals,* St Louis, 2006, Mosby.)

thereby reducing sensitivity of the muzzle and rendering the twitch ineffective

    5. Many horses will attempt to get away or resist the twitch when it is first applied; stay with them by moving with their motions. If they shake you off the first time it will be more difficult to place the twitch again

    6. After the twitch is removed, massage the muzzle to restore circulation

  B. A humane twitch is a hinged pair of long handles that squeeze over the sides of the lip and then can be secured at the bottom

    1. Once applied it need not be held

    2. The pressure is mild and may be ignored by horses

II. A lead shank is a long leather strap with about 2 feet (0.75 m) of flat chain attached to it with a snap on the end

  A. It is used as a distraction device, or if more restraint than just a halter is needed. It is used as a training device and on stallions for added control

  B. There are several ways to use a chain shank (Figure 9-7)

    1. With the halter in place, pass the chain end through the ring on the cheek piece

      a. Pull it across the bridge of the nose to the ring on the other side of the head

      b. Pull it under the jaw. This method is not ideal because this may cause the horse to throw its head up

      c. Place it under the top lip over the upper gum. This is very effective in directing the horse's attention away from other procedures, but it is painful and may inflict injury

      d. Put the chain in the mouth like the bit of a bridle and clip it to the ring on the other side

      C. Be careful not to jerk excessively on the chain shank, because injury may result

III. Eyelid press involves gently placing fingers on the upper eyelid and pressing down; it is a very gentle distraction technique that can be used for injections or to keep the horse still

IV. Shoulder roll is done by grasping a large fold of skin with both hands just over the shoulder and wiggling or moving it from side to side or up and down; it works very well for intravenous injections

V. Caveman pets, or somewhat heavy swats, are excellent ways to distract a horse

VI. Pick up or tie up the opposite foot from the one being radiographed or bandaged

VII. Grasp the base of the ear with the heel of your hand touching the head. Squeeze or rotate the ear in a small circle

  A. It is best to use this only as a last resort

    1. If done incorrectly it could cause the horse to become sensitive and make it afraid of having its ears touched

    2. This can cause the owner of a show animal a lot of frustration when the hair in the ears needs to be trimmed

  B. Do not apply so much pressure to the ear that damage occurs to the cartilage, which can cause the ear to flop over

VIII. A cradle is a device that is placed around a horse's neck to prevent it from chewing or licking at wounds; it prevents the horse from bending or turning the neck

## Tail Tie

I. Always tie the tail to the animal's own body (Figure 9-8)

II. Secure a cord or rope to the hair on the tail using a sheet bend or tail tie knot

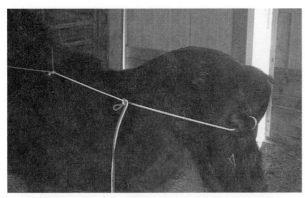

**Figure 9-8** Tail tie on a horse. (From Sheldon CC, Sonsthagen T, Topel JA: *Animal restraint for veterinary professionals,* St Louis, 2006, Mosby.)

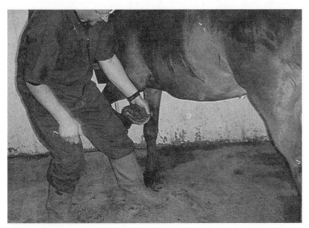

**Figure 9-9** Picking up a front foot on a horse. (From Sheldon CC, Sonsthagen T, Topel JA: *Animal restraint for veterinary professionals,* St Louis, 2006, Mosby.)

III. Pull the tail to the side of the buttocks and pass the rope to the opposite front leg
IV. Use a quick release knot to secure the other part of the rope to the neck or front leg
V. The purpose is to move the tail out of the way for rectal/uterine or obstetric procedures

### Picking Up Feet

I. Front feet (Figure 9-9)
   A. Stand lateral to the shoulder and parallel to the horse, facing the caudal end
   B. Place your closest hand on the horse's shoulder; gently but firmly run it down to the fetlock
   C. Grasp the fetlock by placing your palm on the underside of the fetlock and wrapping your fingers around the joint
   D. Squeeze and lift the foot; at the same time lean into the horse to make it shift its weight to the other three legs
   E. After raising the foot up, bring it slightly out to the side. Position your body close to the horse's body so that your knees are slightly bent. Place the foot between your legs so it rests on top of your knees, allowing both hands to be free. Flex fetlock and hoof toward yourself
II. Rear feet
   A. Approach in the same manner as for the front feet
   B. After you have lifted the foot, extend the leg out to the rear and place it on top of your bent knee closest to the horse

### Foals

I. Capture and restraint
   A. Keep the foal in sight of the mare. Place the mother in a large box stall (the mare often needs to be restrained as well) so that she can see her foal but is not able to get at you
   B. Grasp the foal around the front of the chest with one arm, and around the rump with the other arm, or grasp the tail. Quickly move the foal clear of the dam
   C. Use your arms to form a "mini corral" and keep the foal encircled with your arms
   D. Do not lift the foal off its feet; this makes it very nervous and it will struggle
   E. Always talk to and comfort a foal when handling it

### Casting

I. Laying a horse in lateral recumbency
   A. Anesthetics are used almost exclusively
   B. Key to a smooth drop is to maintain control of the horse's head. Lift it up and to the side when it starts to go down
   C. Once the horse is down, pad the side of the head facing the ground and place a knee on the neck to keep the horse recumbent
   D. Ropes are usually used to secure three of the four legs to prevent kicking
      1. Clove hitch or variations are often used

## CATTLE RESTRAINT
### Danger Potential

I. Head
   A. Horned animals can fatally gore a handler by quick thrusts forward and sideways
   B. Be constantly aware of the swinging arc and the extent of reach from side to side and forward
   C. Butting is done by polled and horned animals
      1. This can be a rushing motion, pinning you against a fence, wall, or ground
      2. It can be a swing of the head, knocking you down and holding you down
II. Body
   A. Cattle can pin restrainers against a wall or fence or between other cows (dairy cows in stanchions)

III. Feet
   A. Front feet are seldom used as weapons
      1. Cattle do paw the ground to show aggression
      2. The split toe can cause serious damage to human toes and feet if they step on you
   B. Hind feet are very dangerous and very accurate
      1. Cattle usually kick by bringing the foot forward, arching out to the side and then backward (cow kicking)
      2. They can kick straight back, like a horse, but seldom do
      3. Usually kick is one legged, not two legged like horses
   C. The safest place to stand is at the shoulder, but remember that bovine can kick past its shoulder
IV. Tail
   A. The tail is useful to cattle for swatting flies and for attending to other twitches
   B. The tail is an annoyance and can cause injury to the restrainer's or examiner's eyes during procedures
      1. To prevent injury, remove awns or burrs from the tail by dipping it in mineral oil
      2. Melt frozen ice and feces by dipping the tail in a warm bucket of water and then tying it up to the cow's body
   C. The tail is very fragile
      1. Never tie the tail to anything but the animal's body
      2. Use the same procedure as with horses; there is not as much hair to work with
V. Cattle seldom bite because they lack upper incisors
   A. If they do bite, it is more of a pinch than a bite and is usually an accident

## Behavioral Characteristics

Cattle differ markedly in their reactions to manipulations and the presence of humans as a result of the breed, handling, and gender.
I. Dairy cows are accustomed to being handled and are the most docile of the bovine breeds
   A. Restraint is usually done in stanchions or by tying to a fence. Talk to and treat dairy cows gently
   B. They may become nervous and vigorously resist handling if not treated gently
II. More so than any other animal, dairy bulls require special restraint techniques because they are extremely unpredictable
   A. If handled correctly, the unpredictability can be minimized
   B. Nose rings, in addition to halters, are often used in bulls for more control while leading
      1. Do not tie the bull fast to stationary objects by the nose ring; the halter and lead rope is used

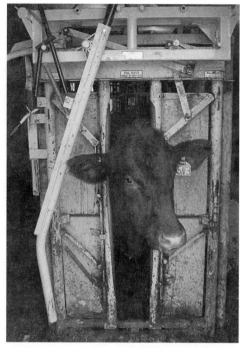

**Figure 9-10** Cow in a head chute. (From Sheldon CC, Sonsthagen T, Topel JA: *Animal restraint for veterinary professionals,* St Louis, 2006, Mosby.)

   C. Beef cows are easily frightened because of little association with people
   D. Restraint involves chutes (with head gates) and alleyways (Figure 9-10)
   E. Beef bulls are handled the same as females; be careful around beef bulls when the females are in heat

## Restraint

I. Approach
   A. Avoid quick movements to prevent startling the animals; use slow, deliberate actions
   B. Talk to them so they are aware of your presence
      1. A low command to move is much preferred over sharp yelling
   C. Do not approach from the front, because it is a natural instinct for cattle to charge. Cattle cannot charge if they are in a squeeze chute and head gate, or tied in a stanchion
      1. Remember, they can still stretch their necks and butt you if you are too close
II. Herding
   A. Flight zone (this is true in cattle, sheep, goats, and horses). Most prey animals have a large field of vision with blind spots directly behind them and a few degrees to the right and left of the rump
   B. To make these animals move forward, walk past the point of their shoulder; this prompts them to move forward

C. If you stand in their blind zone and suddenly talk loudly or slap them with a whip or strap, they may bolt or kick

III. Head

A. If using chutes, always check the operation of the chute before use
   1. Familiarize yourself with the operation
   2. Repair if necessary

B. Rope halters are the basic tool of restraint
   1. The part that tightens is placed around the nose, with the loop down. The lead rope should be on the left side of the cow's head
   2. The head then can be tied to a post, fence, or part of the chute
   3. The position of the head is generally up and to the side
   4. Tie the end of the rope with a snubbing hitch or halter tie
   5. Used for such procedures as blousing, stomach tubing, dehorning, or eye examinations

C. Cattle have a sensitive nasal septum that can be used to produce a mild pain that acts as a distraction technique. Pressure can be applied manually or with instruments
   1. Thumb and index finger can be used for very short periods of time (your fingers will tire quickly)
   2. Nose leads (tongs) are commercially manufactured
      a. Make sure that the balls on the tongs are smooth and not too close together
      b. Close tong handles together to adequately hold onto the nose without pinching too much
      c. Have a holder grasp the tongs or secure it to the halter

D. Examination of eye requires the head to be rotated so that the afflicted eye is parallel with the ceiling
   1. This is usually accomplished with a halter or nose tong

E. Passing a stomach tube requires application of a halter and a mouth speculum (such as a Frick speculum) to hold the jaws apart while passing the stomach tube into the esophagus
   1. If the speculum is not used, the cow may clamp down on the tube

IV. Hobbles

A. Used to prevent kicking—just above the hocks or close to the ankles

B. Place on the back legs
   1. Place on the leg opposite you first, then the one closest to you
   2. Keep the legs square so the cow can maintain its balance

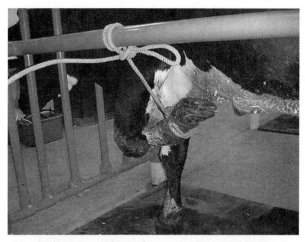

**Figure 9-11**  Front foot of a cow held in place by ropes. (From Sheldon CC, Sonsthagen T, Topel JA: *Animal restraint for veterinary professionals,* St Louis, 2006, Mosby.)

   3. Hobbles can be padded straps held with a chain or an angled piece of metal that slips on the back side of the legs just above the hocks

V. Feet and legs

A. Examination of hind legs or trimming hooves can be performed
   1. Cast the cow in lateral recumbency by using the burley or double half hitch method and administration of a sedative
   2. A hydraulic lift table can be used to place the animal in lateral recumbency—again with the administration of a sedative
      a. Lead the animal in front of the table, strap on, and then lower the table to a lateral recumbency
   3. The legs can be raised with ropes and pulleys, either in a chute or stanchion (Figure 9-11)

VI. Tail

A. "Jacking" the tail up acts as a distraction technique (Figure 9-12)
   1. Is done by lifting the tail straight up and forward from the base
      a. Should be ventral and over the midline so handler can keep balance
      b. Hold the tail about one third of the way down from the base
   2. Pressure on the spinal column removes sensation to the rear
   3. Make sure that the animal is secured from moving forward or from side to side
   4. Used for intravenous venipuncture or rectal examination

B. The jacking should not be performed for more than a few minutes because of possible fracture of coccygeal vertebrae

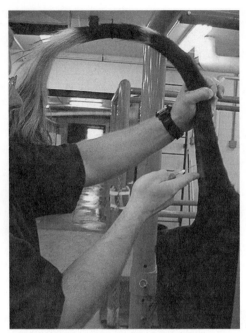

**Figure 9-12** Proper way to "jack" the tail on a cow. (From Sheldon CC, Sonsthagen T, Topel JA: *Animal restraint for veterinary professionals,* St Louis, 2006, Mosby.)

VII. Casting: laying an animal in lateral recumbency
   A. Important for the animal to have a sturdy harness
   B. Avoid incorporating the udder of the cow or testicles of a bull into the flank rope
   C. All knots should be positioned dorsally
   D. Two methods could be used
      1. Burley or half hitch method
         a. A bowline knot around the neck and a set of half hitches distal to the front legs and rear legs, proximal to the flank
         b. Not appropriate for mature cattle, but if used, watch the udder and testicles
         c. One person can easily pull down a cow
      2. Crisscross method
         a. Divide the rope in half and place the middle part of the rope over the neck; then pass it between the front legs near the sternum
         b. Cross the ropes over the back and between the rear legs
         c. Two people are needed
         d. This is appropriate for mature cattle
VIII. Flank restraint
   A. A lariat can be tightened around the flank area just cranial to the tuber coxae to prevent kicking. Avoid excess pressure; otherwise the animal may fall
   B. A metal clamp often known as an antikicker can be placed over the dorsum and along the sides in the same location

IX. Calf restraint
   A. Newborns are guided from place to place by placing one hand under the neck and grasping the tail head or placing the other hand around the hindquarters
   B. Calves up to 200 lb (91 kg) can be put into lateral recumbency by "flanking" or "legging" the calf down. After it is down, apply a three-legged tie: place one knee on its neck and the other knee in front of the closest hind leg to hold it down
   C. Never turn your back to the calf's mother; she is extremely protective of her young and could potentially kill a careless handler

## SHEEP RESTRAINT
### Danger Potential

I. Head is used as a battering ram, with most injuries consisting of serious bruises

### Behavioral Characteristics

I. Sheep have allelomimetic behavior (strong flocking instincts), causing them to move as a group, which makes them easy to handle
II. Move slowly when working with sheep; their first line of defense is speed and flocking to flee, which makes them startle easily

### Anatomy and Physiology

I. Sheep are not the jumpers that goats are, although they can jump up to 1.2 m (4 feet)
   A. Exceptions are range sheep and cheviots (harder to handle)
II. Sheep can have problems when worked in hot weather; normal body temperature can be as high as 104° F (40° C)
   A. Running, struggling, and crowding, plus their heavy wool, can very quickly result in hyperthermia
III. Never grab the wool when restraining sheep because it pulls out easily; damage to the fleece, the skin, and subcutaneous layers can result

### Restraint

I. Trained sheepdogs are your best tool; they save a lot of steps when herding the sheep to specific spots
II. Herding
   A. Flight zone similar to cattle: move as a group
   B. Get one sheep to move in the direction you want, and the rest will follow
III. Crowding the flock into a small pen or area, with portable gates, is usually the best way to work a group or to capture a single sheep
   A. Mark sheep with a wax crayon as it is medicated so that double dosing does not occur

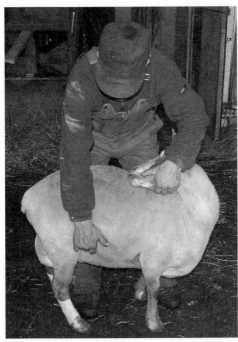

**Figure 9-13** Casting a sheep—starting position. (From Sheldon CC, Sonsthagen T, Topel JA: *Animal restraint for veterinary professionals,* St Louis, 2006, Mosby.)

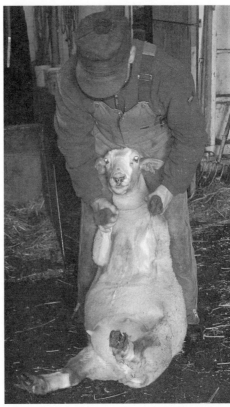

**Figure 9-14** Casting a sheep—final position. (From Sheldon CC, Sonsthagen T, Topel JA: *Animal restraint for veterinary professionals,* St Louis, 2006, Mosby.)

IV. To capture a single sheep
    A. Approach slowly, quietly, and deliberately
    B. Reach down and limit the forward movement with a hand under the chin
    C. Quickly reach for the dock or flank fold with the other hand to stop backward motion
    D. Move wherever you wish by applying pressure on the chin or dock
    E. Turning can be done by grasping the muzzle and turning the head toward the shoulder
 V. A shepherd's crook is a handy tool for catching a sheep
    A. It is used to "snare" a hind leg proximal to the stifle (hock)
VI. "Setting-up" (also referred to as rumping or docking) a sheep allows you to examine the underside of the sheep, shear, vaccinate, or trim the hooves (Figures 9-13 and 9-14)
    A. Move the sheep so it is standing sideways in front of your legs
    B. Plant your left leg by the sheep's shoulder
    C. Grasp the chin with one hand and the flank with the other
    D. Lift up on the flank, turn, and push the sheep's head into its shoulder; pivot on your left leg and move your right leg back. This throws the sheep off balance and onto its dock

    E. Lean the sheep back between your legs and release your hands
    F. Make sure the hocks are off the ground
    G. If done properly, the sheep will not be able to get to its feet. Your hands are free to perform whatever procedure you choose
VII. Halters can be used but the sheep's short nose makes it difficult to prevent the nose piece from sliding down and occluding the nares
VIII. Lambs are held by supporting them beneath their chest with your forearm between their front legs
    A. For castrations and tail docks, the lamb can be held by grasping a front and back leg in one hand and the opposite front and back leg in the other hand, resting the lamb's back against your chest. The head will hang down between the legs

## GOAT RESTRAINT
### Danger Potential

 I. Goats use their heads as battering rams
    A. If annoyed they will rear up on their hind legs and slam into you with their heads

II. Most goats are disbudded or dehorned at a young age
   A. Horned goats do not like to have their horns held and will swing their heads back and forth viciously if held
   B. The horns add power to the butt and can cause injury

## Behavioral Characteristics

I. Goats are very vocal
   A. The kids sound like human babies when handled, and the entire herd will come to investigate any fuss
   B. The herd may try to protect the kid or other members of the herd in danger
II. They respond to gentle treatment and become quite tame if handled a lot
   A. Rough handling may make them nasty
III. Intact males have scent glands at the base of the horns that secrete a very disagreeable long-lasting odor that attracts females during breeding season
   A. When in rut, intact males will mark their territory by urinating on their beards, legs, neck, and body and then rubbing those parts on objects around the farmyard. This odor lasts throughout the breeding season
IV. Goats are good escape artists and will work loose knots and chains
   A. Make sure all gates are properly locked

## Anatomy

I. Their delicate bones are easily fractured and dislocated if grasped incorrectly
II. Goats are very hardy animals that can take a lot of stress
III. They are very good jumpers but will rarely be able to jump over 6 feet (2 m)
   A. If they try to jump over you, you may be hit at chest or shoulder height

## Restraint

I. Capture
   A. To capture a single goat, it is best to place the entire herd in a small pen
      1. Because goats do not have the strong flocking instinct of sheep, it is best to lure them in with grain
      2. After the goats are in the small pen, move slowly and deliberately toward your intended patient
      3. Grasp around the neck or catch by the collar, and place the other hand on the goat's dock to move it
         a. If unable to grasp as above, try capturing by the front leg. This usually makes them stand still

      4. Once caught, grasp the head behind the ears and under the chin and back the goat into a corner
   B. If you are using chain collars, make sure they are the flat chains to prevent the goat from getting caught on fences
   C. It is best to use plastic link breakaway collars
II. Head
   A. To restrain the head with no "neck" wear, you can place both hands on either side of the cheeks and wrap your fingers around the lower jaw
   B. The handler can push the goat sideways against a wall or fence, securing the head by holding the jaws firmly at an upward angle. It works even better if in a corner to prevent the goat from backing up
   C. The beard can be grasped with one hand, with the other hand placed on top of the head
III. Goats cannot be set on their haunches because they are much more agile than sheep and will struggle
   A. They can be flanked similar to a calf, or be placed against a fence and have their legs lifted similar to a horse
   B. Dairy goats can be placed in a milking stanchion for restraint or secured to a fence using a quick-release knot
IV. Dehorning and castration
   A. To disbud kids, hold them like a lamb, then sit down, folding the kid's legs under its body and cradling its head in both hands so the thumbs hold down the ears
   B. To castrate, hold the kid the same as described for lambs
V. Pick feet up as you would pick up a horse's hoof (Figure 9-15)

## PIG RESTRAINT
## Danger Potential

I. Teeth
   A. Newborn piglets have sharp needlelike deciduous teeth (canines and third incisors, called needle teeth) that can damage the sow's udder and handlers
   B. Clipping of the teeth, along with other management techniques, is done soon after birth
      1. Wounds made by the canines (called tusks) are almost always septic
   C. Adults have very strong jaws and can tear flesh easily. A male with tusks is quite dangerous
II. Adult pigs can push and knock down a handler with their head and body

## Behavioral Characteristics

I. Herding instincts are virtually nonexistent, but the entire herd will converge to the rescue of a screaming mate. Sows reacting to perceived danger to their piglets are extremely dangerous

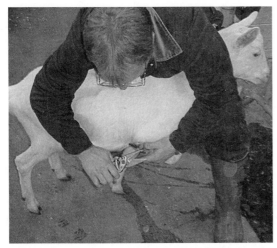

**Figure 9-15** Picking up a front foot for trimming a goat's hooves. (From Sheldon CC, Sonsthagen T, Topel JA: *Animal restraint for veterinary professionals,* St Louis, 2006, Mosby.)

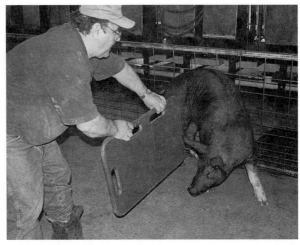

**Figure 9-16** Using a hurdle to move swine. (From Sheldon CC, Sonsthagen T, Topel JA: *Animal restraint for veterinary professionals,* St Louis, 2006, Mosby.)

II. Pigs are stubborn and contrary, but you can use this behavior to your advantage during restraint procedures

III. They are unpredictable and can become aggressive without warning

IV. They enjoy being talked to and petted or scratched gently. Simple procedures can sometimes be done while gently rubbing the ventral abdomen and while they are lying down, but be careful

V. They are extremely vocal

**Anatomy and Physiology**

I. Pigs have streamlined bodies that were designed to run through underbrush, making it very easy for them to slide under objects, such as fences, or between your legs

II. Strong neck muscles developed to root enable the pig to lift with considerable force such items as fencing panels or even a handler

III. Thin legs can easily be fractured or dislocated if held in the wrong manner

IV. Because of a thick layer of subcutaneous fat, pigs overheat easily

**Restraint**

I. Small enclosures are the easiest way to handle large numbers of pigs for injections

A. Each pig is marked with a wax crayon as the injection is administered

II. Squeeze pens and farrowing crates are ideal, but they can be extremely dangerous. Never get into a small pen with a pig (especially a sow and litter) without checking for an escape route with an easy access

III. Moving

A. A cane, light plastic pipe, leather or canvas strap, or flat stick can be used to move or direct the pig

1. A gentle slap on the rear will make a pig move forward; a tap on the side of the head will turn it in the opposite direction

2. Sound, more than pain, is what makes a pig move. Never use any of the objects to inflict pain because it can anger the pig and the pig may attack you

B. A bucket placed over the pig's head will cause the pig to back up

1. You can direct it by grabbing the tail

C. Hog panels or hurdles/shields/barriers are made of solid sheets of plywood, plastic, or aluminum and are used to move and direct pigs (Figure 9-16)

1. The hurdles should be solid and wall-like to prevent the pigs from running through or raising the panel

2. To move a pig using a hurdle, place it between you and the pig and start walking

3. To turn the pig, set the barrier down on the opposite side of the pig's head

4. If a pig charges, set the barrier between you and the pig and tilt the top of it toward you

5. A tap on the snout with a cane or strap may stop a charging pig

IV. Hog snare (Figure 9-17)

A. This is the restraint tool of choice when working with pigs

B. Use of the snare is easy

1. Place the loop in front of the pig's snout

2. Allow the pig to mouth the loop and then quickly slip the noose over the top jaw all the way back to the commissure of the lips

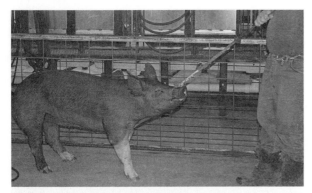

**Figure 9-17** Hog snare in place. (From Sheldon CC, Sonsthagen T, Topel JA: *Animal restraint for veterinary professionals,* St Louis, 2006, Mosby.)

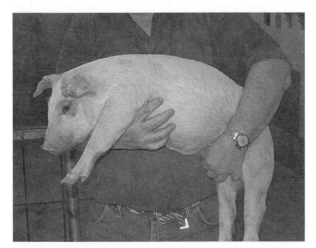

**Figure 9-18** Holding a 50-lb pig. (From Sheldon CC, Sonsthagen T, Topel JA: *Animal restraint for veterinary professionals,* St Louis, 2006, Mosby.)

3. Pull back on the handle, applying pressure to the nose; the pig's response will be to pull back in the opposite direction and squeal. The pig is immobilized by its own stubbornness

C. The snare can be used for restraint when vaccinating, drawing blood samples, or examining pigs

D. Length of time used should be 15 to 20 minutes maximum, because it can have a tourniquet effect on the upper jaw

E. Release of the snare should be quick; if the snare gets caught on a tusk, the pig will jerk the snare out of your hands and start swinging its head until the snare comes loose

V. Lifting

A. Newborns (up to 15 lb [7 kg]) are lifted by a back leg and then held with a hand under the chest and abdomen

1. They will squeal when picked up, so you should move them quickly to your arms or out of the hearing range of the sow (Figure 9-18)

B. Larger pigs (less than 60 lb [27 kg]) can be grasped by a hind leg to capture them

1. Once caught, the other hind leg is held; the pig is held upside down with your legs supporting the back

2. They can then be examined or transported

C. Use the same method for pigs up to 125 lb (57 kg), but two people are necessary, with each holding one leg

VI. Recumbency

A. You can cast a pig a number of ways with the use of ropes; one method is described here

1. Capture pig with hog snare

2. Place a rope on a front and back leg on the same side of the pig

3. Pass the ropes under the abdomen to the opposite side of the pig, moving to that side of the pig

4. Pull the ropes toward you, pulling the legs out from under the pig; the person controlling the hog snare will have to move with the pig so the snare does not injure the upper jaw

5. Use the ropes to tie together three of the pig's legs

6. If the procedure is prolonged, every attempt should be made to make the pig comfortable to prevent nerve and muscle damage

B. V-troughs are made of wood and are V shaped

1. Depending on the size of the trough, a 50- to 70-lb (23- to 32-kg) pig can be placed in the trough on its back, where it will remain until you are finished

2. This may be used for castrations or umbilical hernias

3. The feet are often left untied or just held out of the way because the pig cannot roll out of the trough; however, you can tie with a loop around the foot and a half hitch to the legs

## KNOTS

I. Square knot is a nonslip, noose-forming knot (Figure 9-19)

A. It is important to test the loop to make sure the knot is tied correctly. If it slides open or closed, the knot should be redone

B. There are variations, such as reefer's knot, surgeon's knot (Figure 9-20), and tom fool knot

II. Sheet bend knot can be used to tie together two pieces of rope, one of which can be of different diameter (Figure 9-21)

A. It can be used to tie an animal's tail out of the way

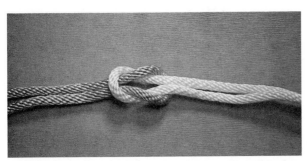

**Figure 9-19** Square knot. (From Sheldon CC, Sonsthagen T, Topel JA: *Animal restraint for veterinary professionals,* St Louis, 2006, Mosby.)

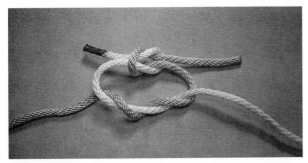

**Figure 9-20** Surgeon's knot. (From Sheldon CC, Sonsthagen T, Topel JA: *Animal restraint for veterinary professionals,* St Louis, 2006, Mosby.)

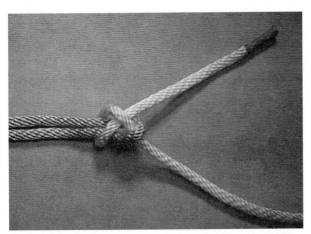

**Figure 9-21** Sheet bend knot. (From Sheldon CC, Sonsthagen T, Topel JA: *Animal restraint for veterinary professionals,* St Louis, 2006, Mosby.)

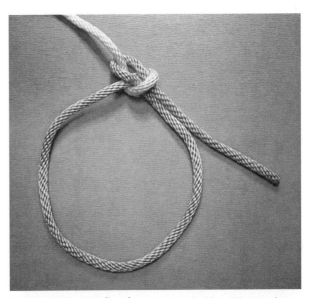

**Figure 9-22** Bowline knot. (From Sheldon CC, Sonsthagen T, Topel JA: *Animal restraint for veterinary professionals,* St Louis, 2006, Mosby.)

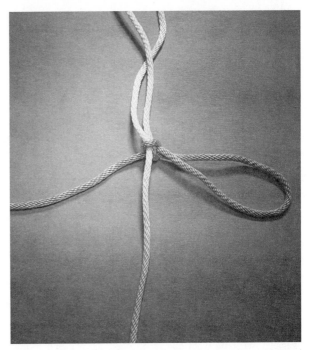

**Figure 9-23** Halter tie. (From Sheldon CC, Sonsthagen T, Topel JA: *Animal restraint for veterinary professionals,* St Louis, 2006, Mosby.)

    B. Use the hair on the tip of the tail as one of the ropes

III. Bowline is the universal knot of restraint (Figure 9-22).

    A. It is a secure knot, yet can be easily untied even after excessive tightening

    B. Can be used around necks or legs as temporary rope halters, casting ropes, and breeding hobbles

IV. Quick release or halter tie is a knot that can be completely undone by quickly pulling on the end (Figure 9-23)

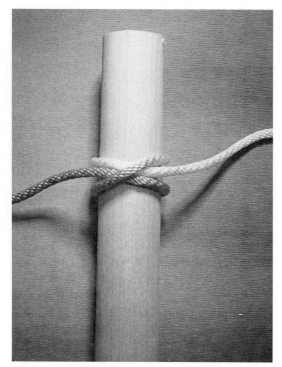

**Figure 9-24** Clove hitch. (From Sheldon CC, Sonsthagen T, Topel JA: *Animal restraint for veterinary professionals,* St Louis, 2006, Mosby.)

    A. This knot is the only one to be used to tie animals to inanimate objects. Any other knot takes too much time to untie and can tighten up so much that the rope has to be cut

  V. Hitches: half hitches are usually stacked one on top of another to hold a rope in place, either on a fence post or around a cleat (Figure 9-24)

    A. Cleats usually associated with sailing and boating are often found on surgery tables

# Glossary

**allelomimetic** Mimicking behavior usually associated with sheep, whereby what one sheep does, the rest will follow; can be used to advantage for restraint

**antikicker** Device shaped like a giant C clamp, which is squeezed over the flank of cattle to prevent them from kicking

**balling gun** Metal or plastic device used to administer pills to large animals, such as sheep and cattle

**bight** Sharp bend in the rope

**breakaway collar** Collar that will release if excessive force is applied

**casting** Laying an animal down on its side for restraint purposes

**caveman pets** Heavy swats usually around the shoulder region of an animal to provide minor distractions

**cradle** Device placed around a horse's neck to inhibit bending of the neck or turning of the head; prevents the horse from licking or chewing at its wounds

**cross tying** Method of securing a horse to two sides of a stanchion or stocks by use of two lead ropes, one attached to each side of the halter. This is used to prevent rearing or movement of the front quarters from side to side

**diastema** Space between two adjacent teeth in the same dental arch; in this case, the large space between the lower incisors and the molars on the lower jaw of a cow

**disbudding** Process of removing horn tissue of young goats or cattle with caustic paste or the use of a hot iron

**dry** An animal that is not lactating; usually in reference to the last 60 days of gestation of dairy cattle

**end** Part of the rope that is the short end or the end that can be freely moved around

**farrowing** In swine, the act of giving birth

**far side** Opposite or right side of the horse

**flanking** Method of restraint usually used in calves. Pressure is applied over the flank region just proximal to the rear legs. Used to cast an animal to the ground into lateral recumbency

**half hitch or loop** Complete circle formed in the rope when tying a knot or hitch

**headgate** Mechanical device at the end of a chute that secures an animal's head on both sides of the neck between the jaws and shoulder

**hitches** Temporary fastening of a rope to a hook, post, or other object, with the rope arranged so that the standing part forces the end against the object with sufficient pressure to prevent slipping

**hobble** Device placed on caudal aspects of the hocks of large animals to restrain hind legs

**hog snare** Device made out of rope, cable, or wire and placed around the pig's upper snout so that the head can be secured

**jacking** Term used in reference to grasping a bovine tail at the base and elevating it dorsally to distract the animal from painful procedures elsewhere on the body

**knot** Intertwining of one or two ropes in which the pressure of the standing part of the rope prevents the end from slipping

**lactation** Period of time during which an animal is producing milk

**lead shank** Lead rope with a snap of some sort attached to the halter of an animal, such as a horse

**near side** Left side of the horse, from which it is accustomed to being handled

**needle teeth** Term applied to the eight deciduous teeth (canines and third incisors) that pigs are born with and that are removed within 1 to 2 days of birth

**overhand knot** Base knot for a number of different knots, made by making a half hitch and then bringing the end through the resulting loop

**poll** Area directly behind the ears on a large animal

**polled** Term used to refer to cattle that are not born with the ability to grow horns

**rut** Annually recurrent state of sexual excitement in males

**setting up** Applied to sheep. Also referred to as docking or rumping; sheep are set up into a sitting position on their hind legs so that they lean against the restrainer's legs

**squeeze chute** Enclosed device into which large animals are individually restrained; these chutes often have various attachments to effectively restrain the head and provide access to other body parts

**stanchion** Area in a barn usually used to tie dairy cattle or goats

**standing part** Part of the rope that is the longer end of the rope or the end attached to the animal

**stocks** A closed-in area used to place a large animal for rectal and head examinations

**throw** When one rope or a section of rope is wrapped around another to make part of a knot

**twitch** Used in horses; a handle with a loop of rope or chain on one end that is tightened over the upper lip or muzzle for restraint

# Review Questions

**1** Which of these behaviors is not a normal behavior for cats?
  a. Hiding under the papers in a cage
  b. Investigating a new room
  c. Being fairly aloof and independent
  d. Rubbing on the leg of a chair

**2** Which of these is not a sign of warning from a cat?
  a. Hissing
  b. Lowering the ears
  c. Swiping at you with a paw
  d. Looking the other way

**3** As a restraint tool, a towel is used to
  a. Wrap up an angry cat
  b. Let the cat curl up and go to sleep
  c. Let the cat hide under
  d. Protect you from bites and scratches

**4** Always muzzle an injured, conscious dog except if it has a
  a. Huge gaping wound on the neck
  b. Spinal injury
  c. Leg injury
  d. Head injury

**5** Horses show many emotions through body language. Which ear movement can mean concentration or anger?
  a. Pricked forward
  b. Constantly moving back and forth
  c. Held erect
  d. Pinned back

**6** Serious injury is most likely to occur from a kick if you are within this range while standing behind a horse
  a. 1 to 2 feet
  b. 3 to 5 feet
  c. 6 to 8 feet
  d. 10 to 12 feet

**7** In a horse, a chain twitch is best applied to the
  a. Upper muzzle
  b. Lower muzzle
  c. Ear
  d. Tongue

**8** A nose lead or tong in cattle is applied to the
  a. Left nostril
  b. Right nostril
  c. Upper muzzle
  d. Nasal septum

**9** "Jacking" the tail is
  a. Twisting it to the side
  b. Bending it straight up
  c. Holding it straight out
  d. Kinking the end of it

**10** To move a newborn calf from one spot to another
  a. Place a halter on its head and neck and lead it
  b. Place your arms around the neck and rump, and guide it
  c. Place a lariat around its shoulder and drag it
  d. Use a whip against its lumbar region and herd it

## BIBLIOGRAPHY

Aanes WA: Restraint of cattle: head restraint, *Mod Vet Pract* 5:498, 1987.

Blanchard S: Here's how to read your horse's body language, *Pet Health News* 5:25, Mission Viejo, Calif, 1989, Fancy Publication.

Crow SE, Sally WO: *Restraint of dogs and cats: manual of clinical procedures in the dog and cat*, Philadelphia, 1997, Lippincott Williams & Wilkins.

Fowler ME: *Restraint and handling of wild and domestic animals*, Ames, 1995, Iowa State University Press.

French DD, Tully TN Jr: Restraint and handling of animals, In McCurnin DM, Bassert JM, editors: *Clinical textbook for veterinary technicians*, ed 6, St Louis, 2006, Saunders.

Leahy JR, Barrow P: *Restraint of animals*, Ithaca, NY, 1953, Cornell University Campus Store.

McBride DF: *Learning veterinary terminology*, ed 2, St Louis, 2002, Mosby.

Sheldon CC, Sonsthagen T, Topel JA: *Animal restraint for veterinary professionals*, St Louis, 2006, Mosby.

Sonsthagen T: *Restraint of domestic animals*, St Louis, 1991, Mosby.

## CHAPTER 10

# Sanitation, Sterilization, and Disinfection

*Teri Raffel*

## OUTLINE

Levels of Microbial Resistance
Degrees of Microbial Control
How Microbial Control Methods
  Work
  Mode of Action
  Efficacy of Microbial Control

Methods of Microbial Control
  Physical Methods
  Chemical Methods
  Autoclave
    Advantages
    Disadvantages

Function
Types
Operation
Quality Control for Sterilization and
  Disinfection
  Sterilization

## LEARNING OUTCOMES

After reading this chapter you should be able to:

1. List the classes of pathogenic organisms in order of their resistance to destruction.
2. Differentiate between sanitation, disinfection, and sterilization.
3. List the different ways that microbial control methods destroy or inhibit pathogenic organisms.
4. List the five categories of physical methods of microbial control.
5. Name and describe the physical methods of microbial control.
6. Identify the level of microbial control achieved with each of the physical methods.
7. State an example of the application of each of the physical methods of microbial control.
8. List the properties of the "ideal chemical agent" for microbial control.
9. Name and describe the classes of microbial control chemicals.
10. Identify the level of microbial control achieved by the chemical classes.
11. State an example of each of the chemical classes of microbial control.
12. List three advantages and two disadvantages of an autoclave in animal care facilities.
13. Explain the function of an autoclave.
14. Compare the gravity displacement autoclave and the prevacuum autoclave.

15. Describe the preparation of each of the following for processing in an autoclave: linen packs, pouch packs, hard goods, liquids, and contaminated objects.
16. List the guidelines for loading an autoclave chamber.
17. Compare the three different autoclave cycles.
18. List and define the five methods of quality control for sterilization.
19. List and define the two methods of quality control for disinfection.

The objective in sanitation, sterilization, and disinfection is to control microorganisms, or pathogens, in the environment, thus protecting patients and staff from contamination and disease, and thereby promoting optimum healing and wellness. Improper application of methods of sanitation, sterilization, and disinfection can lead to microbial resistance and can increase the risk of nosocomial infection.

## LEVELS OF MICROBIAL RESISTANCE

  I. Pathogens are microorganisms that cause disease
 II. Different classes of pathogens vary in their resistance to destruction by chemical methods (Figure 10-1)

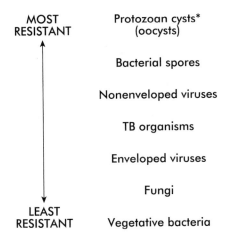

MOST RESISTANT

Protozoan cysts*
(oocysts)

Bacterial spores

Nonenveloped viruses

TB organisms

Enveloped viruses

Fungi

LEAST RESISTANT

Vegetative bacteria

*No chemical disinfectant carries a claim for killing oocysts; the best method for eliminating them is to use heat and agitation (or an autoclave).

**Figure 10-1** Ranking of microorganisms according to resistance to destruction by chemical methods. (Courtesy S. McLaughlin.)

III. Microbial control is achieved by using methods of sanitation, disinfection, and sterilization to a degree that is practical, efficient, and cost effective
   A. Sterilization is used only when necessary
   B. In many situations, sanitation and disinfection create acceptable levels of microbial control

## DEGREES OF MICROBIAL CONTROL

I. Sterilization is the elimination of all life from an object, or complete microbial control
II. Asepsis is a condition in which no living organisms are present; free of infection or infectious material
III. Disinfection, sanitization, and cleaning remove most microorganisms
   A. Most disinfectants are microbicidal; that is, they kill microbes. Some disinfectants are bacteriostatic; they inhibit the growth of microbes
   B. Disinfectants can be classified according to their spectrum of activity as
      1. Bacteriostatic (inhibits growth of bacteria)
      2. Bactericidal (kills bacteria)
      3. Sporicidal (kills bacterial spores)
      4. Virucidal (kills viruses)
      5. Fungicidal (kills fungi)

## HOW MICROBIAL CONTROL METHODS WORK
### Mode of Action

Different physical and chemical methods destroy or inhibit microorganisms in several ways.
   I. Damage cell walls or membranes
   II. Interfere with cell enzyme activity or metabolism

III. Destroy microbial cell contents through oxidation, hydrolysis, reduction, coagulation, protein denaturation, or salt formation

### Efficacy of Microbial Control

The effectiveness of all microbial control methods depends on the following factors.
   I. Time: most methods have minimum effective exposure times
   II. Temperature: most methods are more effective as temperature increases
   III. Concentration and preparation: chemical methods require appropriate concentrations of agent; disinfectants may be adversely affected by mixing with other chemicals
   IV. Organisms: type, number, and stage of growth of target organisms
   V. Surface: physical and chemical properties of the surface to be treated may interfere with the method's activity; some surfaces are damaged by certain methods
   VI. Organic debris or other soils: if present, will dilute, render ineffective, or interfere with many control methods
   VII. Method of application: items may be sprayed, swabbed, or immersed in disinfectants; cotton and some synthetic materials used to apply or store chemicals may reduce their activity

## METHODS OF MICROBIAL CONTROL
### Physical Methods

I. Dry heat (mode of action: oxidation)
   A. Incineration (efficacy: complete sterilization)
      1. Material or object is exposed to a hot fire
      2. Object must become red hot; for example, inoculating loops for microbiology
      3. Used to dispose of tissue or carcasses; must be burned to ashes
   B. Hot air oven (efficacy: complete sterilization)
      1. Sterility requires 1 hour of exposure at 170° C (340° F)
      2. Useful for powders and nonaqueous liquid, such as paraffin or Vaseline
      3. Used in some animal care facilities
      4. Useful for domestic applications (e.g., the kitchen oven)
   C. Drying (efficacy: incomplete sterilization)
      1. Most organisms require humidity to survive and grow
      2. Dry glass bead (efficacy: decontamination)
         a. Glass beads heated to 260° C (500° F)
         b. Tips of the instrument only are decontaminated in 15 seconds

II. Moist heat (mode of action: denatures microbial protein)
   A. Hot water (efficacy: incomplete sterilization)
      1. Used to clean and sanitize surfaces
      2. Addition of detergents increases efficacy by emulsifying oils and suspending soil so they are rinsed away
   B. Boiling (efficacy: may be complete sterilization)
      1. Requires 3 hours of boiling to achieve sterility
      2. Boiling for 10 minutes will destroy vegetative bacteria and viruses but not spores
      3. Addition of 2% calcium carbonate or sodium carbonate will inhibit rust and increase efficacy
      4. Useful for fieldwork
   C. Steam (efficacy: incomplete sterilization)
      1. Similar to boiling because the temperature is the same
      2. Exposure to steam for 90 minutes kills vegetative bacteria but not spores
   D. Steam under pressure (efficacy: complete sterilization)
      1. Autoclave: most efficient and inexpensive method of sterilization for routine use in animal facilities

III. Radiation (mode of action: damages cell enzyme systems and DNA)
   A. Ultraviolet (UV) (efficacy: may be complete sterilization)
      1. Low-energy UV radiation is a sterilant when items are placed at close range; UV radiation has no penetrating ability
      2. Used to sterilize rooms
      3. Very irritating to eyes
   B. Gamma radiation (efficacy: complete sterilization)
      1. Ionizing radiation produced from cobalt-60 source
      2. Good penetrating ability in solids and liquids
      3. Used extensively in commercial preparation of pharmaceuticals, biological products, and disposable plastics

IV. Filtration (mode of action: physically traps organisms that are too large to pass through the filter)
   A. Fluid filtration (efficacy: can be complete sterilization)
      1. Fluid, by means of positive or negative pressure, is forced through a fiber filter or more commonly a screen filter
      2. Used to sterilize culture media, buffers, and pharmaceuticals
      3. Pore size of 0.45 $\mu$m removes most bacteria, but microplasmas and viruses require 0.01- to 0.1-$\mu$m pore size
      4. May be used in conjunction with a prefilter to remove larger particles
   B. Air filtration (efficacy: can be complete sterilization)
      1. Used extensively in animal care facilities in surgical masks, laboratory animal cage tops, and air duct filters
      2. Fibrous filters made of various paper products are effective for removing particles from air
      3. Efficacy is influenced by air velocity, relative humidity, and electrostatic charge
      4. HEPA (high efficiency particle absorption) filters are 99.97% to 99.997% effective in removing particles over 0.3 $\mu$m
      5. Surgical masks are designed to protect the patient from the wearer but not the wearer from the patient; special masks are available for protecting personnel from pathogens in animals
         a. Masks must fit snugly on the face, stay dry, and be changed at least every 4 hours to be effective

V. Ultrasonic vibration (mode of action: coagulates proteins and disrupts cell walls)
   A. Cavitation (efficacy: incomplete sterilization)
      1. High-frequency sound waves passed through a solution create thousands of cavitation bubbles
      2. Bubbles contain a vacuum; as they implode or collapse, debris is physically pulled from objects
      3. Effective as an instrument cleaner

## Chemical Methods

Many chemicals are available to sterilize, disinfect, or sanitize, but none is the "ideal" agent. Chemicals penetrate organism cell walls and react with cell components in various ways to destroy or inhibit growth. Many chemicals are disinfectants with varying levels of activity (Table 10-1); a few are sterilants. Figure 10-2 ranks chemicals in order of their ability to destroy specific classes of microorganisms.

I. Ideal chemical agent
   A. Effective against a broad spectrum of pathogenic organisms
   B. Does not damage or stain surfaces
   C. Stable after application
   D. Effective in a short time
   E. Nonirritating and nontoxic to surfaces and tissues
   F. Inexpensive and easy to store and use
   G. Not affected by organic debris or other soil
   H. Effective at any temperature
   I. Nontoxic, nonpyrogenic, nonantigenic
   J. Residual and cumulative action

II. Chemicals
   A. Soaps
      1. Anionic cleaning agents made from natural oils
      2. Ineffective in hard water

**Table 10-1**  Levels of disinfection

| | Bacteria | | | Viruses | | |
|---|---|---|---|---|---|---|
| Level | Vegetative | Acid-fast | Spores | Lipophilic | Hydrophilic | Example |
| High | + | + | + | + | + | Aldehydes, vapor-phase hydrogen peroxide, chlorine dioxide |
| Medium | + | + | 0 | + | +/− | Alcohols, phenols, seventh-generation quats |
| Low | + | 0 | 0 | +/− | 0 | Quats |

Some manufacturers refer to low-, medium-, and high-level disinfectants. Higher level products are effective against a greater variety of organisms. They must kill hydrophilic and lipophilic viruses. They must also kill spores. Medium-level disinfectants must be tuberculocidal. Low-level products kill vegetative bacteria.

Courtesy S. McLaughlin.

**STERILANTS AND DISINFECTANTS**

HIGH-CIDAL ACTIVITY

Ethylene oxide

Aldehydes

Vapor phase hydrogen peroxide/peracetic acid/chlorine dioxide

Halogens (iodine, chlorine)

Phenols

Seventh-generation quaternary

Alcohols

Chlorhexidine

LOW-CIDAL ACTIVITY

Old generation quaternary

**Figure 10-2** Ranking of chemicals according to *-cidal* activity. (Courtesy S. McLaughlin.)

3. Do not mix well with quaternary ammonium compounds and diminish the effectiveness of halogens
4. Minimal disinfectant capability and are not antimicrobial
B. Detergents
  1. Synthetic soaps
  2. Anionic, cationic, or nonionic; anionic combined with cationic will neutralize both
  3. Anionic and nonionic soaps are good cleansers; cationic soaps are better disinfectants
  4. Most are basic; a few are acidic
  5. Emulsify grease and suspend particles in solution
  6. May contain wetting agents
C. Quaternary ammonium compounds (quats) (e.g., Centrimide, benzalkonium chloride, Zephiran, Quatsyl-D, Germiphene)
  1. Effective against gram-positive and gram-negative organisms and enveloped viruses
  2. Low toxicity and generally nonirritating
  3. Prolonged contact irritates epithelial tissues

4. Inactivated by organic material, soap, hard water, cellulose fibers
5. Ineffective sporicide and fungicide
6. Organically substituted ammonium compounds
7. Bacteria not destroyed may clump together; those inside are protected
8. More effective in basic pH
9. Cationic detergent
10. Deodorize
11. Dissolve lipids in cell walls and cell membranes
D. Phenols (e.g., phenol, carbolic acid, coal tar phenols, cresol)
  1. Active against
    a. Gram-positive bacteria
    b. Enveloped viruses
  2. Developed from phenol or carbolic acid
  3. Synthetic phenols are prepared in soap solutions that are nontoxic and nonirritating
  4. Prolonged contact may lead to skin lesions
  5. Toxic to cats because cats lack inherent enzymes to detoxify
  6. May be toxic to rabbits and rodents
  7. Activity decreased by quats
  8. Not inactivated by organic matter, soap, or hard water
E. Aldehydes (e.g., glutaraldehyde, formaldehyde)
  1. Active against
    a. Gram-positive bacteria
    b. Gram-negative bacteria
    c. Most acid-fast bacteria
    d. Bacterial spores
    e. Most viruses
    f. Fungi
  2. Considered to be a sterilant but may require 12 hours of contact
  3. Glutaraldehyde (Cidex)
    a. Noncorrosive
    b. Supplied as an acid, activated by adding sodium bicarbonate

c. Good for plastics, rubber, lenses in "cold sterilization"

d. Not inactivated by organic material or hard water

e. Irritating to respiratory tract and skin

4. Formaldehyde (Formicide)

a. A vapor phase surface disinfectant that slowly yields formaldehyde

b. Aqueous solution 37% to 40% (w/v) formaldehyde

c. May be diluted with water or alcohol

d. Irritating to tissue and respiratory tract; toxic

5. Biguanide (e.g., chlorhexidine gluconate [Hibitane, Precyde])

a. Active against

(1) Gram-positive bacteria

(2) Most gram-negative bacteria

(3) Some lipophilic viruses

(4) Fungi

b. Efficient disinfectant, used mostly as an antiseptic

c. Some reduction of activity in presence of organic material and hard water

d. Has immediate, cumulative, and residual activity

e. Precipitates to an inactive form when mixed with saline solution

f. Used as a surgical scrub and hand wash

g. Low toxicity

F. Halogens (e.g., chlorine, iodine, fluorine, and bromine)

1. Active against

a. Gram-positive bacteria

b. Gram-negative bacteria

c. Acid-fast bacteria

d. All viruses

e. Fungi

2. Iodine most common; used in solution with water or alcohol

a. Iodophors: iodine plus carrier molecule that acts to release iodine over time

b. Surgical scrub (Betadine): iodophor plus detergent

c. Tinctures and solutions: iodines and iodophors without detergents

d. Inactivated by organic material

e. Aqueous forms are staining, irritating, and corrosive to metals, especially if not diluted properly

3. Chlorine and chlorine-releasing compounds (e.g., chlorine gas, chlorine dioxide)

a. Commonly available as sodium hypochlorite (household bleach)

b. Least expensive and most effective chemical disinfectant

c. Available chlorine equals oxidizing ability

d. Damages fabrics, corrosive to metals

e. Inactivated by organic debris

f. May require several minutes of contact to be effective

g. Skin and mucous membrane irritant if not diluted properly or rinsed well

G. Alcohols (e.g., ethyl alcohol, isopropyl alcohol, methyl alcohol)

1. Active against

a. Gram-positive and gram-negative bacteria

b. Enveloped viruses

2. Most effective when diluted to 60% to 70% (isopropyl), 70% to 80% (ethyl)

3. Used as a solvent for other disinfectants and antiseptics

4. Most commonly used skin antiseptics

5. Low cost and low toxicity

6. Irritating to tissues and painful on open wounds

a. Repeated use dries skin

b. Forms coagulum in presence of tissue fluid

(1) Coagulum consists of layer of tissue fluid whose proteins have been denatured by alcohol

(2) Facilitates survival of bacteria under coagulum

7. Fogs lenses, hardens plastics, dissolves some cements

8. Inactivated by organic debris

9. Ineffective after evaporation

10. Defatting agent

H. Peroxygen compounds (e.g., peracetic acid)

1. Active against

a. Gram-positive and gram-negative bacteria

b. Acid-fast bacteria

c. Fungi

d. Classified as a sterilant; may not kill pinworm eggs

e. No virucidal activity

2. Oxidizing agent

a. Reacts with cellular debris to release oxygen; kills anaerobes

3. Applied as a 2% solution for 30 minutes at 80% humidity when using a chamber

4. Explosive and can damage iron, steel, and rubber

5. Irritating to healthy tissues

I. Ethylene oxide (EO) (EtO)

1. Active against

a. Gram-positive and gram-negative bacteria

b. Lipophilic and hydrophilic viruses

c. Fungi

d. Bacterial spores

e. Classified as a sterilant

2. Effective sterilant for heat-labile objects
3. EO (EtO) is a colorless, nearly odorless gas
   a. Diffuses and penetrates rapidly
4. Flammable and explosive
5. Toxic, carcinogenic, and irritating to tissue
6. Used in a chamber with a vacuum
7. May be mixed with $CO_2$, ether, or Freon
8. Used at temperatures of 21° to 60° C (70° to 140° F) (works more quickly at higher temperatures); exposure times of 1 to 18 hours
9. Requires minimum relative humidity of 30% (40% is optimum)
10. Items must be clean and dry and may be wrapped in muslin, polyethylene, polypropylene, or polyvinyl
11. Sterilized items must be ventilated in a designated area for 24 to 48 hours to remove residual EO
12. Chemical indicators to use as quality control devices are readily available

## AUTOCLAVE

### Advantages

I. Consistently achieves complete sterility
II. Inexpensive and easy to operate
III. Safe for most surgical instruments and equipment, drapes and gowns, suture materials, sponges, and some plastics and rubbers
IV. Safe for patients and personnel
V. Established protocols and quality control indicators are easy to access

### Disadvantages

I. Staff may overestimate the ability of the autoclave; sterility depends on saturated steam of the appropriate temperature having contact with all objects within the autoclave for a sufficient length of time
II. Requires a thorough understanding of techniques to ensure that the criteria just mentioned are met

### Function

I. Heat is the killing agent in the autoclave
II. Steam is the vector that supplies the heat and promotes penetration of the heat
III. Pressure is the means to create adequately heated steam
IV. Complete sterilization of most items is achieved after 9 to 15 minutes of exposure to 121° C (250° F)
V. The temperature of steam at sea level is 100° C (212° F); an increase in pressure results in an increase in the temperature of the steam
VI. The minimum effective pressure of the autoclave is 15 pounds per square inch (psi), which provides steam at 121° C (250° F)

**Table 10-2** Steam sterilization temperature/pressure chart

| Pressure (psi) | Temperature | | Time (min) |
| --- | --- | --- | --- |
| | ° C | ° F | |
| 0 | 100 | 212 | 360 |
| 15 | 121 | 250 | 9-15 |
| 20 | 125 | 257 | 6.5 |
| 25 | 130 | 266 | 2.5 |
| 35 | 133 | 272 | 1 |

Modified from Minshall D: *CALAS training manual*, 1995.

VII. Many autoclaves attain pressures of 35 psi, which creates a steam temperature of 135° C (275° F)
VIII. Exposure times must allow penetration and exposure of all surfaces to 121° C (250° F) steam
IX. Exposure time is decreased by increasing pressure, which increases steam temperature (Table 10-2)

### Types

I. Gravity displacement autoclave
   A. Water is heated in a chamber; the continued application of heat by an electric element creates pressure within the chamber; this pressure raises the boiling point of the water and thus the ultimate temperature of the steam
   B. Known as gravity displacement autoclave because the steam gradually displaces the air contained within the chamber; the air is forced out through a vent
   C. Timing of the cycle begins when the temperature in the chamber reaches at least 121° C (250° F)
   D. After sufficient exposure time, the steam is exhausted through a vent into a reservoir
   E. Air that has been sterilized within the jacket and then filtered is admitted into the chamber to replace the exhausting steam
   F. If the chamber is improperly loaded or there is insufficient steam, there will be air pockets remaining in the chamber that will interfere with steam penetration and result in nonsterile areas
   G. Load must be dried within the autoclave
II. Prevacuum autoclave
   A. Usually a much larger and more costly machine; equipped with a boiler to generate steam and a vacuum system
   B. Air is forced out of the loaded chamber by means of the vacuum pump
   C. Steam at 121° C (250° F) or higher is introduced into the chamber; the steam immediately fills the chamber to eliminate the vacuum
   D. Exposure time starts immediately
   E. At completion of exposure cycle, the steam is vacuumed from the chamber and replaced by hot, sterile, filtered air, which dries the contents

**Table 10-3**   Recommended storage times for sterilized packs

| Wrapper | Shelf-life |
|---|---|
| Double-wrapped, two-layer muslin | 4 wk |
| Double-wrapped, two-layer muslin, heat-sealed in dust covers after sterilization | 6 mo |
| Double-wrapped, two-layer muslin, tape-sealed in dust covers after sterilization | 2 mo |
| Double-wrapped, nonwoven barrier materials (paper) | 6 mo |
| Paper/plastic-peel pouches, heat-sealed | 1 yr |
| Plastic-peel pouches, heat-sealed | 1 yr |

Modified from Pratt PW: *Principles and practice of veterinary technology,* St Louis, 1998, Mosby.
Note that sterilized items from hospitals adopting event-related sterility assurance have an indefinite shelf life.

F. Air pockets are eliminated and processing times are reduced because of use of vacuum

G. Often equipped with readout and/or printout of chamber temperatures and pressures

## Operation

I. Preparation of load
   A. Linen packs
      1. All instruments in packs are scrupulously cleaned with a neutral pH product designed for instrument cleaning rinsed in deionized water, and lubricated
      2. Instruments are disassembled and ratchets are usually left open and unlocked
      3. Appropriate linens are in good repair and freshly laundered
      4. Disposable linens (drapes, wrappers, etc.) are not reused
      5. A chemical sterilization indicator is included in every pack
         a. Chemical sterilization indicators provide verification that the inside of the pack was exposed to appropriate sterilization temperatures for the correct amount of time
      6. The pack is wrapped using at least two layers of material
         a. The shelf-life of the sterilized pack varies with the type of outer wrap (Table 10-3)
      7. Pack is sealed with autoclave tape and labeled with date, contents, and operator
         a. Autoclave tape provides verification that the outside of the pack was exposed to appropriate sterilization temperatures
      8. Pack should not exceed $30 \times 30 \times 50$ cm ($12 \times 12 \times 20$ inches)
      9. Pack should not exceed 5.5 kg (12 lb)
      10. Pack should not exceed 115.3 kg/m$^3$

   B. Pouch packs
      1. Used for single instruments, sponges, etc.
      2. Items should be cleaned as previously described
      3. Instruments should be disassembled and ratchets left open
      4. Multiple piece items (e.g., Tru-cut biopsy needles, Poole suction tips) should be double peel packed to avoid loss of items when the package is opened
      5. Chemical indicators should be placed in the interior of every pack, just as for linen packs
      6. Shelf life should be determined using the event related method, because storage conditions and frequency of handling will affect sterility and package integrity more than time
      7. Previously mentioned guidelines apply (see Linen packs)
      8. Pouches should be heat sealed or self sealed
         a. Ends that are rolled and taped with autoclave or EtO tape do not provide an adequate seal.
      9. Label as previously mentioned
   C. Hard goods
      1. Stainless steel or other hard instruments, trays, bowls, laboratory cages, and other equipment may be autoclaved without wrapping
      2. Must be physically clean and rinsed in deionized water
      3. Syringes and barrels are separated before autoclaving
   D. Liquids
      1. Contained in Pyrex flask three times larger than contents require
      2. Cover with loosely applied lid or paraffin wrapping film, or place a needle through stopper to allow air exchange (the sterility of liquids processed in the autoclave is in question; removing liquids from the chamber is hazardous to personnel)
   E. Contaminated objects
      1. Used before disposal to decontaminate syringes, culture plates, etc., that contain biohazardous waste
      2. Place objects in appropriate container for disposal; special autoclavable biohazard bags are available
II. Loading the chamber
   A. Must allow free circulation of steam; use perforated or wire mesh shelves
   B. Linen packs have 2.5 to 7.5 cm (1 to 3 inch) space between; place multiple packs on a vertical edge instead of horizontal stacking
   C. Paper/plastic pouches are placed in specially designed baskets that support them on edge, with

paper side of each package facing the plastic side of the adjacent package

D. Solid bowls or basins are placed upside down or on edge

E. Mixed loads (hard goods and wrapped goods) have wrapped goods on upper shelf

III. Autoclave cycles
   A. Wrapped goods
      1. Has "dry" cycle that allows wrapped packs to dry
      2. Used for most surgical packs
   B. Hard goods
      1. Has no dry cycle; used for trays, bowls, cages, etc., that will not be maintained in a sterile condition
      2. Also used for "flash autoclave" to quickly sterilize instruments that are needed immediately
   C. Liquids
      1. Exhausts steam more slowly than other cycles
      2. Used for liquids that would be forced from containers during a faster exhaust

## QUALITY CONTROL FOR STERILIZATION AND DISINFECTION

The effectiveness of any method of microbial control must be monitored regularly. Verification of the effectiveness of microbial control should be performed at least monthly.

### Sterilization

I. Recording thermometer
   A. Displays temperature of autoclave chamber; operator observes for correct temperature during cycle
   B. Some autoclaves can provide a printout of the cycle parameters (e.g., chamber temperature, pressure)

II. Thermocouple
   A. Used in steam, dry heat, and chemical sterilization chambers
   B. Temperature sensors are placed in the part of a test pack that is most inaccessible to steam penetration

III. Chemical indicator
   A. Definition: paper strips impregnated with sensitive chemicals that change color when conditions of sterility are met
   B. Used with autoclaves and ethylene oxide systems
   C. Placed deep inside packs before autoclaving

IV. Biological testing
   A. Bacterial spores are exposed to autoclave or ethylene oxide and then cultured
   B. Recommended method for verification of proper autoclave operation in veterinary clinics

V. Bowie Dick test
   A. Tests prevacuumed autoclaves for complete removal of air and uniform steam penetration
   B. Uses a pack made to specific dimensions with a cross of autoclave tape in the center

VI. Surface sampling
   A. Surface to be tested is swabbed with a sterile applicator and transferred to a suitable media plate for growth
   B. Surface or item may be rinsed with sterile solution, which is examined for contaminants
   C. Contact plate of media is touched to surface and incubated
   D. Recommended method for ensuring proper disinfection of surgical suites in veterinary clinics

VII. Serology
   A. The presence of viruses in the environment is monitored by serological testing of animals to determine the presence of viral antibodies
   B. Animals maintained for this purpose are referred to as sentinel animals
      1. Rabbits are commonly used as sentinel animals because of their readily accessible veins for blood collection

## ACKNOWLEDGMENT

The editors and author recognize and appreciate the original work of Pat Carter and Margi Sirois, on which this chapter is based.

# Glossary

**anion** An ion carrying a negative charge

**antiseptic** Antimicrobial chemical that is applied to the skin or mucous membranes

**asepsis** Condition in which no living organisms are present; free of infection or infectious material

**bacteriostat** Agent that stops or inhibits the growth of bacteria but does not necessarily kill the bacteria

**cation** Positively charged ion

**cavitation** Cleaning method that uses sound waves passed through a solution to remove debris from materials

**-cide, -cida** Suffix denoting death or destruction; used after bacteria, virus, spore, etc., to denote "death to"

**cleaning** Physical removal of organic and inorganic soils and many microbial contaminants

**coagulum** Gel-like substance composed of tissue fluid and organic debris formed in the presence of alcohol on an open wound

**disinfectant** An agent, usually chemical, that is applied to inanimate objects to destroy or inhibit the growth of microorganisms

**efficacy** Effectiveness of an agent

**EO or EtO** Ethylene oxide

**fungicide** Agent capable of destroying fungi

**heat labile** Damaged by heat

**HEPA** High efficiency particle absorption filter; removes particles over 0.3 μm in size

**hydrolysis** Addition of water

**hydrophilic** Affinity for water

**lipophilic** Affinity for fat

**microbicidal** Destroying microbes

**microorganism** Microbe, especially pathogenic bacterium

**oxidizing agent** Chemical that releases oxygen when in contact with organic material; usually kills anaerobic organisms

**pathogen** Any disease-producing microorganism

**sanitize** Process of removing infectious material and reducing numbers of pathogens in an environment to promote health; the application of a detergent combined with a disinfectant

**sentinel** Animal that is used for surveillance of an environment

**sporicide** Agent capable of killing bacterial spores

**sterilant** Agent that destroys microorganisms

**sterilize** To eliminate all forms of life, including viruses and spores

**virucidal** Killing or destroying a virus

# Review Questions

**1** The following microorganisms are listed from most to least resistant
   a. Fungi, spores, protozoan cysts, vegetative bacteria
   b. Spores, protozoan cysts, lipophilic viruses, vegetative bacteria
   c. Protozoan cysts, TB organisms, fungi, vegetative bacteria
   d. Spores, protozoan cysts, lipophilic viruses, hydrophilic viruses

**2** Disinfection controls (kills) _____ of the microorganisms on an object
   a. 90%
   b. 99%
   c. 98%
   d. 95%

**3** An agent that stops or prevents the growth of microorganisms but does not necessarily kill them contains the suffix
   a. -cidal
   b. Pathogen
   c. -stat
   d. -biotic

**4** A chemical antimicrobial that is applied to the skin or mucous membranes is a/an
   a. Antiseptic
   b. Disinfectant
   c. Antibiotic
   d. Germicide

**5** The efficacy of boiling as a method of microbial control is increased by adding _____ to the water
   a. Sodium chloride
   b. Calcium chloride
   c. Sodium bicarbonate
   d. Sodium carbonate

**6** Hibitane is an example of which class of disinfectant?
   a. Phenols
   b. Quaternary ammonium compounds
   c. Biguanides
   d. Halogens

**7** The following chemicals are classified as sterilants
   a. Ethylene oxide, peroxygen compounds, alcohols
   b. Ethylene oxide, aldehydes, quaternary ammonium compounds
   c. Aldehydes, peroxygen compounds, halogens
   d. Aldehydes, peroxygen compounds, ethylene oxide

**8** The killing agent in an autoclave is
   a. Steam
   b. Heat
   c. Pressure
   d. Time

**9** The minimum effective pressure in an autoclave is _____
   a. 5 psi
   b. 20 psi
   c. 25 psi
   d. 15 psi

**10** At 135° C (275° F), microorganisms are destroyed in _____ _____ minute(s)
   a. 3
   b. 2
   c. 1
   d. 5

## BIBLIOGRAPHY

Busch SM: *Small animal surgical nursing*, St Louis, 2006, Mosby.

Davidson JR, Burba DJ: Surgical instruments and aseptic technique. In McCurnin DM, Bassert JM, editors: *Clinical textbook for veterinary technicians*, ed 6, St Louis, 2006, Saunders.

Kagan KG: Care and sterilization of surgical equipment, *Vet Tech* 13:65, 1992.

Sirois M: Principles of surgical nursing. In Sirois M, editor: *Principles and practices of veterinary technology*, St Louis, 2004, Mosby.

## CHAPTER 11

# Radiography

*Marg Brown*

## OUTLINE

X-Ray Production
X-Ray Tube
X-Ray Machine
Image Receptors
Darkroom and Processing
   Techniques
   Darkroom Considerations
   Manual Film Processing Pointers
   Automatic Film Processing
Radiographic Quality
   Definition

Radiographic Density
Radiographic Contrast
Radiographic Detail or Definition
Technical Errors and Artifacts
Developing a Technique Chart
Radiation Safety
   Responsibilities
   Hazards of Ionizing Radiation
   Radiation Measurement
   Maximum Permissible Dose
   Safety Practices

Positioning Techniques
   Basic Principles
   Basic Criteria and Principles of
     Positioning and Restraint
Contrast Radiography
   Basic Concepts
   Media
   Patient Preparation
   Positioning and Specific Studies
Digital Radiography

## LEARNING OUTCOMES

After reading this chapter you should be able to:

1. Understand some of the basic principles involved with x-rays and their production.
2. Describe the anatomy of the x-ray tube.
3. Briefly explain the components of the x-ray machine.
4. Understand the principles of accessory x-ray equipment and image receptors used in veterinary practice so that diagnostic radiographs are consistently produced.
5. Properly process radiographs based on your understanding of darkroom principles.
6. Explain what is meant by radiographic quality, including density, contrast, and detail, and the factors influencing these.
7. Identify common technical errors and artifacts and know how to prevent or correct them.
8. Understand the concepts involved with setting up a technique chart.
9. Describe the effects that could occur if proper radiation safety is not practiced.
10. State the units of radiation and the maximum permissible dose allowed.
11. List practical methods that can be used to reduce radiation exposure.
12. List and define proper directional terminology used in radiography.
13. List basic guidelines for veterinary radiographic positioning and restraint.
14. Explain what is meant by contrast media, giving examples.

Radiography is an important diagnostic tool available to veterinary practice. To arrive at a proper diagnosis, high-quality images must be produced. This chapter discusses basic but essential information needed to produce diagnostic radiographs. Radiation physics, positioning and restraint, technique charts, and specialized procedures are discussed briefly and can be further investigated by consulting the excellent texts listed in the Bibliography.

## X-RAY PRODUCTION

  I. Definition of radiation: propagation of energy through space and matter
  II. Three types of radiation

A. Particulate radiation
  1. Particles of the atom
    a. Examples: neutrons, protons, electrons, alpha particles, beta particles
    b. Some particles may have a positive, a negative, or a neutral charge
  2. Cannot reach the speed of light
  3. Process that occurs in the x-ray machine is an example
B. Electromagnetic radiation
  1. Definition: transport of energy through space without matter
  2. Examples: radio waves, television waves, microwaves, x-rays, gamma rays
  3. Has wavelength: defined as the distance from one crest of a wave to the next
  4. Has frequency: the number of crests passing a particular point per unit of time. It is measured in hertz (Hz)
  5. Energy associated with electromagnetic radiation is the ability to do work and is measured in electron volts (eV)
  6. Electromagnetic radiation is measured in frequency, energy, and wavelength
    a. Wavelength and frequency are inversely related
      (1) The shorter the wavelength, the greater the energy
    b. The greater the energy, the greater the ability to penetrate
  7. When matter and electromagnetic radiation interact, wave and particle behavior can be described
  8. X-rays have physical properties similar to those of other forms of electromagnetic radiation
C. Ionizing radiation
  1. Definition: particulate and electromagnetic radiation with sufficient energy to cause ionization
  2. Radiation must have greater energy than the electron binding energy
  3. Ionization damages tissues
III. Definition of x-rays
A. X-rays are a form of radiation that result when the energy of the electrons is converted to electromagnetic radiation
B. X-ray beam is composed of bundles of energy or quanta referred to as photons, which travel in waves
C. Photons have no mass or electrical charge
IV. Production of x-rays
A. X-rays are produced when the fast moving electrons or particulate radiation collide with matter
B. This is best achieved in an x-ray tube. The tube consists of a negative electrode known as the cathode and a positive electrode called the anode

C. A cloud of electrons (negative particulate radiation) forms at the cathode and accelerates across the tube where the electrons interact with the target material at the positive anode
D. This interaction forces the high-speed electrons to lose their energy, resulting in the production of 1% x-irradiation and 99% heat
E. The electrons that travel across the tube have different energies, measured in kilovolt peak or potential (kVp)
F. A setting on the x-ray machine determines the kVp of the electrons and thus the x-ray penetrating power
G. Thus to produce x-rays, one needs a source of electrons, a method of accelerating electrons, a directed path, a target, and an envelope to provide a vacuum, all of which are provided in the x-ray tube
V. Discovery of x-rays
A. Wilhelm Conrad Roentgen on November 8, 1895
B. Used a cathode ray tube (Crookes), which was an evacuated glass tube with two electrodes through which an electrical current was passed
C. X-rays were used almost immediately for medical and surgical diagnoses
D. Changes in skin color, similar to sunburn, due to radiation exposure were reported as early as April 1896

# X-RAY TUBE

I. Cathode (electrically negative portion of the x-ray tube) (Figure 11-1)
A. Provides the source of electrons and a directed path
B. The filament is a coiled wire that emits electrons when heated up
  1. When heated, electrons are held less tightly by the nucleus of the atom. After the binding energy of the electrons is exceeded, an electron cloud available for travel is formed
    a. The flow of current to the filament is controlled by the step-down transformer, which is regulated by the milliamperage (mA) control
  2. The filament is constructed of tungsten, which has a high melting point and atomic number
  3. Most machines contain a small and a large filament
C. The focusing cup is a cavity in which the filaments sit
  1. It is maintained at the same negative potential as the heated filament
  2. Because like charges repel, the electron beam is directed to a small area on the anode
D. Acceleration of the electrons is controlled by the kVp

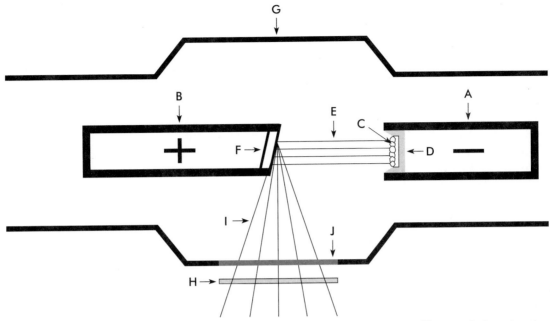

**Figure 11-1** Anatomy of an x-ray tube. *A*, Cathode. *B*, Anode. *C*, Tungsten filament. *D*, Focusing cup. *E*, Accelerating electrons. *F*, Tungsten target. *G*, Glass envelope. *H*, Aluminum filter. *I*, Generated x-rays. *J*, Beryllium window. (From Sirois M: *Principles and practice of veterinary technology*, ed 2, St Louis, 2004, Mosby.)

II. Anode (electrically positive portion of the x-ray tube)
  A. Provides the target for the interaction of the electrons
  B. Composed of the target and a copper stem
  C. Tungsten is used also for the target material to dissipate the high temperatures while the copper stem conducts the heat away from the target
  D. The area on the target that the electrons hit is the focal spot
    1. Size of the spot affects the x-ray image
    2. Size is determined by the filament size chosen
      a. The smaller the focal spot, the sharper the image, but there is less heat dissipation
    3. Because of the target angle, more x-rays leave from the cathode side of the x-ray tube than from the anode side, resulting in an uneven distribution of x-rays on the image (this is known as the heel effect)
      a. Most noticeable when using largest film size, short source-image distance (SID), and low-kVp techniques
      b. May be advantageous to place the thickest part of the animal toward the cathode side
  E. Two types of anodes: stationary anode and rotating anode
    1. Stationary anode
      a. Found in dental units and small portable units for large animals
      b. These units have a small capacity for x-ray production and are unable to withstand heat

  c. Consists of a beveled target angled toward the window embedded on a cylinder of copper
    2. Rotating anode
      a. An approximately 3-inch disk-shaped anode rotates on an axis through the center of the tube
      b. Filament from the cathode directs electron stream against the beveled edge of this tungsten disk mounted on a molybdenum spindle
      c. Position of the focal spot remains fixed while this circular ring rotates rapidly (3350 rpm), using a larger target area for the electrons to dissipate their heat
      d. Can use higher tube currents, shorter exposure time, and smaller filament
III. Tube envelope
  A. Traditionally made of Pyrex glass that has been evacuated to form the vacuum necessary for x-ray production
  B. Window is the thin segment of the glass that allows maximum emission of x-rays and minimum absorption by the glass (also called aperture)
IV. Tube or machine housing
  A. Metallic structure that covers and protects the x-ray tube or, in the case of portable units, the entire machine
  B. Lined internally with lead and contains insulating oil

V. Causes of x-ray tube failure
  A. More than 95% is due to operator error
  B. Most damage is related to heat accumulation in the tube, which may lead to filament evaporating, filament breaking, anode cracking, anode melting or pitting, and bearings burning out or freezing
VI. Tube rating chart
  A. Provided by all manufacturers of x-ray tubes
  B. Composite graph that shows the maximum combination of kVp, mA, and exposure time that can be used safely in a single exposure to avoid injury to the x-ray tube from excessive heat production

## X-RAY MACHINE

I. Electrical circuits for x-ray tube control
  A. High-voltage circuit
    1. Purpose is to provide high electrical potential needed to accelerate the electrons from the cathode to the anode
    2. High potential (kVp peak or potential) generated by a step-up transformer
      a. Incoming wall voltage (110 or 220 V) must be changed to kilovolts (1000× greater)
      b. Most machines have a range of 40 to 120 kVp
    3. kVp selection switch controlled by autotransformer
    4. Line voltage compensator also associated with circuit
  B. Low-voltage (filament) circuit
    1. Purpose is to provide electricity (amperage) needed to heat the filament
    2. Tungsten filament needs minimal energy so a step-down transformer is needed to reduce incoming voltage
    3. Connected to the mA control
  C. Timer switch
    1. Purpose is to control the length of exposure time during which high voltage is applied across the tube
    2. Best to have exposure times of less than one thirtieth of a second (0.03 second) to minimize potential of patient movement
  D. Rectification circuit
    1. Purpose is to change the alternating current coming into the tube into direct current to ensure that there are no negative deflections of the wave when no electrons are generated
    2. Various possibilities exist, depending on the type of x-ray machine
II. Technique selection or control panel
  A. Quality (energy, penetrating ability) of x-rays produced, controlled by kVp potential, whereas mA and time (sec) control the quantity (intensity)
  B. Product of mA and time is milliampere-seconds (mA × sec = mAs)
  C. Depending on the machine, operator can control
    1. kVp, mA, and sec
    2. kVp and mAs
    3. kVp only
III. Tube stand
  A. Apparatus that supports x-ray tube
IV. Accessory x-ray equipment
  A. Filtration
    1. Total filtration is result of inherent (filtering by glass envelope) and added (aluminum disk placed over window) filtration
    2. Purpose is to selectively remove less-energetic, less-penetrating (nondiagnostic) x-rays from primary beam
    3. Filtered primary x-ray beam decreases the amount of undesirable patient exposure by increasing the mean beam energy but decreasing the overall beam intensity. This necessitates increasing the exposure time or mA
  B. Collimation
    1. Beam-restricting device that limits the primary beam
    2. Purpose is to prevent unnecessary patient exposure and to decrease production of scatter (secondary) radiation
      a. This results in greater patient safety, increased operator safety, and an improved quality radiograph
    3. Beam-restricting devices include lead aperture diaphragm, lead cone, lead cylinder, and adjustable lead aperture shutter
    4. Most regulatory agencies require some evidence of collimation on the films
  C. Grids (Figure 11-2)
    1. Series of thin linear strips of alternating radiodense (lead) and radiolucent (plastic or aluminum) materials encased in an aluminum protective cover
    2. Placed between patient and film
    3. Generally used when area radiographed is greater than 9, 10, or 11 cm, depending on the reference source. The author uses 10 cm
    4. Purpose is to prevent scatter radiation from reaching the film. This improves quality of the radiograph
    5. Part of the primary beam is also absorbed, so exposure needs to be increased (usually mA or sec)
    6. Characteristics
      a. Grid ratio: relationship of the height of the lead strips to the distance between them

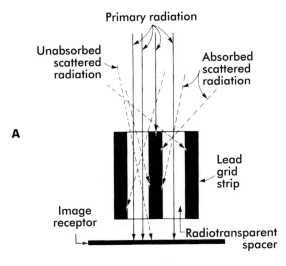

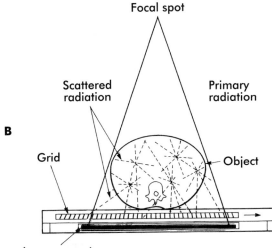

**Figure 11-2** Cross section of a grid. **A,** Diagram of a small section of a grid showing how a large proportion of the scattered radiation is absorbed and image-forming primary radiation passes through to the image detector. **B,** Diagram of focused Potter-Bucky diaphragm being moved toward the right. (From Eastman Kodak Company: *The fundamentals of radiography,* ed 12, Rochester, NY, 1980, Eastman Kodak Company, Radiographic Markets Division.)

(e.g., if the lead strips are eight times as high as the space between them, the ratio is 8:1)
   (1) The greater the ratio, the better the absorption of scatter radiation; but the disadvantages of a higher ratio are greater exposure needed, more perfect centering required, and narrower focusing range permitted
   b. Grid pattern: determined by orientation of lead strips
   (1) Linear grid: lead strips in one direction (most common)
   (2) Crossed grid (crosshatch): two linear grids sandwiched together so that the strips are at right angles to each other

   c. Types of grids
   (1) Parallel grid: strips perpendicular to face of grid and parallel to each other
   (2) Focused grid: strips placed parallel to the primary x-ray beam. Angle begins at 90 degrees to the surface at the center of the grid and progresses to greater angles toward both edges of the film
      (a) Most common
   d. Lines per centimeter or inch (grid frequency)
   (1) As the number of lead strips per centimeter or inch increases, they become narrower, which means the lines will be less objectionable on the radiograph
   (2) The increased frequency also means less absorption of scatter, increased exposure factors, and increased cost
   e. Mode of movement
   (1) Stationary grid: the grid does not move, which means that the grid lines are identifiable on the radiograph
   (2) Moving grid (Potter-Bucky diaphragm): the grid lines move through a mechanical device, so they are not seen
      (a) The image is clearer

## IMAGE RECEPTORS

I. Definition
   A. Mechanisms involved with transferring the invisible ionizing radiation into a visible image
II. Cassette
   A. Rigid film holder designed to keep the intensifying screen and the film in close contact
   B. The front, which is made of plastic, light metal, or carbon fiber, must face the x-ray tube
   C. The back is made of heavy steel to sustain the weight of the patient if necessary
   D. Do not drop the cassette, and keep it clean
III. Intensifying screens; also called scintillating screens
   A. Layers of tiny luminescent phosphor crystals bound together on a plastic base and covered with a protective coating
   B. X-ray film is sandwiched between the two intensifying screens that are positioned on the inner surfaces of the cassette
   C. When the phosphor crystals in the screen are struck by x-irradiation, they fluoresce and emit light
   1. This visible light exposes the light sensitive emulsion of the x-ray film
   2. More than 95% of exposure to film is due to this light emitted from the intensifying screens (indirect imaging)
   D. The primary purpose is to reduce the amount of exposure required to produce a diagnostic image

E. Screen construction
   1. Base material for support
   2. Reflective layer to redirect light toward the film to increase efficiency of film
   3. Phosphor layer composed of calcium tungstate or rare earth crystals to convert the energy of the remnant x-ray beam into visible light
      a. These phosphorescent crystals
         (1) Have a high atomic number
         (2) Have a high level of x-ray absorption
         (3) Must have high x-ray–to–light conversion with suitable energy and color
         (4) Should stop emitting light when the x-ray exposure ceases
   4. Protective coating applied to phosphor to prevent abrasion and allow transmission of light
   5. Screens will deteriorate over time and may need to be replaced
F. Care of intensifying screens
   1. Important to clean regularly (monthly) with a cleaner that is recommended (best) or 70% alcohol
   2. Make sure surface is dry before loading films
   3. Any debris on screen surface will cause artifacts
   4. Avoid "digs and scratches" on the screen surface when loading and unloading film
G. Phosphor types
   1. Calcium tungstate phosphor
      a. Emits blue light
      b. Has good x-ray absorption but lacks efficiency in light conversion
      c. Traditionally used in phosphor layer
   2. Rare earth phosphors
      a. Primarily emit in the green light spectrum
      b. Greater x-ray–to–light conversion, resulting in decreased exposure required
      c. Because of greater absorption and conversion, rare earth screens can produce a better degree of radiographic detail than calcium tungstate with less radiation exposure
H. Screen speed (Figure 11-3)
   1. Relative term referring to the measure of exposure necessary to produce a diagnostic film
   2. Screen speed ratings
      a. Slow (high definition, ultrafine, fine grain): designed for optimal detail with minimal concern for exposure time
      b. Medium (regular, midspeed, normal, par speed): good resolution with relatively low exposures
      c. Fast (high speed) used when reduced exposure time or increased patient penetration required

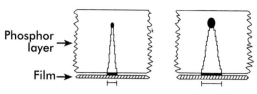

**Light diffusion**

**Figure 11-3** Increasing the size of the phosphor crystals increases the speed of the screen. However, the image appears grainier.

   3. Fast screens
      a. Require less radiation exposure than slower-speed screens to produce the same degree of blackness on the film
      b. Generally have larger crystals to increase the x-ray absorption and light conversion
      c. Usually have a thicker phosphor layer
      d. The larger crystals and thicker layer mean more blurriness (high grain) and less detail
   4. Quantum mottle resulting in a spotty or mottled radiograph is a disadvantage of increased film speed
IV. X-ray film
   A. Purpose is to provide a permanent diagnostic record
   B. Film composition
      1. Transparent polyester base
      2. Adhesive that attaches emulsion to base
      3. Emulsion that consists of gelatin and silver halide crystals (appear as tiny grains under the microscope [billions per mL])
      4. Protective coating to protect emulsion from scratching
   C. Latent image
      1. Definition: an invisible image on the x-ray film after it has been exposed by ionizing radiation or visible light before the film has been processed
      2. On a screen film, the grain of silver halide absorbs the emitted light photon and begins to split apart
      3. The partially split crystals will convert to metallic silver and turn black after the film is developed
      4. The greater the number of converted silver halide crystals, the blacker the film
      5. Unexposed crystals will be cleared away by the fixer
   D. Film types
      1. Screen film
         a. Silver crystals are more sensitive to wavelengths of light emitted from the intensifying screens than from direct ionizing radiation

**Table 11-1**  Comparison of film speed

| Characteristic | Fast film (ultraspeed) | Slow film (high detail) |
|---|---|---|
| Crystal size | Larger crystals | Smaller crystals |
| Exposure required | Lower needed | More needed |
| Film latitude | Less latitude | Greater latitude |
| Image | Grainier image | Less grainy image |
| Definition | Less resolution | Greater resolution |

b. Less exposure needed to produce a diagnostic radiograph
c. Must be sensitive to the light emitted by the intensifying screens
d. Depend on size of the crystal
e. Generally the smaller the crystal, the wider the latitude or exposure factors that can be used without significantly changing the film density (Table 11-1)
    (1) Also, the smaller the crystal, the greater the resolution
f. Medium film represents a compromise between fine grain and speed; it is mostly used in veterinary radiography

2. Nonscreen film
    a. Designed to be more sensitive to direct ionizing radiation
    b. Greater exposure factors required, because there is no intensification of the x-ray beam
    c. Packaged in a light-tight heavy envelope
        (1) Dental film speed that is available is usually designated as D, E, or F
            (a) F film speed is fastest
        (2) Gives greatest detail

E. Film care
    1. Store film boxes on end so film is vertical
    2. Store in a cool (10° to 15° C or 50° to 59° F) room with low relative humidity (40% to 60%)
    3. Use before expiration date to prevent radiographic fogging
    4. Film can be placed in a plastic bag and stored in a refrigerator or freezer to prolong usefulness

V. Film-screen systems
    A. Combined speed determines exposure requirements
    B. Must determine most desirable system for your clinic based on image detail and speed requirement
    C. Numerical value is assigned to each film and screen combination
    D. Numerical value differs for each company, so proper comparisons can be made only for that particular company
    E. As a rule, 300-400 speed is medium speed and considered most versatile

F. Speed of the system is inversely related to the mAs setting: as you increase the speed (higher number), you decrease the mAs
    G. Concept is similar to ISO (ASA) of photographic film

VI. Legal records and identification
    A. Must be properly identified (in film emulsion) to be legal
    B. Identification should include
        1. Patient identification
        2. Owner identification
        3. Date of examination
        4. Name of hospital
    C. Numerical system using a patient case number or file number facilitates record keeping
    D. Methods of labeling a radiograph include
        1. Lead markers
        2. Lead-impregnated tape
        3. Photoimprinting label system
        4. Miscellaneous markers
            a. Right (Rt) or left (Le) is essential
            b. Labeling of front (F) or hind (H) limbs and medial (M) or lateral (L) in equine radiography
            c. Time sequence labels for special procedures
            d. Position markers
            e. Technician identification markers

VII. Film filing
    A. Must be properly labeled and filed for future referral or follow-up examinations
    B. Because these are legal records, provincial and state associations require a minimum file and retrieval period before they are allowed to be discarded
        1. Varies with the state or province

## DARKROOM AND PROCESSING TECHNIQUES ■

Radiography begins and ends in the darkroom, where films are loaded into cassettes and returned for processing into finished radiographs. Most mistakes made in animal radiography are related to the processing of radiographs.

### Darkroom Considerations

I. Cleanliness is absolutely essential
II. Good ventilation and temperature control

III. Lightproof, so that film fogging does not result
IV. Darkroom safelight
   A. Filter must match sensitivity of film used
     1. Amber for blue-sensitive film
     2. Dark red (e.g., Kodak GBX) can be used for blue- and green-sensitive film
   B. Correct wattage (usually 7 to 15 W)
   C. At least 4 feet from working area
   D. Work as quickly as possible
V. Fogging due to light leakage or improper safelight illumination can be evaluated as follows
   A. Place a nonradiographed film on the counter
   B. Cover three fourths of it with a piece of cardboard for 1 minute
   C. Move the cardboard, covering half of the film for 1 additional minute
   D. Shift the cardboard so that only one fourth of the film is covered for 1 additional minute
   E. Remove the cardboard and expose the entire film for 1 additional minute (4 minutes in total)
   F. Process normally
   G. Darkened areas are indicative of fogging
   H. Organize into a wet and dry area to minimize processing artifacts
   I. State, provincial, or federal regulations require proper use of gloves, protective eyewear, eyewash bottle (Workplace Hazardous Materials Information System [Canadian] [WHMIS]/Occupational Safety and Health Administration [United States] [OSHA])

## Manual Film Processing Pointers

I. Basic steps include developing, rinsing or stop bath, fixing, washing, and drying
II. Chemical solutions are usually required by manufacturer to be diluted; follow steps carefully
III. Follow proper OSHA and WHMIS regulations when dealing with chemicals
   A. Wear goggles and protective eyewear, and dispose of fixer and developer properly
IV. Keep all solutions at required temperature
   A. Optimum temperature is 20° C (68° F)
   B. Less activity occurs at lower temperatures; greater activity occurs at higher temperatures
V. Make sure chemicals are well mixed before using
VI. Carefully follow manufacturer's suggestion for time-temperature development
VII. Agitate film intermittently in solutions to prevent air bubbles
VIII. Avoid letting liquid drain back into chemical solutions when removing from the tanks
IX. Keep lids on the solution tanks whenever possible to prevent oxidation
X. Developer: primarily functions to reduce or convert the exposed silver halide crystals of the film to black metallic silver
   A. pH is alkaline in a range of 9.8 to 11.4
   B. Solution needs replacing when it turns brown to green, or when the processed radiographs do not have the expected density or contrast
   C. Maintain level of solution with fresh replenisher
     1. Daily replacement is suggested
XI. Purpose of the rinse bath is to stop the developing process and to prevent contamination of the fixer
   A. Rinse in circulating water for about 30 seconds
XII. Fixer: primary functions are to remove and clear away the unexposed, undeveloped silver halide crystals and to harden the film to make it a permanent record
   A. Fixer consists of clearing or fixing agent, preservative, hardener, acidifier, buffer, and a solvent
   B. pH is acidic
   C. Film can be briefly viewed after it is cleared (about 1 minute but it is safer to wait at least 2 minutes)
     1. Must be returned for complete fixing for about double the development time
     2. This ensures proper hardening
   D. Change fixer when time required for the film to change from cloudy to clear exceeds 2 to 3 minutes
   E. Replenish when solution is low, as evidenced by film artifact (Box 11-1)
XIII. Wash bath: purpose is to remove processing chemicals from the film, thereby preventing film discoloration and fading over time
   A. Wash in clean, circulating water about 15 to 20 minutes
XIV. Drying
   A. Place hanger in drier or hang on rack
   B. Avoid dusty areas
XV. Maintenance and replenishing
   A. Suggestion for optimum chemical efficiency: remove 8 oz (250 mL) of developer and fixer, and replenish with same amount daily
   B. Solutions should be changed at least every 3 months, or when 15 gallons (60 L) of working replenisher has been used

## Automatic Film Processing

I. Mechanized film processing is a more accurate term
II. A roller assembly carries the film through the solutions and dryer
III. Processing times vary from 90 seconds to 8 minutes, depending on temperature
   A. 77° to 96° F (20° to 35° C), with temperature inversely related to length of processing times
IV. Chemicals are more concentrated with similar properties and procedures to the manual processing, but there are a few exceptions

---

**Box 11-1** Artifacts and Other Technical Areas

**BLACK MARKS**
- Film scratches, usually after exposure but before processing
- Crescent marks: rough handling, finger-nail
- Folding of film
- Light leak: defective cassettes, storage in bin
- Static electricity: linear dots or tree pattern from too low humidity or improper handling
- Developer drops before processing
- Fingerprints due to developer on hands during loading or unloading
- Film stuck together while in fixer

Heavy lines due to:
- Grid cutoff: grid out of focal range, upside down, not perpendicular to beam, and not aligned to center of beam
- Damaged grid
- Roller lines of automatic processor
- Film jammed in automatic processor

**YELLOW RADIOGRAPH**
- Exhausted fixer solution
- Fixing time too short
- Inadequate rinsing: residual fixer oxidizes to yellow powder and also destroys image
- Film sticking together during fixer process

**SLOW DRYING**
- Waterlogged films due to: prolonged washing, water too warm, or improper hardening by the fixer
- Air too humid or cool
- Automatic processor
- Thermostat malfunction
- Too low dryer temperatures
- Improper hardening
- Inadequate air venting

**WHITE MARKS OR CLEAR AREAS**
- Film emulsion scratched off, usually before exposure or during processing
- Debris in cassette
- Defective screens (pitted, scratched)
- Smudges of fixer on fingers before developing
- Grit due to remnant fixer not washed
- Increased atomic number of object (e.g., positioning device, lead contrast media on cassette)
- Air bubble on film during developing procedure
- Developing solution low
- Film touching side of tanks during manual developing
- Reticulation due to improper stirring of solutions
- Blank film: unexposed or fixed before development
- Evidence of collimation
- Positive contrast media spilled on table or cassette

**BRITTLENESS OF FINISHED RADIOGRAPH**
- Excessive drying temperature, time
- Excessive hardening in fixer

**GREEN AREAS ON FILMS**
- Processing solutions low
- Two films stuck together during processing

---

A. A hardener is included in the developer
B. No rinsing occurs between developing and fixing
V. Keep processor clean at all times, especially rollers, roller racks, and crossover rollers
VI. Change chemicals as required
VII. As cost of units decrease, automatic processing will become more popular in veterinary clinics

## RADIOGRAPHIC QUALITY

### Definition

I. That "feature of a diagnostic radiograph that describes to what degree the shadows identified on the film clearly depict the anatomical features under investigation"[1]
II. A film of good diagnostic quality should have optimal density, correct scale of contrast, and excellent detail with minimal magnification and distortion
   A. See Table 11-2 for technical errors related to density

## Radiographic Density

I. Definition: the degree of darkness or blackness on the film
II. Determined by the number of photons that have affected the film: the greater the number, the darker the film
III. Influenced by several factors, including
   A. Total number of x-rays that reach the film (mAs)
      1. mAs is a quantity factor that controls the number of x-rays produced (beam intensity)
      2. If more x-rays are produced, the film will be darker
   B. Penetrating power of the x-rays (kVp) (Figure 11-4)
      1. kVp is a quality factor that affects the energy of the x-rays
      2. At higher kVp settings, more x-rays with more energy are produced, there is a better penetration through the tissue, and as a result the film density increases
   C. Developing time and temperature
   D. Forms of beam attenuation, such as filters or grids

**Table 11-2**  Technical errors that will or may cause change in film density if the factors are not compensated for

|  | Decreased film density (film too light) | Increased film density (film too dark) |
|---|---|---|
| Machine factors | Underexposure—too low kVp, mAs<br>Drop in incoming line voltage<br>Equipment malfunction | Overexposure—too high kVp, mAs<br>Surge in incoming line voltage<br>Equipment malfunction |
| Physical factors | Undermeasurement of anatomical part<br>Increased subject density<br>Source-image distance (SID) too great<br>Grid used<br>Positive contrast media used<br>Slow speed screen/film used<br>Cassette not positioned in bucky tray properly<br>Bucky tray not positioned directly<br>   under primary beam | Overmeasurement of anatomical part<br>Decreased subject density<br>SID too short<br>No grid<br>Negative contrast media used<br>Fast speed screen/film |
| Processing factors<br>  Wet tank | Underdevelopment<br>Developer time too short<br>Developer temperature too low<br>Exhausted developer<br>Contaminated developer<br>Diluted developer<br>Defective thermometer<br>Developer improperly mixed | Overdevelopment<br>Developer time too long<br>Developer temperature too high<br>Inaccurate thermometer<br>Solutions too concentrated<br>Bromide missing from developer<br>Defective thermometer |
| Automatic processors | Underreplenishment<br>Developer temperature too low<br>Exhausted developer<br>Developer improperly mixed | Overreplenishment<br>Developer temperature too high<br>Light leak from cover or in darkroom<br>Rollers malfunctioning |

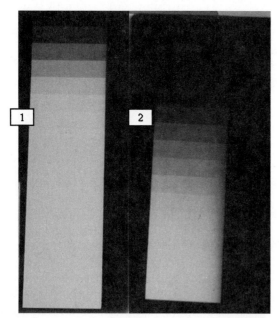

**Figure 11-4**  In this step wedge, number 2 displays more radiographic density than number 1. Both are at the same location of the step wedge. There is considerably more penetration in image 2, which means it was exposed at a higher kVp.

E. Tissue density and patient thickness (Figure 11-5)
  1. Tissue and film density are inversely proportional
  2. Presented in order of increasing film density (white to black) and decreasing tissue density

(most dense to least): metal, bone, water (organs), fat, gas
  F. Other physical factors are film and screen speed, use of contrast agents, and SID (source-image distance, formerly called focal-film distance)
IV. Can be measured with a densitometer

**Radiographic Contrast**

  I. Definition: refers to the visible difference between two adjacent radiographic densities
 II. See Table 11-3 for technical errors related to contrast
III. Can be divided into radiographic contrast and subject contrast
  A. Radiographic contrast
    1. Refers to the various shades of black, gray, and white on a radiographic film, and the differences between them
    2. High contrast film means a very black and white film with few grays
      a. Referred to as having a short latitude or scale of contrast
    3. Fewer, but bigger steps
      a. Preferred for spine and extremity films
    4. Long latitude or scale films have more shades of gray but few differences or contrast between them
      a. More but smaller steps
      b. Preferred for soft tissue

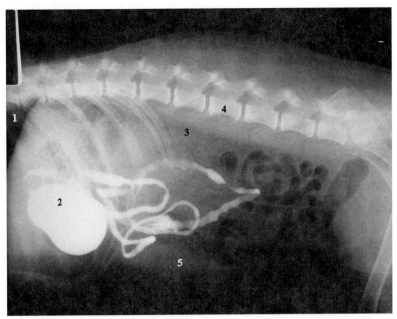

**Figure 11-5** Subject densities: *1*, Air. *2*, Barium. *3*, Fat. *4*, Bone. *5*, Water. Barium is the most dense. Most of the x-rays have been absorbed. Air is the least dense—all of the x-rays have passed through and exposed the film.

5. Kilovoltage has the greatest influence on radiographic contrast
   a. X-ray beam is polychromatic, which means that it contains a spectrum of energies (average energy is one half to one third the peak energy)
   b. At lower kVp there are more lower energy photons and a greater difference in energy levels
   c. As kVp increases, the difference between the energy levels lessens, allowing greater penetration of the x-ray beam through the tissue
   d. The absorption of the x-ray beam by the various tissues at higher kVp is more uniform, resulting in lower radiographic contrast
6. Scatter radiation (non–image-forming radiation that is scattered in all directions resulting from objects in the path of the beam) adds a grayness to the film
   a. Inappropriate areas of the film are exposed, thus decreasing contrast
7. Processing factors and other physical factors (beam attenuation, fogging, etc.) affect radiographic contrast
8. mAs does not affect contrast if sufficient quantity is used, because an increase or decrease in mAs affects the number of x-rays evenly
   a. SID does not affect contrast either, for the same reason

B. Subject contrast is defined as the difference in density and mass between two adjacent anatomic structures
   1. Subject contrast depends on the thickness and density of the anatomic part
   2. Subject contrast affects radiographic contrast
      a. High subject density means high tissue density
      b. The greater the subject density (e.g., bone), the greater the difference between the blacks and whites on the radiograph
      c. High subject contrast then increases radiographic contrast

## Radiographic Detail or Definition (Table 11-4 and Figures 11-6 to 11-8)

   I. Refers to definition of the edge of an anatomic structure
   II. Image sharpness, clarity, distinctness, and perceptibility are synonymous
   III. Lack of detail or penumbra may be due to many factors

## TECHNICAL ERRORS AND ARTIFACTS ▬▬▬

Several errors in handling x-ray film, manipulating exposure factors, or setting up a procedure could result. See Box 11-1 for artifacts and other errors.

## DEVELOPING A TECHNIQUE CHART ▬▬▬

A technique chart is a table with predetermined x-ray machine settings that enables one to select the correct machine settings based on the thickness of the tissue and the anatomical portion to be radiographed.

**Table 11-3** Technical factors affecting radiographic contrast

| | Low contrast (film gray) |
|---|---|
| Machine factors | • Overpenetration from too high kVp |
| Physical factors | • Slower speed screens or film, or those manufactured with lower levels<br>Fog due to<br>• Light leak, such as safelight wattage or filter, while in cassette, or during loading or unloading<br>• Scatter radiation, if not using a grid for thick parts<br>• Direct or scatter radiation, if left lying near machine during other exposures or if film bin exposed<br>• Film stored in too hot or too humid place<br>• Outdated film<br>• No grid used with high kVp exposure<br>• Beam not collimated<br>• Underfiltration<br>• Double exposure<br>• Negative contrast used<br>• Low subject contrast<br>• Excessive pressure on emulsions of unprocessed films |
| Processing factors<br>Wet tank | Chemical fog<br>• Prolonged development<br>• Developer temperature too high<br>• Solutions contaminated or exhausted<br>• Not fixed long enough or turned on light too soon<br>• Luminous clocks and watch faces |
| Automatic processors | • Prolonged development<br>• Developer temperature too high<br>• Exhausted or contaminated solutions |

**Table 11-4** Common errors relating to lack of radiographic detail or definition (penumbra)

| Machine factors | • Too large a focal spot used<br>• Focal spot damaged |
|---|---|
| Physical factors | Motion unsharpness<br>• Motion of patient, cassette, machine<br>• Too slow time used<br>Geometric unsharpness<br>• Poor contact of intensifying screen and film<br>• Increased object-film distance (OFD)<br>• Decreased subject-image distance (SID)<br>• Patient too thick<br>• Rounded area of interest<br>• Poor screen-film contact<br>• Double exposure<br>Geometric distortion and magnification<br>• Patient/part not parallel to the film<br>• Patient/part not perpendicular to the beam<br>• Primary beam not centered over the area of interest<br>• Area of interest not close to the film<br>Radiographic noise<br>• Film graininess (film speed too fast)<br>• Structure mottle (intensifying screen speed too fast)<br>• Quantum mottle (too few photons producing an image) |

I. Each machine requires its own technique chart
II. Several charts may be needed (screen/nonscreen, grid/no grid, species specific, anatomy specific, various film/screen combinations)
III. Can use variable kVp chart, variable mAs chart, or a combination of both
IV. Whatever method is used, certain concepts should be kept in mind
 A. Standardize as many factors as possible (speed of screens, age of screens, speed of film, SID, beam filtration, temperature, age and time of processing, type of grid)
 B. Keep in mind that mAs is directly proportional to film density, but it does not appreciably alter film contrast if the density is correct
 C. Kilovoltage is directly proportional to film density and inversely proportional to film contrast; low kVp means a high scale of contrast
 D. SID squared is inversely proportional to film distance
  1. Change in SID means a change in film density
  2. SID does not alter film contrast if film density is correct
  3. Also referred to as focal-film distance (FFD)
 E. Change in thickness requires a change in kVp setting. For each additional thickness in patient centimeter, add

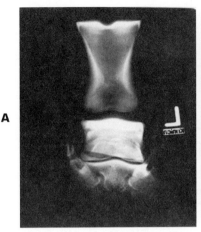
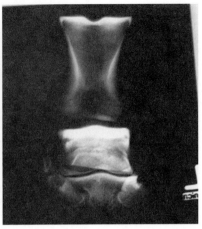

**Figure 11-6** Increasing the object-film distance (OFD), as shown in **B,** increases the magnification and the amount of penumbra, which decreases the radiographic detail as compared with the decreased OFD in **A.**

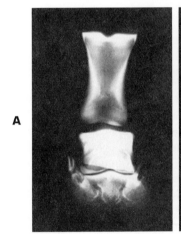
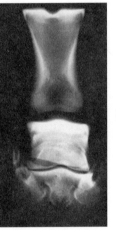

**Figure 11-7** **A,** Increasing the source-image distance (SID) decreases the magnification and the amount of penumbra, increasing the radiographic detail as compared with the decreased SID and increased magnification in **B.**

    1. 2 kVp if less than 80 kVp
    2. 3 kVp if 80 to 100 kVp
    3. 4 kVp if more than 100 kVp
  F. A general relationship exists between mAs and kVp
    1. If film density is too dark, to correct the error
      a. Halve mAs setting, or subtract 10 kVp (in range of 70 to 90)[1]
      b. Decrease mAs 30% to 50%, or kVp 10% to 15%[2]
    2. If film density is too light, to correct error
      a. Double mAs setting, or add 10 kVp (in range of 70 to 90 kVp)[1]
      b. Increase mAs 30% to 50% or kVp 10% to 15%[2]
  G. Exposure factors must also be increased for such conditions as
    1. Pleural fluid/cardiomegaly
    2. Ascites
    3. Obesity
    4. Plaster cast
    5. Special positive radiographic procedures
  H. To determine if kVp or mAs should be changed
    1. If film is too dark but contrast has not significantly been altered (i.e., soft tissue is dark but bones are relatively white), mAs should be decreased
    2. If film is too dark and bones are gray, then the problem is overpenetration or kVp is too high
    3. If film is too light and anatomical parts, especially in cranial abdomen, are not clearly visible, an increase in penetration or kVp will improve density and contrast
    4. If film is too light and anatomical parts, especially in cranial abdomen, are clearly visible, an increase in mAs will improve density

## RADIATION SAFETY

The major objective of a veterinary practice that uses ionizing radiation should be to obtain the maximum amount of information with the minimal exposure to all concerned. "Radiation should be respected, not feared."[2]

### Responsibilities

I. It is the practice owner's responsibility to
  A. Ensure that proper radiation safety measures are observed
  B. Meet state or provincial requirements: dosimetry devices, proper protection devices, registration, room design, etc.
    1. Usually regulated by the Department of Health
  C. Instruct personnel in proper radiation safety and use

### Hazards of Ionizing Radiation

I. All tissues are sensitive to ionizing radiation
  A. *Ionizing radiation* refers to the excitation of orbital electrons in an atom so that the atoms are separated into charged particles

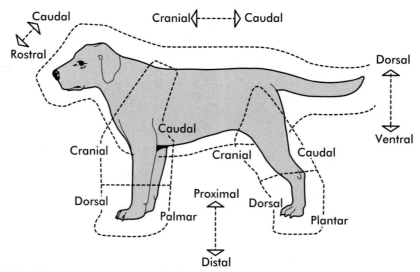

**Figure 11-8**   Veterinary anatomic terminology. (From Han CM, Hurd CD: *Practical diagnostic imaging for the veterinary technician*, ed 3, St Louis, 2005, Mosby.)

**Table 11-5**   Maximum permissible dose: whole body dose for occupationally exposed over 18 years of age*

| Time period | MPD (Sv) | Dose (rem) |
|---|---|---|
| Weekly | 0.001 | (0.1) |
| Quarterly | 0.03 | (3) |
| Calendar year | 0.05 | (5) |
| Accumulated over lifetime | 0.05 (age − 18) | (5 [age − 18]) |

Age for calculation in years.
*ICRP 1986. Some states and provinces have adopted the 1991 schedule, which gives 0.02 Sv (2 rem) as MPD in a calendar year.

1. Molecules may break or alter
2. Charged molecules may function improperly or not at all
   B. Interaction between x-rays and tissues occurs at the atomic level, but it is theorized that visible injury results from molecular derangements of macromolecules and water
   C. Injury to cells, tissues, and organs occurs at the time of exposure, but may require hours, days, or generations to show damage
II. Types of cellular damage in the body
   A. Genetic damage occurs to DNA (genes) of reproductive cells
      1. Manifestation not detectable until future generations
   B. Somatic cell damage occurs in all other cells and becomes evident at some point in the individual's life, although it may never become obvious because of tissue repair
   C. Nucleus of proliferating somatic and genetic cells is considered to be the area of the cell most sensitive to the ionizing effects

D. Greater sensitivity occurs with
   1. Younger tissues and organs
   2. Higher metabolic activity
   3. Greater proliferation rate of cells and growth rate of tissues
E. Organs and tissues considered critical because of their sensitivity are dermis, thyroid gland, eye, lymphatic system, blood-forming tissues, bone, and germinal epithelium or gonads

### Radiation Measurement

I. Absorbed dose is the unit of ionizing radiation that measures the energy transferred by this radiation to a body part
   A. SI unit is gray (Gy) = 100 rad
II. Dose equivalent allows for differences in how ionizing radiation affects each tissue
   A. Current SI unit is sievert (Sv)
   B. Previous unit was rem (1 Sv = 100 rem)

### Maximum Permissible Dose

I. See Table 11-5 for specific maximum permissible dose (MPD)
II. Definition: maximum dose of radiation that a person may receive in a given period
III. Set by the National Council on Radiation Protection and Measurements (NCRP) under the recommendations of ICRP (International Commission on Radiological Protection)
IV. NCRP and most provincial and state regulations allow occupationally exposed persons to restrain and position animals when absolutely necessary, but other states or provinces prohibit any manual restraint
V. Various dosimeters or personal exposure monitoring devices are available, but these and MPD are meaningless unless

A. Each individual involved in taking radiographs properly wears the dosimeter every time he or she takes radiographs

B. Dosimeters are routinely sent to a federally approved laboratory for evaluation

VI. For more information, contact the radiation protection service of the Department of Health of your state or province

## Safety Practices

I. Exposure and damage to tissue can occur from
  A. Primary beam: never allow any part of the body to be in the path of the primary beam even if properly protected
    1. Primary beam will penetrate lead aprons and gloves
    2. Similar to wearing dark sunglasses—light is still emitted
  B. Secondary or scatter radiation that is produced when the primary beam interacts with objects in its path
    1. Amount and direction of scatter depend on kVp level, volume of tissue irradiated, field size, and composition of tissue
  C. X-ray machine leakage

II. Important safety practices
  A. Never permit pregnant women or anyone younger than 18 years in the room during exposure
  B. Remove unnecessary personnel and rotate personnel during procedures
  C. Use nonmanual restraint, such as chemical restraint, sandbags, sponges, tape, and restraining devices whenever possible. A little patience and creativity will go a long way
  D. Always wear protective gloves, thyroid protector, and aprons
    1. Minimum 0.5-mm lead equivalent
    2. Routinely inspect and radiograph protective equipment for signs of damage
  E. Never permit any part of the body, even if it is shielded, to be in the primary beam
    1. Even if shielded, you could still receive 25% of the primary beam
  F. Consider use of protective goggles (0.25-mm lead equivalent) and larger shielding devices
  G. Collimate so there is at least an unexposed border on each film, proving that the primary beam is limited and scatter radiation reduced
  H. Wear dosimeter outside of apron near the collar
  I. Never hand hold an x-ray machine
  J. Do not direct the x-ray beam at any individual or occupied adjacent room
  K. Use 2.5-mm aluminum filter to remove the lower energy portion of the x-ray beam
  L. Have the machine calibrated and checked regularly

  M. Use fastest film-screen systems compatible with obtaining diagnostic radiographs
  N. Plan each procedure carefully to avoid retakes
  O. Keep an exposure log identifying the patient, study, and exposures
  P. Follow state and provincial radiation safety codes

III. Remember the big three methods of radiation safety
  A. Time: avoid retakes, do it correctly the first time, and use the quickest exposure
  B. Distance: keep as far as possible from patient and x-ray beam
  C. Shielding: always wear protective apparel

IV. NCRP developed a program known as ALARA
  A. This stands for "as low as reasonably achievable"
  B. Always keep this policy in mind when restraining animals and taking radiographs

## POSITIONING TECHNIQUES

Proper positioning is essential to obtain diagnostic radiographic examinations. Refer to texts that thoroughly explain specific procedures for various species.

### Basic Principles

I. Common terms and abbreviations used (based on American Committee of Veterinary Radiologists and Anatomists) (Figure 11-9)
  A. Left (Le), right (Rt)
  B. Medial (M), lateral (L)
    1. In reference to limbs
  C. Cranial (Cr)
    1. Toward head
    2. Also for limbs proximal to carpus/tarsus
  D. Cd (caudal), toward tail
    1. Also for limbs proximal to carpus/tarsus
  E. Dorsal (D)
    1. Toward back
    2. Also cranial portion of limb distal to carpus/tarsus
  F. Ventral (V)
    1. Toward abdomen
  G. Palmar (Pa)
    1. Caudal portion of pectoral limb from carpus distally
  H. Plantar (Pl)
    1. Caudal portion of pelvic limb from tarsus distally
  I. Oblique (O)
    1. Less than 90 degrees to axis
    2. Could be in a medial or lateral direction
  J. Rostral (R)
    1. Used for head: toward the nares

II. Beam direction
  A. Lateral: side closest to the film is marked (i.e., side it is lying on)
    1. For example: Rt L = lying on right side

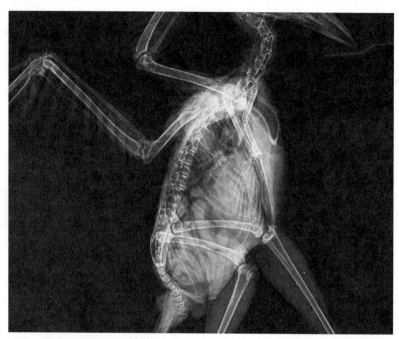

**Figure 11-9** Radiograph exposed with digital radiography unit.

B. Abbreviated term indicates direction of beam: first letter is where the x-rays enter the body, second letter is where x-rays leave the body (part that lies against the film)
  1. For example: VD (ventrodorsal): the x-rays enter the ventral aspect of the animal while the film is against the dorsal aspect
  2. The animal would be lying in dorsal recumbency or on its back
C. Oblique views are usually in reference to limbs
  1. The first two letters indicate where the beam enters the body, the next two letters indicate where it exits (the body part that is specifically against the film)
  2. First letter in each pair describes cranial or caudal; second letter of each pair describes the side of the limb
  3. For example: dorsomedial-palmarolateral oblique (DMPaLO) of the carpus
    a. Carpus is rotated (O) so that the x-ray beam is aimed at the cranial part of the limb (D), toward the medial side (M). This faces the x-ray tube
    b. This means that the beam exits from the caudal portion of the limb (Pa), so that the opposite side (L) faces or is against the film

### Basic Criteria and Principles of Positioning and Restraint

I. Keep comfort and welfare of patient in mind
  A. Be prepared before patient positioning
  B. Use steady, slow, gentle movements
  C. Use minimum restraint through chemical and/or mechanical assistance
II. Minimize exposure to radiation of assistants by using nonmanual restraint whenever possible
  A. When using positioning aids, minimize placing radiopaque devices over the area of interest
  B. Position devices so that the animal has the illusion it is being held
    1. Strategic locations are usually head, shoulders, pelvis, and limbs
    2. Be creative and patient
    3. Stay with the animal until the rotor is depressed and move away quickly
      a. Time is sufficient for most positions, especially laterals
III. Measure the area of interest in centimeters with calipers
IV. Have two views at right angles
  A. Exceptions are thoracic views, contrast studies, and equine radiography, which often require more views
  B. Injury may also allow only one view
V. Have the area of interest as close to the film as possible
VI. Center the beam to area of interest and include specific anatomy for each anatomic area
VII. Keep the area of interest parallel to the film and perpendicular to the x-ray beam
  A. Bisecting angle technique is used in dental radiography (see Chapter 26)
VIII. Collimate using the smallest field size possible to accommodate essential anatomy

IX. When taking radiographs of extremities, include the proximal and distal joints of the long bone being radiographed
    A. If radiographing a joint, include at least one third of the long bones distal and proximal to that joint
X. Make sure patient is adequately prepared
XI. Plan your procedure carefully to avoid retakes

## CONTRAST RADIOGRAPHY

### Basic Concepts

I. Used to enhance the visualization of individual organs and structures that are not adequately visible on the survey radiographs
II. Contrast means density difference

### Media

I. Two classes of contrast media
    A. Positive contrast (radiopaque), such as barium and iodine
        1. Absorb more x-rays than bone, so appear even whiter on a radiograph
        2. May be classified as
            a. Insoluble: barium, which is used mainly for gastrointestinal studies. Never give barium parenterally
            b. Soluble: all other positive contrast media; contains iodine, which can be used for renal, articular, vascular, myelographic, and gastrointestinal studies
            c. Soluble iodinated contrast agents are hyperosmotic and, although rare, may cause toxic reactions
    B. Negative contrast (radiolucent), such as air and carbon dioxide
        1. No x-rays are absorbed, so the medium appears black on the radiograph
    C. Double contrast studies incorporate positive and negative contrast media

### Patient Preparation

I. Depending on the procedure, the patient may have to
    A. Have food withheld 12 to 24 hours
    B. Be given an enema or a cathartic 4 to 12 hours before the procedure
II. Have a survey radiograph completed before the procedure

### Positioning and Specific Studies

Please refer to the excellent references available for positioning as well as further information on special studies.

## DIGITAL RADIOGRAPHY

I. Magnetic resonance imaging (MRI), computed tomography (CT), ultrasound (US), and nuclear medicine (NM) are all digital technologies. Conventional radiography has been slow to evolve, because film radiography is effective and large amounts of digital data are required for digital radiography.
II. Overview of digital radiography
    A. Digital radiography and conventional radiography have the same origins
        1. Production is through a series of analog signals
            a. Light emitted from the intensifying screens
        2. Many available digital radiography systems can use current x-ray machines
    B. Difference is in the conversion of the analog signals to an electronic digital signal
        1. Instead of a film-screen cassette, a reusable image receptor receives x-rays and exposes a digital plate that transforms emitted light to an electrical latent image
        2. Image is transferred to a dedicated digital radiography computer, where images can be adjusted, stored, viewed, and submitted to any other computer or site
        3. Done through an analog-to-digital converter (ADC)
        4. Converted to electronic form that is digitized and numerically encoded into tiny, discrete squares known as pixels
            a. Each pixel displays only one shade of gray
            b. The smaller and more numerous the pixels, the better the spatial resolution
                (1) Spatial resolution is the ability to separate two closely spaced objects
                (2) Efficiency of the imaging plate and other design criteria also affect spatial resolution
        5. Picture archiving and communication system (PACS) is a broad term for computers and components that can capture, transfer, store, and display medical digital information
        6. Proper exposure techniques not as critical as screen-film system, because images can be altered digitally to maximize diagnostic image quality
            a. kVp does not affect the contrast
                (1) Final image can be adjusted
            b. Technique charts do not vary greatly for body parts
            c. Has higher contrast resolution than conventional screen-film radiography
III. Types of digital radiography
    A. Classified as indirect or direct
        1. Indirect systems use a two-part system
            a. X-ray energy is first converted to light and then to an electronic digital signal
            b. Examples include computed radiography (CR), charge-coupled device (CCD), and silicon flat panel receptors

2. Direct digital radiography (DDR) systems convert the x-ray energy directly into an electrical digital signal
   a. Yield highest spatial resolution
   b. Extremely expensive and not as common in veterinary medicine

B. Indirect digital conversion systems: computed radiography
   1. Uses a photostimulable phosphor (PSP) detector screen
      a. Passive (nonelectronic) sensor based on fluorescence
      b. Also called CR imaging plate or storage phosphors
      c. Absorbs and stores latent image to be read later
      d. Various layers, with the phosphor layer being composed of barium fluorohalide
      e. These filmless CR cassettes are used the same way as conventional screen-film cassettes
      f. Once exposed, plate is taken to a laser CR reader unit
         (1) Also referred to as image reader device (IRD) or CR processor
         (2) CR plate removed from the cassette in the reader
         (3) Helium-neon laser beam scans the plate and releases visible light, producing an electrical signal that is digitized and stored on a computer
         (4) Any residual latent image is erased by a bright white light and the CR plate is returned to the cassette, which is then ejected from the CR reader
            (a) Sensitive to secondary radiation, so must be properly stored and erased
            (b) If image not erased within 24 hours, it may show up as ghost artifacts
            (c) Can have image fogging if exposed to scatter radiation
      g. Ensure plate is positioned right side up
   2. Maximum absorption by the PSP screen is 35 to 50 kVp
      a. Radiation efficiency is compared to 200- to 300-speed screen systems of conventional film
   3. Latent image is temporary, so best processed within a few hours
   4. Plates are susceptible to cracking as they bend in the plate reader
      a. Areas without PSP show up white, as does debris in the CR cassette

C. Indirect digital conversion systems: charge-coupled device (CCD)
   1. Equipment is located under the table and is not portable

2. Uses electronic sensor device
   a. Small flat panel that receives and stores incoming light energy from intensifying screens
      (1) Does so as trapped electrons in chips that are coupled to conventional rare earth intensifying screens
   3. Chip is an integrated circuit (IC) composed of crystalline silicon
      a. Photosensitive and divided into tiny electronically isolated pixels
         (1) Referred to as pixilated light detector
   4. Limited by the size of the panel detector
      a. Anatomical areas that have a larger field of view are greater than the current CCD plates available
      b. Need a coupling lens that couples a large intensifying screen onto a smaller CCD
         (1) Called demagnification
         (2) Less than 90% of light energy reaches the CCD
            (a) Results in a grainy appearance known as quantum mottle
            (b) Not enough photons produce a quality image
   5. High quality units not cost effective for most clinics
   6. New similar units use CMOS chips (complementary metal-oxide semiconductor) in place of CCD

D. Indirect digital conversion systems—flat panel detectors
   1. Self contained unit located under the table
      a. Can be used for field work
      b. Is hardwired to digital computer, so not as flexible as CCD
   2. Larger, intimately coupled to rare earth intensifying screens
   3. Contains a light detector (photodiode)
   4. Contains an electronic sensitive layer of silicon that replaces film
      a. Silicon detector consists of matrix that is composed of a large number of individual detector elements
      b. Each detector is an independent element, making it more efficient and less susceptible to manufacturer imperfections
      c. Not as sensitive to ghost image artifacts

# Glossary

**absorbed dose** Amount of energy that tissue receives when it is bombarded by ionizing radiation; measured as gray (Gy) or rad

**actual focal spot** Area on the target bombarded by the electrons to produce x-rays. Because of the angle of the anode, it is viewed from 90 degrees to the target

**amperage** Term used to describe the flow of electrons as current

**analog** A variable signal continuous in both time and amplitude

**anode** Positive electrode in the x-ray tube that contains the target

**artifact** That which decreases the diagnostic quality of a radiograph

**binding energy** Energy that must be surpassed before an electron can be removed from its orbit

**calipers** Measuring device to determine patient thickness

**cathode** Negative electrode in the x-ray tube that supplies the electrons

**caudocranial (CdCr)** Directional term indicating that the x-ray beam enters from toward the tail and exits toward the head. Opposite is CrCd. Usually in reference to limbs, proximal to the carpal and tarsal joints

**CCD** Charge-coupled device. Is a small flat panel device used in digital radiography and photography that converts visual image to an electric signal

**CMOS** Complementary metal-oxide semiconductor. Is a major class of integrated circuits used similar to CCD technology in digital radiography

**CR** Computed radiography. Uses similar equipment to conventional radiography, except that an imaging plate is used and run through a computer scanner to read and digitize the image

**detail** Part of film quality indicating clear resolution and definition of the shadows on the radiographic image

**digital** System uses discrete values (often electrical voltages), especially those represented as binary numbers for data input, processing, transmission, storage, or display, rather than a continuous spectrum of values (i.e., as in an analog system)

**DDR** Direct digital radiography. A digital radiography system that directly converts x-rays into an electronic signal

**DR** Digital radiography

**distal** Farther away from the point of origin; opposite is proximal

**dorsopalmar (DPa)** Directional term that refers to limbs distal to and including the carpus. The beam enters from the front of the limb and exits at the back of the limb; opposite is PaD

**dorsoplantar (DPl)** Directional term that refers to limbs distal to and including the tarsus (see above)

**dorsoventral (DV)** Directional term that indicates that the x-ray beam enters from the back of the animal and exits out its abdomen. The animal would be lying in ventral recumbency (on its abdomen); opposite is VD

**dosimeter** Device used to measure the radiation exposure that personnel receive

**effective focal spot** Area of the focal spot as seen through the x-ray tube window and directed on the film; different from the actual focal spot because of the angle of the anode

**electromagnetic radiation** Propagation of ionizing energy through space in the form of photons

**electron** Negatively charged particle of the atom that circles around the nucleus

**electron beam** Beam of electrons that is accelerated from the cathode to the anode by a high electrical potential in the x-ray tube

**filament** Coiled wire of the cathode that emits the electron beam

**film contrast** Characteristic of the film that influences radiographic contrast. Often, film contrast and latitude are inversely related

**film graininess** Loss of detail caused by the size of the individual silver halide crystals; usually more pronounced in faster speed film; also referred to as radiographic mottle

**film latitude** Exposure range that will produce acceptable density on the film

**focal range** Distance from the grid to the x-ray tube that will minimize grid cutoff

**fogging** Overall grayness that does not contribute to the diagnostic quality of the film; may be caused from chemicals as well as undesirable radiation

**geometric unsharpness** Loss of detail due to geometric distortion; also referred to as penumbra

**grid cutoff** When a grid is not used correctly and the primary beam is absorbed more than normal

**grid ratio** Ratio of the height of the lead strips as compared to the space between them ($r = h/d$)

**heel effect** Owing to the angle of the target, a greater intensity of x-rays is emitted from the cathode side, rather than from the anode side

**ionization** Process of transferring sufficient energy to an atom so that the outer electron is removed; the atom becomes positively charged

**kilovolt peak (kVp)** Maximum energy of the x-ray beam that determines the quality or penetrating power of the beam

**latent image** Invisible image produced on the x-ray film after exposure and before processing

**maximum permissible dose (MPD)** Maximum amount of radiation exposure that an individual is allowed over a given time period

**milliampere-second (mAs)** Amount of current flowing through the tube times the exposure time in seconds; 1 milliampere = 1/1000 ampere

**object-film distance (OFD)** Space between the film and the part being radiographed

**PACS** Picture archiving and communication system. These are computers or networks dedicated to the storage, retrieval, distribution, and presentation of images

**penumbra** Loss of detail due to geometric unsharpness

**photon** Bundle of radiation energy, also known as quanta

**pixel** Short for picture element. A single point in a graphic image

**polychromatic beam** X-ray beam that has a broad spectrum of energies; depends on the kVp: the lower the kVp, the more polychromatic the beam

**quality** Term referring to the average energy of the x-ray beam or its penetrating ability (kVp)

**quantity** Term that refers to the total number of x-ray photons (controlled by mA)

**quantum mottle** Loss of radiographic detail that occurs in faster screens because of the uneven distribution of the phosphor crystals within the screen

**radiodense or radiopaque** Object or tissue that absorbs radiation so that the image on the film is lighter

**radiographic contrast** Variation in degree of darkness between two adjacent areas on the film

**radiographic density** Degree of darkness found on the radiograph

**radiographic quality** How well the shadows on the radiograph are clearly identified

**radiography** Making of radiographs

**radiology** Use of radiant energy in the diagnosis and treatment of disease

**radiolucent** Quality of a tissue or device that allows most of the x-ray beams to pass through unaffected

**rectification** Process of changing alternating current to current flowing in one direction only (direct current)

**remnant beam** Primary radiation emitted from the x-ray tube

**scatter radiation** or **secondary radiation** Caused by interaction of the primary beam with tissue or matter in its path

**scintillating devices** Another name for intensifying screens that emit visible or ultraviolet light when exposed to x-rays

**source-image distance (SID)** Formerly called focal-film distance, it is the distance from the focal spot or source of the x-rays to the image receptor or film

**speed** Exposure required to produce a diagnostic film density

**structure mottle** Loss of radiographic detail that occurs because of phosphor variations found in intensifying screens; more noticeable with fast-speed screens

**subject contrast** Contrast resulting from the difference in density, mass, and atomic number of adjacent tissue structures

**thermionic emission** Heating of the filament so that the energy produced forces the electrons to be released from their atomic orbits

**thermoluminescent dosimeter** Device that personnel wear to indicate dosage of radiation exposure

**x-ray** A short-wavelength, high-energy form of electromagnetic radiation

# Review Questions

1 For your safety when taking radiographs, you should always consider
 a. Increased time, decreased distance, and increased shielding
 b. Increased time, increased distance, and increased shielding
 c. Decreased time, increased distance, and increased shielding
 d. Decreased time, increased distance, and decreased shielding

2 To obtain higher contrast on a film, you should not
 a. Use a grid
 b. Increase the time and temperature of the processing chemicals
 c. Set the collimator aperture so that the field is smaller
 d. Increase the kVp

3 The machine setting is 250 mA and 2.5 mAs. The exposure time that you would use is
 a. 1/10 sec
 b. 2/25 sec
 c. 1/50 sec
 d. 1/100 sec

4 The main purpose of the fixer is to
 a. Reduce exposed silver halide crystals to black metallic silver
 b. Remove unexposed, undeveloped silver halide crystals
 c. Change the calcium tungstate crystals to black calcium
 d. Create a latent image

5 Density is decreased on a film by
 a. Increasing the kVp
 b. Decreasing the tissue density
 c. Decreasing the mAs
 d. Increasing the processing chemical temperatures

6 A higher grid ratio means that
 a. The lead plate is thicker
 b. Less scatter radiation is absorbed
 c. More scatter radiation is absorbed
 d. Less primary radiation is absorbed

7 X-rays
 a. Are a type of electromagnetic radiation
 b. Have less energy than radio waves
 c. Have longer wavelengths than radio waves
 d. Are measured in meters

8 A boxer is lying in left lateral recumbency for an x-ray of its pelvis. The right femur will be:
 a. More magnified because of increased SID and decreased OFD
 b. More magnified because of decreased SID and increased OFD
 c. Less magnified because of decreased SID and increased OFD
 d. Less magnified because of increased SID and decreased OFD

9 A radiograph using 70 kVp and 10 mAs is too dark. Which combination of settings would be most reasonable for the repeat?
 a. 80 kVp and 5 mAs
 b. 85 kVp and 10 mAs
 c. 60 kVp and 20 mAs
 d. 70 kVp and 5 mAs

10 The correct description with screens would be
 a. Large crystals, faster screens, less detail, high graininess
 b. Large crystals, slower screens, less detail, high graininess
 c. Small crystals, faster screens, more detail, low graininess
 d. Small crystals, slower screens, less detail, low graininess

## REFERENCES

1. Health Canada: *Radiation protection in veterinary medicine: recommended safety procedures for installation and use of veterinary x-ray equipment, Safety Code 28*, Ottawa, Canada, 2004, Environmental Health Directorate.
2. NCRP: *Radiation protection in veterinary medicine, #148*. Bethesda, Md, 2006, NCRP.

## BIBLIOGRAPHY

Darby ML, editor: *Mosby's comprehensive review of dental hygiene,* ed 6, St Louis, 2006, Mosby.

Eastman Kodak Company: *The fundamentals of radiography*, ed 12, Rochester, NY, 1980, Eastman Kodak Company, Radiographic Markets Division.

Han C, Hurd C: *Practical diagnostic imaging for the veterinary technician*, ed 2, St Louis, 2005, Mosby.

Lavin L: *Radiography in veterinary technology*, ed 4, St Louis, 2007, Saunders.

Morgan JP: *Techniques of veterinary radiography*, ed 5, Ames, 1993, Iowa State University Press.

Owens JM: *Radiographic interpretation for the small animal clinician*, St Louis, 1998, Ralston Purina.

Partington BP: Diagnostic imaging. In McCurnin DM and Bassert JM: *Clinical textbook for veterinary technicians*, ed 6, St Louis, 2006, Saunders.

Rendano VT, Ryan G: Technician assistance in radiology, part II. Basic consideration and radiation safety, *Comp Contin Educ* 9:547, 1988.

Ryan GD: *Radiographic positioning of small animals*, Philadelphia, 1981, Lea & Febiger.

Smallwood JE et al: A standardized nomenclature for radiographic projections used in veterinary medicine, *Vet Radiol J* 26:2, 1985.

## CHAPTER 12

# Alternative Imaging Technology

*Jane M. Sykes*   *Pierry McLean*

## OUTLINE

Basic Physics of Ultrasound
  Image Production
  Sound Waves
  Attenuation
  Acoustic Impedance
Ultrasound Machine
  Transducers
  Transducer Crystals
  Piezoelectric Effect
  Bandwidth
  Types of Transducers
  Equipment Controls
  Brightness and Contrast
  Gain and Power
  Time-Gain Compensation
Image Physics
  Resolution
  Sound Beam Zones
  Focusing

The Display
  Display Format
Final Image
  Image Characteristics
  Organ Appearance
  Scanning Planes
Artifacts
  Propagation Artifacts
  Attenuation Artifacts
  Other Artifacts
Doppler Imaging
Three-Dimensional Ultrasound
Examination
  Preparing the Patient
Sonographic Appearance of Organs
  Heart
  Spleen
  Liver
  Gallbladder

Kidneys
Bladder
Prostate
Uterus
Stomach and Bowel
Pancreas
Adrenal Gland
Lesions
  Appearance of Lesions
  Classification of Lesions
Other Imaging Techniques
  Introduction to Nuclear Medicine
  Nuclear Scintigraphy
  Positron Emission Tomography
  Computed Tomography
  PET/CT: $^{18}$F-FDG/X-Ray
  Magnetic Resonance Imaging
  Preparing Clients for These
    Procedures

## LEARNING OUTCOMES

After reading this chapter you should be able to:

1. Have a better understanding of the basic physics of ultrasound.
2. Be familiar with the basic functioning of the ultrasound machine.
3. Understand the concepts of image physics.
4. Have an understanding of the concepts of the final image and artifacts.
5. Differentiate between the sonographic appearance of anatomical features and artifacts.
6. Properly prepare a patient for routine ultrasonography.
7. Explain the equipment controls responsible for the images.

Ultrasound is a diagnostic modality used to image various organs in the living body. By noninvasive means, the veterinary technologist may use ultrasound to determine and compare the location, echogenicity, and approximate size of abdominal and thoracic structures. Imaging can be performed easily on most animals without tranquilization, so even the most critically ill patient can tolerate the examination. It is important to understand the basic physics concerning ultrasound. Without this knowledge, it would be difficult to understand the applications and limitations of ultrasound. In this chapter, the ultrasound machine, organ characteristics, artifacts, and patient preparation are discussed.

## BASIC PHYSICS OF ULTRASOUND

Definition: sound waves with a frequency beyond the range of human hearing

## Image Production

I. Waves travel through media, transferring energy from one location to another
II. Sound waves are reflected back to the transducer, analyzed by a computer, and displayed on a screen
III. Pixel placement depends upon the length of time the sound takes to travel into the tissue, be reflected, and return to the transducer

## Sound Waves (Figure 12-1)

I. Wavelength ($\lambda$)
   A. Definition: the distance that a wave must travel in one cycle
   B. Ultrasound has shorter wavelengths than those of audible sounds
   C. Wavelength is determined by the characteristics of the transducer
      1. The shorter the wavelength the higher the frequency transducer, which produces a better quality image
II. Frequency (f)
   A. Definition: the number of cycles per unit of time (seconds)
   B. As frequency increases, the wavelength decreases or becomes shorter
   C. Ultrasound waves are in the 2- to 10-MHz range, compared with human hearing, which is around 20,000 Hz
III. Velocity (v)
   A. Definition: the speed at which sound travels through an object = frequency × wavelength

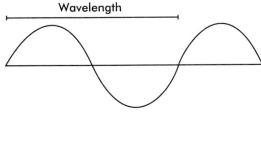

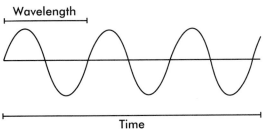

**Figure 12-1** Frequency and wavelength are inversely related. As the wavelength increases, the frequency decreases. (From Han CM, Hurd CD: *Practical diagnostic imaging for the veterinary technician*, ed 3, St Louis, 2005, Mosby.)

B. When the sound wave returns, the computer records the time
C. The computer will use the time taken for the echo to return to calculate the depth at which the sound was reflected
IV. Amplitude: intensity or loudness of a wave
V. Period (T): time needed to produce one cycle

## Attenuation

I. Definition: the loss of intensity of the ultrasound beam as it travels both into and out of tissue; caused by
   A. Absorption: production of heat as sound passes through soft tissue, causing loss of energy
   B. Scattering: sound is reflected in different directions from tissue interfaces and is unable to return to the transducer

## Acoustic Impedance

I. Definition: the ability of tissue to resist or impede the transmission of sound
II. Impedance depends on the density and elasticity of the tissue
III. The greater the difference in acoustic impedance, the more reflective the interface
   A. Air and bone have a large difference in acoustic impedance with other soft tissues, causing almost all the sound to be reflected back to the transducer, creating a barrier to sound transmission
   B. Acoustic impedance allows the sonographer to differentiate one tissue type from another

## ULTRASOUND MACHINE

### Transducers

I. Definition: the part of the ultrasound machine used to scan a patient
   A. Devices that convert sound energy into electrical energy and vice versa
   B. They send out a series of sound pulses and collect the returning echoes
II. Pulsed-wave transducers
   A. A short burst of sound is emitted from this transducer. It waits until the echo comes back before sending another one
   B. Most common
   C. One piezoelectric crystal alternately transmits and receives echoes
III. Continuous-wave transducers
   A. Contains two piezoelectric crystals: one crystal constantly sends sound waves while the other one "listens"

### Transducer Crystals

I. Definition: the active element required to promote the conversion of electrical energy to ultrasound
   A. Natural crystals: quartz, tourmaline, Rochelle salt

B. Synthetics: most common; lead zirconate titanate, barium titanate, and lithium sulfate
C. The crystal produces sound by vibrations through the piezoelectric effect
D. After pulses are sent, the crystals are damped to stop vibrations
E. Struck by the echoes returning, they start to vibrate again
F. Crystals convert echoes into electrical energy

## Piezoelectric Effect

I. Definition: the conversion of electrical energy to pressure energy (ultrasound or acoustic)
II. Piezoelectric means pressure electricity

## Bandwidth

I. Definition: the entire range of frequency
II. A transducer can produce more than one frequency above or below its center frequency

## Types of Transducers

I. Mechanical sector
   A. Consists of one or more crystals mechanically steered to produce a pie-shaped image
II. Linear array
   A. Consists of a small row of crystals sequentially pulsed
   B. Produces parallel lines and allows the image to be rectangular
   C. Ideal for transrectal and equine tendon examinations
III. Phased array sector scanner
   A. Contains about 20 crystals, which are electronically steered through a sector
   B. Commonly used in echocardiography
   C. Usually small and expensive
IV. Broad bandwidth transducer
   A. New type of transducer
      1. Advantages are its lighter weight and lower acoustic impedance
         a. More efficient transmission of sound waves through tissue
   B. The transducer element consists of piezoelectric ceramic and an epoxy material
   C. These transducers have wide frequency bandwidths and therefore can operate at different frequencies or emit pulses of short duration

## Equipment Controls

The ultrasound machine has many controls for adjusting the image. Improper use may decrease quality of the image and possibly produce images of lesions that do not exist.

## Brightness and Contrast

I. Display monitor controls should be adjusted so that black, white, and all different shades of gray can be seen

## Gain and Power

I. Affects brightness of the whole image
II. The higher the overall gain or power, the brighter the image
III. Increasing the power increases the intensity of the sound leaving the transducer and the waves returning to it, because gain amplifies the returning echoes

## Time-Gain Compensation

I. Time-gain compensation (TGC) increases electronic gain of the more distant echoes
II. It enables the returning echoes from different depths to have the same brightness when imaging one tissue type
III. TGC consists of a series of slide pods to control the brightness in different depths of the image

## IMAGE PHYSICS
### Resolution

I. Definition: the ability to separately identify small structures on the ultrasound image or the detail of the image
   A. The frequency of the transducer dictates the resolution of the image
   B. The higher the frequency (i.e., 7.5 MHz), the shorter the wavelength and thus the better the resolution
II. Lateral resolution
   A. The ability of the ultrasound beam to separate two structures lying perpendicular to the sound beam; depends on the beam diameter (width)
   B. The distance between two interfaces must be greater than the beam width for each interface to be identified separately
III. Axial resolution
   A. Ability of the ultrasound beam to separate two structures lying along the path of the beam
   B. Depends on the wavelength of the sound frequency used
   C. The higher the frequency, the shorter the wavelength, the better the resolution

## Sound Beam Zones

The dimensions and design of the transducer determine sound beam zones.
I. Near field
   A. The area of the beam closest to the transducer
II. Focal point
   A. Where the beam reaches its narrowest point
III. Far field
   A. The area of the beam farthest from the transducer

## Focusing

I. Definition: the method of moving the focal point closer to the image, to narrow the width and improve resolution

II. Transducers are focused by shaping the crystal, adding a lens, or combining both methods

## THE DISPLAY
### Display Format

I. Definition: how the returning echo, or the image, appears on the screen
  A. Can be rectangular or sector
II. A-mode (amplitude mode) (Figure 12-2)
  A. One-dimensional graphic display
  B. Returning echoes are viewed as a series of peaks on a graph
  C. The greater the intensity, the higher the peak
III. B-mode (brightness mode) (see Figure 12-2)
  A. Depicts dots or pixels on a screen as a two-dimensional image
  B. Brightness of the pixel depends on the intensity of the returning echo; the higher the intensity, the brighter the pixel
  C. The position of the pixel in the image depends on the depth of the reflecting interface

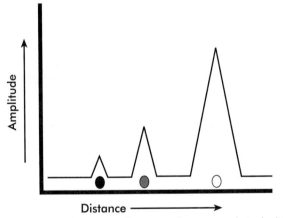

**Figure 12-2** Where A-mode uses peaks on a graph to depict the strength of the returning echoes, B-mode uses bright pixels, or dots, on a monitor. The brighter the pixel, the stronger the returning echo. (From Han CM, Hurd CD: *Practical diagnostic imaging for the veterinary technician*, ed 3, St Louis, 2005, Mosby.)

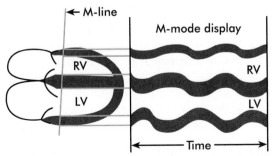

**Figure 12-3** M-mode displays the motion of a thin slice of an organ over time. *LV*, Left ventricle; *RV*, right ventricle. (From Han CM, Hurd CD: *Practical diagnostic imaging for the veterinary technician*, ed 3, St Louis, 2005, Mosby.)

IV. M-mode (motion mode) (Figure 12-3)
  A. A two-dimensional display of a reflector over a time oriented baseline
  B. The position of a reflector is displayed on the vertical axis, and time is displayed on the horizontal axis
  C. Stationary objects result in straight lines, whereas moving objects produce wavy lines
  D. Mainly used in cardiology to assess cardiac valves, walls, and chamber size

## FINAL IMAGE
### Image Characteristics (Figure 12-4)

The format used for ultrasound display is a black background on which echo information appears in white and varying shades of gray. Size, shape, and margins of the organs should be known so that any deviation from normal can be documented.

I. Echogenic (echoic)
  A. Tissue that produces sufficient echoes returning to the transducer for display
  B. Appears bright on the monitor
  C. The greater the difference between two adjacent organs, the greater the echo reflection between them (acoustic impedance)
II. Sonolucent
  A. Tissue that permits the majority of the sound to pass through to deeper regions, with only a few echoes being reflected back
  B. Appears dark on the monitor
III. Anechoic
  A. Describes tissue that transmits all the sound to deeper tissue, reflecting none back to the transducer
  B. Appears black on the monitor
  C. Often is fluid

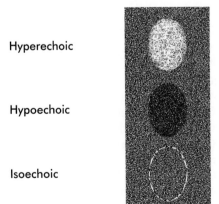

**Figure 12-4** An area within an organ or the whole organ that is brighter or whiter than surrounding tissue is described as hyperechoic. Areas that are darker than surrounding tissue are described as hypoechoic. Areas that are the same as surrounding tissue are described as isoechoic. (From Han CM, Hurd CD: *Practical diagnostic imaging for the veterinary technician*, ed 3, St Louis, 2005, Mosby.)

IV. Hyperechoic
  A. Appears brighter than surrounding tissue
  B. Used to compare tissue types
V. Hypoechoic
  A. Area appears darker than surrounding tissue
  B. Used to compare tissue types
VI. Isoechoic
  A. Tissue equal in appearance to that of surrounding tissue
  B. Used to compare tissue types

## Organ Appearance

I. Contour or architecture
  A. Is the organ outline smooth, rough, or irregular?
II. Texture
  A. Is the organ parenchyma homogeneous?
III. Shape
  A. Does the organ have its proper shape?
IV. Size
  A. Is the size of the organ within normal parameters?

## Scanning Planes

The animal can be scanned in lateral or dorsal recumbency, and the organs should be scanned in two planes.
I. Sagittal (longitudinal) or long axis
  A. Transducer marker should be constantly positioned to the cranial or caudal end of the animal
II. Transverse (short axis)
  A. Transducer marker should be 90 degrees to the longitudinal plane

## ARTIFACTS

Definition: refers to something seen on an ultrasound image that anatomically does not exist
I. Artifacts occur during imaging
II. Some are a direct benefit; others are not
III. It is important to distinguish between artifacts and real structures

## Propagation Artifacts

I. Reverberations
  A. Appear as many linear echoes
  B. Occur when sound is reflected constantly between a strong reflector (e.g., bone or air and the transducer surface)
II. Refraction
  A. Occurs when the sound beam changes direction as it passes from one medium to another
  B. Allows the organ to appear in different positions
III. Mirror image
  A. Appears when an organ lies next to a reflector on the image; the organ appears to be present on both sides of the reflector
  B. Often occurs in the region of the diaphragm and liver

## Attenuation Artifacts

I. Acoustic shadowing
  A. Occurs when sound is totally reflected or absorbed by an object
  B. Prevents sound from traveling to a greater depth
  C. Calculi, bowel gas, etc., can cause this posterior shadowing
II. Distance enhancement
  A. Echoes beside a fluid-filled structure will not be as strong as the echoes from behind it
  B. Enhancement occurs because sound transmitted through fluid is less attenuated than the tissue beside it
  C. This artifact can be used to determine if a lesion is a hypoechoic mass or a cyst

## Other Artifacts

I. Ring down
  A. Similar to reverberation
  B. Produces many parallel echoes
  C. Associated with gas bubbles
II. Comet tail
  A. Similar to reverberation
  B. Caused by a strong reflector
  C. Consists of thin lines with close echoes

## DOPPLER IMAGING

I. Valuable in diagnosing moving structures or fluids, such as blood flow
II. Where there is motion between a sound source and listener, the frequency heard by the listener usually differs from the source
III. The received frequency is either higher or lower than that transmitted by the source
  A. Dependent on whether the listener and source are moving toward or away from each other
  B. Information about the velocity of the structure is provided
    1. Based on a Doppler shift in frequency of a continuous-wave ultrasonic beam reflected from a moving structure
      a. Either by sound audible to the ear or by analysis with an instrument
  C. Variety of uses in veterinary ultrasound
    1. Can determine if a lesion is a mass or a vessel
    2. Helps in the detection of portal systemic shunts
    3. Provides data on cardiac output and structural abnormalities

## THREE-DIMENSIONAL ULTRASOUND

I. State-of-the-art technique
II. Displays the total area rather than sections; therefore has reduced image capture time

III. Improved diagnostic ability with enhanced visualization
IV. Surfaces can be reconstructed with computer capabilities
 V. Useful for surgical applications and imaging horse tendons and prostate glands in small animals

## EXAMINATION

### Preparing the Patient

 I. Shaving
   A. Essential, because the ultrasound beam would otherwise pass through and be reflected by the air-filled hair coat before penetrating the skin
   B. For abdominal ultrasound, the abdomen should be shaved from the xiphoid process to the pubis, and then laterally from the rib cage to the flanks, using a No. 40 clipper blade
   C. For cardiac ultrasound, the cardiac region is shaved using a No. 40 blade
   D. Alcohol can be used to wipe away residual dirt and hair
 II. Positioning
   A. Small animals can be placed in dorsal recumbency in a padded V-shaped trough, or in lateral recumbency for abdominal ultrasounds
   B. Small animal cardiac patients are placed in sternal or lateral recumbency, with the shaved cardiac region situated over a hole in the table so that the transducer may be passed through it
   C. Ultrasound is usually performed with large animals in a standing position
 III. Acoustic coupling gel should be used so that no air is present between the transducer and the skin surface
 IV. Physical and/or chemical restraint should be used as needed
  V. To ensure that all tissues and organs are scanned, each ultrasound examination should be done in systematic order
 VI. Small dogs and cats can be scanned using a 7.5-MHz transducer
   A. It does not penetrate as deeply and signal attenuation is greater, but it provides better detail
 VII. Larger dogs can be scanned with a 5-MHz transducer
   A. The lower frequency increases the depth of penetration and decreases signal attenuation, but results in less detail

## SONOGRAPHIC APPEARANCE OF ORGANS

### Heart

 I. Should use both M-mode and two-dimensional B-mode
 II. Important to obtain both long- and short-axis directional views
   A. Doppler imaging is useful for assessing turbulence and velocity of blood flow

III. Usually examined between the fourth and fifth ribs, or where the acoustic window is the best
IV. Start in right lateral recumbency with an opening to allow the transducer to come from underneath
 V. Heart walls and valves are echogenic

### Spleen

 I. Most hyperechoic of all the organs
 II. Uniform, granular appearance
 III. Surrounded by a bright capsule
 IV. Vessels are seen entering and exiting the hilar surface
  V. Seen best on left side of the patient
 VI. Lies close to the body wall

### Liver

 I. Less echogenic than the spleen
 II. Contains many vessels and bile channels with the parenchyma
 III. Echotexture is coarse
 IV. Contains gallbladder

### Gallbladder

 I. Anechoic with a bright wall
 II. Sometimes contains echogenic debris (sludge)
 III. Can be large in an animal that has fasted

### Kidneys

 I. Scanning in lateral recumbency, kidney is bean shaped. Scanning in dorsal recumbency, it is ovoid
 II. Surrounded by a bright capsule
 III. Cortex is hypoechoic
 IV. Medulla is anechoic
  V. Bright central area is pelvic fat
 VI. A sagittal view can be measured to assess size

### Bladder

 I. Anechoic with a hyperechoic wall
 II. Debris often seen

### Prostate

 I. Can be visualized by following the urethra into the pelvic inlet
 II. Surrounds urethra and is bilobed with a bright appearance
 III. Larger and more echogenic in an intact male

### Uterus

 I. If enlarged, can be seen between the bladder and the colon in the transverse plane
 II. Wall is hypoechoic
 III. Optimal time for pregnancy detection is at 20 days of gestation in small animals and 11 days of gestation in horses
   A. Identify gestational sacs with viable embryos
   B. Hard to determine number of fetuses

## Stomach and Bowel

I. Can be difficult to image because of gas
II. Walls seen as alternating black and white layers
III. Rugal folds can be visualized in the stomach

## Pancreas

I. Adjacent to duodenum on the right side, and between stomach, spleen, and colon on the left

## Adrenal Gland

I. Hypoechoic
II. Uniformly gray
III. Found medial and cranial to or beside the cranial pole of the kidneys
IV. Caudal pole of the adrenal gland is next to the renal artery where it joins the aorta

## LESIONS

Disease can appear as an alteration in echo texture in an organ.

## Appearance of Lesions

I. Focal changes
   A. Readily identified
   B. Can be in one specific area of the organ
II. Diffuse
   A. Can be subtle changes
   B. Can affect the whole organ; thus texture needs to be assessed by comparison with other organs

## Classification of Lesions

I. Cystic
   A. Well-defined borders
   B. No internal echoes
   C. Shows distance enhancement
II. Solid
   A. Contains many echoes, which can be spread throughout
   B. No distance enhancement
III. Mixed
   A. Contains cystic and solid lesions
   B. Borders may be irregular

## OTHER IMAGING TECHNIQUES
## Introduction to Nuclear Medicine

Nuclear medicine is a branch of medicine and medical imaging that uses unsealed radioactive substances in diagnosis and therapy. In diagnosis, radioactive substances are administered to animals and the radiation emitted is measured. Nuclear medicine techniques that are becoming more available in veterinary medicine include gamma scintigraphy, positron emission tomography/computed tomography (PET/CT), and magnetic resonance imaging (MRI). Therapy using radioactive substances includes treating hyperthyroidism in cats with iodine-131.

I. Nuclear medicine procedures are performed after administration of a radionuclide with special affinity to the organ or structure imaged
II. Types of radiation
   A. Beta ray
      1. A particle ray consisting of a fast electron whose mass is nearly 1/2000 of the mass of a proton or neutron
      2. The beta particles emitted are a form of ionizing radiation also known as beta rays
      3. Beta particles are high-energy electrons emitted by certain types of radioactive nuclei
      4. Are produced following spontaneous decay of certain radioactive materials
         a. The production of beta particles is termed beta decay
      5. Beta particles can be used to treat such health conditions as eye and bone cancer, and are also used as tracers
   B. Gamma ray
      1. Gamma ray is also classified as electromagnetic radiation
         a. Has the highest frequency and energy, and also the shortest wavelength, within the electromagnetic radiation spectrum
            (1) Gamma ray's wavelength is far shorter than ultraviolet light
      2. Because of their high energy, they are able to cause serious damage when absorbed by living cells
      3. Gamma rays are produced following spontaneous decay of certain radioactive materials
      4. When administered to a patient, detection of emitted gamma rays can be used to form an image of the radioisotope's distribution
      5. Such a technique can be employed to diagnose a wide range of conditions, such as spread of cancer to the bones
III. Common radionuclides and half-life decay
   A. Definition of half-life: the half-life is the amount of time it takes for half of the atoms in a sample to decay
      1. The half-life for a given radionuclide is always the same; it does not depend on how many atoms you have or on how long they have been sitting around
         a. Iodine-131 has a half-life of 8 days; day 0: 5 mCi, day 8: 2.5 mCi, day 16: 1.75 mCi, etc.

## Nuclear Scintigraphy

I. Small amount of radioactive material or radionuclide is given intravenously, transcolonically, or by aerosol insufflation

II. A gamma scintillation camera is used to detect the gamma emissions from the radionuclide
   A. The radionuclide used most commonly is technetium-99m ($^{99m}$Tc), which can be labeled with different molecules
      1. $^{99m}$Technetium methylene diphosphonate ($^{99m}$Tc-MPD) is used for bone scan and transcolonic portal scintigraphy
      2. Activity is then detected using the gamma camera and images displayed on the computer
      3. A black-and-white image of the selected organ is printed on x-ray film
III. The radiopharmaceutical injected accumulates in the target organ after a certain time; 2 to 4 hours for a bone scan, and immediately for transcolonic portal scintigraphy
IV. Detects functional or physiological, pharmacological, and kinetic data
V. Images generated are different from those produced with other imaging modalities
VI. Clinical applications include thyroid, bone, and liver studies
VII. Often used for horses
VIII. Animals are sedated
IX. Proper radiation protection is required
   A. Excretion of the radiopharmaceutical occurs through the urine and feces
   B. Usually an animal can be discharged 24 to 72 hours after administration of radionuclide
   C. Depends on the each state's or province's safety and protection laws
X. Nuclear medicine images are usually of poor resolution, but provide unique information about specific organs

## Positron Emission Tomography (Figure 12-5)

I. PET images the body's basic biochemistry and function rather than imaging the body's anatomy and structure
II. Useful for detecting conditions affecting the brain and heart, as well as different types of cancer
III. Inverse beta decay of a radioactive tracer isotope is the source of the positrons used in PET
IV. Fluorodeoxyglucose (FDG) is most commonly used in the medical imaging modality
   A. The fluorine in the FDG molecule is chosen to be the positron-emitting radioactive tracer, fluorine-18, to produce $^{18}$F-FDG
   B. After FDG is injected into a patient, a PET scanner can form images of the distribution of FDG around the body
   C. $^{18}$F-FDG is a common tracer. This radioactive material is used as a "tag" when it is attached to other compounds that are familiar to the body, such as glucose, water, and ammonia

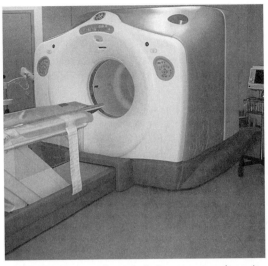

**Figure 12-5** A positron emission tomography unit.

D. Intravenous injection administered approximately 30 to 45 minutes before the imaging
   1. This gives the substance time to travel through the body, allowing it to be absorbed by the tissue that is to be examined
E. The patient is then placed on a reclining table that slides into the middle of an "open-air" scanner
   1. A collection of radiation detectors in the scanner locate and record the energy that the radioactivity in the body emits and sends the data to a computer, where three-dimensional color-coded images are produced
F. Imaging time is 25 to 35 minutes; general anesthesia is required
G. Length of stay is 2 days
H. Used to plan radiation/chemotherapy or surgery

## Computed Tomography

I. CT was originally known as computed axial tomography (CAT or CT scan)
II. One of most expensive diagnostic tests in veterinary medicine
III. Primarily for central and peripheral nervous system diseases
IV. Patient is placed on long movable table
V. Table then moves the patient through the circular gantry that contains the x-ray tube and detectors
VI. X-ray tube and detectors can be moved 360 degrees around the patient
VII. Single cross-sectional pictures or "tomographic slices" of data are obtained with every movement of the scanner
   A. Photons emerging from the patient are absorbed by the scanner
   B. Converted to electronic signals that vary in intensity depending on attenuation

C. Computer reconstructs information into a picture display

VIII. General anesthesia is required

IX. Offers some advantages over other x-ray techniques in diagnosing disease, because it clearly shows the shape and exact location of organs, soft tissues, and bones in any imaged "slice" of the body

X. Can distinguish between a simple cyst and a solid tumor and can aide in determining the stage (extent) of some types of cancer

XI. Used to plan radiation/chemotherapy or surgery

XII. Typical scan time is 30 to 40 minutes; general anesthesia is required

XIII. Length of stay is 2 to 3 hours

### PET/CT: $^{18}$F-FDG/X-Ray

I. A combination of both procedures listed previously

II. Once both studies are completed the images are fused together

III. The CT imaging is performed while waiting for the PET radionuclide to be absorbed by the target organ/region

IV. Total imaging time is approximately 1 hour; general anethesia is required

V. Length of stay is 2 days

### Magnetic Resonance Imaging

I. Similar to CT in that the image is a thin slice of cross-sectional anatomy
  A. Differs in that no ionizing radiation is used

II. Patient is placed in a magnetic field
  A. Signals are transmitted and received by the surrounding coils
    1. Uses a strong magnetic field, pulsed electromagnetic fields known as gradients, and radio waves to stimulate the protons and produce the image in the region of interest
  B. Extraordinary detail of the body or brain with exceptional sensitivity in soft tissue resolution
  C. Greater image resolution, differentiation of anatomy, and sensitivity to distinguish between tissue composition than CT
  D. Primarily used for head and spine evaluation
  E. The distribution of hydrogen nuclei (protons), found in cellular water, depends on the tissue type and whether the tissue is healthy or diseased
  F. Signal intensities provide the optimum difference between light and dark regions of the tissue or organ to help detect lesions, such as a tumor
  G. Does not use ionizing radiation
  H. Most scans take 1 hour; general anesthesia is required
  I. Length of stay is 2 to 4 hours

### Preparing Clients for These Procedures

I. Inform client that when an animal is going to have any radionuclide the animal must remain at the facility for a specified time, governed by
  A. United States Nuclear Regulatory Commission (USNRC)
  B. Canadian Nuclear Safety Commission (CNSC)

II. Determine from the facility what the home care requirements are, for the pet and its owner; all facilities should have a handout with instructions

III. Ensure that the facility has up-to-date records concerning the animal's condition

IV. When general anesthesia is performed, current blood work is mandatory

V. When an animal is being referred to a facility for iodine-131 treatment it is important to have current thyroid hormone ($T_4$) values, renal function assessment, and documentation of the doses of methimazole if the cat has been on this control medication, either long term or on a trial basis

### ACKNOWLEDGMENT

This chapter was reviewed by Connie Han and Cheryl Hurd.

# Glossary

**A-mode** Demonstrates returning ultrasound beam as peaks on a graph; the greater the intensity of the beam, the higher the peak

**acoustic impedance** Ability of tissue to hinder the transmission of sound

**amplitude** Intensity or loudness of an ultrasound wave

**anechoic** Waves are transmitted to deeper tissue; none are reflected back

**attenuation** Loss of intensity of the ultrasound beam as it travels through tissue, caused by absorption or scatter

**axial resolution** Ability of the ultrasound beam to identify separate structures

**B-mode** Uses bright dots or pixels on the screen to identify the intensity of ultrasound echoes; the position of the dot depicts the depth of the reflecting structure

**beta particles** High-energy electrons emitted by certain types of radioactive nuclei. The beta particles emitted are a form of ionizing radiation also known as beta rays

**beta decay** The production of beta particles

**beta ray** A particle ray consisting of a fast electron whose mass is nearly 1/2000 of the mass of a proton or neutron

**computed tomography (CT)** Mode of alternative imaging in which the patient moves through a circular gantry. Photons emerging from the patient are absorbed by the scanner and are converted to electronic signals that vary in intensity depending on attenuation

**cystic lesion** Has a well-defined border with no internal echoes and shows posterior enhancement

**diffuse** Subtle changes that can affect an entire organ

**Doppler shift** Change in perceived frequency of a sound wave due to relative motion between the source and listener or transducer and reflector

**echoic** Tissue that produces enough echoes when it is returned to the transducer and displayed

**focal changes** Readily identified lesions found in a specific area of an organ

**frequency** Number of cycles per unit of time

**gamma rays** Electromagnetic radiations that are of nuclear origin

**gantry** Term applied to a unit that houses the computed tomography x-ray tube and detectors

**half-life** The amount of time it takes for half of the atoms in a sample to decay

**hyperechoic** Tissue that reflects more sound back to the transducer than the surrounding tissues; appears bright

**hypoechoic** Tissue that reflects less sound back to the transducer than the surrounding tissue; appears dark

**isoechoic** Tissue that has the same ultrasonic appearance as that of the surrounding tissue

**lateral resolution** Ability of the ultrasound beam to identify separate structures that lie in a plane perpendicular to the sound beam

**linear scanner** Scanner that produces a rectangular image

**magnetic resonance imaging (MRI)** Type of alternative imaging in which the patient is placed in a magnetic field and radiofrequency signals are transmitted, received, and constructed into detailed cross-sectional images

**M-mode** Mode of ultrasound that displays a two-dimensional image over a timed baseline

**mixed lesion** Borders are irregular and contain cystic and solid areas

**nuclear medicine** A branch of medicine and medical imaging that uses unsealed radioactive substances in diagnosis and therapy

**nuclear scintigraphy** Type of noninvasive imaging procedure that uses radioactive material to obtain an image

**positron emission tomography (PET)** A diagnostic imaging technique used to generate pictures of the patient's biological functions, and the metabolic changes of the cells in the body. PET imaging differs from the more traditional diagnostic imaging techniques, because it images the body's basic biochemistry and function rather than imaging the body's anatomy and structure

**PET/CT** Imaging is accomplished through the integration of two technologies, radiolabeled biologically active compound (tracer) and computed tomography (CT)

**piezoelectric effect** Conversion of electrical energy to ultrasound

**radionuclide** Radioactive material

**sagittal** Transducer marker is held to the cranial or caudal end of the animal; provides a scan of the long axis of an organ

**sector scanner** Scanner that produces a pie-shaped image with a narrow near field and a wide far field

**solid** Contains many echoes spread throughout

**transducer** Part of the ultrasound machine that actually scans the patient, emits pulses of sound, and receives the returning echoes

**transverse** Transducer marker held 90 degrees to the longitudinal plane; provides short-axis view of organs

**ultrasound** Method of sending high-frequency sound waves into tissues and receiving the returning echoes as an image; a noninvasive diagnostic procedure

**velocity** Speed at which sound travels through an object

**wavelength** Length that a wave must travel in one cycle

# Review Questions

**1** A hyperechoic lesion appears
  a. Brighter than surrounding tissue
  b. Darker than surrounding tissue
  c. Dark with posterior enhancement
  d. Same as surrounding tissue

**2** *Piezoelectric* refers to
  a. Acoustic impedance
  b. Pressure electricity
  c. Bandwidth
  d. Time-gain compensation

**3** Bandwidth is best defined as
  a. Attenuation
  b. Half the range of frequency
  c. The entire range of frequency
  d. Image resolution

**4** A Doppler shift is best explained as a change in _____ as a result of motion
  a. Loudness of a perceived sound
  b. Perceived frequency
  c. Loudness of the sound source
  d. Acoustic impedance

**5** The type of transducer that images by transmitting beams in parallel lines is
  a. A broad bandwidth
  b. A phased array
  c. An annular array
  d. A linear array

**6** These extra image artifacts are common next to reflective surfaces
  a. Mirror
  b. Refraction
  c. Acoustic shadowing
  d. Acoustic enhancement

**7** Sound waves have difficulty traveling through
  a. Tissue
  b. Blood
  c. Fluid
  d. Bone

**8** Three-dimensional ultrasound provides
  a. Less visualization
  b. Enhanced visualization
  c. B-mode
  d. M-mode

**9** The normal adrenal glands on ultrasound are best described as
  a. Hyperechoic
  b. Cystic
  c. Hypoechoic
  d. Ceramic

**10** The number of cycles per second is the
   a. Wavelength
   b. Wave period
   c. Doppler shift
   d. Frequency

## BIBLIOGRAPHY

Advanced Veterinary Medical Imaging: Homepage, http://www.avmi.net/. Accessed June 12, 2007.

Centers for the Treatment of Feline Hyperthyroidism: Homepage, http://www.radiocat.com/. Accessed June 12, 2007.

Crump Institute for Molecular Imaging: Homepage, http://www.crump.ucla.edu/. Accessed July 11, 2007.

Department of Physics, University of Colorado at Boulder: *Halflife*, http://www.colorado.edu/physics/2000/isotopes/radioactive_decay3.html. Accessed June 12, 2007.

Han C, Hurd C: *Practical diagnostic imaging for the veterinary technician*, ed 3, St Louis, 2005, Mosby.

Kremkau FW: *Diagnostic ultrasound: principles and instruments*, ed 7, Philadelphia, 2006, Saunders.

Lavin L: *Radiography in veterinary technology*, ed 4, St Louis, 2006, Saunders.

*Let's play PET*, http://www.uib.no/med/avd/miapr/arvid/MOD3_2002/Bildedannelse/lets_play_PET.pdf. Accessed July 12, 2007.

Matheson Boulevard Veterinary Services: Homepage, http://www.mbvs.ca. Accessed June 12, 2007.

Nuclear Medicine Technology Resource Website: Homepage, http://www3.sympatico.ca/lgoodin/pet.htm. Accessed July 11, 2007.

Odwin C, Dubunsky T, Fleischer A: *Appleton and Lange's review for the ultrasonography exam*, ed 3, Norwalk, Conn, 2004, Appleton and Lange.

Partington BP: Diagnostic imaging. In McCurnin DM, Bassert JM, editors: *Clinical textbook for veterinary technicians*, ed 6, St Louis, 2006, Saunders.

Radiation Effects Research Foundation: *What is radiation?* http://www.rerf.or.jp/general/whatis_e/index.html. Accessed July 11, 2007.

Thames Valley Veterinary Services: Homepage, http://www.tvvs.ca. Accessed June 12, 2007.

WebMD: *Bone scan*, http://www.webmd.com/a-to-z-guides/Bone-Scan. Accessed June 12, 2007.

Wikipedia: *Nuclear medicine*, http://en.wikipedia.org/wiki/Nuclear_medicine. Accessed June 12, 2007.

Zagzebski JA: *Essentials of ultrasound physics*, St Louis, 1996, Mosby.

# PART III

# Patient Management and Nutrition

## CHAPTER 13

# Genetics, Theriogenology, and Neonatal Care

*Marianne Tear*    *Margi Sirois*

## OUTLINE

Genetics
  Basic Concepts of Genetics and
    Inheritance
  Predicting Phenotypes
  Inheritance Patterns
  X-Linked Dominant Inheritance
  Breeding Systems and
    Terminology
  Transgenic Animals
  Chromosomal Abnormalities
Theriogenology and Neonatal Care
  Feline
    Puberty
    Breeding Soundness
      Examination
    Semen Collection Techniques
      and Semen Characteristics
    Estrous Cycle
    Signs of Estrus
    Pregnancy Diagnosis
    Gestation/Stages of Parturition
    Causes of Dystocia
    Signs of Dystocia
    Neonatal Care
  Canine
    Puberty
    Breeding Soundness
      Examination
    Semen Collection Techniques
      and Semen Characteristics
    Estrous Cycle
    Signs of Estrus
    Pregnancy Diagnosis
    Gestation/Stages of
      Parturition
    Causes of Dystocia

  Signs of Dystocia
  Neonatal Care
Equine
  Puberty
  Breeding Soundness
    Examination
  Semen Collection Techniques
    and Semen Characteristics
  Estrous Cycle
  Signs of Estrus
  Pregnancy Diagnosis
  Gestation/Stages of Parturition
  Causes of Dystocia
  Signs of Dystocia
  Neonatal Care
Bovine
  Puberty
  Breeding Soundness
    Examination
  Semen Collection Techniques
    and Semen Characteristics
  Estrous Cycle
  Signs of Estrus
  Pregnancy Diagnosis
  Gestation/Stages of Parturition
  Causes of Dystocia
  Neonatal Care
Caprine
  Puberty
  Breeding Soundness
    Examination
  Semen Collection Techniques
    and Semen Characteristics
  Estrous Cycle
  Signs of Estrus
  Pregnancy Diagnosis

Gestation/Stages of Parturition
Causes of Dystocia
Signs of Dystocia
Neonatal Care
Ovine
  Puberty
  Breeding Soundness
    Examination
  Semen Collection Techniques
    and Semen Characteristics
  Estrous Cycle
  Signs of Estrus
  Pregnancy Diagnosis
  Gestation/Stages of Parturition
  Causes of Dystocia
  Signs of Dystocia
  Neonatal Care
Porcine
  Puberty
  Breeding Soundness
    Examination
  Semen Collection Techniques
    and Semen Characteristics
  Estrous Cycle
  Signs of Estrus
  Pregnancy Diagnosis
  Gestation/Stages of Parturition
  Causes of Dystocia
  Signs of Dystocia
  Neonatal Care

## LEARNING OUTCOMES

### After reading this chapter you should be able to:

1. Define common terms related to genetics and inheritance.
2. Use a Punnett square to predict genotypes and phenotypes.
3. Describe commonly used breeding systems.
4. Differentiate between autosomal and sex-linked inheritance patterns.
5. Differentiate between dominance, recessive, co-dominance, incomplete dominance, and epistasis.
6. Describe chromosomal abnormalities.
7. Define the basics of feline, canine, equine, bovine, caprine, ovine, and porcine reproductive characteristics.
8. Define the neonatal feline, canine, equine, bovine, caprine, ovine, and porcine nursing requirements.

This chapter contains the basics of genetics and animal breeding. Students often find genetics difficult. The difficulty could be due to the new terminology that novices must learn to understand the subject. The best suggestion when studying genetics is to approach the genetics parts of this chapter one step at a time and to understand the definitions before continuing on to the next section.

This chapter also briefly describes the reproductive cycles of small and large animals. It includes information on puberty onset, estrous cycles, breeding soundness examinations, semen collection techniques and characteristics, gestation/stages of parturition, pregnancy diagnosis, causes of dystocia, and neonatal care.

## GENETICS

### BASIC CONCEPTS OF GENETICS AND INHERITANCE

I. Genes are segments of the DNA chromosome that provide the code for specific proteins or regulate the expression of other genes
II. Alleles are the forms of a gene that may be present
   A. For most genetic traits, two alleles are possible
   B. For some traits, multiple alleles are possible (e.g., blood groups)
III. Genotype is the term that describes the alleles an organism possesses
IV. Phenotype describes the manifestation of the genotype, (e.g., outward appearance, behavioral characteristics, metabolism)

   A. Some phenotypes are influenced by multiple genes (e.g., behavior)
     1. This is termed polygenic inheritance
V. Higher organisms possess two alleles for most traits
   A. One gene is inherited from the male parent and one from the female parent
   B. The alleles in a gene pair code for the same type of gene
   C. The two alleles of the pair may differ in the phenotype produced
     1. When the two alleles are identical for a given gene, the organism is homozygous for that gene
     2. When the two alleles differ for a given gene, the organism is heterozygous for that gene
   D. Genes for given traits may interact in a number of ways
     1. Dominant genes are those that are always expressed when present
     2. Recessive genes are those that are expressed only when the organism is homozygous for the trait
     3. Some genes exhibit variability in expression
       a. Example: for polydactyly, an extra digit may occur on one or more appendages, and the digit can be full size or just a stub
       b. *Co-dominance* describes a gene pair that are both expressed with a blending of the phenotypes of the two alleles
         (1) Example: a cross between a red carnation and a white carnation produces a pink flower
       c. Epistatic genes are those that modify or prevent the expression of other genes
         (1) Example: the two alleles for Labrador Retriever coat color, brown and black, are both masked when the animal also has homozygous epistatic alleles on a second gene involved in pigment production in different tissues; this produces an animal with a yellow hair coat
       d. Incomplete dominance describes a pair of genes in which both are expressed with both phenotypes visible in the offspring
         (1) Example: A cross between a white chicken and a black chicken produces a chicken with both black and white feathers
   E. The offspring of any purebred parents are described as the first filial ($F_1$) generation

### PREDICTING PHENOTYPES

I. The Punnett square is a genotype diagram used to predict the genotypes of the offspring
   A. Traits are designated with letters; the same letter is used for all alleles of the trait

| Female parent gametes, B or b | Male parent gametes B or b: B | b |
|---|---|---|
| B | BB | Bb |
| b | bB | bb |

**Figure 13-1** Monohybrid cross: predicts the genotype and phenotype of the offspring of two individuals that differ in genotype for a single trait.

| Female parent gametes | Male parent gametes: BS | Bs | bS | bs |
|---|---|---|---|---|
| BS | BBSS | BBSs | BbSS | BbSs |
| Bs | BBSs | BBss | BbSs | Bbss |
| bS | BbSS | BbSs | bbSS | bbSs |
| bs | BbSs | Bbss | bbSs | bbss |

| Phenotype | Genotype(s) | Number of Offspring |
|---|---|---|
| Black short hair | BBSS, BBSs, BbSS, BbSs | 9 |
| Black long hair | BBss, Bbss | 3 |
| Brown short hair | bbSS, bbSs | 3 |
| Brown long hair | bbss | 1 |

**Figure 13-2** Dihybrid cross: predicts the offspring of two individuals that differ in genotype for two traits that are inherited independently.

B. A dominant allele is designated with an uppercase letter; the recessive allele is designated with the same letter in lower case
C. Co-dominant and incomplete dominant alleles are designated with superscripts ($^{i,\ c}$)

II. Monohybrid cross: predicts the genotype and phenotype of the offspring of two individuals that differ in genotype for a single trait
A. Often used to describe the offspring of two monohybrids
B. A monohybrid is the offspring of two parents that are homozygous for alternate forms of alleles for a gene
C. Example (Figure 13-1): in the Siberian Husky, brown eye color is dominant, blue is recessive
D. Heterozygous animals are designated with the genotype Bb
E. The $F_1$ offspring of two heterozygotes can have the genotypes BB, bb, and Bb
F. There is a probability that half (50%) of the offspring will be heterozygous, and half will be homozygous (either bb or BB)
G. There is a probability that 75% of the offspring will have brown eyes (BB and Bb genotypes), and 25% will have blue eyes (bb)

III. Dihybrid cross: predicts the offspring of two individuals that differ in genotype for two traits that are inherited independently
A. In guinea pigs, black hair (B) is dominant to brown (b), and short hair (S) is dominant to long hair (s)
B. If both parents are heterozygous for both traits (BbSs), the gametes that can be produced by each parent are BS, Bs, bS, and bs
C. Phenotypes of offspring produced are in the ratio of 9:3:3:1 (Figure 13-2)

## INHERITANCE PATTERNS

I. Inheritance patterns are described as autosomal dominant, autosomal recessive, sex-linked dominant, or sex-linked recessive, based on the location of the genes and the dominant or recessive nature of the alleles
A. Autosomal refers to all genes that are not located on the sex chromosomes (X and Y)
B. Sex chromosomes: X and Y
1. Females have the designation XX, meaning two X chromosomes
2. Males have the designation XY, meaning one X chromosome and one Y chromosome
C. Genes that are inherited on sex chromosomes are expressed differently in male and female individuals
1. When a male inherits an X-linked recessive allele, it is always expressed, because there is no corresponding allele (even though it is a "single dose")
2. Females must be homozygous for an X-linked recessive allele to express the trait
3. X-linked traits are usually passed from mothers to sons; fathers do not pass an X chromosome to their sons; thus only a Y chromosome is passed from father to son
4. Example: X-linked inheritance in cats
a. Tortoise-shell pattern in cats is an example of X-linked genetics
b. There are very few male tortoise-shell cats; nearly all are female
c. G symbolizes the ginger or orange coat color, which is carried on the X chromosome
d. Male cats have only one X chromosome, so their genotype can be only G (yellow) or g (nonyellow)

e. Female cats have two X chromosomes, so females can be three genotypes

f. GG (yellow), Gg (tortoise-shell), gg (nonyellow)

g. Tortoise-shell is heterozygous and has a unique coat color

h. Color variation is due to the influence of both the G and g genes in different parts of the animal at the same time

i. An important point to remember is that a male can transmit only one gene (G or g) in 50% of the gametes; the other 50% carry a Y chromosome that does not possess a G locus

## X-LINKED DOMINANT INHERITANCE ▬▬▬

I. Normal female will have two X-linked chromosomes; males have only one X-linked gene

II. Because the X chromosome of the male is always transmitted to his daughters, affected males will pass the trait to daughters but not to sons

III. Carrier females are heterozygous for a recessive X-linked gene and therefore will pass it on to 50% of their sons and 50% of their daughters (who will be normal but carriers)

   A. Example: color blindness in humans

IV. X-linked recessive

   A. Disease appears in males whose mothers are unaffected but are heterozygous carriers of the mutant recessive allele

   B. Each son of a carrier female has a 1:1 chance of being affected

   C. Affected male never transmits the gene to his sons; however, he will transmit it to all of his daughters, who will be carriers

   D. Unaffected males never transmit the gene

V. Autosomal dominant

   A. Dominant alleles will transmit disease from one affected individual to their offspring; there will be no skipping of generations unless penetrance is reduced

   B. There will be an approximately equal number of each sex affected with the disease

   C. Fifty percent of the progeny of each affected individual will be affected (because of Aa × aa matings)

   D. Dominant allele can be transmitted by the mother or father

VI. Autosomal recessive

   A. Parents and remote relatives of an affected individual will not be affected (often skips generations)

   B. In matings producing an affected offspring, approximately 25% of the progeny will be affected

   C. There should be an equal number of females and males with the defect or trait

   D. If both parents are affected, offspring will most likely be affected

## BREEDING SYSTEMS AND TERMINOLOGY ▬▬▬

I. Pedigree charts

   A. Diagrams used to track inheritance of specific traits in offspring

   B. Constructing a pedigree allows for identification of recessive allele carriers so that those individuals may be culled from the stock, depending on the trait in question

   C. A variety of configurations are used on pedigree charts to designate specific phenotypes

      1. A number in the symbol indicates the number of individuals

      2. Two symbols joined by a line indicate marriage or mating

      3. Figure 13-3 is an example of a pedigree chart that demonstrates an inheritance pattern for an autosomal recessive trait

II. Test cross: used to determine the genotype of a particular phenotype

   A. Usually the unknown phenotype is crossed with a homozygous recessive individual

      1. Example: black Doberman Pinscher phenotype of either BB or Bb

      2. Genotype B represents black color, and the genotype b represents brown color

      3. Cross will be B_ × bb (a homozygous recessive individual)

      4. If the dog is Bb, the cross will produce 50% bb (brown Dobermans) and 50% Bb (black Dobermans)

      5. If the dog is BB, all of the offspring will be black, or Bb

   B. Backcross: the pairing of an $F_1$ generation hybrid with an organism whose genotype is identical to the parental strain

III. Outbreeding or random breeding

   A. This type of breeding is considered to keep the gene pool as large as possible; mating to other strains maintains an increasing number of heterozygous individuals

   B. This type of breeding keeps all fitness traits, such as resistance to disease, at high levels

   C. In general, this type of breeding is between two animals that are unrelated

IV. Assortative mating is the mating of individuals that are phenotypically similar

   A. Differs from random mating since the individuals are chosen for specific phenotypic characteristics

V. Inbreeding: breeding of closely related individuals to produce ever-increasing similarities in the offspring

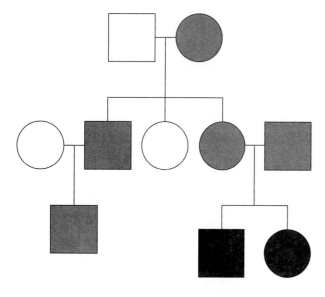

| Male Unaffected | Male Carrier | Male Affected |
|---|---|---|
|  |  |  |
| Female Unaffected | Female Carrier | Female Affected |
|  |  |  |

**Figure 13-3** Pedigree chart.

A. A minimum of 20 or more consecutive brother and sister matings will produce an inbred strain

B. This breeding system is designed to reduce heterozygosity

C. Advantages: the breeding will be "true," and it is possible to fix mutant alleles into a line or strain of animals

D. Disadvantage: recessive alleles may be revealed, such as lethal genes

E. Inbreeding depression: relates to traits of fitness, such as early growth, resistance to disease, or fertility, which are all multifunctional traits

   1. If an individual becomes homozygous, inbreeding depression occurs

   2. To reduce inbreeding depression

     a. Inbreed slowly and be stringent in selection of mating

     b. Do not breed poor phenotypes

   3. If inbreeding depression occurs

     a. Introduce a new sire or male with as many desirable traits as possible

     b. Outcross within your population to minimize inbreeding

     c. Always select healthy animals with good reproductive ability

VI. Heterosis or hybrid vigor

A. An $F_1$ generation is produced by crossing two different inbred strains

B. Heterosis usually results in size increase and weight gain; reproductive ability and resistance to disease are also increased

C. Two individuals from the $F_1$ generation cannot be bred, because this breeding will produce variables in the phenotype

VII. Line breeding: a system of inbreeding of closely related individuals to guarantee similar traits in the offspring

A. Designed to increase the occurrence of genes from one or several exceptional ancestors (i.e., ones with the most desirable traits)

B. This exceptional ancestor may end up as grandfather and great-grandfather in the same pedigree

VIII. Harem mating: a mating in which one male is mated to five females

A. Generally used in some lab animal colonies

B. Intensive system, the male(s) remains with the female(s) continuously.

   1. Several males may be housed with many females

   2. This system also results in somewhat higher stress to females, because they are nearly continuously pregnant or nursing

C. In a nonintensive system, the male(s) and female(s) are housed separately while the female is pregnant

## TRANSGENIC ANIMALS

I. A transgenic strain alters the genetic makeup of a developing embryo by transplanting a specific DNA strand into the morula or by exposing the embryo to mutating factors.

A. DNA may be from another species that has a desirable trait or may be modified from the same species

II. The first generation of a transgenic breeding is referred to as $F_0$. These animals are called the founder animals of the strain

III. Transgenic strains are useful in basic research, because the alterations to the animals' genotypes facilitate specific experimentation

A. Functions absent in a recipient as a result of a bad gene can be corrected by adding it to a vector, which inserts itself into the chromosomes of the recipient, thereby creating a transgenic animal that has been cured through genetics

B. Transgenic plants, fungi, and animals are being used for research because of the added scope that this approach gives to the development of profitable genotypes

## CHROMOSOMAL ABNORMALITIES ▬▬▬

I. Definitions
  A. Mutation: any change in the DNA sequence of a gene
  B. Genetic mutation: any change in the DNA sequence of a gene contained in a gamete
  C. Translocation: the breakage of two chromosomes, resulting in repair in an abnormal arrangement
  D. Deletion: a part or all of a chromosome is missing
  E. Duplication: an allele is duplicated; for example, human trisomy 21 or Down's syndrome—there are three chromosomes rather than two at location 21 in the karyotype
  F. Anomalies: deviations from normal
    1. There are many examples of anomalies in small animal breeding
    2. Many are inherited with multiple genes and also affected by environmental factors
    3. Examples: malocclusions, hip dysplasia, Collie eye, Perthes' disease, hemophilia, diabetes mellitus, microphthalmia, deafness, entropion, and dwarfism
  G. Lethal genes
    1. Definition: a gene that will cause the death of the embryo or serious impairment or death sometime after birth (sometimes called a delayed lethal)
    2. Semilethal gene causes the individual to have abnormal traits
    3. Lethal gene is expressed as a homozygous recessive, usually in the $F_2$ generation
    4. Genotype will be in the ratio of 1:2 instead of 1:2:1 (one individual will die)
    5. Dominant lethal gene is usually expressed only once and cannot be proved to be inherited genetically
    6. However, there are some dominant disorders in which the individual is only impaired and is still able to reproduce
      a. Example: achondroplasia (dwarfism)
    7. Most lethal genes are recessive
    8. An incomplete dominance lethal gene: homozygous dominant individuals will die, but heterozygous individuals will show clinical signs, such as the Manx cat and many human lethal genes
      a. Example: Manx cat
        (1) MM (lethal), Mn (tailless or Manx), mm (normal tail)
        (2) Resulting ratio of the cross Mm×Mm is 25% of the kittens will die (MM), 50% will be the genotype Manx (Mm), and 25% will have genotype normal tail (mm)

## THERIOGENOLOGY AND NEONATAL CARE ▬▬

### FELINE ▬▬▬

### Puberty

I. Queen
  A. Average age, 7 to 12 months
  B. Long-haired cats reach puberty later than short-haired breeds
II. Tom
  A. Sexual maturity about 9 months
  B. Vascular penis (os penis) with spines
  C. Accessory sex glands
    1. Prostate
    2. Bulbourethral gland (Cowper's gland)

### Breeding Soundness Examination

I. Examination of the male
  A. Scrotum and testes
    1. Testes should be symmetrical bilaterally in size and shape, and be firm and smooth
    2. Orchitis can be caused by traumatic injuries or can occur secondary to various viruses or bacteria
    3. Cryptorchidism is not common but may be inherited
    4. Testicular tumors are not common
  B. Penis and prepuce
    1. Major concerns are trauma and feline lower urinary tract disease (FLUTD)
      a. FLUTD can cause penile trauma owing to the obstructive process, licking, and the relieving of the blockage
    2. Mating without penetration may be owing to the accumulation of hair around the glans penis
      a. This can be removed by sliding the hair ring over the glans after retracting the sheath
  C. Semen evaluation
    1. The semen can be collected and evaluated

### Semen Collection Techniques and Semen Characteristics

I. Semen collection
  A. Artificial vagina (AV)
    1. An estimated 20% of tomcats can be trained to use an AV
  B. Electroejaculation
    1. Not commonly used
    2. Teflon rectal probe has been used to collect from tomcats that are under total anesthesia

C. Natural breeding
   1. After natural breeding has occurred, a moistened cotton swab can be placed into the vaginal vault, rolled onto a slide, and examined for sperm
II. Semen characteristics
   A. Volume: 0.03 to 0.09 mL
   B. Concentration: 50 to 60 million/mL
   C. Motility: 80% progressively motile

## Estrous Cycle

I. Seasonally polyestrous, dependent on ovulation occurring
   A. First estrous cycle is usually around 9 months
II. Estrous periods may last 8 to 10 days
III. Ovulation is not spontaneous; it is induced or occurs by reflex after coitus
   A. Ovulation occurs only when a cat is mated or the cervix is stimulated by an instrument, such as a glass rod, cotton swab, or thermometer
IV. Optimal breeding occurs after the third day of estrus. At least three breedings should take place, approximately two hours apart
V. Ovulation can be induced by treatment with hormones, such as human chorionic gonadotropin (hCG), luteinizing hormone (LH), or gonadotropin-releasing hormone (GnRH)

## Signs of Estrus

I. Vocalization
II. Crouching and rolling on the floor; called lordosis
III. Tail deflection

## Pregnancy Diagnosis

I. Abdominal palpation, 15 to 30 days postbreeding
II. Ultrasound
   A. 11 to 16 days: gestational sacs
   B. 16 to 32 days: fetal heartbeats
III. Radiographs as early as 43 days gestation
   A. The only reliable method to determine the size, number and position of kittens in utero

## Gestation/Stages of Parturition

I. Gestation: approximately 63 days
II. Zonary placentation
III. Mammary gland develops during the last week
IV. In the last few days of gestation, milk can usually be expressed from the nipples
V. Stages of parturition (queening)
   A. Stage 1
      1. Restlessness
      2. Vocalization
      3. Nesting behavior can be obvious for up to 48 hours before queening
   B. Stage 2
      1. Few obvious contractions and loud vocalizing by the queen may signal the birth of the first kitten
         a. This may take up to 60 minutes
      2. Between kittens, the queen will remove and eat any placental tissue, sever the umbilical cord, clean the kittens and her vulvar area
      3. Some queens may nurse newborns while continuing with parturition
   C. Stage 3
      1. Placenta is usually expelled after the delivery of each kitten
         a. It is possible for two placentas to be passed after the birth of two kittens
      2. It is uncommon, but parturition may take up to several days
         a. This is not considered abnormal but must be differentiated from dystocia

## Causes of Dystocia

I. Rare
II. Fetal dystocia
   A. May be due to abnormal positioning
   B. Fetal oversize
   C. Fetal deformities
III. Maternal dystocia
   A. May be due to a congenitally small pelvis
   B. Queen may have previously fractured her pelvis
   C. Torsion of the uterus, a single horn, or a portion of a horn
   D. Inguinal hernia
   E. Uterine inertia

## Signs of Dystocia

I. 20 minutes of intense labor with no kitten produced
II. 10 minutes of intense labor with a kitten visible, but not completely expelled
III. Parturition lasting longer than 36 hours

## Neonatal Care

I. Temperature, 38° to 39° C (100° to 102° F); pulse, 140 to 170 beats per minute; respiration, 30 to 50 breaths per minute
II. Tomcats should be kept away from kittens
III. Hand-fed kittens should be fed 15% to 20% of their body weight, divided into three daily feedings
IV. Kittens are unable to thermoregulate for the first 6 days
V. Kittens consume between 5 and 7 mL of milk per feeding by the second week of life and will have doubled their birth weight
VI. Eyes open at 8 to 10 days of age
VII. After each feeding the queen cleans and grooms each kitten. She also stimulates them (by licking) to

urinate and defecate; she then consumes the urine and feces

VIII. By 3 weeks of age, the activity level of the litter has increased, and they are now urinating and defecating some distance from their nest

IX. Solid food is supplemented in the diet by the fourth week

X. Kittens are weaned between 5 and 8 weeks of age

## CANINE

### Puberty

I. Bitch
  A. Average 8 months
  B. Puberty varies by breed and size from 6 to 18 months of age
  C. Smaller breeds reach puberty earlier than larger breeds
  D. Bitch should not be bred during her first estrus; she may be sexually mature but not yet anatomically mature

II. Stud
  A. Approximately 9 months
  B. Vascular penis (os penis)
  C. Accessory sex glands; prostate gland

### Breeding Soundness Examination

I. History
  A. Complete medical history of all organ systems must be obtained before breeding, because infections and neoplasias of other organ systems (e.g., urinary tract) may cause secondary problems
  B. Alteration of secretory patterns of hormones, such as testosterone, follicle-stimulating hormone (FSH), LH, and GnRH, may affect the ability of the male to breed
  C. Administration of drugs (e.g., corticosteroids, cimetidine), stress, trauma, or a history of systemic illness can all affect the overall function of the reproductive tract
  D. All dogs in an active breeding program should be checked for *Brucella canis*
    1. Sexually transmitted disease that can cause abortion, fetal resorption, and infertility
    2. There is no cure. Any infected animal should be removed from breeding pool

II. Examination of the bitch
  A. Vulva
    1. Size and conformity should be evaluated
    2. Discharge, if present, should be evaluated
  B. Vagina
    1. Vagina should be examined for masses, foreign bodies, or inflammation
    2. Vaginal cytology

  C. Mammary glands
    1. Palpate for masses, inverted nipples, or mastitis
  D. Rectal palpation
    1. Injuries or other abnormalities can affect the size of the pelvic canal and prevent pups from passing

III. Examination of the stud
  A. Scrotum
    1. Normal scrotum should be lightly covered with hair, be smooth and soft to the touch, have freely moving skin over the testes, be pain free, and be of consistent thickness
    2. Look for signs of inflammation, trauma, or swelling
  B. Testes
    1. Testes should be palpated for size, shape, and consistency, with the left testicle sitting caudal to the right
    2. Presence of an irregular surface, nodules, or scrotal adhesions may suggest chronic inflammation, infection, or neoplasia
    3. Soft, spongy testes may suggest testicular degeneration, and hard testes may indicate neoplasia or acute orchitis
  C. Epididymis and spermatic cord
    1. Should be palpated for areas of thickening, enlargement, epididymitis, adenomyosis of the epididymis, or an inguinal hernia
  D. Penis and prepuce
    1. Discharge of blood, pus, or urine from the prepuce may be a cause for concern
    2. Penis should be freely movable within the prepuce and can be easily revealed by retracting the prepuce caudal over the bulbus glandis
    3. Penis should be examined for the presence of infection, trauma, foreign bodies, and masses
      a. The mucosa of the penis should be pink, white, and smooth
    4. Os penis should be palpated for congenital deformities and fractures
  E. Prostate gland
    1. Only accessory gland in the dog
    2. Palpate for abnormal size, asymmetry between lobes, and abnormal consistency
  F. Semen evaluation
    1. The semen can be collected and evaluated

### Semen Collection Techniques and Semen Characteristics

I. Semen collection
  A. Teaser bitch
    1. It is easiest to collect semen from a male by allowing him to mount a teaser bitch
    2. Once the male has mounted the female, the penis can be deviated into a collection device or an AV

B. Masturbation
1. Semen can be collected using this technique if there is no teaser bitch
C. Electroejaculation
1. Not commonly used
2. Male must be anesthetized

II. Semen characteristics
A. Volume: total volume about 20 mL, but may vary from as little as 2 mL to 60 mL
B. Concentration of sperm: 10 to 300 million/ejaculate
C. Motility: 60% to 90% motile sperm
D. Intrauterine lifespan is approximately 6 to 7 days

## Estrous Cycle

I. Nonseasonal
A. No true estrous cycle
B. Estrus occurs twice per year
C. Long periods of anestrus
II. Phases of estrous cycle
A. Proestrus: usually lasts 9 to 10 days
1. Hemorrhagic vulvar discharge
2. Vulva is swollen
3. Male will be attracted, but bitch will not allow mating
4. Noncornified squamous epithelial cells predominate in vaginal mucosa
B. Estrus: usually lasts about 9 days
1. Receptive to the male
2. Usually ovulates 24 to 48 hours after the LH surge
3. Clear serous discharge
4. Cornified squamous epithelial cells in vaginal mucosa
C. Diestrus: period following mating
1. Whelping can be predicted from day 1 of diestrus
2. Abrupt decrease in the number of cornified epithelial cells
D. Metestrus average 90 days
1. Occurs in unmated bitches
2. By approximately the tenth day after estrus, all epithelial cells in the vaginal mucosa are noncornified
3. No longer receptive to the male
E. Anestrus: sexual inactivity between cycles
1. Very difficult to differentiate between anestrus and metestrus cytologically
III. Ovulation occurs 2 to 4 days after onset of estrus

## Signs of Estrus

I. Slight swelling of the vulva lips
II. Clear serous discharge
III. Cornified squamous epithelial cells on vaginal cytology
IV. Receptive to the male

## Pregnancy Diagnosis

I. Abdominal palpation: 3 to 4 weeks postbreeding
II. Ultrasound: 24 to 28 days postbreeding
III. Transabdominal ultrasound: 24 to 28 days postbreeding
IV. Hormone assays (relaxin): 28 to 30 days postovulation
V. Lateral abdominal radiographs: as early as 43 days gestation
A. The only reliable method to determine size, number, and position of pups in utero
1. Fetal skeletal elements are present 21 to 42 days postbreeding
VI. Pseudopregnancy is common in the bitch

## Gestation/Stages of Parturition

I. Average gestation: 63 days
II. Zonary placentation
III. Drop in body temperature to less than 37° C (98.6° F) when parturition is imminent
IV. At 12 to 24 hours before whelping, milk can normally be expressed
V. Produce colostrum for up to 3 days postparturition
VI. Stages of parturition (whelping)
A. Stage 1: average 6 to 12 hours; can last 36 hours
1. Starts at the onset of uterine contractions and finishes when the cervix is completely dilated
2. Restlessness, with nesting behavior
3. Nervous anorexia
4. May vomit occasionally
5. Decrease in body temperature (other animals have elevated body temperatures)
B. Stage 2: averages 20 to 60 minutes per pup
1. Starts with full dilation of cervix and ends with the expulsion of the fetus
2. Total delivery period may last from a few hours to 24 to 36 hours. It should take no longer than 2 hours between the delivery of each pup
3. When each pup is passed, the chorioallantoic membrane ruptures, or the bitch removes the membrane by chewing or licking it away
4. Bitch must also remove the amniotic membrane, which the pup is more likely to still have at birth
C. Stage 3
1. Begins with the expulsion of the pup and is completed by the passing of the placenta
2. Placenta is usually passed 5 to 15 minutes after the birth of the pup
D. Dark green discharge during the first 12 to 24 hours after parturition

VII. Average litter size: 4 to 10
   A. Smaller breeds: 1 to 4
   B. Larger breeds: 8 to 12

## Causes of Dystocia

I. Uterus
   A. This may include uterine weakness if there is lack of uterine force to propel the fetus through the birth canal
      1. Primary uterine inertia
      2. Secondary uterine inertia
      3. Miscellaneous causes
         a. A nervous or frightened bitch may actually interfere with whelping
II. Pelvis
   A. Birth canal may be too small
      1. May be a congenital problem where the pelvis is too small
      2. May be acquired, such as a pelvic fracture
III. Fetus
   A. Fetal oversize
      1. Most likely cause is a single fetus
   B. Abnormal fetal presentation
      1. Causes can be a head-first presentation with the legs back, presentation of a single leg, and flexion of the head back along the body
      2. Breech presentation is not abnormal. It does not predispose the bitch to dystocia
   C. Vaginal vault
      1. A puppy wedged in the vaginal vault, owing to fetal oversize or a small pelvis, may be the problem
      2. Vault may be too small because of a vaginal stricture

## Signs of Dystocia

I. Strong contractions for 30 minutes with no pup produced
II. Infrequent contractions for approximately 2 hours with no pup produced
III. Extend period of time between pups

## Neonatal Care

I. Temperature, 38° to 39° C (100° to 102° F); pulse, 120 to 150 beats per minute; respiration, 25 to 50 breaths per minute
II. Should be suckling by 3 hours after whelping to receive optimum amounts of colostrum
III. Pups can be hand-fed three times a day
IV. Newborns can take 10 to 20 mL/feeding, depending on the breed
V. Puppies are unable to thermoregulate for the first 6 days
VI. Eyes open between 5 and 14 days of age, and the external ear canals open 1 to 2 days later

VII. Puppies should gain 2 to 4 g/day/kg of expected adult weight
VIII. After each feeding, the bitch stimulates the puppies to urinate and defecate and cleans each puppy
IX. By 18 days of age, the puppies are moving around and exploring their environment
X. Should be encouraged to consume solid food by 3 to 4 weeks of age
XI. Weaning is at 6 to 8 weeks of age

# EQUINE

## Puberty

I. Mare
   A. Approximately 12 months
   B. Low energy intake may delay puberty
II. Stallion
   A. Seldom used for breeding before 2 years of age
   B. Approximately 12 to 18 months
   C. Libido decreases during winter months
   D. Vascular penis
   E. Accessory sex glands
      1. Seminal vesicles
      2. Prostate
      3. Bulbourethral gland (Cowper's gland)

## Breeding Soundness Examination

I. Conducted mainly to evaluate infertility
   A. Require a complete health history and any drug therapy received during the previous 2 months
II. Examination of the mare
   A. Examination of the external genitalia
      1. Confirmation of the vulva; perineum and anus should be evaluated
      2. Vulvar discharge should be noted
   B. Examination of the internal genitalia
      1. Ovaries, uterus, and cervix should be evaluated
III. Examination of the stallion
   A. Observe stallion in a small corral or pasture to detect any musculoskeletal or other physical problems that may exist
      1. Chronic degenerative joint problems
      2. Chronic laminitis
      3. Back disorders
   B. Penis
      1. Avoid the use of promazine tranquilizer because of risk of penile paralysis
      2. Examine distal portion of penis for trauma or neoplasia (squamous cell carcinoma)
      3. Scarring or injuries may occur farther up the penis but are not common
      4. Swabs can be taken of the penis and prepuce if there is a chance of bacterial infection
   C. Scrotum, testicles, and epididymis
      1. Easily performed postbreeding
      2. Scrotum is rarely affected by disease

3. Note any abnormalities in size, consistency, and symmetry in the testicles and epididymis
   a. It is common for one testicle to be slightly smaller than the other
4. Scrotal circumference is correlated with fertility

D. Accessory sex glands (vesicular and bulbourethral glands, prostate)
   1. There have been few reported pathological changes involving these glands
   2. Can be palpated rectally but may be difficult to locate

E. Stallion's libido, manners, ease of ejaculation, and ability to service the mare should also be taken into consideration

F. Semen evaluation
   1. Semen can be collected and evaluated
      a. Equine viral arteritis (EVA) causes abortions and can be diagnosed on semen evaluation

## Semen Collection Techniques and Semen Characteristics

I. Semen collection
   A. Artificial vagina (AV) and phantom mare
      1. Preferred technique
      2. Most commonly used
   B. Condoms, vaginal collection, and dismount sample
      1. Dismount sample can be collected from the urethra and used, but contamination is common from the vagina and penis and may reduce mobility
         a. The advantage of these techniques is that samples may be collected routinely, preserved, and monitored during breeding season
         b. Samples may be contaminated by bacteria or debris

II. Semen characteristics
   A. Volume: gel free, volumes vary from 20 to 250 mL/ejaculate
   B. Concentration of sperm: 30 to 800 million/mL; average 120 million/mL
   C. Motility: at least 60% progressively motile sperm is desirable

## Estrous Cycle

I. Generally seasonally polyestrous
   A. Cyclic activity from spring to autumn
   B. Estrous activity can be induced by increasing the exposure to light (natural or artificial)

II. Estrous cycle is usually 20 to 33 days, with estrus being 5 to 6 days

III. Estrous cycle is divided into two phases
   A. Follicular phase (estrus): 5 to 6 days
   B. Luteal phase (diestrus): about 14 to 16 days

IV. Most ovulate 1 to 2 days before the end of estrus

V. Approximately 9 days after foaling, mares will have a fertile heat, also called foal heat

## Signs of Estrus

I. Squatting, vulvar winking, raising tail, and urination

II. Usually show signs only in presence of a stallion

## Pregnancy Diagnosis

I. Failure to return to estrus (nonspecific indicator)
   A. A nonpregnant mare should return to estrus 16 to 20 days after ovulation

II. Rectal palpation

III. Transrectal ultrasound: as early as 14 days after breeding
   A. Embryonic vesicle visible as early as 10 to 12 days gestation
      1. 99% accurate by day 15

IV. Progesterone assay: 18 to 21 days postbreeding (nonspecific indicator)
   A. Increased levels indicate presence of the corpus luteum
   B. False positives can result from a persistent corpus luteum or early embryonic death

V. Estrone sulfate: after 80 days postbreeding

VI. Equine chorionic gonadotropin: between 35 to 120 days gestation

## Gestation/Stages of Parturition

I. Gestation: approximately 336 days (11 months)

II. Diffuse and microcotyledonary placentation

III. Corpus luteum maintains pregnancy for 90 to 100 days, then the placenta produces progesterone

IV. Waxing of teats and possible discharge of milk 1 to 4 days before foaling

V. Stages of parturition (foaling)
   A. Stage 1: 30 minutes to 4 hours
      1. Pacing in stall
      2. Abdominal discomfort
      3. Sweating
      4. Pawing
      5. During this stage, the final positioning and posturing of the foal occur
      6. End of stage 1 is indicated by the rupture of the chorioallantoic membrane and the escape of the allantoic fluid
   B. Stage 2: explosive and short in duration (20 to 30 minutes)
      1. Signs are more obvious
      2. May sit up and lay down many times and is generally sweating
      3. When lying down, the legs may be extended and the head may be stretched outward from the rest of the body

4. May urinate/defecate because of the pressure from the contracting uterus, and may roll to try to lessen the pain and/or position the fetus
5. Cervix is completely dilated
6. Stage 2 takes about 20 minutes, from when the chorioallantoic membranes rupture to the delivery of the fetus

C. Stage 3
1. Begins with the foaling and ends with the expulsion of the placenta. This should occur within 3 hours
2. Mare should be allowed to lie quietly for the first hour after parturition

VI. Single births are the most common

## Causes of Dystocia

I. Not common in mares; less than 1% of equine parturition
II. Fetal causes are the most common
A. Primary cause is postural abnormalities because of the fetus's long legs
B. Positional and presentation abnormalities may also occur, but to a lesser degree
III. Round shape of the mare's pelvis, compared with that of a cow, decreases dystocia due to large fetuses
IV. Uncommon causes of fetal dystocia are fetal anasarca, ascites, fetal tumor, hydrocephalic fetus, fetal monster, and mummified fetus
V. Maternal causes of dystocia may be uterine torsion, small pelvis, uterine inertia, immaturity, constriction of the vagina or cervix, and other causes unrelated to the fetus

## Signs of Dystocia

I. If either the first or second stage of parturition is prolonged or not progressive, dystocia is possible
II. The appearance of a red membrane (the chorioallantois) protruding from the vulva is an indication of premature placental separation called red bag
A. This is an emergency situation
1. The chorioallantois must be manually ruptured
2. Delivery must be assisted or the foal will die

## Neonatal Care

I. Foal should be standing and suckling within 3 hours
II. If not suckling by 4 to 5 hours, 250 to 500 mL of colostrum should be administered
III. Physical examination of the foal
IV. Navel should be dipped with 0.5% chlorhexidine diacetate and repeated in 4 to 6 hours
V. Blood sample should be taken at 18 to 24 hours of age to measure IgG level, to make sure there is sufficient immunoglobulin absorption, and treated appropriately by intravenous plasma transfusion

VI. Temperature, 37.5° to 38.5° C (99.5° to 101° F); pulse, 80 to 120 beats per minute; respiration, 14 to 15 breaths per minute
VII. If there are some signs of sepsis, blood cultures should be aseptically collected, and appropriate antibiotic treatment should be started
VIII. Foals will nurse from the mare every 30 to 40 minutes
A. Failure to do so may indicate disease in the foal
B. Healthy foals should gain 1.0 to 2.5 kg/day or 2.2 to 5 lb/day
IX. Foals are susceptible to a variety of problems
A. Constipation due to meconium impaction, abnormal intestinal distention as a result of enterocolitis
B. Ruptured urinary bladder, causing uroperitoneum
C. Profound anemia due to neonatal isoerythrolysis
D. As a result of being premature, they may develop pulmonary insufficiency
E. They are also susceptible to gastric ulcers when placed under stressful conditions

## BOVINE

### Puberty

I. Heifer
A. Approximately 9 to 10 months
B. Age of puberty is directly related to body weight
1. Smaller breeds reach puberty earlier than larger breeds
C. Breed heifer at 15 months of age or 1000 lb (450 kg) of body weight
D. A female is not called a cow until she gives birth to her first calf, at approximately 2 years of age
II. Bull
A. Scrotal circumference is correlated with fertility
B. Accessory sex glands
1. Seminal vesicles
2. Prostate
3. Bulbourethral gland (Cowper's gland)

### Breeding Soundness Examination

I. Breeding capacity test
A. Measure breeding capacity under natural field conditions using ink chin-ball markers and/or constant observation
II. Locomotor abnormalities
A. Any physical abnormality that prevents or limits breeding
1. On the feet, look for corns, hoof cracks, evidence of founder, overgrown hooves, and arthritis
2. Look at structural faults, such as sickle hocks, postlegged conditions, narrow chests, and weak pasterns

a. These faults will make mounting and locomotion more difficult, therefore decreasing breeding capacity

3. Injuries, such as back injuries, sprains, spavins, bruises, and dislocated hips may also affect locomotion and breeding capacity

III. Reproductive abnormalities

A. Penis and prepuce

1. Reproductive organs, such as the penis and prepuce, may be examined by electroejaculation, which will cause the penis to extend, thus allowing a complete external examination

2. Possible penile defects may include hair rings, attached frenulum, lacerations, growths, enlarged glans, scar tissue, deviations, coiled penis, and urethral fistulas

B. Scrotum and testicles

1. Scrotal circumference should be measured because it is related to paired testes weight, and this in turn is related to daily sperm production and semen quality traits

2. With minimal restraint, examine the scrotum for testicular defects

3. Look for testicular firmness, uniform size and shape, lumps, cysts, scar tissue, and excessive heat

4. Epididymis tails can be palpated and should feel full but not swollen and hard

C. Libido

1. Bulls with a high libido are aggressive breeders and are physically fit for high breeding capacity

a. These bulls are considered the dominant breeders

2. Sometimes bulls with a particularly high libido may attempt to breed even after their ability to produce viable sperm is exhausted

3. Bulls with low libido will breed less frequently, are less socially aggressive, and therefore are less likely to become the dominant breeder

IV. Semen evaluation

A. Semen can be collected and evaluated

V. Bull to cow/heifer ratio

A. Length of breeding season, climate, access to feed, and terrain may all affect the conception rates

B. Bulls are expected to breed 25 to 30 cows/heifers over a 60- to 90-day breeding period

VI. Q fever: causes abortions

A. Causative agent: *Coxiella burnetii*

1. Rickettsial organism

B. Clinical signs include later term abortion

C. Zoonotic potential

1. Contact with aborted material, vaginal discharge, and mucous membranes of infected animals

2. Ingesting infected milk

D. Animals suspected of carrying disease should be culled

1. Effects on livestock may be subclinical

2. Diagnosis is based on placental findings, serology, and isolation of the organism

## Semen Collection Techniques and Semen Characteristics

I. Semen collection

A. Electroejaculation

B. Massage

1. Quiet, sexually rested bulls are best candidates

2. This technique may be used if there is an injury of the back, feet, or legs

C. Artificial vagina (AV)

1. Performed almost exclusively at artificial insemination (AI) centers

2. Bulls must be halter broken and nose-ring trained

3. May require a female in estrus to be successful

II. Semen characteristics

A. Volume: 2 to 15 mL

B. Concentration: 300 to 2500 million spermatozoa/mL

C. Motility: rapid vigorous wave motion

## Estrous Cycle

I. Nonseasonal, polyestrous 7 to 18 months

II. 21-Day estrous cycle

III. Estrus: 18 to 24 hours

IV. Ovulates: 12 to 18 hours after the end of estrus, unlike other farm animals, which ovulate during estrus

V. Breeding should occur approximately 12 hours after the first signs of estrus or standing heat

VI. Metestral bleeding occurs about 24 hours after ovulation

## Signs of Estrus

I. Stands still while being mounted by other cows

A. Best indicator for time to breed

II. Trying to mount other cows

III. Bawling

IV. Clear mucus discharge from the vulva (bull stringing)

V. Nervousness

VI. Frequent urination

## Pregnancy Diagnosis

I. Rectal palpation: 30 to 40 days postbreeding

II. Rectal ultrasound: after 24 days postbreeding

III. Abdominal ballottement: after 5 months postbreeding

## Gestation/Stages of Parturition

I. Gestation: 278 days (9 months)

II. Cotyledonary placentation: a combination of maternal caruncles and fetal cotyledons

III. A clear mucous discharge from the vulva can be seen 4 to 5 days before calving

IV. Vulva enlarges the last week of gestation, and sacrosciatic ligaments relax and cause the gluteal muscles to sink

V. Stages of parturition (calving)

  A. Stage 1

    1. Will last from 6 to 24 hours in heifers

    2. Various signs, such as anorexia, restlessness, shifting of weight, and an arched back with an extended tail

    3. If able, most dams will separate themselves from the herd

    4. There may be some minor abdominal straining during the latter portion of stage 1, thus making the change from stage 1 to stage 2 unclear

    5. The end of this stage is marked by the rupture of the chorioallantois and the expulsion of the allantoic fluid

  B. Stage 2

    1. Average length of this stage is 2 to 4 hours in pluriparous cows, and longer in heifers because of the greater effort required to dilate the birth canal tissues

    2. Oxytocin stimulates myometrial contraction, which forces the calf into the cervical canal and stretches the tissues

    3. Appearance of an intact amnion as a fluid-filled sac will usually rupture while the dam is recumbent

      a. This will bring on more forceful and frequent abdominal contractions

    4. When the contractions become more forceful, the dam will roll to lateral recumbency to deliver the calf

      a. Pluriparous dams may deliver their calves while standing, but most deliver while lateral

    5. Much force is required to deliver the calf's head through the vulva

      a. The remainder of the calving should require very little effort

  C. Stage 3

    1. Detachment and expulsion of the placenta

    2. Can occur from a few minutes to 12 hours

    3. Dam may stand and start grooming the calf during this stage

VI. Single births are the most common

  A. Free martin: female twin of male calf

    1. Infertile

    2. Hermaphrodite

## Causes of Dystocia

I. Maternal dystocia is caused by the dam's ability to impede or prevent the delivery

  A. Decreased expulsive force and abnormalities of the birth canal

  B. Primary uterine inertia

  C. Secondary uterine inertia

  D. Birth canal abnormalities

    1. Causes may be inadequate size or deformities of the pelvis

    2. Incomplete dilation of the cervix

    3. Vaginal cystocele; neoplasms of the vulva and vagina

    4. Uterine torsion

II. Fetal causes

  A. Abnormal fetal position, posture, and presentation

    1. Position refers to the dorsum of the fetus versus the quadrants of the maternal pelvis

    2. Posture is the relationship of the extremities to the body of the fetus

    3. Presentation refers to the relationship of the fetal spinal column to that of the dam, and the portion of the fetus that is approaching the birth canal

  B. Fetal monsters

    1. May be caused by schistosomus reflexus and perosomus elumbis

  C. Fetal oversize

    1. Most common cause

    2. Most common in heifers where fetus is normal size but the maternal pelvis is undersize

## Neonatal Care

I. Temperature, 37.5° to 39.5° C (99.5° to 103° F); pulse, 100 to 150 beats per minute; respiration, 30 to 60 breaths per minute

II. Clear mucus from the upper airway

III. Sneezing can be stimulated by tickling the nostrils with straw

IV. Calf should be suckling 2 to 5 hours after birth

V. Colostrum may be administered if calf has not suckled (5% to 8% of its body weight)

VI. Dip umbilical stump in tincture of iodine to prevent navel ill, or omphalitis

VII. Dystocia is the most significant factor affecting perinatal calf survival

  A. Direct losses are from parturient asphyxiation and injury

  B. Indirect loss is that of calves weakened by dystocia

  C. Calves that are hypoxic or injured are not as able to consume adequate colostrum

  D. Trauma may result from excessive use of obstetrical force

    1. Musculoskeletal injuries are common, such as fractures of the metacarpus, metatarsus, femur, ribs, and spine, and luxations of the spine and coxofemoral joints

    2. Neurological damage, such as spinal injuries and trauma to femoral and radial nerves

    3. Soft tissue trauma, such as glossal edema and umbilical evisceration may be encountered

## CAPRINE

### Puberty

I. Doe
  A. Average age 6 to 7 months (pygmy goats could reach puberty as early as 3 months)
  B. Should not be bred until they reach 60% to 70% of their mature body weight
II. Buck
  A. Fertile at 6 to 7 months
  B. Fibroelastic penis
  C. Accessory sex glands
    1. Seminal vesicles
    2. Prostate
    3. Bulbourethral gland (Cowper's gland)

### Breeding Soundness Examination

I. Examination of the doe
  A. A breeding doe should have a body score of 3 to 3.5
  B. External genitalia
    1. Anogenital distance
    2. Vulvar abnormities
    3. Conformation of mammary glands
II. Examination of the buck
  A. Buck should be in good body condition, with a little more flesh than normal because of a possible weight loss during the breeding season
  B. Look for structural faults, because diseases of the hind limbs will decrease the ability of the buck to service the does
  C. Check for foot rot and foot abscesses
  D. Testes
    1. Testes should be examined for size, symmetry, and consistency
    2. Consistency of the testes during breeding is indicated by being firm to the touch, oval, and of equal size
      a. This criterion may change during the non-breeding season or may be an indicator of poor health
  E. Epididymis
    1. Note any changes in the size, form, and consistency. Gross alterations are rare
  F. Penis
    1. Penis can be extended for examination either manually or by electroejaculation
    2. Look for any abnormalities
III. Libido
  A. Libido is difficult to measure during a routine breeding soundness examination
  B. A carefully collected history must be taken to assess libido
IV. Semen evaluation
  A. Semen can be collected and evaluated

V. Q fever
  A. Causative agent: *Coxiella burnetii*
    1. Rickettsial organism
  B. Clinical signs include late-term abortion
  C. Zoonotic potential
    1. Contact with aborted material, vaginal discharge, and mucous membranes of infected animals
    2. Ingesting infected milk
  D. Animals suspected of carrying disease should be culled
    1. Effects on livestock may be subclinical
    2. Diagnosis is based on placental findings, serology, and isolation of the organism
VI. Brucellosis
  A. Causative agent: *Brucella melitensis* or *Brucella ovis*
  B. Clinical signs include abortion, weak kids, mastitis, and localized lesions
  C. *B. melitensis* causes Malta fever in humans
  D. Infected animals may shed the organism in saliva, milk, placenta, and semen

### Semen Collection Techniques and Semen Characteristics

I. Semen collection
  A. Artificial vagina (AV)
    1. No exogenous stimulus is required when using an AV
    2. The buck must be trained to use the AV by using a mount animal
  B. Bailey Ejaculator or electroejaculation
    1. Because of the response by the buck, the Bailey Ejaculator is not used
      a. Use of these machines results in increased vocalization and excessive muscle contractions of the hind limbs
    2. There is a greater volume of semen collected but a lower concentration of sperm using these methods
    3. A combination of rectal massage with the electroejaculator and the use of direct stimulation is usually successful
II. Semen characteristics
  A. Volume: low, approximately 1 mL/ejaculate
  B. Concentration of sperm: very high
  C. Motility: swirling masses of spermatozoa are seen
    1. This swirling mass is called the wave motion

### Estrous Cycle

I. Seasonally polyestrous
  A. Estrous cycle is limited to the fall and winter under natural conditions
  B. Manipulations of light cycles offer year-round breeding capability of does and bucks

II. Estrous cycle is approximately 21 days and is divided into two phases
  A. Follicular phase: 3 to 4 days
  B. Luteal phase: 17 days
III. Estrus (heat) is 24 to 36 hours
IV. Ovulation occurs 24 to 30 hours after the onset of estrus
V. Optimal breeding time is 12 to 24 hours after the onset of estrus
VI. Control of the estrous cycle
  A. Estrus synchronization
    1. Buck effect
      a. Bring odoriferous male near female
    2. Prostaglandins: induce ovulation
    3. Progestins: delay ovulation

## Signs of Estrus

I. Restlessness
II. Vocalization
III. Rapid tail wagging
IV. A "buck jar"
  A. A jar containing a rag that has been rubbed on the scent glands of the buck's horns; may be used to enhance the signs of estrus
V. Attempting to mount other goats

## Pregnancy Diagnosis

I. Failure to return to estrus
II. Progesterone assay: 21 days postbreeding
  A. Serum should be used instead of milk (milk gives false negative results)
  B. Low serum or plasma levels indicate nonpregnancy
III. Estrone sulfate: 50 or more days postbreeding
IV. Pregnancy-specific protein B: 25 days postbreeding
V. External transabdominal ultrasound: 40 or more days postbreeding
  A. Best time for twinning detection: 45 to 90 days postbreeding

## Gestation/Stages of Parturition

I. Gestation: 149 days
II. Maintenance of pregnancy depends on luteal progesterone rather than placental progesterone
III. Cotyledonary placentation
IV. Stages of parturition (kidding)
  A. Stage 1
    1. May last from 2 to 12 hours depending on the age of the dam
    2. Signs exhibited may be those of abdominal discomfort, standing and lying down, pawing at bedding, and frequent bouts of urination and defecation
    3. Appearance of the cervical seal, a thick, yellow-brown mucus that indicates the cervix has relaxed

    4. Fetus, placenta, and fetal fluids are pushed forward to dilate cervix and contact the vagina
  B. Stage 2
    1. Starts with the abdominal press that indicates active labor
    2. This will last 1 to 3 hours
    3. Are routinely in lateral recumbency, but older does may stand to deliver
    4. Chorioallantois ruptures in the vagina
      a. The amnion is pushed through the vulva and ruptures, and the kid is delivered
    5. Doe may rest between kids or may continue to deliver
  C. Stage 3
    1. Delivery of the placenta or placentas and involution of the uterus occur
    2. Placenta should be passed within 1 hour of kidding
    3. After 12 hours, the placenta is considered retained
    4. Involution of the uterus may take up to 12 days
    5. There may be lochia present for up to 3 weeks
V. Twinning common

## Causes of Dystocia

I. Only 3% to 5% of births require assistance
II. Causes
  A. Deviation of position, posture, and presentation
  B. Fetomaternal disproportion
    1. Fetal origin disproportion is when the fetus is too large to pass easily through the pelvis or vaginal canal
      a. Most often encountered with single-fetus pregnancies
    2. Maternal origin is most common in first fresheners that have not grown adequately before parturition
      a. Pelvis is not large enough for the fetus to pass through easily
      b. Other causes may be injury, ankylosis of the tail, and abscesses or tumors around the vagina
  C. Cervical dilation failure
    1. Also known as ringwomb
    2. Common cause of dystocia
    3. Predisposing causes may include hypocalcemia, hormonal or mineral imbalance, twinning, season, and breed
    4. Previously dilated cervix can further complicate dystocia
  D. Uterine torsion
    1. Occasional cause
    2. Typical in single-fetus pregnancies
  E. Uterine inertia

1. Primary uterine inertia
2. Secondary uterine inertia

## Signs of Dystocia

I. Amnion protrusion with no progression through parturition
II. Dam strains without producing a kid for longer than 1 hour

## Neonatal Care

I. Temperature, 38.5° to 40.5° C (101° to 105° F); pulse, 80 to 120 beats per minute; respiration, 12 to 20 breaths per minute
II. Kids should be standing within 15 minutes and nursing within 1 hour postparturition
III. Umbilicus should be dipped several times in 7% tincture of iodine
IV. Observe kids for normal respiration, evidence of respiratory acidosis, and other signs of fetal distress, such as meconium staining
V. Assess adequate colostrum intake
   A. Observe kids nursing from does
   B. Palpate abdomen of kid
   C. Hand feed colostrum if necessary
   D. If using cow colostrum, make sure it is free from *Mycobacterium paratuberculosis*
VI. After treatment with colostrum, kids can be fed pasteurized milk or heat-treated colostrum if available
VII. Doe and kids must have an available, draft-free shelter to protect them from temperature extremes
   A. Shelter decreases the risk of hypothermia, heat stress, or pneumonia
VIII. Concerns for kids
   A. For the first few days, a neonatal kid should be checked for hypothermia, hypoglycemia, and colibacillosis
   B. Cryptosporidiosis and floppy kid syndrome can be seen in kids between 3 and 10 days of age
   C. At 2 to 4 weeks of age, clinical signs of white muscle disease, copper deficiency, *Pasteurella haemolytica* pneumonia, mycoplasmosis, and coccidiosis can occur
   D. Dam-reared kids can be weaned after the age of 3 months

## OVINE

## Puberty

I. Ewe
   A. Average age: 6 to 7 months
   B. Should not be bred until they reach 65% of their mature body weight
   C. Nutrition is important in puberty
   D. Mutton breeds tend to reach puberty earlier than wool breeds
   E. Age of puberty in ewes can be influenced by selecting a ram with a large scrotal circumference
II. Ram
   A. Fertile as early as 7.5 to 9 months, but should not be considered to have adult capacity until they are at least 2 years old
   B. Fibroelastic penis
   C. Accessory sex glands
      1. Seminal vesicles
      2. Prostate
      3. Bulbourethral gland (Cowper's gland)

## Breeding Soundness Examination

I. Examination of the ewe
   A. A breeding doe should have a body score of 2.5 to 3.5
   B. External genitalia
      1. Anogenital distance
      2. Vulvar abnormities
      3. Conformation of mammary glands
II. Examination of the ram
   A. Structural soundness
      1. Refers to the ability of the ram to remain sound during the breeding season
      2. Examine the feet, legs, and teeth for soundness
   B. Physical soundness
      1. Refers to the overall health of the ram
      2. Examine the ram for diseases or conditions that may be transmitted to the ewe or may prevent optimal performance of the ram, such as foot rot, lip and leg ulcerations, and pizzle rot
      3. Body condition score of the ram should be a value of between 2.5 and 3.5
   C. Testes and epididymis
      1. Palpate the testicles for tone and symmetry
         a. Note any swelling, atrophy, and lack of tone or symmetry
      2. Palpate the epididymis for enlargement due to inflammation and fibrosis
         a. *Brucella ovis* is a major infective agent in epididymitis
      3. A scrotal tape should be used to measure the testes and scrotum
         a. This is an estimate of potential sperm production and fertility
         b. It is recommended by the Western Regional Coordinating Committee on Ram Epididymitis
           (1) Ram lambs over 60 kg (132 lb) should have a scrotal circumference of greater than 30 cm (12 inches)
           (2) Yearling rams (12 to 18 months) should have a circumference of greater than 33 cm (13 inches)

(3) Breeding stock rams over 113 kg should have a circumference of greater than 36 cm (14 inches)
    D. Prepuce and penis
       1. Prepuce should be examined for open or ulcerated lesions at the orifice
       2. Penis should be extended and examined for injury or disease
    E. Semen evaluation
       1. Semen can be collected and evaluated
III. Ram to ewe/ewe to lamb ratio
    A. A healthy ram, under most range conditions, can breed 100 females in a 17-day breeding cycle
IV. Q fever
    A. Causative agent: *Coxiella burnetii*
       1. Rickettsial organism
    B. Clinical signs include late term abortion
    C. Zoonotic potential
       1. Contact with aborted material, vaginal discharge and mucous membranes of infected animals
       2. Ingesting infected milk
    D. Animals suspected of carrying disease should be culled
       1. Effects on livestock may be subclinical
       2. Diagnosis is based on placental findings, serology, and isolation of the organism
V. Brucellosis
    A. Causative agent: *Brucella melitensis* or *Brucella ovis*
    B. Clinical signs include abortion, weak kids, mastitis, and localized lesions
    C. *B. melitensis* causes Malta fever in humans
    D. Infected animals may shed the organism in saliva, milk, placenta, and semen

## Semen Collection Techniques and Semen Characteristics

I. Semen collection
    A. Electroejaculation
       1. It is important to collect the semen in as clean a manner as possible
          a. Cells and cellular debris can interfere with proper evaluation
       2. Collection is done by alternating massage with the rectal probe and electrical stimulation
       3. Poor technique, inadequate electroejaculator stimulation, or too much voltage can affect the quality of semen collected
II. Semen characteristics
    A. Volume: low, approximately 1 mL/ejaculate
    B. Concentration of sperm: very high, 3000 million/mL
    C. Motility: swirling masses of spermatozoa are seen and are called the wave motion

## Estrous Cycle

I. Seasonally polyestrous: short day breeders
    A. Estrous cycle is limited to the fall and winter under natural conditions
    B. Manipulation of light cycles offers potential year round breeding of ewes and rams
II. Estrous cycle is approximately 17 days long and is divided into two phases
    A. Follicular phase: 3 to 4 days
    B. Luteal phase: 13 days
III. Estrus (heat): 10 to 30 hours
IV. Ovulation occurs 24 to 30 hours after the onset of estrus
V. Optimal breeding time is 12 to 18 hours after the first signs of estrus
VI. Control of estrus
    A. Shortly before or at the onset of breeding season, a ram is introduced to the ewes, and the ewes will begin cycling 5 to 6 days later
       1. This is known as the Whitten effect
    B. Increasing the dietary intake before ewes are bred can increase the number of follicles that mature and rupture
       1. This is know as flushing

## Signs of Estrus

I. Ewes will seek out the ram and remain immobile while being investigated
    A. A teaser ram on is sometimes used to see if the ewe is in heat
II. Tail wagging
III. Without a ram present, it is almost impossible to tell if a ewe is cycling

## Pregnancy Diagnosis

I. Failure to return to estrus
    A. Use a teaser ram (castrated male) to detect ewes returning to estrus
II. Progesterone assay: 17 to 18 days postbreeding
III. Rectal ultrasound: 30 or more days postbreeding
IV. External transabdominal ultrasound: 40 or more days postbreeding
V. Estrone sulfate: 50 or more days postbreeding
VI. Abdominal ballottement

## Gestation/Stages of Parturition

I. Gestation: 145 to 155 days (5 months)
II. Nutrition should be increased by 50% in the last trimester
III. First third of pregnancy depends on the corpus luteum for progesterone; after 50 days progesterone is mainly produced by the placenta
IV. Cotyledonary placentation
V. Mammary development the last 2 weeks of gestation

VI. Colostrum can be expressed 2 to 3 days before lambing

VII. Body temperature drops 0.5° C (1° to 2° F) during the last 48 hours

VIII. Stages of parturition (lambing)

    A. Labor lasts approximately 1 to 4 hours

    B. Stage 1

        1. Signs of restlessness, decreased appetite, and a swollen vulva

        2. Characterized by increasing myometrial activity and the start of contractions

        3. As the cervix is dilating, myometrial activity is increasing intrauterine pressure and forcing the fetal membranes up to the cervix, causing them to rupture

    C. Stage 2

        1. As the fetus enters the cervical canal and vagina, there is a release of oxytocin, thereby increasing the myometrial contractions

            a. Aided by maternal abdominal contractions, the fetus is expelled and the risk of anoxia is minimized

    D. Stage 3

        1. Fetal membranes should be expelled within 2 hours

IX. Twinning is common

## Causes of Dystocia

I. Maternal causes

    A. Ringwomb

        1. Incomplete dilation of the cervix occurs, often with no known cause

        2. More common in ewe lambs

II. Fetal causes

    A. Head-only presentation

        1. Head may become swollen and edematous because of an extended time in lambing

    B. Fetopelvic disproportion

        1. Large lambs occur more often in ewes that are bred as lambs than in older ewes

    C. Malposition of the head

        1. Lateral deviation of the head and neck is more common in multiple births than in single births

        2. Plastic lamb puller can be used to correct position and deliver the lamb

    D. Elbow lock

    E. Malposition of the forelegs

        1. Important, in multiple births, to determine that the correct fetal appendages are positioned and delivered

        2. Can palpate head and neck to determine fetal appendages

    F. Breech

        1. Possible to rupture lamb's liver and fracture the ribs when delivering in this position

    G. Transverse presentation

        1. Lamb's vertebral column is presented at the maternal opening

        2. Hypoxia and lamb death are common with caudal and transverse presentations

## Signs of Dystocia

I. Only the head appears

II. Water breaks with no further progress for longer than 30 minutes

III. Total parturition lasts for more than 90 minutes

IV. Tail or only one leg is delivered

V. It is imperative to recognize the signs of dystocia because the ewe's cervix will close after 2 to 3 hours of nonproductive labor

## Neonatal Care

I. Temperature, 37.5° to 39.5° C (99.5° to 103° F); pulse, 100 to 150 beats per minute; respiration, 30 to 60 breaths per minute

    A. Spontaneous breathing should occur 20 to 30 seconds after birth

    B. Lambs are susceptible to hypothermia during the first 36 hours after birth. Heat supplementation should be provided to all lambs with a rectal temperature below 100° F

II. Lambs should be given a complete physical examination

III. Common defects

    A. Cleft palate

    B. Umbilical herniation

    C. Entropion

IV. Umbilicus should be dipped in 7% tincture of iodine

V. If lambs have not suckled within 3 hours after being born, they should be given 30 mL of colostrum

VI. Should stand and nurse within 20 minutes of delivery

    A. Maternal factors affecting the lambs attempt to nurse may be a long wool coat, pendulous udder, and enlarged teats

    B. Weak lambs or lambs born after the first of the litter may be ignored by the ewe, therefore increasing the risk of hypothermia and hypoglycemia

VII. Confine ewes and lambs to a claiming pen for the first 24 hours to optimize mothering

VIII. Health management of neonatal lambs

    A. Colostrum

        1. Require 50 mL/kg of body weight of colostrum within the first 2 hours of life and a maximum of 200 to 250 mL/kg within the first 24 hours, split into four or five feedings

    B. Supplemental immunoglobulin

        1. Bovine or caprine colostrum can be used during the first 24 hours

            a. Colostrum should be from herds that are free from pathogenic disease, such as bovine leukosis virus and caprine arthritis encephalitis virus, which may harm sheep

C. Vitamin E and selenium supplementation
   1. If ewes have not been given a selenium supplement and are in a selenium-deficient area, lambs should receive selenium
   2. Ewes may be treated during last trimester of pregnancy if using an injectable selenium, to be repeated at intervals of no less than 14 days to a maximum of four treatments
   3. Supplements used in cattle are not recommended for ewes
   4. Vitamin A and selenium can both be fed to pregnant ewes

D. Lamb identification
   1. Mark at birth
      a. Methods include ear tagging, paint branding, or spraying the lamb with the litter identification

E. Contagious ecthyma vaccination
   1. If there is a history of mastitis, lamb losses, and diminished productivity, vaccinate the lambs at birth
   2. Do not vaccinate a flock if it is unaffected or only mildly affected by the disease

F. Tail dock and castration
   1. Tail docking is ideally performed within the first 24 hours in long-tail breeds, but only after the lamb has received adequate colostrum
      a. Rubber bands
      b. Electric docker
   2. Dock the tail distal to the tail fold
   3. Castrate lambs up to 7 days of age if using rings or cut-and-pull technique, or before 90 days if crushing
   4. Recommend vaccinating lambs with tetanus antitoxin at the time of docking or castration if ewes have inadequate immunity

## PORCINE ▬▬▬▬▬▬▬▬▬▬
### Puberty

I. Sows
   A. Gilts normally reach puberty around 250 lb (114 kg) or about 200 days (4.5 to 6 months) in most breeds

II. Boars
   A. Reach puberty at about 5 to 7 months
   B. They are mature at about 2 years
   C. Fibroelastic penis
   D. Accessory sex glands
      1. Seminal vesicles
      2. Prostate
      3. Bulbourethral gland (Cowper's gland)

### Breeding Soundness Examination

I. Examination in the sow
   A. A complete history should be taken
   B. Examination of mammary glands for defects
   C. Examination of external genitalia for conformation defects

II. Examination in the boar
   A. Sheath
      1. Should be examined for pus and redness (phimosis) and abscesses, which may be noticed on palpation or observation
   B. Testes and epididymis
      1. Size of the testes is related directly to the ability of the boar to produce sperm
      2. Testes should be of equal size with visible epididymal tails
      3. On palpation, testes should be firm to turgid with no hard areas
      4. Tail and lower body of the epididymis should be palpable with a prominent tail
         a. Cysts can be found in the head and body of the epididymis but might not be easily palpated
            (1) These cysts may cause complete or partial occlusion of the epididymal duct
   C. Penis
      1. Can be examined at the time of semen collection
      2. Check for abnormalities such as persistent frenulum, bite wounds, and, rarely, an amputated penis

III. Libido
   A. In situations where there is hand mating and artificial insemination, boars with low libido are usually detected
      1. Poor libido varies from little to no interest in the sow/gilt in standing heat

IV. Semen evaluation
   A. Semen can be collected and evaluated

### Semen Collection Techniques and Semen Characteristics

I. Semen collection
   A. Gloved hand technique
      1. Boar semen is best collected with this technique on a sow in estrus or dummy sow
      2. Sometimes older boars may not collect using hand pressure
      3. Using a sow in heat and letting the boar insert the penis into the vagina until the boar starts to ejaculate will sometimes aid collection

II. Semen characteristics
   A. Volume: 150 to 500 mL ejaculate
   B. Concentration of sperm: $150 \times 10^6$/mL
   C. Motility: 70% to 90% progressively motile sperm

## Estrous Cycle

I. Nonseasonal polyestrous
II. Estrous cycle is approximately 21 days in duration
III. Lasts on average 2 to 3 days (40 to 60 hours)
  A. Standing estrus: 48 to 55 hours
  B. Return to estrus: 4 to 7 days after weaning
IV. Ovulation typically occurs during the second day of estrus
  A. Ovulation occurs from both ovaries
V. Should be bred 24 hours after the onset of estrus and every 24 hours
  A. Gilts should be bred 12 hours after the onset of estrus and repeated at 12-hour intervals

## Signs of Estrus

I. Vulvar swelling
II. Restlessness
III. Alertness
IV. Receptivity to the boar
V. Stationary stance (apply moderate pressure over the loin area with the flat of your hand) with ears still and erect ("popping the ears")
VI. Mounting other animals

## Pregnancy Diagnosis

I. Teasing sow: 18 to 24 days postbreeding
II. Ultrasound: 23 days postbreeding
  A. Transabdominal ultrasound is the primary method
III. Progesterone assay: 17 to 20 days postbreeding
IV. Estrone sulfate: 25 to 29 days postbreeding
V. Failure to return to heat is not a reliable indicator

## Gestation/Stages of Parturition

I. Gestation: 114 days (3 months, 3 weeks, 3 days)
II. Diffuse placentation
III. Main source of progesterone is from the corpus luteum
IV. Abdominal and mammary development as early as 2.5 months gestation
V. Stages of parturition (farrowing)
  A. Signs of impending parturition
    1. 24 hours before parturition: the sow will lie down and rise
    2. 12 hours before parturition: defecation and urination will increase in frequency
    3. Respiratory rate peaks about 6 hours before birth of the first piglet
    4. 3 to 4 hours before parturition, sows become restless and attempt to nest
      a. Crated animals may chew bars
      b. Sow may then rest and resume these activities up until 15 to 60 minutes before the first piglet is born

B. Stage 2
  1. Usually lasts 1 to 5 hours
  2. For the delivery of the piglets, the sow usually remains in lateral recumbency, has mild abdominal contractions, passes a small amount of fluid, and wiggles her tail
  3. Time between piglets is 1 minute to 4 hours, but is usually under 15 minutes, depending on the number of piglets
C. Stage 3
  1. Placenta is usually expelled 21 minutes to 12.5 hours later
    a. Placentas may also be expelled between piglets
  2. Retained placenta may indicate that additional piglets remain in the uterus
VI. Average litter size is 8 to 10

## Causes of Dystocia

I. Less than 1% of sows show signs of dystocia
II. Maternal causes
  A. Primary uterine inertia
  B. Secondary uterine inertia
  C. Uterine deviation
    1. Occurs in older sows with an large number of piglets in the litter
    2. Uterus is pulled ventral to the brim of the pelvis, thereby blocking the passage of piglets
  D. Obstruction of birth canal
    1. Can be caused by constipation, distended bladder, hymen remnant, and swelling of the soft tissues of the birth canal
III. Fetal causes
  A. Oversized piglets
    1. Most common in litters with a small number of piglets
  B. Malpresentations
    1. Account for approximately one third of fetal dystocia
    2. Simultaneous presentation of fetuses in the birth canal or breech presentation is common

## Signs of Dystocia

I. Prolonged gestation
II. Anorexia and lethargy
III. Blood-tinged vulvar discharge or the appearance of meconium without the onset of abdominal straining
IV. Abdominal straining and vulvar discharge without the passing of fetuses
V. Cessation of abdominal straining after the birth of only a few fetuses
VI. Vulvar discharge with a foul smell and discoloration
VII. Parturition longer than 4 hours
VIII. Long interval between piglets

## Neonatal Care

I. Temperature, 36.8° to 39° C (98° to 102° F); pulse, 200 to 250 beats per minute; respiration, 50 to 60 breaths per minute

II. Sows do not lick and clean newborn. If fetus is born with its amnion, the membrane must be removed.

III. Piglets should be placed under a heat lamp and kept warm until all piglets are born; then all are placed with the dam to suckle
   A. Not able to maintain deep body temperature if the environmental temperatures are low

IV. Piglets are born with a limited supply of energy; therefore they must receive food shortly after birth
   A. Should be active and reach a teat within 5 minutes
      1. Area must be draft free and at least 30° C (86° F)
   B. Weak, chilled piglets with poor mobility require tube feeding and warming before being placed with their litter

V. Make sure piglets receive colostrum

VI. Usually weaned at 3 to 5 weeks of age

VII. Castrate young boars not being retained for breeding

VIII. Tasks that should be performed shortly after birth
   A. Dry piglets to decrease heat loss
   B. Cut umbilical cords approximately 5 cm (2 inches) from the body and dip in a mild disinfectant
   C. Clip needle teeth
      1. Teeth are sometimes clipped to prevent the piglet from injuring the dam while nursing
   D. Notch ears
      1. Done as a method of identification
   E. Dock tails
      1. Banding or clipping of the tail is done to prevent piglets from chewing on the tails
   F. Administer 1.0 mL injection of iron dextran
      1. Sow milk is deficient in iron
      2. In confined settings the sow does not receive iron from the environment
      3. The injection should be given in the neck to prevent damage to the meat in the hindquarters

## ACKNOWLEDGMENT

The editors and authors appreciate the original work of Betty Gregan and Karen Anderson, on which this chapter is based.

# Glossary

**abdominal ballottement** Palpation of the fetal head by pushing the fist or fingertips into the abdominal wall, causing the fetus to move away from and then return to the fist or fingers

**adenomyosis** Glandular tissue invading the muscle wall of an organ (e.g., uterus)

**agouti** Brown/gray coat color found in some animals and wolves

**allele** Alternative form of a gene at the same site on a chromosome that determines different traits in an individual. Alleles may code for the same or for alternative forms of the trait

**anasarca** Extensive subcutaneous edema found with such diseases as congestive heart failure

**ankylosis** Abnormal immobilization and solidification of a joint

**artificial vagina** Device that is used for the collection of semen from male animals, consisting of a solid outer tube and lined by a flexible thin rubber sleeve

**ascites** Abnormal collection of a serous, edematous fluid in the peritoneal cavity

**assortative mating** Mating of individuals that are phenotypically similar

**autosomal** Used to describe nonsex chromosomes

**backcross** Pairing of an $F_1$ generation hybrid with an organism whose genotype is identical to the parental strain

**barrow** Male hog that has been castrated before reaching sexual maturity

**boar** Uncastrated male pig

**body condition** Examination of a body by comparison to a chart

**breech** Birth of an animal with buttocks or rear feet first

**chorioallantoic membrane** Extraembryonic membrane consisting of the chorion and the allantois. In several mammals, it forms the placenta

**chromosome** Contains DNA (deoxyribonucleic acid), which transfers genetic information

**co-dominance** Condition in which two alleles of a pair are both expressed equally with the resulting phenotype a blending of the two traits

**colibacillosis** Infection with *Escherichia coli*

**colostrum** Immunoglobulin-rich milk secreted from the mammary gland shortly after parturition: "first milk"

**corpus luteum** Formed in the ovary after ovulation; produces progesterone

**cotyledonary placentation** Attachment of fetal membranes to the endometrium occurring only at projections from the endometrium; found in ruminants

**cryptorchid** Animal with undescended testes

**cryptosporidiosis** Infection with *Cryptosporidium* spp., causing diarrhea

**diffuse placenta** When attachment of the fetal membranes of the endometrium is continuous throughout the entire surface of the fetal membrane; found in horse and pig

**dihybrid cross** Crossing of two traits

**diploid** Two copies of a chromosome in each cell or nucleus

**dominant gene** Gene that produces an effect in an organism regardless of the corresponding allele. A dominant gene masks or suppresses the expression of its corresponding allele. The dominant allele is usually written as a capital letter

**enterocolitis** Inflammation involving the small intestine and colon

**entropion** Turning inward of the eyelid

**epididymitis** Inflammation of the epididymis

**epistasis** Masking of one allele over the genes on another locus

**$F_1$ $F_2$** Family or familial or filial generation

**fetal monster** Fetus with developmental anomalies to be classified as grotesque and often nonviable

**filial** Any generation following the parental generation

**follicular phase** Epithelial lining of the uterus hypertrophies and becomes edematous and congested

**foot rot** Disease involving the foot, mostly caused by bacteria, characterized by dermatitis of the interdigital skin

**flushing** Practice of feeding a higher than normal level of energy at breeding time to increase ovulation rate, especially in the sheep and goat

**frenulum** Small fold of integument that limits the movement of a part

**freshen** Cow or goat that has recently calved and is in its first 2 to 4 weeks of lactation

**gelding** Castrated male horse

**gene** Unit of inheritance

**genetics** Study of similarities and differences that are passed from parent to offspring

**genome** All of the genes carried by a gamete (e.g., chromosomal DNA containing a complete set of hereditary factors)

**genotype** Genetic makeup of an individual

**gestation** Pregnancy

**gilt** A female pig used for breeding that has yet to have a litter of piglets

**glossal edema** Edema involving the tongue

**GnRH** Gonadotropin-releasing hormone; a type of hormone that causes gonads to mature to adult state

**haploid** Having one copy of each chromosome per cell or nucleus

**harem mating** Mating where one male is mated to five or more females

**hCG** Human chorionic gonadotropin; a hormone found in the urine that is used to diagnose pregnancy after implantation of the ovum

**hermaphrodite** An animal that has the reproductive organs, and often the behavior patterns of both sexes

**heterosis** Same as hybrid vigor; a cross performed to produce a better-quality genotype and phenotype

**heterozygous** Different alleles, for example, Bb

**homozygous** Identical alleles, for example, BB

**hybrid** Offspring that are different than the parents

**hydrocephalus** A condition characterized by an abnormal buildup of cerebrospinal fluid in the cerebral ventricular system

**IgG** Type of antibody in plasma that can cross placental barriers

**inbreeding** Mating of closely related individuals to produce ever-increasing similarities in the offspring

**inbreeding depression** Relates to traits of fitness, such as early growth, resistance to disease, or fertility, which are multifunctional traits

**incomplete dominance** Cross in which both alleles of a gene are expressed equally

**inguinal hernia** Hernia occurring in the groin area where the thighs meet the folds of abdominal skin

**intermediate inheritance** Same as incomplete dominance

**karyotype** Photomicrograph of a single cell in the metaphase stage (meiosis) of division that displays chromosomes in descending order and describes the number and morphology of the chromosomes. It is similar to a blueprint or fingerprint. Karyotype is also called diploid chromosome complement

**lethal gene** Gene that will cause the death of the embryo or cause serious impairment or death sometime after birth

**LH** Luteinizing hormone

**line breeding** Breeding of related individuals to guarantee similar traits in the offspring

**lochia** Discharge from the vagina occurring the first or second week after parturition

**locus** Specific site or location of a gene on a chromosome

**lordosis** Downward curvature of the spine

**luteal phase** Portion of the estrous cycle in which the effect of the corpus luteum is dominant and the cow is anestrous because of the increased levels of progesterone in the blood

**malpresentation** Faulty fetal positioning

**meconium** Yellow-orange gummy material contained in the intestine of a term fetus that constitutes the first stool passed by the newborn

**meiosis** Sex cell division that results in haploid cells and independent assortment of chromosomes

**microcotyledonary placentation** Microscopic grouping of villi in the equine placenta where embryo implantation occurs

**mitosis** Method of cell replication that creates cells identical to the parent cells

**monestrus** Experiencing one estrous cycle each year

**monohybrid cross** Crossing of one trait

**mummified fetus** Conversion of the fetus to a dehydrated state, where the soft tissues are reduced in volume, the skin is leatherlike, and the tissues are deeply stained brown

**mutation** Any change in DNA sequence

**myometrial contraction** Contraction of the smooth muscle coat of the uterus

**neonatal** Newborn

**neonatal isoerythrolysis** Condition in which there is an immunity to an alloantigen. This occurs when red blood cells from the offspring enter the maternal circulatory system. If the red blood cell antigens are different from those of the dam, this results in the production of antibodies. If there is more offspring of the same mating combination, where the offspring of the same blood type is produced, a hemolytic anemia will occur in the offspring once it has consumed the maternal antibodies contained within the colostrum

**omphalitis** Inflammation of the umbilicus

**orchitis** Inflammation of the testicles characterized by inflammation of one or both testes, pain, and sensitivity to touch. Chronic orchitis does not involve pain, but the testes may slowly swell and become hard

**outbreeding** Same as random breeding; matings to other strains to increase the amount of heterozygous genes

**ovulation** Release of the egg (ovum) from the ovarian follicle

**parturition** Act of giving birth

**pedigree chart** Chart that shows the ancestry of a particular family

**penetrance** Refers to the appearance in the phenotype of traits determined by the genotype

**perosomus elumbis** Congenital defect most common in calves and lambs. The vertebral column ends at the caudal thoracic region, causing the posterior portion of the body to be joined to the front portion by soft tissue only

**phantom mare** Dummy mare constructed of a padded, hollow device, about the approximate height and width that would suit the stallion. It is used to collect semen for artificial insemination or semen evaluation

**phenotype** Physical characteristics of an individual and/or performance of an individual that is expressed

**phimosis** Condition where the orifice of the prepuce is constricted so that it cannot be pulled back over the glans

**pizzle rot** Condition, found in castrated male sheep, where there is swelling, scabby ulcerations, and inflammation of the interior/exterior of the prepuce and glans penis

**pluriparous** Two or more pregnancies that resulted in living offspring

**polyestrous** More than one estrous cycle in each year

**polygenic traits** Traits that are due to the interaction of several gene pairs

**primary uterine inertia** Sluggishness of the uterine contractions during labor due to an overstretching of the uterus, toxemia, or obesity

**progesterone** Steroid sex hormone that, in pregnancy, protects the embryo and fosters growth of the placenta and, in preparation for lactation, prepares the mammary glands for secretion

**puberty** Physical stage at which sexual reproduction is possible

**Punnett square** Chart used by geneticists to show possible outcomes of specific breeding. Also called a checkerboard

**recessive gene** Gene that produces an effect only when it is inherited from both parents. Usually written in lowercase letters

**ringwomb** Disease of the ewe where the cervix fails to relax so that there is no outward appearance of lambing. Full-term fetuses may die in utero

**schistosomus reflexus** Fetus with a cleft abdomen

**seasonally polyestrous** Occurs in an animal that has several estrous cycles within a breeding season, followed by anestrus until the following breeding season, as in the cat

**secondary uterine inertia** Sluggishness of uterine contractions during labor due to exhaustion or lack of myometrial contractions

**sex chromosomes** X and Y chromosomes, which determine the genetic sex of the individual

**sickle hocks** Abnormal hock joint where the foot and metatarsus are angled forward

**spermatozoa** Sperm

**steer** Male bovine castrated before reaching sexual maturity

**tail deflection** Deflection of the tail to the side

**tail docking** Amputation of the tail

**test cross** Cross performed to determine the genotype of a particular phenotype

**tetanus** Fatal disease of all animal species caused by the neurotoxin of *Clostridium tetani*. The bacterial spores are deposited in the tissue and, under anaerobic conditions, vegetate

**transabdominal ultrasound** Method of examining abdominal contents by using sound waves or ultrasound

**transgenic** An animal whose DNA has been altered so that it contains DNA from another individual

**umbilical evisceration** Pushing out of the internal organs through the umbilicus

**uroperitoneum** Condition in which the urine is free in the peritoneal cavity

**uterine caruncles** Fleshy masses located on the walls of the uterus of pregnant ruminants to which the uterus is attached

**uterine inertia** Sluggishness of uterine contractions during labor

**uterine torsion** Twisting of the body of the uterus in cows and mares, and of the uterine horn in sows, resulting in dystocia

**variable expressivity** Traits that show continuous variation

**wethe** Male sheep or goat castrated before reaching sexual maturity

**whelping** The birthing process

**winking** The opening and closing of the vulva of the mare indicating that she is coming into heat

**zonary placentation** Fetus is attached to the endometrium by a band that encircles the placenta, as in the dog and cat

# Review Questions

**1** Which species ovulates 12 to 18 hours after estrus?
a. Caprine
b. Porcine
c. Equine
d. Bovine

**2** The primary method of pregnancy diagnosis in the sow is
a. Transabdominal ultrasound
b. Rectal palpation
c. Progesterone assay
d. Abdominal radiograph

**3** Which species is an induced ovulator?
a. Canine
b. Bovine
c. Ovine
d. Feline

**4** Which of the following is associated with abortion and infertility in the canine?
a. Q fever
b. Brucellosis
c. *Pseudomonas*
d. *Toxocara*

**5** Stage of the estrous cycle in the canine marked by cornified squamous epithelial cells in the vaginal mucosa
a. Anestrus
b. Diestrus
c. Estrus
d. Metestrus

**6** If a white chicken is bred to a black chicken and the offspring have both white and black feathers, the inheritance pattern is described as
a. Co-dominance
b. Incomplete dominance
c. Variable expression
d. Epistasis

**7** The condition in which two alleles for a gene are expressed equally as a blending of the two traits is described as
a. Co-dominance
b. Incomplete dominance
c. Variable expression
d. Epistasis

**8** Breeding of two individuals that are heterozygous for a given trait will produce
  a. All heterozygous offspring
  b. All homozygous offspring
  c. Half heterozygous offspring, half homozygous offspring
  d. ¾ heterozygous offspring, ¼ homozygous offspring

**9** Breeding of two individuals that are homozygous for alternate alleles for a given trait will produce
  a. All heterozygous offspring
  b. All homozygous offspring
  c. Half heterozygous offspring, half homozygous offspring
  d. ¾ heterozygous offspring, ¼ homozygous offspring

**10** A dominant X-linked gene, B, in the mouse, results in a short, crooked tail; its recessive allele, b, represents a normal tail. If a normal-tailed female is mated to a bent-tailed male, what phenotypic ratio should occur in F1?
  a. Three bent-tailed females/one normal-tailed male
  b. All mice will have a bent tail
  c. Two normal-tailed females/two bent-tailed males
  d. Two bent-tailed females/two normal-tailed males

## BIBLIOGRAPHY

Battaglia RA: *Handbook of livestock management*, ed 4, New Jersey, 2007, Pearson Prentice Hall.

Blanchard TL et al: *Manual of equine reproduction*, ed 2, St Louis, 2003, Mosby.

Blood DC, Studdert VP: *Saunders comprehensive veterinary dictionary*, ed 3, London, 2006, Saunders.

Eales A et al: *Practical lambing and lab care*, ed 3, Ames, Iowa, 2004, Blackwell.

Feldman EC, Nelson RW: *Canine and feline endocrinology and reproduction*, ed 3, St Louis, 2003, Saunders.

Gillespie JR: *Modern livestock and poultry production*, ed 7, Albany, NY, 2004, Delmar.

Griffiths AJF et al: *An introduction to genetic analysis*, ed 8, New York, 2004, Freeman.

Hafez ESE: *Reproduction in farm animals*, ed 7, Ames, Iowa, 2000, Blackwell.

Hanie EA: *Large animal clinical procedures for veterinary technicians*, St Louis, 2006, Mosby.

McKinnon V: *Equine reproduction*, Ames, Iowa, 1993, Blackwell.

Nelson RW: *Canine and feline endocrinology and reproduction*, ed 3, St Louis, 2004, Saunders.

Noakes DE et al: *Arthur's veterinary reproduction and obstetrics*, ed 8, St Louis, 2001, Saunders.

Nussbaum R, McInnes R, Willard H: *Thompson and Thompson genetics in medicine*, ed 6, Philadelphia, 2004, Saunders.

Pineda MH, Dooley MP: *McDonald's veterinary endocrinology and reproduction*, ed 5, Ames, Iowa, 2003, Blackwell.

Pinto CRF, Eilts BE, Paccamonti DL: Animal reproduction. In McCurnin DM, Bassert JM: *Clinical textbook for veterinary technicians*, ed 6, St Louis, 2006, Saunders.

Pugh DG: *Sheep and goat medicine*, St Louis, 2002, Saunders.

Rose RJ, Hodgson DR: *Manual of equine practice*, ed 2, St Louis, 2000, Saunders.

Sutton T: *Introduction to animal reproduction*, ed 2, Vermilion, Alberta, Canada, 2000, EI Sutton Consulting.

Tamarin R: *Principles of genetics*, ed 7, New York, 2002, McGraw-Hill.

Youngquist RS: *Current therapy in large animal theriogenology*, ed 2, St Louis, 2007, Saunders.

## CHAPTER 14

# Companion Animal Behavior

*Emma K. Brown*

## OUTLINE

Normal Canine Behavior
  Behavioral Development
  Social Development
Normal Feline Behavior

Behavioral Development
  Social Development
Applied Animal Behavior
  Preventing Behavior Problems

Common Behavioral Problems
  Canine
  Feline

## LEARNING OUTCOMES

After reading this chapter you should be able to:

1. Describe in chronological order important stages in the behavioral development of both the dog and cat.
2. Describe the social behavior of the dog and the cat.
3. Describe various methods of preventing behavior problems in the dog and the cat.
4. Describe some common behavior problems in the dog and the cat.
5. Identify intervention techniques that may be used to eliminate or modify abnormal behavior.
6. Identify abnormal behavior problems.

It is essential that graduating veterinary technicians have an understanding of companion animal behavior, so that they may assist clients to choose and train their pets. This understanding will ultimately strengthen the human-animal bond and strengthen all of its associated benefits. This chapter is intended to give a basic understanding of the concepts pertaining to cat and dog behavior.

## NORMAL CANINE BEHAVIOR
### Behavioral Development

I. Development by its very nature is a continual and gradual process
  A. Some development we surmise by studying the result of dog behavior
  B. While some we observe in process
  C. Although it is gradual it is a complex process with many contributing factors
  D. Behavioral development can be described in the following stages (Table 14-1)
  E. Development is continual and memory plays an important role in concreting experiences both positive and negative
  F. The last stage is the adult stage. The adult stage begins after sexual maturity
  G. Sexual maturity for dogs occurs anywhere from 6 to 9 months of age, but they are not socially mature until 18 to 36 months of age

### Social Development

Like their wild ancestor, the wolf, dogs value an individual's place in the social group; therefore they will devote much time and effort to secure and maintain that place. An individual dog's place is dependent on how well it interprets its environment and how well it communicates to its fellow group members. The "tool kit" that dogs have to communicate with is composed of elements of

**Table 14-1** Developmental stages of canines

| Stage | Age of commencement | Characterized by |
|---|---|---|
| Neonatal | Birth–2 wk | Complete vulnerability |
| Transitional | 2-3 wk | Rapid maturation of senses |
| Socialization | 3-16 wk | Social relationships |
| | 3-8 wk | Socialize best with other dogs |
| | 5-12 wk | Socialize best with humans |
| | 10-12 wk and 16-20 wk | Adapt to exploring new environments |
| | 8.5 wk | Develop substrate preferences for elimination |
| | 7-10 wk | Dogs experience a fear period where painful and/or traumatic situations should be avoided |
| Juvenile | 10-36 wk | Capacity to learn |
| Adult | After sexual maturity | Continual learning |

From Overall K: *Clinical behavioral medicine for small animals*, St Louis, 1997, Mosby.
Note that Table 14-1 provides only a template, and each dog will vary in its development and time frame.

their normal social behavior, and this in turn is dictated by their senses: visual (and postural signaling), olfactory (smell), and auditory.

I. Vision and postural signaling
 A. The binocular field of view for dogs is poor
 B. Canines have better lateral vision than humans
 C. Herding dogs are capable of discriminating hand signals up to a 1 km distance
 D. Studies have shown that dogs can distinguish colors, but this ability is poor
 E. Canine visual acuity is sufficient for them to use a wide range of postural signals (body language), as both sender and receiver
  1. Dogs rely on their face, muzzle, ears, tail, and body to effectively communicate their intent to others
  2. Common examples include
   a. Dominance signaling
    (1) Eyes are focused, making contact
    (2) Tail is held high
    (3) Mouth is closed
    (4) Ears are rigid and/or erect
    (5) Body is relaxed, with all four feet on the ground
    (6) Tail is held on the horizontal or slightly higher
   b. Subordinance signaling
    (1) Gaze is averted
    (2) Mouth is closed
    (3) Ears and tail are lowered
    (4) The position of the head is lowered
    (5) The overall appearance of body is made to look smaller and nonthreatening
   c. Fearful signaling
    (1) Eyes are darting
    (2) Muzzle becomes loose
    (3) Teeth may be showing

   (4) Head is lowered
   (5) Ears are pulled back, drooping and loose
   (6) Tail hangs in a curve below the horizontal, but may be wagging slowly from side to side
   (7) Note: if the dog is in conflict then it may be showing teeth

II. Olfaction
 A. Dogs are justifiably credited with having the greatest olfactory acuity of any domesticated species
 B. Dogs will leave evidence of their presence (and other information) in a variety of ways, the most common being
  1. Feces, urine, and vaginal and anal sac secretions
  2. Interdigital glands, merocrine glands (pads), sebaceous glands (located on interdigital areas that are covered in hair)
  3. The scratching behavior of dogs while depositing their secretions probably serves two functions
   a. It may disperse the scent over a larger area
   b. It may be a visual display for other dogs in the area

III. Auditory
Auditory or vocal communication in dogs differs from visual and olfactory communication because it is effective over greater distances.

The language of dogs is complex and beyond the scope of this chapter. Karen Overall, in her book *Clinical Behavioral Medicine for Small Animals,* includes an excellent chapter on this topic. For this text we will discuss the following vocalizations used by dogs.
 A. Vocalizations used by dogs
  1. Whimpers and whines: neonatal puppies initially make a mewing sound that gradually progresses to a whimper or whine

**Table 14-2** Developmental stages of felines

| Stage | Age of commencement | Characterized by |
|---|---|---|
| Neonatal | Birth–2 wk | Total dependency |
| Transitional | 2-3 wk | Independence increases |
| | | *Critical period for socialization to humans* |
| Socialization | 3-14 wk | Social relationships |
| | 3 wk | Predatory behavior is taught |
| | 5 wk | Independent predatory behavior |
| | 3-6 wk | Socialization to other cats |
| | 7 wk | Weaning is complete |
| | 7-8 wk | Play with objects |
| | 3-12 wk | Social play (locomotory) |
| | 14+ wk | Social fighting |
| Juvenile | 14-36 wk | No significant changes |
| Adult | 36-52 wk | Continual learning |

From Overall K: *Clinical behavioral medicine for small animals,* St Louis, 1997, Mosby.

a. These sounds are generally considered to indicate need or friendly subordination
2. Growling indicates antagonistic intentions, and is used to signify a threat
3. Barking: this particular vocalization and its frequency of use may directly result from the domestication of the dog, because their wild counterparts do not bark as much
   a. Barks serve to draw attention or to indicate a threat
4. Howling: this is the sound that will travel the greatest distance; domestic dogs howl as a method of seeking attention or as a result of anxiety

## NORMAL FELINE BEHAVIOR

The behavioral development of felines is more complex than that of canines. The domestic cat is an exemplary predator, very territorial, and often falsely accused of being asocial. Individual cats will display a personality that reflects inheritance; specifically, a cat's temperament can be genetically linked to their sire.

### Behavioral Development

I. The developmental stages for cats are described in Table 14-2

### Social Development

Although cats may prefer solitude, they have a very complex social organization. The complexity of the social structure is maintained by effective communication among individuals, and therefore an individual cat's ability to learn and develop effective communication methods is critical to its social well-being. Cats use the same main methods of communication as the dog: visual, olfactory, and auditory.
  I. Vision and postural signaling (Figures 14-1 and 14-2)
    A. The visual capabilities of cats are excellent, the binocular field of view is approximately 120 to 130 degrees, and the monocular field is approximately 80 degrees for each eye
  B. Visual signaling and body posturing are best sent and received over short distances
    1. Eyes and pupils, ears, whiskers, mouth, head and neck, tail (action and position), coat hair, paws (scratching and clawing), and overall body presentation are all used
  C. Research demonstrates that many possible intentions/messages may be conveyed
  D. Some of the changes that occur may be subtle and go unnoticed by us; this often limits our ability to handle cats effectively
  E. Veterinary technicians should develop through observation and memory the ability to quickly gauge the intent of the feline patient
  F. The common posturing signals are:
    1. Friendly relaxed cat
      a. Shoulders and rump on same plane
      b. Tail is horizontal
      c. Hair smooth (no piloerection)
      d. Pupils normal for light conditions
      e. Ears erect
      f. Whiskers outwardly relaxed
    2. Offensive aggression
      a. Rump is elevated
      b. Head and neck are set
      c. Tail is down and hair is piloerected
      d. Pupils are constricted
      e. Pinnae of ears slightly pulled back
      f. Whiskers are tense and forward
    3. Defensive aggression
      a. Head and neck withdrawn to a tense body position (possibly crouching)
      b. Tail is tucked into body
      c. Pupils are dilated
      d. Ears are flattened
      e. Whiskers are flat

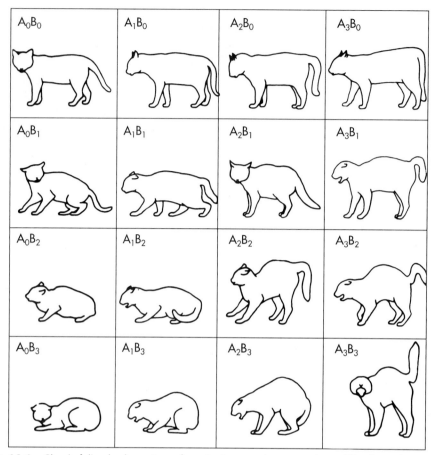

**Figure 14-1** Classic feline body postures from Leyhausen. Interpretations differ from the original, as noted in the text.

$A_0B_0$ represents the basic relaxed, copacetic cat that is monitoring the environment.

As one moves from $A_0B_0$ to $A_3B_0$ (across the X-axis), the cat is becoming more assertive, more confident, and more offensively aggressive. Note that even offensive aggression here is passive and is related more to eliciting deferential behavior than about actual combat. Note the fully extended hind legs, the elevated rump and piloerected tail, the set of the head and neck, and the ears that are slightly pulled back.

Moving from $A_0B_0$ to $A_0B_3$ (down the Y-axis), the cat is becoming more withdrawn, more avoidant of interaction, potentially more fearful, and more defensively aggressive. Aggression will ensue only when the cat can no longer escape.

The cat represented in $A_3B_3$ is exhibiting mixed signals and is in an extremely heightened state of reactivity. The tail is elevated, indicating that interaction is a possibility. The back is arched in a classic fearful posture (note that the back is also arched in $A_0B_3$, but the cat is lying down). The neck is tucked, and the underside of the neck and all teeth are exposed. Full disclosure is a signal that is used to diffuse an undesirable situation. The cat is signaling that he will stand his ground but will not overtly seek aggression unless pursued. It would be inappropriate to call either this posture or that portrayed in $A_0B_3$ as fearful aggression: whereas withdrawal is precluded in the latter, withdrawal and avoidance are the first choices of the former. Note that the cat portrayed in $A_3B_3$ is not confident like the cat in $A_3B_0$. The cat in $A_3B_0$ will back down any challengers and will pursue them if they do not back down; the cat in $A_2B_3$ would neither seek nor choose to interact with a challenger, given the choice. (From Overall K: Clinical behavioral medicine for small animals, St Louis, 1997, Mosby.)

II. Olfaction
   A. The domestic cat has retained the trait of being a solitary predator (i.e., it hunts alone)
   B. This is one of the reasons why cats have an excellent ability to deposit and discriminate scents
   C. The scents that are deposited tell other cats that the territory is claimed, and they do this without the stakeholder having to be present
   D. The scent will last a long time
   E. Scents are also deposited for individual and sexual identification, and in some instances they give

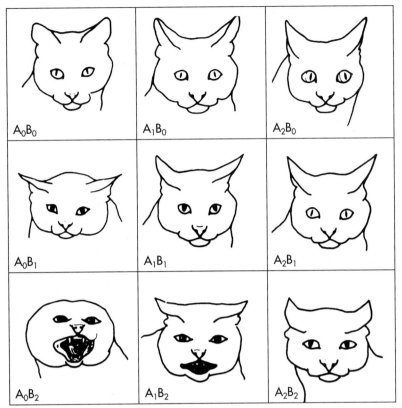

**Figure 14-2** The position of the ears, neck, head, plane of the shoulders, posture of the mouth and nares, and shape and size of the pupils are all important in feline communication.

$A_0B_0$ represents the relaxed cat that is monitoring the environment.

$A_2B_2$ represents a cat that is more offensively and assertively aggressive as represented by body posture $A_3B_0$ in Figure 14-1. Note the set neck and shoulders, slightly lowered head, movement of the pinnae, dilation of the nares, and clamping of mouth. This is a very confident and serious cat.

$A_2B_0$ represents a cat that is fearful and attempting to withdraw. This cat will avoid interaction if possible. Note the positioning of the eyes and the oblique (nondirect) gaze. The cat's ears are back but up, and his neck and head are more withdrawn than set and pushed forward, as in $A_2B_2$. This is the facial expression of the cat in $A_0B_3$ in Figure 14-1.

$A_0B_2$ represents a cat that will pursue aggression, but only as the last resort. Note that the neck, inside of the throat, and the teeth are all exposed, in contrast to $A_2B_2$. Note also that the pinnae are totally swiveled and everted. This is the facial expression of the cat in $A_3B_3$ in Figure 14-1. (Classic feline facial expressions from Leyhausen. Interpretations differ from the original, as noted in the text.) (From Overall K: *Clinical behavioral medicine for small animals*, St Louis, 1997, Mosby.)

the depositor information about that particular locale in the future

F. Cats are equipped with the specialized vomeronasal organ, which helps to receive and interpret scents

G. The common methods of depositing scents
1. Glands: face, flank, tail, and paw pads; sebaceous secretions from these regions are left on humans, other cats, and inanimate objects; scents are deposited in complex sequences, depending on message

H. The scratching deposits scent from the paws and has the added bonus of leaving the scratch marks as a visual cue for other cats

I. Middening: deposition of feces to convey information, generally used at the boundaries of a specific territory

J. Urine: males, females, neutered toms will all urine spray
1. It is either performed by backing up to an object and spraying, or by dispersing urine that was deposited through squatting
2. Information may be about the territory, the reproductive stage of an individual, and willingness to mate

III. Auditory
A. Moelk described the vocalization ability of cats in 1944

B. The names commonly attributed to the sounds are purr, murmur, growl, hiss, meow, and shriek, among others

C. Humans feign an understanding of the most blatant sounds (e.g., a shrieking cat that is being held against its will)

D. Three general categories as described by Bowen and Heath in *Behaviour Problems in Small Animals*

    1. Incite social interactions and amicable encounters

      a. Example: meow

    2. Interactions between mothers and kittens, play, and social interactions with owners

      a. Examples: purr, trill, and chirrup

    3. Strained intensity calls

      a. Examples: hiss, spit, growl, and snarl

## APPLIED ANIMAL BEHAVIOR

Animal behavioral problems are most often a case of mismanagement by humans, and as an increasing number of pet owners seek animal behavior education, we see a decreasing number of animal behavioral problems. Applied animal behavior relies on past and present studies that explain why animals do what they do and assists in applying the information in the context of the human-animal bond.

### Preventing Behavior Problems

Many things affect animal behavior: genetic predispositions, environment, experience and learning, and physiology. Ideally we would have the best of all of these when selecting and raising our companion dogs and cats; realistically we do not. However we do exert influence over most if not all of these factors.

I. Pet selection

  A. Veterinary technicians can be a useful resource for potential owners in selecting an appropriate pet

  B. Species traits

    1. Life span, physical traits, (e.g., long hair, size)

    2. Nutritional requirements

    3. Social needs

    4. Exercise and space requirements

    5. Health care requirements

  C. Owner requirements

    1. Strictly companion

    2. Working component (e.g., herding, guarding, tracking)

    3. Owner's and/or family's lifestyle

    4. Financial and time commitment

II. Pet acquisition

  A. With so many ways for potential owners to acquire pets, a reputable and trusted source should be used whenever possible

  B. The more information we have regarding the pet's genetics and early experiences and environment, the more effective we could be in handling behavioral problems that arise

III. Pet socialization and training

  A. Whether it is a dog or a cat, owners must be made aware of the anticipated development for that animal

  B. References should be given to the owner for both behavioral and social development

  C. Early identification and intervention are critical for the prevention of undesirable behaviors

  D. Many clinics, breeders, and qualified animal trainers offer puppy and kitten classes or series, where much of the needed information can be distributed, explained, demonstrated, and discussed

  E. The benefits of having an experienced individual observe the pet in a nonthreatening environment where conspecifics and owners are also present are invaluable

  F. There are many activities apart from formal obedience training that owners can participate in with their pets

  G. Such activities as agility competitions, fly ball, and animal-assisted therapy will all enhance the bond between animal and human and are lots of fun

IV. Pet health care

  A. Maintaining a healthy pet is a joint effort between the owner and the veterinary clinic

  B. The owner should be aware of the husbandry and disease prevention needs for their pet

  C. If the acquisition of the pet was unexpected and the history of the pet is unknown, then it is equally imperative that the pet be examined by a veterinarian and assessed for behavioral abnormalities

V. Intervention techniques

  A. Sometimes, despite our best efforts to prevent behavior problems, they will develop

  B. Veterinary technicians have a responsibility to act as a first line of defense for owners in recognizing and interpreting emerging behavior problems in their dog and/or cat

  C. A majority of these problems are common and nonthreatening to humans or other animals, and may be rectified using some simple training techniques to regain control or to modify the behavior

  D. In cases judged to be extreme, treatment should be supervised by a professional animal behaviorist; at all times, human safety is most important

  E. The steps and tools to employing effective intervention techniques are as follows:

1. Obtain a complete behavioral history, which includes but is not limited to:
   a. Family and lifestyle
   b. The pet
   c. The behavior problem
2. Family and lifestyle
   a. All aspects must be considered, including age of all family members, information on other or previous family pets, and who is primarily responsible for the pet in question
   b. The living space: the house/apartment, yards, and runs/cages
   c. Level of experience the family has with this species
   d. Any family members with disabilities
   e. The general environment of the neighboring spaces
   f. How many people come and go within the household
   g. How often the animal is left alone and for how long
3. The pet
   a. Signalment of pet, including age, sex (intact vs. neutered/spayed), weight, breed, origin, name
   b. Physical traits, such as information on how the pet spends its time
   c. Level of attention given to pet, level of exercise the pet receives, toys, where the pet sleeps, and restrictions in movement when visitors come
4. The behavior problem
   a. Generally if you ask the client to describe the most recent incident you will get very accurate results; as you ask them to recall previous incidents they will remember more details
   b. Everything is important: where it happened, who was there, what exactly happened, why it happened, when it happened, how often it happens
   c. The information must be highly specific, right down to the physical appearance of the animal when the incident occurred
      (1) Was the incident triggered by anything; have attempts been made to correct the behavior
      (2) If trigger is known, what has been done to correct it
   d. Rule out medical causes for the behavior by completing a physical exam and appropriate diagnostic tests
VI. Correcting the behavior
   A. Environmental modification

1. Examples:
   a. To remove or add an animal, conspecific, or other
   b. To remove or add an inanimate object
B. Physiological modification
   1. Examples:
      a. Neuter, spay
      b. Administer drugs to help modify behavior
         (1) Must be done under supervision of a licensed veterinarian, and to be most effective, in conjunction with other behavior modification techniques
C. Behavior modification using learning theory
   1. Operant conditioning
      a. A behavior that is followed by a pleasant stimulus (e.g., a food treat) increases the likelihood of that behavior being repeated
      b. The pleasant stimulus (e.g., food treat) must quickly follow the behavior, so that the animal will associate the two events; repetition of this method will strengthen the behavior once it is learned; intermittent reinforcement will result in a persistent response
   2. Negative reinforcement
      a. An increase in the frequency of a behavior when an aversive stimulus is avoided
      b. The aversive stimuli precedes the behavior and is withdrawn when the behavior is performed
   3. Negative punishment
      a. A decrease in the frequency of a behavior when a pleasant stimulus is removed
   4. Positive punishment
      a. An aversive stimulus is added to the situation immediately after a behavior is performed; its intent is to decrease the behavior that is being performed (e.g., electric shock is applied)
         (1) This is a poorly understood and ineffectively used method of training, because it teaches the animal only what not to do
   5. Shaping
      a. Occurs when an animal is performing a behavior in part or performs the prelude to a behavior, but it has only a small resemblance to the eventual desired behavior, because steps in the sequence are missing
         (1) When teaching a puppy to sit, initially the puppy will not sit square, but it is rewarded for this behavior anyway
         (2) Over time the puppy will begin to sit square

(3) Each time, the trainer rewards successive attempts that most approximate the desired form

b. Used for naturally occurring behaviors and must proceed in small steps

6. Extinction

a. It is considered an extreme form of negative punishment; it is when a behavior is performed and the reward is taken away or withheld

b. Initially, owners must be cautioned that the behavior may increase in intensity and frequency as the animal seeks the reward that previously reinforced the behavior

c. All individuals that have contact with the animal must be aware that this method is being employed

7. Counterconditioning

a. Conditioning an animal to engage in behavior that is incompatible with the desired behavior (e.g., a dog is taught to sit to prevent it from jumping up on visitors)

8. Systematic desensitization

a. This is the process of exposing an animal to a stimulus, beginning at an intensity that does not evoke the undesirable response, and gradually increasing the intensity in small increments so that the stimulus eventually loses its ability to evoke the undesirable response; often used with counterconditioning and most often used for behaviors that involve fear and anxiety

9. Habituation

a. Learning that involves no rewards

b. An animal is exposed to a stimulus and a behavior follows, but there is no consequence to the animal's response

c. The animal habituates to repeated exposure to the stimulus and eventually there is no response

# COMMON BEHAVIORAL PROBLEMS

## Canine

### Aggression

I. Aggression is the most common behavioral disorder in dogs; there are many forms of aggression that may be demonstrated

II. Some of the common types of aggression are: fear, territorial, redirected, food-related, possessive, play, interdog, predatory, dominance, pain, protective

III. Considerations for aggression in dogs:

A. Contributors to the different forms of aggression are genetics, environment, hormonal influences, and previously learned responses

B. Dogs may have more than one type of aggression

C. Obedience training may help by presenting opportunities to recognize early signs of aggression

D. Attempts to recognize and adhere to the behavioral developmental stages previously mentioned would aid in producing a well-adjusted dog

E. Avoiding the opportunity for the dog to express its aggression, regardless of cause, should be the first step

F. Aggression that is highly specific and isolated in time and place (e.g., maternal and intermale) may be managed by ovariohysterectomy and/or neutering

G. Behavior modification techniques should always constitute a large part of the management in cases of aggression, regardless of type

H. In cases of aggression towards humans (e.g., family members), it is important to remember that an aggressive dog does not have to be a dominant dog

I. Drug therapy as part of the treatment schedule should be considered and is often especially useful in the early treatment stages

J. Punishment is contraindicated in cases of aggression, and will escalate the problem if it is a case of dominance aggression

### Barking

I. Barking is normal canine behavior

II. Permitting excessive barking, whether in the owner's presence or not, is discouraged because the trigger for this behavior is multifaceted and the behavior may heighten or progress to other more destructive behaviors

III. Domestic dogs bark for many reasons, such as defending territory, soliciting play or social interaction, seeking attention, seeking food, and responding to anxiety, it may also be a conditioned behavior or result from cognitive dysfunction

IV. Considerations for barking in dogs

A. Determine exactly what triggers the barking behavior; there may be more than one trigger

B. Identify the stimuli that precede the behavior and prevent exposure to them

1. For example, children or small prey animals that cross the yard may trigger dogs with a view of the yard

C. Owners must be counseled that picking up the dog, cuddling the dog, talking soothingly to the dog, or anything that is perceived as a reinforcer must be avoided

D. Owners should be diligent in recognizing all opportunities to reward quiet behavior, and also to learn how to train the dog to respond to a command to stay quiet

E. Behavior modification techniques, such as desensitization and counter conditioning (as previously discussed), are useful tools for treating this particular behavior

F. Behavior modification aids, such as head halter devices, can be useful

G. Secondary levels of modification, such as electric shock collars, debarking, and drug treatment, should never be instituted unless extensive counseling has been sought

H. Debarking is not a cure-all; often the ability to bark is regained

### House Soiling

I. There are many reasons why a dog may urinate and/or defecate in the house

II. As previously mentioned, medical factors involved in behavioral problems must always be ruled out before embarking on any behavior modification program; this is especially true for suspect cases of house soiling where there may be an underlying urinary tract infection or an anatomical defect

III. Dogs may soil the house because of ineffective housebreaking, anxiety, need to mark territory, excitement, and excessive submission

IV. Considerations for dogs that house soil
   A. The chances of eliminating this behavior are excellent
   B. It must be determined if the presence of the owner is related to the behavior
      1. Territorial marking and incomplete housetraining are not related to the owner's presence
         a. In cases of separation anxiety, the behavior occurs when the owner is absent
         b. Excitement is generally associated with the owner's return
   C. Dogs that soil in the house as a result of ineffective training must be retrained
      1. Owner must learn to identify the body language of the dog before eliminations
      2. Dog should be on a schedule to go outside that reflects the eating and drinking schedule
      3. Dog should be taken outside after periods of play
      4. Dog should always be rewarded when it eliminates outside
      5. Do not punish the dog when it soils in the house
      6. Continual supervision is necessary until the appropriate behavior has been learned
   D. Dogs that soil the house for territorial reasons, usually intact males or females in estrus, should be
      1. Neutered or spayed respectively
      2. Prevented from experiencing the trigger that causes them to mark (e.g., other dogs outside)

3. Startled/distracted with aversive stimuli while in the process of marking,
   a. Do not make stimuli so aversive that it evokes fear; the dog must also not connect the stimuli with the owner
4. An appropriate place to mark should be provided, and a reward should be given every time it is used

E. Dogs that house soil as a result of separation anxiety must be treated for this underlying cause; this includes
   1. Desensitizing the dog to predeparture and departure cues
   2. Slowly getting the dog used to owner's absence
   3. Increasing the amount of exercise the dog receives
   4. Drug treatment may be beneficial early in the modification program
   5. Supervision may also be required in the early stages

## Feline

### Spraying

I. Unfortunately, spraying in felines is one of the most common complaints recorded by cat owners, because it is one of the most complex issues to rectify
   A. Many owners cannot persist when trying to eradicate this behavioral concern

II. Spraying is a normal cat behavior, because it marks the location to communicate with cats already present or cats that venture into that territory later

III. There is also a nonspraying marking behavior of cats
   A. Cats that spray demonstrate a fairly typical posture: they back up to a vertical surface, their tail is held high and they wiggle it at the tip as they spray urine onto the surface; often they will knead with their front paws

IV. Considerations for cats that spray
   A. Generally, vertical surfaces are sprayed, but cats have demonstrated this behavior on horizontal surfaces (e.g., in the middle of owner's bed)
   B. One location or a variety may be chosen
   C. More males than females will demonstrate this behavior
   D. Often, cats that cease this behavior will at some point begin again
   E. Social system of cats is complicated and therefore may be difficult to identify a single eliciting stimulus
   F. It will require modification at all three levels: environmental, behavioral, and pharmacological
   G. Spraying is a result of the cat's social environment

## Inappropriate Elimination

I. Inappropriate elimination must be distinguished from spraying before effective modification can begin

II. Inappropriate elimination is generally due to avoidance of the litter box, substrate, and surface preferences, and the attractiveness of an area away from the litter box

III. Considerations for cats that eliminate inappropriately
A. The litter box plays a pivotal role in this behavior; consider
1. Changing the style of the litter box
2. Changing the type of litter used
3. Keeping the litter box clean at all times
4. Avoiding odors that might be unpleasant to the cat
5. Having as many litter boxes as cats
B. The initial trigger for the behavior may be different than what maintains the behavior (e.g., a cat may learn a location preference)
C. Although extremely difficult to achieve, the undesirable locations used by the cat should be thoroughly clean and odor free
D. Try to put other items (e.g., food bowls, sleeping basket) in the areas that the cat has eliminated in
E. If this does not work, put an aversive smell in the area (e.g., mothballs, citrus scent)

## Scratching

I. Cats that scratch can by a highly divisive issue to many people; it is an innate behavior of cats and is performed to maintain the condition of the claws, deposit scent, leave visual evidence, and explore; they may also scratch during play

II. The quick fix to this problem is viewed as a simple surgical procedure—declawing
A. In many countries this is illegal, and the increasing destructiveness of this behavior presents a significant problem to many cat owners the world over

III. Considerations for cats that scratch
A. Owners need to be counseled that scratching is normal and that kittens will demonstrate this behavior; they should be provided with and encouraged to use a scratching post; to facilitate this
1. Provide more than one post
2. Position posts in prominent areas (e.g., sleeping quarters)
3. Place the kitten's toy on top of post
4. Reward the kitten whenever it approaches post
5. When replacing an old post, replace with the same type, because cats develop preferences

IV. Older cats that are destructively scratching the furniture should be retrained to use an appropriate scratching post; all of the above methods will apply

V. To prevent older cats from scratching the couch and other undesirable locations, try to place things that the cat finds undesirable (e.g., double sided tape, booby traps with noise makers) on these surfaces
A. Do not make any of these so aversive that they evoke fear

VI. Provide attention to the cat when it uses the scratching post in owner's presence

VII. If the owner is using aversive stimuli, then it must be applied in a way that prevents the cat from linking it with the owner

VIII. 100% supervision and dedicated behavior modification techniques must be present when the cat has free access in the house

IX. If supervision is not possible, the cat should be confined where the only acceptable scratching surface is a scratching post

X. Consider allowing the cat outside

XI. Claw sheaths and covers are available to minimize damage

XII. Declawing is an option that necessitates lengthy discussion with a veterinarian

## ACKNOWLEDGMENT

The editors and author recognize and appreciate the original work of Linda Campbell and Patricia Bonnot, on which this chapter is based.

# Glossary

**aggression** Angry and destructive behavior toward another animal or a human

**auditory** Pertaining to the ear or sense of hearing

**aversive** Unpleasant

**behavior modification** Use of various techniques to alter behavior

**conspecifics** Members of the same species

**counterconditioning** Technique used to change undesirable behavior by engaging the animal in a behavior that is different from the undesirable behavior

**extinction** Fading of a conditioned response as a result of nonreinforcement

**habituation technique** Disappearance of a conditioned reflex by repetition of the conditioned stimulus

**merocrine glands** Partly secreting; denoting a secretion where the gland remains intact while forming and discharging the scent

**negative reinforcement** Use of punishment to modify an existing response

**olfaction** The sense of smell

**operant conditioning** Type of learning in which a stimulus produces a response that is rewarded

**piloerection** Erection of hair

**positive reinforcement** Use of a reward to modify an existing response

**psychoactive drugs** Drugs that modify neurological activity

**shaping** Learning technique in which the animal is rewarded for behavior that resembles the desired behavior, and in gradual succession is eventually rewarded for only the exaggerated behavior

**signalment** The part of the patient history that deals with animal's age, sex, and breed

**socialization period** Critical age when young animals establish social relationships

**stereotypical behavior** Anxiety-related disorder, such as obsessive-compulsive disorder

**successive approximation** Consecutively reinforcing a close estimate of the desired behavior

**systematic desensitization** Gradual exposure to stimulus that elicits a response

# Review Questions

**1** What occurs when a behavior that has been previously reinforced is no longer reinforced?
   a. Positive punishment
   b. Negative punishment
   c. Flooding
   d. Extinction

**2** Negative reinforcement involves _____ when a particular behavior occurs
   a. Adding something pleasant
   b. Adding something unpleasant
   c. Subtracting something pleasant
   d. Subtracting something unpleasant

**3** At what age should traumatic experiences be avoided in dogs?
   a. 7 to 10 weeks
   b. The first 6 weeks of life
   c. 11 to 14 weeks
   d. Anytime between 6 and 16 weeks

**4** A hallmark that a dog is dominantly aggressive is
   a. It bites only the young children within the household
   b. Punishment of the dog will escalate the behavior
   c. It ceases the behavior in the absence of food
   d. All of the above

**5** The leading behavioral problem of dogs is
   a. Separation anxiety
   b. Fear of loud noises
   c. House soiling
   d. Aggression

**6** Canines may demonstrate excessive vocalization due to
   a. Play
   b. Separation anxiety
   c. Inherited drive
   d. All of the above

**7** If your cat is scratching destructively because of territorial marking behavior, then one of the best things to do is to
   a. Introduce a new kitten
   b. Keep other cats out of yard
   c. Let him/her mark the whole house first
   d. None of the above

**8** In an attempt to control destructive scratching behavior you should
   a. Place scratching posts away from where the cat sleeps
   b. Place scratching posts close to where the cat sleeps
   c. Scratching posts generally do not help modify this behavior
   d. None of the above

**9** Which of the following is an incorrect statement about cats that spray?
   a. The usual preference for this behavior is a vertical surface
   b. His/her behavior is a result of the social environment of the cat(s)
   c. Females do not demonstrate this behavior
   d. The cat may choose one location or several

**10** A cat that is in its carrier and is terrified to come out would not demonstrate the following
   a. Tail carried upright
   b. Pupils dilated
   c. Ears flattened
   d. Body crouched

## BIBLIOGRAPHY

Beaver V: *Feline behavior: a guide for veterinarians*, ed 2, St Louis, 2003, Saunders.

Borchelt PL: Cat elimination behavior problems, *Vet Clin North Am Small Anim Pract* 21:257, 1991.

Bowen J, Heath S: *Behaviour problems in small animals: practical advice for the veterinary team*, London, 2005, Saunders.

Burghardt WF: Behavioral medicine as a part of a comprehensive small animal medical program, *Vet Clin North Am Small Anim Pract* 21:343, 1991.

Campbell WE: *Behavior problems in dogs*, ed 3, Wenatchee, Wash, 2003, Dogwise Publishing.

Dunbar I: *Dog behavior: why dogs do what they do*, Neptune, NJ, 1979, TFH Publications.

Fox MW: *The dog: its domestication and behavior*, Malabar, Fla, 1978, Garland STPM Press.

Hart BK: *The behavior of domestic animals*, New York, 1985, WH Freeman and Company.

Hetts S: Animal behavior. In McCurnin DM, Bassert JM, editors: *Clinical textbook for veterinary technicians*, ed 6, St Louis, 2006, Saunders.

Jackson J, Anderson RK: *Early learning for puppies to socialize and promote good behavior*, London, Ontario, 1999, Professional Animal Behavior Associates.

Landsberg G, Hunthausen W, Ackerman L: *Handbook of behavior problems the dog and cat*, ed 2, London, 2004, Saunders.

Landsberg GM: Feline scratching and destruction and the effects of declawing, *Vet Clin North Am Small Anim Pract* 21:265, 1991.

Leyhausen P: *Cat behavior: the predatory and social behavior of domestic and wild cats*, New York, 1979, Garland.

Luesher WA, McKeown DB, Halip J: Stereotypic or obsessive-compulsive disorders in dogs and cats, *Vet Clin North Am Small Anim Pract* 21:401, 1991.

Moelk M: Vocalizing in the house cat: a phonetic and functional study, *Am J Psychol* 57:184, 1944.

Overall KL: *Clinical behavioral medicine for small animals*, St Louis, 1997, Mosby.

Pedersen NC: *Feline husbandry, disease and management in the multiple cat environment*, St Louis, 1991, Mosby.

Scott JP, Fuller JL: *Genetics and the social behavior of the dog*, Chicago, 1965, University of Chicago Press.

Thorne C, editor: *The Waltham book of dog and cat behavior*, New York, 1992, Pergamon Press.

## CHAPTER 15

# Small Animal Nutrition

*Frances Cheslo*

---

## OUTLINE

Basic Nutrition
Energy-Producing Nutrients
   Protein
   Carbohydrates
   Fats
Non–Energy-Producing Nutrients
   Water
   Minerals
   Vitamins
Daily Energy Requirements
   Feeding Methods

Nutritional Requirements for Each
   Life Stage of the Dog and Cat
   Gestation and Lactation
   Dogs
   Cats
Feline Lower Urinary Tract
   Disease
Obesity
Critical Care Nutrition
   Enteral Nutrition
   Parenteral Nutrition

Food Allergy or Intolerance
Oral Health
Canine Cancer
Renal Disease
How to Choose a Pet Food
Pet Food
   Pet Food Label
   Guaranteed Analysis
   Ingredient Panel
   Statement of Nutritional
     Adequacy

---

## LEARNING OUTCOMES

**After reading this chapter you should be able to:**

1. Explain the six basic nutrients and their role in supporting life.
2. Understand and calculate a companion animal's maintenance energy requirements based on its particular life stage.
3. Explain why different nutrient levels change with each life stage and what effects excesses or deficiencies may have.
4. Identify key factors that can prevent or help manage FLUTD.
5. Identify, understand, and assist in the management and/or prevention of an obese cat or dog.
6. Understand the role of nutritional management in the aid of the critically ill patient.
7. Identify and describe the various components of a pet food label.
8. Understand the necessary information required to help pet owners make an educated decision of which pet food to feed their animal.
9. Understand a technician's role as a source of information for pet owners about small animal nutrition.
10. Understand and communicate the nutritional options in the management of oral health, canine cancer, and renal disease.

---

The most commonly asked question of a veterinary technician is, "What should I feed my pet?" This chapter will allow a veterinary technician to properly and confidently counsel clients about the dietary requirements of their pets. The importance of small animal nutrition in health management has become increasingly recognized by the veterinary profession. The veterinary technician must be knowledgeable about the commonly used pet foods purchased by the hospital's clients to appropriately respond to questions.

## BASIC NUTRITION

To understand what food is best for a companion animal, one must first understand what nutrients are required by the body for each life stage. A basic understanding of the following six nutrients is essential in discussing small animal nutrition.

## ENERGY-PRODUCING NUTRIENTS ▄▄▄▄▄▄

### Protein

I. Made up of 23 amino acids, the building blocks of proteins
  A. Essential amino acids
    1. Must be present in the food to manufacture a protein
    2. Cats specifically require taurine in their diet
      a. Taurine deficiency could result in dilated cardiomyopathy, retinal atrophy, or infertility
  B. Nonessential amino acids
    1. Amino acids that the animal can manufacture if not available in the body
    2. Dogs can synthesize 10 amino acids; cats can synthesize 11 amino acids
II. Constituent of muscle, hair, blood, organs, etc.; forms hormones and enzymes
III. Excess protein will be burned for energy and can provide 4 kcal/g if energy not obtained from carbohydrates or fat
IV. Only after protein has been used for building body tissues and facilitating certain hormonal processes and other body functions will it be used for energy
  A. This use of protein for energy is less efficient versus energy derived from fats or carbohydrates
V. Biological value
  A. Evaluates protein usability by the body
  B. Relationship between percent of nutrients digested, absorbed, and retained to the percent of nutrients lost
  C. The greater number of essential amino acids in a protein, the greater its biological value and quality
VI. Animal and plant proteins vary in their composition of essential amino acids
  A. Reciprocally, a combination of both sources of protein in a diet can be complementary and result in a higher biological value
VII. Cats are carnivores and have a higher protein requirement than dogs, because they use a certain amount of protein for energy

### Carbohydrates

I. Primary function is for energy
  A. Carbohydrates provide 4 kcal/g, same as protein; however, there are no nitrogenous end products as in protein catabolism
II. Made up of carbon, hydrogen, and oxygen chains
III. Two categories, based on digestibility
  A. Soluble: digestible carbohydrates primarily composed of monosaccharides and disaccharides, such as glucose and sugar beet

1. They supply calories to a diet and can be used immediately for energy
  B. Insoluble: indigestible carbohydrates, primarily composed of polysaccharides, such as starch, lignin, and peanut hulls (fiber)
    1. The portion of a plant that resists digestion and can provide satiety and bulk to a diet
IV. Digested through the digestive tract
  A. Often used in the management of constipation and diarrhea because of their ability to absorb water, stimulate intestinal contractions, and normalize intestinal transit time
V. Fiber and other insoluble carbohydrates aid in regulating blood glucose levels, which is often recommended in managing diabetes
VI. Fiber is also used in pet foods to increase bulk and promote satiety during periods of weight loss and weight control
VII. Body uses carbohydrates primarily in the form of glucose
  A. If not used, carbohydrates are stored as glycogen in the muscle or liver or as body fat

### Fats

I. Provide the most concentrated source of energy at 9 kcal/g of fat
II. Enhance palatability and caloric density of pet foods
III. Required by the fat-soluble vitamins A, D, E, and K for absorption, transportation, and storage
IV. Essential fatty acids (EFAs)
  A. Building blocks of fat
  B. Classified as saturated and unsaturated
    1. Saturated: long carbon chains without a double bond
    2. Unsaturated: one or more double bonds
  C. Essential for maintaining skin and coat
  D. Required for the synthesis of cell membranes, prostaglandins, and sex hormones
  E. Three EFAs are required for normal metabolism
    1. Linoleic acid
    2. Arachidonic acid
    3. Linolenic acid
  F. Dogs require linoleic and linolenic acids in their diet. Although one can be reconstructed from the other, the body's ability to facilitate availability requires a difficult synthetic pathway; therefore both are deemed as essential
  G. Cats require dietary linoleic and arachidonic acids
V. Important in temperature regulation, protection of internal organs, and immune system function
VI. Fatty acid deficiency could cause dermatological problems as well as impair wound healing

VII. Increased dietary fat requirements usually occur during periods of growth, lactation, or increased physical activity

VIII. Excess fat consumption could result in weight gain or obesity if not monitored, and diarrhea or steatorrhea (fatty stools) due to the body's inability to digest or absorb excess fat

## NON–ENERGY-PRODUCING NUTRIENTS

### Water

I. Most essential nutrient required by the body for survival
   A. Needed for almost all body metabolic processes

II. Total daily water requirements equal daily energy requirements in a thermoneutral environment

III. Requirements will vary depending on such factors as environmental temperature, physical activity, metabolism, diet, lactation, and illness

IV. Water makes up approximately 70% of adult body weight

V. Grave illness or death could result if as little as 10% of body water is lost

VI. Essential for absorption of water-soluble vitamins B complex and C

VII. Animals obtain water from metabolic processes or, more important, through ingestion by drinking or eating

VIII. Quantity of water in pet foods varies
   A. Dry kibble: 10% to 12%
   B. Semimoist: 25% to 40%
   C. Canned: 72% to 82%

IX. Animals eating canned food appear to drink less water because they obtain a large portion of daily water requirements from their diet

X. Fresh water must be available at all times
   A. This point must be emphasized to pet owners, especially for dogs housed outside in the winter where there is a risk of water freezing

### Minerals

I. Although the total percent of minerals in the body is less than 1%, they are essential for metabolic processes to take place

II. Macrominerals
   A. Dietary requirements expressed in percentages (%)
   B. Examples: calcium, phosphorus, potassium, sodium, magnesium
   C. Aid in maintaining electrolyte and water balance, skeletal integrity, muscle and nerve conduction, and cellular function

III. Microminerals
   A. Dietary requirements expressed in parts per million (ppm)
   B. Also known as trace minerals
   C. Examples: iron, copper, zinc, iodine

   D. Involved in the majority of biochemical reactions in the body

IV. A close interrelationship exists between minerals
   A. Any excess of one or more minerals could result in the deficiency of others, owing to lack of absorption or imbalance

V. Mineral supplementation is contraindicated if a high-quality, balanced diet is provided

VI. Minerals have many functions; any deficiencies or excesses could be harmful to an animal, as shown in Table 15-1

### Vitamins

I. Function as enzymes, coenzymes, and enzyme precursors

II. Classified by solubility
   A. Water soluble
      1. B complex and C
      2. None stored in the body
      3. Deficiency may occur during periods of excessive water loss, such as polyuria, diarrhea, or gastrointestinal disorders that may alter microfloral populations
         a. Supplementation is recommended during these periods
   B. Fat soluble
      1. A, D, E, and K
      2. Stored in fat or liver
      3. Excesses could be toxic

III. Cats have specific vitamin requirements that dogs do not
   A. In their diet, they require preformed vitamin A, which is found in the highest constituency in animal tissue
   B. Cats also require the B vitamin niacin because they cannot convert tryptophan, an amino acid, to niacin

IV. Dogs can convert beta-carotene derived from plant sources to vitamin A, which is a characteristic of omnivores; cats cannot

V. Vitamin E also functions as an antioxidant, but the amount decreases as the fat is oxidized

VI. Vitamin functions, deficiencies, and possible toxicities are described in Table 15-2

## DAILY ENERGY REQUIREMENTS

How much to feed is as important as what to feed, to ensure that an animal is getting the correct amount and type of food based on its age and lifestyle. Factors that could influence daily energy requirements include growth, lactation, stress, physical exertion, breed, environmental conditions, and age

### Feeding Methods

I. Free choice
   A. Food is available at all times and the animal determines when and how much to eat

**Table 15-1** Mineral functions and effects of deficiency and excess

| Function | Deficiency | Excess |
|---|---|---|
| **CALCIUM** | | |
| Constituent of bone and teeth, blood clotting, myocardial function, nerve transmission, membrane permeability | Decreased growth, decreased appetite, decreased bone mineralization, lameness, spontaneous fractures, loose teeth, tetany, convulsions, rickets (osteomalacia—adults) | Decreased feed efficiency, decreased feed intake, nephrosis, calcium urate stones, lameness, enlarged costochondral junctions |
| **PHOSPHORUS** | | |
| Constituent of bone and teeth; muscle formation; fat, carbohydrate, and protein metabolism; phospholipids and energy production; reproduction | Diminished appetite, decreased feed efficiency, decreased growth, dull hair coat, decreased fertility, spontaneous fractures, rickets | Bone loss, urinary calculi, decreased weight gain, decreased feed intake, calcification of soft tissues, secondary hyperparathyroidism |
| **POTASSIUM** | | |
| Muscle contractility, transmission of nerve impulses, acid-base balance, osmotic balance, enzyme cofactor (energy transfer) | Anorexia, decreased growth, lethargy, locomotive problems, hypokalemia, heart and kidney lesions, emaciation | Rare |
| **SODIUM AND CHLORIDE** | | |
| Osmotic pressure, acid-base balance, transmission of nerve impulses, nutrient uptake, waste excretion, water metabolism | Inability to maintain water balance, decreased growth, anorexia, fatigue, exhaustion, dryness/loss of hair | Occurs only if there is inadequate nonsaline, good quality water available. Causes thirst, pruritus, constipation, seizures, and death. Chronic amounts may induce hypertension resulting in increased heart and renal diseases |
| **MAGNESIUM** | | |
| Component of bone, intracellular fluids, neuromuscular transmission, active component of several enzymes, carbohydrate and lipid metabolism | Muscular weakness, hyperirritability, convulsions, anorexia, vomiting, decreased mineralization of bone, decreased body weight, calcification of aorta | Urinary calculi |
| **IRON** | | |
| Enzyme constituent: activation of $O_2$ (oxidases, oxygenases), $O_2$ transport (hemoglobin, myoglobin) | Anemia, rough hair coat, listless, decreased growth | Anorexia, weight loss, decreased serum albumin |
| **ZINC** | | |
| Constituent or activator of 200 known enzymes (nucleic acid metabolism, protein synthesis, carbohydrate metabolism), skin and wound healing, immune response, fetal development, growth rate | Anorexia, decreased growth, alopecia, parakeratosis, impaired reproduction, vomiting, hair depigmentation, conjunctivitis | Relatively atoxic. Reported cases of Zn toxicity from consumption of die-case Zn nuts |

**Table 15-1** Mineral functions and effects of deficiency and excess—cont'd

| Function | Deficiency | Excess |
|---|---|---|
| **COPPER** | | |
| Component of several enzymes (e.g., oxidases), catalyst in hemoglobin formation, cardiac function, cellular respiration, connective tissue development, pigmentation, bone formation, myelin formation, immune function | Anemia, decreased growth, hair depigmentation, bone lesions, neuromuscular, enzootic ataxia, aortic rupture, reproductive failure | Hepatitis, increased liver enzymes |
| **MANGANESE** | | |
| Component and activator of enzymes (glycosyl transferases), lipid and carbohydrate metabolism, bone development (organic matrix), reproduction, cell membrane integrity (mitochondria) | Impaired reproduction, perosis (poultry), fatty livers, crooked legs, decreased growth | Relatively atoxic |
| **SELENIUM** | | |
| Constituent of glutathione peroxidase and iodothyronine 5'-deiodinase, immune function, reproduction | Muscular dystrophy, reproductive failure, decreased feed intake, subcutaneous edema, renal mineralization | Vomiting, spasms, staggered gait, salivation, decreased appetite, dyspnea, "garlicky" breath |
| **IODINE** | | |
| Constituent of thyroxine and triiodothyronine | Goiter, fetal resorption, rough hair coat, enlarged thyroid glands, alopecia, apathy, myxedema, lethargy | Similar to deficiency. Decreased appetite, listlessness, rough hair coat, decreased immunity, decreased weight gain, goiter, fever |
| **BORON** | | |
| Regulates parathormone action, therefore influences metabolism of Ca, P, Mg, and cholecalciferol | Decreased growth, decreased hematocrit, hemoglobin, and alkaline phosphatase | Similar to deficiency. 150-200 ppm maximum tolerated level |
| **CHROMIUM** | | |
| Potentiates insulin action, therefore improves glucose tolerance | Impaired glucose tolerance, increased serum triglycerides and cholesterol | 1000 mg/day is maximum tolerated level in cats; trivalent form less toxic than hexavalent |

Courtesy Dr. Karen Wedekind, Mark Morris Institute.

B. Advantages
 1. Good for pets that will eat to meet their energy requirements and do not overeat
 2. Recommended method during lactation
 3. Most convenient method for pet owners
C. Disadvantages
 1. Difficult to monitor the pet's consumption, and anorexia may not be noticed immediately
 2. May lead to obesity
 3. Nutritional excesses due to overeating
 4. Economics

II. Time-restricted meal feeding
 A. Unquantified amount of food is available for the pet for a certain period of time, usually anywhere from 10 to 30 minutes
 B. Ideal choice in a multipet household where different diets must be fed
 C. This method can be repeated more than once a day
III. Food-restricted meal feeding
 A. Specific quantity of food offered at specific times during the day

**Table 15-2** Vitamin functions and the effects of deficiency and toxicity

| Function | Deficiency | Toxicity |
|---|---|---|
| **FAT SOLUBLE** | | |
| **Vitamin A** | | |
| Component of visual proteins<br>Differentiation of epithelial cells<br>Spermatogenesis<br>Immune function<br>Bone resorption | Anorexia<br>Retarded growth<br>Poor hair coat<br>Weakness<br>Increased cerebrospinal fluid pressure<br>Aspermatogenesis<br>Fetal resorption<br>Requirement may increase in acute<br>  infection because of urine loss (dog) | Cervical spondylosis (cat)<br>Tooth loss (cat)<br>Retarded growth<br>Anorexia<br>Erythema<br>Long bone fractures |
| **Vitamin D** | | |
| Calcium and phosphorus<br>  homeostasis<br>Bone mineralization | Rickets<br>Osteomalacia<br>Osteoporosis<br>Bone resorption<br>Insulin synthesis<br>Immune function | Hypercalcemia<br>Calcinosis<br>Anorexia<br>Lameness |
| **Vitamin E** | | |
| Biological antioxidant<br>Membrane integrity through<br>  free radical scavenging | Sterility (males)<br>Dermatosis<br>Immunodeficiency<br>Anorexia<br>Myopathy | Minimally toxic<br>Increased clotting time: reversed<br>  with vitamin K |
| **Vitamin K** | | |
| Allows blood clotting protein<br>  formation | Prolonged clotting time<br>Hypoprothrombinemia<br>Hemorrhage | Minimally toxic<br>Anemia (dog)<br>None described for the cat |
| **WATER SOLUBLE** | | |
| **Thiamine ($B_1$)** | | |
| Nervous system | Anorexia<br>Weight loss<br>Ataxia<br>Ventral flexion (cat)<br>Paresis (dog)<br>Cardiac hypertrophy (dog)<br>Bradycardia | Decreased blood pressure<br>Bradycardia<br>Respiratory arrhythmia<br>None described for the cat |
| **Riboflavin ($B_2$)** | | |
| Electron transport in oxidase<br>  and dehydrogenase enzymes | Retarded growth<br>Ataxia<br>Collapse syndrome (dogs)<br>Dermatitis<br>Purulent ocular discharge<br>Vomition<br>Conjunctivitis<br>Coma<br>Corneal vascularization<br>Bradycardia<br>Fatty liver (cat) | Minimally toxic<br>None described for cat and dog |

**Table 15-2** Vitamin functions and the effects of deficiency and toxicity—cont'd

| Function | Deficiency | Toxicity |
|---|---|---|
| **Niacin (B₃)** | | |
| Component of energy-producing biochemical reactions | Anorexia<br>Diarrhea<br>Retarded growth<br>Ulceration of soft palate and buccal mucosa<br>Necrosis of the tongue (dog)<br>Reddened ulcerated tongue (cat)<br>Uncontrolled drooling | Low toxicity<br>Bloody feces<br>Convulsions<br>Death<br>None described for the cat |
| **Pyridoxine (B₆)** | | |
| Neurotransmitter synthesis<br>Niacin synthesis from tryptophan<br>Taurine synthesis<br>Carnitine synthesis | Anorexia<br>Retarded growth<br>Weight loss<br>Microcytic hypochromic anemia<br>Convulsive seizures<br>Renal tubular atrophy, and deposits of calcium oxalate crystals (cat) | Low toxicity<br>Anorexia<br>Ataxia (dog)<br>None described for the cat |
| **Pantothenic acid** | | |
| Protein, fat, and carbohydrate metabolism in the TCA cycle<br>Cholesterol synthesis<br>Triglyceride synthesis | Emaciation<br>Fatty liver<br>Depressed growth<br>Decreased serum cholesterol and total lipids<br>Tachycardia<br>Coma<br>Lowered antibody response | Toxicity is negligible<br>No toxicity described in dog or cat |
| **Folic acid** | | |
| Purine synthesis<br>DNA synthesis | Anorexia<br>Weight loss<br>Leukopenia<br>Hypochromic anemia<br>Increased clotting time<br>Elevated plasma iron<br>Megaloblastic anemia (cat)<br>Sulfa drugs interfere with gut synthesis | Nontoxic |
| **Biotin** | | |
| Component of four carboxylase enzymes | Hyperkeratosis<br>Alopecia (cats)<br>Dry secretions around eyes, nose, and mouth (cat)<br>Hypersalivation<br>Anorexia<br>Bloody diarrhea | No toxicity described in dog or cat |
| **Vitamin C** | | |
| Synthesized from D-glucose in the liver<br>Synthesis of collagen proteins and carnitine<br>Enhances iron absorption<br>Free radical scavenging<br>Biological antioxidant | Liver synthesis precludes dietary requirement, therefore no deficiency symptoms have been described in normal cat and dog | No toxicity described in dog or cat |

*Continued*

**Table 15-2**    Vitamin functions and the effects of deficiency and toxicity—cont'd

| Function | Deficiency | Toxicity |
|---|---|---|
| *Choline* | | |
| Component membranes and neurotransmitter | Fatty liver (puppies)<br>Thymus atrophy<br>Decreased growth rate<br>Anorexia | No toxicity described for dog and cat |
| **QUASI-VITAMIN** | | |
| *Carnitine* | | |
| Transport of long-chain fatty acids into the mitochondria of the cell | Hyperlipidemia<br>Cardiomyopathy<br>Muscle asthenia | No toxicity described for dog and cat |

**Table 15-3**    Calculations for maintenance of energy requirements

| RESTING ENERGY REQUIREMENTS (RER) | | |
|---|---|---|
| $70 \times \text{Weight (kg)}^{0.75}$ or $30 \times (\text{Weight in kg}) + 70$ | | |
| **MAINTENANCE ENERGY REQUIREMENTS (MER)** | | |
| *Canine Feeding Guide* | | |
| Puppies | < 4 months of age<br>> 4 months of age | $3 \times \text{RER}$<br>$2 \times \text{RER}$ |
| Adult | | $1.6 \times \text{RER}$ |
| Senior | | $1.4 \times \text{RER}$ |
| Weight Prevention | | $1.4 \times \text{RER}$ |
| Weight Loss | | $1.0 \times \text{RER}$ |
| Gestation (last 21 days) | | $3 \times \text{RER}$ |
| Lactation | | 4 to $8 \times \text{RER}$ |
| *Feline Feeding Guide* | | |
| Kittens | | $2.5 \times \text{RER}$ |
| Adult | | $1.2 \times \text{RER}$ |
| Weight Prevention | | $1.0 \times \text{RER}$ |
| Weight Loss | | $0.8 \times \text{RER}$ |
| Breeding | | $1.6 \times \text{RER}$ |
| Gestation (gradual increase) | | $2 \times \text{RER}$ |
| Lactation | | $2\text{-}6 \times \text{RER}$ |

Courtesy Hill's Pet Nutrition, Inc.

B. Beneficial for animals that have a digestive disorder where small frequent meals are more tolerable
C. Recommended method for canine breeds prone to gastric dilatation/volvulus (GDV) and for diabetic pets
D. Can still meet desirable growth with this method
E. Best feeding method

IV. Maintenance energy requirement (MER) calculations in Table 15-3 are intended as a starting point and should be adjusted as necessary, based on body condition and lifestyle of the pet
 A. Owners can follow the feeding guidelines on a pet food label as a starting point

## NUTRITIONAL REQUIREMENTS FOR EACH LIFE STAGE OF THE DOG AND CAT

Nutritional requirements vary greatly between each life stage, and proper nutrition will result in a happier, healthier pet over its lifetime.

### Gestation and Lactation

 I. Nutrition is as important before breeding as it is during gestation and lactation
 A. Poor nutrition could result in low birth weight or increased risk of neonatal mortality
 II. Nutritional requirements of a pregnant bitch or queen toward the end of gestation and during lactation are similar to those of a neonate (see Table 15-4 for specific requirements)
 III. Period to begin transition to a high-quality, highly digestible growth diet should be during the last 3 to 4 weeks of gestation in the bitch, and from the second week of gestation in the queen
 IV. It is important to calculate maintenance energy requirements at this stage to ensure that adequate nutrients are being consumed, especially during lactation
 V. Cats begin to gain weight in a linear fashion from the beginning of their pregnancy; dogs have the most weight gain during the last 3 to 4 weeks of gestation
 VI. Offering small frequent meals is the method of choice for dogs; free-choice feeding is recommended for cats

VII. Because of their ability to store and use fat for energy needs, cats tend to eat less postpartum but soon regain their appetite by the third week

VIII. Fresh water should be available at all times

IX. After weaning, the cat or dog should be gradually transitioned back to a good-quality, highly digestible maintenance diet

X. New research suggests the addition of docosahexaenoic acid (DHA), an omega-3 fatty acid, in the food to help in brain, vision, and central nervous system development in the womb

## Dogs

### Young Dogs

I. Neonates and puppies
  A. Neonates should be encouraged to nurse vigorously after birth to ingest colostrum
  B. Colostrum is a special milk that contains maternal antibodies; it is produced within the first 24 to 48 hours after parturition
    1. Colostrum is vital for the neonate, because it provides a passive immunity
  C. After the crucial first 24 to 48 hours, the composition of the bitch's milk begins to change and becomes more complete, to provide all the nutrients that the growing neonate requires until weaning
  D. Nursing should be observed at least four to six times a day
  E. Milk provides all the essential nutrients for growth, and the fluids consumed help to increase the body's total circulatory volume
  F. Neonates should be weighed daily for the first 2 weeks to ensure adequate growth; normal stool should also be observed
    1. Puppies should gain 2 to 4 g/day/kg or 1 to 2 g/day/lb of anticipated adult body weight. Puppies not achieving this growth curve should be closely monitored
  G. Commercial milk replacers are necessary only when supplementing weak or premature neonates, orphans, or large litters, or when a dam is unable to produce sufficient milk

II. Weaning
  A. Should begin at approximately 3 weeks of age, but can be as early as 10 to 14 days if necessary
  B. Commercially available high-quality growth diet should be prepared by blending the diet with water to form a thick, soupy, gruel mixture
    1. This should be offered to puppies three or four times a day
  C. Initially, puppies will walk and play in the food instead of eating it; but it will be ingested as the pups lick each other during play
  D. Puppies should be totally weaned and be eating only a moistened dry or canned growth diet by 5 to 7 weeks for large breeds and 6 to 8 weeks for small breeds
  E. Cow's milk should not be offered because the lactose content is greater than the bitch's milk, and diarrhea and dehydration could result

III. Growth
  A. Growth diet should be fed from weaning until the puppy achieves skeletal maturity, or about 12 months
  B. Characteristics of a growth diet
    1. Palatable
    2. High digestibility, quality, and increased caloric density (this would decrease dietary consumption and stool volume)
    3. Optimum calcium/phosphorus ratio, approximately 1.2:1
    4. New research suggests the addition of DHA, an omega-3 fatty acid, helps in brain, vision, and central nervous system development
  C. Maintenance energy requirements should be calculated for growth (see Table 15-3)
  D. Puppies should be weighed and evaluated every 2 weeks, using body condition scoring as described in Box 15-1, which is the best way to determine whether the amount being offered is optimal
    1. Pet behavior can also indicate whether more or less food is desired
  E. Nutritional characteristics of a growth diet are found in Table 15-4

IV. Feeding large-breed puppies
  A. Most common problem is overfeeding and supplementation, which can result in increased incidence of obesity, hip dysplasia, and osteochondrosis
  B. Excesses or deficiencies in a diet can affect musculoskeletal development
  C. Calcium excesses
    1. Calcium alone is often the offending mineral and not an imbalance with the calcium/phosphorus ratio
    2. The dog may become hypophosphatemic as well as hypercalcemic
    3. May cause retarded bone volume, bone modeling, and cartilage maturation
  D. Recommended levels of calcium are 1% to 1.6% on a dry matter basis
  E. Vitamin D is required in large-breed puppies because
    1. It regulates calcium metabolism and aids in the absorption of calcium and phosphorus
    2. It increases bone cell activity
  F. Food-restricted meal feeding is recommended for large breed puppies based on their MER

## Box 15-1　Body Condition Scoring

**BODY SCORE 1—VERY THIN**
Ribs are easily palpable with no fat cover. Tailbase* has a prominent raised bony structure with no tissue between skin and bone. Bone prominences are easily felt with no overlying fat. In animals older than 6 months, there is a severe abdominal tuck when viewed from the side and an accentuated hourglass shape when viewed from above.

**BODY SCORE 2—UNDERWEIGHT**
Ribs are easily palpable with minimal fat cover. Tailbase* has a raised bony structure with little tissue between skin and bone. Bony prominences are easily felt with minimal overlying fat. In animals older than 6 months, there is an abdominal tuck when viewed from the side and marked hourglass shape when viewed from above.

**BODY SCORE 3—IDEAL**
Ribs are palpable with a slight fat cover. Tailbase* has a smooth contour or some thickening and bony structure is palpable under a thin layer of fat between skin and bone. Bony prominences are easily felt with a slight amount of overlying fat. In animals older than 6 months, there is an abdominal tuck when viewed from the side and a well-proportioned lumbar waist when viewed from above.

**BODY SCORE 4—OVERWEIGHT**
Ribs are difficult to feel with moderate fat cover. Tailbase* has some thickening with moderate amounts of tissue between skin and bone. Bony structures can still be felt. Bony prominences are covered by a moderate layer of fat. In animals older than 6 months, there is little or no abdominal tuck or waist when viewed from the side and the back is slightly broadened when viewed from above. Abdominal fat apron present in cats.

**BODY SCORE 5—OBESE**
Ribs are difficult to feel under a thick fat cover. Tailbase* appears thickened and is difficult to feel under a prominent layer of fat. Bony prominences are covered by a moderate to thick layer of fat. In animals older than 6 months, there is a pendulous ventral bulge and no waist when viewed from the side. The back is markedly broadened when viewed from above. Marked abdominal fat apron present in cats.

*Tailbase evaluation is done only in dogs.

G. A growth diet of poor-quality, cheap, and less calorie-dense food, could result in
   1. Poor appearance
   2. Inferior development
   3. Increased incidence of disease
   4. Overeating in an effort to meet caloric needs
   5. Increase in risk of obesity
   6. Higher stool volume
H. Added L-carnitine increases lean body mass and bone mass and density during growth of large breed puppies. It may also decrease the risk of obesity
I. Goal of feeding large-breed puppies is to decrease the growth rate but still reach the dog's genetic potential at maturity

## Adult Dogs

I. Adult maintenance: lifestyle of the adult dog will determine its nutritional needs
   A. Adulthood ranges from approximately 1 to 7 years, depending on size of the dog
      1. Smaller breeds mature at an earlier age than larger breeds, but they also age slower
   B. Diet and feeding methods should be reviewed with the pet owner; body condition score should be recorded as the dog enters adulthood
   C. Supplementing with treats or table scraps should be discouraged; or, if given, they should not exceed 10% of total energy requirements
      1. Treats can be made from the regular diet as described in Box 15-2, but the quantity per feeding should be adjusted accordingly
II. Active adult dog
   A. Dogs that require increased caloric energy, such as hunting, working, show, and guide dogs, or toy breeds that eat small amounts of food frequently
   B. Increasing a maintenance diet is not always sufficient, because caloric needs may surpass ability to consume the appropriate volume of food (known as bulk limiting)
   C. Offering a highly digestible, calorically dense food that is higher in fat is recommended
   D. If caloric demand is seasonal, such as in hunting or field trial dogs, a transitional period should take place anywhere from 7 days to 3 weeks before the event, with any physical conditioning of the dog
   E. Small frequent meals and fresh water should be offered to avoid dehydration, hypoglycemia, and bingeing due to hunger

## Geriatric Dogs

I. Small breeds begin their geriatric years at about age 7; large and giant breeds begin around age 5
II. Visual, behavioral, and physiological changes begin
   A. Decreased activity level
   B. Cataracts
   C. Graying muzzle

**Table 15-4** Life stage nutritional requirements

| | Protein | Fat | Crude Fiber | Calcium | Phosphorus | Sodium | Chloride | Potassium | Magnesium | Energy | Vitamin E |
|---|---|---|---|---|---|---|---|---|---|---|---|
| **DOG FOOD RECOMMENDATIONS** | | | | | | | | | | | |
| *MMI Recommendations* | | | | | | | | | | | |
| Adult maintenance | 15-30 | 10-20 | 5 max | 0.5-1.0 | 0.4-0.9 | 0.2-0.4 | 0.3-0.6 | 0.4-0.8 | 0.04-0.15 | 3.5-4.5 | 450-1000 |
| Growth (BW < 25 kg) | 22-32 | 10-25 | 5 max | 0.7-1.7 | 0.6-0.3 | 0.3-0.6 | 0.4-0.8 | 0.6-0.9 | 0.04-0.20 | 3.5-4.5 | 450-1000 |
| Growth (BW > 25 kg) | 20-32 | 8-12 | 10 max | 0.7-1.2 | 0.6-1.1 | 0.3-0.6 | 0.4-0.8 | 0.6-0.9 | 0.04-0.20 | 3.0-4.0 | 450-1000 |
| Older | 15-32 | 7-15 | 10 max | 0.5-1.0 | 0.25-0.75 | 0.15-0.35 | 0.3-0.5 | 0.4-0.8 | 0.04-0.15 | 3.0-4.0 | 700-1500 |
| Obesity-prone adult | 15-30 | 7-12 | 5-16 | 0.5-1.0 | 0.4-0.9 | 0.2-0.4 | 0.3-0.6 | 0.4-0.8 | 0.04-0.15 | 3.0-3.5 | 450-1000 |
| High energy | 22-34 | 15 min | 5 max | 0.6-1.0 | 0.4-0.9 | 0.2-0.5 | 0.3-0.6 | 0.45-0.9 | 0.05-0.20 | >4.5 | 450-1000 |
| Gestation/lactation | 22-35 | 10-25 | 5 max | 0.75-1.7 | 0.6-1.3 | 0.35-0.6 | 0.5-0.9 | 0.6-0.9 | 0.04-0.20 | 3.5-5.0 | 450-1000 |
| *AAFCO Nutrient Profiles for Dog Foods* | | | | | | | | | | | |
| AAFCO growth/reproduction | 22 min | 8 min | — | 1.0-2.5 | 0.8-1.6 | 0.3 min | 0.45 min | 0.6 min | 0.04-0.3 | 3.5-4.0 | 50-1000 |
| AAFCO maintenance | 18 min | 5 min | — | 0.6-2.5 | 0.5-1.6 | 0.06 min | 0.09 min | 0.6 min | 0.04-0.3 | 3.5-4.0 | 50-1000 |
| *Common Commercial Dog Foods* | | | | | | | | | | | |
| Average moist grocery (30) | 41 | 27 | 1.8 | 1.7 | 1.4 | 0.9 | 1.1 | 1.1 | 0.11 | 4.5 | Na |
| Average dry grocery (32) | 25 | 12 | 3.1 | 1.4 | 1 | 0.4 | 0.7 | 0.7 | 0.14 | 3.9 | 108 |
| Average dry specialty (93) | 28 | 16 | 3.3 | 1.3 | 1 | 0.4 | 0.7 | 0.7 | 0.12 | 4.2 | 200 |
| Average moist specialty (39) | 32 | 22 | 2.1 | 1.2 | 0.9 | 0.5 | 0.9 | 0.9 | 0.1 | 4.4 | Na |
| **CAT FOOD RECOMMENDATIONS** | | | | | | | | | | | |
| *MMI Recommendations* | | | | | | | | | | | |
| Adult maintenance | 30-45 | 10-30 | 5 max | 0.5-1.0 | 0.5-0.8 | 0.2-0.6 | 0.3 min | 0.6-1.0 | 0.04-0.1 | 4.0-5.0 | 550-1000 |
| Growth | 35-50 | 18-35 | 5 max | 0.8-1.6 | 0.6-1.4 | 0.3-0.6 | 0.45 min | 0.6-1.2 | 0.08-0.15 | 4.0-5.0 | 550-1000 |
| Obesity-prone adult | 30-45 | 8-17 | 5-15 | 0.5-1.0 | 0.5-0.9 | 0.2-0.6 | 0.3 min | 0.6-1.0 | 0.04-0.1 | 3.3-3.8 | 550-1000 |
| Older | 30-45 | 10-25 | 10 max | 0.6-1.0 | 0.5-0.7 | 0.2-0.5 | 0.3 min | 0.6-1.0 | 0.05-0.1 | 3.5-4.5 | 550-1000 |
| Gestation/lactation | 35-50 | 18-35 | 5 max | 0.5-1.0 | 0.5-0.9 | 0.2-0.6 | 0.45 min | 0.6-1.2 | 0.08-0.15 | 4.0-5.0 | 550-1000 |
| *AAFCO Nutrient Profiles for Cat Foods* | | | | | | | | | | | |
| AAFCO growth/reproduction | 30 min | 9 min | — | 1.0 min | 0.8 min | 0.2 min | 0.3 min | 0.6 min | 0.08 min | 4.0-4.5 | 30 min |
| AAFCO maintenance | 26 min | 9 min | — | 0.6 min | 0.5 min | 0.2 min | 0.3 min | 0.6 min | 0.04 min | 4.0-4.5 | 30 min |
| *Common Commercial Cat Foods* | | | | | | | | | | | |
| Average moist grocery (34) | 51 | 27 | 1.5 | 1.8 | 1.5 | 0.9 | 1.3 | 1.1 | 0.09 | 4.3 | Na |
| Average dry grocery (26) | 35 | 12 | 2.2 | 1.3 | 1.2 | 0.4 | 0.8 | 0.7 | 0.12 | 3.8 | 102 |
| Average dry specialty (42) | 35 | 18.5 | 2.4 | 1.1 | 0.95 | 0.5 | 0.7 | 0.7 | 0.09 | 4.3 | 249 |
| Average moist specialty (35) | 26 | 28 | 1.9 | 1.1 | 1 | 0.5 | 1 | 0.9 | 0.1 | 4.7 | Na |

Courtesy Dr. Philip Roudebush, Mark Morris Institute.
Nutrients are expressed as percent dry matter. Energy is expressed as kcal ME (metabolizable energy) per gram dry matter. Vitamin E is expressed as IU/kg dry matter.
Nutrient levels of commercial foods are based on averages of manufacturer's published values or analyticals.
AAFCO nutrient profiles presume 3.5 kcal ME/g in dog food and 4.0 kcal/g in cat food. Levels should be corrected for higher energy density.
*AAFCO*, Association of American Feed Control Officials; *BW*, body weight; *max*, maximum; *min*, minimum; *MMI*, Mark Morris Institute.

---

**Box 15-2** Homemade Treats

**CANNED FOOD**
1. Cut canned food into bite-sized pieces.
2. Place in the microwave on high for 2 to 3 minutes, or bake at 350° F for approximately 25 to 30 minutes until desired texture is reached.
3. Allow to cool before offering to pet, or refrigerate.

**DRY FOOD**
1. Grind kibbles into a flour.
2. Mix enough water to form a dough and shape into cookies.
3. Bake at 350° F on cookie sheet for 25 to 30 minutes until crispy.
4. Allow to cool; refrigerate unused portion.

---

D. Internally, organs cannot tolerate nutrient excesses or deficiencies as before
E. Stiffness; difficulty getting up and climbing stairs
F. Cognitive dysfunction (age-related behavioral changes), such as disorientation, house soiling accidents, changes in interactions with other pets and people, change in sleep patterns
III. Reevaluate the dog's diet and lifestyle with the pet owner. It is important that pet owners understand an aging pet's changing nutritional requirements
IV. Maintenance energy requirements should be recalculated for the geriatric patient (see Table 15-3)
V. Characteristics of a geriatric diet should include
  A. Reduced fat and calories to avoid weight gain
  B. Decreased sodium, protein, and phosphorus, which reduces workload on the cardiovascular system and kidneys
  C. Increased EFAs and zinc for skin and coat
  D. Increased fiber, which slows intestinal transit time, improves nutrient absorption, and regulates bowel movements
  E. Increased palatability and digestibility to compensate for decreases in olfactory senses and appetite
  F. Increased levels of key antioxidants that support brain function and decrease free radical production
    1. Addition of DL-alpha-lipoic acid in the diet can help manage age-related behavioral changes
  G. High levels of omega-3 fatty acids, specifically EPA (eicosapentaenoic acid), found in fish oil
    1. Helps improve clinical signs associated with osteoarthritis
    2. Helps protect cells from free radical damage along with DHA, by supporting cell membrane integrity

VI. Elevated protein quality is crucial when dietary protein restriction is recommended
VII. Owners should be encouraged to continue a daily exercise regimen to maintain muscle tone and circulation
VIII. Avoid supplementing with high-sodium treats and high-fat table scraps
IX. Complete physical examination by the veterinarian should be performed, including oral cavity and dental examination, baseline biochemistry panel, and urinalysis to ensure proper functioning of the internal organs

## Cats

I. Cats are true carnivores; they possess typical dietary characteristics of other carnivores
  A. A cat's protein requirements are much higher than a dog's, because cats catabolize protein for energy
    1. Dogs (omnivores) primarily use fats or carbohydrates
  B. Require two amino acids in their diet: arginine and taurine
  C. Require arachidonic acid (EFA) because, like other carnivores, cats cannot synthesize it from linoleic acid
  D. Require vitamins niacin, pyridoxine (vitamin $B_6$), and preformed vitamin A, of which the two former are found in animal tissue

## Kittens

I. Care and management for kittens are similar to the care and management for puppies
II. Kittens should be observed nursing vigorously after birth to ensure they receive colostrum
III. They should be weighed daily for the first 2 weeks of life and should gain approximately 90 to 100 g (3 oz) per week, which basically means doubling their birth weight
IV. Nutrient requirements of the kitten can be reviewed in Table 15-4
V. A good-quality, highly digestible kitten food can be introduced at approximately 3 weeks of age (in the same fashion as for puppies)
  A. Kittens may not accept the slurry, so offering canned or dry food without water is acceptable
VI. Kittens should be free-choice fed during growth
VII. Kittens should be weaned between 8 and 10 weeks of age, but not earlier than 6 weeks

## Adult Cats

I. Cats by nature are nibblers, but their MER should be calculated and the appropriate amount be left available throughout the day or divided into frequent meals

II. Providing a cat with a premium quality, highly digestible, calorically dense diet will reduce the risk of disease, such as feline lower urinary tract disease (FLUTD)

III. It is important that cat owners understand the phrase, "cats aren't born finicky, they are made finicky"

IV. Consistency is important to avoid behavioral problems or to prevent problems with a cat that is a finicky eater

### Geriatric Cats

I. Cats enter their senior years at approximately 6 years

II. Less information is available about nutritional and physiological changes that occur in aging cats

III. Geriatric work-up should be done to verify organ function and oral health

IV. Most dietary recommendations for cats are based on research on rats, dogs, or humans

V. Lower urinary tract disease and urolithiasis are uncommon in geriatric cats; however, calcium oxalate urolithiasis is more common in older cats

VI. Nutritional requirements for geriatric felines can be viewed in Table 15-4

## FELINE LOWER URINARY TRACT DISEASE

This disease can be frustrating and potentially devastating for cat owners. Prevention is the most important information a veterinary technician can relay to owners.

I. From 1% to 6% of feline cases seen in a veterinary hospital are reported to be due to FLUTD

    A. Incidence of new cases is approximately 0.5% to 1.0% per year

II. Exact etiology of FLUTD has not yet been determined

    A. Cause could be multifactorial but is commonly related to urolithiasis, viral urinary tract infections, or inherited, genital, or acquired disorders

III. Clinical signs include

    A. Dysuria

    B. Hematuria

    C. Pollakiuria

    D. Urethral obstruction

    E. Inappropriate urination (urinating outside the litter box)

    F. Frequent squatting in the litter box

    G. Loss of appetite

IV. Risk factors associated with FLUTD are described in Box 15-3

V. The importance of dietary management with follow-up urinalyses and radiographs must be emphasized to the cat owner to reduce risk of recurrence

VI. Incidence and mineral composition of the most common feline uroliths can be found in Table 15-5

---

**Box 15-3** Some Risk Factors Reported in Cats with Lower Urinary Tract Disease

**AGE**
Uncommon in cats younger than 1 year. Most common between 1 and 10 years, with peak between 2 and 6 years

**SEX**
Urethral obstruction most common in males. Males and females have a similar risk for nonobstructive forms of the disease

**NEUTERING**
Increased risk of disease in neutered males and females, regardless of age of neutering

**DIET**
Consumption of an increased proportion of dry food in the daily ration is associated with increased risk of disease

**FEEDING FREQUENCY**
Increased frequency of feeding associated with increased risk of disease, regardless of diet

**EXCESSIVE WEIGHT**
Obesity associated with increased risk of disease

**WATER CONSUMPTION**
Decreased daily water consumption associated with increased risk for disease

**SEDENTARY LIFESTYLE**
Lazy cats at increased risk of disease

**SPRING OR WINTER SEASON**
Seasonal variation implicated as a risk factor by some investigators, but not others

**INDOOR LIFESTYLE**
Cats using indoor litter boxes for micturition and defecation have increased risk for disease

---

## OBESITY

A veterinary technician has a vital role in helping clients manage and understand obesity in pets. Client education is the key to successful management and, more important, prevention of this condition.

I. Approximately 25% to 44% of companion animals are obese

II. An obese animal is one that weighs more than 20% of its ideal body weight

III. An overweight animal is one that weighs more than 10% of its ideal body weight

IV. The first objective in helping clients deal with this situation is making the pet owner aware that the dog or cat is obese

    A. Pet owner should also be aware of risk factors involved

**Table 15-5**   Mineral composition for 9221 feline uroliths analyzed at the Minnesota Urolith Center in 2005*

| Predominant mineral type | Number of uroliths | % |
|---|---|---|
| Magnesium ammonium phosphate·6H$_2$O | 4435 | 48.10 |
| Magnesium hydrogen phosphate·3H$_2$O | 5 | 0.05 |
| Magnesium phosphate hydrate | 28 | 0.30 |
| Calcium oxalate | 3744 | 40.60 |
| Calcium phosphate | 28 | 0.30 |
| Purines (urate, xanthine) | 428 | 4.64 |
| Cystine | 2 | 0.02 |
| Silica | 7 | 0.08 |
| Other | 9 | 0.10 |
| Urea | 0 | 0.00 |
| Mixed[†] | 81 | 0.88 |
| Compound[‡] | 378 | 4.10 |
| Matrix | 76 | 0.82 |
| Drug metabolite | 0 | 0.00 |
| Total 1/1/05-12/31/05 | 9221 | 100.00 |

Courtesy Dr. Carl A. Osborne, Minnesota Urolith Center, University of Minnesota.
*Uroliths analyzed by polarizing light microscopy and infrared spectroscopic methods. Uroliths composed of 70% to 100% of mineral type listed, no nucleus and shell detected.
[†]Uroliths did not contain at least 70% of mineral type listed; no nucleus or shell detected.
[‡]Uroliths contained an identifiable nucleus and one or more surrounding layers of a different mineral type.

       1. Risk factors can include diabetes mellitus, neoplasia, hypertension, dermatosis, joint disorders, and bacterial and viral infections

V.   In cats, obesity can increase the risk of feline hepatic lipidosis and urinary tract disease

VI.   The veterinary technician can counsel clients about
    A. Benefits of weight loss, including increased activity, health, longevity, and alertness of their companion animal
    B. Identifying any inappropriate feeding behavior that could have been the cause of obesity
    C. Modifying any inappropriate feeding behavior of the pet and the pet owner
    D. Obtaining entire household cooperation and understanding of the pet's situation
       1. This should result in a successful weight loss program

VII.   Another goal of a weight loss program other than having the pet lose weight is to start the pet on an exercise regimen that will improve cardiovascular conditioning and skeletal support

VIII.   Goals should be realistic and achievable to be successful

    A. Subgoals are recommended so that pet owners can see early benefits of their hard work, providing reinforcement to continue until the goal weight is achieved

IX.   Before beginning any weight loss program for a pet, a complete physical examination by the veterinarian should be performed to rule out any medical cause for the obesity
    A. If any illness is identified, it should be treated before a weight loss program is initiated

X.   Determine the ideal weight of the patient and the required kilocalories per day for the patient to achieve that weight. Calorie restriction should be approximately 60% to 70% of the pet's maintenance energy requirements (see Table 15-3)

XI.   Ideal rate of weight loss
    A. Cats: 0.25 lb/wk (115 g)
    B. Small dogs: 0.5 lb/wk (230 g)
    C. Medium-size dogs: 1.0 lb/wk (500 g)
    D. Large dogs: 1.5 lb/wk (750 g)

XII.   Charting weight loss is a useful tool for clients to see the success of their efforts

XIII.   Dogs should be weighed monthly; cats should be weighed bimonthly

XIV.   Have scheduled weigh-in periods in your hospital
    A. Post a chart on all patients involved in a weight loss program
    B. Plan weekly meetings that allow pet owners to discuss with other owners how their pets are doing
       1. Ensure that clients use a standard 8-oz measuring cup to measure out daily food requirements
       2. Place one day's food in a separate container to avoid accidental overfeeding
       3. Any family member can feed the pet from the daily allowance storage container or remove a few kibbles to use as a treat
       4. Once empty, the container should not be refilled until the next morning
       5. Divide the daily allowance into several meals for the most efficient weight loss
       6. Keep your pet in another room when preparing or eating your own meals
       7. Offer only recommended low-fat treats
    C. Competition tends to encourage pet owners to stick with the program and your recommendations
    D. Cat owners should be cautioned about too quick a weight loss, because cats can develop hepatic lipidosis

XV.   Feeding small, frequent meals throughout the day reduces begging

XVI. Acceptable treats while on a reducing diet include ice cubes; ice chips; low-calorie vegetables, such as carrots or celery; or homemade treats made from a portion of the prescribed diet, as described in Box 15-2.

XVII. Recording a cat's or dog's body condition score (see Box 15-1) throughout its life is the best way to prevent obesity or to identify it in a new client

XVIII. Characteristics of a weight loss food
A. High in fiber and low in fat and calories, which is an option for both cats and dogs
B. High in protein and low in carbohydrates, which is a relatively new option for cats only. This option helps alter the cat's metabolism, promoting weight loss
C. Addition of high levels of L-carnitine
1. >300 ppm (DMB) for dogs, and >500 ppm (DMB) for cats
2. Helps convert fat into energy
3. Helps maintain lean muscle mass during weight loss by ensuring that the energy is fat and not protein

XIX. The Association of American Feed Control Officials (AAFCO) regulates use of terms for the calorie and fat content
A. On a pet food label, manufactures may use such terms as lite, low calorie, weight control, reduced calorie, and reduced fat
1. Be aware that these products may in fact be higher in calories and fat, and may cause weight gain in pets that should be maintaining or losing weight
B. AAFCO guidelines indicate that only products that meet the following ME/kg can use the term *light* on their label
1. Dog foods: 3100 kcal ME/kg (dry), 900 kcal ME/kg (canned)
2. Cat foods: 3250 kcal ME/kg (dry), 950 kcal ME/kg (canned)
3. You can feel confident recommending or endorsing any pet food that claims it is light on the label

## CRITICAL CARE NUTRITION

The need for nutritional therapy is emerging as an important factor in treating critically ill patients.

I. Trauma, disease, sepsis, and stress will increase an animal's metabolism, therefore increasing its energy requirements

II. Protein-energy malnutrition may deplete energy stores, inhibit wound healing, and affect pulmonary, cardiovascular, and gastrointestinal function

III. The body eats 24 hours a day, regardless of whether the gut is fed

IV. After a patient is identified as requiring nutritional therapy, the simplest method for administering it should be chosen

## Enteral Nutrition

I. Coaxing: warming the food, feeding by hand, etc.
II. Drugs can be used as an appetite stimulant
III. Force feeding by syringe
IV. Orogastric intubation
V. Nasogastric/nasoesophageal intubation
VI. Esophagostomy tube feeding
VII. Gastrostomy tube feeding
VIII. Enterostomy tube feeding

## Parenteral Nutrition

I. Direct intravenous infusion with basic constituents of dextrose, crystalline amino acids, and lipid emulsion

II. Option if enteral nutrition is unsuccessful or contraindicated

III. Calculating illness energy requirements (IER)
A. MER is rarely met if pet is in a debilitated state
B. Canine IER = 1.25 to 1.50 × MER
C. Feline IER = 1.10 to 1.25 × MER

IV. If the diet chosen is tolerated, the product should be introduced gradually
A. Suggested guidelines
1. One third total calories on day 1
2. Two thirds of the total on day 2
3. Total calories on day 3
B. If human products are used, nutritional supplementation is required

## FOOD ALLERGY OR INTOLERANCE

Cats and dogs may exhibit abnormal responses to the food or food additives they ingest. These responses could manifest as gastrointestinal or dermatological signs.

I. Antigenic responses occur at the highest level when food is ingested

II. Clinical cases related to food allergy or food intolerance have been poorly documented or reported

III. Risk factors
A. Specific foods or ingredients
B. Proteins that are not easily digested
C. Any disease that affects intestinal mucosal permeability
D. Breed
E. Age: less than 1 year
F. Concurrent immunological disease

IV. Adverse food reactions could be
A. Immunological: allergy
B. Nonimmunological: intolerance

V. Common food allergens reported in North America
A. For cats: beef, dairy products, fish

B. For dogs: beef, dairy products, wheat, lamb, chicken egg, chicken, soy

VI. Protein (glycoprotein) is often the nutrient of concern in adverse reactions to food

VII. Factors that contribute to a food reaction
   A. Previous exposure to the protein or offending nutrient
   B. Number of different protein sources found in the pet's diet
   C. Digestibility of the protein: poor-quality protein
   D. Protein level

VIII. Identifying the food allergen is key to managing or preventing recurrence
   A. Elimination diet trials can be used for identification of allergens

IX. Trial period should be approximately 4 to 10 weeks

X. A complete diet history, including homemade foods and treats, must be obtained from the pet owner

XI. Ideal elimination diet
   A. Contains a limited number of novel protein sources or a protein hydrolysate
      1. Hydrolyzation breaks down the protein into tiny molecules
      2. Hydrolyzed protein goes undetected by the animal's immune system, avoiding an allergic reaction, but is used by the animal
   B. Highly digestible
   C. Avoids protein excess
   D. Avoids additives
   E. Nutritionally balanced for the animal's life stage and body condition score
   F. Avoid treats, supplements, toys, other food sources, chewable medications during trial
   G. Have clients maintain a diet log during the trial, and ensure that everyone in the household follows the strict regimen

XII. If no clinical improvement is evident after the trial period, then something other than food must be the cause of the animal's clinical signs

XIII. If clinical signs do improve, reintroduce original diet or individual proteins, one at a time, to monitor for a recurrence in the signs

XIV. If a food allergy or intolerance is identified, the veterinary technician can now find a commercially prepared, nutritionally balanced diet that does not contain the offending nutrient or ingredient

XV. Protein hydrolysate diets are an excellent option as both an elimination diet and a long-term maintenance diet
   A. Potential for an adverse food reaction is significantly reduced, because the body's immune system does not recognize the protein as an allergen (if the protein's molecular weight is less than 10,000 daltons)

## ORAL HEALTH

As discussed in Chapter 26, home care is key to prevention of oral disease. Daily brushing is the ideal, but pets aren't always compliant and neither are their owners. Feeding a food specially created to prevent and/or remove plaque and tartar (calculus) is extremely beneficial to the oral health of your patients.

I. Goal is to control plaque and tartar buildup

II. Nutrition plays a key role in maintaining oral health along with daily brushing

III. Characteristics of an oral health diet should include
   A. Veterinary Oral Health Council (VOHC) seal of approval on the bag
      1. VOHC was established in 1997 to recognize and establish preset standards of plaque and tartar prevention in cats and dogs
      2. Daily use of diets or treats carrying the VOHC seal will reduce the severity of periodontal disease
      3. For a list of VOHC approved products, visit www.vohc.org
   B. Larger kibble that resists crumbling and has mechanical cleaning properties
   C. Addition of sodium hexametaphosphate (HMP) for dogs and sodium polyphosphate for cats
      1. Deters calcium deposition on teeth, thereby preventing tartar formation
      2. Plaque leads to gingivitis and periodontal disease
      3. Limiting tartar formation through the use of HMP or polyphosphate does not prevent dental disease, but it may slow it down
   D. Prevention of plaque is key to preventing dental disease, because plaque can lead to gingivitis and periodontal disease without tartar formation

## CANINE CANCER

Nutrition can have a very beneficial role in helping manage dogs with cancer, while improving their quality of life.

I. Dogs with cancer undergo changes in their metabolism that could be managed through proper nutrition

II. Nutritional support helps in the healing process, may decrease side effects of chemotherapy, and prolong the disease-free state and survival time

III. Characteristics of a cancer diet should include the following:
   A. Low carbohydrate, high fat, additional omega-3 fatty acids, and arginine to help manage metabolic changes
   B. Tumor cells use carbohydrates for energy, so a food with limited carbohydrates may reduce tumor formation

C. Cancer cachexia can be avoided by feeding a higher fat diet. As well, tumor cells cannot use fat as efficiently as carbohydrates for growth

D. Added fish oil, which supplies specific omega-3 fatty acids, DHA and EPA, may inhibit tumor formation and enhance immune function

E. Owing to altered protein metabolism and increased risk of cachexia, protein levels should be significantly higher than for healthy dogs
   1. Dietary protein should be between 30% to 45% on a dry matter basis

## RENAL DISEASE

Chronic renal disease (CRD) is progressive and can affect patients of any age, but primarily it is diagnosed in older pets

I. Nutrition can play a very important role in helping manage the clinical signs associated with CRD, as well as reduce uremic episodes, reduce mortality, and improve quality of life

II. Characteristics of a renal diet should include the following:
   A. Reduced protein and phosphorus to help slow the progression of the disease and reduce the clinical signs
   B. Increased levels of omega-3 fatty acids and lower sodium to improve blood flow to the kidneys
   C. Lower sodium and chloride to reduce renal hypertension
   D. Increased buffering capacity to counteract the effects of metabolic acidosis
   E. New research indicates that renal diets supplemented with antioxidants may be beneficial to cats with renal disease by reducing blood urea nitrogen level

III. With advanced renal failure, it is sometime difficult to get the patients to eat

IV. Ways to encourage eating include
   A. Offering a canned alternative
   B. Warming the food to room temperature
   C. Feeding small, frequent meals
   D. Serving it in a different dish or in a different room
   E. Offering the food by hand and showing patience and encouragement

## HOW TO CHOOSE A PET FOOD

I. Pet owners often seek knowledge and guidance from a member of the veterinary health care team about the best diet for their companion animal

II. It is important to be familiar with premium pet foods sold in the area, as well as products sold or endorsed by the hospital

III. Remember that the pet food label will never truly reflect the quality or nutritional value of its contents

**Table 15-6** Calculating daily feeding costs

| Step | Description | Diet A | Diet B |
|------|-------------|--------|--------|
| A | Cost per 40-lb bag (640 oz) | $29.00 | $45.00 |
| B | Cost per pound of diet (A/40) | $0.73 | $1.13 |
| C | Cost per ounce (B/16 oz) | $0.05 | $0.07 |
| D | Ounces/cup (by weighing one cup of food) | 3.5 oz | 3 oz |
| E | Feeding amounts in ounces/day (based on maintenance energy requirement or feeding guide on bag) | 17.5 oz (5 cups) | 7.5 oz (2.5 cups) |
| F | Days bag will last (640 oz bag/E) | 37 | 85 |
| G | Cost per day (C × E) | $0.79 | $0.53 |
| H | Cost per year (G × 365 days) | $289.43 | $135.00 |

IV. Calculating the daily feeding cost (Table 15-6) is beneficial when comparing a poor-quality, low-density product with a premium-quality, calorically dense product
   A. Often the cost per day is less for the premium food, and the food lasts longer because of the caloric density and digestibility

## PET FOOD

### Pet Food Label

I. A pet food label should include
   A. Product name
   B. Designation: cat or dog food
   C. Net weight
   D. Name and address of manufacturer
   E. Guaranteed analysis
   F. Ingredient panel
   G. Nutritional adequacy statement or purpose of product
   H. Feeding guidelines
   I. Date of manufacture or expiration code

II. In Canada, Consumer Packaging and Labelling Act and Regulations dictate that only product identity, product net quantity, dealer's name, and principal place of business be on the label

III. In the United States, regulation is by the Food and Drug Administration, Department of Agriculture
   A. U.S. law dictates that the following must be on the label: product name, designator, net weight, ingredients, guaranteed analysis, nutritional adequacy statement, feeding guide, and manufacturer or distributor

---

**Box 15-4** How to Calculate the Dry Weight Analysis

**GUARANTEED ANALYSIS FROM CAN**
Water 75%
Protein 10%
Other dry matter 15%

**CALCULATION OF DRY WEIGHT ANALYSIS**
1. Dry matter % = 100% − % moisture
   = 100% − 75% = 25%
2. % Nutrient ÷ % dry matter × 100
   EXAMPLE: Protein = 10/25 = 0.4 × 100 = 40% protein

**THUS DRY WEIGHT ANALYSIS IS**
Protein 40%
Other dry matter 60%

---

IV. American Association of Feed Control Officials (AAFCO) is an association established by animal feed control officials as a regulating body to develop standards for uniformity of definitions, policies for manufacturing, labeling, distribution, and sale of animal feeds

V. National Research Council (NRC) is a nonprofit organization that was the recognized authority for substantiation of pet food claims for nutrient requirements before 1990

## Guaranteed Analysis

I. Guaranteed analysis (GA) provides minimum or maximum percentages of certain nutrients that the manufacturer claims the product meets

II. The following nutrients are required to be on the GA. Other nutrients added to the label are at the discretion of the manufacturer
  A. Crude protein: expressed as minimum %
  B. Crude fat: expressed as minimum %
  C. Crude fiber: expressed as maximum %
  D. Moisture: expressed as maximum %

III. Crude: term used to describe the analytical procedure used to estimate the nutrients

IV. GA should not be used to compare products, because values indicated do not reflect exact amounts, only minimums or maximums of a nutrient

V. GA also includes the moisture content of the product; therefore the nutrient value indicated is diluted in moisture, so a canned food may appear to have a lower percent of nutrients than a dry product because of the amount of water

VI. Dry weight analysis
  A. Approximate percent of a nutrient based on dry matter of the product
  B. Converting nutrients to dry matter allows for a more accurate comparison of products with different moisture levels (Box 15-4).

C. Manufacturers should provide nutrients listed on a dry matter basis (DMB) for comparison and accurate values

## Ingredient Panel

I. Listed in descending order by weight, beginning with heaviest ingredient

II. Ingredients with a high water content will appear higher on the panel, even if they are of poor nutrient value, than one with less water content

III. Terms used must be common in the feed industry or be assigned by AAFCO

IV. Manufacturers can alter ingredients so that a more desirable ingredient will appear higher on the ingredient panel

V. The same ingredient may be described in various forms, such as wheat broken down into wheat middling, cracked wheat, whole wheat, and flaked wheat
  A. This can make an ingredient appear to be in smaller quantities in the diet, even though, when combined, it forms a large percentage of the diet

VI. AAFCO determines what is meant by terms such as meat byproducts, but it is difficult to know what ingredients were actually used, unless one contacts the manufacturer directly
  A. Meat byproduct could be anything, such as liver, lungs, udders, or tongues

VII. Ingredient panel should not be used as a mode of comparison, because two ingredient panels could be identical and there is no way to determine the quality or digestibility of the ingredients that each manufacturer uses

VIII. Formulas can be fixed or variable
  A. Fixed formula: every bag purchased has the same ingredients as the previous
    1. Products in this category tend to be of higher quality and more expensive and have more digestible ingredients
  B. Variable formula: ingredients may change from batch to batch based on ingredient availability and market price

## Statement of Nutritional Adequacy

I. AAFCO established guidelines that U.S. manufacturers attempt to meet for nutrient profiles for cats and dogs (see Table 15-4)

II. "Complete and balanced" refers to a diet that contains all essential nutrients in concentrations that are proportional to the energy density of the food

III. Nutritional adequacy statements are based on feeding trials, such as that of AAFCO or through a calculation method

IV. Veterinary technicians should recommend products that have undergone feeding trials

V. Statements about meeting or exceeding standards without feeding trials are based on a chemical analysis and do not verify the digestibility or true adequacy of a product. Statements help determine if the product is for a specific purpose, as in "Complete and balanced for puppies," or all purpose, as in "Meets the requirements for the life of your cat"

   A. A product with the latter statement on it could have nutrient deficiencies or excesses for a particular life stage, because it was formulated for every life stage

VI. Snacks, treats, and therapeutic diets do not require nutritional statements

# Glossary

**AAFCO** American Association of Feeding Control Officials, the regulating body of pet food manufacturers in the United States

**aspermatogenesis** Inability to form male gametes (sperm)

**ataxia** Incoordination or wobbliness

**calcinosis** A condition that results in calcium deposits in any soft tissue in the body, such as muscles, tendons, and nerves

**carbohydrate** Organic compound composed of carbon, hydrogen, and oxygen that provides energy for body tissues

**cognitive dysfunction** Age-related changes in brain function, causing certain behavioral changes

**dry matter basis** Describes nutrient amounts in percentages as found in the dry weight of a product when the moisture is removed

**encephalomalacia** Means "softening of the brain"; usually used to denote degenerative brain diseases

**enteral** Administered through the alimentary canal (mouth, esophagus, stomach, small intestine)

**essential amino acids** Amino acids that the body requires through diet because the body cannot manufacture them

**FLUTD** Feline lower urinary tract disease

**free radicals** Are highly reactive unpaired electrons that are common by-products of normal chemical reactions. These molecules can cause damage to cells throughout the body

**glycoprotein** Class of compounds consisting of a protein conjugated to a carbohydrate

**goiter** Enlargement of the thyroid gland

**guaranteed analysis (GA)** Describes nutrients in minimum or maximum percentages that a pet food manufacturer claims are met by the product

**hepatic lipidosis** Another term for fatty liver disease

**hydrolysate** Compound that is produced through hydrolysis

**hydrolysis** Process of breaking a chemical bond of a molecule by the addition of water

**hyperkeratosis** Increased thickness of the horny layer of the skin

**ingredient** A raw or processed agricultural product or other element that delivers nutrients to the body. Some ingredients may be nonnutritive and may be added as a preservative, thickening agent, flavoring, etc.

**keratomalacia** Softening and necrosis of the cornea due to a vitamin A deficiency

**lipoic acid** Occurs naturally in plants and animals and is vital to cell energy production

**MER** Maintenance energy requirements; estimated number of calories required per day for maintenance of a particular life stage

**myopathy** Inflammation of the muscle

**nitrogenous** Molecule that contains nitrogen

**novel** New or not resembling something formerly known

**NRC** National Research Council

**nutrient** Food component that provides nourishment to the body

**osteoarthritis** A noninflammatory, degenerative joint disease. It is due to the deterioration of the cartilage that cushions the ends of bones within joints. It occurs primarily in older animals

**osteomalacia** Softening of bones

**osteoporosis** Condition of marked loss of bone density

**parakeratosis** Appearance of thickened skin with scale formation and underlying raw red surface, often due to zinc deficiency

**parenteral** Administered via some other route than the alimentary canal

**pollakiuria** Abnormally frequent urination

**protein** Nutrient composed of up to 23 amino acids

**steatitis** Inflammation of fatty tissue

**taurine** Essential amino acid that only cats require in their diet

**uremic** Term used to define the presence of abnormal quantities of urine in the blood

**urolithiasis** Formation of urinary stones

# Review Questions

**1** Energy-producing nutrients are
   a. Protein, fats, water
   b. Carbohydrates, fats, protein
   c. Fats, protein, vitamins
   d. Vitamins, minerals, water

**2** Biological value
   a. Pertains to the value of carbohydrates in the diet
   b. Describes the quantity of plant and animal protein sources in a diet
   c. Evaluates protein usability by the body
   d. Pertains to the value of fat in the diet

**3** Which nutrient aids in the management of diarrhea and constipation?
   a. Minerals
   b. Fat
   c. Water
   d. Carbohydrates

**4** The maintenance energy requirements (MER) for an 8-month-old, 22-kg (48.5-lb) Mastiff is
   a. 1460 kcal/day
   b. 740 kcal/day
   c. 2190 kcal/day
   d. 3140 kcal/day

**5** Characteristics of a canine geriatric diet include
   a. Low fiber and sodium; higher fat
   b. Decreased sodium and essential fatty acids
   c. Restricted protein and phosphorus; increased fiber
   d. Increased fiber and calories; restricted essential fatty acids
**6** Possible clinical signs associated with FLUTD may include
   a. Frequent defecation
   b. Increased hunger
   c. Weight gain
   d. Hematuria
**7** An animal is considered obese when its weight exceeds what percentage of its ideal weight?
   a. 5%
   b. 10%
   c. 15%
   d. 20%
**8** Manufacturers are required to include which percentage of the following ingredients in the guaranteed analysis?
   a. Maximum crude protein and fat
   b. Minimum crude protein and fat
   c. Minimum minerals and ash
   d. Minimum crude fiber and moisture
**9** A pet food claim that it is formulated to meet the AAFCO cat food nutrient profile for growth and lactation means that the food
   a. Also meets the nutrient profile for adult maintenance
   b. Meets NRC standards
   c. Has undergone AAFCO feeding trial testing growth and lactation
   d. Has been chemically analyzed only to meet the standards
**10** The best way to compare the actual nutrients of two pet food labels is by
   a. Guaranteed analysis
   b. Ingredient panel
   c. Nutritional adequacy statement
   d. Dry weight analysis
**11** Which nutrient helps convert fat into energy and promotes lean muscle mass?
   a. Hexametaphosphate
   b. Polyphosphate
   c. L-Carnitine
   d. Beta-carotene
**12** Tumor cells are efficient in using which nutrient as an energy source?
   a. Protein
   b. Carbohydrates
   c. Essential fatty acids
   d. Fat
**13** Increased levels of omega-3 fatty acids in a renal diet
   a. Improve blood flow to the kidneys
   b. Decrease blood flow to the kidneys
   c. Improve blood flow through the bladder
   d. Decrease blood flow through the bladder

## BIBLIOGRAPHY

American Association of Feed Control Officials, Official Publication, Atlanta, Ga, 2001.

Case LP, Carey DP, Hirakawa DA: *Canine and feline nutrition, a resource for companion animal professionals*, ed 2, St Louis, 2001, Mosby.

Colgan M, Brune C: *Hill's healthcare connection*, Topeka, Kan, 1999.

DHA: Brain food for puppies and kittens, Technical Information Services Nutritional Nuggets #NN0044, Hill's Pet Nutrition Inc, 2006.

Dodd CE et al: Omega-3 fatty acids in canine osteoarthritis: a randomized, double-masked, practice-based, six-month feeding study, unpublished data, Hill's Pet Nutrition Center, Topeka, Kan, 2004.

Ettinger SJ, Feldman EC: *Textbook of veterinary internal medicine*, ed 6, St Louis, 2005, Saunders.

Gross KL, Zicker SC: L-Carnitine increases muscle mass, bone mass and bone density in growing large breed puppies, *J Anim Sci* abstract #746, 2000.

Hand MS et al: *Small animal clinical nutrition*, ed 4, Topeka, Kan, 2000, Mark Morris Institute.

Hoffman L, Kelley R, Waltz D: For smarter more trainable puppies: effect of docosahexaenoic acid on puppy trainability, ADSB#07356100, Research and Development Division, The Iams Company, Lewisburg, Ohio.

Loeffler et al: Dietary trials with a commercial chicken hydrolyzate diet in 63 pruritic dogs, *Vet Rec* 154:519, 2004.

Lund EM et al: Prevalence and risk factors for obesity in adult cats from private US veterinary practices, *Intern J Appl Res Vet Med* 3:88, 2005.

Milgram NW et al: Dietary enrichment counteracts age-associated cognitive dysfunction in canines, *Neurobiol Aging* 23:737, 2002.

Osborne CA et al: Feline lower urinary tract disease: relationships between crystalluria, urinary tract infection, and host factors. In August JR: *Consultations in feline internal medicine*, ed 2, St Louis, 1994, Saunders.

Osborne CA, Finco DR: *Canine and feline nephrology and urology*, Philadelphia, 1995, Lippincott Williams & Wilkins.

Roudebush P: Ingredients associated with adverse food reactions in dogs and cats, *Adv Small Anim Med Surg* 15:1, 2002.

Tefend M, Berryhill S: Companion animal clinical nutrition. In McCurnin DM, Bassert JM: *Clinical textbook for veterinary technicians*, ed 6, St Louis, 2006, Saunders.

Yu S, Paetau-Robinson I: Dietary supplements of vitamins E and C and beta-carotene reduce oxidative stress in cats with renal insufficiency, *J Vet Res Commun* 30:403, 2006.

Zicker SC et al: Safety of long-term feeding of dl-alpha-lipoic acid and its effect on reduced glutathione: oxidized glutathione ratios in beagles, *Vet Ther* 3:167, 2002.

## CHAPTER 16

# Large Animal Nutrition and Feeding

*James A. Topel*

## OUTLINE

Feeding Large Animals
  Large Animal Nutrition
    Concepts
Ruminant Digestion
  Basic Anatomy and Physiology
  Feeding Dairy and Beef Cattle
    Feed Sources
    Special Nutritional Requirements
    Life Stages
    Disease Related to Improper
      Nutrition
  Feeding Sheep and Goats
    Feed Sources
    Special Nutritional Requirements

Life Stages
  Disease Related to Improper
    Nutrition
Feeding Camelids
  Feed Sources
  Special Nutritional
    Requirements
  Life Stages
  Disease Related to Improper
    Nutrition
Monogastric Digestion
  Basic Anatomy and
    Physiology
Feeding Swine

Feed Sources, Preparation, and
    Feeding of Grains
  Special Nutritional
    Requirements
  Life Stages
  Disease Related to Improper
    Nutrition
Feeding Horses
  Feed Sources
  Special Nutritional
    Requirements
  Life Stages
  Disease Related to Improper
    Nutrition

## LEARNING OUTCOMES

After reading this chapter you should be able to:

1. Define the nutrient needs of large animals.
2. Identify the elements that influence nutrient requirements.
3. Identify the parts and functions of large animal digestive systems.
4. Learn of the different feedstuffs in large animal diets.
5. Identify the various life stage nutritional requirements of large animals.
6. Identify the relationship of disease to improper nutrition.

Improper nutrition can be related to as much as 90% of health-related disease in large animals. Reasons for improper nutrition include owners' inadequate training, improper emphasis on prevention and prophylaxis, and lack of consultation. It is advantageous for the veterinary team to combine preventive feeding with herd health. The increased requirements for growth, breeding, and lactation are different from those for maintenance. Ration formulation, a science best left to specially trained individuals in that field, is not covered in this unit.

## FEEDING LARGE ANIMALS

### Large Animal Nutrition Concepts

I. Livestock nutrition basics
   A. The livestock producer's greatest challenge is producing or purchasing feed that can be consumed by the animal at the least cost, with the best financial return
   B. Nutrients are used for homeostasis, developing body tissues (growth, repair, and finishing), replenishing body tissues (maintenance), reproduction, lactation, and wool and meat production
   C. Maintenance nutrient requirements (MNRs) are the levels of nutrients needed in the large animal diet to maintain body weight without a gain or loss
      1. About one half of consumed and absorbed nutrients are needed to meet the MNRs

D. The National Research Council has established feeding standards for the different production or use purposes for each large animal species

II. Nutrients

A. Protein

1. Contains nitrogen, sulfur, carbon, hydrogen, and oxygen. Some contain phosphorus
2. Protein is the main constituent of the soft tissues and organs of the animal body
3. Amino acids are the building blocks of proteins
   a. Twenty amino acids are used in varying combinations to make proteins
   b. Twenty-three amino acids are known to exist
   c. Amino acids are classified as either essential or nonessential
4. Used for growth; reproduction; lactation; repair of body tissues; the formation of enzymes, antibodies, and certain hormones; and energy production
5. Depending on life stage, protein quality may not be important. However, even though total protein intake may be adequate, digestible protein may be insufficient
   a. Dietary protein requirements are highest in the young, growing animal
6. Protein supplements (soybean, cottonseed, and linseed meals) are highly digestible protein sources. Common grains (corn, oats, wheat, and barley) and legumes, such as alfalfa, are good protein sources. Grass hay has the least amount of digestible protein
   a. Highly digestible proteins are considered high in total digestible nutrients (TDNs) and low in fiber
   b. Grass hay is high in fiber but low in TDNs
7. Nonprotein nitrogen (NPN) (e.g., urea) is a nitrogen source that can be converted to protein by rumen microbes
8. Deficiencies may result in limited growth, anemia, decreased milk production, infertility, reduced synthesis of certain hormones and enzymes, and depressed appetite with weight loss and unthriftiness
9. Excesses may also affect reproduction

B. Fats

1. Fats provide dietary energy, source of heat, insulation, and body protection and serve as a carrier for absorption of fat-soluble vitamins
2. Fat has 2.25 times more energy per gram than carbohydrates or proteins
3. Fats are classified as
   a. Simple lipids: esters of fatty acids with glycerol or alcohol

   b. Compound lipids: phospholipids, glycolipids, and lipoproteins
   c. Derived lipids: fatty acids and sterols
      (1) Linoleic acid and linolenic acid are essential
      (2) Arachidonic acid is considered essential only if linoleic acid is absent
      (3) Arachidonic acid can be synthesized from linoleic acid

C. Carbohydrates

1. Carbohydrates are the primary energy source in large animal rations
2. Carbohydrates are the building blocks for other nutrients (fats)
3. Carbohydrates are stored in the animal's body after being converted to fats
4. Cereal grains and forages are high in carbohydrate content
5. Carbohydrates (sugars and starches) are broken down into simple sugars so they can be absorbed from the digestive tract
6. Microflora in the rumen of ruminants and the cecum of some nonruminants can convert fiber (cellulose, hemicellulose, pectins, and gum) into energy
   a. Lignin is a fiber but is considered to be the indigestible portion found in forages of poor quality
7. Feed concentrates (grains and high-starch compounds) and forages (grasses and legumes) generally supply all the energy needed in the diet

D. Minerals

1. Minerals are made of inorganic, solid, and crystalline chemical elements
   a. Total mineral content of animals and plants is called ash
   b. Minerals make up 3% to 5% of the animal body dry weight
2. A highly complex relationship exists among the minerals
   a. Calcium, iron, and copper can interfere with the metabolism of other minerals and nutrients
3. Minerals that are lacking in the diet can be force fed in supplements combined with common salt
4. Other than common salt, animals apparently do not have any ability to select needed minerals
   a. A mineral block or granular mineral supplement is vitally important for health and should be offered as a free-choice part of the diet
5. Minerals are grouped as macrominerals and trace minerals, based on their need in the diet

a. See Chapter 15 for general mineral functions and effects of deficiencies and excesses. Also see Table 16-1

6. Macrominerals include sodium, chloride, potassium, phosphorus, calcium, magnesium, and sulfur
   a. Calcium and phosphorus
      (1) Make up more than 70% of the minerals in the body
      (2) Generally, a calcium/phosphorus ratio of 1.4:1 to 2:1 should be provided by the ration
      (3) Common supplements are bone meal, defluorinated phosphates, and dicalcium phosphate
      (4) Calcium and phosphorus are closely tied to vitamin D and the parathyroid gland
      (5) A large excess of either calcium or phosphorus interferes with absorption of the other, so a balance is necessary
      (6) In Europe, bone meal and other animal-based byproducts have been considered the likely carriers of the infectious protein that causes bovine spongiform encephalopathy ("mad cow disease")
   b. Sodium and chloride
      (1) Hydrochloric acid, a substance rich in chloride that is obtained from salt, is essential in the digestive processes
      (2) Salt must always be supplied to animals in addition to the amounts contained in the usual well-balanced ration
      (3) Good livestock managers provide free access to salt at all times
      (4) Increased salt intake results in increased water intake
      (5) In severe deficiencies, animals may experience muscle cramps, weight loss, decrease in milk production, and rough hair coat
      (6) Most animals will tolerate large excesses of salt if the water supply is adequate. If the water is contaminated with excess salt, this can cause anorexia, weight loss, and eventually physical collapse (salt toxicosis)
   c. Magnesium
      (1) Magnesium is allied with calcium and phosphorus in the body
      (2) Care must be taken to avoid a magnesium-deficient diet
      (3) Lactating cows are more susceptible, although other stock can be afflicted
      (4) Magnesium-deficient cattle exhibit anorexia and reduced dry matter (DM) digestibility
      (5) Young stock may have defective bones and teeth when deficiencies occur
      (6) Toxicity is rare
   d. Sulfur
      (1) Sulfur is a component of amino acids, biotin, and thiamine
      (2) A deficiency of sulfur leads to reduced growth. Toxicity is unlikely
   e. Potassium
      (1) Potassium is the major intracellular cation and is involved in maintaining osmotic pressure, acid-base balance, and muscle activity
      (2) Deficiencies lead to lethargy, diarrhea, untidy appearance, coma, and even death
      (3) Toxicities can reduce magnesium absorption, which in turn reduces potassium retention

**Table 16-1** Body condition scoring classification for livestock

| Body condition scoring scale* | | | Generalized animal description† |
|---|---|---|---|
| 1.0 | 1 | Emaciated | All bones obviously protruding; no subcutaneous fat is evident |
| 1.5 | 2 | Very thin | Bones visible and easily palpated; minimal subcutaneous fat |
| 2.0 | 3 | Thin | Thin, flat musculature; prominent ribs, pelvic bones, and spinal processes |
| 2.5 | 4 | Moderately thin | Minimal subcutaneous fat; individual ribs not obvious |
| 3.0 | 5 | Moderate | Smooth musculature; bones not visible but palpable |
| 3.5 | 6 | Moderate fleshy | Fat palpable; soft fat over ribs and covering pelvis |
| 4.0 | 7 | Fleshy | Fat visible; ribs difficult to palpate; rounded appearance to pelvis |
| 4.5 | 8 | Fat | Thick neck; ribs difficult to palpate; rounded appearance to pelvis |
| 5.0 | 9 | Grossly obese | Bulging fat all over, patchy pads around tailhead |

From Grosdidier SR et al: Nutrition. In Sirois M, editor: *Principles and practice of veterinary technology*, ed 2, St Louis, 2004, Mosby.
*The body condition scoring scale used depends on the species. Dairy cattle, sheep, pigs, and goats are generally scored on a scale of 1 to 5. Beef cattle and horses are usually scored on a scale of 1 to 9.
†Base the body condition score on the amount or lack of fatty tissue over the neck, ribs, spine, and pelvis without reference to body weight and frame size.

7. Trace minerals include zinc, selenium, manganese, iodine, fluorine, chromium, copper, iron, silicon, molybdenum, and cobalt
   a. Trace minerals and macrominerals have profound interactions. Deficiencies or toxicities of one may lead to deficiencies or toxicities of another
   b. See Special Nutritional Requirements section for deficiencies and toxicities of trace minerals for each large animal species
E. Vitamins (see Chapter 15, Table 15-2 for vitamin function, deficiency, and toxicity)
   1. Fat-soluble vitamins are A, D, E, and K
   2. Water-soluble vitamins include ascorbic acid (vitamin C) and the B complex vitamins
   3. Ruminants require water-soluble vitamins when they are ill, because of a reduced ability to synthesize them
   4. Fat-soluble vitamins are stored in the body fat in large amounts; therefore excess in one or more of them can result in a toxic effects
   5. Deficiency in any of these vitamins can result in severe health problems
   6. Normal, healthy ruminants do not require a dietary source of vitamin B complex, vitamin C, and vitamin K, because the rumen microflora or tissues synthesize them
      a. If insufficient vitamin $B_1$ (thiamine) is produced, polioencephalomalacia will result
   7. Vitamin A deficiency may occur if limited or poor-quality forages are fed. Deficiency signs include reproductive failure, night blindness, skin ailments, and weak offspring
   8. Vitamin E deficiency along with a selenium deficiency may result in white muscle disease, especially in calves
   9. Sun-cured hay is the only natural food with a high vitamin D content—the leafier the better
      a. An hour-a-day exposure to direct sunlight is sufficient to meet daily vitamin D needs
F. Water
   1. Adequate water intake is essential for life. Potable water should always be available
   2. Water makes up 65% to 85% of an animal's body weight at birth, and 45% to 60% of body weight at maturity
   3. A loss of 10% of total water content seriously distresses the animal; a loss of more than 12% will lead to shock with death imminent
   4. All nutrients must be dissolved before the body can use them
      a. Waste products of the body are removed by water as urine. Waste of the digestive tract cannot be removed until it has been softened by water

5. Except for newborn calves, water should be offered free choice
   a. Calves should be offered free choice water by two weeks of age
   b. Calves that are limit fed milk replacer are at risk of water intoxication when water is suddenly offered free choice
6. Because of rumen fermentation, cattle need two to three times more water per day than horses
III. Elements that influence nutrient requirements
A. Environment
   1. Temperature variations
      a. Cold stress requires more energy
      b. Warmer temperatures decrease appetite
   2. Wind, precipitation, and sun exposure
   3. Consult district agrologist for specific area requirements
B. Location concerns
   1. Soil nutrient leaching and increased animal population leading to overgrazing will affect the quality of the feed that is consumed
      a. Soil and feed tests will provide valuable information
      b. Consult a nutritionist and use services of the district agrologist for specific area requirements
C. Other factors influence nutrient requirements
   1. Genetics, body size, gender, breed, reproductive status, health status, stress, exercise, behavior, and availability of nutrients

# RUMINANT DIGESTION

## BASIC ANATOMY AND PHYSIOLOGY

I. Cattle, sheep, goats, and camelids are ruminants
II. Ruminants are herbivores with a diet composed mainly of plants with high fiber (cellulose) content
III. Ruminants can convert forage unfit for direct human consumption into a consumable product
A. Accomplished through symbiotic relationship with bacteria and protozoa
   1. Byproducts of anaerobic fermentation are volatile fatty acids, amino acids, vitamins, methane, and $CO_2$
      a. Methane and $CO_2$ are eructated (belched), and the remaining byproducts are used for body maintenance and production
IV. True ruminants, such as cattle, have a prehensile tongue for gathering foodstuffs
V. Functional ruminants, such as llamas, use their lips to carefully select the foodstuff and then crop the forage short by shearing the plant stems with their lower incisors and upper dental pad
VI. The stomach of true ruminants is multicompartmented. In cattle, the stomach is composed of four

chambers: reticulum, rumen, and omasum, which make up the forestomach, and the abomasum

  A. Reticulum: (honeycomb) forces ingested feed material into the rumen or omasum and regurgitates ingesta during rumination

  B. Rumen: (paunch) main fermentation vat; the microbial products are available for digestion and absorption

  C. Omasum: (manyplies) filled with muscular laminae or "leaves" to squeeze fluid out of the ingesta

  D. Abomasum (true or glandular stomach)

    1. Corresponds to stomach of monogastrics

    2. Process of peptic digestion of proteins begins here

VII. Functional ruminants, such as llamas, have a three-compartment stomach (C-1, C-2, C-3)

  A. Compartments 1 and 2 support microbial anaerobic fermentation (similar to the rumen of cattle)

VIII. Sugars and starches (e.g., concentrates) are fermented more rapidly than cellulose (e.g., forages)

IX. Intraruminal pH is generally between 6.2 and 7.2, depending on the diet

  A. A more acidic rumen is noted in animals fed a high grain diet

X. Conversion of protein, starches, and lipids by microorganisms results in usable nutrients for the host

XI. Microorganisms can use poor-quality protein and NPN compounds (e.g., urea) to make amino acids and energy

  A. Microbial protein passes into the abomasum and is digested the same way as other dietary protein

  B. Microbial protein can form a significant amount of ruminant dietary protein, but the intake of NPN compounds should be carefully monitored

  C. Dietary fiber is required to keep the microbial fermentation chambers active

  D. Microorganisms also synthesize vitamins B and K

XII. To ensure proper microbial population, ruminants require proper feed, appropriate feeding intervals (fermentation is continuous), regurgitation of cud (bolus of food), rechewing (remastication), ensalivation, reswallowing (deglutition), continuous churning, eructation (belching), outflow to the rest of the digestive tract, and ingestion of sufficient water

XIII. Anatomy and physiology of the small and large intestines in ruminants is similar to those of swine

## FEEDING DAIRY AND BEEF CATTLE

### Feed Sources (Boxes 16-1 and 16-2)

I. Roughages or forages include pastures, range plants, plants fed green ("green-chop"), silages, and dry forages, such as hay (alfalfa, clover, brome, timothy, native grasses, etc.), straw, and chopped corn stalks

---

### Box 16-1 Typical Roughages Fed to Ruminants

**LEGUMES**
Alfalfa, red clover, Alsike clover, white clover, sweet clover, birdsfoot trefoil, crown vetch

**GRASSES**
Kentucky bluegrass, smooth bromegrass, orchard grass, timothy, reed canary grass, tall fescue, redtop, perennial rye grass, southern grasses, Sudan grass, native grasses

---

### Box 16-2 Concentrates Fed to Ruminants

**CARBONACEOUS CONCENTRATES**
Corn, oats, sorghum, barley, rye, wheat

**PROTEINACEOUS CONCENTRATES**
Urea, biuret, diammonium phosphate, monoammonium phosphate, ammonium sulfate, soybean meal, cottonseed meal, linseed meal, sunflower meal, safflower meal

---

  A. Forages generally have large amounts of fiber, low TDNs and energy density, and high bulk (low weight per unit volume)

    1. This is due to the plant cell wall material of cellulose, hemicellulose, lignin, and other compounds

  B. Protein content depends on the type of plant and stage at harvesting

    1. The more mature the plant, the greater the fiber content, but mature plants have less protein and energy and are not as easily digested

  C. Hays are divided into legumes (e.g., alfalfa, clover, birdsfoot trefoil) and grasses (e.g., timothy, brome, sorghum, bluegrass, and native grasses)

    1. Legumes have higher protein content and a higher protein biological value compared with grass hays

    2. Some legumes, such as alfalfa and clover, are more likely to cause bloat in cattle

    3. Hay quality is determined by

      a. Mixture of grasses (e.g., brome, alfalfa or bluegrass, and clover)

      b. Stage of maturity when cut (50% bloom, 75% bloom, or full bloom)

      c. Method and speed of harvesting

      d. Spoilage and loss during storage and feeding

  D. Silage is roughage that is preserved by ensiling, which undergoes anaerobic fermentation

    1. Most common silages are corn silages and grass or legume silages (also called haylage)

2. Silage with a water content of 55% to 75% retains the most nutrients through harvesting and storage

II. Concentrates or cereal grains include corn, barley, wheat, oats, and screenings (left over from grain processing)
   A. The way a grain is processed affects its digestibility
   B. Concentrates are fed primarily for energy and/or protein
   C. Grains contain 60% to 80% starch
   D. Fats and oils of plant or animal origin have 2.25 greater energy density than carbohydrates
   E. Corn is the most commonly fed grain
   F. Other than cereal grains, molasses, root crops, and milling byproducts can also be used as energy concentrates

III. Any concentrates that are more than 20% crude protein are classified as protein supplements
   A. Concentrates are classified as carbonaceous (grain) or proteinaceous (processed byproducts)

IV. Cattle (and other ruminants) should not be fed material derived from mammalian sources, such as meat, bone meal, and other animal by-products
   A. The FDA (Food and Drug Administration) implemented this rule in August 1997
   B. This ban on feeding mammalian tissue to ruminants was implemented to eliminate the potential of ruminants acquiring and spreading TSEs (transmissible spongiform encephalopathy)

## Special Nutritional Requirements

An adequate diet should include water and feeds containing energy, proteins, minerals, and vitamins.
   I. Water
      A. Ad libitum for mature animals
         1. Mature nonstressed cattle generally drink 10 to 14 gallons (38 to 53.2 L) per day
      B. Dairy cows require 3 to 5 gallons (11.4 to 19 L) of water to produce 1 gallon (3.8 L) of milk
      C. A cow at peak lactation may need up to 45 gallons (171 L) per day, depending on various factors
   II. Energy
      A. Energy requirements are greatest during lactation
      B. This requirement must be met with a good grain source and high-quality forage for lactation
   III. Protein
      A. Good-quality pasture and forage balanced with grains and topped up high-protein supplements will usually provide adequate protein in the diet during growth and lactation
      B. Maintenance requirements can be supplied with just fair- to good-quality pasture and forage

C. In cattle, rumen microbes have the ability to convert fair- to poor-quality feedstuff protein into a higher-quality protein
      D. In contrast, rumen microbes may actually reduce higher-quality feedstuff proteins through microbial degradation and synthesis of proteins

   IV. Minerals
      A. Includes the macrominerals (sodium, chloride, calcium, phosphorus, magnesium, sulfur, and potassium) and the trace minerals (zinc, selenium, manganese, iodine, fluorine, chromium, copper, iron, silicon, molybdenum, and cobalt). All minerals should be balanced in the diet: neither deficient nor in excess
         1. Sodium and chloride
            a. Best fed free choice to cattle
            b. Salt is important for general thriftiness
         2. Calcium
            a. A deficiency in calcium can occur with high-grain diets
            b. Balance grains with forages. Legumes and high-quality forages are high in calcium
            c. Calcium deficiencies are more rare, but can be corrected with the addition of limestone to the feed
            d. Calcium imbalances during the late dry period may lead to fever (parturient paresis)
               (1) Bone calcium reserves are then not readily available at onset of lactation
         3. Phosphorus
            a. Phosphorus availability is influenced by content in the soil
            b. Mature brown summer forage and winter range can be deficient in phosphorus
            c. Phosphorus deficiency results in slow growth, poor appetite, and unthriftiness in young animals. In lactating animals, milk production declines, bones become fragile, and feed intake is poor
            d. Phosphorus deficiencies can be corrected with a phosphorus supplement
         4. Iodine
            a. Feeding stabilized iodized salt will prevent deficiencies
            b. Most important in pregnant animals; deficiencies may lead to an increase in stillbirths
         5. Cobalt
            a. Cobalt is an essential component of vitamin $B_{12}$
            b. Feed with the trace mineralized salt
            c. Deficiency develops rapidly, because very little is stored
            d. Deficiency shows up as ocular discharge, listlessness, anemia, decreased skin and

hair coat quality, abortions, decreased milk production, ketosis, and decreased appetite

   e. Signs of toxicity include decreased growth rates, incoordination, rough hair coat, and elevated hemoglobin and packed cell volume levels

6. Copper
   a. Signs of deficiency include neurological disorders, anemia, lameness, and diarrhea
   b. Signs of toxicity include gastroenteritis, hemorrhagic diarrhea, liver and kidney disease, and increased incidence of respiratory disease in calves
   c. A balance of sulfates and offering trace mineralized salt with copper will generally correct a deficiency

7. Selenium
   a. Growing cattle fed low-protein diets require more selenium and vitamin E in the diet to prevent deficiencies
   b. Cattle fed selenium-deficient diets have increased incidence of reproductive problems, immunosuppression; calves are born weak and have reduced growth weights (white muscle disease)
   c. Levels vary in soil based on region and geological phenomenon
   d. A trace mineralized salt should include selenium and should also supply adequate vitamin E

8. Zinc
   a. Higher levels are required for normal testicular development
   b. High calcium intake increases the need for zinc
   c. Deficiency signs include reduced conception rates, reduction in growth, reduced immune response, decreased appetite, bone irregularities, decreased wound healing, hoof problems, and hair loss
   d. Zinc can be added to trace mineralized salt to prevent deficiencies
   e. Calves are most susceptible to toxicities, with signs including polydipsia, polyuria, diarrhea, pica, anorexia, pneumonia, arrhythmias, and ultimately death

9. Iron
   a. Iron is an essential component of hemoglobin
   b. Deficiencies rarely occur in adults, but may be an issue in calves fed an all-milk diet
   c. Treatment for deficiencies includes iron dextran injections in calves and iron sulfate added to a mineral mix in adults

V. Vitamins
   A. Vitamin A
      1. Important for vision, growth, and reproduction
      2. Deficiencies should be addressed immediately by supplementation
   B. Vitamin D
      1. Essential for the absorption of calcium and phosphorus
      2. Deficiency leads to rickets
      3. Deficiency is extremely rare, because vitamin D requirements are met by 1 to 2 hours of sunlight a day
   C. Vitamin E
      1. Oxidation rapidly destroys vitamin E
      2. Old hay or ground grains are poor sources
      3. Deficiency is recognized as a common cause of white muscle disease
      4. This vitamin is of practical importance only to the young
      5. Vitamin E interacts with selenium
   D. Vitamin K
      1. Synthesized by rumen microorganisms
   E. B-complex vitamins
      1. Not necessary when the rumen is functioning properly
      2. Milk replacers should be fortified
   F. Vitamin C
      1. Not required; ruminants synthesize their own vitamin C

## Life Stages

I. Nutrient requirements for maintenance energy levels of beef and dairy animals
   A. Maintenance energy level requirements relate to instances where there is no loss or gain in body energy

II. Nutrient requirements of pregnant and lactating beef and dairy animals
   A. Factors to consider before a ration is developed include availability, quality, and cost of feedstuffs
   B. Energy source is the most important part of the ration
      1. Until the energy requirement is met, protein, minerals, and vitamins may not be well used
   C. Cow size does not seem to have much effect on the efficiency of milk production, so it is more important to feed cows on the basis of their potential
      1. Referred to as challenge feeding
   D. Judge individual cow or heifer requirements by body score
      1. A condition score of 3 is desirable before calving to help with the birth and the subsequent rebreeding (see Table 16-1)

E. It is desirable in the last trimester for the cow to gain an amount of weight equal to what will be lost at calving

F. An obese animal is as undesirable as an underweight animal, because cows may be predisposed to ketosis, along with other problems

G. Last trimester and lactation are the most important stages, with lactation often exerting the most severe strain

H. Beef cows can use poor-quality forage fairly well, if they are supplemented to meet nutrient requirements for the stage of pregnancy

  1. In cow/calf management systems, cows produce calves that form part of the breeding herd or are sent to feedlots

    a. They are usually fed forages with supplements as needed

  2. Same considerations apply for pregnant dairy cattle, especially during lactation

    a. Cows in good condition fed good-quality hay or pasture require no extra concentrates until 2 weeks before calving

  3. For lactating cattle, a fully balanced ration with the proper dry matter intake (DMI) is essential for optimum milk production

    a. Concentrates supply the highest level of energy, but a proper proportion is important to prevent obesity, digestive problems, and decreased milk production

    b. Cow's body type and ability to achieve maximum milk production are considered

    c. Generally, dairies use good-quality forages and grains at the correct mixture to achieve the best production that they can, without losing body condition on the cow

III. Feeding replacement/breeding animals

A. Replacement animals are those used in the breeding herd after they come of age

B. First calf heifers will still be growing at the time of first parturition

C. Energy intake of breeding animals, males and females, should be controlled so they will not become obese

D. In calves, adequate colostrum intake is critical within the first 18 hours, to ensure maximum absorption of colostral antibodies

  1. Calves should receive 10% to 12% of their body weight in colostrum within the first 18 hours, preferably half the total volume within 4 to 6 hours of birth

E. Beef calves should be "creep fed," which is feeding small amounts of grain in a location the dam does not have access to

  1. This aids in lowering weaning stress and enables the calves to start to digest foodstuff they will be eating in their postweaning life stage

  2. Beef calves are usually weaned at 6 to 8 months

  3. Creep fed calves will generally show a 50-lb (22.5-kg) weight advantage at weaning

F. Dairy calves should be pail- or bottle-fed whole milk or milk replacer until at least 1 month of age

  1. Good-quality calf starter rations and good-quality forages should be fed to encourage rumen development while receiving milk

  2. Longer periods (up to 2 months) of liquid feeding may be beneficial under some conditions, because it results in decreased disease and death losses

  3. Proper sanitation of pails and bottles is important to prevent scours

G. Forages and concentrates should be fed in large enough amounts to ensure continuous growth

IV. Animals fed for consumption

A. Slaughter usually occurs between 13 and 18 months of age

B. Beef animals not raised as breeding stock can be fed two ways

  1. Weaned calves can be "backgrounded": the calves are fed sufficient feed to gain between 1 and 1.5 lb (0.45 to 0.68 kg) a day through the winter, and fed on pasture through the summer as yearlings

    a. Then they are slowly fed a ration increasing in grain until they reach slaughter weight

  2. Weaned calves can also be put directly on a ration increasing in grain until slaughter

    a. This is usually done in a feedlot, although some ranchers keep them on the range

    b. Feedlots usually hire a nutritionist for ration consulting; ranchers will sometimes use whatever feed is readily available and not necessarily in the correct amounts

  3. Weather (drought) and availability of feedstuffs are factors to consider in choosing which method is best for feeding beef calves

  4. Economics is the overriding factor in this decision

V. Nonbreeding dairy calves

A. Can be raised as "dairy beef"; usually not pastured and fed a ration in a feedlot to finish operation

B. Can be fed as veal; fed a total liquid diet to keep the meat low in hemoglobin so that it stays white (anemia)

There is no "magic" amount of food that can be calculated to feed each life stage of cattle. Nutritionists factor quality and type of food and available nutrient levels into the ration for each cow in the herd. This has to be done by calculations, using some of the terms listed in the Glossary.

## Disease Related to Improper Nutrition

I. Bloat
   A. Bloat is the increase of froth or free gas in the rumen
   B. Allowing cattle to graze on lush (rapidly growing) legume pasture, feeding legume greenchop, or feeding a low-roughage feedlot ration increases the risk
   C. To reduce the risk of bloat, feed cattle dry forages before allowing them to graze on new pasture or consume green-chop

II. Enterotoxemia
   A. Rare in cattle, but most commonly caused by overeating milk, milk replacer, or a high-carbohydrate diet in fast-growing juveniles
   B. *Clostridium perfringens* is the contributing agent, which causes neurological signs and death
   C. To prevent enterotoxemia in cattle, avoid overfeeding and vaccinate for *C. perfringens*

III. Failure of passive transfer (FPT)
   A. FPT occurs when a calf does not receive adequate colostral antibodies
      1. Calves are noted to be less vigorous and are more prone to disease, because they do not have the antibodies available to fight disease
   B. Reasons for inadequate colostral antibody absorption include poor-quality colostrum nursed or fed, inadequate colostrum consumed, and first colostrum intake postponed
   C. To prevent FPT, ensure that the calf receives adequate high-quality colostrum within the first hours and days of life

IV. Fatty liver disease
   A. Disease occurs when high dietary fat or cholesterol intake is not properly metabolized in the liver, or fats are pulled from the adipose tissue in a negative energy state
      1. This leads to an accumulation of lipids in the liver and alters liver function
   B. In a healthy animal, fatty liver disease may be avoided through adequate energy intake

V. Grass tetany (hypomagnesemic tetany)
   A. Most likely to occur in mature cattle and during early lactation in high-producing dairy cattle
   B. Cattle that graze on pastures that are magnesium deficient may become anorexic and may exhibit muscle fasciculations (twitching) or even convulsions
   C. Grass tetany can be prevented by supplementing magnesium in the diet before and during early lactation of at-risk animals

VI. Milk fever (parturient paresis)
   A. Milk fever is most often seen after calving in high-producing cows
   B. Decreased blood calcium leads to a decreased appetite; often an animal collapses. These cows are sternally recumbent and turn their head back toward their flank. Cows are often hypothermic and rumen motility is decreased
   C. By balancing calcium and phosphorus levels during the "dry period" and preventing obesity, milk fever can be prevented

VII. Displaced abomasum (DA)
   A. When the abomasum is filled with gas, it may be displaced dorsally, to either the left (LDA) or right (RDA) side
   B. A cow with a DA will become anorexic, milk production will drop, and on auscultation of the right or left abdomen, an area of resonance (ping) will often be noted
   C. There are many known causes for DAs, but a common thread seems to be the high-producing animal that is fed a high-grain/low-forage diet
   D. Preventive measures include feeding adequate long-stem forages and avoiding moldy feeds

VIII. Ketosis (acetonemia)
   A. Insufficient energy intake in high-producing cattle causes the catabolism of body fats to supply the needed energy. When fat catabolism does not occur properly, ketone levels build up in the bloodstream
   B. Ketosis occurs most often in early lactation and often leads to decreased milk production and appetite
   C. It is confirmed by noting sweet "acetone" breath and testing for urine ketone levels
   D. Ketosis is preventable by maintaining a leaner, healthier animal, and by increasing energy intake in early lactation

IX. Thiamine-deficiency polio (polioencephalomalacia)
   A. Polio of ruminants is a noninfectious disease that is characterized by cerebrocortical necrosis
   B. Cause appears to be thiamine deficiency, but has not been completely confirmed. There seems to be an association with animals that are fed imbalanced diets
      1. These imbalances include a high-carbohydrate diet, selenium/cobalt/sulfate imbalances, and evidence of mycotoxins or poisonous plants in the diet
   C. Preventive measures include improving roughage quality, balancing grain intake, and giving thiamine injections

X. Rickets
   A. Rickets results from an imbalance of calcium, phosphorus, and vitamin D in the diet and tends to occur more in young animals

B. Animals with rickets often have enlarged joints and have difficulty in moving

C. To prevent rickets in cattle, a proper balance of calcium and phosphorus is critical but should also include the animal's having access to direct sunlight and sun-cured hay

XI. Rumen acidosis

A. Overfeeding of grains may lead to a decrease in rumen pH

B. Rumen becomes acidic

C. Rumen function is significantly altered, because rumen microbes cannot survive in the lower pH environment

D. Preventive measures include limiting or balancing concentrate intake with forage intake, and if necessary, may require repopulating the ruminal microbes (transfaunation)

XII. Indigestion in calves

A. Ruminal drinking can cause indigestion in young calves

B. Cause of this indigestion is insufficient closure of the reticular groove, which allows milk to pool in the undeveloped rumen and not bypass directly to the abomasum

1. Affected calves become unthrifty

C. Affected calves can be treated by allowing them to suck on the herdsman's fingers before feeding to facilitate the closure of the reticular groove

XIII. Urea toxicity

A. Overconsumption of urea leads to toxic levels of ammonia in the bloodstream, which can make cattle sick or result in death

B. Be sure to balance NPN intake with conventional high-protein concentrates

XIV. Water belly

A. Urinary tract obstruction from urinary calculi leads to rupture of the urethra or urinary bladder

B. Castrated males are most susceptible

C. Carbonate calculi are most common

D. Cattle on high-grain diets develop struvite crystals

E. Silicate calculi may be seen in animals out on open range in certain geographical areas

F. Preventive measures are limited to economically feasible feed management practice changes when an increased incidence of urethral obstructions occurs in an individual herd

XV. White muscle disease

A. White muscle disease is a polysystemic disease caused by vitamin E and selenium deficiencies

B. Juvenile cattle are the most susceptible

C. Clinical signs in ruminants include swollen painful muscles, stiffness, and muscle weakness

D. Preventive measures include supplementing vitamin E and selenium in the late gestation cow

## FEEDING SHEEP AND GOATS

The numbers of veterinarians in sheep practice are few; there are fewer sheep than cattle. Goats are becoming more popular as a source of meat and milk. Wool sheep and meat goats are managed similarly to beef cattle. Dairy goats are managed more intensely because of high nutritional requirements for milk production.

I. Adequate nutrition is important for the economical soundness of sheep and goat rearing. As with cattle, definitions for nutritional requirements in all life stages can be difficult, because of the wide variety of environmental conditions in which sheep and goats are maintained

A. Different stages include

1. Increased lamb and kid crop

2. Continuous and rapid growth of lambs and kids

3. Heavy weaning weights

4. Heavy fleece weights

5. Milk production

### Feed Sources (see Boxes 16-1 and 16-2)

I. Good hay is a highly productive feed; poor hay, no matter how much is available, is suitable only for maintenance

II. Grains/concentrates can include barley, oats, wheat, bran, beet pulp, soybeans, and corn

III. Goats must be allowed to consume "browse" (brushy plants) and "forbs" (leafy plants)

### Special Nutritional Requirements

An adequate diet should include water and feeds containing energy, proteins, minerals, and vitamins.

I. Water

A. Ad libitum for mature animals

1. Generally drink 1 to 1.5 gallons (3.8 to 5.7 L) per day

B. One-half gallon (~2 L) per day for fattening lambs and kids

II. Energy

A. Maintenance energy requirements can be met by feeding good-quality forages with access to browse and forbs

B. Energy requirements are greater 8 to 10 weeks after start of lactation

1. This requirement must be met with a good grain source and high-quality forage for lactation

III. Protein

A. Good-quality pasture and forage will usually provide adequate protein

B. Sheep digest poor-quality proteins as well as or better than cattle do

C. Sometimes a supplement is indicated. Concentrates or NPN may be an option

IV. Minerals
  A. Include sodium, chloride, calcium, phosphorus, magnesium, sulfur, potassium, and the trace minerals (cobalt, copper, iodine, iron, manganese, molybdenum, zinc, and selenium)
  1. Salt
    a. Best fed free choice
    b. Adults will consume 10 g of salt daily
    c. Salt is important for general thriftiness
  2. Calcium
    a. Legumes and high-quality forage are high in calcium
    b. A deficiency in calcium can occur on high-grain diets (e.g., corn silage)
    c. Calcium deficiencies are more rare, but can be corrected with the addition of limestone to the feed
  3. Phosphorus
    a. Phosphorus availability is influenced by content in the soil
    b. Mature brown summer forage and winter range can be deficient in phosphorus
    c. Phosphorus deficiency results in slow growth, poor appetite, and unthriftiness in young animals. In lactating animals, milk production declines, bones become fragile, and feed intake is poor
    d. Phosphorus deficiencies can be corrected with a phosphorus supplement
  4. Iodine
    a. Deficiencies can be prevented by feeding stabilized iodized salt
    b. Most important in pregnant animals
  5. Cobalt
    a. Feed with the trace mineralized salt
    b. Deficiency develops rapidly because very little is stored
    c. Deficiency shows up as anemia, loss of appetite, retarded growth, general emaciation, rough hair coat, and a loss of milk production
  6. Copper
    a. Sheep require a minimum of 5mg/kg of dry matter intake
    b. Molybdenum and inorganic sulfates can affect copper absorption
    c. Signs of deficiency include anemia, brittle or fragile bones, and loss of wool or hair pigment
    d. A balance of sulfates will usually correct a deficiency problem
    e. Copper can be added to the trace mineralized salt
    f. Sheep are susceptible to copper toxicity
      (1) With acute toxicity, a severe gastroenteritis develops with hemorrhagic diarrhea as the typical sign
      (2) Chronic toxicity leads to liver and kidney disease, resulting in death
  7. Selenium
    a. Levels vary in soil
    b. Supplementation can be provided by injections, oral feeding, or addition of trace mineralized salt
    c. Deficiency can cause nutritional muscular dystrophy, white muscle disease in lambs, and periodontal disease of the molars
    d. Toxicity results in loss of appetite, loss of hair, sloughing of hoofs, and eventual death
  8. Zinc
    a. Higher levels are required for normal testicular development
    b. High calcium intake increases the need for zinc
    c. Signs of deficiency include slipping of wool, swelling and lesions around hooves and eyes, excessive salivation, anorexia, wool eating, general listlessness, reduced food consumption, reproductive problems, and reduction of growth
    d. Zinc can be added to trace mineralized salt
V. Vitamins
  A. Vitamin A
  1. Very low levels are present at birth
  2. If dams are deficient, young may be born dead or so weak they die within a few days; females may abort during the latter stage of pregnancy
  3. Injury to the optic nerve may occur in growing animals, cerebrospinal fluid pressure is elevated, and a staggering gait may develop
  4. Immediate action is required in the form of vitamin A injections and a corrective diet
  B. Vitamin D
  1. Essential for the absorption of calcium and phosphorus
  2. Deficiency leads to swollen leg joints and beaded ribs (rickets)
  3. Deficiency is extremely rare, because vitamin D requirements are met by 1 to 2 hours of sunlight a day
  C. Vitamin E
  1. Oxidation rapidly destroys vitamin E
  2. Old hay or ground grains are poor sources
  3. Deficiency is recognized as a common cause of white muscle disease
  4. This vitamin is of practical importance only to the young
  5. Vitamin E has a direct relationship with selenium
  D. Vitamin K
  1. Synthesized by rumen bacteria
  2. Becomes toxic in moldy sweet clover

E. B complex vitamins
1. Milk replacers should be fortified
2. Deficiency may result if animal goes "off feed" for a long time
a. Death will likely occur if deficiencies are not corrected
F. Vitamin C
1. Not required; ruminants synthesize their own vitamin C

## Life Stages

I. Breeding and pregnant animals
A. Period from weaning to breeding is critical, because a high rate of twinning and milk production is desired
B. Females should not be allowed to become excessively fat
C. There should be a slight daily weight gain from weaning to breeding
D. After mating, females can be maintained on good pasture
E. During the last 6 to 8 weeks of pregnancy, growth of the fetus is rapid; therefore nutrition should be increased gradually. This can be achieved by the addition of supplements
II. Lactating animals
A. Good pasture is fine for grazers (sheep)
1. Dairy goats are browsers and should be offered high-quality hay and a complete grain ration to maximize milk production
B. If it is winter and the animal is confined, a good grain and forage ration with the addition of trace mineralized salts should be fed
III. Feeding lambs and kids
A. Newborns should nurse within several hours of birth to ensure colostrum intake. Neonates can then nurse or be fed milk or milk replacer for approximately 2 months
B. At 2 weeks of age, they should have free access to creep feed (ground coarse or rolled grain and hay)
C. They should be creep fed until pasture comes available
D. If they are not to be pastured, they should be finished in a dry lot
E. Slowly convert to whole grain in small amounts at first, then increase until the animal is on full feed
F. In addition to grain, the animal is fed a complete diet of hay with a supplement
G. Market weight is reached in 3 to 4 months of age
IV. Orphaned young
A. Orphans should be raised on extra milk or milk replacers
B. Ensure they receive adequate colostrum
1. Keep an extra supply of frozen colostrum for orphans

C. Give water to drink in addition to the milk when they are put on creep at 9 to 10 days of age
D. They can be weaned at 4 to 5 weeks of age if consumption of creep feed is at a reasonable level

## Disease Related to Improper Nutrition

I. Bloat
A. Disease similar to that in cattle
B. Sheep and goats fed on mature pasture with available browse are unlikely to bloat
II. Enterotoxemia
A. Disease similar to that in cattle, except it is more common in sheep and goats
B. Preventive measures are similar to cattle; other measures in lambs include vaccination with *C. perfringens* type D, and types C and D in breeding ewes
C. If an outbreak occurs in lambs, an enterotoxemia antiserum may also be administered
III. Failure of passive transfer (FPT)
A. Similar to that in cattle
IV. Grass tetany
A. Disease similar to that in cattle
V. Ketosis (lambing paralysis)
A. Seen most commonly in ewes (during the last trimester) carrying twins or triplets
B. Preventive measures include feeding the ewe a higher-energy diet supplied through increased grain intake
VI. Thiamine-deficiency polio
A. Disease similar to that in cattle
B. Goats (doe) may be affected while nursing the kids
VII. Rickets
A. Disease similar to that in cattle
VIII. Rumen acidosis
A. Disease similar to that in cattle
IX. Urea toxicity
A. Disease similar to that in cattle
X. Water belly
A. Disease similar to that in cattle
B. Most common in castrated pygmy goats, although there is an increased incidence in all males
C. Other preventive measures in sheep and goats include increasing salt availability and avoiding vitamin A deficiency
XI. White muscle disease
A. Disease similar to that in cattle
B. White muscle disease is most common in the rapidly growing individuals of a flock

Raising sheep and goats can be a relatively low maintenance operation if done properly; however, it is important to find the best feedstuff available in your area. Keep in mind that because of the size and constitutions of sheep and goats, deficiencies or toxicities can develop rather quickly; death rates can be high as a result.

## FEEDING CAMELIDS

Llamas, alpacas, vicunas, and guanacos are part of the group known as South American camelids. Camelids are not classified taxonomically as ruminants but are considered to be functional ruminants. Functional ruminants, like true ruminants, have the ability to convert roughage to usable nutrients. Camelids consume both grass and legume forages and browse and forbs with equal interest. In South America, camelids never need concentrates or supplements and are rarely fed cured hay because they thrive well on the native grasses and forbs. This section on camelid nutrition discusses the feeding and nutrition of camelids in North America to maintain proper health.

### Feed Sources

I. Forages
  A. Although camelids are native to South America and thus have evolved to thrive on forages of that region, they still have the ability to thrive on native grasses of North America
  B. Typical grasses and legumes grown in North America that are fed to true ruminants can be fed to camelids
    1. Camelids are extremely efficient in their ability to convert forages to energy
      a. Obesity is a concern in overfed camelids
    2. Camelids do best when they are allowed to graze on pasture
  C. Feed consumption is based on a percentage of body weight and is higher in the smaller animal and lower in the larger animal
    1. A 50-kg (110-lb) camelid will consume feed at 1.4% of its body weight on an "as-fed" basis
    2. A 150-kg (330-lb) camelid will consume feed at 1.1% of its body weight on an as-fed basis
II. Browse and forbs
  A. Browse and forbs are an extremely important part of the camelid's diet. Camelids are selective consumers of shrubs and leaves. Camelids should be allowed free access to these food sources when available
III. Concentrates
  A. Because camelids are such efficient converters of forage to usable nutrients, concentrates are rarely, if ever, needed
  B. Concentrates may be useful in cases where increased energy and protein are necessary
  C. Mixtures of grains and protein supplements can be used as concentrates

IV. Supplements
  A. Minerals and vitamins can be supplied in block or granular form if the extra nutrients are needed in the diet
    1. Llamas prefer to chew on salt blocks instead of licking them

### Special Nutritional Requirements

I. Water
  A. Camelids should have access to and be allowed to consume clean water ad libitum
    1. Camelids are less likely than other animals to consume contaminated water
  B. If water intake is restricted, feed consumption will be decreased, lactation will be decreased or may cease, and in some extreme cases the camelid may become hyperthermic
  C. Camelid erythrocytes may be more resistant to osmotic pressure changes when the animal consumes large volumes of water. This is a characteristic of camelids; their oval erythrocytes can swell up to 240% of normal size without rupturing
    1. In other species, the round erythrocytes can swell to only 150% of normal size before rupturing
  D. Water requirements of camelids are approximately 9% to 13% of body weight (kg) when on pasture
  E. Camelids living in cold climates need to have a heated waterer because they will not break through the ice to get water
  F. Trail llamas frequently do not drink during the day even if they have access to water
II. Energy
  A. Camelids may be able to convert fiber to energy more efficiently than other ruminants
  B. In comparison to cattle, camelids have a lower metabolizable energy (ME) requirement
  C. Like other ruminants, energy sources include forages and the grains/concentrates that are consumed
III. Protein
  A. Protein requirements are directly related to energy requirements and similar to those of sheep and goats
    1. Protein requirements are 31 g protein per Mcal DE
  B. Camelids can convert poor-quality low-level protein as efficiently as sheep can
  C. Crude protein intake of 10% is adequate for maintenance, and crude protein intake of 16% is required for growth, lactation, and late pregnancy
    1. Crude protein requirements are calculated on a 100% DM basis

IV. Minerals
  A. Calcium and phosphorus
    1. A camelid's final diet should contain more than 0.3% calcium on a DM basis
    2. Calcium/phosphorus ratio should not be less than 1.2:1
    3. Calcium and phosphorus levels are rarely deficient in temperate climate pasture, but tropical climate pastures may be deficient in phosphorus
  B. Sodium and chloride
    1. Camelids should have free access to a mineral block
  C. Cobalt
    1. Need for cobalt is similar to that of other domestic large animals
    2. A deficiency of cobalt eventually leads to thiamine and ascorbic acid deficiency and reduced glucose and ATP levels
      a. Signs of deficiency include ocular discharge, lethargy, weakness, poor weight gain, anemia, ketosis, rough hair coat, and decreased conception rates
    3. Signs of toxicity are similar to those of deficiencies
  D. Copper
    1. Signs of deficiency and toxicity are similar to those of cattle and sheep
      a. Camelids are quite sensitive to copper toxicity
    2. Llamas and alpacas fed side-by-side with sheep in copper-deficient areas did not develop deficiencies
  E. Iron
    1. Iron deficiency in llamas and alpacas is thought to be a factor in the failure to thrive syndrome seen in the cria (neonate)
      a. Camelid milk contains little iron, much like other domestic large animals
    2. Signs of deficiency and treatment methods are similar to those of other domestic large animals
  F. Selenium
    1. As in other animals, selenium and vitamin E must be balanced
    2. Signs of deficiency are similar to signs in cattle and sheep
    3. Selenium supplementation is best offered in a grain mix or as part of a trace mineralized salt block
  G. Zinc
    1. Zinc has close interactions with calcium, copper, iron, and vitamin A
    2. Zinc deficiency in llamas and alpacas may present as a dermatitis
    3. Signs of toxicities have not been observed or reported in llamas and alpacas
    4. Zinc should be incorporated into trace mineral mixes to prevent deficiencies
  H. Iodine
    1. Llamas and alpacas are at risk when raised in iodine-deficient areas in North America
    2. Prevention of deficiencies is easily accomplished through iodine supplementation in the mineral mix or grain mix
    3. Iodine toxicity is rare but is readily prevented by avoiding excessive therapy with iodine-containing medications and preventing overconsumption of iodized salts
V. Vitamins
  A. Microbes in the first compartment of camelids synthesize B-complex vitamins, vitamin C, and vitamin K
    1. Deficiencies occur when first compartment microbial activity is altered
    2. Importance of vitamins B complex, C, and K is similar to that for other ruminants
  B. Species-specific data for vitamins A, D, and E are limited in camelid medicine
    1. Signs of deficiency/toxicity and treatment methods are best taken from other ruminant species data and applied to camelids
    2. Importance of vitamins A, D, and E is similar to that for other ruminants

## Life Stages

Although specific life stage nutrition resources are not available, a practical guide to each stage can be extrapolated from that for other large animal species. These guidelines include the following.
  I. Ensure that the cria (neonate) receives adequate colostrum from the dam within the first 18 to 24 hours after birth
 II. Juveniles will need extra energy and a high-quality protein source for growth. A balanced source of minerals and vitamins will also be important in growth
III. The adult should be fed for maintenance to avoid issues with obesity
IV. Pregnant dams will need more energy and protein in the last trimester for growth of the fetus
 V. Lactating dams will need higher energy and protein levels to nurse the cria

## Disease Related to Improper Nutrition

  I. FPT
    A. Similar to cattle
 II. Failure to thrive/wasting syndrome
    A. Some llamas have been observed to become anorectic, lose weight, and die

B. This condition is a complex syndrome that may be caused by many factors, but may partly be due to poor nutrition

C. Proper nutrition plays a major role in prevention of this syndrome

III. Metabolic bone disease (rickets)

A. As seen in other mammals, metabolic bone disease is caused by inadequate levels of calcium, phosphorus, and vitamin D

1. Other factors that may cause this disease include protein deficiency and primary diseases of the kidney, liver, and intestine

B. In addition to these factors, some camelid owners suspect that the high calcium content in alfalfa disrupts the absorption of phosphorus, thus leading to rickets. This has not been proven

C. Clinical signs and preventive measures are the same as those in other animals

IV. Obesity

A. Overfeeding of concentrates leading to obesity is a frequent problem

B. Feeding camelids to excess is not only costly but also leads to health problems, such as infertility and hyperthermia

C. All nutritional requirements should be balanced to fit the individual animal

1. Feed more energy to underweight animals and decrease energy in overweight animals

V. Starvation/inanition

A. Camelids that are underweight because of starvation may be a common problem among inexperienced owners

1. Other factors that should be considered in underweight animals are infectious and parasitic diseases

B. Identifying marked weight loss in camelids may be difficult for the owner, because the thick fiber coat of camelids obscures the view of the backbone

1. Camelid owners should be instructed to evaluate body weight and body condition by

a. Weighing and recording body weights on a regular basis

b. Performing a body score on the animal (see Table 16-1 as a guide)

(1) Locations for evaluating body conditions on camelids are over the withers, the fiberless area behind the elbow, between the rear legs, the chest between the front legs, and the perineum

C. Prevention of starvation is more a management issue that is simply addressed by frequently observing and weighing animals and feeding an adequate, well-balanced diet

## MONOGASTRIC DIGESTION

### BASIC ANATOMY AND PHYSIOLOGY ■■■■■■

I. Mouth and esophagus

A. Tongue, teeth, and salivary glands are important for proper prehension, mastication, mixing, and deglutition

1. Lips of horses are important in prehension of foodstuffs

2. Swine saliva acts as a lubricant and as a buffer to regulate stomach pH, and contains salivary amylase to break down carbohydrates

3. Equine saliva contains no enzymes

4. Horses cannot regurgitate because of one-way esophageal peristalsis

II. Stomach

A. Stomach of swine is a muscular organ that causes the physical breakdown of food through powerful contractions

1. Hydrochloric acid, pepsin, and rennin are the digestive enzymes secreted by the stomach

2. Swine stomachs maintain a pH of 2 and have a strong bactericidal effect on ingested microorganisms

B. Equine stomach is smaller relative to that of other animal species

1. Horses should be fed small portions more frequently per day

2. Equine stomach does not mix foodstuffs well, so digestive disorders often originate in the stomach

III. Small intestine

A. Small intestine of swine and horses is divided into the duodenum, jejunum, and ileum, like all monogastric animals

B. Small intestine is important because digestive enzymes are mixed with chyme (food mixture from the stomach), digestion continues, and nutrients are absorbed

C. A unique characteristic of horses is that they have no gallbladder, so bile is constantly secreted into the duodenum

IV. Large intestine

A. Cecum

1. The cecum of swine has minimal function in digestion

2. The cecum of horses, however, is quite large (up to 8-gallon capacity in mature animals) and breaks down cellulose and synthesizes nutrients via microbial fermentation, much like the rumen of cattle

B. Colon

1. Function of the colon in swine and horses is resorption of water, bacterial fermentation of vitamins B and K, synthesis of protein, some breakdown of fiber, and limited nutrient absorption

2. Water is absorbed primarily from the small colon in horses
   C. Rectum
      1. Serves to store waste before defecation

## FEEDING SWINE

I. Swine are omnivores and as such can accommodate some dietary fiber
II. Swine exhibit a better rate of weight gain from concentrates, which are fortified with energy, protein, and mineral and vitamin supplements to form the normal diet
III. Advanced technology is highly evident in many swine operations today
   A. Formulation of diets is more precise and economical, with synthetic nutrients, high-quality byproducts, and new feeds
   B. Swine operations use the technology of their feed supplier to meet the nutritional needs of all pigs in the herd
   C. Feeding a premix in their regular grain ration will meet nutritional needs
   D. Nutrient deficiencies of these grains are corrected by the premix
   E. All life stages are met with different premix formulations

### Feed Sources, Preparation and Feeding of Grains

I. Improvements in gain and feed efficiency can be expected from grinding grain, but if grain is ground too fine, digestive problems can be created
II. Grain should be reduced to a medium-fine particle size
III. Common grains are corn, oats, wheat, barley, and sorghum

### Special Nutritional Requirements

I. Water
   A. Best given free choice with easy access
II. Energy (chiefly carbohydrates and fat)
   A. Energy content in a diet controls the amount eaten
   B. Fiber corresponds directly to fat
   C. High-energy diets are fed during lactation
III. Protein and amino acids
   A. Amino acids are essential for maintenance, growth, gestation, and lactation
   B. Amino acids indispensable for growing pigs are arginine, histidine, isoleucine, leucine, lysine, methionine, phenylalanine, threonine, tryptophan, and valine
      1. Three of greatest importance are lysine, tryptophan, and threonine
IV. Minerals
   A. Calcium and phosphorus
      1. Primarily for skeletal growth
      2. Important for metabolism

3. Adequacy is essential to gestation and lactation
4. Easily supplied by use of tankage, meat meal, meat and bone and fish meal, limestone, and oyster shell
   B. Sodium chloride
      1. Recommended salt allowance is 0.25% of the total diet
      2. Supplied by animal and fish byproducts in the diet
   C. Iodine
      1. Used by the thyroid gland to produce thyroxine
      2. Supplied as iodized salt
   D. Iron and copper
      1. Necessary for hemoglobin formation and to prevent nutritional anemia
      2. Sow's milk is severely deficient in iron
      3. Feeding lactating sows increased levels of iron does not seem to pass sufficiently high levels to piglets
   E. Cobalt
      1. Present in vitamin $B_{12}$
   F. Manganese
      1. Essential for normal reproduction and growth
   G. Potassium
      1. Requirements are met in the feedstuffs
   H. Magnesium
      1. Essential for growing swine
   I. Zinc
      1. In swine nutrition, zinc is interrelated with calcium
      2. Supplemented zinc is recommended to prevent parakeratosis
   J. Selenium
      1. Vitamin E is interrelated with selenium
      2. Selenium requirement depends on soil conditions where crop for feed is grown. Most swine today are raised in total confinement
V. Vitamins
   A. Vitamin A
      1. Use of stabilized vitamin A is common
      2. Natural vitamin A is degraded under normal environmental conditions
   B. Vitamin D
      1. Necessary for proper bone growth and ossification
      2. Vitamin D needs can be met by exposing pigs to direct sunlight for a short time each day
      3. Sources: irradiated yeast, sun-cured hays, activated plant or animal sterols, fish oils, and vitamin A and D concentrates
   C. Vitamin E (tocopherol)
      1. Required by swine of all ages
      2. Interrelated with selenium
      3. Green forage, legume hays, and cereal grains all contain appreciable amounts of vitamin E

D. Vitamin K
  1. A fat-soluble vitamin, necessary for blood clotting to convert fibrinogen to fibrin
  2. Supplement vitamin K for added insurance
E. Thiamine, riboflavin, and niacin
  1. Thiamine is not of practical importance in the diet
  2. Riboflavin is a requirement of breeding stock and lightweight pigs
    a. Crystalline form of riboflavin (and niacin) is added to premixes
  3. Riboflavin is naturally found in green forage, milk byproducts, and brewer's yeast
  4. Natural sources of niacin include fish and animal byproducts
F. Pantothenic acid
  1. Especially important for females (reproduction)
  2. Crystalline form is added in premixes
  3. Natural sources include green forage, legume meals, milk products, and brewer's yeast
G. Pyridoxine (vitamin $B_6$)
  1. Plentiful in ingredients of swine feed
H. Choline
  1. Essential for normal functioning of liver and kidneys
  2. Supplementing choline has been shown to increase litter size
  3. Naturally found in fish solubles, fish meal, and soybean meal
I. Vitamin $B_{12}$
  1. Required by the young pig for growth and normal hemopoiesis
  2. Present in animal, marine, and milk products
  3. Crystalline form is added to premixes
J. Biotin, folic acid, and ascorbic acid
  1. Biotin and folic acid are essential for growth
  2. There is no evidence to indicate the need to supplement

## Life Stages

I. Management of breeding sows and litters
  A. Breeding sows are limit fed from breeding up to the last trimester
    1. Sows are fed 4 to 6 lb (1.8 to 2.7 kg) of a complete ration supplying 6000 to 7000 kcal ME
  B. In the last trimester, feed is increased to supply additional energy to the rapidly growing fetuses
    1. Sows are fed a complete ration that supplies 9000 to 10,000 kcal ME per day
    2. The sow should not be overfed, because this will directly affect milk production during lactation
    3. The more vigorous a baby pig is, the better is its chance for survival. To produce healthy pigs, the gestation diets must be adequate in all nutrients
  C. During lactation, energy intake will be increased to 15,000 to 20,000 kcal ME per day
    1. Fat may be added to the diet to improve feed palatability and energy density
II. Management of piglets
  A. Care should be taken to ensure that each piglet has nursed regularly
    1. Keep the sow's teat line clean so the piglets are less likely to develop scours
      a. Scouring leads to poor gains or even death
  B. An anemia prevention program should be in place
    1. Injection or oral iron dextran should be given within 3 days of birth
  C. A palatable pig starter diet should be available from 2 weeks of age until weaning
III. Starter pigs
  A. Piglets are weaned at 3 to 5 weeks of age and are fed as starters until they weigh 40 to 50 lb (18 to 22.7 kg)
    1. Starter pigs are fed ad libitum
  B. Starter rations are high in protein (20% to 24%), nutrient dense, supplied as a pellet, and often purchased from a commercial feed supplier because of the feed complexity
  C. Starter ration is eventually changed to a ground feed in the last couple weeks of the starter period
IV. Management of growing/finishing market hogs
  A. For today's market hog, higher levels of protein and less energy are fed to develop the leanest animal
    1. Feeds are evaluated on their amino acid content
    2. Protein sources supplied in the growing/finishing ration are usually soybean meal, meat and bone meal, and synthetic amino acids
      a. Synthetic amino acids are lysine, methionine, threonine, and tryptophan
  B. Grower/finishers are fed ground cereal grains (corn, wheat, sorghum, and barley), which make up to 85% of a typical ration
  C. Growing/finishing rations are fortified with numerous minerals and vitamins
    1. Calcium and phosphorus should be properly balanced during this period
  D. Housing and space are important aspects in growing/finishing swine. A veterinary technician's role in a swine facility involves herd health and piglet care. Nutritional needs and problems are met by the feed supplier with premixes and rations tailored to individual operations and life stages of the pigs.

## Disease Related to Improper Nutrition

I. Anemia
  A. Anemia is a regularly diagnosed problem in baby pigs

B. Baby pigs should be given iron dextran by injection (150 to 200 mg) or as an oral solution

C. Iron can also be supplied in the prestarter ration of piglets that are creep fed

D. Vitamin E should be given just before the iron injection to prevent iron toxicity

II. FPT

   A. Similar to that of other livestock

   B. Runt piglets within a litter fail to thrive and may need special attention

III. Parakeratosis

   A. Metabolic disturbance due to a deficiency of zinc and an excess of calcium in the diet

   B. Disease is characterized by changes in the skin, mainly skin lesions. The skin lesions are areas of excessive growth and keratinization of the skin epithelium

   C. Parakeratosis is prevented and treated by balancing zinc and calcium in the diet

## FEEDING HORSES

Horses are herbivores and are classified as hindgut fermenters. The stomach has a relatively small capacity (5 to 15 L) and contributes little to the digestion of the feed. Horses must eat frequently. Enzymatic digestion similar to that of dogs and cats occurs in the small intestine. Any ingested food that reaches the cecum and large intestine undergoes microbial fermentation. There is no gallbladder for storage, and bile is excreted continuously.

### Feed Sources

I. A horse consumes most of its nutritional requirements in the form of forages, such as hay and pasture

   A. Quality of dry roughage depends greatly on the stage of maturation at harvesting and weather conditions during harvest

   B. Soil quality also has an effect on forage quality

   C. Ensiled forage is not generally fed because of the sensitivity of horses to molds and mycotoxins that may be in silage

II. Ideal forages include grass hay (bromegrass, orchard grass, Bermuda grass, and timothy), legume hay (alfalfa and clover), and grazing pastures

   A. Straw and corn stalks are not recommended as a feed, because they have low nutritional value and there is a risk of compaction if too much is consumed

   B. Hay and grasses contain varying amounts of cellulose and starch, depending on their maturity

   C. It is important for horses that all forages be clean and dry with no mold or dust present. Forages should be leafy, have a green color, and be harvested earlier so plant fiber can be easily digested

      1. Horses fed moldy sweet clover are at risk of developing sweet clover poisoning. Horses

with sweet clover poisoning develop multisystemic hemorrhages owing to the impact on blood coagulation

      2. Horses grazing on pastures with fescue grass are at risk of developing fescue grass toxicosis

         a. The endophyte *Acremonium* is known to infect fescue grass

         b. Significant reproductive problems may be noted with the mare fed contaminated fescue grass

III. Grains are used as a supplement to any forage feeding program

   A. Amount of grain will be indicated by horse's life stage and/or workload

   B. Corn, barley, wheat, and oats are common grain supplements

   C. Protein supplements, such as linseed meal, soybean meal, and milk protein (foal diet), can be offered to improve feed protein values

   D. Horses should be fed forages before grains to ensure proper and complete digestion of the grain

      1. If grains are fed before or with forages, the grains are passed in the feces before they can be adequately digested

   E. Fat and vegetable oil supplementation has been suggested to provide energy for growing, lactating, and working horses

   F. Fermentable fiber byproducts, such as rice, wheat bran, and beet pulp, are becoming more popular

      1. Wheat bran is often used in conjunction with psyllium to improve fiber bulk to prevent or treat sand colic in horses

IV. Horses should be kept free from disease and dewormed on a regular basis to fully benefit from good nutritional practices

### Special Nutritional Requirements

I. Carbohydrates supply 80% to 90% of dietary energy for horses and are available in the forms of grains, forages, and supplements. The interaction of minerals and vitamins and their availability in the grains and grasses grown can be complex

II. Minerals and vitamins

   A. Amount required for all minerals vary according to age, weight, and work of the horse

   B. Minerals and vitamins for the horse are essentially the same as for cattle (see earlier section)

   C. If feedstuff is deficient in minerals, a mineral supplement may be fed free choice

      1. If a mineral deficiency is suspected, do not overlook the resources of the local diagnostic laboratory

      2. Deficiencies are often the result of anorexia or poor-quality feed

D. Oversupplementation generally occurs inadvertently by well-meaning owners
E. For ease of definition for horse feeding, minerals can be divided into two groups: macrominerals and microminerals
   1. Macrominerals
      a. Macrominerals are constituents of bones and structural proteins
      b. Expressed as parts per hundred
      c. Potassium: most forages have this available
      d. Calcium and phosphorus: for bone and cell function
         (1) Ratio is about 1.7:1 in foals and 1 to 1.3:1 in adults
         (2) Deficiency can cause abnormal bone growth and thin weak bones. Mild deficiencies may cause subtle lameness
         (3) Excess calcium may impair trace mineral and phosphorus absorption. Excess phosphorus can cause a secondary nutritional hyperparathyroidism
      e. Magnesium
         (1) Deficiency is very uncommon, but if present will cause staggering, nervousness, and convulsions
      f. Sodium chloride (salt) is necessary for cell function and water balance
         (1) Salt is typically fed in a block
         (2) Horses lose 30 grains of salt in every pound of perspiration; working horses require additional salt in their grain rations
         (3) Salt added to a ration does not compensate for the other minerals if the forage and grain are deficient
   2. Microminerals
      a. Referred to as trace minerals; only small amounts needed by the horse
      b. Measured as parts per million (mg/kg)
      c. Iodine
         (1) Produces the hormone thyroxine, which is needed in fetal development
         (2) Deficiencies can cause serious fetal abnormalities
         (3) Foals will be born weak and prone to infections and may not suckle or stand; thyroid glands can be enlarged
         (4) Mares may have goiter, a longer gestation, and retained placenta
         (5) Excess can cause same symptoms as deficiency
      d. Copper
         (1) Important for cartilage, bone, and pigment formation and for use of iron
      e. Iron
         (1) Necessary to form hemoglobin
         (2) Deficiency causes anemia
         (3) Overuse of injectable iron can cause iron toxicity
      f. Manganese and zinc
         (1) Zinc deficiency may cause hair loss and poor wound healing
         (2) Zinc excess can cause bone problems and lameness
      g. Selenium
         (1) Needed with vitamin E
         (2) Deficiency causes white muscle disease. Foals are born weak and unable to stand, suckle, or breathe normally. Mares have reduced fertility and increased incidence of retained placentas
         (3) Excess causes serious health problems. Overdose can cause sudden excitability and difficulty breathing. Chronic high intakes cause lameness, loss of mane or tail hair, and hoof deformity

III. Protein
   A. Feeding excess protein is wasteful. A strong ammonia odor exists in stables where horses are fed excess protein
      1. Alfalfa hay will cause stronger ammonia smell than grass hay because of its increased nitrogen
   B. Protein-deficient diets are very harmful
      1. Signs can be low weight gains or weight loss and skeletal stunting in young horses

IV. Water
   A. Water is vital
   B. Horse's body is made up of 70% water
   C. Horses drink 2 to 4 L water/kg DM feed eaten (1 gallon/2 lb of dry feed). A 1000-lb (455-kg) horse fed hay will drink about 40 to 50 L (10.5 to 13 gallons) daily
   D. Intake also depends on size of horse, amount and type of diet fed, outdoor temperature, and amount of work being done

## Life Stages

I. Feeding programs are based on the following
   A. Age (weanling, yearling, 2-year-old, mature adult, senior)
   B. Current weight and ideal for age
   C. Function: idle, working, or breeding
   D. Feeds available in the area
   E. Management, including housing conditions and overcrowding
II. Feed consumption
   A. A proper horse-feeding program provides adequate water and energy to ensure proper body condition (see Table 16-1)

B. Calculations are generally based on a horse's weight and the amount of feed required per 100 lb (45 kg) of horse
   1. Adult at maintenance requires about 1.2% to 1.5% of body weight of forage DM per day
      a. Example: A 1000-lb (455-kg) horse requiring 1.5% dietary forage would receive 15 lb (7 kg) of hay per day, or, in practical terms, three 5-lb (2.3-kg) "flakes" of hay per day
   2. Energy levels need to be increased when exercise or work increases, and it is generally supplied by grains and concentrates
   3. Pregnancy demands an increase in energy of 20% to 30%, depending on the stage
   4. Peak lactation may require 75% increase in energy
   5. Ribs should be felt but not seen in young horses

III. Feeding the horse
   A. Feeding suckling foals and weanlings
      1. Suckling foals
         a. Ensure that the foal stands within 2 hours of birth and begins nursing. Adequate colostrum intake is critical within the first 18 hours to ensure maximum absorption of colostral antibodies
            (1) Healthy foals will nurse from the mare 25 to 30 times per day and ingest 20% or more of their body weight in milk
         b. Foal will obtain the majority of its nutrients from nursing for the first several months of life
            (1) Make sure the mare is adequately fed high-quality feedstuffs while nursing the foal
         c. Offer small amounts of creep feeds and high-quality forages beginning as early as 1 to 2 weeks of age
            (1) Commercial concentrate mixtures (sweet feed) supplying 16% crude protein are recommended
            (2) Young foals may be offered creep feeds top dressed with milk protein/milk replacer if they are not gaining weight adequately
         d. Starting at 2 to 3 months of age, feed 1 lb (0.45 kg) of grain concentrate per day and increase to 1 additional lb of grain concentrate for every month of age through weaning, with a maximum of 7 to 9 lb (3.2 to 4 kg) of grain concentrate
         e. Start deworming foals at 2 to 3 months of age
            (1) Continue a deworming schedule of every 30 to 60 days throughout life

   2. Weanlings
      a. Weanlings should be fed 6 to 8 lb (2.7 to 3.6 kg) of concentrate per day, and at least 1 lb of high-quality forage for every 100 lb (45 kg) of body weight through 12 months of age
      b. DM intake should equal 3% of body weight
   B. Feeding yearlings and 2-year-olds
      1. Yearlings can be fed free choice high-quality hay and pasture at this stage
      2. Yearlings and 2-year-olds should still be receiving an adequate supply of protein, vitamins, and minerals to ensure proper growth and development of the body tissues and skeleton
         a. Trace mineralized salt blocks should be available
      3. A 13% crude protein concentrate can be fed at this stage
      4. DM intake should equal 2.5% of body weight
   C. Feeding the mature horse, dry mare, and gelding
      1. A mature animal that is idle or ridden or worked infrequently can be maintained on hay or pasture alone
         a. DM intake should equal about 1.75% of body weight
      2. A calcium/phosphorus and salt supplement should be offered to these animals
      3. Concentrates can always be offered in small amounts or can be increased based on the amount of work. Make changes in diet slowly, preferably over 7 to 10 days
         a. Concentrate protein levels may be fed at 8.5% to 10% crude protein
   D. Feeding for reproduction
      1. Gestation
         a. A mare can be fed at maintenance levels until the last 90 days of gestation
         b. During late pregnancy, the mare needs 20% more energy and an increase to an 11% crude protein level
         c. During the last 3 weeks of gestation the mare needs 30% more energy, more calcium and phosphorus, and 1.75 to 2.0 lb (0.7 to 0.9 kg) of legume hay per 100 lb (45 kg) of body weight
            (1) If nutrient intake was adequate during gestation, the mare should have gained an extra 10% body weight
            (2) Lactation
               (a) Same ration type fed to yearlings can be used for the lactating mare
               (b) Bring the mare to a full feed regimen providing 1 to 1.5 lb (0.45 to

0.7 kg) of concentrate per 100 lb of body weight within 7 to 10 days postpartum

    (c) If rebreeding the mare while she is still lactating, be sure to consider the total energy requirements needed for maintenance, lactation, and rebreeding. Offer additional feed to allow the mare to gain weight to get her in breeding condition

E. Feeding the working or performance horse
1. Exercise increases a horse's need for energy, but not necessarily the protein and mineral requirements
2. A hardworking horse may require more concentrate than forage to supply the needed energy
    a. Be sure to feed at least 1 lb (0.45 kg) forage per 100 lb (45 kg) of body weight to minimize digestive disturbances
    b. A light working horse on 8.5% crude protein concentrate needs 0.5 to 1.5 lb (0.2 to 0.7 kg) of grain per hour of activity per day
    c. A moderate working horse on 8.5% to 10% crude protein concentrate needs 2 to 3 lb (0.9 to 1.4 kg) of grain per hour of activity per day
    d. A heavy working horse on 8.5% to 10% crude protein concentrate needs at least 4 lb (≥1.8 kg) of grain per hour of activity per day
3. After heavy exercise, be sure to cool the horse down before allowing the horse to drink. A hot horse is more likely to have digestive disturbances and to founder if allowed to drink immediately after exercise

F. Feeding stallions
1. Feed stallions at maintenance levels when not used for breeding
2. Offer some additional grain during the breeding season to keep the stallion in good breeding condition

G. Feeding hospitalized horses
1. A sick horse has the same nutritional deficits, stresses, and catabolic wasting problems that small animals have when they are sick. Major gastrointestinal disturbances (e.g., colic and colitis), including decreased gastrointestinal motility, often lead to an animal that is unwilling to eat
2. It may be necessary to administer a slurry of feedstuffs by a nasogastric tube to ensure that the animal receives some nutrients until it is ready to eat on its own

**Disease Related to Improper Nutrition**

I. Rhabdomyolysis (myositis, azoturia, Monday morning sickness)
  A. Acute inflammatory disease of muscle
    1. Clinical signs of disease include excessive sweating, nervousness, abdominal distress, reluctance to walk or move, stiff gait, and coffee-colored urine (myoglobinuria)
  B. True cause of rhabdomyolysis is unclear, but it is associated with a feeding schedule in which high-grain or concentrate diet is fed throughout the week, followed by rest for 1 to 2 days; this is when they develop clinical signs
  C. Preventive measures include reducing feed intake when a horse is not working and exercising the animal during the rest period

II. Colic
  A. There are many causes of colic. Potential nutritional issues include inadequate water intake, overfeeding, overeating on new pasture, and improper feeding
  B. Preventive measures for colic include proper feeding and deworming practices, free access to salt to encourage adequate water intake, and limiting exposure to new pasture

III. Choke
  A. Choke is not considered a true nutritional disease, but can be attributed to improper feeding practices
  B. Most common causes of choke are inadequate water intake, feedstuffs that are fed too dry, feedstuff particle sizes that are too large, and greedy eating habits
  C. Preventive measures include encouraging adequate water intake, soaking feedstuffs before feeding (e.g., beet pulp and alfalfa cubes), and using hay nets or restrictive muzzles to slow feed intake of greedy eaters

IV. Diarrhea (colitis)
  A. Nutritional diarrhea is uncommon in the equine foal or adult, and not all cases can be associated with specific diseases or nutritional imbalance
  B. Any change in feed or feeding regimen and nutritional imbalances could change the gastrointestinal environment and lead to diarrhea
  C. It is best to offer only good-quality feedstuffs and balanced diets and to change feeds or feeding regimens slowly over 7 to 10 days

V. Failure of passive transfer (FPT)
  A. Similar to that in livestock
  B. Foals nursing mares that came into milk early and were leaking colostrum, and foals later diagnosed with neonatal maladjustment syndrome ("dumby-foal") tend to be at the greatest risk

**Table 16-2** Relative nutrient content of various feedstuffs for livestock

| Feedstuff group | Protein | Energy | Minerals | | Vitamins | | Fiber |
| | | | Macro | Micro | Fat-Sol. | B complex | |
|---|---|---|---|---|---|---|---|
| High quality roughage | +++ | ++ | ++ | ++ | +++ | + | +++ |
| Low quality roughage | + | + | + | + | – | – | ++++ |
| Cereal grains | ++ | +++ | + | + | + | + | + |
| Grain millfeeds | ++ | ++ | ++ | ++ | + | ++ | ++ |
| Fats and oils | – | ++++ | – | – | – | – | – |
| Molasses | + | +++ | ++ | ++ | – | + | – |
| Fermentation products | +++ | ++ | + | ++ | – | ++++ | ± |
| Oil seed proteins | +++ | +++ | ++ | ++ | + | ++ | + |
| Animal proteins | ++++ | +++ | +++ | +++ | ++ | +++ | + |

From Grosdidier SR et al: Nutrition. In Sirois M, editor: *Principles and practice of veterinary technology,* ed 2, St Louis, 2004, Mosby.

C. Prevention is similar to that in livestock. Taking a proactive role in ensuring that the foal stands and nurses within the first few hours of life is critical

VI. Heaves

A. Essential cause of heaves is unknown, but it is associated with the consumption of moldy or dusty feeds at times of challenge (e.g., upper respiratory disease, pneumonia)

B. Incidence of heaves may be decreased by feeding good-quality, dust-free feedstuffs or by moistening dusty feeds

VII. Laminitis and chronic founder

A. Laminitis is often associated with consumption of excess grain, lush pasture, or water

B. By providing a proper ration and monitoring consumption of feedstuffs, most instances of nutritionally induced laminitis and chronic founder can be prevented

VIII. Moon blindness (periodic ophthalmia, equine recurrent uveitis)

A. Occurrence of moonblindness appears to be associated with a lack of riboflavin and with bacterial or viral disease

B. By feeding rations that contain at least 40 mg of riboflavin per day (green grass and green leafy hay), incidences of moonblindness may be reduced

IX. Rickets

A. As in other large animals, rickets is associated with imbalances of calcium, phosphorus, and/or vitamin D

B. By balancing the minerals and vitamins in the ration, rickets can be prevented

X. Water belly

A. As in other large animal species, males are most often affected

B. Clinical signs, cause, and prevention of water belly are similar to those of other large animal species

Consult the district agrologist or university extension agent for types of feeds and nutrient levels in your area. There usually are pamphlets available on the care and feeding of horses that pertain to the climate and area where you live. All horses are individuals, and feeding programs should stress that. The diet must be balanced for proteins, minerals, and vitamins.

Ruminant, swine, and equine feeding is a science that should be practically met whenever possible in agricultural operations. Large animal veterinarians who have a herd health practice will rely heavily on nutritional diagnosis. The importance of the technician is to be able to take accurate descriptions of feeding programs, know where discrepancies may occur, and know what mineral and vitamin deficiencies occur in the area. A technician in a large animal practice will have to answer questions regarding feeding programs, and it helps to have some common knowledge of basic nutrition (Table 16-2).

### ACKNOWLEDGMENT

The author and editors recognize and appreciate the original work of Sandy Hass, on which this chapter is based.

# Glossary

**additive** Ingredient or combination of ingredients added to the basic feed to fulfill a specific need

**ad libitum** Means "as needed"; also thought of as free choice

**anorexia** Lack or loss of the appetite for food

**background** Feed a calf to gain 1 to 1.5 lb (0.45 to 0.7 kg) of body weight a day

**biological value** Percentage of true absorbed protein that is available for productive body functions

**bloom** Stage of flowering in legumes. Usually classified as early, 50% bloom, 75% bloom, or full bloom

**browse** Brushy plant, a shrub, a bush, or a tree of small stature

**carbonaceous** High in energy; some feedstuffs are naturally high in energy

**choke** Obstruction of the esophagus with feedstuffs or foreign bodies. Seen most often in the horse and cattle

**colostrums** First milk from postparturient animal that is high in antibodies and rich in nutrients

**concentrates** Classification of a feedstuff. Concentrate feeds include corn, milo, cottonseeds, barley, and wheat. Concentrates are feeds that are low in fiber. A concentrate is divided into two categories: protein and energy

**cri** Neonatal llama and alpaca

**deglutition** Act of swallowing

**digestible energy (DE)** Gross energy of a food minus the energy lost in the feces. This measurement may overestimate the available energy of high-fiber feedstuffs

**digestion** Process of breaking down proteins, carbohydrates, and fats into absorbable nutrients

**dry matter intake (DMI)** Percentage of dry matter that an animal consumes. A very important criterion for formulating rations

**ensiling** Harvesting process by which a forage is chopped and placed in a storage unit (e.g., silo) that excludes oxygen. Through fermenting, lactic acid is produced

**eructation** Belching of rumen gas

**feedlot** Where a beef or dairy animal is fed to slaughter. Feed resources must be known to calculate a balanced ration

**feedstuff** Also called feed; any dietary component that provides some essential nutrient

**forbs** Leafy plant

**founder** Inflammation of the tissue that attaches the hoof to the foot; also called laminitis. Founder is considered to be a more chronic condition, whereas laminitis is either acute or chronic

**FPT** Failure of passive transfer

**gross energy (GE)** Related to chemical composition. It has no real value in assessing feed, but has to be used in determining the energy value of feedstuffs

**haylage** Ensiled chopped alfalfa

**herbivore** Species of animal that depends entirely on plants for food

**inanition** Condition of exhaustion caused by inadequate nutrition

**legumes** Leafy hay, such as alfalfa, red and white clover, birdsfoot trefoil, and vetch

**maintenance nutrient requirements (MNRs)** Levels of nutrients needed to sustain body weight without gain or loss

**mastication** Reduction in feed particle size by chewing

**Mcal** Megacalorie; 1 Mcal is equal to 1000 kcal

**metabolizable energy (ME)** Measure of the dietary energy available for metabolism after energy losses that occur in the urine (UE) and the combustible gases are subtracted from digestible energy. DE and ME are correlated

**NPN** Nonprotein nitrogen includes compounds (e.g., urea and biurates) that are not proteins but contain nitrogen and can be converted to protein through bacterial action in the rumen of livestock

**nutrient** Substance that can be used as food

**parakeratosis** In swine, it is caused by a zinc deficiency and is characterized by excessive growth and keratinization of the skin

**pica** A depraved appetite characterized by a craving for unnatural articles (dirt, sand, hair, feces, etc.)

**potable water** Clean, fresh water suitable for drinking

**premix** Total ration mixed with various feedstuffs at the feed mill

**proteinaceous** High in protein value. Some feedstuffs have a naturally high protein value

**ration** Amount of total feed provided to one animal during a 24-hour period for the desired productive purpose

**regurgitation** Casting up of undigested material (cud); cud is remasticated and reswallowed

**replacement heifer** Female calf placed in the breeding herd at 24 to 30 months of age, when she has her first parturition

**rhabdomyolysis** Severe muscle damage that can occur when horses are fed a high-grain or high-concentrate diet throughout the week and then are rested for 1 to 2 days. They develop clinical signs that include myoglobinemia and myoglobinuria (coffee-colored urine)

**roughages or forages** Consist of most or all of the plant, such as pasture and hay

**scours** Neonatal diarrhea

**silage** Ensiled chopped corn

**springing heifer** Pregnant (first calf) heifer

**tankage** Act or process of storing or putting in a tank; animal residues left after rendering fat in a slaughterhouse, used for fertilizer or feed

**tocopherol** Vitamin E

**total digestible nutrients (TDNs)** Attempts to measure digestible energy in weight units. The basis is rather simple: every feed has a total energy. After it has been through the animal, measure what comes out. What is left over is the TDN

**total mixed ration (TMR)** Practice of weighing and blending all feedstuffs into a complete ration

**transfaunation** Repopulation of healthy rumen microbes in one ruminant into another ruminant with poor rumen function or decreased rumen microbial population. This is most often accomplished through siphoning the healthy rumen microbes from a donor animal (microbe-rich liquid or transfaunate) via a stomach tube and then placing an orogastric tube in the recipient's distal esophagus or rumen and administering the transfaunate

# Review Questions

1 Ketosis in the cow and lambing paralysis in the ewe can be prevented by
   a. Feeding poorer quality proteins during gestation
   b. Increasing energy intake when energy needs are highest for each species
   c. Increasing calcium intake
   d. Fortifying the diet with vitamin C
2 The "fermentation vat" in ruminants is the
   a. Omasum
   b. Abomasum
   c. Rumen and reticulum
   d. None of the above

**3** In sheep, an acute toxicity of this trace mineral can lead to a severe gastroenteritis with hemorrhagic diarrhea
   a. Cobalt
   b. Copper
   c. Selenium
   d. Zinc

**4** The purpose of creep feeding is to
   a. Allow young animals access to grain that the dams are denied
   b. Allow dams access to grain that the young are denied
   c. Increase ovulation before breeding
   d. Improve lactation capacity of dairy cattle

**5** Vitamin A deficiency in cattle can result in all except
   a. Rickets
   b. Reproductive failure
   c. Night blindness
   d. Poor hair coat

**6** White muscle disease is related to
   a. Overconsumption of urea in the diet
   b. Consuming moldy feeds
   c. Vitamin E and selenium deficiencies
   d. Insufficient energy intake

**7** The greatest energy demand for most animal species occurs during
   a. First trimester of pregnancy
   b. Last trimester of pregnancy
   c. Peak lactation
   d. Growth as a yearling

**8** An injection given routinely to piglets at birth is
   a. Seven-way clostridial injection
   b. Iron
   c. Vitamins A, D, and E
   d. Selenium

**9** In young ruminants, enterotoxemia is caused by
   a. Feeding roughages too early in life
   b. Overeating milk or milk replacer
   c. Inadequate colostrum intake within 18 hours of birth
   d. Grazing on magnesium deficient pastures

**10** An example of a legume commonly fed to cattle is
   a. Corn
   b. Oats
   c. Barley
   d. Alfalfa

## BIBLIOGRAPHY

Aiello SE et al: *The Merck veterinary manual*, ed 9, Rahway, NJ, 2005, Merck.

Church D, Kellems R: *Livestock feeds and feeding*, ed 5, Portland, Ore, 2001, Prentice-Hall Career & Technology.

Fowler ME: *Medicine and surgery of South American camelids*, ed 2, Ames, Iowa, 1998, Blackwell.

Grosdidier SR: Nutrition. In Sirois M, editor: *Principles and practices of veterinary technology,* ed 2, St Louis, 2004, Mosby.

Jurgens MH: *Animal feeding and nutrition*, ed 9, Dubuque, Iowa, 2001, Kendall/Hunt.

National Research Council: *Nutrient requirements of beef cattle*, ed 7, Washington, DC, 1996, National Academy Press.

National Research Council: *Nutrient requirements of dairy cattle*, ed 6, Washington, DC, 1988, National Academy Press.

National Research Council: *Nutrient requirements of goats: angora, dairy, and meat goats in temperate and tropical countries*, ed 5, Washington, DC, 1996, National Academy Press.

National Research Council: *Nutrient requirements of horses*, ed 5, Washington, DC, 1996, National Academy Press.

National Research Council: *Nutrient requirements of sheep*, ed 6, Washington, DC, 1985, National Academy Press.

National Research Council: *Nutrient requirements of swine*, ed 9, Washington, DC, 1988, National Academy Press.

Naylor J, Ralston S: *Large animal clinical nutrition*, St Louis, 1991, Mosby.

Radostits O et al: *Veterinary medicine: a textbook of the diseases of cattle, sheep, pigs, goats, and horses*, ed 10, St Louis, 2007, Saunders.

Schoenherr WD: Large animal clinical nutrition. In McCurnin DM, Bassert JM: *Clinical textbook for veterinary technicians*, ed 6, St Louis, 2006, Saunders.

## CHAPTER 17

# Laboratory Animal Medicine

*Mary E. Martini*

## OUTLINE

Mouse
  Origin and Uses in Research
  Characteristics: Behavioral and
    Physiological
  Handling and Restraint
  Breeding Considerations
  Sampling
  Signs of Pain and Distress
  Health Conditions
Rat
  Origin and Uses
    in Research
  Characteristics: Behavioral and
    Physiological
  Handling and Restraint
  Breeding Considerations
  Sampling
  Signs of Pain and Distress
  Health Conditions
Syrian Hamster
  Origin and Uses in Research
  Characteristics: Behavioral and
    Physiological
  Handling and Restraint
  Breeding Considerations
  Sampling

Signs of Pain and Distress
  Health Conditions
Mongolian Gerbil
  Origin and Uses in Research
  Characteristics: Behavioral and
    Physiological
  Handling and Restraint
  Breeding Considerations
  Sampling
  Signs of Pain and Distress
  Health Conditions
Rabbit
  Origin and Uses in Research
  Characteristics: Behavioral and
    Physiological
  Handling and Restraint
  Breeding Considerations
  Sampling
  Signs of Pain and Distress
  Health Conditions
Guinea Pig
  Origin and Uses in Research
  Characteristics: Behavioral and
    Physiological
  Handling and Restraint
  Breeding Considerations

Sampling
  Signs of Pain and Distress
  Health Conditions
Chinchilla
  Origin and Uses in Research
  Characteristics: Behavioral and
    Physiological
  Handling and Restraint
  Breeding Considerations
  Sampling
  Signs of Pain and Distress
  Health Conditions
African Clawed Frog
  Origin and Uses in Research
  Characteristics: Behavioral and
    Physiological
  Handling and Restraint
  Breeding Considerations
  Sampling
  Signs of Pain and Distress
  Health Conditions
Fish
  General Caging and Housing
Zoonosis
Laboratory Animal Allergy

## LEARNING OUTCOMES

After reading this chapter, you should be able to:

1. List the research uses and behavioral characteristics of mice, rats, hamsters, gerbils, rabbits, guinea pigs, chinchillas, and frogs.
2. Describe the handling and breeding consideration, signs of pain and distress, and health conditions of the above species.
3. List suggested sites and volumes for injection and sampling.
4. Suggest appropriate housing conditions for each species.
5. Discuss zoonotic diseases and their effect on research and personnel.
6. Discuss laboratory animal allergens and their effects on personnel.

Laboratory animals have been used in research for many years. In the past couple of decades, growing concern from the public over the use of animals in research has led to the establishment of guidelines to promote better care and responsible use of laboratory animals. The information provided in this section is also useful in a clinical setting when dealing with these species as pet animals. In addition to the information provided in this text, an excellent reference handbook for laboratory animals is the *Formulary for Laboratory Animals*, Second Edition, 1999, by C.T. Hawk and S.L. Leary in association with the American College of Laboratory Animal Medicine, Iowa State University Press. This formulary covers analgesics, sedatives, anesthetics, antiinfectives, and parasiticides and is an invaluable resource.

## MOUSE *(Mus musculus)*
### Origin and Uses in Research

I. The laboratory mouse today is purposely bred for research
II. The different strains of mice in laboratories are defined by ecological and genetic characteristics
III. Outbred, inbred, congenic, and transgenic stock are strains defined by genetic characteristics
    A. Outbred strains are the result of random mating to achieve genetic variations. An example of an outbred mouse is the CD-1
        1. Outbred mice are considered to express heterozygosity and to represent the diversity of the human population
    B. Inbred strains are the result of brother/sister, father/daughter, mother/son matings for a minimum of 20 consecutive generations
        1. An example of an inbred mouse is the BALB/c strain
        2. Inbred mice are genetically homozygous and therefore are very useful in transplantation research
    C. Congenic strains are animals that genetically differ at one particular locus
    D. Transgenic strains are the result of microinjection of DNA into mouse eggs for the production of very specific disease models; particularly useful in studying some forms of cancer
IV. The strains of mice defined by ecological characteristics can be divided into axenic, gnotobiotic, specific pathogen free, barrier sustained, and conventional
    A. Axenic, or germ-free, animals are derived from hysterectomy, free from infection by any microorganisms, and maintained in a germ-free isolation housing system
    B. Gnotobiotic mice are germ-free mice that have been introduced to one or more known nonpathogenic microorganisms. They are housed in isolators or barrier units
    C. Specific pathogen–free (SPF) and viral antibody–free (VAF) animals are those free from specific pathogenic organisms
    D. Barrier-sustained animals are gnotobiotic animals maintained under sterile conditions in a barrier unit. All air, bedding, and water must be sterilized; staff usually shower and aseptically scrub and dress before entering
    E. Conventional animals are those housed with no special precautions. They are typically SPF/VAF in origin
    F. In both a barrier-sustained and conventional housing facility, sentinel animals are used to ensure that the animals maintain their expected health status
V. Mice are the most widely used vertebrate in toxicology studies and biomedical research

### Characteristics: Behavioral and Physiological

I. Mice are social animals and can usually be housed in small groups if they are compatible
II. Males that have reached puberty may fight
III. Occasionally the dominant mouse in a group will remove the facial hair from all the other mice in the cage
    A. This is called barbering and can be a source of stress to the submissive mice, so the "barber" should be removed from the cage
IV. Mice are nocturnal animals
V. A unique anatomical feature of mice is the bone marrow of the long bones, which is functional throughout their lives
VI. Mice have a highly developed sense of smell and an acutely sensitive sense of hearing. They can respond to a range of ultrasonic frequencies and are more likely to be disturbed by high-pitched sounds and ultrasound than by lower frequencies
VII. Mice have an expected life span of 1 to 2 years
VIII. Rectal temperature: 36.5° to 38.0° C (97.5° to 100.5° F)

### Handling and Restraint

I. Mice should be picked up by the base of the tail. Never pick up a mouse by the middle or tip of the tail, because you may cause degloving or sloughing of the outside of the tail
II. For assistance in restraining a mouse, the mouse can be placed on a wire grid, such as the cage lid, so that its front feet grip the bars
    A. The handler should then carefully grasp the loose skin on either side of the neck and over the back with the thumb and forefinger

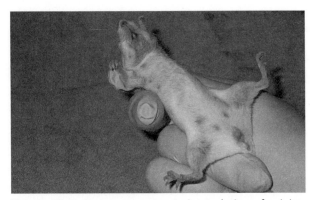

**Figure 17-1** Proper mouse restraint technique for injections, gavaging, and examination.

    B. The body of the mouse is laid across the palm of the hand, and the tail is restrained under the little finger (Figure 17-1)

III. Tubular restraining devices can be used for blood collection and other procedures

IV. The best methods of permanent identification of mice are microchip insertion, tail tattooing, and ear punching, along with cage card identification. For all of these procedures, the pain level involved must be considered; anesthesia may be appropriate for tattooing and microchip insertion; for ear punching, use of a topical analgesic, such as EMLA cream, is recommended

### Breeding Considerations (Table 17-1)

    I. If a group of female mice are exposed to a male mouse, the majority of these female mice will be in estrus the third night. This is known as the Whitten effect

    II. The Bruce effect is a pregnancy block that occurs when a pregnant female is exposed to a strange male within 48 hours of copulation

       A. The female will return to estrus in 4 or 5 days

    III. From 12 to 36 hours after mating, a waxy postcopulatory plug can be found in the vagina

    IV. Postpartum estrus occurs within 24 hours of parturition

    V. A male can be set up with two females; separate the male into his own cage for 1 week, then bring females to his cage (or it may affect his dominance and inhibit breeding)

    VI. Typically the female will have her pups during the dark hours. She will walk around the cage during labor and delivery and then carry the pups to the nest

### Sampling

For injection routes, sites, needle sizes, and volumes, see Table 17-2.

    I. Gastric gavage can be done by placing a bulbed, curved dosing needle over the tongue, into the esophagus, and then into the stomach

    II. Simple blood sampling procedures (e.g., from saphenous vein) can be done on awake but restrained mice

    III. Cardiac puncture is considered a terminal procedure because of potential complications

    IV. Before blood collection, always calculate the maximum safe volume that can be withdrawn

       A. One of the easiest routes for collection is via the saphenous vein

       B. Mice have approximately 70 to 80 mL/kg total blood volume

          1. Of this, 10% to 15% can be safely withdrawn every 2 to 3 weeks

    V. Collection of urine and feces can be done by placing the animal in a metabolic cage, or by collecting the samples as the animal is restrained, because it will often urinate and defecate

       A. A hematocrit tube can be used to collect the urine

### Signs of Pain and Distress

    I. The following are signs of pain and distress in mice

       A. Weight loss, dehydration, sunken eyes, and change in urine and fecal output and consistency due to decreased food and water intake

       B. Hunched posture

       C. Lethargy, depression, and withdrawal from the group

       D. Change in locomotion

       E. Decreased grooming and ruffled hair coat

       F. Ocular and nasal discharge may be seen along with increased and labored breathing

       G. Change in behavior, particularly when handled or manipulated. May vocalize or try to bite handler

       H. Scratching excessively, licking, or biting at painful areas, which may lead to self-mutilation

    II. Analgesics, such as buprenorphine and butorphanol, are appropriate to administer to a mouse in pain

### Health Conditions

    I. Respiratory disease

       A. Sendai virus causes pneumonia, is often latent and becomes apparent in young weanling, stressed mice, or in combination with bacterial infections. It is self-limiting in immunocompetent mice

       B. Bacteria that may contribute to respiratory infections include *Pasteurella pneumotropica*, *Klebsiella pneumoniae*, *Mycoplasma pulmonis*, and *Corynebacterium kutscheri*

       C. Clinical signs are weight loss, ruffled hair coat, hunched posture, anorexia, dyspnea, chattering, and sudden death

       D. Treat with antibiotics (e.g., tetracycline in drinking water) for secondary bacterial infections

    II. Mouse hepatitis virus

       A. Caused by a coronavirus. It is often a latent infection that can lead to encephalitis and/or hepatitis in mice

**Table 17-1** Reproductive data

| Litter size | Weight at birth (g) | Weaning age | Puberty | Breeding age | Estrous cycle | Mating | Gestation |
|---|---|---|---|---|---|---|---|
| **MOUSE** | | | | | | | |
| 6-12 | 1 | 21 days | 4-6 wk | 6 wk | 4-5 days, Whitten and Bruce effects | Harem 1:4 | 19-21 days |
| **RAT** | | | | | | | |
| 7-14 | 5-6 | 21 days | 4-6 wk | 10-12 wk | 4-5 days, Whitten and Bruce effects | Harem 1:6 | 20-22 days |
| **GUINEA PIG** | | | | | | | |
| 2-6 | 60-200 | 21 days | 3-4 wk | 12 wk | 16 days, polyestrous | Harem 1:5-10 | 63 days |
| **HAMSTER** | | | | | | | |
| 4-12 | 1-2 | 21 days | 4-6 wk | 6-7 wk | 4 days, polyestrous, female will exhibit lordosis | Monogamous or harem 1:4 | 16 days |
| **GERBIL** | | | | | | | |
| 4-5 | 3-4 | 21-28 days | 10 wk | 10-12 wk | 4-6 days, polyestrous | Monogamous (mate for life) or harem 1:3 | 24-26 days |
| **RABBIT** | | | | | | | |
| 6-10 | 40 | 6-8 wk | 5-9 mo | 6-9 mo | Induced polyestrous | Hand mating, 1:10-15 | 28-34 days |
| **CHINCHILLA** | | | | | | | |
| 1-2 | 30-60 | 6-8 wk | 8 mo | 8 mo | 38 days, polyestrous, vaginal closure membrane | Harem 1:12 | 111 days |

    B. Causes wasting disease in immunosuppressed animals, such as severe combined immunodeficiency disease (SCID) mice

    C. Clinical signs include dehydration, weight loss, diarrhea, and sudden death

    D. To control disease in a colony, stop breeding, consider hysterectomy derivation, and place filter tops on cages

III. Tyzzer's disease

    A. *Clostridium piliformis* is the causative bacterium

    B. Most commonly affects immunosuppressed animals and those kept in poor housing

    C. Causes dehydration, weight loss, diarrhea, and sudden death

    D. These bacteria are spore formers that are highly infectious to a number of laboratory animals

       1. Isolation is imperative; culling or hysterectomy derivation of the colony should be considered

IV. Epizootic diarrhea of infant mice (EDIM)

    A. A disease caused by a rotavirus that affects suckling mice

    B. Clinical signs include soft yellow feces or fecal staining of the anogenital area in mice less than 2 weeks of age

    C. Filter top cages should be used to prevent the spread of this disease

    D. Cull affected litters

V. Pinworm

    A. Two strains: *Aspicularis tetraptera* and *Syphacia obvelata*

    B. Both strains can be observed on fecal floatation test, but *S. obvelata* can also be detected by making a cellophane tape impression of the perineal area

    C. Use anthelmintic, such as ivermectin or pyrantel palmate, and carefully sanitize the environment because these eggs are "sticky"

    D. Unapparent infection, but may decrease growth rate

VI. Mites

    A. Several species of mites can affect mice, including *Myobia musculi* and *Myocoptes musculinus*

**Table 17-2**  Recommended needle sizes and sites and maximum volumes for injection/sampling

| SQ | IM | IP | IV | Sampling (nonlethal)* |
|---|---|---|---|---|
| **MOUSE** | | | | |
| < 23 Gauge<br>2-3 mL<br>Scruff | 25 Gauge<br>0.05 mL/site<br>Quadriceps, posterior thigh | 25 Gauge<br>< 3 mL<br>Lower right quadrant | < 25 Gauge<br>0.2 mL<br>Lateral tail vein, saphenous | Saphenous vein, lateral tail vein, jugular, retro-orbital sinus[†]: 100 µL<br>Cardiac[†]: 1-2 mL<br>Tail nick: 50 µL, DO NOT REMOVE VERTEBRAE |
| **RAT** | | | | |
| < 23 Gauge<br>5-10 mL<br>Scruff, back | 23-25 Gauge<br>0.3 mL/site<br>Quadriceps, posterior thigh | 22-23 Gauge<br>5-10 mL<br>Lower left quadrant | < 23 Gauge<br>0.5 mL<br>Lateral tail vein, saphenous vein, dorsal penis vein, sublingual | Saphenous vein, lateral tail vein or artery, retro-orbital sinus[†]: 1 mL<br>Cardiac[†]: 3-5 mL<br>Jugular vein[†]: 2-3 mL |
| **HAMSTER** | | | | |
| 23 Gauge<br>3-5 mL<br>Scruff | 23 or 25 Gauge<br>0.1 mL/site<br>Quadriceps, posterior thigh | 23 Gauge<br>3-4 mL<br>Lower right quadrant | 25 Gauge<br>0.3 mL<br>Difficult, cutdown to jugular, cephalic, tarsal, lingual | Retro-orbital sinus[†]: 0.5 mL<br>Jugular cutdown[†]: <2 mL, 23 Gauge<br>Cephalic, tarsal, lingual: 0.5 mL, 25 Gauge<br>Cardiac[†]:<2 mL, 23 Gauge |
| **GUINEA PIG** | | | | |
| < 21 Gauge<br>5-10 mL<br>Scruff, back<br>*Tough skin | 23-25 Gauge<br>0.3 mL/site<br>Quadriceps, posterior thigh | < 21 Gauge<br>10-15 mL<br>Lower abdominal quadrant | < 23 Gauge<br>0.5 mL slowly<br>Marginal ear vein, saphenous, penile | 23 Gauge<br>Anterior vena cava: 2-3 mL<br>Ear vein: 0.5 mL<br>Cardiac[†]: 0.5 mL<br>Penile, saphenous, jugular: 2-3 mL |
| **RABBIT** | | | | |
| 21-23 Gauge<br>30-50 mL<br>Scruff, flank | < 21 Gauge<br>0.5-1.0 mL/site<br>Lumbar, quadriceps | (Not recommended)<br>21 Gauge<br>50-100 mL | 23 Gauge<br>1-5 mL, slowly<br>Marginal ear vein, saphenous | 21 Gauge<br>Marginal ear vein, 2-3 mL<br>Central ear artery: 30 mL<br>Cardiac[†]: use only for terminal bleeds, 100+ mL |
| **GERBIL** | | | | |
| 23 Gauge<br>2-3 mL<br>Scruff | 25 Gauge<br>0.1 mL/site<br>Quadriceps, posterior thigh | 23 Gauge<br>2-3 mL<br>Lower abdominal quadrant<br>*See notes in text | 25 Gauge<br>0.2-0.3 mL<br>Lateral tail vein | 23-25 Gauge<br>Lateral tail vein, saphenous, retro-orbital sinus[†]: 0.2-0.4 mL<br>Cardiac[†]: 1 mL |

*Continued*

**Table 17-2** Recommended needle sizes and sites and maximum volumes for injection/sampling—cont'd

| SQ | IM | IP | IV | Sampling (nonlethal)* |
|---|---|---|---|---|
| **CHINCHILLA** | | | | |
| < 21 Gauge<br>5-10 mL<br>Scruff, back | 23-25 Gauge<br>0.3 mL/site<br>Quadriceps, posterior thigh | < 21 Gauge<br>10-15 mL<br>Lower abdominal quadrant | 25 Gauge<br>1 mL slowly<br>Saphenous, cephalic | < 23 Gauge<br>Jugular: 2-3 mL<br>Cranial vena cava: 2-3 mL<br>Cephalic, saphenous: 1 mL |
| **FROG** | | | | |
| < 23 Gauge<br>2-3 mL | 23-25 Gauge<br>0.5 mL<br>Thigh | 23 gauge | Difficult | Cardiac puncture |

*Before collecting any blood sample, always calculate the amount that can be safely drawn based on body weight and blood volume for that particular species and the health status of the animal. Generally, 4% to 7% of blood volume, dependent on species, can be safely drawn. Consider replacing equal amounts of fluid (i.e., physiological saline).

†Cardiac and jugular cutdown bleeding must be done under anesthesia. Because of the risk of postprocedural complications, cardiac puncture is generally only used for a terminal procedure. Retro-orbital sinus bleeding must be done under anesthesia or sedation.

B. The most obvious signs of mite infection are alopecia, pruritus, and dermatitis

C. Mites can be diagnosed by close examination for mites in the fur; pluck or scrape and examine findings under magnification

D. Easiest and most economical control of mites is through exposure to the vapors from pest strips (dichlorvos)

# RAT (Rattus norvegicus)

## Origin and Uses in Research

I. The rat is a rodent of the family Muridae

II. Rats were being used as experimental animals by the early 1800s

III. Uses in biomedical research include cardiovascular disease, metabolic disorders (e.g., diabetes mellitus), organ transplantation, toxicology, neurobehavioral studies, cancer susceptibility, and renal disease studies

IV. Rats are raised and maintained in ecological classes similar to mice

V. Common outbred strains include Wistar, Sprague-Dawley, Long Evans, Kyoto, and Wistar- Kyoto

VI. Through selective breeding and mutations, more defined and inbred strains can be produced to suit a specific study
   A. Examples
      1. CAR/CAS: caries resistant/susceptible
      2. BB: spontaneously develop diabetes
      3. Brattleboro: diabetes insipidus
      4. Zucker: obesity

## Characteristics: Behavioral and Physiological

I. Rats are generally docile and may become tame and easily trained if handled frequently

II. Rats can be communally housed and may share raising of their young

III. Rats are omnivorous, feed primarily at night, and are generally fed a commercially prepared laboratory rodent diet

IV. Rats have a life expectancy of 2.5 to 3 years; a restricted protein and fat diet will extend life expectancy for months

V. They display a range of behavioral traits and are intelligent, making them suitable for behavioral studies

VI. Rats do not have a gallbladder

VII. Rats, like other rodents, have a layer of brown fat distributed over their back and neck. In a young rat this plays a role in thermoregulation, but its significance decreases with age

VIII. Rats have continually erupting incisors, called hypsodontic

IX. The harderian gland is a lacrimal gland located behind the rat's eyeball; its secretion is rich in lipids and proteins, and it lubricates the eye. In some disease conditions and in times of stress, these red secretions, called porphyrin, will overflow the eye and stain the face

X. Albino rats have very poor vision and rely on their facial whiskers and sense of smell for orientation

XI. Rats will practice coprophagy

XII. Rectal temperature: 35.9° to 37.5° C (96.6° to 99.5° F)

## Handling and Restraint

I. Rats should not be picked up by their tail, because it could result in degloving of the tail, exposing the coccygeal vertebrae

II. Two commonly used methods of picking up and restraining a rat
   A. Place hand over the shoulder and back area, with the mandibles just in front of the thumb and forefinger

B. Place hand over the shoulder and back area with the head between the first two fingers and the thumb behind the rat's foreleg

C. With both of these restraint techniques, it is important to use your other hand to secure the hind limbs and tail (base of tail can be held in these secure positions)

III. Rats can be identified by using cage cards, coat color, and/or placement of markings, placement of a microchip, or tattooing the tail or ear pinna (under anesthesia)

## Breeding Considerations

See Table 17-1 for reproductive data.

I. Female rats are polyestrous and can breed year round

II. The Whitten effect (see mouse) is less pronounced in rats than in mice

A. The Bruce effect (see mouse) does not affect rats as it does mice. Pseudopregnancy in rats is rare

III. A white, waxy, postcopulatory plug is present in the vagina for 12 to 24 hours after mating

IV. Females have a postpartum estrous cycle within 48 hours. Because of this, usually the male is removed just before parturition and placed back in with the female(s) after weaning

## Sampling

For injection routes, sites, needle sizes, and volumes, see Table 17-2.

I. Gastric gavage can be performed by placing a ball-tipped, curved dosing needle over the tongue, into the esophagus, and then into the stomach

II. For blood collection, oral dosing, physical examinations, and injections, it is important to have one person restrain the rat while the other performs the technical procedure

III. Before blood collection, always calculate the maximum safe volume that can be withdrawn

A. Rats have approximately 50 to 65 mL/kg total blood volume

B. Of this, 10% to 15% can be safely withdrawn every 2 to 3 weeks

C. One of the easiest collection routes is via the saphenous vein

## Signs of Pain and Distress

See mouse section. Clinical signs are similar. Rats in pain should also be treated with analgesics, such as butorphanol and buprenorphine.

## Health Conditions

I. Parvovirus

A. Three main serogroups include rat virus (RV), H-1 virus, and rat parvovirus (RPV)

B. Can cause a wide range of symptoms varying with the viral strain and the age and immune status of the rat

1. Young rats can display tremors, ataxia, jaundice, stunted growth, and oily hair coats

2. Mature rats tend to have asymptomatic latent infections and can exhibit signs of paralysis, scrotal cyanosis, and hemorrhage if they are stressed or if they become immunocompromised

C. Because these viruses are shed in urine, feces, saliva, and milk and are vertically transmitted through direct contact and fomites, they are highly contagious

1. Parvoviruses may severely interfere with research

II. Coronaviruses

A. Although there are several coronaviruses that affect rats, the primary three are considered to be sialodacryoadenitis virus (SDAV), rat coronavirus (RCV), and the causative agent of rat sialoadenitis virus (CARS)

B. Intramandibular and/or ventral cervical swelling is a common clinical sign, as well as red porphyrin staining of the face and paws, sneezing, anorexia, photophobia, bilateral or unilateral suborbital or periorbital swelling, squinting, blinking, bulging eyes, and occasional self-mutilation of the eyes

C. Disease is self-limiting with high morbidity and low mortality rates, but has the potential to interfere with research

D. These viruses are highly contagious via respiratory aerosol or direct contact

III. Sendai virus

A. An RNA virus of the family paramyxovirus (parainfluenza virus type 1)

B. Usually asymptomatic but depends on the host's immune status, age, and so on

1. High morbidity and low mortality rates

C. Clinical signs include respiratory difficulty, chattering, wheezing, weight loss, decreased breeding efficiency, and anorexia

D. Can have a dramatic effect on research, particularly reproductive, respiratory, and nutritional studies

IV. Murine mycoplasmosis

A. Disease caused by *M. pulmonis*

B. Very common in pet and conventionally housed rats

C. Carried in the upper respiratory tract and transmitted via aerosol, direct contact, and in utero transfer, making it a highly contagious disease; affected animals should be quarantined

D. There are two major areas that can be affected by an infection with *M. pulmonis*

E. The respiratory system clinical signs include sniffling, moist rales, sneezing, chattering, weight loss, rough hair coat, and torticollis (head tilt)

F. The genital infection will cause breeding inefficiencies and infertility

G. Tetracycline hydrochloride in the drinking water will suppress clinical signs

V. Mammary tumors

A. Neoplasms in the mammary tissue are common in most strains of rats

B. Tumors can be large but rarely metastasize

C. They may be surgically removed but often grow back

VI. Endoparasites and ectoparasites (see mouse)

# SYRIAN HAMSTER
## (Mesocricetus auratus) ▬▬▬▬
## Origin and Uses in Research

I. The Syrian (or golden) hamster is a rodent of the family Cricetidae. The origin of the golden hamster is the Middle East, where, unfortunately, the natural habitat is being destroyed

II. The Syrian hamster is popular as both a pet and a research model

III. The hamster has a unique evertable pouch used to transport food, but it also very useful for research on tumor induction, tissue and organ transplant, and microcirculation

IV. Hamsters are also of use in hypothermia studies because they are able to go into short periods of pseudohibernation when temperatures are under 48° F (10° C) and daylight hours shorten

V. Inbred strains of hamsters have been produced as animal models of epilepsy, muscular dystrophy, and heart failure

## Characteristics: Behavioral and Physiological

I. Female hamsters are generally larger, stronger, and more aggressive than males

II. Hamsters are burrowers and like to hoard their food

III. They are solitary animals under natural conditions and are best kept separate

IV. They are expert escape artists; cages should not be made out of wood, aluminum, or soft plastic, and must have a tight fitting lid

V. Flank glands or sebaceous glands are used to mark territory. Although both males and females have them, they are quite prominent in the males

VI. Hamsters are omnivores; diets can be supplemented with fresh fruits and vegetables

VII. They are nocturnal animals that will put many kilometers on a running wheel through the course of one night

VIII. Hamsters will choose different areas of their cage for food storage, nesting, defecation, and urination

IX. Urine has a high pH of 8, which is full of crystals, giving it a turbid, milky appearance

X. Hamsters have a life expectancy of about 2 years

XI. Rectal temperature, 37.0° to 38.0° C (98.6° to 100.4° F)

## Handling and Restraint

I. Hamsters are extremely deep sleepers and can be aggressive if awakened and startled, so it is important to wake up the hamster before handling

II. Hamsters can be gently scooped up in the palm of the hand or in a plastic/metal container

A. To restrain for a physical examination or technical procedure, they can be grasped by the loose skin over the neck and shoulder area using the whole hand (hamster should appear to be smiling when effectively restrained)

## Breeding Considerations

See Table 17-1 for reproductive data.

I. During the winter months, hamsters will exhibit a normal decrease in fecundity, and mortality in litters will increase; this effect can be only partially reduced by maintaining the housing at temperatures between 22° and 24° C (71° to 75°F) and a light cycle of 12 to 14 hours

II. Monogamous pairs are frequently established before sexual maturity to avoid the possible fighting that can occur when a male is placed in a cage with a strange female

III. In a harem set-up, bring the male to the receptive female 1 hour before the dark light cycle, observe them closely for fighting, and separate if this occurs. Separate also after breeding has occurred to avoid injury to the male

IV. The estrous cycles last about 4 days; on the second day of estrus the female has a vaginal discharge that has a distinctive pungent odor that attracts the male. The female will usually approach the male for breeding within 3 days of this postovulatory discharge

V. The gestation period for the hamster is only 16 days. It is advisable to not disturb the female and her litter until at least 7 days postpartum, or she may cannibalize her offspring

## Sampling

For injection routes, sites, needle sizes, and volumes, see Table 17-2.

I. The hamster has few accessible veins for blood collection and injection. The cephalic vein, tarsal vein, lingual vein (requires anesthesia), or jugular vein (requires anesthesia and surgical cutdown) can be used

II. Most of the techniques for injection and gavage are the same as those used for the rat and mouse

III. Oral medication can be placed in the cheek pouch
IV. Collection of urine and feces can be done by placing the hamster in a metabolic cage; often when they are restrained, they will urinate or defecate
V. Before blood collection, always calculate the maximum safe volume that can be withdrawn
   A. Hamsters have 65 to 80 mL/kg total blood volume
   B. Of this, 10% to 15% can be safely withdrawn every 2 to 3 weeks

## Signs of Pain and Distress

I. The hamster is usually a healthy and hardy animal. Clinical signs of pain are the same as those listed for the mouse
II. Ocular discharge is commonly associated with stress and may be accompanied by an increase in respiratory rate
III. It is unusual for a hamster to be constipated. Diarrhea, when it occurs, is profuse liquid, staining the perineal area
IV. Lateral recumbency is unusual and indicative of an unwell hamster
V. Analgesics are appropriate to administer to a hamster in pain; the selection and use of these agents should be in consultation with a veterinarian.

## Health Conditions

I. Wet tail (proliferative ileitis or transmissible ileal hyperplasia)
   A. The causative agent is unknown, but several types of bacteria have been cultured from hamsters with proliferative ileitis, including *Campylobacter* spp., organisms similar to *Campylobacter, Escherichia coli*, and an organism similar to *Lawsonia intracellularis*
   B. Clinical signs include profuse watery diarrhea, lethargy, weight loss, severe depression, irritability, anorexia, and sudden death within 3 days of clinical signs
   C. May be predisposed by stresses of confinement and weaning, with highest mortality in nursing or newly weaned animals between 3 and 8 weeks of age
   D. Erythromycin in the drinking water has been shown to effectively decrease the mortality rate
   E. Best method of control is prevention through a high level of hygiene and avoidance of stress
II. Tyzzer's disease *(Clostridium piliforme)*
   A. Not commonly seen in hamsters, but this may be due to lack of diagnosis, because the clinical signs are similar to those of wet tail and the causative organism is difficult to culture
   B. Treatment for Tyzzer's disease with tetracycline has been successful in other rodents

C. *C. piliformis* is a spore-forming bacteria; thorough decontamination of the housing facility is imperative after an outbreak to prevent reinfection
III. *Salmonella* spp.
   A. Hamsters may be more susceptible to *Salmonella* spp. than other rodents
   B. Clinical signs include lethargy, rough hair coat, weight loss, distended abdomen, and increased respiratory rate
   C. Zoonotic disease; strict hygiene protocols should be adhered to when working with suspect animals
IV. Lymphocytic choriomeningitis virus (LCM)
   A. LCM is a zoonotic disease that causes meningitis in humans
   B. Clinical signs of the disease in hamsters are difficult to detect because they usually are asymptomatic
   C. May present as a chronic wasting disease
   D. Virus is shed in the urine
V. Antibiotic sensitivity
   A. Hamsters have predominantly gram-positive intestinal flora and tend to develop a fatal gram-negative enterotoxemia when given certain antibiotics
VI. Pneumonia
   A. This is a relatively common health concern with hamsters
   B. Commonly associated with *P. pneumotropica*
   C. Clinical signs include respiratory distress and ocular discharge
   D. Sendai virus may produce pneumonia in suckling hamsters
      1. Hamsters are susceptible to the pneumonia virus in mice
VII. Endoparasites and ectoparasites
   A. Pinworms and mites can affect hamsters similarly to other rodents (see mouse section)

## MONGOLIAN GERBIL *(Meriones unguiculatus)*

### Origin and Uses in Research

I. Gerbils are desert dwellers and can be found in northern Africa, India, Mongolia, northern China, and some sections of eastern Europe
II. The gerbil is a rodent of the Cricetidae family. Although the Mongolian gerbil is by far the most commonly used research and pet strain, there are many varieties of gerbils with a wide range of sizes and colors
III. Gerbils are useful in radiation studies because they are more resistant to radiation than other common laboratory animals. They are also used in studies relating to epilepsy, infectious disease, endocrinology, and lipid metabolism

## Characteristics: Behavioral and Physiological

I. Gerbils are gentle and friendly. They are curious animals that will explore all new environmental enrichment thoroughly, particularly tubes and other devices that mimic their natural burrows

II. Gerbils are active throughout the day, with their peak of activity occurring during the dark hours

III. They are incredibly driven to burrow and will occasionally damage caging and cause self-mutilation with their intense burrowing activities

IV. Some strains can be susceptible to epileptiform seizures after excitement, stress, and sudden noises, with spontaneous recovery and no noted ill effects

V. Gerbils have a greater capacity than most laboratory animals for temperature regulation and can tolerate temperatures between 0° and 32° C (32° and 92° F)

VI. Relative humidity should be lower for these animals (30% to 50%) than most laboratory animals
    A. When the humidity is over 50%, the fur will stand away from the body and appear to be matted, as opposed to the sleek, smooth appearance

VII. Gerbils are herbivorous and granivorous. Care should be exercised when feeding seeds because gerbils are extremely fond of sunflower seeds and will eat them to the exclusion of all other foods. Standard laboratory rodent diet should be fed
    A. Gerbils hoard food, with the female exhibiting this behavior more than the male

VIII. Feces are tubular, dry, and almost black in color

IX. Gerbils have a low to moderate requirement for dietary water (but must always be supplied with clean, fresh water) and in turn put out very little urine, keeping odors down in comparison with other laboratory animals

X. Gerbils tend to nonaggression and can be group housed in large numbers (in accordance with housing density standards) by sex, at weaning

XI. Like rats, gerbils have a harderian gland in the orbit of the eye
    A. Red coloring may appear around the eyes and neck if excessive secretion occurs

XII. Like most laboratory rodents, gerbils have a sensitivity to cedar bedding that is enzyme induced

XIII. Average life expectancy in the gerbil is 3 years

XIV. Rectal temperature: 37.0° to 38.5° C (98.6° to 101.3° F)

## Handling and Restraint

I. Gerbils tolerate handling well, and there are generally no problems associated with the handling of young litters and newborn pups

II. To move a gerbil from cage to cage, scoop the gerbil up gently with both hands, ensuring that it cannot jump out of your hand. They can also be transferred by securing one hand over the back, with the gerbil's head between the first two fingers

III. To restrain a gerbil for a physical examination or technical procedure, grip the base of the tail with one hand and the loose skin around the neck and shoulder area with the other hand
    A. Extreme care should be taken to avoid grasping the tail away from the base because this could cause degloving of the tail
    B. Gerbils do not tolerate being turned on their backs; they will struggle

## Breeding Considerations

See Table 17-1 for reproductive data.

I. Gerbils are monogamous and will mate for life. Care should be taken if introducing a new mate, because this quite often results in severe fighting

II. Male gerbils will aid in the care of the young, but if separated to avoid postpartum mating, he should be returned to his mate within 2 weeks of separation

III. Harem mating systems can be set up in production facilities with one male to two or three females

IV. The estrous cycle lasts about 4 to 6 days with spontaneous ovulation

V. Matings tend to occur during the dark hours

## Sampling

For injection routes, sites, needle sizes, and volumes, see Table 17-2.

I. Sampling procedures are similar to those performed in mice and rats

II. Because gerbils dislike being placed on their backs, the intraperitoneal injections are given with the animal carefully restrained (described earlier) but held vertically, with head slightly declined, while the needle is placed into the lower left or right abdominal quadrant

III. Before blood collection, always calculate the maximum safe volume that can be withdrawn. Gerbils have 65 to 85 mL/kg total blood volume. Of this, 10% to 15% can be safely withdrawn every 2 to 3 weeks

## Signs of Pain and Distress

The clinical signs of pain and distress in the mouse apply to gerbils.

I. Gerbils are normally extremely active and nervous, and under severe stress may temporarily collapse

II. Analgesics are appropriate to administer to a gerbil in pain; the selection and use of these agents should be in consultation with a veterinarian

## Health Conditions

I. Tyzzer's disease *(C. piliforme)*
  A. Gerbils are highly susceptible to infection by *C. piliforme* and are commonly used in laboratories as sentinels for this organism, because transmission readily occurs through contact with soiled bedding
  B. The disease causes high morbidity and mortality rates in weanling-age gerbils
  C. *C. piliforme* is a spore-forming bacterium that can be spread to other animals in a research facility. Thorough decontamination must occur after an outbreak of this disease
  D. Clinical signs of Tyzzer's disease include acute death, lethargy, rough hair coat, and diarrhea
  E. Treatment may be successful with the addition of oxytetracycline in the drinking water and fluid therapy for dehydrated individuals
II. Nasal dermatitis, or "sore nose"
  A. This disease is seen to be a byproduct of stress and anxiety. In high-stress situations, gerbils will attempt to alleviate their stress by excessive burrowing.
    1. Porphyrins secreted during stress-induced chromodacryorrhea may be irritating to the skin
    2. The lesions resulting are commonly contaminated with *Staphylococcus aureus* and/or *Staphylococcus xylosus*, which is an opportunistic pathogen
  B. Clinical signs include facial or nasal dermatitis that can progress into chronic moist dermatitis
    1. In very severe cases, and where the underlying cause has not been rectified, the disease can lead to wasting, anorexia, and possibly death
  C. Treatment must address evaluating and eliminating the cause of the stress. The lesions can be cleaned and then topically treated with appropriate antibiotic ointments
    1. Clay bedding material can be used instead of shavings or chips
III. *Salmonella*
  A. Outbreaks cause diarrhea, perineal staining, anorexia, weight loss, and sudden death
  B. Typically, animals will recover after a short bout of diarrhea
  C. Zoonotic potential; when dealing with these animals, exercise good personal hygiene
IV. Malocclusion and overgrowth of incisors are fairly common and require regular trimming of the teeth
V. Gerbils over the age of 2 show a high incidence of tumors
  A. Malignancies appear as spontaneous neoplasms involving the ovaries, ventral sebaceous glands, kidney, adrenal gland, and skin

VI. Although dehydration is uncommon, gerbils that do not have access to fresh water (due to blocked sipper tube, immature animals that cannot reach the sipper tube, etc.) could have lower fertility rates, decreased body weights, and possibly higher mortality

## RABBIT *(Oryctolagus cuniculus)* ▬▬▬
## Origin and Uses in Research

I. The rabbit is a lagomorph of the family Leporidae
II. Present breeds are derived from the wild European rabbit. These wild rabbits still exist today in northwestern Africa and Europe
III. Breeds of rabbit are divided by size, shape, and color variations
  A. Large breeds (6.4 to 7.3 kg, or 14 to 16 lb) include the giant chinchilla and the Flemish giant
  B. Medium breeds (1.8 to 7.3 kg, or 1 to 14 lb) include the New Zealand white and Californian
  C. Small breed (0.9 to 1.8 kg, or 2 to 4 lb) include the Dutch and Polish
IV. The New Zealand white is the most common specific pathogen–free (SPF) rabbit produced commercially for research
V. Rabbits are useful in biomedical research for alimentary, aging, cancer, cardiovascular, genetic, immunology, virology, and toxicology studies, as well as many other areas
  A. Rabbits are commonly used to produce antibodies

## Characteristics: Behavioral and Physiological

I. Rabbits are docile, alert, gregarious burrowers
  A. They are generally a social animal but may be housed singly in laboratories to avoid fighting and to prevent ovulation and pseudopregnancy in females
II. Rabbits are crepuscular, meaning that they are most active at twilight
III. Aggressive or nervous rabbits may stomp their hind feet and may spray urine
  A. If they panic or are handled roughly, they may vocalize with a high pitched scream
IV. Rabbits are herbivorous. They should be fed a commercially prepared, pelleted, high-fiber rabbit diet and supplemented with good quality grass hay and fresh vegetables; fruits can be given as treats
V. Rabbits have a higher requirement for fiber than other species; a high-fiber diet will decrease the incidence of hairballs
VI. Rabbits have highly vascularized ears, allowing for easy intravenous and intraarterial access; they serve as the rabbit's heat regulatory organ
VII. Rabbits have two pairs of upper incisors; a smaller pair (peg teeth) is found behind the larger pair

A. Both pairs grow continuously (open rooted) and may need to be trimmed if not naturally worn down, otherwise leading to health conditions, such as malocclusion

B. Enamel is found on the entire tooth surface

VIII. Rabbits have a chin gland, which is more obvious in males

IX. Rabbit urine is unlike that of other species; it is quite thick and cloudy and contains crystalline material

A. Suckling babies and fasting adults have clear, crystal-free urine

X. Daytime feces are usually hard and dark-green, round pellets. Rabbits tend to eat most of their food at dusk; the first 4 hours after eating goes toward the production of these fecal pellets

A. Night feces (cecotroph) are moist, stronger in odor, brighter green, and mucus covered

1. Coprophagy of these cecotrophs, directly from the anus, is normal behavior in rabbits; it helps increase the digestibility of proteins and maintain adequate nutrition and intestinal flora

2. These pellets are formed in the 4 hours after the day pellets are formed

XI. Average life expectancy of a rabbit is 5 to 6 years

XII. Rectal temperature: 38.5° to 40.0° C (101.3° to 104° F)

## Handling and Restraint

I. Approach rabbits slowly and talk to them softly to avoid startling them

II. Rabbits can be picked up

A. By grasping the loose skin over the neck area with one hand and supporting the hind limbs with the other, taking care that the nails do not get caught in the caging

B. To transport the rabbit, place the rabbit on your forearm with its head tucked in your elbow and your same hand supporting the hind limbs. The other hand should be over the rabbit's shoulder, being prepared to grasp this skin again in case it struggles

C. Rabbits must never be picked up by their ears

III. To handle rabbits for physical examination or technical procedure (Figure 17-2)

A. Place the rabbit on a nonslip surface (examination table with a mat) and carefully restrain with both hands to prevent it from jumping off the table. If possible (i.e., during ear bleeds), wrap the rabbit in a towel or laboratory coat to comfort and protect it from hurting itself

B. Rabbits can be carefully laid on their backs, on the handler's lap

1. Start by sitting on a stool or on the floor with rabbit on your lap with its head toward your abdomen

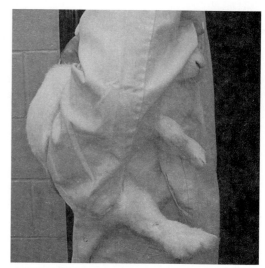

**Figure 17-2**    Appropriate technique for transporting a rabbit.

2. Cover the rabbit's eyes with one hand and hold the scruff of skin over the shoulders with the other

3. Gently roll the rabbit so that its feet are closely tucked into your abdomen and its head rests near your knees; if the rabbit struggles, make sure that your hand is still covering its eyes

a. Once it has quieted, resume slowly

IV. Place hind end into cage first. This prevents the rabbit from jumping into a cage and possibly injuring itself

V. Rabbits are generally easy to handle, with training, but be aware that they have powerful bites and can charge and scratch

## Breeding Considerations

See Table 17-1 for reproductive data.

I. Rabbits are induced ovulators and do not have an estrous cycle, but they do have a period of receptivity that lasts between 7 and 10 days

II. Pregnant rabbits should be provided with a clean, dry, well-bedded nest. They will also hair pluck to line the nest

III. Does will not retrieve kits that leave the nest. If kits are found outside the nest, they will need to be warmed immediately

IV. Do not disturb the doe during parturition

V. Cannibalism is rare in rabbits

VI. Cross-fostering works well with rabbits, so large litters should be decreased in size by cross-fostering to another doe with a similar age litter

VII. As in rodents, thermoregulation is regulated by brown fat in young rabbits

## Sampling

For injection routes, sites, needle sizes, and volumes, see Table 17-2.

I. Collection of feces and urine can be done by placing the rabbit in a metabolic cage

II. Liquid oral medications can be given by introducing the dosing syringe into the interdental space and pointing the tip toward the back of the mouth. Pills can also be given by pushing them through the interdental space and back toward the molars

III. If nasogastric tubes are necessary, it is recommended to obtain a radiograph of the rabbit after tube placement, because rabbits will not cough when saline is introduced directly into the lungs

IV. Before blood collection, always calculate the maximum safe volume that can be withdrawn. Rabbits have 57 to 65 mL/kg total blood volume. Of this, 10% to 15% can be safely withdrawn every 2 to 3 weeks

## Signs of Pain and Distress

I. Difficult to identify signs of pain because rabbits often hide their symptoms

II. Rabbits that appear to be unwell should have a full physical examination that includes temperature, respiration rate, heart rate, and body weight
   A. Careful examination of the animal may reveal decreased muscle mass, dehydration, ocular discharge, debris in ears, nictitating membranes, inappetence, staining of perineal area, lesions, limited movement, and other signs
   B. Careful examination of the cage will be helpful in determining if the rabbit is unwell
      1. Look for leftover feed, diarrhea, uneaten cecotrophs, lack of feces, unconsumed water (sipper tube may be faulty)

III. Rabbits in pain may be lethargic, remain at the back of the cage, and face away from sources of light

IV. Analgesics are appropriate to administer to a rabbit in pain; the selection and use of these agents should be in consultation with a veterinarian.

## Health Conditions

I. Pasteurellosis: *Pasteurella multocida*
   A. Rabbits under stress (such as during and after shipping) and in poor health conditions are more susceptible
   B. The major causative agent is "snuffles," or upper respiratory tract infections in rabbits. The other organisms that are cultured include *Bordetella bronchiseptica* and *Moraxella catarrhalis*
   C. Rabbits with pasteurellosis could have the following on clinical presentation: upper respiratory tract infection, otitis, pleuropneumonia, bacteremia, and abscesses
      1. Clinical signs include nasal discharge, ocular discharge, dermatitis, torticollis, vaginal discharge, and abscess formation
   D. Antibiotic therapy is indicated as treatment, but watch for gastrointestinal upset
      1. In cases of torticollis, it may also be appropriate to administer analgesics, corticosteroids, and an antinausea/vertigo drug
      2. Abscesses may require lancing and then flushing
   E. Pasteurellosis is quite contagious, through direct and indirect transmission; sick animals must be isolated or culled

II. Trichobezoars (hairballs)
   A. This disease is associated with feeding a diet that is low in fiber
   B. Suspect a hairball in an anorexic rabbit
   C. The hairball can sometimes be palpated, or radiography can assist in diagnosis
   D. Nonsurgical treatment should be attempted first. Force feeding a slurry of high-fiber chow, offering free choice hay and fresh vegetables, and giving the proteolytic enzymes bromelin and papain

III. Coccidiosis
   A. Rabbits can be infected with hepatic coccidia *(Eimeria stiedae)* or intestinal coccidia (several different types)
   B. Clinical signs of intestinal coccidiosis include diarrhea and possibly death in cases of heavy infections
   C. Clinical signs of hepatic coccidiosis include diarrhea, abdominal swelling, weight loss, anorexia, icterus, and sudden death
   D. Diagnosis through identification of oocysts on fecal examination
   E. Prevention must consist of isolation of infected rabbits and a thorough cleanup of the environment daily to remove sporulated oocysts
      1. Treatment with sulfonamides is effective in controlling heavy infections

IV. Dermatitis/alopecia
   A. Can be caused by a number of agents, including fur and ear mites, dermatophytes, malocclusion, and possibly barbering
      1. Mites can be confirmed through skin scraping/fur plucking or careful examination of the ear
      2. Dermatophytosis causes alopecia and will require a culture for fungal organisms to diagnose
      3. Malocclusion can cause scalding around the mouth and chin due to excess salivation; teeth will need to be trimmed regularly using a dental unit or a Dremel tool, or the incisors can be permanently removed
      4. Barbering usually occurs due to lack of dietary fiber: increase fiber in diet and provide rabbit with chewing material, such as branches and wood blocks

## GUINEA PIG (*Cavia porcellus* [CAVY]) ▬▬▬▬

### Origin and Uses in Research

I. Wild caviae still exist in Peru, Argentina, Brazil, and Uruguay
II. Member of the rodentia suborder Hystricomorpha; other rodents in this suborder include the chinchilla and the porcupine
III. The most common strains of guinea pig used in research today include the Duncan-Hartley, Hartley, and inbred strains 2 and 13
IV. The most common pet strains include the Peruvian (long haired), Abyssinian (short haired with rosettes), and the English (short haired)
V. Primarily used in genetics, anaphylaxis, microbiology, immunology, nutrition, and audiology studies. Diagnostic tests for infectious diseases use guinea pig serum

### Characteristics: Behavioral and Physiological

I. Nervous but tame and easily handled
II. They may freeze at unexpected sounds or stampede at unexpected movements
III. Group-housed guinea pigs rarely fight except when overcrowded or if strange males are in the presence of a female in estrus
IV. Have poor jumping/climbing abilities and may be housed in low-walled, open-topped pens
V. Guinea pigs have constantly erupting (hypsodontic) teeth, which may lead to malocclusion and "slobbers" (see Health Conditions)
VI. Guinea pigs lack the L-gluconolactone oxidase enzyme, involved in the synthesis of ascorbic acid (vitamin C) from glucose; therefore it is extremely important that sufficient amounts of vitamin C be provided in the diet (also see Health Conditions, Scurvy)
   A. Commercially prepared laboratory guinea pig diets contain a form of vitamin C that is stable for approximately 90 days (or longer; see product information)
   B. Guinea pig food available in pet stores is notoriously deficient; guinea pigs fed this diet will need supplemental ascorbic acid at a rate of 5 mg/kg daily for a mature adult and 30 mg/kg daily for pregnant and immature animals
   C. Guinea pigs are monogastric herbivores and cecal fermenters. In addition to their pelleted diet, they should be offered free choice hay and some fresh vegetables and fruit (but not more than 10% to 15% of the weight of the pelleted food) as treats
   D. Guinea pigs respond poorly to diet change. They tend to establish their eating preferences early in life and will chose not to eat as opposed to eating new food. Introduction of novel feedstuffs early in life diminishes this response
VII. Guinea pigs respond poorly to stress and antibiotic therapy
VIII. Both males and females have two nipples. Females have no difficulty raising litters of more than four offspring
IX. Guinea pigs are considered to be quite messy and often play with the sipper tubes of their water bottles and drain the bottle
X. They are coprophagic, eating cecotrophs throughout the day
XI. Average life span is 2 to 4 years
XII. Rectal temperature: 37.2° to 39.5° C (99° to 103.1° F)

### Handling and Restraint

I. Lift by grasping firmly and gently over their shoulders, with two fingers behind and two fingers in front of the forelimbs. The rump must always be supported with the other hand
   A. It is important for the safety of the guinea pig that all technical procedures be performed with one person holding the animal while the other performs the task

### Breeding Considerations

See Table 17-1 for reproductive data.

I. Females should be bred before the age of 6 months (preferably between 2.5 and 3 months), because of the risk of fusion of the pubic symphysis, leading to failure of the fetus to pass and thus dystocia
II. Guinea pigs can be successfully mated monogamously or as a harem
   A. They are spontaneous ovulators; ovulation occurs 10 hours after estrus and 2 to 3 hours postpartum
III. Guinea pigs have a vaginal closure membrane that seals off the vagina when the sow is not in estrus
   A. Closes after estrus or copulation and the expulsion of the vaginal plug, and ruptures shortly before parturition
IV. During the latter stages of pregnancy, the sow becomes extremely heavy. Care must be taken to provide adequate support when handling and to ensure easy access to food and water
V. Sows do not build nests
VI. Newborn guinea pigs are precocious and relatively mature with hair, erupted teeth, and open eyes

### Sampling

For injection routes, doses, needles sizes, and blood volumes, see Table 17-2.

I. Accessing veins for injections or bleeding requires sedation or anesthesia

II. Oral dosing can be achieved using a ball-tipped dosing needle

III. Urine and fecal samples can be obtained by placing the guinea pig in a metabolic cage

IV. Before blood collection, always calculate the maximum safe volume that can be withdrawn

    A. Guinea pigs have approximately 65 to 90 mL/kg total blood volume

    B. Of this, 10% to 15% can be safely withdrawn every 2 to 3 weeks

## Signs of Pain and Distress

I. Key signs of pain and distress include withdrawal, vocalization, rough coat, and unresponsiveness

II. Acceptance to capture and restraint

III. Lethargy

IV. Sunken dull eyes, dehydration

V. Increased, and possibly labored, respiratory rate

VI. Weight loss, diarrhea, decreased food and water consumption

VII. Tendency toward barbering under dietary stress, hair loss, scaly skin

VIII. Group aggression

IX. Excessive salivation

X. Change in locomotion, lameness, careful gait

## Health Conditions

I. Scurvy (hypovitaminosis C)

    A. Clinical signs include lameness, lethargy, weakness, anorexia, rough hair coat, diarrhea, weight loss, change in teeth and gums, nasal and ocular discharge

        1. The limb joints are often affected and may be enlarged and painful to the touch

    B. Treatment should include daily dosing with ascorbic acid (5 to 10 mg/kg for maintenance) in the food, water, per os or parenteral injection

        1. This should reverse the effect of deficiencies

    C. Prevention is key

        1. Always provide fresh (within 90 days of milling) pellets that have been stored in an airtight container in a cool, dark storage area

        2. Supplement feed with vitamin C–rich fruits and vegetables, such as oranges, kale, red pepper, or cabbage

II. Antibiotic-associated enterotoxemia

    A. Intestinal flora in guinea pigs is predominantly gram positive, and when treated with antibiotics that act on gram-positive organisms (penicillin, ampicillin, chlortetracycline, lincomycin, erythromycin, tylosin), the intestinal flora will be drastically altered, leading to an overgrowth of gram-negative organisms

    B. Clinical signs include diarrhea, dehydration, hypothermia, and anorexia

    C. Treat symptomatically and with supportive care

        1. Fluids should be administered; *Lactobacillus* spp. can be used to reestablish normal flora

    D. Prevention through use of appropriate antibiotics

        1. Guinea pigs seem to tolerate trimethoprim-sulfa, chloramphenicol, and enrofloxacin (Baytril) well

III. Malocclusion

    A. Guinea pigs have open-rooted incisors, premolars, and molars

    B. Clinical signs include anorexia, weight loss, and excess salivation ("slobbers") that can lead to dermatitis

        1. Thorough examination of the entire mouth is necessary; use of a vaginal speculum or otoscope and sedation or anesthesia may be helpful to observe the molars and oral mucosa

    C. Trim teeth with a dental tool, Dremel tool, or rongeurs

    D. As with most animals that are prone to malocclusion, there is a genetic predisposition and therefore all animals with this problem should not be selected as breeders

IV. Cervical lymphadenitis

    A. "Lumps" is a disease caused by *Streptococcus zooepidemicus* and occasionally *Streptobacillus moniliformis*, bacteria normally found in the conjunctiva and nasal cavity that enter the bloodstream through abrasions in the oral mucosa

    B. This disease is easily recognizable; the guinea pig will present with cervical masses that contain pus

    C. Treatment includes surgical excision of the affected cervical lymph nodes or draining and flushing abscess followed by systemic antibiotic treatment

    D. Because guinea pigs seem to be more prone to this disease in a stressful environment, prevention includes removal of overt sources of stress and access to a healthy balanced diet

V. Bacterial pneumonia

    A. Commonly caused by *B. bronchiseptica* and *Streptococcus pneumoniae*

    B. Clinical signs include depression, anorexia, nasal and ocular discharge, and dyspnea

    C. Diagnosis may be made on clinical signs, radiography, and culture and sensitivity of nasal exudates. It is difficult to collect blood from guinea pigs without causing stress, but a complete blood cell count could also help in the diagnosis

    D. Treatment options include fluid and antibiotic therapy

VI. Salmonella

    A. Was once the most frequently reported bacterial infection in guinea pigs; common serotypes include *Salmonella typhimurium* and *Salmonella enteritidis*

B. Clinical signs include anorexia, dull and ruffled hair coat, lethargy, and sudden death

C. Diagnosis through culture of blood or spleen

D. Antibiotic treatment will eliminate clinical signs but will not eliminate *Salmonella* spp. from the colony. Prevention includes thorough hand washing and ensuring that all vegetables and fruit are properly washed before feeding

E. This organism has zoonotic potential

VII. Anesthetic complications/considerations

A. Ketamine must be given as a deep muscular injection, because if it is given subcutaneously it will cause sloughing of the tissue

B. It is important to use atropine

C. Muscular movement may occur during surgical anesthesia

VIII. Dermatitis and alopecia (see Rabbit, Health Conditions)

## CHINCHILLA *(Chinchilla langier)* ▬▬▬
### Origin and Uses in Research

I. Chinchillas are in the same family as guinea pigs; they are both hystricomorph rodents from South America. The chinchilla is a native of Peru, Bolivia, Chile, and Argentina

II. Hunted for their prized pelts in the early 1900s, they are very rare in the wild and may be extinct

III. Used almost exclusively for hearing research

### Characteristics: Behavioral and Physiological

I. Chinchillas are easy to handle and curious, and have a curled and tufted tail that is carried high

II. They are monogastric herbivores and cecal fermenters

III. Chinchillas and guinea pigs are very similar in their anatomical and physiological characteristics, but unlike the guinea pigs, chinchillas do not require a dietary source of ascorbic acid

IV. Chinchillas require a dust bath frequently (daily to every other day is optimal)

A. One recommendation is to make your own using 9 parts silver sand with 1 part Fuller's earth, or it can be purchased commercially. Do not use playground sand

B. A round fishbowl makes an excellent dust bath container because it retains the sand

C. They will dust bathe for up to 1 hour. Afterwards, remove dust bath from cage to keep cage clean

V. Chinchilla teeth, like those of the guinea pig, are all open rooted and continually erupt

A. They are naturally yellow in color

B. To help avoid malocclusions, provide with chew toys, pieces of clean wood, fruit tree branches (unsprayed, of course), and porous rock to gnaw

VI. They should be fed a commercially prepared chinchilla diet and free choice high-quality grass hay

A. Alfalfa hay can be used short term but is not preferable because it is very rich and could cause digestive disturbance

B. Hay is important because it provides them with the chewing that they need, it reduces their stress, and it provides them with a low-energy roughage that will not promote obesity

C. Fresh, clean fruits and vegetables can also be given as treats. They love raisins, but eating too many has been reported to cause dental caries

VII. Their coat is extremely luxurious and contains more fur per square inch than any other animal

VIII. They are virtually odorless

IX. They love to climb and jump; caging should provide areas in which to hide and to climb

X. In nature they tend to be most active around dawn and dusk, but in a home or research environment they are active throughout the day

XI. They have four toes on front and rear feet

XII. They are coprophagic and tend to consume their cecotrophs in the morning and early afternoon

XIII. Expected life span is 10 years

XIV. They can be quite comfortable in cool temperatures, but do not tolerate temperatures over 26° C (79° F) and high humidity

XV. Rectal temperature: 38.0° to 39.0° C (100.4° to 102.2° F)

### Handling and Restraint

I. If the chinchilla has been hand raised, it will probably come out of the cage quite willingly and onto your open hands

II. If you must remove it from its cage, the chinchilla can be grasped around the scruff of the neck/shoulders with one hand and the base of the tail with the other

A. Rough or inexperienced handling could frighten the chinchilla and cause fur slip (loss of a large patch of fur)

B. If the tail is grasped anywhere but the base, it might slough off

III. It is appropriate, and safer for the chinchilla, to have one person restrain while the other person performs the technical procedure or physical examination

### Breeding Considerations

See Table 17-2 for reproductive data.

I. Females have a vaginal closure membrane, similar to that of guinea pigs, that is open only during estrus and parturition

II. They have three pairs of mammary glands

III. Like guinea pigs, they are placentophagic

IV. Females do not build nests but will use a nesting box, which can help keep the kits warm

V. Young are born precocious with teeth and open eyes and ears

VI. Can set up polygamous or monogamous matings. In commercial chinchilla farms, the male will be permitted to access a number of females' cages by a back runway to which only he has access. The females wear collars to prevent them from leaving their cage

VII. Cross-fostering and hand raising are usually successful

## Sampling

For injection routes, doses, needles sizes, and blood volumes, see Table 17-2.

I. Can be very sensitive to injectable medications; whenever possible, give medications orally

A. Chinchillas will often take pills and chew them up

B. Medications can be given in raisins or on bread, or by crushing and adding to food

## Signs of Pain and Distress

I. Indifference to human attention, lethargy

II. Dull hair coat and eyes

III. Perineal staining

IV. Weight loss

V. Change in locomotion

VI. Anorexia

VII. Excess salivation

## Health Conditions

Although chinchillas have been used in research and raised as pets and for their fur, there are few reference materials about their disease problems. They are similar in many aspects, including health concerns, to the guinea pig. Fortunately there is an abundance of reference materials on guinea pig diseases, and these can be followed when trying to diagnose, treat, and prevent diseases in the chinchilla.

I. Malocclusion (see guinea pig health concerns)

II. Choke and bloat

A. Chinchillas cannot vomit

B. Clinical signs of choke include retching, drooling, dyspnea, and anorexia. Animals that are bloated will lie on their sides with swollen abdomens

C. Important to decompress the abdomen by passing a gastric tube or inserting a needle or trocar

D. Similar to rabbits, chinchillas can also get trichobezoars; cause and treatment are basically the same as for the rabbit

III. Constipation

A. Caused by feeding a diet that is too rich in concentrated food and not enough roughage

B. Clinical signs of constipation are straining to defecate and producing small, dry fecal pellets

IV. Fur ring and paraphimosis

A. Caused by a ring of fur around the penis that eventually stops the penis from retracting into the prepuce

B. Clinical signs include excessive grooming, straining to urinate, passing only small volumes of urine, and an engorged penis resulting in paraphimosis

C. Ring will need to be cut or rolled (lubricate first) off the penis

D. All males should be checked on a regular basis (weekly)

V. Alopecia

A. Can be caused by *Trichophyton mentagrophytes* (ringworm), particularly if seen on the nose or front feet or behind the ears

B. Diagnosis and treatment similar to those for other species

C. Zoonotic potential

## AFRICAN CLAWED FROG *(Xenopus laevis)* ■■■■

### Origin and Uses in Research

I. Animals used in biomedical research on embryonic development studies, and eggs used for research into diseases involving ion channels

II. Historically, frogs were used primarily for studies on physiology, ecology, and behavior

III. The use of amphibians in biomedical research continues to rise. When amphibians were initially introduced, *Rana pipiens* were the most frequently used frog, but they have been recently surpassed by the hardier, easier to care for *X. laevis*

### Characteristics: Behavioral and Physiological

I. Xenopus are a totally aquatic amphibian

A. In their natural habitat, xenopus are pond dwellers

B. In a research environment they seem to do quite well in tanks with both flowing and non–flow-through systems

II. They are carnivorous

A. Frogs can be fed commercially produced frog brittle or small pieces of organ meat, such as heart and liver

III. Xenopus are secretive, and hiding is an integral part of their behavior

IV. Xenopus, like all reptiles, amphibians, and fish, are ectotherms. This means that they are unable to generate enough metabolic heat to raise their body temperatures above the ambient level of their environment

V. Unlike most toads and frogs, xenopus lacks a tongue

VI. The average life span of the African clawed frog is 15 years

VII. Xenopus readily regenerate lost limbs

VIII. Xenopus have unique colors and patterns on their skin; therefore photography can be used to identify individuals

IX. Adult amphibians respire through the lungs, skin, and buccopharyngeal cavity, and larvae breathe with external gills

## Handling and Restraint

I. Xenopus are very mucoid and slippery. Great care should be taken to avoid disruption of this protective layer of mucus. Always use a good quality net to remove frogs from their tank

II. Frogs should always be carefully examined in their housing tank before removal. Observe for activity level, posture, appetite, response to stimuli, and skin and body condition

III. For short procedures or for transferring frogs from one tank to another, manual restraint in a soft net will be adequate. Use two hands and moisten before manipulating

## Breeding Considerations

I. Males are approximately 20% smaller than females and have slimmer bodies and legs. Males do not have a cloaca. At sexual maturity the males develop black nuptial pads on their forearms, which they use to grasp the female during mating or amplexing

II. The females are plump, with pear shaped bodies. They have a cloaca through which eggs and waste are passed. Females do not develop nuptial pads

III. Xenopus become mature in about 14 weeks and become sexually mature at a body length greater than 7.5 cm

IV. Environmental factors appear to induce reproduction
   A. With xenopus, removing approximately 30% of their water and replacing it with cooler water seems to be effective

V. Eggs are externally fertilized
   A. Breeding is referred to as amplexing
   B. The male will mount the female from behind and, clasping his front legs just in front of her thighs, will squeeze the female to release the eggs
   C. She will release hundreds of eggs
   D. Unless eggs are removed, they will likely be eaten

VI. Females should be bred no more than four times per year

VII. Eggs develop into the typical larval or tadpole stage and metamorphose into the adult

## Sampling

I. Any manipulation that might take longer than a minute or two and that could potentially be painful should be done under anesthesia

II. Typically, MS222 (tricaine methanesulphonate) is used at a dose of 1 to 2 g/L for anesthetizing adult frogs
   A. This dose must be buffered with sodium bicarbonate, 23 mEq/L
   B. The frog is placed in the solution until anesthetized, which can take up to 15 minutes

III. Respiratory rate is markedly decreased or absent during deep levels of anesthesia. Percutaneous respiration appears to carry the load during these brief periods of lack of visual respirations

IV. Skin scrapings or a sample of the mucus can be obtained by gently scraping the affected area with a coverslip or spatula
   A. Samples can be viewed directly and with new methylene blue staining
   B. Suspect bacterial lesions should be cultured with a sensitivity performed

V. Peripheral venous access is difficult, but cardia puncture seems to be quite well tolerated
   A. Frog is anesthetized and placed in dorsal recumbency
   B. The heart is located dorsal to the xiphoid
   C. A small gauge needle is inserted at an angle of 10 to 20 degrees to the body

VI. For quick radiographic images, the anesthetized frog can be placed in damp towels and taped between two sections of foam

VII. If a disease appears to be affecting more than one animal, it may be advisable to sacrifice one of the affected animals and perform a postmortem examination
   A. Note that frogs autolyze very rapidly and must be examined immediately after euthanasia

## Signs of Pain and Distress

I. Environmental stresses can induce ill health and distress in frogs
   A. Changes in water quality, transportation, overcrowding, poor nutrition, temperature extremes, and ammonium buildup can all contribute to distressed and potentially immunosuppressed frogs

II. Assessment of pain and distress in frogs should include a thorough evaluation of their environment and a knowledge of their normal behavior and relevant history

III. Frogs in the laboratory should be weighed regularly. Weight loss can be an indicator of pain and distress. Frogs can lose up to 50% of their body weight before death

IV. Typical signs of distress and pain include
   A. Frog stays at the surface of the water when approached
   B. Presence of sloughed skin clouds the water

C. Tremors in extremities
D. Heavy mucoid excretion

## Health Conditions

I. *X. laevis* are considered to be very hardy frogs and can be raised and maintained relatively easily in the laboratory
II. When a disease outbreak occurs or animals appear to be distressed, it is important to look beyond the treatment of the symptoms of the disease and fully assess the environment
III. Disease outbreaks will occur when the frogs are stressed by inappropriate handling, a change in the quality of the water, overcrowding, and poor nutrition
IV. Frogs are very susceptible to chemicals in the water, including chlorine, copper, and ammonia
V. To prevent the spread of infection, animals displaying symptoms of illness should be removed from the group and placed in isolation during treatment and recovery
VI. Red leg
  A. Caused by bacterial infection, typically *Aeromonas hydrophila, Proteus hydrophilus*, and *Pseudomonas hydrophilus*
  B. Causes high morbidity and mortality in frogs
  C. Clinical signs include hemorrhage in extremities, excessive mucus production, anorexia, lack of response to stimuli
  D. If caught early, the disease can be treated with oral antibiotics. Antibiotics, such as trimethoprim sulfa, can be injected into beef heart and fed to affected frogs
  E. Skin hemorrhage has also been associated with gas bubble disease, poor water quality, and chemical toxins
VII. Parasitic infections
  A. As with most frogs, xenopus can be host to a wide variety of parasites
    1. Fecal analysis can reveal flagellates, ciliates, strongyle and strongyloid eggs, and cestode and trematode eggs
    2. Epidermal desquamation and irritation may be caused by *Capillaria* spp. infestation
    3. This 2- to 4-mm nematode can be diagnosed by skin scraping and treatment with 0.2 to 0.4 mg/kg ivermectin orally or subcutaneously. Ivermectin can be very successful if caught in the early stages
  B. Skin protozoa, such as *Trichodina, Costia*, and *Vorticella*. Symptoms include skin irritation and cloudiness, and excessive mucus production
VIII. Fungal infections
  A. Fungal infections are relatively common in frogs and are often secondary to bacterial infections and trauma; they can occur following the use of antibiotics

B. Symptoms include skin ulcers, skin nodules, black spots, and weight loss
C. Diagnosis by skin scraping and cultures of lesions
D. Treatment typically consists of topical antifungals, such as mecurochrome, methylene blue, or benzalkonium chloride
IX. "Dropsy" or "bloat"
  A. Characterized by subcutaneous fluid accumulation
  B. Symptoms include loose skin on thighs, bloated appearance, and food regurgitation
  C. Some sources recommend aspirating the fluid and treating the wound topically with peroxide

## FISH

I. The use of fish in research has been steadily on the rise. The increase globally of aquaculture of fish for human consumption has brought with it many challenges
  A. The primary focus in this area has been addressing the nutritional challenges of these intensive systems
  B. In biomedical science research, the use of the small zebra fish has been on the rise for the past decade
    1. These diminutive fish have been used extensively for developmental and genetic analysis
    2. More recently, researchers have developed a transgenic fish model for the study of environmental toxicology
II. For more specific information about the care and use of fish in research, please consult the Canadian Council on Animal Care website (http://www.ccac.ca) or the American Association of Laboratory Animal Science website (http://www.aalas.org)

## GENERAL CAGING AND HOUSING

I. Select the size of cage appropriate to the species; see Table 17-3
II. Animals should be confined securely with comfort and safety ensured, permitting normal postural and behavioral adjustments
III. Environmental enrichment should be provided for social and behavioral needs
IV. Animals that are social in nature should not be housed singly unless necessary for research protocol and approved by the appropriate body (animal care committee)
  A. When social animals must be housed singly, they should be able to see, hear, and smell their conspecific
V. Provide adequate ventilation, viewing, and easy access to animal

**Table 17-3**  Housing data

| Temperature* (° C,/° F) | Relative humidity†(%) | Ventilation‡ (air changes/hr) | Lights (hr) | Caging | Other conditions§ |
|---|---|---|---|---|---|
| **MOUSE** | | | | | |
| 22-25/72-78 | 50-70 | 8-12 | 12-14 nocturnal | Shoebox or suspended mesh | Can be group housed in same-sex groups; occasionally males of certain strains will fight and need to be separated. Barbers should be removed. Provide nesting material and places to hide, such as plastic pipe sections |
| **RAT** | | | | | |
| 20-25/68-76 | 50-55 | 10-20 | 12-15 nocturnal | Shoebox or suspended mesh | Can be group housed in same-sex groups. Provide nesting material; places to hide, such as cardboard boxes; exercise wheels |
| **GUINEA PIG** | | | | | |
| 18-22/66-72 | 50-60 | 4-8 | 12-15 crepuscular | Shoebox, floor pens or stalls, suspended mesh | Light changes should be gradual. Not necessary to have a lid on cages that are taller than 40 cm. Group house females |
| **HAMSTER** | | | | | |
| 21-24/70-78 | 45-65 | 6-10 | 12 nocturnal | Shoebox | House in groups if raised and weaned together, otherwise separate at puberty. Hibernation brought on by decrease in temperature and light hours |
| **GERBIL** | | | | | |
| 15-24/60-78 | 40-50 | 8-10 | 12-14 nocturnal/ diurnal | Shoebox | Burrowers, produce less urine (therefore less ammonia) and have dry fecal pellets |
| **RABBIT** | | | | | |
| 16-20/62-70 | 40-50 | 10-20 | 12-14 crepuscular | Floor pens or stalls, suspended mesh | Group house compatible females; mature males will fight. Provide raised platforms for resting on or hiding under |
| **CHINCHILLA** | | | | | |
| 15-22/60-70 | 40-70 | 8-10 | 12-14 nocturnal | Solid bottom or suspended mesh | Important to allow dust bathing at least twice per week. Provide chewing devices or wood |
| **FROG** | | | | | |
| 15-23C | N/A | N/A | 12:12 | Plastic tanks | 4-5 L water/frog, nonabrasive area to hide |

Information from Canadian Council on Animal Care (CCAC): *Guide to the care and use of experimental animals, Volume 1*, Ottawa, Canada, 1993.
*Information from National Research Council: *Guide for the care and use of laboratory animals*, Institute of Laboratory Animal Resources, National Academy Press, 1996 (suggests that the range of temperature for all listed species be between 64° and 79° F [18° and 26° C]).
†The range of humidity for each is 30% to 70%.
‡The CCAC is gradually increasing their expectations regarding ventilation for most laboratory animals to 15 to 20 air changes/hr.
§Noise greater than 50 dB or ammonia levels greater than 22 ppm are detrimental to most laboratory animals.

VI. Food and water delivery systems
   A. Must provide easy access to all ages and sizes of animals within the microenvironment
   B. Must not be contaminated with excrement
   C. Must be thoroughly cleanable, and in some cases they must be able to withstand sterilization in an autoclave
   D. Guinea pigs often play with their watering systems, which may flood the cage

VII. Housing design and material must facilitate cleaning and disinfection. Although ease of cleaning is important, this should not be the factor that determines which style of housing is used
   A. For example: wire-bottom cages with excreta pans for rabbits are perhaps easier to clean than solid-bottom pens with shavings, but the floor pens are preferable for many other reasons and are cleanable, too, with a bit more effort

VIII. Consider light intensity, noise level, ventilation, and temperature effects on the animal's microenvironment and ensure that they are within recognized guidelines

IX. All ceiling, wall, and floor surfaces in a laboratory animal facility must be made of a sealed, nonporous material to facilitate thorough disinfection

## ZOONOSIS

From an occupational health standpoint as well as for animal colony management, be aware of the diseases that can be transmitted from one species to another, including humans (Table 17-4).

## LABORATORY ANIMAL ALLERGY

I. Laboratory animal allergy (LAA) is the most common health condition that affects people working in a research animal facility
   A. At risk are the technicians, investigators and their staff, and facility support staff, such as front office administrative personnel
   B. From 10% to 30% of people working in this field will develop allergy symptoms

II. LAA is a hypersensitivity to certain substances, such as the proteins found in dander, urine, serum, and saliva
   A. Does not cause a reaction in a nonallergic person
   B. The immune system produces antibodies to the specific proteins, and this results in observable signs

III. Observable symptoms
   A. Rhinitis
   B. Conjunctivitis
   C. Contact urticaria (hives)
   D. Asthma
   E. Anaphylaxis

IV. Risk of exposure should be assessed; there are certain tasks, such as cage cleaning, cage changing, animal handling, and sweeping that increase exposure
   A. Once the risk of the task has been assessed, the appropriate control method should be chosen
   B. Engineering controls
      1. Are the most appropriate controls in the long term

**Table 17-4** Zoonosis

| Causative organism/distribution | Laboratory species | Means of spread, vectors | Outcome of infection, to humans |
|---|---|---|---|
| **SALMONELLOSIS** | | | |
| Bacteria Worldwide | Mice, rats, guinea pigs, hedgehogs, chinchilla | Ingestion, inhalation, contact | Gastroenteritis (vomiting, diarrhea), headache, and fever |
| ***Campylobacter*** | | | |
| Bacteria Worldwide | Hamsters | Ingestion | Abdominal pain and severe diarrhea |
| **LYMPHOCYTIC CHORIOMENINGITIS** | | | |
| Arenavirus Worldwide | Hamsters, rodents | Contact, inhalation, congenital transmission, tissue culture transmission | Aseptic meningitis, encephalitis or meningoencephalitis: temporary illness with nervous symptoms or permanent disability associated with the central nervous system |
| **RINGWORM** | | | |
| Fungus: *Microsporum, Trichophyton* Worldwide | Guinea pigs, rodents, rabbits, chinchilla | Direct contact, soil may be a reservoir | Progressively itchy, weeping, chronic dermatitis |

*Continued*

**Table 17-4** Zoonosis—cont'd

| Causative organism/distribution | Laboratory species | Means of spread, vectors | Outcome of infection, to humans |
|---|---|---|---|
| **TULAREMIA/RABBIT FEVER** | | | |
| *Francisella tularesis* Circumpolar in northern hemisphere | Rabbits, rodents | Inhalation, contact, tick and insect bites, ingestion of contaminated food and water | Without antibiotic treatment, fatal in 5% of cases; diagnosis by antibody identification via blood testing; signs are fever, lethargy, anorexia, coughing, diarrhea |
| **PLAGUE** | | | |
| *Yersinia pestis* Western United States, South America, Asia, Africa | Rodents | Flea bites, inhalation | Fever, shivering, severe headaches, swollen lymph glands Pneumonic plague may be a complication; coughing produces bloody frothy sputum, labored breathing |
| **PSEUDOTUBERCULOSIS (YERSINIOSIS)** | | | |
| *Yersinia pseudo-tuberculosis* Northern Hemisphere | Rodents | Contact, contaminated food and water, ingestion | Coughing, chest pain, shortness of breath, fever, sweating, poor appetite, weight loss |
| **RAT BITE FEVER** | | | |
| *Streptobacillus* and *Spirillum minus* Worldwide | Rodents | Rodent bites, ingestion | Inflammation at site of bite, swollen lymph nodes, bouts of fever, rash, painful joints |
| **LEPTOSPIROSIS (WEIL'S DISEASE)** | | | |
| *Leptospira* spp. Worldwide | Rodents | Contact, urine contaminated soil and water | Fever, chills, headache, muscle aches, eye inflammation, skin rash |
| **HANTAVIRUS** | | | |
| Hantavirus | Mice | Contact, inhalation | Fever and muscle aches (1-5 wk postexposure), shortness of breath, coughing |
| **SALMONELLA** | | | |
| Bacteria Worldwide | Rodents, frogs | Ingestion | Diarrhea, dehydration, chills |

2. Consider substituting bedding for less dust, providing better localized ventilation, and using HEPA vacuums
C. Administrative controls: switching jobs within the facility, cross-training
   1. Improve personnel hygiene
   2. Institute medical surveillance program
D. Personal protective equipment: respirators (must be fit tested), facility-specific clothing, eye protection
   1. Do not wear street clothes into the animal facility, because allergens can be carried home on clothing
   a. Avoid taking facility clothing home, because this exposes members of your family to allergens
   2. Avoid wearing soiled clothing into the common facility areas, such as the lunch room; this will decrease the exposure of the administrative staff

## ACKNOWLEDGMENT

The editors and author recognize and appreciate the original work of Amanda Hathaway and Jodilynn Pitcher, on which this chapter is based.

# Glossary

**amplexus** Occurs when the male frog grasps the female with his front legs, inducing her to release hundreds of eggs which he fertilizes with a fluid containing sperm

**axenic** Also referred to as germ free; these animals are hysterectomy derived, free from all microorganisms, and maintained in germ-free isolation housing

**barbering** Occurs when one animal clips or chews the fur of another, usually around the muzzle or head to show dominance

**barrier sustained** Gnotobiotic animals that are maintained under sterile conditions in a barrier unit

**Bruce effect** Pregnancy block that occurs when a pregnant female is exposed to a strange male within 48 hours of copulation

**cecotrophs** Soft night and early morning fecal pellets ingested directly from the anus

**chromodacryorrhea** Secretion of dark red fluid from the harderian gland

**congenic** Animals that genetically differ at one particular locus; having similar genotypes

**conspecific** Member of the same species

**coprophagia** Eating of one's stools or feces

**crepuscular** Becoming active at twilight or just before sunrise

**degloving** Removal of the skin from its underlying structures

**denuding** Stripping or laying bare of any part

**diurnal** Becoming active through the day

**fecundity** Ability to produce offspring frequently and in large numbers

**gavage** Force feeding/medicating usually through a tube passed into the stomach

**gnotobiotic** Germ-free animals that have been introduced to one or two known nonpathogenic microorganisms

**harderian gland** Lacrimal gland located behind the rat's eyeball that secretes a lipid- and protein-rich secretion that lubricates the eye

**harem mating** Mating one male with two or more females

**high-efficiency particulate air (HEPA filter)** Used in clean rooms, biological safety cabinets, laminar flow units, etc., to filter out contaminating particles as small as 0.3 µm in diameter

**hypsodontic** Teeth that continuously erupt

**immunosuppressed** Diminished immune response

**inbred** Inbreeding resulting from mating between closely related animals for at least 20 generations

**latent infection** Condition or infection that may not be clinically noted in the animal, but under stress or poor health conditions it develops into a recognizable disease state

**lordosis** Abnormal curvature of the spine; may be shown by a female as a sign of receptiveness to a male

**malocclusion** Genetic or dietary related condition in which the opposing teeth do not meet when the jaw is closed

**mantle** Thick muscle layer running along the back and supporting the spine

**metabolic cage** Caging that allows separation of the urine and feces from the direct animal environment

**microenvironment** Isolated habitat, usually within a cage

**monogastric** Refers to having a single-chambered stomach

**nocturnal** Becoming active at night

**outbred** Result of random breeding to achieve genetic diversity

**paraphimosis** Inability to retract penis due to swelling

**phenotype** Outward visible expression of the hereditary constitution of an organism

**placentophagia** Practice of consuming the placenta

**SCID** Severely compromised immune deficient animal

**sentinel** An animal used to monitor disease in other animals

**SPF** Specific pathogen–free

**transgenic animals** Animals whose hereditary DNA has been augmented by the addition of DNA from a source other than parental germplasm, usually from another animal or a human, using recombinant DNA techniques

**trichobezoar** Mass of hair found in the gastrointestinal tract, caused from animals licking themselves. Often called a hairball

**VAF** Viral antibody free

**Whitten effect** Response observed in mice whereby a majority of a group of females will be in estrus the third night after exposure to a male

# Review Questions

**1** Which animal requires a dust bath?
a. Rabbit
b. Chinchilla
c. Gerbil
d. Hamster

**2** Which species does not practice coprophagy as a necessary nutritional supplement?
a. Mouse
b. Chinchilla
c. Guinea pig
d. Rat

**3** Which species is unable to synthesize vitamin C?
a. Rabbit
b. Degu
c. Guinea pig
d. Hamster

**4** Which of the following are zoonotic diseases?
a. *Salmonella,* ringworm, lymphocytic choriomeningitis
b. *Salmonella,* ringworm, chromodacryorrhea
c. Ringworm, chromodacryorrhea, lymphocytic choriomeningitis
d. Ringworm, scurvy, chromodacryorrhea

**5** Inbred strains are the result of at least how many generations of brother × sister mating?
a. 10
b. 20
c. 30
d. 40

**6** Which species is known to go into pseudohibernation if housing temperatures are decreased?
a. Hamster
b. Guinea pig
c. Gerbil
d. Mouse

**7** Intramandibular swelling and red porphyrin staining on face and paws of a rat could indicate signs of what disease?

a. Mite infestation

b. Sialodacryoadenitis virus

c. Sendai virus

d. *M. pulmonis*

**8** Chromodacryorrhea is commonly referred to as red tears and is

a. A zoonotic viral condition

b. A bacterial condition

c. Caused by porphyrin secretions from the harderian gland

d. Caused by a secretion from the hibernating gland

**9** Many outbreaks of diseases in frogs are secondary to

a. Environmental stress

b. Bacterial infections

c. Fungal infection

d. Malnutrition

**10** A rabbit presents with torticollis. What could be causing this?

a. A hairball

b. May have been improperly handled and has now fractured its vertebrae

c. An infection caused by *Pasteurella multocida*

d. Malocclusion

## BIBLIOGRAPHY

Animals for Research Act, 1983, Government of Ontario.

Bell JC, Palmer SR, Payne JM: *The zoonoses: infections transmitted from animals to man*, London, 1988, Edward Arnold.

Brown SA: *Rabbit medicine*, Proceedings of the 21st Waltham's/Oklahoma State University Symposium, Oklahoma.

Buckland MD et al: *A guide to laboratory animal technology*, London, 1981, William Heinemann Medical Books.

Canadian Association for Laboratory Animal Science: *CALAS training manual*, Ottawa, Canada, 1995, CALAS.

Canadian Council on Animal Care: *Guide to the care and use of experimental animals,* vol 1, Ottawa, Canada, 1993, CCAC.

Canadian Council on Animal Care: *Guide to the care and use of experimental animals*, vol 2, Ottawa, Canada, 1980-1984, CCAC.

Crawshaw GJ: *Medicine and diseases of amphibians,* Proceedings from The Care and Use of Amphibians, Reptiles and Fish in Research conference, New Orleans, La, 1991.

Field KJ, Sibold AL: *The laboratory hamster and gerbil*, Boca Raton, Fla, 1999, CRC Press.

Fine J, Quimby FW, Greenhouse DD: Annotated bibliography on uncommonly used laboratory animals: mammals, *ILAR News* XXIX:4, 1986.

Flecknell PA: *Laboratory animal anaesthesia*, ed 2, San Diego, 1996, Academic Press.

Harkness JE, Wagner JE: *The biology and medicine of rabbits and rodents*, ed 4, Philadelphia, 1995, Lea & Febiger.

Harris JC: *Chinchillas: a complete introduction*, Neptune City, NJ, 1987, TFH Publications.

Harrison DJ: *Innovative methods for controlling exposure to laboratory animal allergens*. Notes from workshop presented at the American Association for Laboratory Animal Science Conference, Baltimore, Md, October 2001.

Hawk CT, Leary SL: *Formulary for laboratory animals*, ed 2, Ames, 1999, Iowa State University Press.

Hrapkiewicz K, Medina L, Holmes DD: *Clinical laboratory animal medicine: an introduction*, ed 2, Ames, 1998, Iowa State University Press.

Kraft H: *Diseases of chinchillas*, Neptune City, NJ, 1959, TFH Publications.

Krinke GJ: *The laboratory rat*, San Diego, Calif, 2000, Academic Press.

Laber-Laird K, Swindle M, Flecknell P, editors: *Handbook of rodent and rabbit medicine,* Tarrytown, NY, 1996, Pergamon Press.

Marcus LC: *Veterinary biology and medicine of captive amphibians and reptiles*, Philadelphia, 1981, Lea & Febiger.

Maronpot RR: *Pathology of the mouse*, Vienna, Ill, 1999, Cache River Press.

National Research Council: *Occupational health and safety in the care and use of research animals*, Washington, DC, 1997, National Academy Press.

National Research Council, Committee on Rodents, Institute of Laboratory Animal Resources: *Rodents*, Washington, DC, 1996, National Academy Press.

National Research Council, Institute of Laboratory Animal Resources: *Guide for the care and use of laboratory animals*, Washington, DC, 1996, National Academy Press.

Plunkett SJ: *Emergency procedures for the small animal veterinarian*, ed 2, Oxford, England, 2001, Saunders.

Poole T et al: *The UFAW handbook on the care and management of laboratory animals, vol 1, terrestrial vertebrates*, ed 7, New York, 1999, Blackwell Science.

Quesenberry KE, Carpenter JW: *Ferrets, rabbits and rodents: clinical medicine and surgery*, ed 2, St Louis, 2004, Saunders.

Sirois M, editor: *Laboratory animal medicine: principles and procedures*, St Louis, 2005, Mosby.

Wagner JE, Manning PJ: *The biology of the guinea pig*, New York, 1976, Academic Press.

Waynforth HB, Flecknell PA: *Experimental and surgical technique in the rat*, ed 2, London, 1992, Academic Press.

## CHAPTER 18

# Exotic Animal Medicine

*Geraldine Higginson*

## OUTLINE

Avian Medicine
  Classification
  Anatomical and Physiological
    Comparison of Avians and
    Mammals
  Housing
  Restraint and Handling
  Nursing Care
  Anesthesia and Analgesia
  Nutrition: Diets and Problems
  Noninfectious Diseases and
    Conditions
  Infectious Diseases
    Bacterial Diseases
    Viral Diseases
    Mycotic Diseases
  Parasites
    Ectoparasites
    Endoparasites
Reptilian Medicine
  Classification
  Anatomical and Physiological
    Comparison of Reptiles and
    Mammals
  Housing

Restraint and Handling
Nursing Care
Anesthesia and Analgesia
Nutrition: Diets and Problems
  Snakes
  Chelonians
  Lizards
Clinical Conditions and Diseases
Infectious Diseases
  Bacterial Diseases
  Viral Diseases
  Protozoal Diseases
  Mycotic Diseases
Parasites
  Ectoparasites
  Endoparasites
Hedgehog Medicine
  Origin
  Characteristics: Behavioral and
    Physiological
  Housing and Nutrition
  Restraint and Handling
  Breeding Considerations
  Nursing Care
  Signs of Pain and Distress

Anesthesia and Analgesia
Health Conditions
Degu Medicine
  Origin
  Characteristics: Behavioral and
    Physiological
  Housing and Nutrition
  Restraint and Handling
  Breeding Considerations
  Nursing Care
  Signs of Pain and Distress
  Anesthesia and Analgesia
  Health Conditions
Ferret Medicine
  Origin
  Nomenclature
  Characteristics: Behavioral and
    Physiological
  Housing and Nutrition
  Restraint and Handling
  Breeding Considerations
  Nursing Care
  Anesthesia and Analgesia
  Health Conditions

## LEARNING OUTCOMES

After reading this chapter you should be able to:

1. Describe the anatomical and physiological differences in reptilian and avian species compared with mammals.
2. Describe optimum housing and husbandry for reptilian and avian species.
3. Describe restraint and handling for reptilian and avian species.
4. Describe nursing care and procedures for reptilian and avian species.
5. Describe anesthesia techniques and common concerns for reptilian and avian species.
6. Describe common analgesics for both reptilian and avian species.
7. List optimum nutritional requirements for various avian and reptilian species.
8. Identify common clinical conditions and infectious diseases by describing their etiology, clinical signs, and pathology.
9. Describe ectoparasitic and endoparasitic diseases in reptilian and avian species.

10. Compare the anatomy and physiology of the hedgehog, degu, and ferret.
11. Describe the nursing care, restraint, handling and nutritional requirements of the hedgehog, degu, and ferret.
12. Identify common clinical conditions and infectious diseases of the hedgehog, degu, and ferret by describing their etiology, clinical signs, and pathology.

# AVIAN MEDICINE

## CLASSIFICATION

I. Class Aves
   A. Order Psittaformes (psittacines: parrots, cockatoos, macaws, budgies, cockatiels)
   B. Order Passeriformes (songbirds: swallows, finches, canaries)
   C. Order Anseriformes (waterfowl: ducks, geese, swans)
   D. Order Ciconiiformes (waterbirds: cranes, storks, herons)
   E. Order Falconiformes (raptors: falcons, hawks, eagles, osprey)
   F. Order Galliformes (fowl: poultry, pheasants, peafowl, quail)
   G. Order Columbiformes (doves: pigeons, mourning doves)
   H. Order Strigiformes (owls: barn owls, typical owls)

## ANATOMICAL AND PHYSIOLOGICAL COMPARISON OF AVIANS AND MAMMALS

There is a reduction and modification of organs and organ systems to obtain the capacity for flight. Lack of teeth, hollow bones, shortened gastrointestinal tract, air sacs, higher rate of metabolism, oviparity, and feathers are all adaptations for weight reduction and flight ability.

I. Integument
   A. Thinner and more delicate than in mammals
   B. Consists of the epidermis, dermis, and subcutaneous layers
   C. Modifications may include the legs, feet, beak, cere, or cheek patches
   D. The ventral surface of the female bird can change during breeding season to form a brood patch
   E. The dermal layer contains the feather follicles arranged in rows called pterylae, separated by featherless tracts called apteria
   F. Smooth muscles attach to the follicles and are responsible for feather fluffing to conserve heat (similar to piloerection of hair in mammals)
   G. Deficient of glands with the exception of the meibomian glands of the eyelid, uropygial gland above the tail base, and holocrine gland of the external ear canal
   H. Feathers are epidermal structures analogous to mammalian hair and are used for insulation, thermoregulation, courtship displays, and flight
   I. Feather types
      1. Contour (e.g., body and flight feathers)
      2. Plume (e.g., down and powder down)
      3. Semiplume (e.g., bristles and hairs)
   J. Molting is the process of shedding and regrowing of feathers, influenced by season, temperature, nutrition, stress, species, and sex. Molting occurs at least yearly systematically, and does not usually leave the bird flightless. In waterfowl, some species will molt all primary feathers simultaneously after the nesting season is complete. Heavy molting may occur twice yearly in pet birds

II. Sensory: senses of smell and taste are poorly developed; visual senses are extremely well developed
   A. Color vision: rods and cones are present, the numbers dependent on diurnal or nocturnal habits
   B. Three functional eyelids: upper, lower, and nictitating
   C. Eyeballs are fixed in their sockets; however, the bird is able to rotate its head almost 360 degrees
   D. Movement of one eye is independent of the other (no consensual reflex)
   E. Sclerotic ring is the bony ring around the eye, where the cornea joins the sclera
   F. Pecten: a brown vascular fringe that projects from the fundus into the vitreous toward the lens; assumed to help the choroid provide oxygen and nutrients to the retina

III. Skeleton: extreme adaptations for flight
   A. Some bones are pneumatic (hollow): lightweight (e.g., humerus, femur)
   B. Some of the air sacs are in direct communication with the proximal bones (e.g., the interclavicular with the humerus)
   C. Fusion of bones: furcula (paired clavicles), carpometacarpus, tarsometatarsus, and the pelvic girdle (synsacrum)
   D. Pectoral girdle consists of a tripod of bones: clavicle, coracoid, and scapula

IV. Digestive system varies with gross anatomical differences and short transit time (3 to 12 hours)
   A. Psittacines, galliformes, and passeriformes possess a true crop
   B. Falconiformes have a poorly developed crop; strigiformes (owls) lack a crop

C. Ciconiiformes and other fish-eating birds lack a crop

D. Beak is epidermal tissue: its characteristics vary based on the species feeding habits

E. Oral cavity is made up of the tongue, glottis (no epiglottis), and pharynx

F. Proximal esophagus leads to crop (if present), distal esophagus leads to stomach (proventriculus and ventriculus)

G. Associated organs: liver and spleen

H. Small intestine: duodenum, jejunum, and ileum

I. Pancreas and gallbladder (presence varies among species) empty into the terminal segment of the duodenal loop (rather than the proximal segment as in mammals)

J. Large intestine; presence of paired ceca is variable among species (absent in psittacines); rectum

K. Cloaca: coprodeum (digestive), urodeum (urinary), and proctodeum (collection chamber)

V. Respiratory: unique anatomy

A. No diaphragm

B. Trachea: complete tracheal rings

C. Larynx: at anterior end of the trachea; unlike mammals, no vocal cords

D. Syrinx: usually at base of the trachea (varies among species); sound producing organ

E. Bronchi: bifurcates caudal to syrinx with a primary bronchus leading to each lung

F. Lungs: the most efficient gas exchange system among the vertebrates

1. Compressed dorsally against the ribs, fixed, and do not expand during inspiration

2. Unidirectional flow through the lungs; takes two breaths for air to move through system:

a. First inhalation: air moves through to abdominal air sacs; first exhalation: air is forced to the lungs with abdominal contraction, gas exchange occurs here

b. Second inhalation: air leaves the lungs to the cranial air sacs (interclavicular and cranial thoracic); second exhalation: cranial air sacs contract and drive the air into the trachea

G. Air sacs

1. Eight to nine air sacs: single interclavicular, single or paired cervical, and paired cranial thoracic, caudal thoracic, and abdominal

2. Communicate with the proximal pneumatic bones (humerus, femur)

3. Thin walled, one cell thick, epithelial tissue

4. Connect to the lung directly by the primary or secondary bronchus

5. Connect indirectly by the parabronchi

6. Act as a bellows system, using the sternum to push air through the lungs

VI. Circulatory: endurance for flight

A. Four-chambered heart

1. Larger than the mammalian heart relative to size

2. Faster heart rate

3. Greater arterial pressure

4. Lower peripheral resistance

B. Blood cells

1. Nucleated erythrocytes

a. Large in comparison to mammalian cells

b. Life span of 28 to 45 days (shorter than mammals)

c. Rapid turnover rate

d. High polychromatic index

2. Thrombocytes (analogous to mammalian platelets)

3. Heterophils (analogous to mammalian neutrophils)

4. Eosinophils

5. Basophils

6. Lymphocytes

7. Monocytes

VII. Urogenital

A. No urinary bladder

B. Metanephric kidneys

C. Renal portal system: blood from the caudal portion of the body passes through the kidneys via the renal portal system before entering the main vascular system

D. Kidneys have three lobes: cranial, middle, and caudal

E. Urine excreted as uric acid; voided with feces through the cloaca

F. Female reproductive system

1. Only one functional ovary and oviduct on the left, the right being vestigial in most species

2. Oviduct consists of five sections: infundibulum (receives ovum from follicle), magnum (adds albumen), isthmus (adds two shell membranes), uterus (lays down calcium shell), and vagina (directs egg to cloaca through muscular expulsion)

G. Male reproductive system

1. Paired testes: increase dramatically in size during the breeding season

2. Vas deferens

3. Seminal vesicles (end of ductus deferens): store sperm and pass them into urodeum of cloaca

4. Phallic organ is present in proctodeum of some birds (waterfowl, ostriches, rheas, emus, herons, flamingos); acts as an intromittent organ during copulation

H. Age of sexual maturity varies with species; budgies are active at 1 year (life span, 8 to 10 years), canaries at 1 to 4 years (life span, 4 to 8 years), cockatiels at 2 years (life span, 10 to 15 years), and larger parrots at 3 to 7 years (life span, 30 to 50 years for an Amazon parrot)

## HOUSING

I. Clinic caging
   A. Incubators (with oxygen source available)
   B. Stainless steel dog kennels
   C. Commercial wire bird cages
II. Home caging
   A. Constructed of nontoxic materials (caution with lead or zinc compounds)
   B. Safe and easy for cleaning
   C. Sturdy, nontoxic food and water bowls
   D. Variety of perch diameters and form (hardwood, cement, rope), set at different heights in cage
   E. Substrate lining: newspaper, paper towel, paper liner (avoid corncob bedding because of possible fungal contamination and ingestion)
   F. Large enough to allow full body extension (as large as space allows)
   G. Strong enough to resist dismantling by the bird
   H. Stimulating toys and environment
III. Quarantine
   A. A new bird should be quarantined for 30 to 45 days in a separate facility or area before introducing it into the home or existing flock; allow no cross contamination from handling birds, food bowls, or supplies in this time

## RESTRAINT AND HANDLING

I. Restraint: do not restrict movement of the sternum (birds breathe by sternal movement); hold wings to body to prevent injury
   A. Small psittacines and songbirds can be caught from behind with a small towel or barehanded; hold the head between the middle and index finger, with the hand enveloping the wings and body
   B. Large psittacines should be caught from behind with a towel (gloves are not recommended); hold the head between the thumb and index finger and the other hand holding the feet; the towel should drape around the body, restraining the wings
   C. Waterfowl can be restrained with the body under one arm and the other hand holding the head
   D. Waterbirds (e.g., herons, grebes) can inflict nasty injuries with their pointed beaks; wear eye protection and restrain similar to method used for waterfowl
   E. Raptors can be captured from behind with a towel; grasp both legs high above the talons with one hand, and restrain the head and body as with psittacines

## NURSING CARE

I. Physical examination
   A. The physical examination should be performed with the minimum amount of stress to the patient
   B. Before handling, a complete history should be obtained from the owner, including: age, sex (if known), place of purchase and length of ownership, any clinical complaints, any prior medical history, and a detailed description of the diet
   C. The bird should be assessed during this time for its posture, respiratory rate, activity level, and general attitude while perched in the cage or carrier; any feces present in the carrier should be assessed for consistency and color
   D. Accurate body weights are critical for health monitoring and for safe drug administration
      1. Perch gram scale, accurate to within 1 gram
      2. Triple beam balance with a basket
      3. Weigh carrier with and without the bird
   E. Physical examinations should follow a thorough, consistent manner, assessing symmetry and palpating for abnormalities
      1. Cere and nostrils should be clear of discharge
      2. Crop should not be palpable unless the bird has recently eaten
      3. Body condition is scored through palpation of the keel (sternum) and pectoral muscles:
         a. An emaciated bird will have a sharp keel with little muscle present; obese birds will appear to have cleavage over the keel
      4. The abdomen is difficult to evaluate unless there is an abnormal mass or lesion in the intestinal peritoneal cavity; occasionally the caudal border of the ventriculus may be palpated
      5. The vent should be clean and free of fecal debris
      6. The skin and feathers can be examined by blowing on the feathers or wetting down with alcohol
         a. The skin is usually clear/white with visible blood vessels and muscle beneath
         b. The presence of blood feathers should be noted
         c. All feathers should be symmetrical, smooth edged, and free of defects
      7. When examining the wings and legs, all joints must be supported (especially in the wing) to avoid iatrogenic injury
      8. Heart rate, respiration rate, and temperature
         a. Auscultate with a pediatric stethoscope
         b. Heart rates: 100 to 300+ beats per minute, dependent on species size

c. Respiration rate: 20 to 60+ breaths per minute, dependent on species size and stress level

d. Temperature: 40° to 44° C (104° to 111° F); typically not taken except for hypothermic situations or during anesthetic monitoring

II. Beak trimming

A. Birds may need their beaks trimmed if there is evidence of overgrowth or retained keratin (usually due to lack of proper chewing wear) or if the beak is malaligned

B. A nail file or Dremel tool can be used to reshape the beak (method dependent on beak size)

C. The beak has a central blood supply

1. Trimming the beak too short may cause bleeding; stop with hemostatic powder application

III. Nail trimming

A. Birds may occasionally need nails trimmed

1. Use a Dremel tool, scissor trimmers, or a nail file to reshape

2. If perch diameters are not correct for species, may see curling of nails, particularly in back toes

3. If trimmed too short, the quick may bleed; stop with application of hemostatic powder

4. Any blood loss in birds is considered serious; therefore each nail should be examined after trimming

IV. Wing clipping

A. Wing clipping is used to limit the bird's flying ability (for safety and as an aid in training and taming)

1. The wing trim should allow the bird to safely glide a short distance down from a height but not attain any height

2. The most common wing clip is where primary feathers are trimmed bilaterally from the outside primary (#10) inward (height is gained from most distal primaries); feather is clipped just beneath coverts; removing the feathers from one wing can cause the bird to circle and crash

3. The number of primaries removed is dependent on the size and species of the bird (smaller birds often require more feathers trimmed to restrict flight)

4. During the wing trim, the underside of the wing should be examined for immature or growing blood feathers

a. If a blood feather is accidentally cut, the feather must be pulled out immediately to prevent blood loss

5. A bird with newly trimmed wings should be placed at a low height until it is acclimated to the change

V. Blood collection

A. Sites

1. Right jugular vein (the right is slightly larger than the left)

2. Brachioulnar or cutaneous ulnar veins (wing)

3. Medial tibiotarsal or medial metatarsal veins (leg)

4. Toenail clipping is not recommended

B. Blood is collected using a 22- or 25-gauge needle

1. A sample can be collected in a syringe and transferred to a small volume heparinized tube

2. Pressure should be applied directly to the site of the collection after removal of the needle, particularly if using ulnar and leg veins

3. The site should be evaluated for bleeding before releasing the bird

4. Able to collect less than 1% of accurate body weight in milliliters

VI. Blood analysis

A. Coulter counters cannot be used for avian blood because of the nucleated red blood cells

1. Complete blood cell count can be obtained by combining the Unopette system or hemocytometer count, which give an absolute heterophil and eosinophil count, with a differential count from a smear

2. Biochemical profile: uric acid is used to assess renal function in birds

VII. Intravenous catheters are placed most commonly in the wing or leg veins

A. Difficult to maintain except during anesthesia or in moribund birds

1. Awake psittacines with IV catheters must be monitored continuously, because they are capable of chewing through bandages and catheters

VIII. Intraosseous catheters placed in the proximal tibia or distal ulna (preferred)

A. More stable and difficult for bird to remove than IV catheters

B. The site must be aseptically prepared

C. Confirm placement with saline flush (watch brachioulnar vein blanch)

D. Injections and fluid infusion rates are similar to IV use

E. Important technique for use in smaller species or if the bird is in shock or dehydrated

IX. Intramuscular injections are generally performed in the pectoral muscle (potential nephrotoxicity via renal portal system if leg muscles are used)

A. Wet down the feathers with alcohol to visualize the skin and ensure accurate placement in the muscle

B. Needle size should be appropriate for size of patient

X. Subcutaneous (SC) injections are used mainly for fluid administration
  A. SC fluids can be administered in the inguinal region, over the pectoral muscles, or the interscapular area; avoid cervical region because of air sacs
  B. Fluids should be warmed before administration
XI. Oral drug administration/gavage feeding is performed using rigid, curved, stainless steel (for psittacines or raptors) or rubber (waterfowl species) feeding tubes
  A. The bird must be restrained upright with the neck extended
  B. The tube is gently inserted over the tongue, angling to the bird's right side, into the esophagus, and then crop (if present) at thoracic inlet
    1. There is risk of perforation of the esophageal/crop wall if the placement is too aggressive or if the bird is not adequately restrained
  C. Ensure proper placement by palpating for the tube before injecting any liquid, because injection of liquid into the trachea will likely kill the bird

## ANESTHESIA AND ANALGESIA

I. Isoflurane anesthesia is the method of choice
  A. Anesthesia is helpful for diagnostic imaging, sample collection, and some procedures to improve techniques and reduce patient stress
  B. Ensure that the crop is empty to prevent regurgitation and aspiration
  C. Use appropriately sized face mask (modified small animal masks, syringe cases) and mask down at 5% isoflurane; induction will take 1 to 2 minutes
  D. Intubate with uncuffed endotracheal (ET) tubes (2.0 to 5.5 mm); use ET tube or cotton swab to pull tongue forward for visualization of glottis and secure to mandible with tape
  E. Maintain on 1.5% to 3.0% isoflurane if intubated or 3% to 5% if on mask; for oxygen flow rates 0.5 to 1.0 L/min, using Bain circuit
II. Monitoring
  A. Heart rate: Doppler flow meter, and esophageal or pediatric stethoscope
  B. Pulse rate: palpate ulnar artery at elbow
  C. Respiration rate and depth, intermittent positive pressure ventilation (IPPV) regularly
  D. IV access ideal
III. Analgesics
  A. Opioids most commonly used (butorphanol 1 to 3 mg/kg, meperidine 3 to 5 mg/kg)
  B. Nonsteroidal antiinflammatory drugs (NSAIDs) (meloxicam 0.3 to 0.5 mg/kg SID to BID)

## NUTRITION: DIETS AND PROBLEMS

I. Proper psittacine diet
  A. Approximately 80% of dietary intake should consist of a commercial psittacine pelleted ration

  B. Nuts and seeds should be restricted because of the high fat component
  C. Budgies do not synthesize iodine and thus require iodine in their diet (usually as vitamin-enriched seeds)
  D. Grit is not necessary as a supplement
II. Waterfowl diet: commercially available pellets
III. Poultry diet: commercially available pellets
IV. Ciconiiformes are carnivorous: feed fish and frogs
V. Raptorial species are carnivorous: feed mice, rats, quail, and chicks
VI. Dietary deficiencies
  A. Hypovitaminosis A: unhealthy mucous membranes and epithelium
  B. Hypocalcemia: "metabolic bone disease" and nutritional hypoparathyroidism; hypocalcemic tetany observed in psittacines, problems with egg-binding; usually due to inadequate calcium intake from diet
  C. Thiamine deficiency: stargazing and opisthotonos
  D. Hypovitaminosis E and selenium deficiency: cause degeneration of skeletal muscles; referred to as white muscle disease

## NONINFECTIOUS DISEASES AND CONDITIONS

I. Predisposing factors, such as immunosuppression, dehydration, malnutrition, starvation, poor hygiene, suboptimal environmental conditions, and stress, can leave the bird susceptible to disease
II. Trauma: dislocations, fractures, soft tissue damage, and pododermatitis
III. Feather abnormalities: behavioral ("feather-picking"), hypoparathyroidism, stress, improper molting, skin allergies, possible viral etiology or, less commonly, ectoparasites
IV. Egg-binding and chronic egg-laying: abdominal distention, dyspnea, and hypocalcemic seizures
V. Regurgitation/vomiting: normal courtship behavior, lead poisoning, foreign body ingestion, or a gastrointestinal problem
VI. Toxins
  A. Inhalants from household appliances or products, paints, pesticides
  B. Toxic plants
  C. Heavy metals (lead or zinc)
    1. Clinical signs of lethargy, depression, green diarrhea, paresis, paralysis, and convulsions
    2. Sources for pet birds include stained glass, old paint, solder, wine foil, galvanized wire, batteries, pellets, antique jewelry
    3. Waterfowl ingest cast lead shot from feeding at bottom of ponds
    4. Raptorial species ingest waterfowl with lead shot in their muscle (secondary lead toxicity)

5. Treatment includes chelation therapy with calcium disodium versenate and supportive care (removal of the object is often difficult)

# INFECTIOUS DISEASES

## Bacterial Diseases

I. Normal gastrointestinal flora of psittacines is predominately gram positive

II. Normal gastrointestinal flora for raptors and other carnivorous species is predominately gram negative

III. Common diseases in psittacines, poultry, raptors, and waterfowl

A. Chlamydiosis (psittacosis, ornithosis)
1. Common species: psittacines, poultry, waterfowl
2. Cause: *Chlamydophila psittaci*
3. Clinical signs: include green diarrhea, pneumonia, nasal and ocular discharge, lethargy; sometimes totally asymptomatic
4. Blood work: usually elevated heterophil count in acute disease
5. Lesions: splenomegaly, hepatomegaly, pericarditis, air sacculitis, and pneumonia
6. Zoonotic: can cause flulike symptoms in humans
7. Diagnosis: polymerase chain reaction on feces, blood, and choanal swab; antigen capture ELISA; serology
8. Treatment: doxycycline, azithromycin, or chlortetracycline, and supportive care

B. Avian mycobacteriosis
1. Common species: psittacines, poultry, waterfowl, raptors
2. Cause: *Mycobacterium avium-intracellulare* complex
3. Clinical signs: chronic weight loss and lethargy
4. Blood work: marked increase in heterophilic leukocytes, monocytosis
5. Zoonotic: potential infection of immunosuppressed humans
6. Diagnosis: acid-fast smears of feces, biopsy of the infected liver or intestinal mucosa, presence of granulomas
7. Treatment: long-term combination antibiotic therapy

C. Coryza: upper respiratory disease
1. Common species: poultry
2. Cause: *Haemophilus* spp. and *Mycoplasma* spp.
3. Clinical signs: rhinitis, sinusitis, and upper respiratory signs
4. Diagnosis: culture and sensitivity of respiratory tract

D. Pneumonia and air sacculitis: lower respiratory tract infections
1. Common species: psittacines, poultry, waterfowl, raptors
2. Cause: gram negatives (e.g., *Escherichia coli*, *Pseudomonas* spp.)
3. Clinical signs: hyperpnea, dyspnea, abdominal breathing, cyanosis, or no symptoms
4. Diagnosis: culture and sensitivity

E. Avian cholera or pasteurellosis
1. Common species: waterfowl
2. Cause: *Pasteurella multocida*
3. Clinical signs: diarrhea, dehydration, ataxia, septicemia, and sudden death

F. Bacterial enteritis
1. Common species: waterfowl, poultry; psittacines and raptors less commonly
2. Cause: various bacteria, including *Clostridium perfringens*
3. Clinical signs: diarrhea, dehydration, death

G. Bacterial toxemia
1. Common species: waterfowl
2. Cause: *Clostridium botulinum*
    a. Botulism from ingestion of toxins produced by the bacteria
3. Clinical signs: weakness, "limberneck," paresis, paralysis, and death in waterfowl (often by drowning)
4. Treatment: supportive care and botulism antitoxin

## Viral Diseases

Table 18-1 contains a list of common viruses that occur in psittacines. A variety of other viral diseases affect waterfowl, passerines, and poultry.

## Mycotic Diseases

I. Aspergillosis
A. Cause: *Aspergillus fumigatus*
B. Clinical signs: lethargy, droopy wings, anorexia, respiratory distress, death
C. Common in: stressed or weak patients, primarily a secondary disease or heavy environmental contamination

II. Candidiasis
A. Cause: *Candida albicans* (opportunistic yeast)
B. Clinical signs: gray to white plaque lesions in the oral cavity, esophagus, and crop
C. Common in: columbiformes, raptors, and psittacines

III. Megabacteria/avian gastric yeast
A. Cause: *Macrorhabdus ornithogaster*
B. Clinical signs: weight loss, failure to thrive, abnormal GI motility, asymptomatic
C. Common in: budgerigars
D. Diagnosis: direct fecal smear

**Table 18-1**  Common viral diseases affecting psittacines

| Etiology | Clinical signs/occurrence |
| --- | --- |
| **NEWCASTLE'S DISEASE (PARAMYXOVIRUS)** | |
| Paramyxovirus (9 virus types currently identified) | Ataxia, opisthotonos, and seizures<br>Occurs in poultry, columbiformes, psittacines occasionally |
| **PACHECO'S DISEASE** | |
| Herpesvirus | Anorexia and sudden death<br>Occurs in outbreak/stress conditions |
| **POLYOMA** | |
| Polyomavirus | Subcutaneous hemorrhage, hepatomegaly, acute death<br>Occurs in young psittacines, often outbreaks |
| **PSITTACINE BEAK AND FEATHER DISEASE** | |
| Circovirus | Clubbing of feather shafts, feather atypia, beak lesions, feather loss<br>Diagnosed by a feather biopsy and histology |
| **PROVENTRICULAR DILATION DISEASE** | |
| Possibly due to unidentified virus | Abnormal gastrointestinal transit and function, neurological deficits, and death. Definitive diagnosis difficult except on necropsy, because of the segmental nature of the disease. History, clinical signs, radiographic and fluoroscopic examination, and crop biopsy may suggest presence of disease |

# PARASITES

## Ectoparasites

I. Lice
   A. *Mallophaga* spp. only
II. Mites
   A. Scaly leg and face mites: *Knemidocoptes* spp.
      1. Common in budgerigars and poultry; rarely in other psittacines
      2. Lesions on the beak, eyelids, and legs
   B. Tracheal mites: *Sternostoma tracheacolum*
      1. Common in: finches and canaries
      2. Clinical signs: sneezing, open-mouth breathing, dyspnea, and loss of voice

III. Flies
   A. Hippoboscid flies often seen on raptorial birds
IV. Treatment: most ectoparasites are easily treated with ivermectin or dilute carbaryl dusting powders

## Endoparasites

I. Nematodes
   A. Ascarids
   B. Microfilaria
   C. Gapeworm (*Syngamus trachea* in galliformes, and *Cyathostoma* spp. in waterfowl)
   D. Several species of capillaria
II. Cestodes: uncommon
III. Trematodes: uncommon
IV. Protozoa
   A. Coccidiosis
      1. Cause: *Eimeria* spp., *Isospora* spp.
      2. Common species: important disease in poultry; also seen in finches waterfowl, and raptors
      3. Clinical signs: anorexia, lethargy, diarrhea, dehydration, and wasting
   B. Histomoniasis
      1. Cause: *Histomonas meleagridis*
      2. Clinical signs: "blackhead" in turkeys and game birds; lesions on liver and intestines
   C. Trichomoniasis
      1. Cause: *Trichomonas* spp.
      2. Common species: columbiformes, raptors, psittacines
      3. Clinical signs: oral plaques similar to candida and capillaria
   D. Hemosporidia
      1. Cause: blood protozoans *Hemoproteus* spp., *Leucocytozoon* spp., and *Plasmodium* spp.
      2. Common species: wild caught psittacines and most waterfowl and raptors in small densities
      3. Problem occurs only at high densities or under stress

# REPTILIAN MEDICINE

## CLASSIFICATION

I. Class: Reptilia
   A. Order: Chelonia (turtles and tortoises)
   B. Order: Crocodilia (crocodiles, alligators, and caimans)
   C. Order: Rhynchocephalia (tuatara)
   D. Order: Squamata
      1. Suborder: Serpentes (snakes)
      2. Suborder: Sauria (lizards)

## ANATOMICAL AND PHYSIOLOGICAL COMPARISON OF REPTILES AND MAMMALS ▬

I. Lifestyle
   A. Terrestrial
   B. Aquatic (freshwater)
   C. Marine
   D. Arboreal

II. Life span: wide range among species but very dependent on captive conditions
   A. Approximately five years for a panther chameleon
   B. One hundred fifty years or more in a Galapagos tortoise

III. Growth and metabolism
   A. Slow metabolic rate
   B. Continual growth; growth rate slows nearing maturity

IV. Integument
   A. Scales or scutes
      1. Chelonians have a superficial layer of keratin shields, which make up the carapace dorsally and the plastron ventrally
      2. Some lizards have bony plates in the dermis called osteoderms
   B. The skin is made up of the dermis and epidermis
   C. Periods of ecdysis (shedding of the skin)
   D. Autotomy: the ability of a lizard to shed its tail when captured; the new tail will lack vertebrae
   E. Healing is much slower than in mammals, because of the decreased metabolic rate

V. Sensory
   A. Lizards have a movable eyelid, but the nictitating membrane is reduced and nonfunctional
   B. The eye in snakes is covered by a transparent protective membrane called a spectacle; it does not touch the cornea and is shed during ecdysis

VI. Skeletal
   A. Appendages as limbs (most species)
   B. Appendages modified as flippers (aquatic turtles)
   C. Appendages entirely lacking (snakes)
   D. Pythons and boas possess vestiges of hind limbs, evident as spurs on either side of the cloaca
   E. Chelonians have their entire limb girdles housed within their rib cage (shell)
   F. In snakes and some lizards, the quadrate bone's articulation with the maxilla and the lack of a mandibular symphysis allow the ingestion of large prey
   G. Lizards and chelonians possess a tympanic membrane, whereas snakes do not; snakes do not possess a middle ear cavity
   H. Some snakes have infrared receptors that are extremely sensitive to changes in heat; the receptors also help determine distance and direction in finding prey

VII. Digestive
   A. Well-developed epiglottis in some lizards; other reptiles without
   B. Glottis is usually located at the tongue base and can be moved forward to allow breathing while ingesting large prey
   C. Esophagus, stomach, small intestine, large intestine, rectum
   D. Cloaca: copredeum (fecal), urodeum (urinary and reproductive), proctodeum (storage)

VIII. Respiratory
   A. Diaphragm absent
   B. Lizards and snakes: tidal volume controlled by expansion and contraction of the ribs
   C. Chelonians: respiration controlled by alternating body cavity pressure during locomotion and pharyngeal pumping
   D. Left lung in snakes is reduced or absent
   E. Lizards have two saccular lungs
   F. Chelonians have two saccular lungs compressed dorsally against the carapace

IX. Thermoregulation
   A. Poikilothermic: rely on environmental temperature to maintain their own body temperature and metabolic processes

X. Circulatory
   A. The crocodile is the first vertebrate to develop the complete interventricular septum and, therefore, a four-chambered heart
   B. All other reptiles have a three-chambered heart
      1. Two atria
      2. One ventricle
      3. Incomplete interventricular septum that partially prevents the mixing of blood
   C. Blood cells
      1. Nucleated red blood cells
      2. Thrombocytes (analogous to mammalian platelets)
      3. Heterophils (analogous to mammalian neutrophils)
      4. Eosinophils
      5. Basophils
      6. Lymphocytes
      7. Monocytes
      8. Azurophils: unique to reptiles; have azurophilic cytoplasm but believed to be monocytes, because they have similar cytochemical and structural characteristics

XI. Urogenital
   A. Metanephric kidneys
   B. Some species possess a bladder
   C. Terrestrial species excrete uric acid
   D. Aquatic species excrete urea and ammonia
   E. Renal portal system filters blood from caudal portion of the body through the

kidneys before entering the main vascular system

F. Chelonians have single extrudable penis

G. Lizards and snakes have two hemipenes

H. Reproduction by oviparity in caiman, alligators, turtles, and some lizards and snakes

I. Reproduction by viviparity or ovoviviparity in some lizards and snakes

## HOUSING

I. Clinic housing
  A. Incubators
  B. Stainless steel dog kennels
  C. Full spectrum UV (especially UVB) light source for vitamin D synthesis and calcium metabolism
  D. Basking/heat lamp to provide thermal gradient in tank

II. At home
  A. Aquarium
  B. Terrarium
  C. Custom-made cage
  D. Controlled temperature and humidity
    1. Each species has its own preferred optimal temperature range (POTR): for most common tropical pet species, it is 26° to 37° C (80° to 98° F), and for most temperate species, it is 24° to 29.5° C (75° to 85° F); thermometer should be used to monitor tank temperature
    2. Provide a basking area or "hot spot" with a direct heat source, where temperature is higher
    3. Low environmental temperatures can lead to anorexia and increase susceptibility to infection
    4. Humidity is an important factor, 50% to 70% is the optimum for most species
    5. Heated rocks are not recommended owing to risk of thermal injury
    6. Maintaining temperature at upper range of POTR during illness will optimize metabolism, immunity, and appetite/digestion
  E. Full spectrum ultraviolet light source is necessary for synthesis of vitamin D for calcium absorption
    1. In warm climates or during the summer months, some reptiles may be housed outdoors to obtain natural ultraviolet radiation
    2. Photoperiod of 12 hours daylight is suitable for all reptiles
  F. Clean, shallow water dish
    1. Chameleons will not drink from a water dish; use a dripping water bottle or mister
  G. Environmental enrichment appropriate to species (e.g., arboreal species need climbing trees, burrowing species need deep litter, shy and nocturnal species need a hide box)

H. Substrate can be newspaper, aquarium gravel, corncob bedding, or sand litter, as long as substrate is made of digestible fibers in case of ingestion

## RESTRAINT AND HANDLING

I. Restraint
  A. Venomous snakes: should be restrained only by experienced herpetological personnel
  B. Nonvenomous snakes: restrain from behind at the mandible and support the body
    1. Large constrictors should be handled by two people
  C. Lizards: grasp behind the head at the mandible and hold the pelvis and tail base with the other hand
    1. Be aware of claws and tail lashing in defense
    2. Never restrain by the tail only, because it may break off in a natural defense mechanism
  D. Chelonians: restrain by carapace, anterior to the hind legs
  E. Restraint for radiographs: applying mild digital pressure to the eyes; this causes a quiescent state that can last for a few minutes (vasovagal response) in some species

## NURSING CARE

I. Physical examination
  A. Annual physical examinations to determine baseline values
  B. Basic signalment should include correct species ID, age, weight, sex, husbandry, diet management, and any previous medical history
    1. Length of ownership and place of purchase should also be noted
  C. A thorough examination and palpation (as is possible) of body structures should be conducted in a routine manner
    1. Examine the oral cavity by use of nonabrasive mouth gags (e.g., rubber spatula, tongue depressor, tape strips)
  D. Temperature, pulse, and respirations
    1. Cloacal temperature values are not useful because reptiles are ectothermic
    2. Respiration: range from 4 to 30 breaths per minute
    3. Heart rate: auscultation can be difficult because of irregular skin surface; can place a wet gauze under bell of a pediatric stethoscope over cardiac region
    4. Peripheral pulses not easily palpated

II. Blood collection
  A. Can be challenging in some species
  B. Ventral tail vein (lizards, chelonians)
    1. Restrain in either dorsal recumbency with the ventral aspect of the tail facing up, or in ventral recumbency with the tail hanging off the end of the table

2. Insert needle/butterfly catheter perpendicular to the tail along the midline to the depth of the vertebrae
C. Dorsal and ventral buccal veins of the mouth (snakes)
D. Right jugular vein (chelonians)
   1. Introduce needle in a craniocaudal direction with the head restrained
E. Dorsal venous sinus of tail (chelonians)
F. Dilution with lymphatic fluids common from tail and venous sinus locations
G. Nail clip is not recommended

III. Blood analysis
A. Coulter counter cannot be used because of nucleated red blood cells
B. Complete blood cell count can be obtained by combining the Unopette system or hemocytometer count, with a differential count from a smear
C. Biochemical profile: uric acid level is used to assess renal function

IV. Intraosseous catheterization
A. Site: proximal tibia (trochanteric fossa) or femur in species with limbs
   1. Must be aseptically prepared
   2. Most drugs licensed for IV use can be infused safely into bone marrow
   3. Important technique because IV access can be challenging in some species

V. Intravenous injection
A. May require a skin cutdown
B. Chelonians: right jugular or coccygeal vein
C. Lizards: ventral abdominal or tail vein
D. Snakes: coccygeal or right jugular vein (via cutdown)

VI. Intramuscular injection
A. Chelonians and lizards: front legs
B. Snakes: dorsal epaxial muscles in cranial half
C. Nephrotoxicity or premature elimination of some drugs given in the hind limbs is a possible risk because of renal portal system

VII. Fluids
A. Because of limited IV access, SC fluid administration often used
B. Can be given intracoelomically in the right or left lower quadrants in snakes and chelonians, or right lower quadrant in lizard
C. Should be warmed before administration

VIII. Oral administration of meds/stomach feeding is performed using rigid stainless steel or rubber feeding tubes
A. Anorexia is common in ill reptiles
   1. Normal feeding patterns vary between species (e.g., some snakes can go months without eating)

B. Protect oral mucosa and teeth with use of rubber spatulas or tongue depressors as speculum
   1. Glottis in reptiles is cranial (at the base of the tongue) and is easily visualized when the mouth is open
   2. Insert tube to level of distal esophagus or stomach

## ANESTHESIA AND ANALGESIA

I. Inhalant
A. Isoflurane is anesthetic of choice
B. Will hold their breath, so they are difficult to mask down
C. Intubate with uncuffed ET tubes; can intubate some species awake and manually IPPV until anesthetized
D. Maintain at upper end of POTR before, during, and after anesthesia for quicker induction and recovery
E. Exhibit respiratory depression under anesthesia (apnea or bradypnea); require manual or automated ventilation

II. Injectable
A. Used for induction or to maintain anesthesia
B. Propofol is preferred for induction or short procedures, but requires IV access
C. Ketamine only or ketamine (lower dose) in combination with midazolam or medetomidine are commonly used

III. Monitoring
A. Heart rate: Doppler flow meter probe over the cardiac region, carotid artery, ventral tail artery; esophageal or pediatric stethoscope
B. IPPV if intubated
C. Maintain at high end of POTR for faster recovery
D. Give fluids if possible

IV. Analgesia
A. Opioids (butorphanol or buprenorphine) commonly used
B. NSAIDs (meloxicam, ketoprofen) commonly used
C. Access to exotics formulary is important, because doses range widely among different species and at different environmental temperatures

## NUTRITION: DIETS AND PROBLEMS
### Snakes

I. All snakes are carnivorous; diet preference is species dependent
A. Rats, mice, gerbils, chicks, fish
II. Feed once weekly up to once monthly (or less), depending on body size and species

### Chelonians

I. May be carnivorous, omnivorous, or herbivorous
A. Carnivorous: trout chow, fish, or pinkie mice
B. Omnivorous: a balanced mix of the two diets

C. Herbivorous: salad of leafy greens, especially foods rich in calcium and vitamin A
II. Feed daily for most species

## Lizards

I. Insectivorous species (geckos, chameleons, anoles, and skinks): crickets, silkworms, and mealworms gutloaded or supplemented with calcium powder; feed daily
II. Carnivorous species (monitors): whole prey diet; feed a few times weekly
III. Omnivorous species: vegetables, fruit, crickets, silkworms, mealworms; feed daily
IV. Herbivorous species (green iguana): calcium-rich vegetables (broccoli, squash), leafy greens (escarole, endive); feed daily
V. May need to use a calcium and vitamin supplement

## CLINICAL CONDITIONS AND DISEASES ▬▬▬

I. Poor husbandry: temperature, humidity, or management
   A. Anorexia
   B. Hypothermia
   C. Trauma
   D. Rodent bites
   E. Dysecdysis (improper shedding)
II. Nutritional problems
   A. Herbivorous and insectivorous species commonly have dietary problems
   B. Metabolic bone disease or hypocalcemia
      1. Common in green iguana and chameleons
      2. Occurs with inadequate calcium in the diet and not enough UVB exposure to synthesize vitamin D for calcium metabolism
      3. Clinical signs: pathological fractures of long bones; poorly mineralized cortices on radiographs; thickened, swollen jaws and thighs because of fibrous osteodystrophy; problems with egg laying, seizures
      4. Treatment: calcium therapy, broad-spectrum ultraviolet light supplementation, and diet correction
   C. Hypovitaminosis A
      1. Common in pet red-eared slider turtles
      2. Clinical signs: palpebral edema, swollen eyes, anorexia
      3. Treatment: vitamin A injection initially, followed by diet correction
   D. Hypovitaminosis E or steatitis: occurs when rodent food source is stored too long
III. Treat for secondary bacterial infections, because sepsis is common in ill and injured reptiles

## INFECTIOUS DISEASES ▬▬▬
## Bacterial Diseases

The bacterial diseases are listed by clinical problem rather than by specific pathogen.
   I. Stomatitis or mouth rot

A. Cause: suboptimal temperature and humidity, poor management, malnutrition, trauma
B. Common bacteria isolated include *Pseudomonas* spp. and *Aeromonas* spp.
C. May progress to osteomyelitis of the jaw if left untreated
II. Pneumonia
   A. Cause: usually poor husbandry and management
   B. Often seen in snakes and chelonians
   C. Clinical signs: dyspnea, open mouthed breathing, abnormal tilt when swimming
   D. Commonly bacterial but also viral, fungal, and parasitic causes
III. Septicemia
   A. Cause: a variety of bacteria (e.g., *Pseudomonas* spp. and *Aeromonas* spp.)
   B. Clinical signs include pinpoint focal necrosis of the skin, SC abscesses or granulomas, and lethargy
   C. Treatment: broad-spectrum antibiotics with gram negative coverage, surgical excision or debridement
IV. Septicemic cutaneous ulcer disease (SCUD)
   A. Identified in aquatic turtles
   B. Cause: variety of gram negative bacteria (e.g., *Citrobacter* spp.)
   C. Clinical signs: cutaneous ulceration, anorexia, septicemia, and death
V. Salmonellosis
   A. Cause: *Salmonella* spp., normal bacterial flora of many reptiles
   B. Zoonotic: significant concern; causes bloody diarrhea and severe enteritis in humans

## Viral Diseases

Viral diseases are uncommon.
   I. Paramyxovirus in snakes
   II. Viral encephalitis in snakes (inclusion body disease)
   III. Herpesvirus in iguanas and turtles

## Protozoal Diseases

I. Cryptosporidium
   A. Concern for snakes: causes regurgitation, anorexia, and death; enteric in geckos and some other lizards
   B. Zoonotic: causes diarrhea and lethargy in humans

## Mycotic Diseases

I. Pneumonia caused by variety of fungi, including *Aspergillus* spp.

## PARASITES ▬▬▬
## Ectoparasites

I. Ticks: common on snakes, tortoises
II. Mites: common on snakes and iguanas

## Endoparasites

I. Coccidia

II. Entamoeba

III. Cestodes

IV. Trematodes

V. Nematodes

    A. Cestodes, trematodes, and nematodes may affect the oral, respiratory, gastrointestinal, and circulatory systems

# HEDGEHOG MEDICINE

## ORIGIN

I. From the insectivore family, Erinaceidae

    A. Hedgehogs are small insectivores native to England, parts of Europe, Africa, and Asia

    B. The hedgehog that is typically kept as a pet in North America is the African pygmy hedgehog *(Atelerix albiventris)*, native to equatorial and central Africa

## CHARACTERISTICS: BEHAVIORAL AND PHYSIOLOGICAL

I. Hedgehogs are generally solitary, nocturnal animals

    A. The hedgehog will roll into a protective ball when it hears a loud noise or is touched by an unfamiliar person

II. Both back and sides are covered with barbless spines; the underside is covered in normal mammalian hair

III. Possess 36 to 44 teeth

IV. Males have a conspicuous prepuce located midabdomen; no scrotal sacs (testes located in perianal recess)

V. Females have little space between the urogenital opening and the anus; possess 2 to 5 pairs of mammae; may be induced ovulators

VI. Hedgehogs have highly developed senses of smell and hearing; vision is limited

    A. Hedgehogs can occasionally be seen "self-anointing," which is triggered by a novel scent

        1. The hedgehog will lick at the novel item and produce large amounts of saliva, which it then spreads over its back and flank with its tongue

VII. Toenails may need trimming on a regular basis

VIII. Expected life span is 6 to 8 years

IX. Heart rate: 180 to 280 beats per minute; respiratory rate: 25 to 50 breaths per minute; rectal temperature: 36.6° to 37.4°C (97.9° to 99.3° F)

## HOUSING AND NUTRITION

I. Cages should have a solid bottom (to avoid catching feet in wire); a hide box (made from PVC tubes, flower pots, cloth bags); an exercise area (e.g., exercise wheel, climbing area); deep bedding (avoid corncob or cedar chips); and a litter pan

    A. Hedgehogs can be trained to use a litter box

    B. Because they are natural foragers, deep bedding will encourage their inquisitive nature

    C. If caging is large enough, a warm water swimming area could be added

II. Environmental temperatures should ideally be maintained at 24° to 29° C (75° to 85° F); temperatures that are too high or low can cause torpor

III. Humidity levels should be low (< 40%)

IV. Supervised outside playtime is recommended for exercise and to stimulate foraging behavior

V. Natural diet of the African pygmy hedgehog would include snails, slugs, spiders, small reptiles, carrion, fruits, and seeds

VI. In captivity, hedgehogs should be fed a commercially prepared hedgehog diet (< 2 tbsp)

    A. Hedgehogs fed dry cat food may develop cystitis or urolithiasis

    B. Small amounts of fruits and vegetables can be offered (< 1 tsp of grapes, berries, banana, beans, cooked carrots, leafy greens, etc.)

    C. Also, small amounts (1 to 2 tsp) of moist food (e.g., canned cat food, cooked egg or meats) may be offered

    D. The diet should include small numbers of crickets, waxworms, or mealworms hidden in their bedding to stimulate normal foraging behaviors

    E. Hedgehogs are prone to obesity; offer two smaller meals per day, and remove any uneaten food after a few hours

## RESTRAINT AND HANDLING

I. Physical examination

    A. For complete physical examination, most hedgehogs will require inhalant anesthesia unless they are extremely tame or very ill. Most will roll into a tight ball as soon as you need to have a look at them. See anesthesia section for more specific details. This technique is probably less stressful than trying to get them to uncurl

        1. Sometimes getting them to walk into a clear plastic tube or tank will allow you to have a general look at them

II. A few methods have been documented for uncurling and restraining an awake hedgehog

    A. With an assistant holding a towel directly below the table edge, push the hedgehog toward the edge of the table. It will probably uncurl to protect itself from falling over the edge; when it does, quickly grasp it by the hind legs

    B. Placing the hedgehog in a pan of shallow water (about 1 inch) will usually entice it to uncurl; then grasp the hind legs

C. Hedgehog can be placed on its back on the examination table; wait until it tries to right itself and then grasp the hind legs

D. Once you have the hedgehog uncurled, you can "mantle scruff" it with a gloved hand. One person should restrain while the other performs the procedures

## BREEDING CONSIDERATIONS

I. Females can conceive as young as 8 weeks of age, but should not be bred until they are at least 6 months

  A. They will be healthily productive until about 2.5 years of age

II. Move the female to the male's cage; females can be quite territorial and attack the male. Watch carefully for fighting and remove her if this occurs. Otherwise, she should be left in the cage for at least 3 days

III. It is quite common for hedgehogs to cannibalize their young, especially if they are disturbed

  A. Do not handle the sow or the litter for at least the first 7 to 10 days

IV. Young are born blind with a membrane covering their spines

V. Once the young have left the nest at about 21 days, they are ready to be habituated to humans and should be handled daily

## NURSING CARE

I. Intramuscular injections can be given into the mantle or thigh region; subcutaneous injections can be given between the spines or in furred areas; for both types of injections, use small gauge needles (23 to 27 gauge)

II. Blood can be collected from the jugular vein, cranial vena cava, saphenous vein, and cephalic vein; IV access can be difficult to maintain long term; IO catheters in the femur or tibia are preferred

III. Fecal and urine samples can be collected using a metabolic cage for a brief period

## SIGNS OF PAIN AND DISTRESS

I. Weight loss, sunken sides

II. Lethargy/reduced activity (e.g., lack of wheel running)

III. Changes in fecal pellets

IV. Decreased appetite/anorexia

V. Changes in locomotion

VI. Will roll self into ball if frightened; if distressed, will erect spines and sometimes hiss or scream

## ANESTHESIA AND ANALGESIA

I. Isoflurane is anesthesia of choice

  A. "Tank" mask induction at 5% isoflurane (use large dog mask as tank);

  B. Maintain by small nose cone mask 2% to 3% isoflurane, or intubate (1.5 mm uncuffed ET tubes or 18- to 20-gauge catheters)

  C. Injectable drugs can be used (ketamine, diazepam/midazolam, medetomidine) but will prolong recovery

  D. Keep warm via heating pads or blankets

  E. IV access ideal but challenging because of their small size

  F. Important to minimize stress preinduction and perform required techniques quickly

  G. Monitoring

    1. Heart rate: pediatric stethoscope, Doppler flowmeter if possible

    2. Respiration rate: observational, should be regular; auscultate for tracheal mucus obstruction (if present, manipulate head position; or clean oropharynx with cotton tip applicators) if maintained by mask; if intubated, IPPV regularly and monitor expirations for signs of a mucus plug due to narrow size of tube

II. Analgesia

  A. Opioids (butorphanol, oxymorphone) and NSAIDs (meloxicam) commonly used, often in combination for longer coverage

## HEALTH CONDITIONS

I. Respiratory disease

  A. Bacterial agents (e.g., *Bordetella bronchiseptica*, *Mycoplasma* spp., and possibly *P. multocida*) noted more commonly in European hedgehogs

  B. Lungworm infection through ingestion of the intermediate host (slugs or snails);

  C. Lung threadworm

  D. Neoplasia

  E. Cardiac disease

  F. Environmental stress (from suboptimal temperatures, dusty bedding)

  G. Clinical signs: coughing, wheezing, lethargy, dyspnea, increased lung sounds, inappetence, and nasal discharge

  H. Diagnosis: by culture and sensitivity; cytology; endoscopy, ultrasound or radiography; auscultation

  I. Treatment includes

    1. Supportive care (e.g., increase environmental temperatures with incubator); flow by oxygen

    2. Initiate antibiotic therapy, bronchodilators, anthelmintics, and others as needed, in least possible stressful manner

II. Dermatitis and alopecia

  A. Cause: hedgehogs can get fleas, ticks, mite infestations, and dermatophyte infections

    1. Common mite species seen include *Caparinia tripilis, Sarcoptes* spp., and *Demodex* spp.

  B. Clinical signs: cutaneous lesions, particularly around the head; scratching; anemia; loss of spines (denuding); and visualization of the ectoparasite

C. Diagnosis: cytology of skin scrapings; skin biopsy (if mites are suspected); fungal culture of skin scrapings, and visual assessment for presence of fleas and ticks

D. Treatment: varies with cause

 1. Ivermectin (at 200 to 500 µg/kg) has been used successfully in hedgehogs to eliminate mites

III. Cardiac disease

 A. Dilated cardiomyopathy is quite common in older hedgehogs

 B. Clinical signs: lethargy, dyspnea, weight loss, heart murmur, ascites

IV. Miscellaneous diseases

 A. Zoonoses: hedgehogs may carry *Salmonella* organisms; clinical presentations can include diarrhea, decreased appetite and dehydration

 B. Obesity is quite common and can be controlled by restricted feeding and increased exercise

 1. Hedgehogs are often fed ad libitum and housed in cages that are too small for natural activities (e.g., digging, foraging, and running on a wheel)

 C. Prone to wide range of internal parasites, including *Crenosoma striatum* (lungworm) and threadworms

 D. Human herpes simplex virus 1 can cause chronic hepatitis

 E. High incidence of neoplasia: oral squamous cell carcinoma; mammary gland and uterine adenocarcinoma

 F. Clinical signs can include inappetence, weight loss, lethargy

 G. Periodontal disease can be quite common because of gingivitis and tartar buildup; may see pawing at the mouth or decreased appetite

 1. Feline tartar control treats and regular dental cleaning may prevent serious problems

## DEGU MEDICINE

### ORIGIN

I. The degu is a rodent of the Octodontidae family

II. A native of Chile, it ranges the western slopes of the Andes

III. Has been referred to as the trumpet-tailed rat or brush tail rat

### CHARACTERISTICS: BEHAVIORAL AND PHYSIOLOGICAL

I. Degus are very social animals. In nature they live in large colonies very similar to the prairie dog and are considered to be agricultural pests in native region

II. They are diurnal and active throughout the year

III. Probably because of their social structure, degus make a wide variety of vocalizations, specific to certain stimuli or behaviors

 A. Degus quite openly acknowledge familiar people and other degus. When someone they recognize enters the room, they will stand up on their hind legs and squeak quite loudly

IV. Degus can be intensely active for short periods of time

 A. They can climb trees

 B. For these reasons, their ideal cage should allow enough space for rambunctious play, social interactions, a running wheel, and climbing areas

 C. They tend to sleep in short cycles of about 20 minutes

V. Similar to chinchillas, degus need to have access to a dust bath a few times weekly

VI. Degus have large orange incisors and open-rooted teeth

VII. They are hind-gut fermenters

VIII. They produce urine that is normally thick and yellow

IX. Average life span is 5 to 8 years in captivity; average body weight is 170 to 300 g

X. Can develop spontaneous diabetes mellitus

XI. Normal body temperature approximately 37.9° C (101.8° F)

## HOUSING AND NUTRITION

I. Caging should have solid bottoms; be multilayered with deep bedding; have hiding spots; have platforms and apparatus on which to climb; and have a running wheel

II. Degus may play with their watering system, which can flood their cage

III. Dust baths are required a few times a week

IV. Should not be housed singly because of their social nature

V. Degus are herbivorous and granivorous; in the wild they would eat variety of plants, roots, seeds, fruit, and livestock droppings

 A. In captivity, feed a commercially prepared laboratory rodent diet

VI. Monitor intake of sugary food, because of the possible development of diabetes mellitus

 A. Avoid feeding fruit or any vegetable high in sugar (e.g., carrots)

 1. Preferred vegetable treats can include beet greens, sweet potatoes, turnips, Brussels sprouts, bok choy, and kale

VII. Limit access to raw peanuts and sunflower seeds, because they have been linked to fatty liver disease. Degus are also prone to obesity

VIII. Degus should be offered free choice high-quality grass hay

## RESTRAINT AND HANDLING

I. Hand-tamed degus can be picked up by presenting an open hand and allowing them to walk on. Once they are on your hand, use both hands to secure them

II. For physical examination or technical procedure
   A. Grip the base of the tail with one hand and the scruff (the loose skin around the neck and shoulder area) with the other hand, similar to a gerbil
      1. Degus can also be restrained similarly to rats by placing fingers on both sides of the head behind the mandibles
      2. Extreme care should be taken to avoid grasping the tail away from the base, because this could cause degloving of the tail
      3. Two people should be involved in any technical procedure

III. Degus rarely bite, but they will if frightened or startled. They tend to emit a loud warning squeak when handled improperly or frightened before biting

## BREEDING CONSIDERATIONS

I. Females have four pair of teats (eight mammae)

II. Males do not have a true scrotum; the testes are contained within the inguinal canal or abdomen

III. The relatively long gestation period (90 days) means that newborn degus are fairly well formed. They are born fully furred with open eyes

IV. The male will assist in caring for the young, and whenever possible should be left with the female

V. Young degus can be handled after 7 days of age; early habituation has a positive impact on handling by humans in the future

VI. Degus are thought to be induced ovulators

## NURSING CARE

I. Techniques used for other members of the rodent family are applicable to degus

## SIGNS OF PAIN AND DISTRESS

I. Isolation from the group

II. Lack of interest in socializing with familiar people

III. Lethargy

IV. Change in consistency of fecal pellets

V. Weight loss, inappetence

VI. Polyuria/polydipsia

VII. Alopecia/dermatitis

VIII. Lameness

## ANESTHESIA AND ANALGESIA

I. Isoflurane is anesthesia of choice
   A. Tank mask induction at 5% isoflurane (use large dog mask as tank); maintain by small nose cone mask 2% to 3% (due to small size, very difficult to intubate)
   B. Injectable drugs can be useful but will prolong recovery
   C. Keep warm via heating pads or blankets
   D. IV access ideal but challenging due to size
   E. Important to minimize stress preinduction and perform required techniques quickly
   F. Monitoring
      1. Heart rate: pediatric stethoscope, Doppler flow-meter if possible
      2. Respiration rate: observational, should be regular, auscultate for tracheal mucous obstruction (if present, manipulate head position; or clean oropharynx with cotton tip applicators)

II. Analgesia
   A. Opioids (butorphanol, oxymorphone) and NSAIDs (meloxicam) commonly used, often in combination for longer coverage

## HEALTH CONDITIONS

I. There is a profound lack of scientific documentation on health conditions in degus. This is apparently due to the fact that few infectious lesions have been noted in this animal

II. Reported naturally occurring infections include *Echinococcus granulosus* (tapeworm) and *Trypanosoma cruzi* (protozoa)

III. Commonly seen lesions that are associated with diabetes mellitus include cataracts, amyloidosis, and hyperplasia of the islets of Langerhans

# FERRET MEDICINE

## ORIGIN

I. From the family Mustelidae, along with skunks, weasels, mink, otter, marten and badger; the "musk" pertaining to their two scent or anal glands

II. Ferrets are thought to have been domesticated for at least 2000 years and to be derived from the European polecat
   A. Were historically often used for rodent control and hunting rabbits
   B. They were introduced in New Zealand in the late 1800s to control rabbit populations; feral populations still exist and prey on other native wildlife

III. In many municipalities in North America, keeping ferrets is illegal

## NOMENCLATURE

I. Male ferrets are referred to as hobs; female ferrets are referred to as jills

II. Castrated males are called hobbles or gibs, and neutered females are referred to as sprites

III. Young ferrets are referred to as kits

## CHARACTERISTICS: BEHAVIORAL AND PHYSIOLOGICAL

I. Have long tubular body with short stubby legs and long tail; the spine is very flexible, allowing the ferret to contort into variety of positions
  A. Ferrets have a simple stomach and short small intestine
    1. Ferrets have no cecum
II. In the wild, mustelid hair coats, body weights, and reproductive cycles are affected seasonally by amount of daylight; in domestic ferrets, similar seasonal body weight and hair coat changes are noted
  A. There are two common hair coat colors
    1. Fitch (wild) or sable: buff-colored coat with black mask, limbs, and tail
      a. Mutations of the fitch color include: silver-mitt, cinnamon, and ginger
    2. Albino: white with pink eyes
      a. As an albino ferrets matures, its coat becomes more yellow
III. Similar to all mustelids, the unneutered male ferret is approximately twice the size of a female (can weigh about 2 kg)
  A. Most pet ferrets in North America are neutered and descented at 5 to 6 weeks of age at breeding farms, and the sexes are more similar in size (males may weigh 1 to 1.4 kg; females may weigh 0.8 to 1.1 kg)
IV. Have poorly developed sweat glands and are prone to heat prostration
V. Musky body odor and yellowing of undercoat is due to very active sebaceous glands, not their anal glands
VI. Ferrets are naturally inquisitive and playful; can enjoy communal living where aggressive play behavior is common (neck biting); will perform territorial marking (urination/defecation) in new cages or environments
VII. Ferrets are nocturnal animals and therefore spend 15 to 20 hours per day sleeping
VIII. Ferrets can be easily trained to use a litter box to urinate and defecate in one place
IX. Life span is 5 to 10 years

## HOUSING AND NUTRITION

I. Cages should be fairly large with solid bottoms, and narrow wire sides (to prevent escape); litter box; heavy dishes for food and water (or water bottles); sleeping area (e.g., hammocks, pillow cases, old shirts, tents)
  A. Ferrets back up to urinate or defecate, so litter boxes should have raised sides
  B. In clinic settings, ferrets may escape between the bars of standard cat and dog cages; a Plexiglas cage front can be used to prevent escape
II. Play area should be completely ferret-proofed
  A. No access to water pipes, heating ducts, and other fixtures, because they can easily escape
  B. Couches, chairs, and mattresses should be covered on the bottom with thin wood to prevent burrowing
  C. No access to foam or latex toys, shoes, rubber bands, head phones, and similar objects, because ferrets appear to have a natural attraction to these items and are often the cause of foreign body obstructions, particularly in younger ferrets
  D. PVC pipes and climbing apparatus create fun entertainment
III. Ferrets are strict carnivores, so their diet should be high in fat (15% to 20%) and good quality protein (30% to 35%) and low in carbohydrates and fiber
  A. Most pet ferrets are now fed a commercial ferret kibble
  B. Vegetables can be offered as treats; foods with high sugar content, such as fruit, should be avoided

## RESTRAINT AND HANDLING

I. Most pet ferrets are easily handled and held still with light restraint; scruffing the back of the neck is usually required for more active ferrets or those requiring injections, blood collection, or other procedures
  A. Scruffing the ferret will allow examination of the oral cavity (they tend to yawn initially); auscultation of the chest; and abdominal palpation
  B. Offering products such as Ferratone or Nutri-Cal to lick will often distract the ferret during injections, ear cleaning, and some diagnostic procedures
  C. For radiographs, blood collection, and catheter placement, inhalant anesthesia is often used to shorten the procedure time and reduce stress to the patient

## BREEDING CONSIDERATIONS

I. Ferrets reach their sexual maturity at approximately 9 to 12 months of age
II. Females are induced ovulators and are seasonally polyestrous
  A. Some can remain in estrus if not bred and die of hyperestrogenism or estrogen toxicity; this is uncommon now, because most females are spayed before reaching the pet trade
III. Male ferrets have a preputial opening on the ventral abdomen; have a palpable os penis
IV. The breeding season usually lasts from March to August. This is dependent on light cycles, and therefore artificial light can be used to induce the breeding season
V. Male breeding season is from December to July. This precedes the female breeding season to allow for spermatogenesis and maturation of the sperm

A. The male testicles enlarge and descend into the scrotum, marking the time when sexual activity will begin

VI. Mating should take place 2 weeks after the onset of vulvar swelling

VII. The female's vulva should decrease to normal size after 2 to 3 weeks postmating if she is pregnant

VIII. The average gestation is 42 days
  A. Fetuses can be palpated at 14 days
  B. Litter sizes range from 2 to 17 kits
  C. Ferrets can produce 2 litters per year

IX. Young kits weigh approximately 7 to 10 g when born and are hairless and blind
  A. Eyes and ears open at 21 to 37 days of age, and they begin eating solid food at about 3 weeks of age
  B. Weaning begins at 6 to 8 weeks, and they reach their adult weight at about 4 months of age

## NURSING CARE

I. Blood collection
  A. The jugular vein and cranial vena cava are the most common sites for blood collection in the ferret; for small samples (e.g., PCV/TP), the cephalic or saphenous veins can be used
    1. For jugular blood collection, the ferret is positioned similarly to a cat; the vein is located more laterally than in dogs and cats
    2. For cranial vena cava collection, the ferret must either be anesthetized (preferable if performing the technique for the first time) or be restrained on its back by two people, one scruffing the neck and extending the forelegs, the other holding the pelvis
      a. The 25-gauge needle is inserted to the hub at a 30° angle between the manubrium and the first rib, angled toward the opposite hip
        (1) Slowly draw the needle out until blood flows into the syringe
        (2) This site should not be used in awake fractious ferrets, because of the risk of lacerating the vein
    3. For cephalic and saphenous veins, use a 25-gauge needle and 1 mL syringe to prevent collapsing the vein
  B. Blood collected under inhalant anesthesia should be drawn immediately after induction, because isoflurane can cause false depressions of the hematocrit, hemoglobin, and plasma protein concentrations
  C. Intramuscular injections are given in the quadriceps muscle using small gauge needles (23 to 25 gauge)

D. Intravenous catheters can be placed in cephalic and lateral saphenous veins (24-gauge over-the-needle catheters); jugular catheters rarely used

E. Intraosseous catheters can be placed in the proximal femur of very small or shocky ferrets; this site is also used for bone marrow collection

F. Ferrets lack detectable blood groups and as such can be safely transfused without risk of a transfusion reaction

II. Fluid therapy
  A. Crystalloid and colloid solutions are used with methods similar to those used for dogs and cats
    1. Cat fluid maintenance requirements can be used as a reference
  B. Infusion pumps are useful for short-term procedures because of the small volumes of fluids required

III. Other concerns
  A. Older ferrets are at risk for hypoglycemia due to insulinomas; avoid fasting longer than 3 hours; if possible, check blood glucose before any surgery and supplement surgical fluids with 2.5% dextrose as needed
  B. Male urinary catheter placement can be difficult, because urethral blockage is usually due to prostatitis from adrenal disease, rather than urinary calculi
    1. The prepuce and penis tip are often swollen
    2. The urethral opening is located ventrally on the penis and is very small

## ANESTHESIA AND ANALGESIA

I. Isoflurane is the most commonly used anesthetic
  A. Anesthesia is helpful for accurate diagnostic imaging, sample collection, and other procedures to improve techniques and reduce stress
  B. Premedication with drugs such as acepromazine, diazepam or midazolam, glycopyrrolate or atropine and opioids, is commonly used for longer periods of surgical anesthesia
    1. For short procedures, such as radiographs or catheter placement, mask induction with no premedication is often used
      a. This allows for quick recovery from anesthesia
  C. Induction via mask anesthesia with 5% isoflurane is common; most ferrets will need to be wrapped in a towel for restraint; they are usually relaxed in 1 to 2 minutes
  D. Ferrets are easily intubated but will retain strong jaw tone even at moderate anesthetic planes
    1. Use of tape stirrups for the upper jaw and a laryngoscope blade will facilitate intubation
      a. Use lidocaine gel on the tip of the ET tube (2.5 to 3.5 mm uncuffed/cuffed ET tube)

2. The ET tube can be tied using gauze around the tube, then under the arms and tied across the back

E. Maintain on 1% to 3% isoflurane; oxygen flow rates 0.5 to 1.0 L/min flows, using a nonrebreathing circuit

II. Monitoring

A. Heart rate and pressures: Doppler flow meter, esophageal or pediatric stethoscope, ECG

B. Respiration rate and depth; IPPV as needed

C. IV access and fluid therapy for long procedures is ideal

D. Core body temperature: at risk for hypothermia because of their small size; monitor with esophageal thermometers; keep warm via warmed fluids, heating pads, convective heat source

III. Analgesia

A. Opioids and NSAIDs are most commonly used for ferrets

1. Buprenorphine (0.01 to 0.03 mg/kg), butorphanol (0.2 to 0.5 mg/kg) most common opioids; high end doses will cause significant sedation in ferrets

2. Meloxicam (0.2 to 0.3 mg/kg SID) most common NSAID (PO, SC)

## HEALTH CONDITIONS

I. Hyperadrenocorticism (adrenal disease)

A. Etiology due to hyperplasia of adrenal tissue and resulting secretion of sex hormones (versus cortisol in the dog and cat)

1. Very common in middle-aged and older ferrets

2. Prevalence is thought to be linked to early spay/neuter

B. Clinical signs: symmetrical alopecia (often starts at tail), muscular atrophy, pruritus, vulvar enlargement in females, increased aggression and musky odor, prostatitis (causing dysuria/anuria) in males

C. Diagnosis: history, clinical signs, abdominal ultrasound (assessing adrenal gland size), adrenal hormone panel (measures estradiol, androstenedione and 17-hydroxyprogesterone)

D. Treatment: leuprolide acetate (synthetic gonadotropin releasing hormone or GnRH analog); melatonin implants; surgical removal of affected gland

II. Lymphoma

A. Etiology: possible infectious etiology, genetics, or environmental factors

B. Clinical signs: anorexia, weight loss, lethargy, palpable lymph nodes or nodules on liver and spleen (vary depending on the affected organ system); may see mild anemia and lymphopenia on blood work

C. Diagnosis: radiographs, ultrasound, fine needle aspirate cytology, histology

D. Treatment: chemotherapy (prednisone, vincristine, cyclophosphamide, etc.)

III. Insulinoma (pancreatic beta cell tumors)

A. Etiology: insulin-secreting pancreatic islet cell tumor; most common neoplasia in ferrets

B. Clinical signs: episodic signs of weakness, ataxia, seizures, sudden collapse, with subsequent quick recovery; will usually increase in duration as tumor grows

C. Diagnosis: history, blood glucose monitoring, surgical exploration

D. Treatment

1. Surgical excision (can be difficult to locate early on because of small size)

2. Dietary management (small frequent meals)

3. Prednisone therapy manages clinical signs but does not stop tumor growth

4. Hypoglycemic episodes can usually be initially managed by the owner through rubbing corn syrup or honey on oral mucosa

IV. Proliferative bowel disease

A. Etiology is possibly *Campylobacter* spp. or *Desulfovibrio* spp.

B. Characterized by intermittent diarrhea for long periods of time

1. Signs also include weight loss, rectal prolapse, and dehydration

C. Treatment includes antibiotics and supportive fluid therapy

V. Human Influenza

A. Ferrets are susceptible to strains of human flu virus

1. Signs include listlessness, anorexia, pyrexia, sneezing, and nasal discharge

B. Treatment usually includes antihistamines, cough suppressants, and antibiotics

C. Humans can be infectious for ferrets and ferrets can be infectious to humans

VI. Aleutian disease (AD), viral enteritis

A. Etiology: parvovirus that causes Aleutian disease in mink

B. Clinical signs include slow wasting disease, melena, splenomegaly, pyrexia, posterior paresis, tremors, and eventually leading to death

C. Diagnosis is made by serological testing and histological findings

D. There is no treatment or vaccine to prevent Aleutian disease

VII. Aplastic anemia

A. Female ferrets that are not bred and undergo prolonged periods of estrus contribute to this disease

B. This condition is not as common as it once was, because most pet ferrets are spayed before leaving the breeding facility

C. Clinical signs include swollen vulva, alopecia, petechial hemorrhage, anorexia, pale mucous membranes, and marked depression

D. Hematological findings include thrombocytopenia, granulocytopenia, severe anemia, abnormally low packed cell volume (PCV), and bone marrow depression

E. Treatment includes: ovariohysterectomy, B vitamins and iron supplements, steroids, force feeding, and hormone therapy

VIII. Other health concerns

A. Ferrets should be vaccinated yearly against rabies and canine distemper

1. Anaphylactic vaccine reactions have been noted in ferrets after some distemper vaccines; premedicate with diphenhydramine

2. Only killed rabies vaccine should be administered. Some sources also state that the vaccine should be of chicken embryo origin

B. Foreign body ingestion and obstruction is common, particularly in young ferrets

1. Avoid access to rubber or sponge objects, rubber bands, and similar objects

C. Splenomegaly is a common finding on physical examination; often due to idiopathic extramedullary hematopoiesis, but can also be related to lymphosarcoma

D. Renal cysts are a common finding on ultrasound, which are thought to be of no apparent significance

E. Dental disease is common; regular dental cleaning is recommended

F. Gastritis can be due to coccidia, eosinophilic gastroenteritis, *Helicobacter mustelae* infection

G. Respiratory disease can be due to pneumonia, mediastinal lymphoma, cardiac disease

H. Ferrets are susceptible to fleas, heartworm, ear mites *(Otodectes cynotis)*, and sarcoptic mange, similar to dogs and cats

## ACKNOWLEDGMENT

The editors and authors recognize and appreciate the original contribution of Rebecca M. Atkinson and Mary Martini, on which this chapter is based.

# Glossary

**Aleutian disease** A slow, progressive disease of mink and related species caused by a type of parvovirus infection. Death is generally related to kidney failure

**apteria** Featherless tract on a bird

**arboreal** Living in trees

**autotomy** Ability of a lizard to shed its tail when captured

**carapace** Dorsal shell of chelonians

**carnivorous** Eats primarily flesh

**cere** Area at the base of a bird's beak

**clubbing of feathers** Feathers have a coiled structure due to improper eruption from the feather sheath

**convective heat source** Transmission of heat in a liquid or gas by circulation of heated particles

**degloving** Removal of the skin from its underlying structures

**denuding** Stripping or laying bare of any part

**diurnal** Becoming active throughout the day

**dysecdysis** Improper shedding in reptiles

**ecdysis** Shedding of the superficial keratin layer of skin in reptiles

**fibrous osteodystrophy** Clinical condition in which fibrous tissue replaces bone

**granivorous** Feeding on grain

**habituation** Gradually adapting to a stimulus or environment

**hemipenes** Two vascular structures, which act as a penis in snake and lizards

**herbivorous** Eats plants and plant products

**herpetology** Branch of zoology dealing with reptiles

**holocrine** Type of secretion that is formed by the entire gland

**idiopathic** Occurring without a known cause

**intracoelomic** Into the body cavity or coelom

**intraosseus (IO)** Into bone

**IPPV** Intermittent positive pressure ventilation—via compression of rebreathing bag

**limberneck** Paralysis of the neck

**mantle** Thick muscle layer running along the back and supporting the spine

**manubrium** The most cranial portion of the sternum

**mediastinal** Pertaining to the mediastinum; between the sternum and the vertebral column

**meibomian gland** Sebaceous follicle between the cartilage and conjunctiva of the eyelids

**melena** Dark tarry stool

**metanephric** Embryo-like kidney

**nictitating** Third eyelid in animals; a fold of conjunctiva attached at the medial canthus of the eye

**nocturnal** Becoming active at night

**omnivorous** Eating any sort of food

**opisthotonos** Form of spasm in which the body is bowed downwards and the head and tail are bowed upwards

**osteomyelitis** Inflammation of the bone, usually due to a pyogenic infection

**oviparous** Producing eggs in which the embryo matures outside of the maternal body

**ovoviviparous** Producing live young that hatch from eggs inside the maternal body

**parabronchus** Tertiary branch in the avian lungs

**paresis** Slight or incomplete paralysis

**pectin** Brown vascular fringe projecting from the fundus into the vitreous which is thought to help the choroid provide nutrients and oxygen to the retina

**piloerection** Erection of the hair

**plastron** Ventral shell of chelonians

**pododermatitis** Inflammation of the skin of the foot

**poikilothermic** Animal relies on the environmental temperature to maintain body temperature and metabolic rate

**POTR** Preferred optimum temperature range

**preputial** Pertaining to the prepuce

**prostatitis** Inflammation of the prostate gland

**pterylae** Feather tracts on birds

**pyrexia** A fever

**spectacle** Snakes possess fused eyelids that form a protective transparent membrane over the globe that is shed during ecdysis

**steatitis** Inflammation of the fatty tissue

**stomatitis** Inflammation of the mucosa of the mouth

**tetany** Continuous spasm of a muscle; steady contraction of a muscle without twitching

**torpor** Sluggishness in reference to activity level

**uropygial** Gland located dorsally to the tail that secretes oil to aid in feather conditioning

**vasovagal response** Arising as a result of efferent and afferent impulses through the vagus nerve

**viviparous** Bearing live young

# Review Questions

1 The digestive system in the bird includes the following anatomical structures, moving from cranial to caudal
   a. Crop, glottis, proventriculus, gizzard
   b. Beak, glottis, esophagus, proventriculus, ventriculus
   c. Crop, ventriculus, gizzard
   d. Beak, glottis, esophagus, crop, gizzard

2 The bird has _____ air sacs that make up the respiratory system
   a. 4 pairs of
   b. 6 to 8
   c. 8 to 9
   d. 13

3 The heterophil can be compared with a (an) _____ in mammals
   a. Eosinophil
   b. Neutrophil
   c. Lymphocyte
   d. Monocyte

4 Female birds have only one functional _____ and a slightly larger _____ vein
   a. Left ovary and oviduct; right jugular
   b. Right ovary and oviduct; left jugular
   c. Right kidney; left medial tibiotarsal vein
   d. Left kidney; right medial tibiotarsal vein

5 Blood analysis in avian and reptilian species cannot be run on a Coulter counter because of the
   a. Presence of nucleated red blood cells
   b. Small size of the cells
   c. Presence of heterophils
   d. Large size of the cells

6 Some reptiles may be restrained for radiography by
   a. Manual restraint
   b. Pressure on their eyes
   c. Holding their tail in position
   d. Inhalation anesthetic only

7 Vitamin D synthesis and calcium absorption in reptiles depends on
   a. Optimum temperatures
   b. A broad-spectrum ultraviolet light source
   c. A heating pad or hot rock under the substrate
   d. Optimum humidity in the enclosure

8 Septicemic cutaneous ulcer disease
   a. Affects iguanas mainly and is caused by poor diets
   b. Is an infection with *Citrobacter* spp. and causes cutaneous ulceration and anorexia
   c. Affects aquatic turtles with a gram-positive bacterial infection
   d. Affects all reptiles

9 Birds and terrestrial species of reptiles excrete
   a. Urine
   b. Ammonia
   c. Urea
   d. Uric acid

10 A cause of denuding (loss of spines) in hedgehogs can include
   a. Sarcoptic mange
   b. Demodectic mange
   c. Dermatophyte infections
   d. All of the above

## BIBLIOGRAPHY

Abou-Madi N: Avian anesthesia. In Heard D, editor: *The veterinary clinics of North America—exotic animal practice: analgesia and anesthesia,* Philadelphia, 2001, Saunders.

Altman RB: Perching birds, parrots, cockatoos, and macaws (psittacines and passerines). In Fowler ME, editor: *Zoo and wildlife medicine,* ed 5, St Louis, 2003, Saunders.

Altman RB, Clubb SL, Quesenberry K, editors: *Avian medicine and surgery,* Philadelphia, 1997, Saunders.

Cantwell S: Ferret, rabbit and rodent anesthesia. In Heard D, editor: *The veterinary clinics of North America—exotic animal practice: analgesia and anesthesia,* Philadelphia, 2001, Saunders.

Delong GL, Okumura S: Nursing care of cage birds, reptiles and amphibians. In Sirois M, editor: *Principles and practice of veterinary technology,* ed 2, St Louis, 2004, Mosby.

Evans HE: Reptiles, introduction and anatomy. In Fowler ME, editor: *Zoo and wildlife medicine,* ed 5, St Louis, 2003, Saunders.

Fox JG: *Biology and diseases of the ferret,* ed 2, Baltimore, 1998, Lippincott Williams & Wilkins.

Frye FL: *Biomedical and surgical aspects of captive reptile husbandry,* ed 2, Melbourne, 1991, Krieger.

Harrison GJ, Harrison LR: *Clinical avian medicine and surgery,* Philadelphia, 1986, Saunders.

Hernandez-Divers S et al: Reptile clinical anesthesia: advances in research, *Exotic DVM* 6(3):64, 2004.

Hrapkiewicz K, Medina L, Holmes DD: *Clinical laboratory animal medicine,* ed 2, Ames, 1998, Iowa State University Press.

Jackson OF, Lawrence K: Chelonians. In Cooper JE et al, editors: *Manual of exotic pets,* Gloucestershire, England, 1985, British Small Animal Veterinary Association.

Jacobsen ER: Diseases in reptiles. In Johnston DE, editor: *Exotic animal medicine in practice. The compendium collection,* Newark, NJ, 1986, Veterinary Learning Systems.

Jacobsen ER, Kolias GV: *Exotic animals,* New York, 1988, Churchill Livingstone.

Johnson D: What veterinarians need to know about degus, *Exotic DVM* 4(4):39, 2002.

Lichtenberg M: Shock, fluid therapy, anesthesia and analgesia in the ferret, *Exotic DVM* 7(2):26, 2005.

Mader D, editor: *Reptile medicine and surgery,* ed 2, St Louis, 2006, Saunders.

Marcus LC: *Veterinary biology and medicine of captive amphibians and reptiles,* London, 1981, Lea & Febiger.

McDonald SE: Anatomical and physiological characteristics of birds and how they differ from mammals. In Association of Avian Veterinarians Proceedings, 1990.

McKay J: *Complete guide to ferrets,* Shrewsbury, England, 1995, Swan Hill Press.

Proctor NS, Lynch PJ: *Manual of ornithology: avian structure and function,* London, 1993, Yale University Press.

Quesenberry KE, Carpenter JW, editors: *Ferrets, rabbits and rodents: clinical medicine and surgery,* ed 2, St Louis, 2004, Saunders.

Ritchie BW, Harrison GJ, editors: *Avian medicine: principles and application,* Lake Worth, Fla, 1994, Wingers Publishing.

Rosskopf WJ, Woerpel RW, editors: *Diseases of cage and aviary birds,* ed 3, Baltimore, 1996, Lippincott Williams & Wilkins.

Samour J, editor: *Avian medicine,* London, 2000, Harcourt.

Smith DA: Common dosages in avian medicine. In Allen DG, Pringle JK, Smith DA, editors: *Handbook of veterinary drugs,* ed 3, Philadelphia, 2005, Lippincott-Raven.

Smith DA: Common dosages in ferret medicine. In Allen DG, Pringle JK, Smith DA, editors: *Handbook of veterinary drugs,* ed 3, Philadelphia, 2005, Lippincott-Raven.

Smith DA: Common dosages in reptile medicine. In Allen DG, Pringle JK, Smith DA, editors: *Handbook of veterinary drugs,* ed 3, Philadelphia, 2005, Lippincott-Raven.

Smith DA: Common dosages in rodents and rabbit medicine. In Allen DG, Pringle JK, Smith DA, editors: *Handbook of veterinary drugs,* ed 3, Philadelphia, 2005, Lippincott-Raven.

Smith DA, Taylor WM: Exotic/small animals. In Matthews KA, editor: *Veterinary emergency and critical care,* ed 3, Guelph, Ontario, 2006, Lifelearn.

Storer P, Vriends MM: *Hedgehogs: a complete owner's manual,* Hauppauge, NY, 1995, Barron's Educational Series.

Sykes L, Durrant J: *The natural hedgehog,* London, 1995, Gaia Books.

Taylor WM: Companion bird management and nutrition. In Association of Avian Veterinarians Proceedings, 1990.

Tully TN: Care of birds, reptiles and small mammals. In McCurnin DM, Bassert JM, editors: *Clinical textbook for veterinary technicians,* ed 6, St Louis, 2006, Saunders.

Turner T: Cagebirds. In Cooper JE et al, editors: *Manual of exotic pets, Gloucestershire,* England, 1985, British Small Animal Veterinary Association.

# PART IV

# Anesthesia and Pharmacology

## CHAPTER 19

# Anesthesia

*Lucy Siydock*

## OUTLINE

Preanesthetic Assessment
Preanesthetic Agents
Classifications of Preanesthetic
  Agents
  Anticholinergics
  Tranquilizers and Sedatives
  Opioids
  Neuroleptanalgesics
Injectable Anesthetic Agents
Classifications of Anesthetic Agents
  Barbiturates
  Cyclohexamines
  Etomidate
  Fentanyl
  Guaifenesin
  Propofol
Inhalation Anesthetic Agents
Classifications of Inhalants
  Methoxyflurane
  Halothane

Isoflurane
Sevoflurane
Desflurane
Nitrous Oxide
Anesthetic Equipment
  Anesthetic Machine
  Components of an Anesthesia
    Machine
Breathing Systems
  Rebreathing System
  Nonrebreathing System
Breathing Circuits
Health Hazards and Environmental
  Concerns
Equipment Maintenance and
  Concerns
Monitoring Techniques
  Central Nervous System
  Cardiovascular System
  Ventilation

Oxygenation
Fluids
Temperature
Equipment
Stages of Anesthesia
Analgesia
Muscle Relaxants
Ventilation
Fluid Therapy
  Blood Loss
  Acid-Base Balance
Oxygenation and
  Anesthetic Equipment
  Problems

## LEARNING OUTCOMES

After reading this chapter you should be able to:

1. Understand the indications, advantages, disadvantages, effects on the body, and the associated adverse side effects of the commonly used preanesthetic drugs.
2. Explain the rationale, effects on the body, and advantages and disadvantages of the commonly used intravenous, intramuscular, and inhalation anesthetic agents.
3. Identify or describe the components of general anesthesia, including the various stages and planes.
4. Define the rationale for and the various parameters that should be monitored during anesthesia, and describe why blood pressure is important to monitor.
5. Understand the differences between advantages and disadvantages of rebreathing and nonrebreathing systems.

6. Be familiar with the various parts of the anesthetic machine.
7. Differentiate between a precision and a nonprecision vaporizer, and recognize the advantages and disadvantages of each.
8. Understand the important concepts of analgesics and muscle relaxants.
9. Understand the techniques of assisted and controlled ventilation.
10. Understand the principles involved with providing proper fluid therapy and for maintaining the acid-base balance.
11. Identify oxygenation problems that might occur.

Anesthesia is a broad subject and could involve extensive reading. This chapter condenses the information by discussing the commonly used anesthetic agents, equipment, and procedures. Although much of this chapter could pertain to any species, the emphasis is on domestic dogs and cats.

## PREANESTHETIC ASSESSMENT

The following assessments will determine if there are any potential problems or concerns for the procedure scheduled and/or anesthesia administered

I. Patient identification
   A. A hospital band includes the patient's name and hospital number
   B. The patient signalment includes the species, breed, age, sex, body weight, and temperament
II. Patient history
   A. The patient's history will reveal the following information:
      1. The duration and nature of the illness
      2. Any concurrent diseases (e.g., vomiting, diarrhea, heart murmur, renal failure, epilepsy)
      3. The patient's activity level or exercise tolerance
      4. Previous or current medication and drug history
      5. Any previous anesthesia problems (e.g., prolonged recovery or excitement)
      6. The patient's last feeding
      7. Vaccination history
III. Physical examination
   A. To obtain information on the patient's health
   B. What is the general body condition of the patient (e.g., obese, cachexia, dehydrated)?
   C. Cardiovascular system (e.g., heart rate, rhythm)
   D. Pulmonary system (e.g., respiratory rate, mucous membrane color, breath sounds)
   E. Hepatic function is important for metabolism and excretion of anesthetic drugs
   F. Renal disease (e.g., anuria, oliguria, or polyuria/polydipsia)
   G. Gastrointestinal disease (e.g., diarrhea, vomiting)
   H. Neurological dysfunction (e.g., seizure history)
IV. Diagnostic tests
   A. Diagnostic tests are selected based on the history and physical examination of the patient
   B. Each veterinary clinic will have policies that stipulate certain tests, which are based on the preoperative condition of the patient, are to be completed before anesthesia
   C. Diagnostic tests that will provide information for anesthetic assessment include complete blood count (CBC), blood chemistries, urinalysis, blood clotting tests, electrocardiogram, and radiographs (possibly magnetic resonance imaging, computed tomography scan, and/or ultrasound)

V. Anesthetic risk
   A. After the preanesthetic assessment is completed, a classification of the patient's physical status can be determined
   B. The American Society of Anesthesiologists (ASA) integrates a scale system that categorizes a patient into classes based on the evaluation of anesthetic risk
      1. Each class defines the anesthetic risk involved with the anesthesia and/or procedure (Table 19-1)
VI. Selection of the anesthetic protocol
   A. The final preparation for anesthesia is selecting an anesthetic protocol that is based on the information collected from the preanesthetic assessment. It is important to judge the anesthetic drug, dose, and route based on the assessment information

## PREANESTHETIC AGENTS

I. Indications
   A. Preanesthetic agents are drugs administered before general anesthesia
II. Advantages
   A. Reduces anxiety and calms patients by producing mild to moderate sedation
   B. Induction and recovery are smoother
   C. Decreases the amount of induction agent and inhalant anesthesia agent required
   D. Provides analgesia for preoperative, intraoperative, and postoperative phases
   E. Provides muscle relaxation
   F. Reduces secretions
   G. Tranquilizes/sedates patient for safe handling
III. Disadvantages
   A. Disadvantages are minimal
   B. Cost is a common concern. However, the higher cost can be offset by the reduction in amounts of induction and inhalant agents
   C. Time constraints can be a factor. However, depending on the route of administration, the time frame may not be a factor, considering the advantages just mentioned to administrating preanesthetic drugs
      1. For example, preanesthetics given subcutaneously (SC) usually take 20 minutes to reach peak effect but can last up to 2 hours
      2. Most premedication can be given intramuscularly (IM) or with caution intravenously (IV)
   D. Some drugs have been associated with temporary behavior and personality changes (e.g., xylazine, acepromazine, opioids, and benzodiazepines)
IV. Examples
   A. Preanesthetic agents include
      1. Anticholinergics
      2. Tranquilizers and sedatives
      3. Opioids
      4. Neuroleptanalgesics

**Table 19-1** American Society of Anesthesiologists (ASA) scale

| Category | Description | Examples |
|---|---|---|
| **I**<br>Minimal risk | Normal, healthy patient | Ovariohysterectomy, castration |
| **II**<br>Slight risk | Mild systemic disturbances | Ruptured cruciate ligament, neonate, geriatric patient |
| **III**<br>Moderate risk | Moderate systemic disturbances or disease with mild clinical signs | Anemia, fever, heart murmur, moderate dehydration |
| **IV**<br>High risk | Severe systemic disturbances that are life threatening | Shock, severe dehydration, fever, gastric torsion with arrhythmias |
| **V**<br>Extreme risk/moribund | Submitted for surgery in desperation but little chance of survival<br>Patient not expected to live 24 hr | Advanced multiple organ failure, shock, severe trauma |
| **E**<br>Emergency | Any of the above classes presented for immediate surgery | — |

## CLASSIFICATIONS OF PREANESTHETIC AGENTS
### Anticholinergics

I. Anticholinergics are sympatholytic drugs that exert their effects by blocking the actions of the parasympathetic neurotransmitter acetylcholine at the muscarinic receptors
  A. Two examples are atropine and glycopyrrolate
  B. Both drugs can be administered IV, IM, or SC
II. Indications and effects
  A. Prevent or treat bradycardia by suppressing stimulation of the vagal nerve
  B. Administered in combination with opioids
  C. Reduce salivary and tear secretions
  D. Promote bronchodilation
  E. Dilate pupils (mydriatic)
  F. Thicker mucous secretions in the airway may occur, especially in the cat and horse
  G. Reduce gastrointestinal activity by inhibiting peristalsis
  H. Contraindications
    1. Patients with preexisting tachycardia
    2. Possibly with geriatric patients or those with other conditions, such as congestive heart failure, that could not handle a potential tachycardia
    3. Conditions, such as constipation or ileus, which would further reduce peristaltic action of the intestine (e.g., endoscopy procedures and upper gastrointestinal [GI] barium series)

III. Atropine
  A. More potent and faster acting than glycopyrrolate
  B. Will cross the placental barrier in pregnant patients
  C. Atropine overdose can be reversed with physostigmine. Signs of atropine toxicity include drowsiness, excitement, or potential seizures
IV. Glycopyrrolate
  A. Slower onset of action and generally has less potential for producing tachycardia or cardiac arrhythmias than atropine
  B. Lasts longer than atropine
  C. Will not cross the placental barrier in pregnant patients

### Tranquilizers and Sedatives

I. A tranquilizer is a drug that calms an anxious patient by reducing anxiety but will not necessarily reduce awareness
II. A sedative is a drug that reduces excitement or irritability by causing sleepiness and decreased mental activity
  A. Examples of tranquilizers and sedatives are phenothiazines, benzodiazepines, butyrophenones, and $\alpha_2$-agonists
III. Tranquilizers and sedatives are used in anesthetic protocols to:
  A. Sedate and reduce anxiety
  B. Smoothen inductions and recoveries
  C. Reduce anesthetic induction and inhalant drugs
IV. Examples of tranquilizers and sedatives

A. Phenothiazines
1. Examples include acepromazine, chlorpromazine, and triflupromazine
2. The mechanism of action involves the blockade of D2 dopamine receptors in the brain
3. Indications
   a. Acepromazine is most commonly used in veterinary medicine
   b. Used as a tranquilizer and sedative
   c. Skeletal muscle relaxation
   d. Antiarrhythmic effect
   e. Antiemetic effect
   f. Lowers the seizure threshold
   g. Antihistamine effect
   h. Hypothermia through depressing the thermoregulator center
   i. Hypotension (dose dependent) through peripheral vasodilation
   j. No analgesic properties
   k. May cause excitement rather than sedation
   l. Personality changes that usually subside within 48 hours
B. Contraindications
1. Shock, hypovolemia, and hypothermia, which has existing peripheral vasodilation that can further exacerbate hypotension
2. Convulsing/epileptic patients, seizure history, or head trauma
3. Depressed patients
4. Caution with geriatric and pediatric patients; use a lower dose or consider alternative agents, such as benzodiazepines
5. Use with caution in patients with liver or kidney disease
6. Allergy testing because of its antihistamine effect

V. Benzodiazepines
A. Examples of benzodiazepines are diazepam (Valium), midazolam (Versed), lorazepam (Ativan), and zolazepam
B. The mechanism of action involves binding to a specific site on the γ-aminobutyric acid (GABA) receptor in the brain
C. Indications: tranquilizer
1. Calming effect
2. Minimal cardiovascular and respiratory effects, therefore indicated for use in geriatric, pediatric, and other moderate to high risk patients
3. Anticonvulsant
4. Muscle relaxant
5. Sometimes given IV to sedated patients to enhance sedation or reduce the dose of induction agent
6. Combined with ketamine and works effectively as an induction agent
7. Ideal for older, depressed, or anxious patients
D. Contraindications
1. Normal, excitable, healthy animals may not be sedated or tranquilized with benzodiazepines; therefore it may cause excitement in some patients
2. Drugs are metabolized in the liver, therefore should be avoided in patients with poor hepatic function

VI. Butyrophenones
A. The two butyrophenones commonly used in veterinary medicine are droperidol (Inapsine) and azaperone (Stresnil)
1. Butyrophenones structurally resemble and evoke pharmacologic effects similar to those of the phenothiazines
2. The main effects in the central nervous system (CNS) are by the blockade of D2 dopamine receptors in the brain
B. Indications and side effects
1. Dopamine antagonist
2. Reduces anxiety
3. Reduces movement and response to stimuli
4. Very high doses can cause rigidity and seizures
5. Hypotension effects
6. Bradycardia
7. Increases respiratory rate or sometimes causes panting
8. Produces salivation
C. Droperidol
1. Available with opioid fentanyl citrate: Innovar-Vet (Canada only)
2. Innovar-Vet is a neuroleptanalgesia that combines an opioid with a sedative/tranquilizer
3. Reports of dogs experiencing long-lasting changes in behavior following Innovar-Vet administration
D. Azaperone
1. Has similar physiological effects to those of droperidol
2. It is primarily used to treat aggression in swine

VII. α₂-Agonists
A. Examples of α₂-agonists commonly used in veterinary medicine are xylazine (Rompun, AnaSed), romifidine (Sedivet), detomidine (Dormosedan), and medetomidine (Domitor)
B. The drug stimulates α₂-adrenoceptors, causing a decrease in the release of norephinephrine
C. Indications

1. Reduction in dose of induction and inhalant agents when used as a preanesthetic drug
2. Moderate analgesia
3. Causes sedation
4. Muscle relaxation
5. Side effects include
   a. Profound cardiovascular effects include bradycardia, decreased cardiac output, and second-degree heart block
   b. Initial increase in total peripheral resistance with hypertension followed by a longer period of hypotension
   c. Hypothermia
   d. Other side effects may include:
      (1) Vomiting (up to 50% of dogs and 90% of cats)
      (2) Slight muscle tremors
      (3) Excitement
      (4) Reduced intestinal motility
      (5) Diuresis
6. $\alpha_2$-Agonists inhibit insulin release; therefore they may cause hyperglycemia, which may be harmful in dehydrated patients
7. Associated with temporary behavior and personality changes

D. Addition of an opioid with an $\alpha_2$-agonist will enhance sedation and analgesia

E. Contraindications
1. Cardiac arrhythmias
2. Coronary insufficiency
3. Respiratory disease
4. Hepatic or renal disease
5. Gastric dilation and torsion (dehydration)

F. Xylazine
1. Most commonly used tranquilizer in veterinary medicine for both large and small animals until the early 1990s
2. Sedative effects last 1 to 2 hours
3. Analgesic effects last approximately 30 minutes
4. Generally used for large animals
   a. Caution in ruminants: may cause decreased oxygen exchange
   b. Used in ruminants but in much lower doses

G. Romifidine
1. More potent than xylazine
2. Used in horses
3. Provides 50% longer sedation than xylazine with less ataxia
4. More profound bradycardia and second-degree heart block than with xylazine

H. Detomidine
1. Chemically similar to xylazine

2. Potent sedative and analgesic (50 to 100 times more potent than xylazine)
3. Analgesia lasts as long as sedation
4. Approved for use in horses
5. Bradycardia and hypotension are more severe compared to xylazine
6. May cause more ataxia than xylazine

I. Medetomidine
1. Newest $\alpha_2$-agonist approved for veterinary use; has greater affinity for the $\alpha_2$-adrenoceptors (mediates the sedation effects)
2. More potent and effective than other drugs is this class
3. For small animal use as sedative analgesic
4. Similar to xylazine but cardiovascular problems may be less significant because of recommended lower doses used

J. $\alpha_2$-Agonist reversal agents
1. Yohimbine (Yobine) and tolazoline (Priscoline) can reverse the effects of xylazine and detomidine
2. Atipamezole (Antisedan) is specific to medetomidine

## Opioids (Table 19-2)

I. Opioids can be classified based on which opioid receptor they act on
   A. Opioid receptors include mu, delta, kappa, and sigma, which are located in the CNS mainly in the presynaptic membrane of pain pathways, cough center, and centers associated with respiration and nausea
   B. Their stimulation inhibits the release of neurotransmitters from the presynaptic cell

II. Classified as a narcotic in Canada and a Schedule II drug in the United States, with strict regulations

III. Classification of opioids
   A. Pure (mu) agonists include morphine, meperidine, oxymorphone, hydromorphone, and fentanyl, which stimulate all opioid receptors
      1. There is a full range of physiological responses that occur with each opioid drug; however, responses depend on the type of drug, dose, and species of patient
   B. Mixed agonists-antagonists include butorphanol, buprenorphine, and pentazocine, which block one type of receptor and stimulate another type of receptor
   C. Pure antagonists, such as naloxone, will reverse the effects of pure and mixed agonists with very little clinical effect on their own
      1. Reversal occurs because of the competition with the opioid for the specific receptor

2. It is possible to titrate naloxone dose to remove side effects while keeping the analgesic properties of the opioid

IV. Clinical effects of opioids
A. Act by reversible combination with one or more specific receptors in the brain and spinal cord
B. Produce a variety of effects, such as analgesia, sedation, dysphoria, euphoria, and excitement
C. Can be combined with a tranquilizer to induce neuroleptanalgesia (e.g., morphine plus acepromazine)
D. Commonly used as an analgesic in premedication, as an induction agent, or postoperatively for balanced anesthesia and preemptive pain control
   1. Decrease amount of general anesthetic needed
   2. Have minimal cardiovascular depressant effects
E. The physiological effects are reversible with narcotic antagonists
F. Analgesic effect is mild to profound, based on the classification of the opioid
G. Can cause bradycardia
H. Respiratory effects include panting in dogs; opioids cause the thermoregulatory center in the brain to reset itself
   1. Respiratory depression is dependent on dose and whether it is combined with other potent respiratory depressants during general anesthesia
I. May lower body temperature
J. Nausea, vomiting, and defecation (dose dependent)
K. Constipation may occur from prolonged gastrointestinal stasis
L. Mild muscle relaxation
M. Cough suppression
N. Addiction
O. Salivation
P. Miosis (dog and pig) and mydriasis (cat and horse)
Q. Increased responsiveness to noise
R. Sweating, particularly in the horse
S. Morphine and meperidine may cause histamine release when administered IV. This results in vasodilation and hypotension
T. Excitement occurs if given rapidly IV
   1. Horse and cat are particularly susceptible to the excitatory effects. Give morphine at very low doses in cats
V. All opioids are water soluble
VI. Contraindications
A. Previous history of excitement
B. Morphine has higher incidence of inducing vomiting (depending on the dose). Therefore avoid use with cases of gastrointestinal obstruction or diaphragmatic hernia

VII. Route of administration: IV, IM or SC
A. Other routes for opioids include oral, transdermal patch (e.g., fentanyl), epidural (e.g., morphine), and constant rate infusions (CRIs) (e.g., fentanyl, morphine)
B. Transdermal routes of administration: fentanyl patch
   1. Fentanyl is highly lipid soluble, therefore it can be absorbed through the skin
   2. Fentanyl is available in various concentrations (e.g., 25 µg, 50 µg, 75 µg)
   3. Provides continuous steady-state analgesia for 3 to 5 days
   4. Takes 8 to 12 hours to become effective
   5. Very few cardiovascular effects and does not significantly contribute to vasodilation or hypotenson
   6. Contraindications include:
      a. Hypersensitivity to fentanyl or adhesives
      b. Avoid use if suspected or have increased intracranial pressure
      c. Central hypoventilation
      d. Renal or hepatic dysfunction
      e. Fever
   7. Precautions and concerns
      a. Heating pads can increase transdermal uptake
      b. Use caution when placing fentanyl patches in areas that may come in contact with heat (overdose can occur)
      c. Accidental exposure of humans to the fentanyl in the patch; therefore wear gloves to apply and remove patch
      d. Suboptimal dose due to poor skin contact, and unexpected high dose, which can cause marked sedation, narcosis, or inappetence (e.g., from high body temperature or a patch that is too large for patient)

## Neuroleptanalgesics

I. Any combination of an analgesic (e.g., morphine, meperidine, hydromorphone, butorphanol) and a tranquilizer (e.g., acepromazine, medetomidine, diazepam)
A. This combination will enhance the CNS depressant effects of each drug
II. Drugs can be mixed in same syringe or administered separately (IM or IV)
A. Commercially made drugs used to induce neuroleptanalgesia, such as Innovar-Vet (fentanyl/droperidol) are available in some countries
III. Opioid component can be reversed with opioid antagonist (e.g., naloxone) or mixed agonist/antagonists (e.g., butorphanol can reverse the effects of morphine)

**Table 19-2** Summary of opioids

| Drug | Analgesic potency relative to morphine | Receptor | Classification | Duration of analgesia | Analgesic effects |
|---|---|---|---|---|---|
| Morphine | 1× | Mu | Agonist | 3-6 hr | Moderate to severe pain |
| Codeine | 0.1× | Mu | Agonist | 3-6 hr | Moderate to severe pain |
| Hydromorphone | 5× | Mu | Agonist | 3-6 hr | Moderate to severe pain |
| Oxymorphone | 10× | Mu | Agonist | 3-6 hr | Moderate to severe pain |
| Meperidine | 0.1× | Mu | Agonist | 1-2 hr | Mild to moderate pain |
| Fentanyl | 100× | Mu | Agonist | 20-30 min | Moderate to severe pain |
| Butorphanol | ~3-5× | Kappa, mu | Agonist-antagonist | 1-2 hr | Mild to moderate pain |
| Buprenorphine (unavailable in Canada) | 30× | Partial mu | Partial agonist | 6-8 hr | Mild to moderate pain |
| Pentazocine | ~1/3× | Partial mu and kappa | Agonist-antagonist | 1-2 hr | Mild to moderate pain |

A. Some of the other tranquilizer components cannot be reversed (e.g., phenothiazines, thiazine derivatives, and other nonopioid drugs)

IV. Indications
   A. Need heavier sedation (depending on dose) for short procedures (e.g., wound suturing, porcupine quill removal)
   B. Cardiac or shock cases

V. Contraindications
   A. Patient will become hyperactive to auditory stimulus. Need a quiet environment
   B. Respiratory depression (opioid dose dependent)
   C. Some patients may pant (temperature-regulating center of the brain interprets that the normal body temperature is being elevated) because of opioid effect
   D. Opioid may cause defecation, vomiting, or flatulence
   E. Bradycardia (dose-related effect of the opioid)
   F. Morphine and meperidine injected intravenously may cause histamine release
   G. Miosis in dogs and mydriasis in cats
   H. Excessive salivation

## INJECTABLE ANESTHETIC AGENTS

I. Indications
   A. Administration of anesthesia followed by inhalant agents
   B. As an anesthetic agent for short, minor procedures (e.g., suturing, radiographs)
   C. Administered by repeated boluses or by infusion, such as total intravenous anesthetic (TIVA)
   D. Supplement to inhalant agents
   E. Can provide long term sedation (e.g., patients in ICU)

II. Advantages
   A. Rapid onset and recovery of drug
   B. Simple, requires little equipment (except for infusions)
   C. Drugs do not irritate airways
   D. Minimal adverse effects to cardiovascular and respiratory systems (dose dependent)
   E. Provides analgesia and good muscle relaxation

III. Disadvantages
   A. Difficulty in catheterization (patient has fibroses in peripheral veins)
   B. Intravenous drug therefore may be difficult to maintain if there is no IV catheter in place
   C. Some drugs are irritants if given perivascularly
   D. Drug cannot be removed once it is injected
   E. Cumulative effect of the drug
   F. Risk of airway complications if the patient is not intubated (e.g., aspiration)
   G. May cause induction apnea
   H. May cause hypotension
   I. May cause excitement on induction or recovery

## CLASSIFICATIONS OF ANESTHETIC AGENTS
### Barbiturates

I. Classification of barbiturates
   A. Based on the chemical substitutions on the barbituric acid molecule and the duration of action

II. Chemical classifications

A. Oxybarbiturates: pentobarbital (Nembutal or Somnotol), phenobarbital (considered as an anticonvulsant, not an anesthetic), barbital, and secobarbital

B. Thiobarbiturate: thiopental (Pentothal)

C. Methylated oxybarbiturates: methohexital (Brevital)

1. Duration of action
   a. Long acting (e.g., phenobarbital): 8 to 12 hours
   b. Short acting (e.g.,pentobarbital): 45 to 90 minutes
   c. Ultrashort acting (e.g., thiopental): 5 to 15 minutes

III. Indications

A. Sedation

B. Anticonvulsants

C. General anesthesia

1. Commonly used as an induction agent to allow endotracheal intubation followed by maintenance with an inhalant anesthetic, such as isoflurane or halothane
2. Causes unconsciousness at an adequate dose
3. Depresses respiration and cardiovascular system to varying extents
4. Give to effect (amount necessary to induce anesthesia)
5. Give a bolus (usually one third to one half of the calculated dose given rapidly)

D. Nonreversible

E. Protein binding

1. Level of plasma protein can alter the rate and amount of absorption of the barbiturates
2. Barbiturates will bind to protein; therefore the amount of barbiturate free in the circulation and not bound to protein will increase if the patient is hypoproteinemic
3. More barbiturate will be available to penetrate the central nervous system and cause unconsciousness

F. Lipid solubility

1. Increases in the barbiturates from the long acting to the ultrashort acting
2. There is a quicker onset of action with the shorter-acting barbiturates, because they cross the blood-brain barrier faster. This also accounts for the quicker recovery of the shorter acting barbiturates
3. Recovery from these drugs depends on a combination of redistribution (to muscle and fat) and hepatic metabolism
   a. If a drug has low lipid solubility, there is little or no redistribution and recovery depends mostly on metabolism (a slow process)
   b. If a drug has high lipid solubility, it is readily redistributed from the blood to the muscle and fat tissues where it is not available to act on the brain. Therefore, recovery from a highly lipid-soluble drug is much faster
   c. As the blood levels decline because of metabolism, small quantities of the redistributed drug (from muscle and fat) reenter the circulatory system to also be metabolized
   d. The low levels that arise from the muscle and fat stores are not sufficient to clinically alter the level of consciousness
4. Barbiturates are eliminated from the body through liver metabolism, and their metabolites are excreted into the urine

IV. Examples of barbiturates

A. Phenobarbital

1. Used mostly as a sedative for excitable dogs or as an anticonvulsant for epileptic seizures
2. Sedation can last up to 24 hours (dose dependent)

B. Pentobarbital

1. Once used commonly for anesthetic inductions, it now has been replaced mostly by the ultrashort-acting barbiturates
2. It can also be used to control seizures (although electroencephalographic seizure activity may persist)
3. It can be administered IM for sedation without tissue reaction
4. With IV induction, there is a significant effect at 1 minute after injection (maximum effect is in 5 minutes)
5. Recovery by metabolism is slow and rough in all animals except sheep (recovery is smoother and faster)

C. Thiopental

1. Found as a crystalline powder in multidose vials that can be reconstituted into various concentrations
2. Limited stability once reconstituted
3. Avoid injecting air that may cause premature precipitation
4. Has a high lipid solubility
5. Enters the brain rapidly
6. Redistribution from the brain to other tissues; therefore initial recovery is fairly quick
   a. It is redistributed to muscle and fat tissue and metabolized very slowly
7. Avoid in sight hounds; low body fat will result in a prolonged recovery
8. Problems with recovery will occur if subsequent doses have been given for maintenance of anesthesia and if the muscle and fat tissues are saturated

a. Cumulative effect with repeated administration
b. Recovery will be slow and rough
c. Best to use for induction only or a maximum maintenance of 30 minutes
9. Significant effect is noted 30 to 60 seconds after injection
10. There is a transient arrhythmogenic potential with this drug, especially if given rapidly
   a. Transient apnea may occur if given rapidly
11. If given perivascularly at a concentration of greater than 2.5% (25 mg/mL), it can cause extreme tissue irritation and may lead to tissue sloughing
   a. If this accidentally occurs, DILUTE the perivascular thiopental by injecting small amounts of normal saline around the site
12. Poor relaxation and analgesia when used alone
13. Can be used in combination with propofol for induction

D. Methohexital
1. Highly lipid soluble and rapidly metabolized
2. It has the quickest onset, shortest duration, and quickest recovery (even if used for long-term maintenance)
3. Good choice of barbiturates for sight hounds or other patients with excessively lean body
   a. These patients seem to be extremely sensitive to barbiturates (because of poor ability to metabolize and a lack of fat storage), and they have prolonged recoveries
   b. Liver metabolism is more rapid, therefore additional administration is not cumulative
4. Good choice for brachycephalics to obtain quick and smooth intubation and rapid recoveries without hangover effects
   a. Induction effect is noted 15 to 60 seconds after injection
5. Induction and/or recoveries may be rough and accompanied by convulsions. Effect minimized if good sedation given
6. Lethal dose is only 2 to 3 times the anesthetic dose
7. Methohexital can cause profound respiratory depression
8. No longer available in Canada

## Cyclohexamines

I. Classified as dissociative anesthetics (e.g., dissociation from one's environment). Examples include ketamine HCl (Ketalar, Ketaset, Vetalar), phencyclidine HCl (Sernylan, Sernyl) and tiletamine HCl (Telazol)

II. Indications
   A. Produce a cataleptic state through CNS excitement (and not through depression)
   B. Inhibits $N$-methyl-D-aspartate (NMDA), resulting in analgesia
   C. Analgesic properties: selective superficial analgesia
   D. Visceral pain not abolished
   E. Pharyngolaryngeal reflexes are partially intact
   F. Produces cardiovascular stimulation (increased blood pressure, decreased cardiac contractility and increased heart rate)
   G. Increases muscular rigidity, which can be minimized by prior administration of tranquilizers, sedatives, or benzodiazepines
   H. Apneustic breathing pattern
   I. Respiratory rate may increase (decrease in arterial $CO_2$ especially after administration)
   J. Hyperresponsive and ataxic during recovery
   K. Small percentage of cats will show convulsive behavior, especially with large doses
   L. Minimally sensitizes the heart to catecholamine-induced arrhythmias
   M. Tissue irritation
   N. Increased salivation and lacrimation
   O. Increase in intracranial pressure
   P. Immobilization of patient
   Q. Amnesia properties
   R. Open eyes with central dilated pupils
   S. Nystagmus (repetitive side-to-side motion of the eyeball)
   T. Increase in intraocular pressure
   U. Temporary personality changes
   V. Excitement on recovery
   W. Can administer via mouth (mucous membrane absorption is effective in nasty cats)
   X. Effects partially reversed by adrenergic and cholinergic blockade
   Y. Metabolized by the liver and excreted somewhat in an unchanged form through the kidneys in dogs
   Z. Excreted primarily by the kidneys in the cat
   AA. Can be used in cats with urethral obstruction, provided that renal disease is absent and the obstruction has been eliminated

III. Contraindications
   A. May induce pulmonary edema or acute heart failure in animals with preexisting heart conditions
   B. Use with caution in animals with hepatic or renal disease
   C. Never use alone in cats (increased muscle rigidity)
   D. Used alone in dogs may cause seizurelike activity; therefore ketamine should be combined with a tranquilizer (e.g., acepromazine or diazepam) when used with dogs

E. Avoid as a preanesthetic medication in dogs

F. Avoid in animals with seizure history (may cause convulsions with high doses)

G. Provides poor visceral analgesia but fair to good peripheral analgesia

H. Increases intracranial pressure: DO NOT use in neurological cases (e.g., possibility of brain herniation or tumor) or if you suspect increased intracranial pressure (e.g., head trauma in patient that was hit by car)

I. Increases ocular pressure; therefore do not use in cases if there is a suspicion of glaucoma or perforation of the eye chamber

J. Prolonged and unreliable recoveries

IV. Ketamine

A. Commonly combined with diazepam or other benzodiazepines as an induction agent

1. This provides muscle relaxation and smoother recoveries than with ketamine alone

B. In species where IV administration is not possible or easily accessible, ketamine can be combined with midazolam and given IM

V. Tiletamine

A. Tiletamine and zolazepam are combined commercially in Telazol for use in all animal species

B. Same action as ketamine/diazepam but can be given IM or SC; therefore it is good for exotic and aggressive animals

## Etomidate (Amidate)

I. Very safe, rapid-acting, ultrashort-acting, rapidly distributing, noncumulative induction agent

II. Interacts with $GABA_A$ receptors as with barbiturates

III. Very popular for animals with cardiac disease because it has little to no effect on cardiac output, respiratory rate, and blood pressure

IV. Can be given as repeated bolus or continuous infusion

V. Occasionally may cause vomiting, diarrhea, excitement, and apnea on induction and recovery. Can be inhibited with proper preanesthetic medication

VI. Mild respiratory depressant

VII. Does not produce a histamine release

VIII. Produces excessive muscle rigidity and seizures in horse and cattle

IX. Rapidly metabolized in the liver

X. Does cross placental barrier, but effects are minimal because of rapid clearance

XI. Injection may be painful and may cause phlebitis, especially in the smaller veins

## Fentanyl

I. Considered primarily an analgesic

II. It can produce unconsciousness

III. Used as an injectable induction agent, often in combination with a tranquilizer, sedative, or benzodiazepine

IV. Referred to as a neuroleptanalgesic

V. It is safe for high-risk patients, because it does not cause apnea and does not affect contractility or cardiac output

## Guaifenesin (Glycerol Guaiacolate)

I. Available as a powder and reconstituted with warm sterile water or dextrose

II. This is a common decongestant and antitussive, and is commonly used for its effect as a central muscle relaxant, mostly in large animals

III. Minimal effects of the diaphragm at relaxant dosages

IV. Induction and recovery are excitement free

V. Minimal respiratory and cardiac effect

VI. Does cross placental barrier, but effects on fetus are minimal

## Propofol

I. Used for sedation, induction, and/or anesthesia maintenance by repeated bolus injections or CRI

A. Rapid acting with smooth, excitement-free induction

B. Rapid smooth recovery, because of redistribution and rapid metabolism due to redistribution to vessel-rich areas, such as the brain rather than to muscle or fat

C. More easily and rapidly biotransformed by the liver than barbiturates; therefore it has reduced or possibly no hangover effect

D. First choice for inductions in sight hounds and other lean-body patients

E. Ideal for injectable maintenance of anesthesia, because there is no accumulation

F. Minimal cardiovascular effects, but may cause tachycardia, bradycardia, transient arterial and venous dilation, and depressed cardiac contractility

1. However, use with caution on most cardiac patients

G. Good anticonvulsant

H. Nonirritating with incidental perivascular injection

I. Some muscle relaxation occurs, but analgesia is poor

J. Will support bacterial growth because of soy content (no preservative). Opened vials should be discarded within 6 hours to avoid contamination

II. Contraindications and cautions

A. Transient apnea has been reported after rapid IV injection

B. Apnea is very dependent on how quickly the drug is given, and it has caused respiratory arrest in some cases

C. Avoid in animals that are hypotensive (e.g., blood loss, dehydration, recent trauma, or severe illness)

D. May see transient excitement and muscle tremors

## INHALATION ANESTHETIC AGENTS ▰▰▰▰

I. General considerations
   A. Are vapors or gases that are directly absorbed into the system through the lungs
   B. Are absorbed from the alveoli to the brain relatively rapidly
   C. Primarily eliminated unchanged by the lungs
      1. Biotransformation of inhalation anesthetics to metabolites does occur to some degree
   D. Metabolism is generally by hepatic microsomal enzymes
   E. Factors that affect the brain concentrations of volatile anesthetic include
      1. Delivery of suitable concentrations of agent, which depends on the vapor pressure, boiling point, and anesthetic system
      2. Factors responsible for delivering the anesthetic from the lungs, which include the alveolar partial pressure of the anesthetic, the inspired concentration, and the alveolar concentration
      3. Factors that affect the lung, brain, and tissue uptake, such as solubility, tissue and arterial blood flow, anesthetic concentration, type of tissue, and its blood supply, among other factors
         a. Increased solubility leads to slow induction and slow recovery
         b. There is a relatively high blood-gas partition coefficient, which is the solubility of an inhalant anesthetic between the blood and the gas
            (1) The higher the coefficient, the greater the solubility of the anesthetic
            (2) Larger amount of anesthetic has to be taken in before anesthesia results

II. Potency of inhalant anesthetics
   A. Expressed as MAC; this is the minimum alveolar concentration of an induction that produces no response in 50% of patients exposed to a painful stimulus
      1. The lower the MAC, the more potent the anesthetic. A lower concentration is thus required to maintain a similar anesthetic depth
      2. Values vary among species and are affected by age, temperature, disease, other CNS-depressant drugs, and pregnancy
      3. Tables 19-3 and 19-4 describe physical and pharmacological properties of selected inhalation agents

III. Advantages over injectable anesthesia
   A. Easier to control and change depths of anesthesia
   B. Excreted mainly by respiration; therefore recovery is fairly rapid and there is little metabolism
   C. Requires administration of oxygen ($O_2$) to the patient, which provides a patent airway (endotracheal tube placed)
   D. Respiratory and cardiovascular depression is minimal at safe concentrations
   E. Provides some analgesia and muscle relaxation
   F. Less accumulation and recoveries are rapid

## CLASSIFICATIONS OF INHALANTS ▰▰▰▰
## Methoxyflurane

I. Physical and chemical properties
   A. Methyl-ethyl-ether, which is nonflammable and nonexplosive at commonly used concentrations
   B. High solubility in the blood, tissues, and rubber components (endotracheal tubes, circuit hoses, and reservoir bags)
   C. MAC: 0.23%
   D. Most potent inhalation anesthetic because of the MAC %

**Table 19-3**  Physical properties of the common inhalation anesthetics

|  | Nitrous oxide | Halothane | Methoxyflurane | Isoflurane | Sevoflurane |
|---|---|---|---|---|---|
| Formula | $N_2O$ | $CF_3CHClBr$ | $CH_3OCF_2CHCl_2$ | $CF_3CHClOCHF_2$ | $CFH_2COCF_3CF_3$ |
| Molecular weight | 44 | 197 | 165 | 184 | 200 |
| Date of first clinical use | 1845 | 1956 | 1959 | 1981 | 1981 |
| Trade name | — | Fluothane | Metofane Penthrane | Forane Aerrane | SevoFlo |
| Saturated vapor pressure (mm Hg) | 800 | 243 | 22.5 | 261 | 160 |
| **SOLUBILITY** | | | | | |
| Blood | 0.47 | 2.4 | 13 | 1.4 | 0.6 |
| Oil | 1.4 | 224 | 825 | 60 | 53 |
| Rubber | 1.2 | 120 | 635 | 62 | |
| Minimum alveolar concentration in dogs (%) | 188 | 0.87 | 0.23 | 1.2 | 2.1-2.3 |

E. Lower vapor pressure compared to halothane and isoflurane; therefore more difficult to vaporize (from liquid to gas form)
F. Maximum amount of vapor that is produced from methoxyflurane is ~3% at room temperature
G. Low vapor pressure; therefore can use with out-of-circuit precision vaporizers or nonprecision in-the-circle vaporizers
H. Requires preservative, butylated hydroxytoluene, to prevent acid formation
I. Highly reactive to metal

II. Pharmacological effects
A. CNS depressant
B. Increased solubility, therefore slower induction, recovery, and responses to changes in concentration
C. Good analgesia and muscle relaxation
D. Minimal arrhythmogenicity
E. Hypotension is dose related and primarily due to decreased cardiac output if it occurs
F. Methoxyflurane may decrease renal blood flow and cause vasoconstriction, therefore affecting the renal function
G. Possible renal toxicity, which is directly related to the length of anesthesia, the concentration of inhalant delivered, and whether the patient is obese
   1. The toxicity is due to the by-products of methoxyflurane rather than methoxyflurane itself
H. Respiratory depression is dose related
I. Slow response to changes in concentration, which may be a concern in an emergency situation (e.g., if surgical bleeding occurs)
J. Not suitable for mask inductions because of excitement that may occur
K. Due to concerns over safety of personnel administering methoxyflurane, as well as documented increase in birth defects and impairment of kidney and liver function, this is no longer a commonly used inhalation agent
L. If used, an ACTIVE scavenger system must be in place, systems should be leak tested and maintained meticulously, and all reasonable precautions taken to avoid inhalation by personnel
M. Can cross placental barrier
N. Majority of inhalant is exhaled from the lungs; however, up to 50% of inspired concentration can be metabolized by the liver

## Halothane

I. Physical and chemical properties
A. Halogenated hydrocarbon
B. Nonflammable and nonexplosive at commonly used concentrations
C. Much less soluble in blood, tissues, and rubber anesthetic components than methoxyflurane
D. Moderate solubility means rapid induction and recovery times
E. Depth of anesthesia with halothane can be changed fairly rapidly if compared to methoxyflurane
F. MAC: 0.8%, which is a moderate anesthesia potency (between isoflurane and methoxyflurane)
G. Preservative, thymol, is used as an antioxidant; therefore UV light can oxidize thymol instead of halothane
H. Highly reactive to metal
I. High vapor pressure; therefore halothane will vaporize very easy. For safe use, an out-of-circle precision vaporizer is required
J. Using a nonprecision vaporizer could result in concentrations over 30%, which is extremely dangerous

II. Pharmacologic effects
A. CNS depressant
B. Respiratory depression (dose related)
C. Lower solubility than methoxyflurane, therefore faster induction, recovery, and responses to changes in concentration
D. Not nephrotoxic
E. Can induce by mask
F. Cardiovascular depression (dose related): myocardial depression through decreasing contractility
G. Arrhythmogenic potential
H. Hypotension (dose related)
I. Decreases peripheral resistance, which results in vasodilation (may lead to hypothermia and hypotension)
J. Little analgesia
K. Muscle relaxation varies with depth of anesthesia
L. Hepatotoxic
M. About 60% exhaled through the lungs; 40% metabolized in the liver to toxic products that damage liver and kidneys
N. Crosses the placenta

## Isoflurane

I. Physical and chemical properties
A. Halogenated ether
B. Volatile
C. Chemically similar to sevoflurane and methoxyflurane
D. Higher margin of safety compared to halothane or methoxyflurane
E. Vapor pressure is close to that of halothane
F. High vapor pressure (easily vaporized); therefore precision out-of-circle vaporizers used
G. Least soluble of volatile inhalant anesthetics in blood, tissues, and anesthetic components
H. MAC: 1.2% in dogs and 1.6% in cats
I. Very stable compound; no preservative required

J. Does not react to metals
K. More expensive

II. Pharmacological effects
 A. CNS depressant
 B. Minimal to moderate effects on the cardiovascular system: reduced arrhythmogenicity and better cardiac output (dose related)
 C. Vasodilation and hypotension, which is dose related (as with halothane)
 D. Respiratory effects are dose related
 E. Muscle relaxation
 F. Minimal hepatic metabolism
 G. Low solubility in the tissues: rapid changes in anesthetic depth (faster than halothane)
 H. Low solubility: rapid induction and recovery times
 I. Better suited for mask or chamber inductions when compared to halothane or methoxyflurane
 J. Faster recoveries could result in occasional stormy recoveries

## Sevoflurane

I. Physical and chemical properties
 A. Halogenated ether that is nonflammable and non-explosive
 B. Blood solubility is similar to desflurane: rapid induction and recovery times
 C. Nonpungent and nonirritating odor; therefore mask or chamber inductions are easier
 D. MAC: 2.4% in dogs and 2.6% in cats
 E. Will react to soda lime or Baralyme and produce a nephrotoxic compound called olefin
 F. Does not require a preservative
 G. High vapor pressure, therefore highly volatile agent; used only in agent-specific out-of-circle precision vaporizers

II. Pharmacological effects
 A. Rapid anesthetic depth is achieved because of its low solubility in the blood
 B. Produces dose-dependent CNS depression
 C. Low solubility; therefore extremely rapid induction and recoveries
 D. Low solubility; rapid changes in anesthetic depth can be achieved
 E. Dose-dependent cardiovascular effects of decreased cardiac output and blood pressure
 F. Produces good muscle relaxation and analgesia
 G. Nonarrhythmogenic (does not sensitize the myocardium to catecholamine)
 H. Respiratory depression similar to that of isoflurane
 I. Rapidly crosses placenta and will cause fetal depression
 J. Much more expensive than isoflurane or halothane
 K. Excellent choice of inhalant for avian species, because of its smooth rapid induction and recovery, which minimizes stress on these patients
 L. Slight hangover that is present with other inhalants is lessened or absent with sevoflurane
 M. Excretion of sevoflurane is through exhalation. Approximately 3% of sevoflurane is metabolized

## Desflurane

I. Physical and chemical properties
 A. Halogenated ether
 B. At commonly used concentrations, it is nonflammable and nonexplosive
 C. Extremely low solubility; very rapid inductions and recoveries. It is the most rapid-acting of all inhalation agents
 D. Pungent and produces airway irritation, which provokes coughing and breath holding; therefore mask induction is very difficult
 E. MAC: 7.2% in dogs and 9.79% in cats
 F. Stable compound; therefore does not require a preservative
 G. Does not react to metals
 H. Low boiling point; therefore temperature greatly influences the vapor pressure. It requires an electrically heated vaporizer, which is very expensive

II. Pharmacological effects
 A. CNS depression is dose-related
 B. No hepatotoxicity or nephrotoxicity
 C. Dose-related depression of cardiovascular system. Effects are similar to those of isoflurane
 D. Nonarrhythmogenic (does not sensitize the myocardium to catecholamine)
 E. Excretion primarily through exhalation; however, 0.02% of inhalant is metabolized
 F. Can cause malignant hyperthermia in some species
 G. Recovery may be too rapid and/or unpleasant, which may require resedation

## Nitrous Oxide (N$_2$O)

I. Physical and chemical effects
 A. Inorganic gas that is colorless, nonirritating, and sweet-smelling
 B. Nonflammable but will combust in the absence of oxygen
 C. Liquid form, but is compressed to gas form and supplied in cylinders
 D. Very insoluble in blood, body tissues, and rubber anesthetic components
 E. Has lowest solubility of any of the inhalant agents

F. Low solubility; rapidly diffuses from alveoli into the blood then into the tissues

G. MAC: 188 to 297% in dogs and 250% in cats

H. Very stable; does not react to metals or soda lime

II. Pharmacological effects

A. Extremely high MAC, which means it is a weak CNS depressant; therefore it cannot produce general anesthesia on its own

B. To produce general anesthesia using $N_2O$ alone would require more than 100% inspired $N_2O$, which would result in hypoxia and death

C. Can be used to speed inhalation induction by the "second gas effect"

D. Used to reduce the amount of other inhaled anesthetic (e.g., reduces the percent of halothane or isoflurane) that is needed to produce general anesthesia

E. Provides additional analgesia

F. Minimal cardiovascular and respiratory effects

G. No significant physiological effects on hepatic or renal systems

H. Inductions and recoveries are rapid

I. Drug compatible (e.g., narcotics, inhalants)

J. Majority of $N_2O$ is excreted through exhalation, unchanged in the lungs (0.0004% $N_2O$ is metabolized)

III. Precautions in using $N_2O$

A. Danger of hypoxia if not used properly

B. The second gas effect is accomplished by increasing the speed and uptake of other anesthetic gases (e.g., isoflurane) into the bloodstream, therefore caution regarding toxicity

C. Risk of hypoxia

1. 50% is the minimum amount of $N_2O$ needed to effectively achieve analgesia

a. The recommended values are closer to 60% to 66% $N_2O$, which then reduces the inspired $O_2$ levels to 33%

2. Avoid use in patients with respiratory problems, such as pneumonia, lung tumors, pulmonary edema, diaphragmatic hernia, or other conditions that compromise the patient's ability to oxygenate

D. Low solubility

1. $N_2O$ can diffuse into air pockets

a. $N_2O$ cannot be used with animals with gas-occupying cavities (e.g., gastric dilation, intestinal obstruction, pneumothorax) or where bloat is a problem (e.g., ruminants) because it will diffuse faster than the rate at which resident gases leave

(1) This results in increased distention and pressure within these cavities

E. Should not be used in a closed anesthetic system, because of the low inspired $O_2$ and the patient removing $O_2$ through metabolism. $N_2O$ levels could increase to dangerous levels

F. Diffusion hypoxia: $N_2O$ diffuses out rapidly into the lungs, which can displace $O_2$ molecules in the alveoli. This limits the $O_2$ available to the patient

1. To prevent this from happening, the patient should remain on high $O_2$ flow for a minimum of 5 minutes

IV. Clinical use

A. For mask induction: initially use 100% $O_2$ with gradual increases in percentage of inhalant anesthetic agent. When the high level of inhalant agents is reached, turn on $N_2O$ at a $N_2O:O_2$ ratio of 2:1 to continue induction. This provides 66% $N_2O$ and 33% $O_2$

B. If you plan to use $N_2O$ as part of your anesthetic maintenance, continue with the 2:1 ratio

C. To ensure adequate oxygenation of the patient: never have $O_2$ levels below 500 mL/min, because some flowmeters may not be accurate below this

D. Patient should be provided with a pulse oximeter (measures percentage of $O_2$ saturated hemoglobin)

E. Never have $O_2$ levels below 30 mL/kg/min (three times metabolic requirement) when using a rebreathing system (circle system)

F. When using $N_2O$ with a partial rebreathing or nonrebreathing system (e.g., Bain), make sure that the total fresh gas flow ($N_2O$ and $O_2$ combined) is at least 130 mL/kg/min, of which 33% should be $O_2$ (see Breathing Systems)

G. If the patient's $O_2$ saturation or mucous membrane color deteriorates (gray, cyanotic) at any time throughout the procedure, it is best to discontinue $N_2O$ use in case hypoxia is impending

H. When the procedure is complete, turn off the $N_2O$ at the same time as the inhalant anesthetic

I. If $N_2O$ is turned off too soon, you may be withdrawing a necessary analgesic source and therefore will have to increase the inhalant anesthetic agent to continue the procedure

J. After $N_2O$ is turned off, increase the $O_2$ flow rate to 100 mL/kg/min with a rebreathing system or 300 mL/kg/min with a nonrebreathing system

1. Keep the patient on this increased $O_2$ flow rate for at least 5 minutes to prevent diffusion hypoxia

2. Observe the patient for at least 5 minutes after the $O_2$ source is removed to ensure that the patient is oxygenating well on room air

K. On recovery, especially note mucous membrane color and capillary refill time

1. Supplemental $O_2$ by a face mask should be used if needed

**Table 19-4** Pharmacological properties of selected agents

| Property | Methoxyflurane | Halothane | Isoflurane | Sevoflurane |
|---|---|---|---|---|
| Muscle relaxation | Excellent | Fair | Good | |
| Effect on nondepolarizing muscle relaxants | None | Increased | Greatly increased | Probably increased |
| Analgesia | Excellent | Slight | Slight | Slight |
| Effect on respiration | Marked depression of rate and depth | Some depression | Depression | Depression |
| Effect on heart | Mild depression | Severe depression | Slight | Slight |
| Potential for causing cardiac arrhythmias | Some | Very common | None reported | None reported |
| Effect on blood pressure | May decrease | Decrease | Decrease | Decrease |
| Elimination from the body | Metabolism 50% Respiration 50% | Metabolism 20% Respiration 80% | Respiration 99% | Respiration 97% |
| Effect on the liver | Rare toxicity reported in humans | May rarely cause hepatitis in humans | None reported | |
| Effect on the kidneys | Toxicity reported in humans and animals | None reported | None reported | Possible risk of toxicity |
| Lipid solubility | High | Moderate | Low | Low |
| Maintenance range | 0.25%-1% | 0.5%-2% | 1%-3% | |

Modified from McKelvey D: Halothane, isoflurane and methoxyflurane, *Vet Tech* 12(1):25, 1991.

## ANESTHETIC EQUIPMENT

### Anesthetic Machine

Inhalant anesthetic agents are delivered to the patient through the respiratory system. The inhalants are liquids that are vaporized and delivered with $O_2$ to the breathing system and ultimately to the patient. The anesthetic machine is designed to deliver inhalant agents with $O_2$ and eliminate waste gases from the environment.

### Components of an Anesthesia Machine

Figure 19-1 has corresponding labeled numbers to the roman numerals that pertain to the following description of the components.

I. Gas supply
   A. Consists of compressed gas cylinders and/or bulk sources of medical gases, which can supply both $O_2$ and $N_2O$
   B. Cylinders: made of a steel, steel alloy or aluminum
   C. Cylinders: strictly regulated with labels that are color-coded, displaying the name of the gas, hazards associated with the content, and the name and address of manufacturer or distributor
   D. Oxygen and nitrous oxide are contained in compressed gas metal cylinders. They are found as E-sized cylinders that are usually attached to the machine (portable sources of medical gases) via yokes that are equipped with a specific pin system. Primarily used for transport and emergencies (e.g., if central or bulk supply fails)
   E. E cylinders have a specific pin spacing for each gas; therefore you cannot accidentally attach the wrong gas (e.g., cannot put an $O_2$ cylinder on a $N_2O$ yoke)
   F. Tanks also come in large G or H cylinders, which can be attached to a manifold to provide an economical way of supplying medical gases
   G. Bulk and bank sources of medical gases require a pipeline system, which delivers the gas to stations within the hospital/clinic. The stations are color-coded and fitted with noninterchangeable, gas-specific connectors (e.g., diameter-indexed safety system, or DISS)
   H. DISS connectors are specific to each gas (i.e., cannot connect an $O_2$ line into an $N_2O$ connector or vice-versa)
   I. Sources of bulk $O_2$ and $N_2O$ include tanks of liquid $O_2$, or bank of G or H compressed gas cylinders
   J. Figure 19-1 shows both $O_2$ line and E $O_2$ tank
II. Check valve
   A. Situated in the E tank yokes of the anesthetic machine, pipeline (to and from the bulk source), and in the regulators
   B. Ensures a one-way flow of gas from the tank, regulator, or pipeline. Therefore when you disconnect the $O_2$ line from the bulk system while the E tank is on, $O_2$ will not come out of the $O_2$ line
   C. Also, if the machine is connected to the bulk system when the E tank is disconnected and removed, the $O_2$ cannot come out of the yoke
III. Pressure gauge
   A. It is attached to the cylinder

B. Indicates the cylinder pressure when the valve on the tank is open

C. Gauges are labeled and color-coded with their specific gas symbol

D. The pressure in a full $O_2$ E cylinder is approximately 2200 pounds per square inch (psi), or 15,000 kilopascals (kPa)

   1. Oxygen tanks should be changed when the pressure drops below 100 to 200 psi (680 to 1360 kPa)

   2. The volume of an $O_2$ E tank can be calculated by multiplying the psi by 0.3

   3. A full tank of 2200 psi will contain 660 liters of $O_2$ ($2200 \times 0.3 = 660$ L)

E. Nitrous tanks are stored at lower pressures than $O_2$ tanks. A full $N_2O$ tank is 770 psi (5170 kPa)

   1. $N_2O$ tanks should be changed when pressure gauge drops to less than 500 psi (3400 kPa)

   2. Both liquid and gas states are present, but the gauge reads only the pressure of the gas state

     a. Liquid evaporates to more gas as soon as the gas leaves the tank; therefore the pressure in the tank will not change until all of the liquid has evaporated

IV. Pressure-reducing valve or regulator

A. Pressures in the cylinders are high and therefore must be reduced and regulated to provide a safe, constant pressure and flow of gas to the flowmeter

B. Reduces the high pressure of the $O_2$ or $N_2O$ leaving the tank to a low pressure of approximately 50 psi (340 kPa)

V. Flowmeters

A. Measure and indicate the rate of gas flow to the common gas outlet

B. Measures $O_2$ and/or $N_2O$ in liters per minute (L/min). The machine in Figure 19-1 has only one flowmeter, which is $O_2$

C. Allows the anesthetist to set the $O_2$ or $N_2O$ flow rates that will be delivered to the patient

D. As the gases pass through the flowmeter, gas pressure is reduced further from 50 psi (340 kPa) to 15 psi (100 kPa)

E. Newer machines have improved their accuracy by designing flowmeters that can deliver low flows of $O_2$ less than 1 L/min and high flows of $O_2$ greater than 5 L/min

F. Ensure appropriate amount of $O_2$ delivered to meet the patient's metabolic demands and ensure sufficient $O_2$ concentration for proper hemoglobin saturation

VI. Vaporizers

A. Vapor pressure is characterized by the amount of vapor related to its liquid in a closed container. The pressure exerted by the gas is called the vapor pressure and will increase with temperature. Because most anesthetics vaporize at a concentration higher than necessary for clinical anesthesia, a vaporizer is used to deliver diluted anesthetics to patients

B. Converts the liquid anesthetic into a gas state and controls the amount of vaporized anesthetic to the carrier gases ($O_2 \pm N_2O$)

C. Most are agent specific

D. Most have an indicator window that shows amount of liquid anesthesia agent in the vaporizer

E. If the machine and/or vaporizer are tipped or shaken, the anesthesia liquid could enter the bypass area of the vaporizer. This could increase the amount of anesthesia delivered to the next patient

F. Vaporizers are categorized based on their location relative to the breathing system

   1. VOC: vaporizer out-of-circle

     a. The vaporizer sits outside the breathing circuit between the $O_2$ flowmeter and circle

   2. VIC: vaporizer in-the-circle

     a. The vaporizer is placed inside the breathing system, usually between the inspiratory valve and the patient. VICs are always nonprecision

   3. The position of the vaporizer is based also on the resistance that it has to the gas flows

     a. Nonprecision vaporizers have a low resistance with respect to gas flows

     b. Precision vaporizers have a high resistance with respect to gas flows

G. Vaporizers are classified as either precision or nonprecision

   1. Precision vaporizers

     a. Gas flow, temperature, and back-pressure are compensated

     b. Graduated dial with percent concentration (e.g., 1.5%, 2%)

     c. Percentage dialed is the exact output amount of anesthetic agent

     d. Percentage of anesthetic is determined by dial, chart, or mathematical calculation

     e. Are complex and expensive; however, they have the advantage of being able to control the anesthetic agent closely

     f. Not affected by changes in the flow rates or ventilation of the patient

g. VOC
  (1) Because of internal resistance, precision vaporizers must always be placed out-of-circle, because the patient cannot physically draw gases through them
h. Easy to control anesthesia depth and make adjustments based on MAC values
i. Examples include Tec series (3 up to 6) (Ohmeda, Drager, Ohio), concentrated-calibrated vaporizers, measured-flow vaporizers (copper kettle)
j. Require servicing every 6 to 12 months (clean and recalibrate)

2. Nonprecision vaporizers
  a. Much simpler in design and less expensive than the precision vaporizers
  b. Are affected by
    (1) Fresh gas flow rates, temperature, ventilation changes, liquid and wick surfaces, amount of liquid anesthetic in vaporizer, and back-pressure
  c. VIC
    (1) Little internal resistance, therefore can be used in-the-circle
  d. Not delivered as a percent, but rather a lever control setting (setting from 1 to 10)
  e. Although they can be used out-of-circle, the nonlinear concentrations delivered make anesthesia depth hard to control
  f. Example: Ohio 8, which is a glass jar with a wick
    (1) Methoxyflurane is commonly used because of its low vapor pressure
    (2) The carrier gas ($O_2$) passes over the surface of the anesthetic liquid or past the wick. Incoming gases mix with warmed exhaled gases from the patient
    (3) Better vaporization of liquid is obtained when low fresh gas flows are used
    (4) High flows cool the liquid and reduce vaporization
  g. Can use isoflurane or halothane when a controlled low-flow technique is used and the wick is removed
    (1) Patient should be monitored carefully and connected to a gas analyzer (measures % inhalant in the breathing system)

h. Simple and less expensive and require less servicing

VII. Circle system or breathing system
  A. See Breathing Circuits
  B. Delivers the inhalant anesthetic(s), supplies the $O_2$, removes the $CO_2$, and provides a way to assist or control the patient's ventilation

VIII. Unidirectional valves
  A. Also known as inhalation/exhalation flutter valves
  B. Ensures a unidirectional flow of gas to and from the patient when delivering anesthesia through a circle system (breathing system)
  C. Also used while monitoring rate of breathing

IX. Reservoir bag
  A. Also known as the rebreathing bag (Figure 19-1 shows both circle and Bain system reservoir bag)
  B. Allows the patient to breathe easier from a reservoir of gas
  C. Allows for flexibility in the system
  D. The reservoir bag can also be used to deliver $O_2$ (with or without anesthetic gas) and manually assist respirations, which is commonly called bagging
  E. Bags should have a minimum volume of 60 mL/kg of patient weight

X. Pop-off valve (pressure relief valve)
  A. Also known as the exhaust valve or pressure relief valve (Figure 19-1 shows both circle and Bain pop-off valves)
  B. Exhaust gases leave the system via the exhaust valve and into the scavenging system
  C. The valve can be fully or partially open when a patient is connected to the machine
  D. The valve is closed for leak tests or when filling the reservoir bag for assisted respirations or ventilation

XI. Carbon dioxide absorber
  A. Used in the rebreathing systems to remove carbon dioxide ($CO_2$) from the expired gases
    1. Exhausted gases enter a canister containing soda lime or barium hydroxide
    2. $Na^+$, $K^+$, $Ca^{2+}$, and $Ba^{2+}$ hydroxide reacts with the exhaled $CO_2$ and water to form carbonate
    3. Heat is liberated and the pH decreases
  B. A pH color indicator turns blue or purple on consumption
  C. When the soda lime or barium hydroxide granules turn color or the granules become hard instead of crumbly, they are saturated with $CO_2$ and should be replaced
  D. When in use, granules will produce heat and condensation inside the canister

E.  The color reaction is time limited, so exhausted crystals should be removed immediately and replaced with new granules
   1.  Should be changed after 6 to 8 hours of use, depending on the size of the patient and the gas flow rate
   2.  If the machines are left standing for longer than 30 days, granules should be replaced before using the machine
   3.  New type of soda lime called Amsorb Plus
      a.  Made with two color indicators: white to violet or pink to white
      b.  Unlike conventional soda lime products, once exhausted will not revert back to the original color

XII.  Common gas outlet
   A.  Where the mixture of anesthetic gases (including $O_2$) exits the anesthetic machine through a conduit tube (rubber or Silastic tubing) and enters into a breathing system (circle or Bain circuit)

XIII.  Oxygen flush valve
   A.  Oxygen bypasses the vaporizer, delivering 100% $O_2$ to the breathing system
   B.  Enables the anesthetist to flush the system with pure $O_2$
   C.  Fills the reservoir bag and system to check for leaks (leak test the breathing system)
   D.  Also flushes anesthetic gases out of the circuit and replaces it with 100% $O_2$
   E.  Never use the $O_2$ flush valve with the Bain system when it is attached to a small animal
      1.  It produces too much pressure, which could cause significant lung damage and possible death

XIV.  Bain mount (Bain system)
   A.  See next section on breathing systems circuits
   B.  Delivers the inhalant anesthetic(s), supplies the $O_2$, removes the $CO_2$, and provides a way to assist or control the patient's ventilation
   C.  This metal block (see Figure 19-1) is fitted for the following components
      1.  Coaxial (Bain) hose
      2.  Reservoir bag
      3.  Manometer
      4.  Pop-off valve
      5.  Scavenge tubing

XV.  Pressure manometer
   A.  Not to be confused with the tank pressure gauge
   B.  Sits on top of or near the $CO_2$ absorber or on the Bain mount

C.  Measures the pressure in the circle or Bain system in millimeters of mercury (mm Hg) or centimeters of water (cm $H_2O$)
D.  Generally is calibrated from −30 to +50 cm $H_2O$
E.  Gauge reflects the pressure of gas in the animal's airways and lungs
F.  The pressure should be at 0 with the patient spontaneously breathing
G.  When providing positive assisted ventilation, the pressure should not exceed 15 to 20 cm $H_2O$ (11 to 15 mm Hg)

XVI.  Scavenging systems
   A.  Minimize exposure of personnel, which could be a potential health hazard if they are continually exposed to inhalant anesthetics
   B.  Attached to the exhaust valve (pop-off valve)
   C.  A basic scavenger system consists of tubing that collects waste gases and directs them outside of the building or to a charcoal canister that absorbs waste anesthetic gases
   D.  Scavenger systems can be active or passive
   E.  Active scavenging systems require a vacuum pump or fan to eliminate waste gases from the anesthetic machine
   F.  Passive scavenging systems can vent gases by placing tubing through a hole in an exterior wall of a building or attach tubing onto an activated charcoal canister
      1.  Activated charcoal canisters must be weighed after each use and discarded as needed
         a.  There will be an increase in the canister's weight as the charcoal absorbs the waste gases

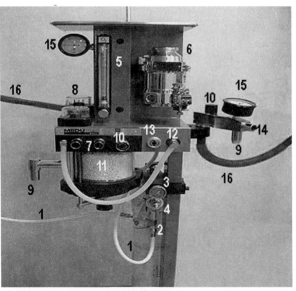

**Figure 19-1**  Components of an anesthesia machine. (Courtesy D. Dyson, DVM, Ontario Veterinary College, University of Guelph.)

XVII. Negative pressure relief valve (not on Figure 19-1)
   A. Some newer machines have this safety valve
   B. If negative pressure is created in the system, the valve will open and allow room air into the circuit
   C. Negative pressure could be caused by an active scavenger system (too high vacuum rate) or low $O_2$ supply

## BREATHING SYSTEMS

### Rebreathing System

I. Also called circle system
II. Rebreathing refers to breathing a mixture of expired gases and fresh gases
III. The amount of $CO_2$ in inhaled gases depends on whether the breathing system has a $CO_2$ absorber or on the flow rate of fresh gases
   A. The higher the fresh gas flow rate, the more expired gas is pushed out the scavenging system and not rebreathed
IV. Depending on the flow rate of fresh gas, the system is classified as
   A. Closed system (total rebreathing of expired gases)
   B. Semiclosed system (partial rebreathing of expired gases)
V. Closed system: fresh gas flow rate does not exceed the patient's metabolic $O_2$ consumption, which is 5 to 10 mL/kg/min
   A. The system may be used with a closed pop-off valve and a fresh gas flow of approximately 5 to 10 mL/kg/min
   B. The expired gases are recirculated (after $CO_2$ removal from absorber) with incoming fresh gases
   C. There is a danger of increased $CO_2$ accumulation if the $CO_2$ absorber is not working efficiently
   D. It is economical and there is minimal pollution
      1. However, it takes longer to change planes of anesthesia
         a. $O_2$ depletion and $N_2O$ buildup are common, so $N_2O$ should not be used with this system
         b. This system requires constant monitoring (should not leave patient unattended) to ensure that pressures do not build up in the system if the $O_2$ flow delivered exceeds the metabolic requirement
   E. It is recommended that the pop-off valve be left slightly open to prevent increased pressures in the system and to adjust the $O_2$ flow rate accordingly, to prevent the rebreathing bag from collapsing
      1. If the bag does not collapse, you can be confident you are delivering sufficient $O_2$ to meet the patient's metabolic requirements

VI. Semiclosed system: also known as partial rebreathing system
   A. The fresh gas is delivered in excess of the metabolic consumption at 25 to 50 mL/kg/min
   B. The gas escapes through the pop-off valve to the scavenge system or after having the $CO_2$ removed by the soda lime, and then recirculates with fresh gases
   C. Higher flows can be used
      1. Then less rebreathing will occur
VII. $N_2O$ can be safely used in the semiclosed system
   A. $N_2O$ flow is calculated 2:1 ratio with $O_2$ as previously mentioned
   B. $N_2O$ buildup is less of a concern with higher flow rates
   C. Important to flush the system to prevent nitrogen buildup from the expired gases

### Nonrebreathing System

I. There is no mixing of inhaled and exhaled gases and no rebreathing of expired gases; all expired gas goes to the scavenging system
II. $CO_2$ absorber not required
III. Fresh gas flow rates required at 130 to 300 mL/kg/min
IV. Induction and recovery $O_2$ flow rates 200 to 300 mL/kg/min
V. Maintenance $O_2$ flow rates 130 mL/kg/min
VI. At or below 130 mL/kg/min flow rate, there will be some rebreathing of exhaled gases

## BREATHING CIRCUITS

I. There are many kinds of breathing circuits available. The most common in veterinary medicine are circle systems, universal F-circuits, and Bain systems
II. Circle system
   A. Consists of a $CO_2$ absorber (e.g., soda lime canister) with inspiratory and expiratory unidirectional valves, two breathing hoses connected with a Y piece to the patient's endotracheal tube, rebreathing bag, pop-off valve (exhaust valve), and scavenger
   B. Can be used as a nonrebreathing system (200 mL/kg/min), partial rebreathing system (25 to 50 mL/kg/min), or total rebreathing system (5 to 10 mL/kg/min)
   C. An advantage is the mixture of expired gases with incoming gases, which humidifies and warms the incoming gases
   D. The main disadvantages of the circle system occur with smaller patients
      1. Excess weight and bulk of hoses
      2. Excess dead space (Y piece)
      3. Resistance to breathing through unidirectional valves
III. Universal F-circuit

A. Basically a modified circle system where the inspiratory hose is placed within the expiratory hose

B. Still requires a $CO_2$ absorber, rebreathing bag, unidirectional valves, pop-off valve, and scavenger

C. Incoming fresh gas is warmed also by expired gases

D. The advantage is lighter weight and less bulk than the circle system (Y piece and circuit hoses)

E. A disadvantage is that if the circuit is stretched when in use, the end of the inspiratory hose pulls away from the end of the expiratory hose. This is considered a safety feature to prevent breakage of hoses, but it increases the amount of dead space
   1. When not stretched, the dead space is less than that of the circle system

IV. Bain system (coaxial)
   A. Consists of one tube inside another tube
   B. Fresh gases flow through the inner tube, and the unused fresh gases and exhaled gases flow through the outer tube
   C. Bain circuit is attached to a metal mount device, which consists of a reservoir bag, pop-off valve, scavenger hose, and connection to the common gas outlet
   D. Between breaths, the fresh gases flow through the inner tube toward the patient and then back through the outer tube toward the scavenger
   E. When the patient inspires, the gases are drawn from the inner tube, which will be 100% fresh gases ($O_2$ plus inhalant agent), or a mixture of fresh gases and expired gases ($O_2$, $CO_2$, plus inhalant agent), depending on the fresh gas flow rate
   F. This system can be used as a nonrebreathing system with fresh gas flow rates of 130 to 300 mL/kg/min
      1. The high flow rates push exhaled gases away so that there is no rebreathing of exhaled gases
   G. This system can also be used as a partial rebreathing system with flow rates at or below 130 mL/kg/min
      1. Flow rate pushes most of the exhaled gases away but there is partial rebreathing of some exhaled gases
   H. Bain system is ideal for small patients (< 10 kg) because of its light weight, minimal dead space, and little resistance to breathing
   I. This system is good for small animals in general, but is not economical when patients weigh more than 10 kg. Increased costs are associated with increased $O_2$ flow rates
   J. Limiting factor is the size of the patient
      1. The $O_2$ flowmeter must provide flow rates required for a partial or nonrebreathing system
      2. Total volume of the Bain hose must be greater than the tidal volume of respiration of the patient to effectively prevent rebreathing
   K. Good for procedures involving the head (less tubing in the way) or requiring much manipulation (taking radiographs)
      1. However, the universal F-circuits can be used now for larger patients for these procedures
   L. Warming and humidification are minimal with partial rebreathing
   M. Requires a precision vaporizer

## HEALTH HAZARDS AND ENVIRONMENTAL CONCERNS

I. Health hazards
   A. Health hazards to personnel exposed to waste anesthesia gases. There are potential toxic metabolites produced by the inhalant anesthetic's biodegradation
   B. Occupational Health and Safety Administration (OHSA) recommendations
      1. Halogenated anesthetic agents (i.e., halothane, methoxyflurane, isoflurane, enflurane) should not exceed 2 ppm (parts per million) dose per day
      2. $N_2O$ usage should not exceed 25 ppm per day
   C. Reproductive problems
      1. Studies show that of personnel who work with waste gases (hospital setting: OR nurses, doctors, anesthesiologists), there is a statistically significant increased risk of spontaneous abortion among women
   D. Hepatotoxicity and increased risk of liver disease in personnel who work in operating rooms that are exposed to halothane and methoxyflurane
      1. Evidence does not exist for exposure to enflurane, isoflurane, or $N_2O$
   E. Other reported abnormalities
      1. There is evidence that methoxyflurane use can result in renal dysfunction in patients as well as operating room personnel
      2. There have been reports of personnel with CNS dysfunction that results in headaches, nausea, fatigue, and irritability
      3. There are reports of myeloneuropathies in people who have been chronically exposed to $N_2O$

II. Environmental concerns
   A. There are ways or methods to reduce waste anesthetic gas exposure
      1. Scavenging waste gases from the patient and anesthesia machine is probably the single most important method
         a. The different systems all have interfaces (scavenger tubing coming from the

anesthetic and attached to a disposal system) that can channel or capture the waste gas
  b. Scavenging/disposal systems as previously mentioned include active (central vacuum) or passive (through the wall or charcoal absorbers)
  c. Detection and correction of equipment leaks will decrease the amount of waste anesthetic gas exposure
    (1) See equipment high pressure versus low pressure leaks
B. Preventative maintenance on the anesthetic machine and vaporizer can be performed by a certified biomedical technician. During this annual maintenance check, any major equipment leaks or concerns can be addressed
C. Monitor the waste anesthesia gases by wearing a dosimeter badge for the day. The badge is sent to a laboratory for analysis. Analysis will determine the ppm of anesthetic gas that the individual was exposed to
D. Vigilant anesthesia techniques include
  1. Do not forget to attach the scavenger hose
  2. Do not turn vaporizer or $N_2O$ on until the patient is connected to the delivery system
  3. Use proper sized cuffed endotracheal (ET) tubes (uncuffed ET tube in avian species, because they have complete cartilage rings in contrast to dogs and cats)
  4. Empty the reservoir bag to the scavenger instead of into the room air
  5. Minimal use of mask or chamber inductions
  6. Avoid spilling of anesthetic agents; wear a specific respirator when filling or emptying all vaporizers
  7. Everyone, especially pregnant women, should avoid exposure to waste anesthetic gases, either by not being present or by wearing a specific respirator mask
  8. Vaporizers and $CO_2$ absorbers should be filled with minimal personnel in the room and in a well-ventilated area; personnel should wear specific respirator mask and gloves
  9. In recovery, keep the patient on 100% oxygen as long as possible and scavenge any expired gases

## EQUIPMENT MAINTENANCE AND CONCERNS

I. Before use, the machine should be checked for both high and low pressure leaks
  A. High pressure leaks
    1. On high pressure system, check for leaks from the tanks or bulk gas supply to the anesthetic flowmeter

  2. Leaks can occur between the tank and flowmeter, DISS connectors on the central lines, tank yoke connectors, regulators, manometers, and so on. These can be checked by
    a. Turning on the tank, noting the tank pressure gauge reading and turning the tank off again. The flowmeter should be set at zero so that there is no line evacuation of gas
    b. In 1 hour, the tank pressure gauge should still have the same reading
    c. Possible leaks can also be found by putting 10% detergent solution on any tank connections or joints
      (1) Bubble formation will indicate a leak
B. Low pressure leaks
  1. On a low pressure system, check for leaks from the flowmeter of the anesthetic machine to the patient
  2. Leaks can occur at the connection between the flowmeter and vaporizer, unidirectional valves, soda lime canister, endotracheal tube, rebreathing bag, delivery hoses, and pop-off valve. To check for low pressure leaks:
    a. Turn the tank on (or connect to bulk system), close the pop-off valve, and occlude the end of the hose so the gas cannot escape
    b. Turn the flowmeter on, allowing the bag to fill gradually until there is 20 cm $H_2O$ pressure (look at manometer) in breathing system
    c. Turn flowmeter off
    d. Maintain the pressure for minimum 10 seconds
    e. If the pressure stays at 20 cm $H_2O$ there is no leak
      (1) If the gauge on the manometer slowly falls (does not hold at 20 cm $H_2O$), there is a leak
      (2) Turn flowmeter on to 300 mL/min flow
      (3) If the gauge stops falling, the leak is considered acceptable. If the gauge continues to fall again, the leak is unacceptable. Therefore, look for leaks in all areas as previously described
  3. If there is no manometer on your breathing system, observe and listen for any hissing of escaping air or use a detergent solution as described earlier
C. Anesthetic machine concerns
  1. Oxygen tanks must be turned off to prevent excess pressure on the regulators
  2. Flush remaining $O_2$ to minimize damage to pressure gauge and reducing valves
  3. Turn flowmeter off to prevent sudden rush of $O_2$ into the flowmeter when $O_2$ is turned back on.

Do not overtighten, because the knobs can be easily twisted off

4. After each anesthesia induction, removable machine parts and anesthetic equipment that have come in contact with the animal should be washed in a mild soapy solution, soaked in a cold disinfectant, thoroughly rinsed, and air dried

5. The flutter valves and absorbent canister should be occasionally disassembled and wiped dry. The unidirectional valves need periodic removal and cleaning with alcohol or disinfectant to prevent adherence to the machine housing

6. Vaporizers should be turned off when not in use and periodically emptied to prevent buildup of the preservative and other residue
   a. Best to clean and recalibrate by authorized personnel every 6 to 12 months

7. Barium hydroxide or soda lime granules found in the $CO_2$ absorbers need replacing when the granules have changed color or cannot be easily crumbled. Do not tightly pack canister when filling, and leave about 2 cm (1 inch) of air space from the top
   a. Most canisters will have a fill line on them
   b. Avoid having dust enter tubing or hoses of the machine

8. Rubber items (degradation from halogenated substances) will likely need to be replaced after prolonged use

## MONITORING TECHNIQUES

### Central Nervous System

I. The objective of monitoring the CNS is to observe the patient's reflex activity and to monitor the degree of CNS depression. The signs you observe from monitoring may differ depending on the species and the anesthetic agents being used. The following signs are general for domestic small animals (e.g., cat and dog).
   A. Eye position
      1. Eye position will rotate ventromedially during Stage III, plane 2 of anesthesia
      2. Eye will return to central when the patient is too light or too deep
   B. Palpebral reflex (blink)
      1. Stimulated by lightly touching the medial or lateral canthus of the eyelids
      2. Lateral palpebral reflex is eliminated before the medial palpebral reflex as the patient becomes deeper
      3. Reflex will become slow, weak, and then absent in stage III, plane 2 with most inhalant agents
      4. If an analgesic has been given or injectable anesthesia alone or methoxyflurane is used, then a mild medial palpebral reflex is acceptable

C. Corneal reflex
   1. Stimulated by lightly touching the cornea of the eye
   2. This reflex should be present under anesthesia
   3. Absence of this reflex indicates anesthesia overdose
   4. Considering the potential damage that can be inflicted on the cornea, there is a wide range of other monitoring options available. Use only as your last resort
D. Pupil size
   1. Generally dilated when the patient is in a light, nonsurgical plane
   2. Constricted in a light surgical plane
   3. Dilated in a deep plane
   4. Note that the sympathetic responses such as pain or certain drugs (e.g., atropine) will dilate the pupils
E. Pedal reflex (pain response):
   1. Stimulated by pinching the skin between the toes
   2. Normal response is to withdraw the leg
   3. This response should become slower and weaker to absent as the anesthetic plane becomes deeper, being completely eliminated by a light surgical plane
F. Jaw tone (muscle tone)
   1. Stimulated by attempting to spread the jaws apart two to three times
   2. Normal response is to resist
   3. A good reflex to check before intubation
   4. This response should become weaker as the anesthetic plane becomes deeper and should be absent in a light surgical plane
   5. If a good analgesic or methoxyflurane has been used, mild jaw tone can remain if all other monitoring signs indicate an appropriate plane of anesthesia
   6. Some breeds will appear to have increased jaw tone because of increased muscle mass in this area (e.g., Rottweiler)

### Cardiovascular System

I. The objective of monitoring the cardiovascular system is to measure the heart rate and blood pressure and to ensure that blood flow to the tissues is adequate
   A. Heart rate (HR)
      1. Most accurately measured with a stethoscope
      2. Can also be measured by digital readout of mechanical monitoring equipment (e.g., ECG)
      3. Normal rate under anesthesia is 70 to 140 beats per minute for dog and 110 to 160 beats per minute for cat. Minimal acceptable heart rate in anesthetized dogs is generally 60 beats per minute

4. Heart rate may decrease with deepening anesthetic plane but may also stay constant or increase with a dangerously deep plane and/or with hypotension

5. Bradycardia (decreased heart rate) is not always a sign of deep anesthesia. Causes of bradycardia include
   a. Drug effect (e.g., opioids, xylazine)
   b. Anesthetic depth
   c. End-stage hypoxia (e.g., respiratory obstruction)
   d. IPPV (intermittent positive pressure ventilation)
   e. Hypertension
   f. Vagal nerve stimulation (e.g., surgically induced, intubation, pressure on eye)
   g. Hypothermia
   h. Hyperkalemia
   i. Myocardial ischemia
   j. Hypoxemia (late sign)
   k. Fluid overload
   l. Tachycardia (increased heart rate) is not always a sign of light anesthesia
   m. Pain
   n. Hypoxemia
   o. Hypercarbia
   p. Ischemia
   q. Anaphylaxis
   r. Anemia, hypovolemia
   s. Drug effects (e.g., ketamine, thiopental)
   t. Fever

B. Pulse rate
   1. Measure by palpation of an artery
   2. Pulse deficits (difference between heart rate and pulse rate) should be noted

C. Rhythm
   1. Arrhythmias can be monitored by arterial palpation but are not accurately monitored with an electrocardiogram
   2. Methods for monitoring HR: direct palpation, esophageal stethoscope, Doppler monitor, and ECG

D. Blood pressure
   1. Palpation of a peripheral pulse can indicate drastic increases or decreases in blood pressure but not actual values
   2. Blood pressure is more accurately measured by an indirect or direct arterial blood pressure monitoring system. There are many commercially available monitoring devices
      a. Most will measure systolic, diastolic, and mean pressures and can be set to read at regularly timed intervals
      b. Commonly, pressures are read every 1 to 2 minutes

3. Direct blood pressures can be monitored through placement of arterial line and provide a constant reading
   a. Superior to indirect monitoring but may not be practical in regular practice, because of the specialized equipment (e.g., arterial transducer, monitor) that is necessary for this type of monitoring

4. Doppler monitor is affordable. It can give a fairly accurate systolic pressure reading as well as audible heart sounds

5. Using an inappropriate cuff size on any blood pressure monitor will give you distorted or false readings; therefore ensure that you have a proper cuff size for the patient
   a. For example, if the cuff is too big, it will give lower readings. Conversely, if the cuff is too small it will give higher readings

6. Generally blood pressure will decrease as the anesthetic plane deepens
   a. Mean blood pressure in dogs should not be allowed to drop under 60 mm Hg
   b. Kidneys will become inadequately perfused below this level
   c. This may result in renal impairment after anesthesia

7. Normal blood pressures
   a. Systolic: 100 to 160 mm Hg
   b. Mean: 80 to 120 mm Hg
   c. Diastolic: 60 to 100 mm Hg

8. Causes of hypotension
   a. Hypovolemia
   b. Shock
   c. Drug effect (e.g., thiopental, inhalants)
   d. Depth of anesthesia

9. Causes of hypertension
   a. Pain
   b. Hypercarbia
   c. Fever
   d. Drug effect (e.g., ketamine)

10. Methods for monitoring blood pressure
    a. Direct palpation
    b. Mucous membrane color
    c. Capillary refill time (CRT)
    d. Oscillometric blood pressure monitor
    e. Doppler monitor and direct arterial catheterization

E. Capillary refill time
   1. Acquired through digital compression on any unpigmented mucous membrane. Time between release of pressure and return of blood flow to the area
   2. Normal CRT is less than 2 seconds
   3. Good indication of how well cardiac output is affecting peripheral perfusion. It is important

to monitor this in conjunction with blood pressure

4. CRT will generally become longer with deepening anesthetic planes and hypovolemia

## Ventilation

I. The objective of monitoring the ventilation/respiratory system is to ensure that the patient's ventilation is adequately maintained

II. Monitor rate and depth (character) of the ventilation

III. Under anesthesia, normal rate is 8 to 20 breaths per minute, and normal tidal volume is 10 to 15 mL/kg

IV. All induction drugs have the potential to cause a transitory apnea. One must monitor the patient's respiratory rate and $O_2$ saturation carefully, immediately on induction to ensure smooth transition to stage 3

   A. In a very light plane of anesthesia, the ventilation will be irregular in depth and rate in response to stimulation

   B. In a surgical plane, the rate and depth are generally regular

   C. In a deep plane of anesthesia, breathing may become shallow and rapid, or both the rate and depth may decrease

   D. As the plane gets deeper, there will be some thoracic muscle paralysis, producing paradoxical breathing (abdomen rises and chest falls during an inspiration)

V. Blood gas levels can also be monitored. The $O_2$ levels will define the patient's oxygenating ability and the $CO_2$ levels will define the ventilation status

VI. Hypoventilation is indicated by increase $CO_2$ levels (respiratory acidosis)

VII. Hyperventilation is indicated by decreased $CO_2$ levels (respiratory alkalosis)

VIII. Monitoring $O_2$ levels may be performed using a pulse oximeter. However, this monitor will display only $O_2$ saturation and not $CO_2$ levels

IX. Tachypnea (rapid breathing) may be a result of the following:

   A. Anesthetic depth

   B. Hypoxemia

   C. Hypercapnia

   D. Hyperthermia

   E. Postoperative pain

   F. Drug induction (e.g., hydromorphone)

   G. Individual variation (e.g., obesity, body position)

X. Hypercapnia (increased $CO_2$) may be a result of the following:

   A. Excessive depth of anesthesia

   B. Airway obstruction

   C. Thoracic or abdominal restrictive disease

   D. Pulmonary disease

   E. Dead space breathing

XI. Ventilation/respiration system monitoring can be done using the following methods

   A. Observation of chest wall and/or rebreathing bag movement

   B. Auscultation of breath sounds

   C. Respiratory monitors

   D. Capnography (mainstream or sidestream)

   E. Blood gas analysis

## Oxygenation

I. The objective of monitoring oxygenation is to ensure adequate $O_2$ concentration in the patient's arterial blood

II. Hypoxemia can be a concern

III. Cause of hypoxemia

   A. Decreased inspired $O_2$ concentration (e.g., $O_2$ flow too low, especially when using $N_2O$), hypoventilation while inspiring 21% $O_2$ (which is room air), or venous admixture (e.g., bronchoconstriction, atelectasis, shunting)

IV. Mucous membrane color

   A. Generally pink in unpigmented areas

   B. Mucous membranes may change color to a gray tinge or blue with decreased $O_2$ levels in the blood

     1. However, this change may be delayed and is not considered a good forewarning

   C. High $CO_2$ due to hypoventilation may produce a very bright pink, vasodilated, mucous membrane

   D. Pale mucous membranes may occur with anemia, hypothermia, or with light planes of anesthesia when pain is occurring

V. Oxygenation monitoring can be done using the following methods:

   A. Observation of mucous membrane color

   B. Pulse oximetry

   C. Oxygen analyzer

   D. Blood gas analysis

## Fluids

I. The objective of monitoring fluids during anesthesia is to ensure adequate blood volume, cardiac output, and to replace insensible losses

   A. Furthermore, to maintain IV access in case you have an emergency situation

II. See Fluid Therapy

## Temperature

I. The objective of monitoring a patient's temperature is to ensure that the patient's natural homeostasis is adequately maintained

   A. Decreases in body temperature and slow metabolism can reduce the amount of anesthetic agent required

   B. It is very important to monitor and support body temperature from the time of sedation through to recovery

II. Hypothermia: develops when the thermoregulation fails to control the balance between metabolic heat production and environmental heat losses (< 35° C). All patients are at risk
   A. Concerns with hypothermia include: decreased metabolic rate, bradycardia, and further CNS depression; therefore, it is important to quickly warm up the patient
   B. Hypothermic patients should be actively re-warmed to 37.5° C (99° F), after which heat sources should be removed to prevent hyperthermia
   C. It is very important in nursing care to help your patient to fully recover with SAFE warming tools (e.g., water bottles, Bair Hugger)
      1. Placing a recovering animal on a heating pad unattended is not recommended
      2. To prevent burning the patient, any heat source used should not produce heat over 42° C (107.6° F)
      3. Physical sources of heat should be wrapped in a towel before placement against the patient
      4. Continual postoperative monitoring of the heating sources is also needed to make sure that the patient does not become cold and further cause temperature issues
III. Hyperthermia: increased temperature (> 40° C) has harmful effects that are primarily related to high metabolic activity and cellular $O_2$ consumption
   A. Causes of hyperthermia include excessive heat application, drug interaction, or genetic defect (e.g., malignant hyperthermia syndrome)
IV. Temperature monitoring can be done using either a thermometer (monitor rectal or axillary peripheral temperature) or an esophageal probe (monitor core temperature)

### Equipment

I. The objective of anesthesia equipment monitoring is to ensure that the equipment used to support and monitor the patient is in good working order and properly calibrated
II. Review section on health hazards and environmental concerns
III. Review section on equipment maintenance and concerns
IV. Equipment monitoring include
   A. Knowing your machine thoroughly, so that you can trouble shoot in an emergency or after common mishap (e.g., exhausted soda lime, $O_2$ depleted, $O_2$ flowmeter accidentally turned off, accidentally closed pop-off, leaky ET tube, leak in anesthetic machine)
   B. Pressure testing (e.g., anesthetic machine, bags, hoses, ET tubes)

   C. Routine maintenance on the anesthetic machine (e.g., servicing vaporizer)
   D. Proper equipment monitoring will prevent some common mishaps as previously mentioned

## STAGES OF ANESTHESIA

I. Ideally, a smooth induction goes from Stage 1 to Stage 3, quickly bypassing Stage 2
II. Stage 1
   A. Induction stage, stage of analgesia, and altered consciousness
   B. From beginning to loss of consciousness
   C. Sensations become dull
   D. Loss of pain
   E. Pupils are normal in size, then begin to dilate when entering stage 2
   F. Blood pressure may be elevated
   G. Respiration rate is generally increased, may be irregular
   H. Vomiting, retching, and coughing may occur
III. Stage 2
   A. Stage of delirium or excitement, loss of consciousness
   B. Excitement and involuntary muscular movement
      1. May appear to struggle
   C. Eyes closed, jaw set
      1. Reflexes present, may be exaggerated
   D. Pupils dilated, light reflex still present
   E. Respiration irregular
      1. Panting or breath holding is common
   F. Vomiting may occur
IV. Stage 3
   A. Stage of surgical anesthesia
   B. Respiration full and regular
   C. Pupils begin to constrict
   D. Palpebral blink is absent (or minimal with methoxyflurane)
   E. Four subplanes
      1. Subplane I
         a. Eyeball begins to roll, pupil is light-responsive, and medial palpebral still present
         b. Muscle tone still present
         c. Pain reaction still present
         d. Respiration is half thoracic and half abdominal
         e. Blood pressure and heart rate are normal
      2. Subplane II
         a. Ideal surgical plane
         b. Respiration becomes deep and regular
         c. Fixed eyeball, often rotated ventrally; sluggish pupillary response
         d. Increase in heart and respiratory rate is mild in response to surgical pain
         e. Peripheral reflexes (e.g., pedal, palpebral) are absent

3. Subplane III
   a. Increased abdominal respiration, delayed thoracic inspiratory effect (intercostal paralysis)
   b. Respiration rate decreases, breaths are no longer deep and regular
   c. Eyeballs fixed and usually centrally rotated
   d. Pupils begin to dilate
   e. Pulse fast and faint
   f. Blood pressure decreased; fails to respond to surgical pain stimulation
4. Subplane IV
   a. Progressive respiratory paralysis
   b. Tidal volume decreased
   c. Palpebral and corneal reflexes absent
   d. Pupils dilated and not light responsive
   e. Heart rate decreased, blood pressure significantly low
   f. Apnea or jerky inspirations
   g. Pale mucous membranes and prolonged CRTs
F. Stage 4
1. Stage of medullary paralysis
2. Apnea
3. Cardiac arrest

## ANALGESIA

I. Why do we treat pain or use analgesics?
   A. There are many issues surrounding pain management that affect the patient's physiological signs (increased heart rate and blood pressure). But there are also pathological effects that result in the following consequences: delayed tissue/wound healing (prolonged hospital stay), inappetence, immobilization, not sleeping, increased risk of infection, and possible behavioral changes
      1. Therefore it is a humane and ethical responsibility to manage pain
II. Depending on the individual patient and the procedure, consider
   A. Which agent to use
   B. Timing (preprocedure, intraprocedure, or postprocedure) of administration
   C. Length of analgesia required
   D. Potency of analgesia required
   E. Choice of route of administration (e.g., systemic [SQ, IM, IV], local, regional, or epidural)
   F. If the patient is in pain, analgesics should be provided in the preanesthetic medication to help alleviate pain and provide for a smoother induction
   G. Administration of analgesics preoperatively and intraoperatively will allow reduction of induction and/or maintenance anesthetic agents required by the patient and maintain a level plane of anesthesia with proper analgesia
   H. Analgesics should be provided during and/or after any surgical or otherwise painful procedure
   I. Timing is important, because if given postoperatively before swallowing reflex is present, extubation may be prolonged significantly
   J. Application of analgesia before conscious awareness of pain will have a positive influence on the effect of the analgesia
   K. It has been proven that pain is much easier to prevent if analgesics are given before surgical procedures and before the animal shows signs of pain
   L. By decreasing pain of recovery, stress of the patient is decreased and therefore a quicker, more successful recovery is promoted
III. Examples of analgesic agents and techniques
   A. Nursing care
      1. Handling your patient using excellent nursing care is very important. For example, making sure that they are comfortably positioned after surgery will positively aid the healing process
IV. Local anesthetics
   A. Can be applied topically, epidurally, regionally, or infiltrated in an area (e.g., declaw blocks, intercostal blocks, intraarticular)
   B. Type of local anesthetic drug will depend on the procedure; therefore select the drug based on its efficacy, potency, onset of action, and duration of action
   C. Lidocaine: commonly used for local anesthesia
      1. Indicated for procedures that are minimally invasive, short in duration, and cover a small surface
      2. The onset occurs within 5 minutes and lasts up to 2 hours
   D. Bupivacaine: more potent than lidocaine
      1. The onset occurs within 10 to 15 minutes and lasts 4 to 6 hours
   E. Local anesthetics in an epidural injection into the spinal cord will block both motor and sensory function
      1. An epidural is an excellent preemptive analgesia
      2. It decreases the amount of maintenance anesthesia, provides intraoperative analgesia, and will provide postoperative analgesia for the patient
      3. Opioids (e.g., morphine, hydromorphone) can be added to the local anesthetic and injected epidurally
      4. The advantage of adding an opioid is the long duration of analgesia

5. Given epidurally, morphine has a duration of 12 to 24 hours, and hydromorphone has a duration of 6 to 8 hours

V. Opioids
   A. There are several different opioid receptors in the CNS that are primary for pain relief. Opioids can be used systemically, epidurally, or orally
   B. Review previous section on opioids

VI. α₂-Adrenergic agonist
   A. Affect receptors in the CNS that are part of the pain modulation system
   B. Examples of α₂-agonists: xylazine, detomidine, romifidine. and medetomidine
   C. Review previous section on α₂-adrenergic agonists

VII. Nonsteroidal antiinflammatory drugs (NSAIDs)
   A. Act peripherally by reducing the prostaglandin production in the area of tissue damage
   B. Used for acute and chronic pain control
   C. Long-term use of these drugs for arthritis and other joint diseases is common, but care must be taken to monitor kidney function regularly, because they can be nephrotoxic
   D. They appear to be excellent for use in musculoskeletal pain
   E. They are commonly used in conjunction with opioids, because it is safe to do so
   F. Common NSAIDs used include meloxicam, carprofen, aspirin, deracoxib, ketorolac, ketoprofen, and acetaminophen
   G. Phenylbutazone, flunixin, meclofenamic acid, aspirin, ketorolac, ketoprofen, acetaminophen, and tolfenamic acid are associated with the following side effects:
      1. Gastric ulceration and hemorrhage
      2. Renal failure can result when the NSAIDs are used in patients that are dehydrated or in shock
      3. Drugs could interfere with blood flow control to the kidneys and the stomach
      4. Acetaminophen must never be used in cats and is rarely used in dogs
      5. Meloxicam is less nephrotoxic and is better tolerated for long-term use

VIII. Other therapies
   A. Need to look at the benefits, mechanisms involved and concerns with each therapy before considering pain management
   B. Some of these therapies are for chronic pain rather than preoperative, intraoperative, and postoperative pain
   C. Few controlled studies have been conducted; therefore there is controversy due to the unknown efficacy of these therapies

1. Examples include
   a. Acupuncture
   b. Physiotherapy (e.g., ultrasound, manipulation via rehabilitation techniques)
   c. Chiropractic therapy
   d. Massage therapy
   e. Topical products (e.g., local anesthetics, DMSO)
   f. Neutraceuticals

## MUSCLE RELAXANTS

I. Neuromuscular blocking agents
   A. Relax skeletal muscles for better manipulation during surgery
   B. Used to obtain better surgical exposure
   C. Control ventilation
   D. Assist in tracheal intubation
   E. Immobilize the eyes for ocular surgery (very common use)
   F. Reduce the amount of anesthetic agent used when deep anesthesia will not be tolerated by the patient
      1. However, NOTE that muscle relaxants do not have analgesic properties
   G. Require ventilation of the animal at all times (the drugs cause striated-muscle paralysis, which includes the intercostal and diaphragmatic muscles)
   H. Requires some form of analgesia
   I. Requires close monitoring for depth of anesthesia, because several monitoring signs will be eliminated
   J. Use a nerve stimulator to aid in the assessment of the effect of the neuromuscular block. Indicates the time to give subsequent doses and when to reverse the blocking agent
   K. Neuromuscular agents eliminate signs such as jaw tone, eye position, palpebral reflex, spontaneous breathing
   L. Blood pressure monitoring technique that is recommended is the direct (arterial) method
   M. There is no CNS depression
   N. Doses, duration of effect, side effects, and reversal agents differ
      1. The larger the dose, the longer the duration
   O. Some agents are excreted by the kidney; therefore if the patient has renal dysfunction there will be a prolonged effect of the drug
   P. Hypothermia causes a decrease in metabolism (e.g., decreased enzyme activity); therefore the effect of the agent will be prolonged
   Q. Certain electrolyte imbalances will cause a decrease or prolonged effect of the muscle relaxant
   R. Some agents require hepatic metabolism; therefore if the patient has liver disease, there may be a prolonged effect of the agent

S. Classification of neuromuscular blocking agents
   1. Acetylcholine agonists
      a. Depolarizing drugs which include succinylcholine
      b. They act similarly to acetylcholine by causing depolarization (contraction of the muscles)
   2. Acetylcholine antagonists
      a. Nondepolarizing drugs which include D-tubocurarine (curare), vecuronium, gallamine, pancuronium, and atracurium
      b. Nondepolarizing muscle relaxants compete with acetylcholine at the postjunctional receptors
      c. They act by competitive inhibition, which results in flaccid muscle paralysis (and not muscle contraction as seen in the depolarizing drugs)
T. Adverse side effects
   1. Bradycardia due to stimulation of cardiac muscarinic receptors
   2. Tachycardia due to inhibition of cardiac muscarinic receptors
   3. Hypotension due to autonomic ganglia blockade
   4. May cause bronchial constriction
   5. Increased salivary secretions
   6. Can cause release of histamines and norephinephrine

## VENTILATION

I. Assisted (occasional sigh or additional breaths) or controlled (IPPV)
II. Manual or mechanical
III. Goal is to maintain near normal acid-base status and oxygenation, and to counteract $CO_2$ retention
IV. In some cases, only assistance is needed (e.g., obese patient, patient in head-down recumbency, hypothermia, pulmonary disease)
V. Occasional "sighing" or "bagging" the patient (e.g., once or twice a minute) may achieve these goals
   A. To properly bag an animal, close the pop-off valve, apply steady pressure to the bag, release and IMMEDIATELY reopen the pop-off valve
   B. When squeezing the bag, it is important to make sure that the manometer reading stays below 20 cm $H_2O$
VI. In many cases, it is necessary to control the ventilation using IPPV
   A. Use with neuromuscular blocking agents; with thoracic surgery, diaphragmatic hernia, or gastric torsion; or with any patient that is obviously hypoventilating

VII. Observe guidelines and reassess results continually
   A. Rate: 8 to 12 breaths per minute
   B. Inspiration to expiration ratio should be 1:2
   C. Tidal volume: 15 to 20 mL/kg (30 mL/kg for open chest)
   D. Inspiratory pressure: 12 to 20 cm $H_2O$ (30 cm $H_2O$ with open chest)
   E. The goal of using these parameters is to decrease $CO_2$ levels to slightly below normal, thereby eliminating spontaneous breathing and allowing control of ventilation
VIII. In most cases, it is not necessary to use a neuromuscular blocking agent to perform IPPV
IX. A $CO_2$ monitor (i.e., capnograph) is a useful device that measures end-tidal $CO_2$
   A. A normal reading should be between 35 and 55 mm Hg
   B. $CO_2$ should never be allowed to go above 60 mm Hg
   C. Hyperventilation in cases involving possible brain herniation, tumor, or intracranial pressure increases should be adjusted so that the $CO_2$ readings are below 30 mm Hg
X. Double check all ventilation with visualization for "normal" chest movement
   A. Reassess the patient's other parameters
      1. Mucous membrane color, CRT, heart rate, pulse strength, and blood gases when available
XI. Concerns with ventilation
   A. Ventilation has a larger tidal volume than a patient's normal spontaneous tidal volume, therefore more anesthetic agent will be delivered. Generally the percentage of inhalant anesthetic is decreased
   B. If the patient breathes spontaneously while IPPV is performed, it is an indication of the following:
      1. Underventilation: an indication for you to increase the minute volume by increasing the rate and/or volume of breaths
         a. Patient is in pain: increase the level of inhalant anesthetic if possible, add $N_2O$, or give intraoperative analgesics (e.g., opioids)
         b. Patient is at a light anesthetic plane
         c. If you are ventilating adequately, the patient will not attempt to breathe spontaneously
      2. Overventilation
         a. Overventilation has potential to damage an animal's lungs
            (1) Rupture of alveoli, leading to pneumothorax or mediastinal emphysema
         b. Decreased cardiac output and venous return

c. Excessive decrease in $CO_2$, leading to respiratory alkalosis
C. Patient with a pneumothorax will have to be ventilated with caution
   1. This means ventilating with a smaller tidal volume, lower pressures, and higher rates (breaths per minute)
   2. Be prepared for the development of a tension pneumothorax
D. Tension pneumothorax is indicated by increased pressures with chest expansion, which is seen on the pressure manometer (anesthetic machine or ventilator manometer) and/or may be felt when squeezing the rebreathing bag becomes more difficult
E. When removing the patient from the ventilator, continue to ventilate for several minutes after turning off the inhalant anesthetic
   1. This will help eliminate the inhalant from the patient's system and speed recovery
   2. Also, decrease the minute volume (rate and/ or tidal volume) to allow the $CO_2$ levels to increase slightly in the patient's system and to stimulate the patient to breathe spontaneously

## FLUID THERAPY

If time allows, possible fluid imbalances, electrolyte imbalances, anemia, and hypoproteinemia should be stabilized before proceeding with anesthesia.
I. Fluid characteristics
   A. Most anesthetic cases are maintained on an IV replacement crystalloid, such as Normosol R, Plasmalyte 148, or P-LA, as opposed to a maintenance crystalloid, such as Normosol M or Plasmalyte 56
   B. Replacement crystalloids should have a high sodium and chloride levels and low potassium levels, similar to plasma
   C. Replacement crystalloids are administered at 5 to 10 mL/kg/hr for routine, healthy anesthesia or surgery
   D. It is common to run long procedures at 10 mL/kg/hr for the first hour, decreasing to 5 mL/kg/hr for subsequent hours if there are no significant surgical loses
   E. Having a patient on IV fluids allows you to
      1. Replace fluid loss because of preoperative water and/or food restriction, evaporation from open body cavities, and/or breathing dry gases
      2. Maintain hydration, tissue perfusion, and organ function (especially renal). This is monitored by keeping blood pressure values within normal ranges

3. Replace blood loss
4. Maintain patent IV access in case of an emergency situation

II. Fluid calculations
   A. For dehydrated patients, if time does not allow hydration status to be fully stabilized before anesthesia, 50% of the fluid deficit can be replaced IV over the 20 to 30 minutes required for effective premedication
   B. Total volume to treat dehydration is calculated as follows:
      1. [% Dehydration × weight (kg) × 1000] ÷ 100 = _____ mL of fluid to administer; example: a 20-kg dog that is 7% dehydrated: [7 × 20 kg × 1000] ÷ 100 = 1400 mL
      2. Give 700 mL of fluid 20 to 30 minutes before anesthesia induction
      3. Recognize that instability may persist until the entire deficit is replaced
         a. To maintain adequate blood pressure, continue at an increased fluid administration rate of 20 to 90 mL/kg/hr during the remainder of anesthesia or until the deficit is replaced
         b. Once the volume of deficit is finished, maintain patient on surgical fluid rate (10 mL/kg/hr)
   C. A maximum fluid rate of 60 mL/kg/min (cats and older dogs) to 90 mL/kg/min (other dogs) to replace the calculated fluid loss is a safe rapid administration rate in awake and anesthetized patients
      1. Other abnormal losses, such as surgical bleeding, are also replaced

### Blood Loss

I. Anemia from acute blood loss is more critical than chronic anemia
II. Patients with chronic anemia will tend to compensate and may tolerate a lower packed cell volume (PCV)
III. If PCV is less than 25% in dogs or 20% in cats, whole blood or packed red blood cells should replace the surgical fluids and be started before anesthesia if possible
   A. Oxyglobin may also be used when available
IV. If PCV is normal but the total protein (TP) is less than 3.5 g/dL, plasma or synthetic colloids (e.g., dextrans, hetastarch) should replace surgical fluids
V. Total volume to improve PCV or TP is calculated as follows:
   A. Volume needed
      1. [Desired PCV (TP) − Recipient PCV (TP)] × Wt (kg) × 50 ÷ Donor PCV (TP) = _____ mL
      2. When blood or plasma is used to correct anemia or hypoproteinemia during surgery, the rate of administration is 3 to 10 mL/kg/hr

B. Test dose of the colloid (blood product) should be completed
   1. Test dose = 0.25 mL/kg over 15 minutes to observe for a transfusion reaction
C. Observe for transfusion reaction signs
   1. Hypotension, tachypnea, tachycardia, poor CRT, vomiting (if awake), pallor, and urticaria
D. When blood products or synthetic colloids are given to treat chronic anemia, the rate of administration should not exceed 20 mL/kg/hr (cats and older dogs) to 30 mL/kg/hr (other dogs)
E. For acute intraoperative blood loss, 10% to 15% of the patient's total blood volume can be replaced with replacement crystalloid fluids, provided that the PCV and TP were normal to begin with
F. To calculate the volume lost, consider that the total blood volume is approximately 100 mL/kg in dogs and 75 mL/kg in cats
   1. Example calculation: 10-kg dog with a 10% blood loss
      a. 10 kg × 100 mL/kg = 1000 mL of dog's total blood volume
      b. 1000 mL × 10% (0.1) = 100 mL (volume of blood the dog lost)
G. When replacing a 10% to 15% blood loss with crystalloids, replace at two to three times the volume lost (in addition to the surgical fluid rate)
H. Only one third of the crystalloid volume will stay in the vascular compartment
   1. The remaining two thirds of the crystalloid volume will move into the interstitial space
   2. Using the example calculation: 100 mL blood loss would be replaced with 200 to 300 mL of crystalloid
I. If greater than 15% blood loss is replaced with crystalloid, there is a risk of hemodilution
J. Any blood loss over 15% of the total body blood volume may require replacement with whole blood or packed red blood cells
K. Unlike crystalloids, the whole volume of colloids administered will remain in the vascular compartment; therefore the volume of colloid administered will be equal to the volume of blood loss
L. If the condition of the patient allows, begin with a test dose and watch for transfusion reaction. Then continue administration of the remainder of the colloid as fast as the loss occurs
   1. In an emergency situation, the test dose may not be possible; the need for fast administration of blood may outweigh the risk of a transfusion reaction
M. In cases where acute ischemia is present (e.g., GDV or equine colic) or blood supply to important structures is impaired or occluded, oxyglobin is indicated to replace blood loss and combat hypovolemia and shock
   1. Oxyglobin has much smaller molecules than regular blood, so it can oxygenate these areas when regular blood cannot
   2. Oxyglobin is very valuable in cases such as these; however, it is extremely expensive and hard to obtain

**Acid-Base Balance**

Acid-base balance is defined by pH, which is the result of processes in the body tending toward acidosis or alkalosis.

I. Mechanisms that regulate pH are respiratory or metabolic in nature and are maintained by three systems
   A. Chemical buffers
      1. Bicarbonate (carbonic acids)
      2. Phosphate (red blood cells, kidneys)
      3. Hemoglobin
   B. Respiratory system
      1. By breathing and alternating the $CO_2$, the lungs can regulate the concentration of carbonic acid
   C. Renal system
      1. Elimination of excess acid or bases: carbonic acid—$CO_2$ equilibrium
      2. $CO_2 + H_2O = H^+ + HCO_3^-$ (respiratory) (metabolic)
II. Four categories of acid-base disturbances
   A. Respiratory acidosis
      1. $CO_2$ production is greater than $CO_2$ excretion
      2. Indicated on blood gas analysis by an increase in $CO_2$ levels
      3. Caused by anything that depresses ventilation (hypoventilation) and impairs excretion of $CO_2$ (e.g., deep anesthesia, pulmonary disease, respiratory obstruction)
      4. May also be caused by increased $CO_2$ production with malignant hyperthermia
      5. Increase in $CO_2$ level causes a gain in acids; therefore the pH decreases
      6. Other signs: increased cardiac output (hypertension), vasodilation, and ventricular arrhythmias
      7. Natural compensation of the body with time through the kidneys (although chronic hypercapnia is rare)
      8. Respiratory acidosis can be treated by:
         a. Ventilating the patient with a higher minute volume (increase the tidal volume and/or respiratory rate) than what the patient was breathing spontaneously to help remove some of the $CO_2$
         b. Treatment of the underlying disease (e.g., pneumonia)

B. Respiratory alkalosis
1. $CO_2$ excretion is greater than $CO_2$ production
2. Indicated on blood gas analysis by decrease in $CO_2$ levels
3. Caused by excessive controlled ventilation (IPPV) or anything that stimulates spontaneous hyperventilation (such as pain and excitement)
4. Causes excess loss of $H^+$ and gain in bases
5. Other signs: may produce tachycardia and electrocardiographic changes
6. Natural compensation of the body with time through the kidneys, although chronic hypocapnia is rare; therefore compensation is seldom seen
7. Respiratory alkalosis can be treated by
   a. Decreasing the minute volume if the patient is being ventilated
   b. If the patient is breathing spontaneously and hyperventilating, assess and treat the cause of hyperventilation (e.g., light anesthesia plane, pain)

C. Metabolic acidosis
1. Indicated on blood gas analysis by low adjusted base excess (ABE) or low $HCO_3^-$
2. Common causes are lactic acid gain (commonly caused by decreased tissue perfusion), renal failure, body secretions rich in $HCO_3^-$ that are lost and not reabsorbed (e.g., from diarrhea)
3. Causes loss of $HCO_3^-$, which means an $H^+$ gain
4. Natural compensation by rapid response of respiratory system by hyperventilating
5. Metabolic acidosis can be treated
   a. For mild imbalance, give an alkalinizing IV solution (containing lactate, glaciate, acetate)
   b. For more severe imbalances, treat with sodium bicarbonate:
      (1) Dose is calculated as follows: ABE (value) $\times$ Wt (kg) $\times 0.3 =$ ___ mEq of $Na^+$ bicarbonate
      (2) This volume should be given slowly IV (over 15 to 30 minutes)
      (3) Deaths have occurred during fast administration of sodium bicarbonate in dehydrated animals
         (a) $HCO_3^-$ combines with $H^+$ to produce $CO_2$ and $H_2O$
         (b) $CO_2$ will rapidly enter the brain
         (c) $HCO_3^-$ will take longer to enter into cells
         (d) Excess $CO_2$ in the brain will drop the pH of the CNS further, resulting in coma and death
         (e) Paradoxical CNS acidosis

D. Metabolic alkalosis
1. Indicated on blood gas analysis by high ABE or high $HCO_3^-$
2. Caused by vomiting (loss of $H^+$), hypochloremia (increased renal absorption of $HCO_3^-$)
3. Natural compensation through the respiratory system by hypoventilation, resulting in a mild respiratory acidosis
4. Metabolic alkalosis can be treated, if severe, by replacing the missing element
   a. Potassium replacment may be necessary if patient is hypokalemic
   b. Chloride replacement may be necessary in the vomiting patient

III. Interpretation of blood gas results
A. Normal values
1. pH: 7.35 to 7.45
2. $P_{O_2}$
   a. 400 to 500 mm Hg (arterial, 100% inspired $O_2$)
   b. 150 to 250 mm Hg (arterial, $N_2O$: $O_2$ mix inspired)
   c. 90 to 100 mm Hg (arterial, 21% $O_2$ inspired room air)
   d. 50 to 200 mmHg (venous, 100% inspired $O_2$)
   e. 30 to 60 mm Hg (venous, 21% $O_2$ inspired room air)
3. $P_{CO_2}$: 35 to 45 mmHg (arterial, will increase by 6 mmHg with venous sample)
4. $HCO_3^-$: 20 to 24 mEq
5. ABE: $-4$ to $+4$

B. When interpreting values from a blood gas sample, there may be two disorders: a primary disorder and a secondary (compensating) disorder
1. First look at the pH
   a. pH less than 7.35 indicates an acidosis
   b. pH greater than 7.45 indicates an alkalosis
2. Then look at the $P_{CO_2}$ and ABE to determine respiratory and metabolic conditions respectively
3. Generally the pH will vary in the direction of the primary disorder
4. Generally the component with the greatest change is the primary disorder
   a. Natural compensation is usually not 100% and seldom will there be an overcompensation
      (1) $P_{CO_2}$ greater than 45 mm Hg indicates respiratory acidosis
      (2) $P_{CO_2}$ less than 35 mm Hg indicates respiratory alkalosis
      (3) ABE less than $-4$ mm Hg indicates metabolic acidosis
      (4) ABE greater than $+4$ mm Hg indicates metabolic alkalosis

(5) ABE considers any alteration in $P_{CO_2}$ and adjusts, so even if the $CO_2$ is abnormal, the ABE can be relied on to determine the metabolic state

(6) $HCO_3^-$ can be used as an indication of metabolic state if the $CO_2$ is normal:

(7) $HCO_3^-$ less than 20 mEq indicates metabolic acidosis

(8) $HCO_3^-$ greater than 26 mEq indicates metabolic alkalosis

## OXYGENATION AND ANESTHETIC EQUIPMENT PROBLEMS

I. If the patient seems to be poorly oxygenating, it may be from something as simple as a mechanical problem, such as a detached endotracheal tube, disconnected or leaking rebreathing bag, or a kinked or blocked breathing hose or endotracheal tube

A. The correction for such problems is obvious once the problem is isolated

1. If the rebreathing bag is empty, the flow rate could be too low or the flowmeter could be off

2. An overdistended bag could be because of a pop-off valve that was inadvertently closed, a flow rate that was too high, or poor scavenging

3. A leak in the system may be because of a hole in the rebreathing bag or tubing, disconnected or leaking tubes or rebreathing bags, or a problem with the scavenging system

II. If a patient's anesthesia level seems light, the problems may be because of the following

A. An empty vaporizer, one that is not working properly, or an inadequate setting

B. Hoses or attachments that are not properly placed

C. There may be excessive $CO_2$ buildup because of an exhausted $CO_2$ absorbent or sticky unidirectional valves

D. If the nitrous oxide is set too high relative to the $O_2$ flow, the patient may be receiving a hypoxic mixture

III. If a patient's anesthesia level seems deep, the problems may be because

A. The vaporizer may be set too high or not working properly

B. Patient may be severely hypercapnic or hypoxic or may be hypotensive

IV. Other problems may be clinical problems, such as pneumonia, lung pathology, diaphragmatic hernia, and pulmonary edema

A. These cases may best be handled anesthetically with a neuroleptanalgesic, in which case supplemental $O_2$ is required, through either a nasal catheter or face mask

B. If a general anesthetic is used on these cases, oxygenation may be improved by assisting or controlling the ventilation

## ACKNOWLEDGMENT

The author and editors recognize and appreciate the original work of Cynthia Stoate and Kathleen Goucher, on which this chapter is based.

# Glossary

**acidosis** Increase in acid pH in blood and body tissue

**adjusted base excess (ABE)** Measures the change in $HCO_3^-$ when the effects of $CO_2$ are eliminated

**agonist** Drug that has an affinity for a receptor, thereby producing an effect

**alkalosis** Increase in base pH in blood and body tissue

**analgesia** Relief of pain

**anemia** Decrease in erythrocytes

**antagonist** Substance that blocks a specific action by binding with the receptor so that the agonist cannot do so

**antisialogogic** Drug that prevents salivation

**apnea** Cessation of breathing

**arrhythmia** Any variation from the normal rhythm of the heartbeat

**brachycephalic** Breeds with short, wide heads

**bradycardia** Decreased heart rate

**bronchodilators** Agents that cause dilatation of the lungs

**hypoventilation** Decreased rate and/or depth of ventilation leading to an increased $CO_2$ level

**hypovolemia** Decreased volume of plasma in the body

**hypoxia** Low $O_2$ levels in the blood

**inotropic** Agent that affects the force of cardiac muscular contractions

**IPPV** Intermittent positive pressure ventilation

**minimal alveolar concentration (MAC)** Concentration that prevents 50% of patients from responding to painful stimulus

**miosis** Decreased pupil size

**mydriasis** Increased pupil size

**preemptive** Often used in relation to analgesia, whereby an agent is given before the procedure to minimize pain and discomfort

**subarachnoid** Space between the arachnoid and the pia mater. Nerve transmission blocks are produced by injecting local anesthetic into this space around the spinal cord

**synergist** Agent that acts with or enhances the activity of another

**tachycardia** Increased heart rate

**tachypnea** Increased respiration, usually shallow and rapid

**urticaria** Vascular reaction in the skin resulting in red, slightly raised patches

**vasodilation** Dilation of a vessel

# Review Questions

1 Acepromazine is contraindicated in epileptics because it can
   a. Cause hypotension
   b. Lower the seizure threshold
   c. Not be combined with anticonvulsants
   d. Cause catatonia

**2** Injectable diazepam is soluted with
  a. Hydrogen peroxide
  b. Calcium carbonate
  c. Propylene glycol
  d. Ethyl alcohol

**3** If propofol is given to a patient too rapidly, it may cause
  a. Profound transient apnea
  b. Irritation of the vein
  c. A long-lasting excitement phase
  d. Seizures

**4** A popular induction drug for patients with cardiac disease is
  a. Thiopental
  b. Lidocaine
  c. Innovar-Vet
  d. Etomidate

**5** This inhalant agent requires a special, electrically heated vaporizer
  a. Halothane
  b. Isoflurane
  c. Sevoflurane
  d. Desflurane

**6** Nitrous oxide is contraindicated in
  a. Orthopedic procedures
  b. Painful procedures
  c. Pneumothorax
  d. Exotics

**7** Flowmeters on newer machines have
  a. Numbers in imperial and metric
  b. A pop-off valve attached to the flowmeter
  c. Low and high flowmeters for greater accuracy
  d. Alarms for hypoxia

**8** Minimally acceptable systolic pressures are
  a. 80 mm Hg in dogs and 90 mm Hg in cats
  b. 60 mm Hg in dogs and 120 mm Hg in cats
  c. 40 mm Hg in dogs and 80 mm Hg in cats
  d. 120 mm Hg in dogs and 60 mm Hg in cats

**9** Ideally, a smooth induction should bypass
  a. Stage 1
  b. Stage 2
  c. Stage 3
  d. Stage 4

**10** Which of the following is NOT true of a Doppler monitor?
  a. Affordable
  b. Can measure systolic pressure
  c. Can measure direct arterial pressure
  d. Can provide accurate heart rate

## BIBLIOGRAPHY

Dyson D: *Veterinary anesthesia (VETM*3470 course manual)*, Guelph, 2004, University of Guelph.

Kirk RW, Bistner SI: *Handbook of veterinary procedures and emergency treatment*, ed 8, St Louis, 2006, Saunders.

McKelvey D, Hollingshead KW: *Veterinary anesthesia and analgesia*, ed 3, St Louis, 2003, Mosby.

Muir WW, Hubbell JAE: *Handbook of veterinary anesthesia*, ed 3, St Louis, 2000, Mosby.

Paddleford RR: *Manual of small animal anesthesia*, ed 3, Philadelphia, 1999, Saunders.

Pettifer G: Veterinary anesthesia. In McCurnin DM, Bassert J, editors: *Clinical textbook for veterinary technicians*, ed 6, St Louis, 2006, Saunders.

Sawyer DC et al: *Anesthetic principles and techniques*, ed 6, East Lansing, 1981, Michigan State University.

Short CE: *Principles and practice of veterinary anesthesia*, Baltimore, 1987, Lippincott Williams & Wilkins.

Thurman J et al: *Lumb and Jones' veterinary anesthesia*, ed 3, Oxford, 1996, Blackwell.

## CHAPTER 20

# Pharmacology

*Elizabeth Warren*

## OUTLINE

Definitions and Basic Terminology
Pharmacokinetics
Classes of Drugs
Antimicrobial Drugs
Analgesic/Antiinflammatory Drugs
Anesthetic Drugs

Other Nervous System Drugs
Cardiovascular Drugs
Respiratory Drugs
Gastrointestinal Drugs
Antiparasitic Drugs
Hormones and Endocrine Drugs

Immunological Drugs
Topical Drugs
Chemotherapeutic Drugs
Antidotes and Reversal Agents

## LEARNING OUTCOMES

### After reading this chapter you should be able to:

1. Understand basic classifications of drugs and general characteristics of each type.
2. Understand the importance of proper drug administration and problems associated with incorrect administration.
3. Explain common, yet potentially serious, adverse effects that can occur with certain drugs.
4. Explain the processes of drug absorption, distribution, metabolism, and excretion.
5. List potential human health hazards associated with the handling of certain drugs.

**P**harmacology is a science that deals with the origin, nature, chemistry, effects, and uses of drugs. This chapter will review the basic concepts of pharmacology by exploring definitions, pharmacokinetics, and distinctive characteristics of common drugs.

Although veterinary technicians do not, by law, prescribe drugs, they are often responsible for the administration of drugs to animals in the hospital and for dispensing drugs per the veterinarian's prescription. In the hospital ward, the veterinary technician is often the person calculating the amount of drug to give, preparing the dosage, administering the drug, and observing its effects. In the exam room, the veterinary technician often has the first and last contact with the client and patient and should therefore be a source of current drug information.

The tables in this chapter contain examples of common drugs in use in veterinary practice at the time of publishing. For supplementary information, consult a formulary, which contains complete lists of drugs, their major effects, indications, contraindications, and dosages.

## DEFINITIONS AND BASIC TERMINOLOGY

I. A drug is "any chemical compound used on or administered to humans or animals as an aid in the diagnosis, treatment, or prevention of disease or other abnormal condition, for the relief of pain or suffering, or to control or improve any physiologic or pathologic condition"[1]

II. A poison is "a substance that, on ingestion, inhalation, absorption, application, injection, or development within the body, in relatively small amounts, may cause structural or functional disturbance"[2]

   A. The drugs we use in veterinary medicine to help our patients could very easily become poisons if used inappropriately. All drugs are potential poisons

III. Drugs have a generic name usually derived from the chemical structure of the drug. A single generic drug can have several trade or proprietary names

   A. For example, the drug neomycin is the active ingredient in the brand name products Biosol, Tritop, Panalog, and Tresaderm

IV. In the United States, drugs are approved by regulatory agencies after rigorous testing and development
   A. Approval is given for the specific doses, indications, and species that are tested
   B. Using a drug in any way other than the approved way is called extra-label use
      1. Veterinarians must often resort to extra-label use when there is no drug available that is specifically labeled to treat the condition diagnosed in a particular patient
   C. The Animal Medicinal Drug Use Clarification Act of 1994 (AMDUCA) provides legal guidelines to veterinarians for extra-label drug use, and the American Veterinary Medical Association (AVMA) has produced a brochure explaining those guidelines
V. Drugs are manufactured in many dosage forms
   A. Capsules, tablets, solutions, suspensions, ointments, semisolids, and extracts are all examples of dosage forms
   B. Some drugs, particularly suspensions, are labeled "shake well" because of the likelihood of particulates settling out of solution during storage
      1. In general, it is a good idea to gently mix all solutions by rotating and rocking before administration to ensure proper distribution of the drug particles, unless otherwise specified by the manufacturer
VI. Drugs stored in the veterinary hospital must be maintained and handled correctly to ensure their safety and efficacy as well as the safety of staff working with them
   A. Drugs must be stored according to the environmental conditions (temperature, humidity, light exposure), expiration date, and reconstitution recommendations on the label or package insert
   B. A Material Safety Data Sheet (MSDS) must be on file in the hospital for every chemical used in the facility
      1. Some drugs are considered hazardous and have special handling procedures prescribed by the Occupational Safety and Health Administration (OSHA). There are numerous sources for obtaining information about the correct storage, use, and disposal of hazardous drugs
VII. Drugs that have the potential to be abused are called controlled drugs and are under both Food and Drug Administration (FDA) and Drug Enforcement Administration (DEA) regulation
   A. These drugs are classified by the DEA according to their abuse potential and are denoted by the symbols C-I (most abuse potential) through C-V (least abuse potential). Schedule I drugs have no current acceptable medical use and will not be found in veterinary practices
   B. Schedule II drugs are highly regulated drugs that have restricted medical uses, stringent record keeping standards, and specific storage requirements
      1. C-III to C-V drugs are generally treated in the same way in terms of required record keeping and storage facilities
   C. Canadian Food and Drug Act Schedules specify which drugs are over-the-counter (OTC), prescription, controlled, and narcotic
      1. Medications requiring prescriptions fall under three Federal Drug Schedules: F (part 1), G (controlled substances), and N (narcotics)
VIII. Drug withdrawal times are important in food animal medicine
   A. Any drug given to a food animal can potentially be transferred to people through ingestion of animal products
   B. Drugs dispensed for food animals have the withdrawal time listed on the label
   C. Many books listing withdrawal times are available to the practitioner
   D. Rules regarding extra-label use of drugs in food animals are more stringent than in companion animals because of withdrawal time regulations
IX. Important information that can be obtained from the package insert or other drug references include
   A. Indications: the approved uses of the drug
   B. Precautions: usually mild side effects or adverse effects (any effect other than the intended effect) that may occur with normal usage
   C. Contraindications: situations in which the drug should NOT be used
   D. Overdose: this section will describe the toxic effects that can occur when too much drug is given or when drug accumulates in the body
   E. Dosage and administration: the recommended amount and route by which the drug should be given
X. Compounded drugs
   A. Compounding is a manipulation of a drug that is not provided for in an FDA approved drug label
      1. When a therapeutic need cannot be fulfilled by an FDA approved drug, compounded drugs may play an important role in therapy
   B. Reasons for compounding drugs
      1. To provide a drug concentration more appropriate for the patient
      2. To add flavoring to increase client and patient compliance

3. Alternative routes of administration
    a. Injectable products may be compounded to make topically applied forms, oral products, or transdermal gels
C. Concerns with compounding
    1. Slight changes can impact the drug's action
    2. The efficacy and safety of a compounded drug is not scientifically tested
    3. Alteration of a drug may change its performance in the patient, including residual depletion in food animals
    4. The veterinarian may be held liable if the compounded drug has an adverse reaction or therapeutic failure

## PHARMACOKINETICS

I. A drug must reach its target tissue in the correct amount (within the therapeutic range), which must be maintained for the correct amount of time, to exert the desired effect
II. Proper administration of a drug is critical and must include administering the right drug, at the right time, by the right route, in the right amount, to the right patient. These "five rights" should be verified whenever a drug is administered or dispensed
    A. If at any time the medication orders are unclear, double-check them with the attending veterinarian
    B. Vials and containers of different drugs and different concentrations of the same drug may have a similar label design. It is best to use the "three checks" system when preparing drugs
        1. Look at the drug name and concentration as you pull the bottle off the shelf
        2. Look again as you are preparing the dose
        3. Check a third time as you are returning the drug to the shelf
    C. Watch concentrations carefully. Many drugs come in small animal and large animal concentrations
        1. Administering the correct amount of the incorrect concentration of drug could be a fatal mistake
    D. Drugs must be administered at specific time intervals that may vary by route of administration to maintain a therapeutic level
        1. For example, ingesta interferes with the absorption of some drugs, so timing doses around mealtimes becomes important
    E. Drugs labeled for one route of administration may not be absorbed, and may be dangerous, if administered via other routes
        1. Never give a drug intravenously (IV) unless it is specifically labeled for IV use, or the attending veterinarian has verified that route of administration

2. Drugs are generally administered either orally (PO), by injection (subcutaneously [SC or SQ], intramuscularly [IM], and intravenously [IV] most commonly), topically (skin, eye, ear), or by inhalation
III. Therapeutic index (TI) is "the relationship between a drug's ability to achieve the desired effect compared with its tendency to produce toxic effects"[3]
    A. TI is the comparison between a drug's ability to reach the desired effect and its tendency to produce toxic effects
        1. TI is expressed as a ratio between the $LD_{50}$ (dose of a drug that is lethal in 50% of the animals in a trial) and the $ED_{50}$ (dose of a drug that is effective in 50% of the animals in a trial): $TI = LD_{50}/ED_{50}$
        2. The larger the number for the TI, the safer is the drug. Drugs with lower TI numbers, such as those used to treat cancer, tend to be more toxic
        3. The more toxic drugs are usually also more hazardous for veterinary staff to handle
IV. After administration (except topical), a drug must make its way to the bloodstream (absorption) and then into the intended tissues (distribution)
    A. Absorption and distribution depend on several factors in the body and certain characteristics of the drug
        1. $pK_a$ (ionization tendency) of the drug
        2. pH (acidity or alkalinity) of the tissues
        3. Solubility of the drug
        4. Perfusion of the tissues
        5. Vd (volume of distribution)
        6. Other factors, such as the blood-brain barrier
    B. Orally administered drugs travel to the liver before reaching the systemic circulation and may be removed before they are able to affect the rest of the body
        1. This is called the first-pass effect
V. When a drug reaches its target tissues it has either a receptor-mediated or a non–receptor-mediated effect
    A. Binds to a receptor site and causes the cell to react (agonist) or prevents a reaction (antagonist)
    B. Interacts with ions in the body to create a chemical reaction
    C. Physical presence of the drug facilitates a reaction
VI. Process of eliminating a drug from the body usually requires biotransformation (metabolism) and excretion
    A. Changes in the chemical structure of drugs are caused by the liver and, to a lesser degree, other organs
        1. Resulting drug components are termed metabolites
            a. The metabolites of a drug may be pharmacologically active

b. In some instances the metabolites may be toxic to the animal

B. Circulating metabolites are usually filtered into the urine through the kidneys, although they may also be excreted in the feces, sweat, or through respiration

1. Monitoring hydration status becomes critical with such drugs as aminoglycosides, which are nephrotoxic and excreted by the kidneys

2. Patients with decreased liver or kidney function may not be able to eliminate drugs efficiently

C. Oral drugs that are not absorbed pass through the intestine unchanged and are excreted in the feces

## CLASSES OF DRUGS

I. Drugs are divided into different classes according to the effect they have on the body; drugs will often have multiple effects on different body systems

II. One drug may have multiple indications for use

A. For example, diazepam (Valium) is used for sedation, appetite stimulation, and for short-term seizure control

## ANTIMICROBIAL DRUGS (Table 20-1)

Antimicrobials are drugs that kill or inhibit the growth of microorganisms, such as bacteria, viruses, and fungi. Antimicrobials are classified by the type of organism they fight and whether they kill (-cidal) the organism or only prevent its replication (-static). Table 20-1 provides details about some commonly used antimicrobial drugs.

I. Antimicrobials are the most commonly prescribed drugs in veterinary medicine

A. For an antimicrobial to be effective

1. Organism must be susceptible to the drug selected

2. Drug must be able to penetrate the site of infection at an effective concentration for an appropriate length of time to kill or inhibit the organisms

3. Patient must be able to tolerate the treatment

B. Bacterial resistance to antibiotics is a major problem in human and veterinary medicine and can make successful treatment of a bacterial infection very difficult

1. Resistance is created when bacteria develop the ability to survive in the presence of an antibiotic drug; they pass on this resistance to subsequent generations of bacteria

2. When treatment with an antibiotic is insufficient to kill off a bacterial population, resistance can result

C. Technicians must educate clients about the importance of administering medications at home as directed and for the entire course prescribed—even if the animal appears to be better after a few days

II. Antimicrobial agents work via one of five mechanisms

A. Disruption of the development of microbial cell wall (e.g., penicillins)

1. Interfering with the formation of the cell wall causes the cell to lyse during the growth stage

2. Giving a bacteriostatic antibiotic (thus stopping bacterial growth) concurrently with this type of medication would prevent it from working

B. Damaging the cell membrane in static/adult populations (e.g., polymyxins)

1. Change in permeability allows

a. Drugs to diffuse into the bacterial cell

b. Bacterial structures to diffuse out, collapsing the cell

C. Interference with microbial protein synthesis

1. Aminoglycosides are bactericidal

a. They make their way into the bacteria and attach to the ribosomes, rendering the bacteria unable to produce vital proteins

2. Tetracyclines, lincosamides, chloramphenicol, and macrolides use the same method but are bacteriostatic

D. Inhibition of nucleic acid production

1. Because this method interferes with DNA and/or RNA synthesis, the potential exists for mutations and birth defects to occur in patients receiving these drugs

2. Griseofulvin, ketoconazole, and metronidazole are drugs that work via this mechanism

3. Enrofloxacin (Baytril) works via this method, but is selective for bacterial DNA

E. Disruption of microbial metabolic activity (e.g., sulfa drugs)

1. This usually prevents bacteria from dividing; therefore such drugs are bacteriostatic.

## ANALGESIC/ANTIINFLAMMATORY DRUGS (Table 20-2)

I. These drugs are two separate classes but are used for a similar purpose: pain control

II. Examples are opioid (narcotic) analgesics, corticosteroids, and nonsteroidal antiinflammatory drugs (NSAIDs)

A. Opioid analgesics include morphine, meperidine, oxymorphone, butorphanol, and codeine

1. These drugs block the pain impulse in the brain, and therefore reduce the perception of pain, but do not address the cause or source of the pain

B. Opioids are used frequently as perianesthetic agents because of their analgesic and concurrent sedative effects

1. A common side effect is respiratory depression, although panting may be seen initially

C. Dexamethasone and prednisone are two commonly used corticosteroids

*Text continued on p. 375*

**Table 20-1** Antimicrobials

| Generic | Trade name(s) | Route(s) | Notes |
|---|---|---|---|
| **AMINOGLYCOSIDES** | | | |
| Amikacin | Amiglyde-V | IV, IM, SC, intrauterine | Keep animal well hydrated; possible nephrotoxic, ototoxic effects |
| Gentamicin | Gentocin, Garasol | IV, IM (stings), SC (stings), PO (water additive), topical | Keep animal well hydrated; possible nephrotoxic, ototoxic, neurotoxic effects |
| Neomycin | Biosol | IV, IM, SC, PO, topical | Not absorbed well systemically; highly nephrotoxic when given parenterally |
| Tobramycin | Tobrex ophthalmic; no veterinary approved parenteral products in United States | Ophthalmic, IV, IM, SC | Systemic use: nephrotoxic, ototoxic, neurotoxic effects |
| Kanamycin | Ingredient in Amforol | PO | Amforol also contains gastrointestinal (GI) protectants; bactericidal activity within gut only (not absorbed) |
| **PENICILLINS** | | | |
| Amoxicillin | Amoxi-Tabs, Amoxi-Inject, Biomox, Amoxi-Mast | IV, IM, SC, PO, intramammary | Give with food if GI upset occurs |
| Amoxicillin with clavulanic acid | Clavamox | PO | An alternative for bacteria that have developed resistance to amoxicillin |
| Ampicillin | Polyflex | IV (slow), IM, PO | Do not give orally to rabbits |
| Carbenicillin | Geocillin | PO | Antipseudomonal |
| Penicillin G | Crystacillin, Flocillin, Dual-Pen | IV, IM, SC, PO | Route of administration depends on drug form (potassium, procaine, benzathine, etc.)<br>Check label and do NOT give cloudy solutions intravenously unless specifically instructed |
| Penicillin VK | Veetids<br>Pen-Vee K | PO | Best penicillin for oral administration |
| Ticarcillin, ticarcillin with clavulanic acid | Ticar, Timentin | IV, IM, topical, intrauterine | Injectable form often used in combination with aminoglycosides; they should not be mixed in the same syringe |
| Cloxacillin, dicloxacillin, oxacillin | Cloxacillin: Cloxapen, Dri-Clox, Dari-Clox | PO, intramammary; oxacillin: IV, IM, SC, PO | Therapeutic equivalent penicillinase-resistant penicillins |
| **CEPHALOSPORINS** | | | |
| Cefadroxil | Cefa-Tabs, Cefa-Drops | PO | First-generation cephalosporin; cephalosporins should not be used in patients with known allergy to penicillin |
| Cefazolin | Ancef, Kefzol | IV (slow), IM, SC | First-generation cephalosporin |
| Cephalexin | Keflex | PO | First-generation cephalosporin |
| Cephapirin | Cefadyl, Cefa-Lak | IV, IM, SC, intramammary | First-generation cephalosporin |
| Cefoxitin | Mefoxin | IV, IM, SC | Second-generation cephalosporin |
| Cefaclor | Ceclor | PO | Second-generation cephalosporin |
| Cefotaxime | Claforan | IV, IM, SC | Third-generation cephalosporin |
| Ceftiofur | Naxcel | IM | Third-generation cephalosporin; do not use if precipitate forms that does not dissipate with warming |
| Ceftriaxone | Rocephin | IV, IM | Third-generation cephalosporin; long half-life; achieves high concentration in central nervous system (CNS) |

*Continued*

**Table 20-1** Antimicrobials—cont'd

| Generic | Trade name(s) | Route(s) | Notes |
|---|---|---|---|
| Ceftazidime | Fortaz | IV, IM, SC | Third-generation cephalosporin; especially useful in reptiles |
| Cefpodoxime | Vantin, Simplicef | PO | Oral third generation cephalosporin; once daily dosing |
| Cefixime | Suprax | PO | Oral third generation cephalosporin |
| Cefepime | Maxipime | IV, IM | Fourth generation cephalosporin; reserve for highly resistant organisms |
| **TETRACYCLINES** | | | |
| Tetracycline | Panmycin | IV (slow), IM, PO | Tetracyclines may cause tooth discoloration in prenatal and neonatal animals |
| Doxycycline | Vibramycin, Doxy 100, Doxirobe Gel | IV, PO, periodontal gel | Longer half-life, better CNS penetration than tetracycline |
| Oxytetracycline | Oxytet, Liquamycin, Terramycin | IV, IM, PO | Many veterinary products and uses, including feed additive |
| **QUINOLONES** | | | |
| Ciprofloxacin | Cipro | IV, IM, SC, PO | Rarely used in veterinary medicine; quinolones as a class should not be used in growing animals because of risk of damage to cartilage |
| Difloxacin | Dicural | PO | Veterinary drug; approved for use in dogs, may cause GI upset in cats |
| Enrofloxacin | Baytril, Baytril Otic | IM, PO, topical | Veterinary drug; similar to ciprofloxacin with better bioavailability in animals; avoid use in renal failure patients |
| Orbifloxacin | Orbax | PO | Veterinary drug |
| Marbofloxacin | Zeniquin | PO | Newest veterinary-approved fluoroquinolone |
| Moxifloxacin, norfloxacin, ofloxacin | | Ophthalmic | For corneal infections with gram-negative organisms |
| **LINCOSAMIDES/MACROLIDES** | | | |
| Clindamycin | Antirobe | IM (stings), SC, PO | Do not administer to rabbits, hamsters, guinea pigs, and horses |
| Lincomycin | Lincocin | IV, IM, PO | Clindamycin is usually chosen over lincomycin because it is more bioavailable and less toxic |
| Erythromycin | Erythro-100, 200 | IV (slow), IM (stings), PO | Enters prostate but not CNS; also used as a prokinetic to facilitate gastric emptying |
| Azithromycin | Zithromax | PO | Better absorption, longer half-life, and better tolerated than erythromycin |
| Tylosin | Tylan Soluble Powder | IM, PO (in food) | Powder form may be used for management of chronic colitis |
| **SULFONAMIDES** | | | |
| Sulfadiazine/ trimethoprim | Tribrissen, Di-Trim | IV, SC, PO | Can precipitate in the kidneys of dehydrated animals; can cause keratoconjunctivitis sicca |
| Sulfadimethoxine | Albon | IV, IM, SC, PO | Sulfas are coccidiostatic |

**Table 20-1** Antimicrobials—cont'd

| Generic | Trade name(s) | Route(s) | Notes |
|---|---|---|---|
| Sulfasalazine | Azulfidine | PO | Used for inflammatory bowel disease (antibacterial and antiinflammatory) |
| **MISCELLANEOUS** | | | |
| Chloramphenicol | Chloromycetin | IV, IM, SC, PO | Penetrates CNS; may cause aplastic anemia in humans; do not give to food animals (banned by the FDA) |
| Florfenicol | NuFlor | IM, SC | May be used when chloramphenicol is contraindicated |
| Imipenem-cilastatin | Primaxin | IV, IM | May be useful for serious infections when other antibiotics have failed; must be given parenterally; chloramphenicol may antagonize; read insert for potential adverse effects and contraindications |
| Metronidazole | Flagyl | IV, PO | Antiprotozoal; may be neurotoxic and immunosuppressive at higher dosages |
| **ANTIFUNGALS** | | | |
| Amphotericin B (AMB) | Fungizone, Abelcet | IV (rapid or slow bolus) | Can cause severe toxicity; should be used to treat potentially life-threatening disease only (systemic mycoses); lipid-based formulation recommended |
| Flucytosine | Ancobon | PO | Used in combination with AMB for *Cryptococcus* |
| Fluconazole | Diflucan | IV, PO | Fungistatic; probably most useful for CNS infections |
| Griseofulvin | Fulvicin U/F | PO | Known teratogen in cats |
| Itraconazole | Sporanox | PO | Information on safety and toxicity limited |
| Ketoconazole | Nizoral | PO | Much less toxic than AMB; used for similar systemic fungal infections; also used in conjunction with cyclosporine to reduce dose required |
| Nystatin | Panalog, Derma-vet, Quadritop Mycostatin | PO, topical | Used to treat GI and skin *Candida* infections |
| Miconazole | Monistat, Conofite, Micaved | Topical | Used to treat fungal ophthalmic infections |
| Terbinafine | Lamisil | PO, topical | Used to treat dermatophytosis, avian mycoses |
| **ANTIVIRALS** | | | |
| Acyclovir | Zovirax | IV, PO, topical | Used for feline herpes infection and Pacheco's disease in birds |
| Idoxiuridine, trifluridine | | Topical | Ophthalmic antivirals for feline herpes infection |
| Interferon-alpha 2a | Roferon-A | PO | For treatment of nonneoplastic feline leukemia virus infections in cats |
| Oseltamivir | Tamiflu | PO | Used anecdotally in treatment of parvoviral enteritis and other mucosal superinfections |

**Table 20-2**  Analgesics and antiinflammatories

| Generic | Trade name(s) | Route(s) | Notes |
|---|---|---|---|
| **NSAIDS (NONSTEROIDAL ANTIINFLAMMATORY DRUGS)** | | | |
| Acetaminophen | Tylenol | PO | Analgesia; do not use in cats; causes methemoglobinemia and liver damage |
| Acetylsalicylic acid | Aspirin | PO | Analgesic, antiinflammatory, and antipyretic; use with caution in cat; enteric coating can prevent gastric irritation |
| Carprofen | Rimadyl | IV, IM, SC, PO | Labrador Retrievers may be more prone to severe adverse effects |
| Deracoxib | Deramaxx | PO | Cyclooxygenase (COX)-1 sparing; approved for dogs only |
| Etodolac | EtoGesic, Lodine | PO | COX-2 selective; approved for dog only |
| Firocoxib | Previcox | PO | COX-2 selective; chewable tablets; approved for dogs only |
| Flunixin meglumine | Banamine | IV, IM, PO | May cause gastric ulceration, nephrotoxicity; keep patient hydrated |
| Ketoprofen | Ketofen, Orudis | IV, IM, SC, PO | |
| Meloxicam | Metacam | IV, SC, PO | COX-2 selective; used for chronic or acute musculoskeletal disorders; approved for use in cats |
| Phenylbutazone | Many | | Analgesic, antiinflammatory, and antipyretic |
| Piroxicam | Feldene | PO | Use in cat is as an antineoplastic |
| Tepoxalin | Zubrin | PO | COX and LOX (lipoxygenase) inhibitor; rapidly disintegrating tabs for dogs |
| Tolfenamic acid | Tolfedine | IM, SC, PO | Pharmacologically similar to aspirin; approved for dogs and cats in Canada, Europe |
| Dimethyl sulfoxide (DMSO) | | IV, topical | Teratogenic in some species; wear gloves when applying |
| **CORTICOSTEROIDS** | | | |
| Betamethasone | Betasone | IM | Long acting |
| Dexamethasone | Azium, Dexasone | IV, IM, SC, PO | Long acting |
| Methylprednisolone | Medrol, Depo-Medrol | IM, SC, PO | Intermediate acting |
| Triamcinolone | Vetalog | IM, SC, PO | Intermediate acting |
| Prednisone | Meticorten, Deltasone | IV, IM, SC, PO | Intermediate acting |
| Hydrocortisone | Cortef | IV, IM, PO | Short acting |
| **GLYCOSAMINOGLYCANS** | | | |
| Glucosamine | Many | PO | Often combined with chondroitin, these agents are considered nutraceuticals, not drugs |
| Hyaluronate (hyaluronic acid) | Hycoat | IA (intraarticular) | For synovitis |
| Polysulfated glycosaminoglycan | Adequan | IM, IA | Postinjection inflammation possible when administered into the joint |
| Pentosan polysulfate | Cartrophen-Vet (outside United States), Elmiron | IM, SC, PO | Used for osteoarthritis and interstitial cystitis (cats) |
| **MUSCLE RELAXANTS, OPIOID (NARCOTIC) ANALGESICS** | | | |
| Methocarbamol | Robaxin-V | IV, PO | Skeletal muscle relaxant, may cause sedation |
| Butorphanol | Torbutrol, Torbugesic, Dolorex | IV, IM, SC, PO | Partial agonist/antagonist; poorly absorbed from gastrointestinal tract; also used as an antitussive |
| Buprenorphine | Buprenex | IV, IM, SC, TM (transmucosal) | Partial agonist; may cause respiratory depression; TM administration in dogs is unreliable |

**Table 20-2**  Analgesics and antiinflammatories—cont'd

| Generic | Trade name(s) | Route(s) | Notes |
|---|---|---|---|
| Hydromorphone | Dilaudid | IV, IM, SC, rectal | Mu agonist; may cause panting, then respiratory depression; Class II controlled substance |
| Morphine | Many | IV, IM, SC, PO, rectal, epidural | Mu agonist; may cause panting, then depression; use preservative-free form for epidural; Class II controlled substance |
| Oxymorphone | Numorphan | IV, IM, SC | May cause respiratory and cardiac depression; Class II controlled substance |
| Fentanyl | Duragesic, Sublimaze | IV constant rate infusion, transdermal | Patch gives about 3 days of analgesia; injectable is short-acting; Class II controlled substance |
| Tramadol | Ultram | PO | Synthetic mu agonist and serotonin, norepinephrine reuptake inhibitor |
| **LOCAL ANESTHETICS** | | | |
| Lidocaine, mepivacaine, procaine, tetracaine | Many | Local infusion, topical, transdermal, epidural | These drugs are used to block nerve impulses from local or regional areas; they are available in injectable and topical forms; epinephrine is sometimes added to extend the effects |
| **MISCELLANEOUS** | | | |
| Amantadine, dextromethorphan | Symmetrel, Robitussin | PO | *N*-methyl-D-aspartate receptor antagonists; adjunct to analgesia use is experimental |
| Gabapentin | Neurontin | PO | Analgesic and anticonvulsant adjunct; experimental |

1. Corticosteroids act as analgesics by reducing tissue inflammation
2. Corticosteroid drugs can have significant effects on the endocrine and immune systems; therefore extra care must be taken with their use

D. Phenylbutazone, aspirin, ibuprofen, etodolac, and carprofen are examples of NSAIDs
   1. NSAIDs will not produce sufficient analgesia to counteract pain associated with organs or broken bones
   2. Most NSAIDs work by blocking prostaglandin production from within the inflammatory process. They are safer but less effective than steroidal antiinflammatory drugs
   3. Cats lack the ability to metabolize many NSAIDs; therefore they should be used only with extreme caution on the direction of a veterinarian

E. Narcotic agonist drugs are competitively antagonized by naloxone (Narcan) and naltrexone (Trexan)

## ANESTHETIC DRUGS (Table 20-3)

See also Chapter 19.

I. General anesthetics cause the loss of all sensation

II. General anesthetics are available as injectables and inhalants

III. Overdoses of some general anesthetics are used for euthanasia, although an overdose of any general anesthetic can be fatal
   A. Pentobarbital sodium is the most common euthanizing agent
   B. By itself, pentobarbital is a C-II drug in the United States (DEA) and a controlled drug in Canada; but some euthanasia agents contain additives, such as phenytoin in Beuthanasia-D or lidocaine in FP3. These additives act as cardiac depressants and change the DEA status to C-III in the United States
      1. Pentobarbital sodium can cause necrosis if injected perivascularly
      2. Perivascular injection will delay or inhibit death
      3. Animals in pain may require a tranquilizer before pentobarbital sodium administration
      4. These products must not be used in food-producing animals
      5. The carcass will be toxic to scavengers that ingest tissues

## OTHER NERVOUS SYSTEM DRUGS
(See Table 20-3)

I. Many types of drugs have various effects on the nervous system. They can affect both the central (brain and spinal cord) and the peripheral (autonomic) nervous systems

II. Drugs that affect the central nervous system include anesthetics, analgesics, tranquilizers, sedatives, anticonvulsants, stimulants, and psychoactive drugs.

**Table 20-3** Anesthetics and other central nervous system (CNS) drugs

| Generic | Trade name(s) | Route(s) | Notes |
|---|---|---|---|
| **BARBITURATES** | | | |
| Pentobarbital | Nembutal | IV (slow to effect) | Used for induction of general anesthesia and to manage status epilepticus; can be used as a single agent for euthanasia; Class II controlled substance; short-acting |
| Pentobarbital with phenytoin | Beuthanasia-D | IV | For euthanasia only |
| Thiopental | Pentothal | IV only | May adsorb to plastic intravenous bags and lines; ultra–short-acting |
| **TRANQUILIZERS/SEDATIVES** | | | |
| Acepromazine | PromAce, Atravet | IV, IM (stings), SC, PO | Do not use in conjunction with organophosphates; may cause paradoxical CNS stimulation, hypotension |
| Diazepam, midazolam | Valium, Versed | IV, IM, PO, rectal | Used as anxiolytic, muscle relaxant, appetite stimulant, perianesthetic, and anticonvulsant |
| Oxazepam, alprazolam | Serax, Xanax | PO | Used primarily in behavior modification programs |
| Medetomidine | Domitor | IV, IM | Alpha-2 agonist used for sedation/analgesia in young, healthy animals; adverse effects, such as bradycardia, can be treated by reversing the drug |
| Xylazine | Rompun, Anased | IV, IM, SC | Alpha-2 agonist used for sedation/analgesia in young, healthy animals; available in 20 and 100 mg/mL; check concentration before administering; respiratory depression and vomiting are common side effects and can be treated by reversing the drug |
| **INHALANTS** | | | |
| Halothane | Fluothone | Inhalant | Causes increased cerebrospinal fluid pressure; rarely may cause malignant hyperthermia, hepatotoxicity |
| Isoflourane | Aerrane, Forane | Inhalant | Rapid induction and recovery; noxious odor |
| Sevoflurane | SevoFlo | Inhalant | Very rapid induction and recovery; no odor |
| **MISCELLANEOUS ANESTHETICS** | | | |
| Ketamine | Ketaset, Vetalar | IV, IM | Dissociative anesthetic; most reflexes and muscle tone are maintained; no somatic analgesia |
| Propofol | Rapinovet, PropoFlo, Diprivan | IV only | Rapid induction and recovery; drug is carried in an egg lecithin/soy base, which supports bacterial growth |
| Tiletamine/ zolazepam | Telazol | IV, IM | Tiletamine is a dissociative anesthetic; zolazepam is a tranquilizer; most reflexes are retained |
| Etomidate | Amidate | IV | Minimal effects on cardiovascular and respiratory system; given alone causes myoclonus |
| Guaifenesin | Guailaxin | IV, PO | Muscle relaxant perianesthetic when given parenterally; expectorant when given orally |
| **ANTICONVULSANTS** | | | |
| Phenobarbital | Luminal | IV (slow), IM, PO | Usual first drug of choice for idiopathic epilepsy; may be used for status seizure; long acting |
| Bromides | (Potassium, sodium) | PO | Used as an adjunct in management of idiopathic epilepsy |
| Diazepam | Valium | IV, rectal, intranasal | Used to control seizures in progress |
| Pentobarbital | Nembutal | IV | Used in status epilepticus, for intractable seizures |

**Table 20-3** Anesthetics and other central nervous system (CNS) drugs—cont'd

| Generic | Trade name(s) | Route(s) | Notes |
|---|---|---|---|
| OTHERS | | | |
| Edrophonium, pyridostigmine | Tensilon, Mestinon | IV, PO | Anticholinesterase agents used to diagnose and treat myasthenia gravis |
| Succinylcholine, pancuronium | Anectine, Pavulon | IV | Neuromuscular blocking agents; paralytics |

Most of these drugs are federally controlled substances

A. Tranquilizers and sedatives, such as benzodiazepines and phenothiazine drugs, reduce anxiety, produce a tranquil mental state, and cause sleepiness

B. Anticonvulsants used to control seizures in progress are administered in the hospital for relatively short durations (e.g., diazepam and pentobarbital)

C. Anticonvulsants used for long-term management of seizure-prone patients are usually given orally at home on a long-term basis (e.g., phenobarbital and potassium bromide)

D. Doxapram is used to stimulate the respiratory center in the brain

E. Other stimulants, such as caffeine, theobromine, and amphetamines, are frequently toxic to animals

F. Drugs are sometimes used to treat behavioral problems in animals
  1. Many of these are human psychiatric medications that have not been approved for use in animals
  2. They may have undesirable side effects and can take a long time to work
     a. Clomipramine (Clomicalm) is a veterinary-labeled tricyclic antidepressant used to treat separation anxiety in dogs
     b. Selegiline (Anipryl) is a veterinary-labeled antidepressant used in the treatment of canine cognitive dysfunction

III. Drugs that affect the autonomic nervous system can be simply classified by the system they affect
  A. Cholinergics produce parasympathetic effects; anticholinergics block them
     1. These drugs work by stimulating or blocking different receptors and/or stimulating or blocking the effects of various neurotransmitters
        a. Examples of cholinergic agents include
           (1) Pilocarpine, which reduces intraocular pressure
           (2) Metoclopramide, which stimulates the gastrointestinal (GI) system
           (3) Urecholine, which stimulates the urinary system

IV. Adverse side effects of cholinergics are related to overstimulation of the parasympathetic nervous system
  A. Anticholinergics have the opposite effects including
     1. Slowing GI motility (aminopentamide)
     2. Drying secretions, dilating the pupil, and speeding the heart (atropine sulfate, glycopyrrolate)
        a. Adverse side effects are dose related
           (1) For example, care must be taken not to confuse the large animal concentration with the small animal concentration of atropine sulfate
  B. Adrenergics produce sympathetic effects; adrenergic blockers inhibit them
     1. Adrenergic agents have many diverse effects according to the receptors stimulated
        a. Some of the most common include
           (1) Epinephrine stimulates the heart to beat
           (2) Dopamine is used to treat hypotension/shock
           (3) Phenylpropanolamine is used for urinary incontinence
           (4) Terbutaline and albuterol are used for bronchodilation
           (5) Xylazine and medetomidine are analgesic and sedative agents
     2. Similarly, adrenergic blockers are a diverse group. Some of the more common α-blockers include
        a. Phenoxybenzamine, to reduce urethral sphincter tone
        b. Acepromazine and droperidol, which are tranquilizers
        c. Yohimbine, the reversal agent for xylazine, and atipamezole (Antisedan), the reversal agent for medetomidine
     3. Of the β-blockers, propranolol, used for cardiac arrhythmias and cardiomyopathy, and timolol, used to treat glaucoma, are most commonly used in veterinary practice

## CARDIOVASCULAR DRUGS (Table 20-4) ▬▬

Cardiovascular drugs affect the heart. They include anti-arrhythmics, diuretics, positive inotropic drugs, catecholamines, and vasodilators. The cardiovascular system is regulated by the autonomic nervous system, and many of the drugs that affect it work by stimulating or blocking nervous impulses.

I. Antiarrhythmics
   A. When arrhythmias occur in the heart, antiarrhythmics restore normal electrical activity
   B. Drugs that work by controlling $Na^+$ flow include lidocaine and procainamide
   C. Drugs like propranolol, a negative inotrope, work by blocking β-receptors
   D. Verapamil and diltiazem are calcium channel blocker antiarrhythmics

II. Diuretics
   A. Furosemide and mannitol are examples of diuretics
   B. Diuretics create an osmotic force in the renal tubules, thus drawing in water and increasing urine output
      1. Removing water decreases cardiac workload
      2. Use cautiously in hypovolemic or hypotensive animals

III. Positive inotropes and catecholamines
   A. These drugs increase the strength of contraction of the heart
      1. Positive inotropes, such as digoxin, are used for long-term maintenance of contractility by increasing the amount of calcium available in the heart
      2. Catecholamines, such as epinephrine and dobutamine, are used for management of short-term increased contractility; they act by mimicking the sympathetic nervous system (adrenergics)

IV. Vasodilators
   A. Nitroglycerin, hydralazine, and enalapril are vasodilators
   B. Vasodilators cause an expansion in the diameter of blood vessels
      1. This increase in diameter allows blood to flow more easily, which in turn reduces the workload of the heart

V. Other cardiac drugs
   A. Aspirin helps to reduce the formation of blood clots
   B. Bronchodilators enable the animal to increase oxygen intake
   C. Sedatives can calm anxious patients, especially those having trouble breathing
   D. Oxygen is almost always an indicated treatment for patients with cardiac disease, but as with all drugs, it can be toxic in excess

## RESPIRATORY DRUGS (Table 20-5) ▬▬

I. Antitussives, such as butorphanol and hydrocodone, are mild narcotics that suppress the cough reflex
   A. These drugs are indicated only for patients with a hacking, unproductive cough; dogs with infectious tracheobronchitis (kennel cough) may be treated with cough suppressants
   B. Antitussives may be contraindicated with productive coughs because of the risk of accumulation of mucus and debris in the airways

II. Expectorants increase the fluidity of respiratory mucus, making it easier to expel; mucolytics break up mucus, decreasing its viscosity
   A. Guaifenesin is available in OTC cough medications
      1. Human OTC expectorants are of little benefit to animal patients
   B. Acetylcysteine is a mucolytic that is often administered via nebulization
   C. Humidification of inspired air can also increase mucus fluidity

III. Bronchodilators expand the bronchioles in the lungs, making it easier to breathe
   A. Terbutaline, albuterol, and metaproterenol stimulate $β_2$-receptors in the lung, which in turn cause bronchodilation
   B. Theophylline and aminophylline cause relaxation of smooth muscles in the lungs and, in turn, bronchodilation

IV. Other drugs used to treat respiratory problems include antihistamines, corticosteroids, diuretics, and oxygen
   A. Antihistamines also cause bronchodilation if given prophylactically, by preventing histamine from affecting the respiratory tract
   B. Corticosteroids are given when inflammation of the airways is severe
   C. Diuretics help to remove fluid from the lungs
   D. Oxygen administration is indicated whenever perfusion is compromised

## GASTROINTESTINAL DRUGS (Table 20-6) ▬▬

I. Emetics cause vomiting
   A. Used when noncaustic poisons are eaten or to empty the stomach before anesthesia
   B. Some emetics act locally (cause irritation to the GI tract), such as syrup of ipecac and hydrogen peroxide, and others act centrally (stimulate vomiting center in central nervous system), such as apomorphine

II. Antiemetics prevent or decrease vomiting; the choice of antiemetic depends on the cause of the vomiting
   A. Chlorpromazine, diphenhydramine, and dimenhydrinate may be used when vomiting is related to motion sickness or vestibular disturbance

**Table 20-4** Cardiovascular drugs

| Generic | Trade name(s) | Route(s) | Notes |
|---------|---------------|----------|-------|
| **INOTROPIC** | | | |
| Digoxin | Lanoxin, Cardoxin | IV, PO | Toxic and therapeutic doses may overlap; Dobermans tend to be sensitive to digoxin |
| Dobutamine | Dobutrex | IV infusion | Use diluted solutions within 24 hr |
| Pimobendan | Vetmedin | PO | Used to manage congestive heart failure; available in Canada and Europe |
| **ADRENERGICS** | | | |
| Epinephrine | Adrenalin | IV, IM, SC | Available in several sizes for various uses |
| | | IT (intratracheal) | 1:100 (1% or 10 mg/mL) topical, inhalation |
| | | IC (intracardiac) | 1:1000 (0.1% or 1 mg/mL) IV, IM, SC, IT |
| | | Inhalation | 1:10,000 (0.01% or 0.1 mg/mL) IV, IC |
| Isoproterenol | Isuprel | IV (infusion), rectal, sublingual | Do not use with epinephrine |
| Dopamine | Intropin | IV (infusion) | Effects are dose dependent |
| **ANTICHOLINERGICS** | | | |
| Atropine | Many | IV, IM, SC | Used for cardiac support |
| Glycopyrrolate | Robinul-V | IV, IM, SC | Used for cardiac support; not suitable for emergency use |
| **β-BLOCKERS** | | | |
| Atenolol | Tenormin | PO | Sympathomimetic drug effects |
| Propranolol | Inderal | IV (slow), PO | Can be blocked by β-agonists |
| Metoprolol | Lopressor, Toprol | PO | Similar to propranolol, safer for patients with bronchoconstriction |
| **CALCIUM CHANNEL BLOCKERS** | | | |
| Amlodipine | Norvasc | PO | Use cautiously in animals with heart failure |
| Diltiazem | Cardizem | PO | Toxicity may be treated with calcium infusion |
| Verapamil | Isoptin | IV | High first-pass effect; watch for toxicity in animals with hepatic disease |
| **ANGIOTENSIN-CONVERTING ENZYME (ACE) INHIBITORS** | | | |
| Benazapril | Lotensin | PO | For adjunctive treatment of heart failure |
| Captopril | Capoten | PO | Use cautiously in animals with renal disease |
| Enalapril | Enacard, Vasotec | IV, PO | Give on an empty stomach |

*Continued*

**Table 20-4**   Cardiovascular drugs—cont'd

| Generic | Trade name(s) | Route(s) | Notes |
|---|---|---|---|
| **VASODILATORS** | | | |
| Hydralazine | Apresolene | IM, PO | Use cautiously in patients with severe renal disease |
| Nitroglycerin | Nitro-Bid, Nitrol | Topical | Wear gloves when applying ointment |
| Nitroprusside | Nitropress | IV infusion | Adverse effects are due to drug's hypotensive effects |
| Prazosin | Minipress | PO | Also used to treat functional urethral obstruction |
| **ANTIARRHYTHMICS** | | | |
| Lidocaine | Xylocaine | IV | Do not use lidocaine with epinephrine preparations for intravenous solutions |
| Procainamide | Pronestyl, Procan | IV, IM, PO | Use with caution with other antiarrhythmics |
| Quinidine | Quinidex | IV, IM, PO | Use with caution with other antiarrhythmics |
| **DIURETICS** | | | |
| Furosemide | Lasix, Disal, Diuride, Salix | IV, IM, PO | Veterinary preparations are normally slightly yellow; if human preparations turn yellow, do not use |
| Spironolactone | Aldactone | PO | Potassium-sparing diuretic |
| Chlorothiazide, hydrochloro-thiazide | Diuril, Hydrodiuril | PO | Thiazide diuretics |
| Mannitol | Osmitrol, Mannitrol | IV infusion | Primary use is to decrease intracranial pressure |
| **ANTICOAGULANTS** | | | |
| Heparin | Many | SC | Used in disseminated intravascular coagulation and in IV flush solutions |
| Dalteparin, enoxaparin | Fragmin, Lovenox | SC | Low molecular weight heparin used to prevent thromboembolisms |

B. Metoclopramide causes increased gastric motility

C. Aminopentamide is an antispasmodic

III. Antidiarrheals are used to control frequent loose stools

  A. Diarrhea has various causes, and treatment depends on the cause

  B. These drugs work by modifying intestinal motility; adsorbing enterotoxins, and preventing intestinal hypersecretions

    1. Mild narcotics, such as loperamide and diphenoxylate, are often very effective antidiarrheals

    2. Antispasmodics, such as aminopentamide, are sometimes indicated

    3. Protectants and adsorbents, such as bismuth, kaolin, pectin, and activated charcoal, are generally benign and are sometimes recommended for home use

IV. Laxatives are used to relieve constipation and to clear the lower intestinal tract

  A. Hyperosmotics, such as lactulose and magnesium hydroxide, draw water to the bowel, where it softens the stool

    1. Fleet enemas should NOT be used in cats

  B. Bulk-producing agents (fiber) help to increase the water content of the stool and stimulate peristalsis in the GI tract

  C. Lubricants, such as mineral oil and petroleum jelly, make the passage of stool easier

  D. Stool softeners (docusate) allow water to penetrate GI contents

V. Antacids increase gastric pH, reducing irritation

**Table 20-5** Respiratory drugs

| Generic | Trade name(s) | Route(s) | Notes |
|---|---|---|---|
| **BRONCHODILATORS** | | | |
| Albuterol | Ventolin, Proventil | PO, inhalation | Most adverse effects are dose related and generally transient |
| Terbutaline | Brethine | SC, PO, inhalation | |
| Metaproterenol | Alupent | PO, inhalation | |
| Aminophylline | Many | IV, IM (painful), PO | Do not inject air into multidose vials; $CO_2$ causes drug to precipitate; narrow therapeutic index |
| Theophylline | | IV, IM, PO | Available in sustained-release oral dose form |
| **INHALED STEROIDS** | | | |
| Fluticasone | Flovent | MDI (multiple dose inhaler) | Use a spacer for administration |
| Beclomethasone | Vanceril, QVAR | MDI | Use a spacer for administration |
| **ANTIHISTAMINES** | | | |
| Chlorpheniramine | Many | PO | Do not allow time-released capsules to dissolve before oral administration |
| Cyproheptadine | Periactin | PO | Also used for appetite stimulation in cat |
| Diphenhydramine | Benadryl | IV, IM, PO | Intravenous form used to counteract anaphylactic reactions |
| Hydroxyzine | Atarax | PO | All antihistamines may cause sedation |
| Clemastine | Tavist | PO | Do not use the over-the-counter product Tavist-D |
| Trimeprazine (with prednisolone) | Temaril-P | PO | Combination antihistamine/corticosteroid |
| **ANTITUSSIVES** | | | |
| Butorphanol | Torbutrol, Torbugesic | IV, IM, SC, PO | Narcotic cough suppressant |
| Codeine | Many | PO | Cough syrups containing codeine are usually combination drug products |
| Hydrocodone | Hycodan, Tussigon | PO | Narcotic cough suppressant |
| Dextromethorphan | Robitussin | PO | Nonnarcotic cough suppressant; available over the counter |
| **DECONGESTANTS** | | | |
| Phenylpropanolamine | Propagest, Proin | PO | Most common use in veterinary medicine is to treat urinary incontinence |
| **MUCOLYTICS** | | | |
| Acetylcysteine | Mucomyst | IV, PO, inhalation | Also antidote for acetaminophen toxicity |
| **STIMULANTS** | | | |
| Doxapram | Dopram | IV, SC, sublingual | Use in newborn resuscitation is controversial |

A. Systemic antacids block gastric acid production by one of several means
  1. H-blockers, such as cimetidine, ranitidine, and famotidine, prevent the production of hydrochloric acid
  2. Omeprazole is a proton pump inhibitor that prevents hydrogen ions from being pumped into the stomach
  3. Misoprostol inhibits the release of hydrogen ions and stimulates production of bicarbonate and mucus in the stomach

VI. Antiulcer medications are used to treat defects in the stomach lining
  A. Nonsystemic antacids directly neutralize acid in the stomach; are usually salts of aluminum, calcium, or magnesium (Maalox, Amphogel, Mylanta, etc.)

**Table 20-6** Gastrointestinal (GI) drugs

| Generic | Trade name(s) | Route(s) | Notes |
|---|---|---|---|
| **ANTIEMETICS** | | | |
| Chlorpromazine | Thorazine | IV, IM, PO, rectal | Protect from light; may discolor urine to pink or red-brown |
| Dimenhydrinate | Dramamine | PO | Used primarily for motion sickness |
| Dolasetron | Anzemet | IV, IM, SC | Similar to ondansetron with once daily dosing |
| Meclizine | Antivert | PO | Primarily used for motion sickness |
| Metoclopramide | Reglan | IV (slow), IM, SC, PO | Promotility agent; inhibits gastroesophageal reflux |
| Ondansetron | Zofran | IV, PO | Indicated for refractory vomiting, chemotherapy sickness, and other hard to treat nausea |
| Prochlorperazine | Compazine | IM, SC, PO, rectal | Rectal suppositories available for at home use in vomiting animals |
| Maropitant citrate | Cerenia | SC, PO | Labeled for motion sickness, intractable vomiting in dogs |
| **ANTIULCER** | | | |
| Antacids | Amphogel, Maalox, Basalgel, Tums | PO | Neutralize acid; can affect absorption rates of other oral medications |
| Cimetidine | Tagamet | IV, IM (stings), SC, PO | Oral form available over the counter (OTC); do not refrigerate injectable form |
| Famotidine | Pepcid | IV, IM, SC, PO | Oral form available OTC |
| Nizatidine | Axid | PO | Similar to ranitidine with prokinetic activity |
| Ranitidine | Zantac | IV (slow), IM (stings), SC, PO | Reduces gastric acid output |
| Sucralfate | Carafate | PO | Forms a protective barrier at gastric ulcer site; give 30 min before other antacids |
| Misoprostol | Cytotec | PO | May cause GI side effects such as diarrhea |
| Omeprazole | Prilosec | PO | A proton-pump inhibitor, may affect absorption rates of drugs requiring a low stomach pH |
| **APPETITE STIMULANTS** | | | |
| Cyproheptadine | Periactin | PO | Appetite stimulation in cat; may take more than one dose to be effective |
| Diazepam | Valium | IV | Appetite stimulation in cats; effective immediately after injection; dose is a fraction of that used for sedation |
| Oxazepam | Serax | PO | Appetite stimulation in cats |
| **ANTISPASMODICS** | | | |
| Aminopentamide | Centrine | IM, SC, PO | Hypomotility drug; if urine retention noted as a side effect, discontinue |
| **STIMULANTS** | | | |
| Metoclopramide | Reglan | IV (slow), IM, SC, PO | Do not use if GI obstruction is suspected |
| Cisapride | | PO | Has been removed from U.S. market; used in management of feline chronic constipation |
| **LAXATIVES** | | | |
| Magnesium salts | Milk of Magnesia | PO | Hyperosmotic; holds water in GI tract and softens stool |
| Bisacodyl | Dulcolax | PO, rectal suppository | Stimulant laxative |
| Lactulose | Enulose | PO | Hyperosmotic; also used to reduce blood ammonia levels in hepatic disease |
| Docusate | Colace, DSS | PO, enema | Stool softener; watch hydration status |

**Table 20-6**  Gastrointestinal (GI) drugs—cont'd

| Generic | Trade name(s) | Route(s) | Notes |
|---|---|---|---|
| **ANTIDIARRHEALS** | | | |
| Diphenoxylate/atropine | Lomotil | PO | Opiates reduce gut motility; a small amount of atropine reduces other narcotic effects |
| Kaolin/pectin | Kaopectate, K-P-Sol | PO | Kaopectate also contains salicylates; use with caution in cats |
| Bismuth subsalicylate | Pepto-Bismol | PO | May discolor the stool to black; use salicylates with caution in cats |
| **EMETICS** | | | |
| Apomorphine | | IV, IM, SC, topically in conjunctiva | If vomiting does not occur with initial dose, subsequent doses are not likely to be effective and may induce toxicity; wear gloves when handling |
| **MISCELLANEOUS** | | | |
| Ursodiol | Actigall | PO | Used to increase the flow of bile |
| S-adenosyl methionine (SAMe) | Denosyl | PO | Nutraceutical used as an adjunct to treatment of liver disease |
| Pancreatic enzymes | Viokase, Pancrezyme | PO | Products contain lipase, amylase, protease; cats strongly dislike the taste of powder forms |
| Activated charcoal | Toxiban, Liquichar | PO | Adsorbent used to prevent absorption of toxic elements in the GI tract |

B. Sucralfate is a protectant that binds to the surface of gastric ulcers

## ANTIPARASITIC DRUGS (Table 20-7)

I. Antiparasitics kill or inactivate internal and/or external parasites
   A. They may be drugs or insecticides
II. Rotating the antiparasitic used can help prevent parasite resistance

## HORMONES AND ENDOCRINE DRUGS (Table 20-8)

I. Most reproductive drugs are hormones; these include the estrogens, progestins, prostaglandins, and oxytocin
   A. Estrogens
     1. May be used after mismating to prevent pregnancy
     2. Interfere with ova by not letting them reach the uterus
     3. Aplastic anemia is one of many rare but serious side effects
   B. Progestins
     1. Used for estrous cycle regulation
       a. If a mare is in transitional anestrus, progestins can return the animal to proestrus
       b. If an animal is in proestrus, progestins can prevent estrus
     2. Liquid progestins can be absorbed through the skin; technicians should use caution and wear gloves when preparing and administering

C. Prostaglandins
     1. Lyse the corpus luteum
       a. Can initiate a new estrous cycle for animals in diestrus
       b. May cause abortion in pregnant animals and humans
     2. Prostaglandins are easily absorbed through skin; use caution and wear protective apparel
       a. See MSDS or package insert for handling precautions
   D. Oxytocin
     1. Causes uterine contraction and milk letdown
     2. Contraindicated if cervix is not dilated
II. Examples of commonly used endocrine drugs are insulin and thyroid supplements
   A. Insulin
     1. Insulin is measured as international units (IU) per milliliter
     2. Only insulin syringes should be used to measure insulin
     3. Each mark on an insulin syringe is equal to 1 IU
     4. Insulin is available in U-100 and U-40 concentrations
       a. Each concentration has its own syringe type that must be used to measure that particular concentration. If U-100 insulin is measured in a U-40 syringe the animal will receive an overdose that is $2.5\times$ the desired dose
     5. Insulin removes glucose from circulation and stores it in tissues

**Table 20-7** Antiparasitics

| Generic | Trade name(s)* | Route(s) | Efficacy | Notes |
|---|---|---|---|---|
| Ivermectin | Ivomec, Heartgard Plus, Iverheart Plus | IM, SC, PO | Effective against most internal parasites except cestodes and liver flukes; used as a heartworm preventative and microfilaricide | Collies and similar breeds may be sensitive to ivermectin; use with caution and observe for adverse reactions |
| Selamectin | Revolution | Topical | Dog: adult and developing fleas, heartworms, ear mites, sarcoptic mange<br>Cat: also controls hookworm and roundworms | Safe for ivermectin-sensitive Collies |
| Moxidectin | Proheart, Advantage Multi | SC, topical | Heartworm preventive | Injectable has been removed from the U.S. market indefinitely |
| Milbemycin oxime | Interceptor, Sentinel | PO | Heartworm preventive also effective against hookworms, roundworms, and whipworms | May cause shocklike reaction in dogs with large numbers of microfilaria |
| Lufenuron | Program, Sentinel | SC, PO | Interrupts flea life cycle | Inhibits chitin production; does not kill adult fleas |
| Nitenpyram | Capstar | PO | Adult fleas | Kills 98% of adult fleas on pet within 6 hr of administration and for about 24 hr |
| Fipronil | Frontline | Topical | Adult fleas and ticks | Transient irritation may occur at site of spot-on administration |
| Imidacloprid | Advantage, Advantage Multi | Topical | Adult fleas | Advantage may be used weekly for severe infestations |
| Pyrethrins (permethrin) | Many insect sprays and over-the-counter (OTC) flea/tick spot-ons | Topical | Insects | Neurotoxin insecticide; many permethrin toxicity cases in cat are due to inappropriate application |
| Organophosphates | Many (home and yard, area, and pet products) | PO, topical | Many internal and external parasites | Use of or exposure to more than one organophosphate at a time greatly increases the possibility of toxicity; signs of toxicity include salivation, lacrimation, urination, defecation, dyspnea, and emesis |
| Amitraz | Mitaban, Preventic Collar, Taktic, ProMeris Duo | Topical | *Demodex* mites, other ectoparasites | Avoid contact with skin; avoid breathing fumes; can be toxic to cat and rabbit; may cause transient sedation and central nervous system depression, and may interact with antidepressant medications |
| Benzimidazole (mebendazole, fenbendazole, albendazole, etc.) | Panacur, Telmin, Valbazen | PO | Roundworms, hookworms, tapeworms (except *Dipylidium caninum*), some lungworms, large and small strongyles | |
| Epsiprantel | Cestex | PO | Tapeworms | |
| Metronidazole | Flagyl | IV, PO | Antiprotozoal | See Table 20-1 |
| Piperazine | Pipa-Tabs (OTC) | PO | Roundworms | |
| Praziquantel | Droncit, Drontal Plus | IM/SC (stings), PO | Tapeworms | |

**Table 20-7** Antiparasitics—cont'd

| Generic | Trade name(s)* | Route(s) | Efficacy | Notes |
|---------|----------------|----------|----------|-------|
| Pyrantel | Nemex, Strongid, Heartgard Plus, Iverheart Plus | PO | Roundworms, hookworms | Piperazine antagonizes the effects of pyrantel |
| Melarsomine | Immiticide | IM only (stings) | Heartworm adulticide | Swelling at injection site common; posttreatment thromboembolism is possible with adulticide therapy; minimize activity after treatment to reduce this risk |
| Methoprene (precor), nylar, fenoxycarb | Adams, Defend, Ectokyl, ProTICall, Knockout | Topical, environmental applications | Fleas | Insect growth regulators are added to many flea control products; interrupt flea life cycle |
| Metaflumizone | ProMeris, ProMeris Duo | Topical | Fleas | Reported to be effective up to 6 wk |

*Of products containing this ingredient. Many antiparasitics are combination formulas that may contain two or more drugs.

6. Insulin is available in three forms
  a. Regular insulin (short acting) is used when a rapid drop in blood sugar is needed
  b. NPH insulin (intermediate acting) is used to control diabetes mellitus on a daily basis
  c. Protamine zinc insulin (long-acting) is used in animals, usually cats, that need a slower release of insulin to carry them through 24 hours
B. Thyroid medications
  1. The pituitary gland secretes thyroid stimulating hormone (TSH), which tells the thyroid gland to produce and secrete the hormones triiodothyronine ($T_3$) and thyroxine ($T_4$)
  2. These hormones regulate the metabolic rate for the rest of the body
  3. Two common conditions associated with the thyroid gland are hypothyroidism (usually seen in dogs) and hyperthyroidism (usually seen in cats)
  4. Hypothyroidism occurs when thyroid function is decreased
    a. This can happen when the thyroid gland is diseased (primary hypothyroidism) or when the pituitary gland is diseased (secondary hypothyroidism)
    b. Hypothyroidism slows metabolic processes
    c. Thyroid supplementation is the treatment of choice for hypothyroidism
    d. Synthetic $T_3$, synthetic $T_4$, and thyroid extract are the supplementation choices available
      (1) Thyroid extract is highly variable in its effectiveness
      (2) Oversupplementation is common with $T_3$ administration
      (3) $T_4$ supplements are usually indicated in animals
  5. Hyperthyroidism occurs when thyroid function is increased, thus speeding up metabolic processes

    a. Thyroidectomy is usually an option for hyperthyroid treatment
    b. Two other courses of treatment are also available
      (1) Methimazole (Tapazole), which interferes with the production of $T_3$ and $T_4$
      (2) Introduction of radioactive iodine, which is taken up by the thyroid gland and destroys any tumor cells (and most of the normal thyroid cells) that are present

# IMMUNOLOGICAL DRUGS (Table 20-9) ■■■■

Also see Chapter 8.
I. The sheer number of vaccines available to induce active immunity limits their discussion in this chapter to general characteristics
  A. Vaccines are used to prevent disease or to reduce the virulence of diseases that animals may contract
    1. Vaccines cannot cure a disease process that is present before vaccination
  B. Vaccines stimulate an animal's immune system by introducing an antigen derived from pathogenic agents and encouraging an anamnestic response
    1. Vaccines are described as live, modified live, or killed
    2. Killed vaccines are safest but tend to be less effective than the other forms
    3. Modified live and live vaccines tend to be more effective, but are also more likely to induce disease and may be dangerous to pregnant animals
  C. Vaccines are available in many forms, including injections, intranasal solutions, powdered feed additives, aerosol sprays, and water additives
  D. Vaccine efficacy depends on several factors, including dose given, route of administration, age of animal, storage conditions, health/immune status of animal, and breed/species of animal

**Table 20-8** Hormones and other endocrine drugs

| Generic | Trade name(s) | Route(s) | Notes |
|---|---|---|---|
| **ESTROGENS** | | | |
| Estradiol | ECP | IM | Primarily used to induce estrus; prevents pregnancy after mismating in dog and cat (rare use); toxic to bone marrow; contraindicated in pregnancy |
| Diethylstilbestrol (DES) | | PO | Used to treat estrogen-responsive urinary incontinence and other conditions in dog and cat; toxic to bone marrow; contraindicated in pregnancy; banned in food animals |
| **PROGESTINS** | | | |
| Megestrol | Ovaban, Megace | PO | For false pregnancy, control of estrous cycle; contraindicated in pregnancy; can induce hypoadrenocorticism, personality changes, transient diabetes, and many other possible side effects |
| Altrenogest | Regu-Mate | PO | Used primarily in horses to synchronize estrus or maintain pregnancy; many handling warnings |
| Medroxy-progesterone | Depo-Provera | IM, SC, PO | Used in treatment of some behavioral and dermatologic conditions; many side effects |
| **ANDROGENS** | | | |
| Testosterone | | IM, SC | Testosterone products are now Class III controlled substances with limited use in veterinary medicine |
| Mibolerone | | PO | Prevention of estrus and treatment of pseudocyesis in adult dog; not recommended for cats |
| **PROSTAGLANDINS** | | | |
| Dinoprost | Lutalyse | SC | Causes uterine contents to be expelled; pregnant women and asthmatics should handle only with extreme caution |
| Fluprostenol | Equimate | SC | For large animal use |
| Cloprostenol | Estrumate | SC | For large animal use |
| **PITUITARY HORMONES** | | | |
| Desmopressin | DDAVP | SC, intranasal | An antidiuretic hormone used in control of diabetes insipidus |
| Oxytocin | Pitocin | IV, IM, SC | Induction/enhancement of uterine contractions at parturition |
| Corticotropin | Cortrosyn | IV, IM | Used in the adrenocorticotropic hormone stimulation test |
| **STEROIDS** | | | |
| Fludrocortisone | Florinef | PO | Mineralocorticoid for treatment of hypoadrenocorticism |
| Desoxycortico-sterone (DOCP) | Percorten-V | IM | Mineralocorticoid for treatment of hypoadrenocorticism |
| Stanozolol | Winstrol | PO | Anabolic steroid; rarely used; controlled substance in United States |
| Nandrolone | Deca-Durabolin | IM | Anabolic steroid; rarely used; controlled substance in United States |
| **STEROID INHIBITORS** | | | |
| Mitotane, trilostane | Lysodren, Vetoryl | PO | For treatment of pituitary-dependent hyperadrenocorticism; trilostane must be imported into United States |
| Selegiline (L-deprenyl) | Anipryl, Eldepryl | PO | For treatment of hyperadrenocorticism; also used in the treatment of canine cognitive dysfunction |

**Table 20-8** Hormones and other endocrine drugs—cont'd

| Generic | Trade name(s) | Route(s) | Notes |
|---|---|---|---|
| **ANTIDIABETICS** | | | |
| Insulin | Many | SC | Store in refrigerator; mix gently—do not shake before using; clients should be given thorough instructions on the use of insulin |
| Glipizide, glyburide | Glucotrol, Micronase | PO | Oral hypoglycemic agents |
| **DRUGS AFFECTING THYROID HORMONE** | | | |
| Levothyroxine | Soloxine, Thyrozine | PO | $T_4$ thyroid hormone supplement |
| Liothyronine | Cytobin | PO | $T_3$ hormone supplement; may be useful in hypothyroid cases that do not respond to $T_4$ |
| Methimazole | Tapazole | PO | Used in the medical management of hyperthyroidism |

E. It is not known when passive immunity via maternal antibodies ceases to protect neonates; therefore multiple doses of vaccine are required at regular intervals to optimize protection for young animals

F. Most vaccines are not effective immediately after administration

   1. Some take 2 weeks or more to reach maximum efficacy

G. Warming vaccines just before use reduces pain of administration

II. Vaccines that produce passive immunity by providing the animal with a short-term supply of ready-made antibodies come in two basic forms

A. Antitoxins contain antibodies to specific toxins (e.g., *Clostridium, Tetanus*)

B. Antiserums contain antibodies to specific microorganisms (e.g., *Escherichia coli, Salmonella*)

III. Drugs such as Acemannan (derived from aloe vera), Staphage Lysate, and Immunoregulin may help stimulate the immune system in certain conditions

IV. Immunosuppressants are used to treat diseases in which the animal's immune system is responding inappropriately

A. Drugs such as azathioprine, cyclosporine, cyclophosphamide, and corticosteroids are used for various immunosuppressive effects

## TOPICAL DRUGS

I. Topical drugs are applied to the skin surface, including mucous membranes, and may be administered into or onto the ear, eye, nose, mouth, prepuce, or vulva

A. Generally, topical drugs are not absorbed well systemically

   1. Drugs labeled for transdermal (TD) or transmucosal (TM) administration are formulated for systemic absorption

B. Because veterinary patients tend to lick their wounds, read package instructions carefully

   1. Extra caution is warranted when using human products, because they are more likely to be toxic if consumed

C. Wear proper protective clothing when applying topical drugs that are meant to be absorbed systemically (e.g., nitroglycerin and pour-on preparations)

II. Ophthalmic agents are usually in drop or ointment form and may require multiple applications to be effective. Read the package inserts and advise clients accordingly

A. Mydriatics, such as atropine, are used to dilate the pupil

   1. Tropicamide is a rapidly acting mydriatic used in the veterinary hospital to prepare a patient for ocular fundus examination

B. Miotics, such as pilocarpine, cause pupillary constriction

C. Several drugs are used to reduce intraocular pressure; they work by either reducing aqueous humor production or having a diuretic effect on the eye

D. Proparacaine and tetracaine are ophthalmic anesthetics

E. Cyclosporine stimulates increased tear production

F. There are numerous ophthalmic antiinfective agents and antiinflammatory agents

   1. Preparations containing steroids should NOT be used if a corneal ulcer could be present

III. Otic preparations are most often either antiinfective (antibacterial, antifungal, antiparasitic), antiinflammatory, or both

A. Many of these drugs should NOT be used in the presence of a ruptured eardrum, so an examination is necessary before they can be dispensed

**Table 20-9** Chemotherapeutic and immunological agents

| Generic | Trade name(s) | Route(s) | Toxicity/notes |
|---|---|---|---|
| **ALKYLATING AGENTS** | | | |
| Carboplatin | Paraplatin | IV | Bone marrow, gastrointestinal (GI) |
| Cisplatin | Platinol | IV | Bone marrow, GI; do not use in cats |
| Chlorambucil | Leukeran | PO | Bone marrow, GI |
| Cyclophosphamide | Cytoxan | IV, PO | Bone marrow, GI, hemorrhagic cystitis |
| Dacarbazine | DTIC-Dome | IV | GI; do not use in cats |
| Lomustine | CCNU, Ceenu | PO | Bone marrow, GI, hepatopathy |
| **ANTIMETABOLITES** | | | |
| Cytarbarine | Cytosar-U | IV, SC | Bone marrow, GI |
| Methotrexate | | IV, PO | Bone marrow, GI, renal |
| 5-Fluorouracil | | IV | Bone marrow, GI, central nervous system (CNS); do not use in cats |
| **ANTIBIOTICS** | | | |
| Doxorubicin | Adriamycin | IV | Bone marrow, GI, cardiac, urticaria, alopecia, vesicant |
| **MITOTIC INHIBITORS** | | | |
| Vincristine | Oncovin | IV | GI, peripheral nervous system, vesicant; skin contact causes irritation |
| Vinblastine | Velban | IV | Bone marrow, GI, alopecia; vesicant; skin contact causes irritation |
| **MISCELLANEOUS CHEMOTHERAPEUTICS** | | | |
| Asparaginase | Elspar | IV, SC | Anaphylaxis, coagulation disorder |
| Hydroxyurea | Hydrea | PO | Bone marrow, GI, alopecia, dysuria |
| Mitoxantrone | Novantrone | IV | Bone marrow, GI |
| Piroxicam | Feldene | PO | GI ulceration |
| **IMMUNOSUPPRESSANTS** | | | |
| Azathioprine | Imuran | PO | Bone marrow, immunosuppression |
| Cyclophosphamide | See above | | |
| Cyclosporine | Sandimmune, Neoral, Atopica | Ophthal-mic, PO | Used for immune suppression, treatment of atopy, and stimulation of tear production |
| Corticosteroids | See Table 20-2 | | |
| Metronidazole | See Table 20-1 | | |
| **IMMUNOSTIMULANTS** | | | |
| Acemannan | | | Aloe vera derived |
| *Staphylococcus* phage lysate | SPL | | Lethargy, fever, chills, injection site Irritation; used in treatment of pyoderma |
| *Propionibacterium acnes* | Immunoregulin | IV | Lethargy, fever, chills |
| *Mycobacterium* cell wall fraction | Regressin | Intratu-mor | Fever, lethargy |
| Interferon alpha-2a (human), omega (feline) | Roferon, Virba-gen Omega, Trental | SC, PO | Feline interferon not yet available in United States |

**Table 20-9** Chemotherapeutic and immunological agents—cont'd

| Generic | Trade name(s) | Route(s) | Toxicity/notes |
|---|---|---|---|
| **OTHERS** | | | |
| Pentoxifylline | | PO | GI, CNS; used in treatment of immune-mediated dermatosis (dogs), endotoxemia and navicular disease (horses) |
| Erythropoietin | Epogen, Procrit | SC | Autoantibody formation may limit usefulness in treatment of nonregenerative anemia |
| Filgrastim (granulocyte colony-stimulating factor) | Neupogen | SC | Autoantibody formation/immune response to human DNA-origin drug may worsen neutropenia |

**Table 20-10** Antidotes and reversal agents

| Generic | Trade name(s) | Uses/indications |
|---|---|---|
| Acetylcysteine | Mucomyst | Acetaminophen toxicity |
| Antivenin (Crotalidae) polyvalent | Antivenin | Poisonous snake envenomation (United States) |
| Atipamezole | Antisedan | Reversal of medetomidine (Domitor) |
| Atropine | Many | Organophosphate toxicity |
| Calcium EDTA | Calcium Disodium Versenate | Lead poisoning |
| Crotalidae polyvalent immune FAB (ovine) | Crofab | Crotalid snake envenomation |
| Cyproheptadine | Periactin | Serotonin syndrome (selective serotonin reuptake inhibitor toxicity) |
| Dantrolene | Dantrium | Malignant hyperthermia |
| Dimercaprol | BAL in Oil | Arsenic, lead, mercury, gold toxicity |
| Ethanol | Many | Ethylene glycol toxicity |
| Flumazenil | Romazicon | Reversal of benzodiazepines (Valium) |
| Fomepizole (4-MP) | Antizol-Vet | Ethylene glycol toxicity |
| Methylene blue | Urolene Blue | Nitrate, chlorate toxicity in ruminants |
| Naloxone | Narcan | Opioid agonist reversal |
| Pamidronate | Aredia | Cholecalciferol toxicosis |
| Neostigmine | Stiglyn | Neuromuscular-blocking agent toxicity (pancuronium, succinylcholine) |
| Penicillamine | Cuprimine | Lead, copper toxicity |
| Pralidoxime (2-PAM) | Protopam | Organophosphate toxicity |
| Yohimbine | Yobine | Reversal of xylazine (Rompun) |

B. Many are also ineffective in the presence of debris, so the ear canals must be cleaned before medications are used

IV. Drugs used on the skin come in several forms
  A. Shampoos, conditioners, and sprays
  B. Wound-healing agents, such as cleansers, protectants, and healing stimulators

## CHEMOTHERAPEUTIC DRUGS
(See Table 20-9)

I. Antineoplastic agents kill cells. They do not discriminate between "good" cells and "bad" cells, or between animal cells and human cells. Therefore it is extremely important to wear protective clothing when administering or preparing these agents
  A. Consult the MSDS, package insert, and hospital procedures manual for information about the safe handling of chemotherapeutic drugs

B. These drugs target rapidly dividing cells, such as those in tumors, bone marrow, GI tract, and reproductive tract
  1. They can cause permanent alterations to DNA

C. Doses are administered according to body surface (measured in meters squared, not body weight)

D. There are five basic types of antineoplastic drugs: alkylating agents, antimetabolites, plant alkaloids, antibiotics, and hormonal agents
  1. Chemotherapy is often a scheduled combination or alternation of two or more of these agents, depending on the cancer type and stage
  2. This complicated treatment system is often best left to cancer specialists

II. Hematinics are substances that promote an increase in the oxygen-carrying capacity of the blood

A. Iron, copper, and B vitamins support the formation of hemoglobin
B. Erythropoietin is a growth hormone produced by the kidneys that stimulates red blood cell production
   1. A synthetic form is available for injection
C. Androgens (anabolic steroids), although rarely used because of the problems associated with them, may be beneficial in treating certain chronic anemias
D. Blood substitutes, such as Oxyglobin, can increase oxygen-carrying capacity temporarily while the body grows new red blood cells
III. Anticoagulants, such as heparin and coumarin derivatives, are sometimes used to treat thrombotic disease in vivo, but anticoagulants in general are more commonly used to preserve blood samples in vitro
IV. Thrombolytics, such as streptokinase, have largely proved minimally effective and cost-prohibitive in the treatment of thromboembolic disease in animals

## ANTIDOTES AND REVERAL AGENTS
(Table 20-10)

## SUMMARY

Pharmacology is an inexact science. Any given drug may affect different animal species, or even individual animals within one species, unpredictably. Remember to treat each patient as an individual and pay attention to any abnormal behavior displayed by an animal being treated with any pharmaceutical. Used correctly, drugs are a great benefit to veterinary medicine; used incorrectly, they can be detrimental.

## ACKNOWLEDGMENT

The editors and author recognize and appreciate the original work of Cathy Painter, on which this chapter is based.

# Glossary

**absorption** Movement of drug from the site of administration to the bloodstream
**adrenergic** Agent that acts like adrenaline (epinephrine)
**adverse effect** Any effect that a drug causes other than the intended effect; may be mild to severe or fatal
**agonist** Drug that binds to a specific receptor site and causes the cell to react
**alkylating agent** Compounds that combine readily with other molecules and are used in chemotherapy of cancer
**α-blockers** Agents that inhibit the activities of α-receptors in the sympathetic nervous system

**analgesics** Pain relievers
**anamnestic response** A secondary immune response; occurs following a subsequent exposure to an antigen
**antagonist** Drug that binds to a specific receptor site and prevents a cell reaction
**antiarrhythmic** Agent that prevents or stops cardiac arrhythmias
**anticholinergics** Drugs that block stimulation of the parasympathetic nervous system; also called parasympatholytics
**antiemetic** Agent that relieves vomiting
**antimetabolite** Substance that interferes with the use of an essential metabolite
**antimicrobial** Suppression of microorganism either by killing it or stopping its multiplication or growth
**antineoplastic** Agent that inhibits the maturing and growth of tumor cells
**antispasmodic** Preventing or relieving spasms
**antitussive** Cough suppressant
**bactericidal** Kills bacteria
**bacteriostatic** Prevents the growth or reproduction of bacteria
**β-blocker** A drug that blocks the action of adrenaline at beta-adrenergic receptors; effects include increased heart rate and contractions, vasodilation of the arterioles that supply the skeletal muscles, and relaxation of the bronchial muscles
**biotransformation** See Metabolism
**bronchodilator** Agent that causes dilation of the bronchi
**catecholamine** Chemical released by the body to respond to stress
**cholinergics** Drugs that stimulate the parasympathetic nervous system; also called parasympathomimetics
**compounded drugs** Manipulation of a drug that is not provided for in an FDA approved drug label
**contraindications** Situations in which a drug should NOT be used
**DEA, Drug Enforcement Administration (United States)** Controls drugs that have the potential for abuse
**diffusion** Process of spreading, especially from areas of greater concentration to areas of lesser concentration
**distribution** Movement of drug from the bloodstream into tissues
**diuretic** Drug that promotes water loss via increased urine formation and excretion
**drug** Any substance used in the diagnosis, treatment, or prevention of disease or other pathological condition
**$ED_{50}$** Dose of a drug that is effective in 50% of the animals to which it is administered in a trial
**efficacy** Ability of a drug to create its intended effects
**emetic** Substance that promotes vomiting
**excretion** Elimination of circulating drug metabolites from the body, usually in urine, but also in feces, sweat, or breath
**expectorant** Agent that promotes coughing or swallowing material from the trachea, bronchi, or lungs
**extra-label** Use of a drug for any other than its indicated uses
**first-pass effect** Orally administered drugs travel to the liver before reaching the systemic circulation and may be removed before getting into the general circulation
**generic** Nonproprietary drug name, usually derived from its chemical structure
**helminthic** Pertaining to a parasitic worm

**indication** An approved use of a drug

**ingesta** Stomach contents

**inotropic** Affecting the force of the cardiac contraction

**LD$_{50}$** Dose of a drug that is lethal to 50% of the animals to which it is administered in a trial

**metabolism** Changes in the chemical structure of a drug caused by the liver and, to a lesser degree, other organs from the form in which it was administered to one that can be eliminated from the body

**miotic** Drug that contracts the pupil

**mucolytic** Destroying or dissolving mucus

**mydriatic** Drug that dilates the pupil

**OTC (over-the-counter)** Drugs that do not require a prescription for purchase

**overdose** Condition of having too much drug in the body, due to incorrect administration or drug accumulation, which leads to toxicity

**parasympathetic** Part of the nervous system concerned with maintaining homeostasis

**perfusion** Passage of blood through the vessels of a tissue

**perianesthetic** Period of time before, during, and after an anesthetic episode

**pH** Degree of acidity or alkalinity

**pharmacokinetics** Study of drug actions and effects on the body

**pK$_a$** Specific pH at which a drug is equally composed of ionized and nonionized molecules

**poison** Substance that may cause structural damage or functional disturbance within the body

**precautions** A list of usually mild side effects or rare adverse reactions that can be found on a drug label or package insert

**proprietary** Drug name assigned and owned by a particular manufacturer

**psychoactive** Affecting mental state

**resistance** Ability of an organism to adapt and survive in an environment containing an antimicrobial to which it was previously susceptible

**solubility** Ability of a solid to dissolve in a liquid

**susceptibility** Vulnerability of an organism to an antimicrobial

**suspension** Solid particles suspended in but not dissolved in a liquid

**therapeutic range** Ideal range of drug concentration in the body, where it is effective but not toxic

**thrombolytic** Agent that dissolves a blood clot

**thyroidectomy** Removal of the thyroid gland

**TI (therapeutic index)** Relationship between ability of a drug to achieve its desired effect compared with its tendency to produce toxic effects

**vasodilator** Causing dilation of blood vessels

**Vd (volume of distribution)** Body space in which a drug will be distributed; a calculated number representing the amount of drug/amount of body space

**withdrawal time** Time after administration of a drug to a food-producing animal during which the products of that animal cannot be sold for human consumption

# Review Questions

**1** Insulin is dosed in what unit of measurement?
a. mL
b. tsp
c. IU
d. g

**2** In what class of drugs are nephrotoxicity, neurotoxicity, and ototoxicity problems?
a. Barbiturates
b. Aminoglycosides
c. Phenothiazine tranquilizers
d. Dissociative anesthetics

**3** With what group of animals is withdrawal time especially important?
a. Food animals
b. Exotics
c. Equids
d. Pets

**4** What is the primary organ involved in excretion of drugs?
a. Liver
b. Intestine
c. Kidney
d. Spleen

**5** A cow is accidentally dosed with an equine dose of xylazine. What drug should be immediately administered?
a. None: the cow cannot survive that amount of xylazine
b. Epinephrine followed by naloxone
c. Yohimbine
d. Do nothing

**6** The therapeutic index is
a. The comparison between the ability of a drug to reach the desired effect and its tendency to produce toxic effects
b. The dose of a drug that produces the lethal dose in 50% of the animals tested
c. The comparison between the ability of a drug to reach a toxic effect and a lethal effect
d. The dose of a drug that produces the effective dose in 50% of the animals tested

**7** The "first-pass effect" is
a. Blood-brain barrier
b. Metabolization of drugs containing proteins
c. Reduction of drugs reaching the systemic circulation by the liver
d. Ionization of drugs

**8** Which drug requires protective clothing when handled?
a. Xylazine
b. Torbugesic
c. Prostaglandin
d. Lidocaine

**9** Vaccines may fail because
a. Animal is too young for the vaccine to be effective
b. Vaccine was improperly stored
c. Animal was febrile at the time of administration
d. All of the above

**10** A dog is seen eating battery acid
   a. Emesis should be induced as soon as possible
   b. Emesis should not be induced
   c. The veterinarian may prescribe a laxative to relieve the dog of the GI upset
   d. The veterinarian may prescribe an antacid, such as Magnolax or Maalox

## REFERENCES

1. Taylor EJ, editor: *Dorland's illustrated medical dictionary,* ed 30, Philadelphia, 2003, Saunders.
2. O'Toole MT, editor: *Miller-Keane encyclopedia and dictionary of medicine, nursing, and allied health,* ed 7, Philadelphia, 2005, Saunders.
3. Wanamaker BP, Massey KL: *Applied pharmacology for the veterinary technician,* ed 3, St Louis, 2004, Saunders.

## BIBLIOGRAPHY

Allen DG et al: *Handbook of veterinary drugs,* ed 3, Ames, Iowa, 2004, Blackwell.

Augustus M, Boss SB: Pharmacology and pharmacy. In McCurnin DM, Bassert JM, editors: *Clinical textbook for veterinary technicians,* ed 6, St Louis, 2006, Saunders.

Bill R: *Pharmacology for veterinary technicians,* ed 3, St Louis, 2006, Mosby.

Line S, Kahn CM, editors: *The Merck veterinary manual,* ed 9, Hoboken, NJ, 2005, John Wiley and Sons.

Muir W et al: *Handbook of veterinary anesthesia,* ed 3, St Louis, 2002, Mosby.

O'Toole MT, editor: *Miller-Keane encyclopedia and dictionary of medicine, nursing, and allied health,* ed 5, Philadelphia, 1992, Saunders.

O'Toole MT, editor: *Miller-Keane encyclopedia and dictionary of medicine, nursing, and allied health,* ed 7, Philadelphia, 2005, Saunders.

Plumb D: *Veterinary drug handbook,* ed 5, Ames, Iowa, 2005, Blackwell.

Rawlings CA, McCall JW: Melarsomine: a new heartworm adulticide, *Compend* 18:373, 1996.

Samuelson S: Pharmacology and pharmacy. In Sirois M, editor: *Principles and practice of veterinary technology,* ed 2, St Louis, 2004, Mosby.

Taylor EJ, editor: *Dorland's illustrated medical dictionary,* ed 27, Philadelphia, 1988, Saunders.

Taylor EJ, editor: *Dorland's illustrated medical dictionary,* ed 30, Philadelphia, 2003, Saunders.

Wanamaker BP, Massey KL: *Applied pharmacology for the veterinary technician,* ed 3, St Louis, 2004, Saunders.

## CHAPTER 21

# Pharmaceutical Calculations

*Monica M. Tighe*

## OUTLINE

Metric System
   Metric Conversions
   Metric Time
   Metric Date
   Metric Temperature

Metric Mass
Dosage Calculations
Dilutions/Solutions
Parts per Million
Drip Rates

Prescriptions
   Guidelines
   Veterinary Technician's Role in
      Dispensing Medications
   Prescription Labels

## LEARNING OUTCOMES

After reading this chapter you should be able to:

1. Describe the rules for writing metric, dates, and symbols.
2. Perform conversion of numbers to various metric units.
3. Calculate dosages.
4. Calculate dilutions.
5. Calculate concentrations of solutions.
6. Describe parts per million and calculate a parts per million dose.
7. Calculate drip rates.
8. Define the technician's role in dispensing medication.
9. Define the information that must be included on a prescription label.

This chapter contains basic information on the metric system, including the conversion of metric units. Formulas for calculating dosages, preparing solutions and dilutions, and estimating drip rates are also included with examples. This chapter also includes a brief section on prescription labels, an abbreviations list, and an equivalence chart. Check appendixes for further information.

## METRIC SYSTEM

The metric system can also be referred to as the SI system, or Système International d'Unités.

## Metric Conversions

I. Abbreviations of commonly used units are shown in Table 21-1. The prefix and a base unit are also shown
II. Metric unit conversion methods
  A. Step method
    1. Move the decimal place to the right if converting to a smaller unit, and to the left if converting to a larger unit
    2. Example: to convert 500 milligram (mg) to gram (g)
      a. As shown in Table 21-2, 500 mg is 0.001 of a gram (1000 mg = 1 g)
      b. Therefore the decimal must move 3 decimal places
      c. Also, 1 g is larger than 1 mg; therefore the decimal place must move to the left
      d. The answer is 0.5 g
  B. Proportion equation
    1. Example: to convert 500 mg to g
      a. According to the chart, 1 g = 1000 mg
      b. Therefore $x$ g/500 mg = 1 g/1000 mg
      c. ($x$ = unknown number)

$$\frac{x \, g}{500 \, mg} = \frac{1 \, g}{1000 \, mg}$$

$$1000 \, mg \times x \, g = 500 \, mg \times 1 \, g$$
$$x \, g = 500 \, mg \times 1 \, g \div 1000 \, mg$$
$$x \, g = 0.5 \, g$$

**Table 21-1** Prefix, abbreviation, and a base unit for metric units

| Prefix | Symbol | Value |
|--------|--------|-------|
| giga | G | base unit × $10^9$ (largest unit) |
| mega | M | base unit × $10^6$ |
| kilo | k | base unit × $10^3$ |
| hecto | h | base unit × $10^2$ |
| deca | dk | base unit × 10 |
| Base unit | | |
| gram | g | |
| meter | m | 1 |
| liter | L | |
| deci | d | base unit × $10^{-1}$ |
| centi | c | base unit × $10^{-2}$ |
| milli | m | base unit × $10^{-3}$ |
| micro | μ | base unit × $10^{-6}$ |
| nano | n | base unit × $10^{-9}$ |
| pico | p | base unit × $10^{-12}$ (smallest unit) |

**Table 21-2** Common medical units and conversions

| Unit | Value |
|------|-------|
| liter (L) to milliliter (mL) | 1 L = 1000 mL |
| gram (g) to milligram (mg) | 1 g = 1000 mg |
| milliliter (mL) to microliter (μL) | 1 mL = 1000 μL |
| meter (m) to centimeter (cm) | 1 m = 100 cm |
| kilometer (km) to meter (m) | 1 km = 1000 m |
| microgram (μg) to milligram | 1 μg = 0.001 mg |

## Metric Time

I. Measured in hours, minutes, and seconds using a 24-hour clock
   A. The 24-hour clock expresses the time in four digits beginning at midnight with 00:00 or 24:00
      1. The first two digits express the number of hours since midnight, and the second two digits express the number of minutes in that hour
   B. Example: The time at 2:53 PM is written 14:53
      1. There is no need to write AM or PM because it is expressed in the value of time

## Metric Date

I. A metric date is written in the following format: year/month/day/time (24-hour clock)
   A. Example: January 24, 2003, 5:50 PM, is written 2003/01/24 17:50
II. There may be a slash, dot, or space between the numbers
III. In the United States the date is commonly written month/day/year
   A. Example: 01/24/2003

## Metric Temperature

I. Celsius or C (capital C)
   A. Freezing point = 0° C at 1 atmospheric pressure
   B. Boiling point = 100° C at 1 atmospheric pressure
II. Fahrenheit or F
   A. Freezing point = 32° F at 1 atmospheric pressure
   B. Boiling point = 212° F at 1 atmospheric pressure
III. To convert from ° C to ° F use the formula
   A. $° F = ° C × \frac{9}{5} + 32$
IV. To convert from ° F to ° C use the formula
   A. $° C = ° F - 32 × \frac{5}{9}$

## Metric Mass

I. Gram (g) is the standard unit
II. Nonmetric unit is the pound (lb)
III. 1 kg = 2.204 lb
IV. To convert lb to kg
   A. kg = lb ÷ 2.204
V. To convert kg to lb
   A. lb = kg × 2.204
VI. One ton = 1000 kg or 2204 lb

## DOSAGE CALCULATIONS

I. Definitions
   A. Dose is the amount of medication measured (e.g., mg, mL, units)
   B. Dosage is the amount of medication based on units per weight of animal (e.g., 50 mg/kg, mL/kg, or tablets/kg)
   C. The concentration of a drug is calculated by the manufacturer (e.g., mg/mL, mg/tablet)
II. To calculate the dose in milligrams (mg) use the following formula
   A. Dose (mg) = weight (kg) × dosage (mg/kg)
   B. Example: What is the dose if a patient weighs 30 kg and the dosage is 10 mg/kg?
   C. Dose (mg) = 30 kg × 10 mg/kg
   D. Therefore dose = 300 mg
III. To calculate the dose in mL use the formula
   A. Dose (mL) = dose (mg) ÷ concentration (mg/mL)
   B. Example: What is the dose in milliliters (mL) of a drug, if the dose is 300 mg and the concentration of the drug is 50 mg/mL?
   C. Dose (mL) = dose (mg) ÷ concentration (mg/mL)
   D. Therefore dose = 300 mg ÷ 50 mg/mL = 6 mL
IV. To calculate the dose in tablets use the formula
   A. Dose (tablets) = dose (mg) ÷ concentration (mg/tablet)
   B. Example: What is the dose (in tablets) of a drug if the required dose is 100 mg and the concentration of the drug is 50 mg/tablet?
   C. Dose (tablets) = dose (mg) ÷ concentration (mg/tablet)
   D. Dose = 100 mg ÷ 50 mg/tablet = 2 tablets

V. Because drugs are manufactured in various concentrations, the milligram dose of a drug should always be recorded on the patient file (rather than the administered dose or mL/tablets)
   A. Example: 1 mL of acepromazine maleate is administered to a patient. If the concentration of acepromazine maleate is 10 mg/mL, the patient will receive 10 mg of the drug. However, if the concentration of acepromazine maleate is 25 mg/mL, and the patient was given 1 mL, the patient would have received 25 mg, or 2.5 times the prescribed amount

## DILUTIONS/SOLUTIONS

I. Definitions
   A. Solution: mixture of substances made by dissolving solids in liquids or liquids in liquids
   B. Solvent: solution capable of dissolving other substances
   C. Solute: substance that is dissolved in a liquid
   D. Dilution: reduction of a concentration of a substance
   E. Diluent: agent that dilutes
II. When working with solutions/dilutions, the concentration of the substance is the amount of solute dissolved in the solvent
III. Concentrations may be expressed as
   A. Volume per volume (or v/v) for liquids: percent volume in volume expresses the number of milliliters of solute in 100 mL of solution
   B. Weight per volume (or w/v): percent weight in volume expresses the number of grams (g) (weight) of solute in 100 mL of solution (volume)
   C. Weight per weight (or w/w) for solids: percent weight in weight expresses the number of grams (g) of a solute in 100 g of solution
IV. Calculating the percent strength of a solution (w/v)
   A. Use the formula: concentration (g/mL) = mass (g) ÷ volume (mL)
   B. Example: What is the strength of a solution if 20 g of powder is dissolved in 500 mL of liquid?
      1. Concentration (g/mL) = mass (g) ÷ volume (mL)
      2. Concentration = 20 g ÷ 500 mL = 0.04
      3. To find percent multiply the concentration by 100 (0.04 × 100 = 4%)
   C. Any of the quantities can be substituted in the equation (e.g., mass or volume or percent)
      1. Variations in the formula include
         a. Mass (g) = volume (mL) × concentration (g/mL)
         b. Volume (mL) = mass (g) ÷ concentration (g/mL)
   D. Percent (w/v) means that there are a number of grams of solute in 100 mL of solution

1. Example: A 5% (w/v) solution means that there are 5 g of solute in 100 mL of solution
2. A pure solution is assumed to be 100%, or 100 g of solution in 100 mL of solution
E. Concentration of a solution can also be expressed as a ratio
   1. 1:100 = 1 g/100 mL = 1% = 10 mg/mL
V. Calculating the strength of diluted solutions (v/v)
   A. If a pure solution is diluted, the result is a stock solution
   B. A weaker solution can be made by diluting it with solvent; however, a stronger solution requires the preparation of a new solution or the addition of pure solution
   C. Use the formula

Concentration of desired solution × volume of desired solution = concentration of stock × volume of stock

   D. Example: Prepare 2 L of a 25% solution given a 50% solution and sterile saline
      1. Substitute all known quantities and solve for the unknown $(x)$
         a. Concentration of desired solution is 25%
         b. Volume of the desired solution is 2000 mL or 2 L
         c. Concentration of the stock solution is 50%
         d. Volume of stock solution needed to prepare the solution is the unknown $(x)$

concentration of desired solution × volume of desired solution = concentration of stock × volume of stock

$$25\% \times 2000 \text{ mL} = 50\% \times x$$
$$25 \times 2000 = 50x$$
$$50,000 = 50x$$
$$50,000 \div 50 = x$$
$$1000 \text{ mL of the 50\% solution} = x$$

         e. To calculate the amount of sterile saline or diluent to add to the 1000 mL of 50% solution to make 2000 mL of 25% solution
            (1) Use the formula: Diluent = volume of desired solution − volume of stock solution

$$2000 \text{ mL} - 1000 \text{ mL} = 1000 \text{ mL}$$

            (2) Thus 1000 mL of 50% solution is added to 1000 mL of diluent to prepare 2000 mL of 25% solution

## PARTS PER MILLION

I. Parts per million (ppm) is defined as the number of parts of solute contained in 1 million parts of solution. One part per million is 1 g solute in 1,000,000 mL or 1 part/$10^6$

A. Example: What is the ppm for a 0.6% solution?
B. Knowing that a 0.6% solution = 0.6 g/100 mL = $x$/1,000,000
   1. 0.6 g × 1,000,000 = 100 mL × $x$
   2. $x$ = 0.6 × 1,000,000 ÷ 100
   3. $x$ = 6000 ppm

## DRIP RATES

I. Use this formula

$$\text{Drip rate} = \frac{\text{Volume of solution (mL)} \times \text{drops/mL}}{\text{time (seconds)}}$$

A. Volume of solution (mL) is the amount of solution to be administered
B. Drops/mL is the calibrated amount of an administration set determined by the company that produces it
   1. The drop/mL value is usually written on the administration set package
C. Time (seconds) is the amount of time that the fluids are to be administered
   1. Time could be expressed as seconds, minutes, or hours; however, the drip rate is usually expressed as drops/min
   2. To calculate how many minutes there are in a value expressed in seconds, divide the seconds by 60
D. Drip rate (drops/min) is the number of drops that are administered per 1 minute
E. Example: What is the drip rate if the volume of the solution is 1 L, the drops/mL = 20, and the time is 4 hours?

$$\text{Drip rate} = \frac{1000 \text{ mL} \times 20 \text{ drops/mL}}{4 \text{ hours} \times 60 \text{ minutes}}$$
(There are 60 minutes in 1 hour)
$$= \frac{20,000 \text{ drops}}{240 \text{ minutes}}$$
$$= 83.33 \text{ drops/min}$$

II. Variations on the formula include
A. Time = (volume × drops/mL) ÷ drip rate
   1. Example: How long will it take for 2 L of normal saline to be administered to a patient if the drops/mL is equal to 20 and the drip rate is 60 drops/min
   2. Time = 2 L × 20 drops/mL ÷ 60 drops/min
   3. Before continuing, 2 L must be converted to 2000 mL
   4. Therefore time = 2000 mL × 20 drops/mL ÷ 60 drops/min
   5. Time = 40,000 drops ÷ 60 drops/min
   6. Final answer is time = 666.666 minutes = 11.11 hours = 11 hours, 6.6 minutes
B. Volume = (drip rate × time) ÷ drops/mL

   1. Example: How much normal saline can be administered if the drip rate is 60 drops/min, the veterinarian would like the patient to receive the fluids in 4 hours, and the drops/mL is equal to 20?
   2. First convert the time of 4 hours to 240 minutes
   3. Volume = 60 drops/min × 240 minutes ÷ 20 drops/mL
   4. Volume = 14,400 drops ÷ 20 drops/mL
   5. Volume = 720 mL = 0.720 L

## PRESCRIPTIONS

### Guidelines

I. The American Veterinary Medical Association (AVMA) has approved the following guidelines
A. "A prescription drug can only be dispensed by or upon the lawful written order of a licensed veterinarian within the course of his or her professional practice where a valid veterinarian-client-patient relationship (VCPR) exists
   1. A VCPR exists when the following conditions have been met
      a. The veterinarian has assumed the responsibility for making clinical judgments regarding the health of the animal(s) and the need for medical treatment, and the client has agreed to follow the veterinarian's instructions
      b. The veterinarian has sufficient knowledge of the animal(s) to initiate at least a general or preliminary diagnosis of the medical condition of the animal(s)
      c. The veterinarian is readily available for follow-up evaluation or has arranged for emergency coverage in the event of adverse reactions of failure of the treatment regimen
B. All veterinary prescription drugs must be properly labeled when dispensed"[1]

### Veterinary Technician's Role in Dispensing Medications

I. The technician should not issue or refill medications without the veterinarian's approval
A. If medication is dispensed by a technician, this is in violation of federal law
II. The ultimate responsibility for any medication dispensed lies with the prescribing veterinarian
A. Technicians may only prepare labels, count tablets, pour medication, attach labels, and price the dispensed medication

### Prescription Labels

I. Even though most prescription labels are now generated by a computer, the label should be checked for accuracy before dispensing the drug

**Table 21-3** Abbreviations commonly used in veterinary medicine

| Abbreviations | Definition |
|---|---|
| ad lib. | Freely; as much as is wanted |
| $\overline{aa}$ | Of each |
| a.c. | Before meals |
| aqua | Water |
| aqua dist. | Distilled water |
| at diet. | As directed |
| b.i.d. | Twice daily |
| caps | Capsules |
| chart. | Powder |
| $\overline{c}$ | With |
| cc | Cubic centimeter |
| d.t.d. | Give such doses |
| $D_5W$ | 5% dextrose in water |
| gtt | A drop; drops |
| h | Hour |
| h.s. | Hour of sleep; at bedtime |
| IM | Intramuscular |
| IV | Intravenous |
| K | Potassium |
| M | Mix |
| non. rep. or N.R. | Do not repeat |
| No. | Number |
| o.h. | Every hour |
| O.D. | Right eye or overdose |
| O.S. | Left eye |
| os | Mouth |
| per os | Oral |
| pil. | Pill |
| p | After |
| p.c. | After meals |
| p.o. | By mouth |
| p.r.n. | According to circumstances; occasionally |
| q.2h | Every 2 hours |
| q.s. | A sufficient amount |
| q.i.d. | Four times a day |
| Q.R. | Quantity required |
| $R_x$ | Dispense |
| SC | Subcutaneous |
| SQ | Subcutaneous |
| SS | One-half |
| s.i.d. | Once daily |
| sig. | Write on label |
| s | Without |
| $S_x$ | Surgery |
| stat | Immediately |
| $T_x$ | Treatment |
| tab | Tablet |
| t.i.d. | Three times a day |
| Tr. | Tincture |
| Ung. | Ointment |

Sometimes these abbreviations are written without periods: for example, bid or po.

II. The label should contain the following information
  A. Name, address, and telephone number of the clinic
  B. Prescribing veterinarian's name
  C. Name of patient and client's last name and the species in some provinces/states
  D. Name of drug
  E. Concentration of drug and amount of drug dispensed
  F. Date
  G. The drug identification number (DIN) (check provincial/state regulations to determine if required)
  H. Refills should be noted
  I. Specific instructions (sig)
    1. No abbreviations should be used (Table 21-3)
      a. Example: b.i.d. should be written out as two times a day or every 12 hours
    2. If the medication is for the left or right eye, it should be noted on the label
    3. If the drug should be administered with food or without food, it should also be noted
    4. The instructions should be clearly typed
  J. The vial may also need additional labels, such as
    1. *For veterinary use only*
    2. *Keep refrigerated*
    3. *Keep out of reach of children*
    4. *Withdrawal time*
    5. *Shake well*
    6. *Do not use after* [date]
    7. *Poison*
    8. *External use only*
  K. A childproof container may be necessary to comply with state/provincial laws
    1. The vial may also need to be amber in color to prevent the breakdown of some drugs due to ultraviolet light
III. Also see Appendixes A and B for further information

# Review Questions

**1** How much sterile water is needed to make a 4% solution using 1 g of drug?
  a. 25 mL
  b. 400 mL
  c. 100 mL
  d. 50 mL
**2** Convert 6 mm to m
  a. 0.006 m
  b. 0.000006 m
  c. 6000 m
  d. 600 m

**3** Given a 45% solution and sterile diluent, how would you prepare 3 L of 15% solution? Take
  a. 200 mL of 45% and add 2000 mL of sterile diluent
  b. 1000 mL of sterile diluent and add 2 L of 45% solution
  c. 1000 mL of 45% solution and add 2 L of sterile diluent
  d. 2 L of water and add 4.5 L of 45% solution

**4** A previous client calls to report that her new pet needs some antibiotics. She will be by in 1 hour to pick up the prescription. What should the technician do?
  a. Explain to the client that a veterinarian must examine the animal before any medication can be dispensed
  b. Explain to the client that a technician cannot dispense medication and suggest that the client speak with the veterinarian
  c. Explain to the client that antibiotics require a prescription to be dispensed
  d. All of the above

**5** Given the following information: 1987 mL of saline at 15 drops/mL over an 8 hour period, the approximate drip rate should be
  a. 10.3/10 sec
  b. 1.05/10 sec
  c. 20/10 sec
  d. 1.92/sec

**6** Given a pure solution, how would you make 500 mL of 50% solution?
  a. Add 500 mL of 100% solution to 500 mL of water
  b. Add 100 mL of sterile water to 400 mL of pure solution
  c. Add 5000 mL of sterile water to 500 mL of 50% solution
  d. Take 250 mL of pure solution and add 250 mL of sterile water

**7** What is the concentration (mg/mL) and percentage of the following solution (w/v): 5 g added to 200 mL of sterile water
  a. 25 mg/mL, 2.5%
  b. 250 mg/mL, 2.5%
  c. 50 mg/mL, 5%
  d. 4 mg/mL, 40%

**8** What is the percent of the final solution (v/v) if 30 mL of solution is added to 70 mL of water?
  a. 30%
  b. 100%
  c. 10%
  d. 3%

**9** A dog weighs 20 kg, the dose rate is 5 mg/kg, and the tablet size is 50 mg. The prescription reads "100 mg bid for 10 days a.c." How many tablets are needed for 1 dose and for a 24-hour period?
  a. 2 tablets, 8 tablets
  b. 1 tablet, 2 tablets
  c. 2 tablets, 4 tablets
  d. 4 tablets, 8 tablets

**10** How would you prepare 1.5 L of a 1:200 (w/v) solution given a 12% solution and sterile water? Take
  a. 625 mL of the 12% solution and add 875 mL of sterile water
  b. 1437.5 mL of the 12% solution and add 62.5 mL of sterile water
  c. 62.5 mL of the 12% solution and add 1 437.5 mL of sterile water
  d. 875 mL of 12% solution and add 635 mL of sterile water

## REFERENCE

1. Augustus M, Boss SB: Pharmacology and pharmacy. In McCurnin DM, Bassert JM, editors: *Clinical textbook for veterinary technicians*, ed 6, St Louis, 2006, Saunders.

## BIBLIOGRAPHY

Ansel HC, Stoklosa MJ: *Pharmaceutical calculations*, ed 11, Philadelphia, 2001, Lippincott Williams & Wilkins.

Augustus M, Boss SB: Pharmacology and pharmacy. In McCurnin DM, Bassert JM, editors: *Clinical textbook for veterinary technicians*, ed 6, St Louis, 2006, Saunders.

Bill RL: *Clinical pharmacology and therapeutics for the veterinary technician*, ed 3, St Louis, 2006, Mosby.

Bill RL: *Medical mathematics and dosage calculations*, Ames, 2000, Iowa State University Press.

McConnell VC, Ritchie BW: *Calculations for the veterinary professional*, Ames, Iowa, 2000, Blackwell.

Petrie A, Watson P: *Statistics for veterinary and animal science*, Oxford, England, 1999, Blackwell Science.

Samuelson S: Pharmacology and pharmacy. In Sirois M, editor: *Principles and practice of veterinary technology*, ed 2, St Louis, 2004, Mosby.

# PART V

# Medical and Surgical Nursing

## CHAPTER 22

# Surgical Preparation and Instrument Care

*Rachael J. Higdon*

## OUTLINE

Surgical Instruments
  Scissors
  Forceps
  Needle Holders
  Retractors
  Common Orthopedic Instruments

Miscellaneous Instruments
  Needles and Suture Material
Instrument Care and Pack Preparation
  Instrument Care
  Preparing Instrument Packs and
    Linens

Patient Preparation
Draping
Surgeon and Sterile Assistant
  Surgical Scrub
Operating Room Conduct

## LEARNING OUTCOMES

After reading this chapter you should be able to:

1. Recognize common surgical instruments and define their intended use.
2. Identify types of surgical needles.
3. Identify suture material.
4. Understand the sizing of suture material.
5. Describe proper instrument care.
6. Describe pack preparation for sterilization.
7. Understand the principles of sterilization monitors.
8. Describe aseptic technique when performing a patient surgical preparation and when positioning a patient.
9. Describe how to maintain asepsis in a surgical suite.
10. Describe correct surgical scrubbing and conduct in the operating room.
11. List possible duties of a sterile surgical assistant.

---

This chapter contains basic information on instrument identification, instrument care, and sterile technique. The chapter also includes a summary of aseptic patient preparation, pack preparation, and surgical suite preparation.

Acting as sterile assistant to a surgeon or as a circulating nurse during surgery is an important aspect of the veterinary technician's role in a veterinary hospital. These concepts are not only learned and memorized, but by experience become second nature.

## SURGICAL INSTRUMENTS

The veterinary technician should be familiar with basic surgical instruments and their intended use (Figure 22-1). The following are some common instruments used in veterinary surgery.

### Scissors

I. Operating scissors are generally for cutting suture, drape material, or other inanimate material. They are classified in three ways
  A. Type of point (e.g., blunt/blunt, sharp/blunt, or sharp/sharp)
    1. Blunt scissors have a rounded edge
    2. The most common operating scissors has the sharp/blunt point
  B. Shape of the blade (e.g., straight or curved)
  C. Cutting edge (e.g., plain or serrated)
II. Mayo scissors work well for cutting and dissecting dense tissue (Figure 22-2)
  A. Tips are blunt
  B. Blades can be straight or curved
III. Metzenbaum scissors have fine tips and long handles for cutting and dissecting more delicate tissue
  A. Tips can be blunt or pointed
  B. Blades can be straight or curved

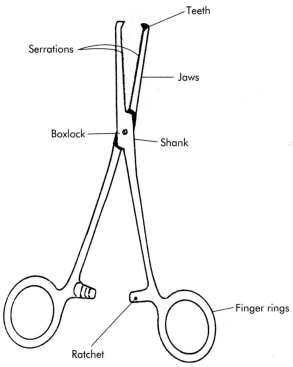

**Figure 22-1** Parts of surgical instruments. (Courtesy The Ohio State University. From Tracy DL: *Small animal surgical nursing,* ed 3, St Louis, 2000, Mosby.)

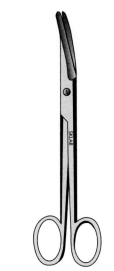

**Figure 22-2** Mayo dissecting scissors.

IV. Iris scissors are small, sharp, delicate scissors commonly used for intraocular surgery
V. Wire-cutting scissors have short, thick jaws with serrated edges for cutting wire suture material
VI. Littauer and Spencer suture removal scissors are used to cut and remove sutures postoperatively
   A. Have blunt tips with one blade terminating into a thin curved hook
   B. Spencer scissors are smaller than Littauer scissors

VII. Lister bandage scissors are used to cut under a bandage without puncturing the patient's skin (Figure 22-3)
   A. One blade has a flat, thick edge and a blunt tip
   B. Available in various sizes

**Forceps**

I. Thumb forceps are hand held in a pencil grip to hold tissue
   A. Rat-tooth thumb forceps are used to grasp skin and are commonly used to place sutures
      1. They have large teeth
      2. The teeth intermesh (one tooth fits in between two teeth on the opposite tine when closed)
   B. Adson tissue forceps provide good tissue grip with minimal damage to tissue because they have very fine "rat tooth" tips. They are used on delicate tissues
   C. Brown-Adson tissue forceps have multiple fine intermeshing teeth on edges of the tips (Figure 22-4)
      1. The sides of the blades are wider for ease of handling
      2. They are also used with delicate tissue
   D. Dressing forceps have serrations but no teeth on the jaws; they are useful for handling dressing material
   E. Russian tissue forceps have rounded tips and are used for holding hollow viscera
II. Self-retaining forceps use a ratchet-locking device to grasp and retract tissue
   A. Allis tissue forceps have intermeshing teeth that ensure a secure grip, but they can cause trauma to delicate tissue
   B. Babcock intestinal forceps are similar to the Allis forceps but have no gripping teeth, which enables them to be used on delicate tissues
   C. Doyen intestinal forceps are useful for holding bowel
   D. Ferguson angiotribe forceps assist in holding large bundles of tissue
   E. Sponge forceps have a hole in the center of its circular tips and hold gauze to provide hemostasis during surgery or when performing patient preparation
   F. Backhaus towel clamps are considered forceps and are used to secure drapes to the patient's skin (Figure 22-5)
   G. Roeder towel forceps are similar to the Backhaus towel forceps, but have a metal bead on each tip that does not puncture the skin as deeply and helps keep the drape from sliding
III. Hemostatic forceps (commonly referred to as hemostats) can be straight or curved and are used for ligating vessels and tissues

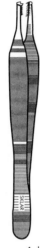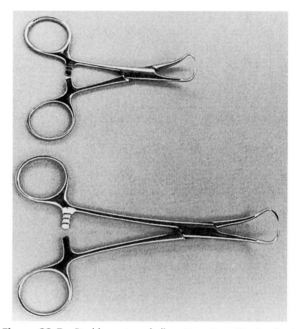

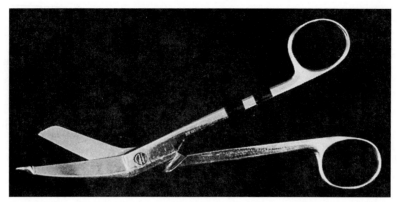

**Figure 22-3** Lister bandage scissors. (From Tracy DL: *Small animal surgical nursing,* ed 3, St Louis, 2000, Mosby.)

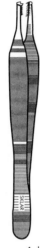

**Figure 22-4** Brown-Adson tissue forceps.

A. Halsted mosquito forceps control capillary bleeders (Figure 22-6)
 1. Length: up to 10 cm (4 inches)
 2. Transverse serrations cover the entire jaw length
B. Kelly and Crile forceps are used to grasp intermediate-size vessels
 1. Standard length: 12.5 cm (4.5 inches)
 2. Kelly forceps have distal transverse grooves
 3. Crile forceps have complete transverse grooves
C. Rochester-Pean and Rochester-Carmalt forceps clamp large tissue bundles that contain blood vessels; they are commonly used in stump and pedicle ligation (Figure 22-7)
 1. Larger forceps 20 cm (9 inches)
 2. Rochester-Carmalt forceps have longitudinal grooves and distal transverse grooves
 3. Rochester-Pean forceps have transverse grooves
D. Rochester-Ochsner forceps are similar to Rochester-Pean forceps, but in addition have 1:2 teeth at the tips

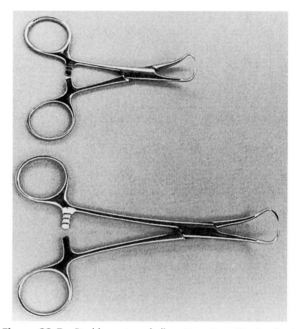

**Figure 22-5** Backhaus towel clips. (From Tracy DL: *Small animal surgical nursing,* ed 3, St Louis, 2000, Mosby.)

 1. 1:2 means that one tip has one tooth and the other tip has two teeth, and the teeth mesh when the tips are closed
 2. The teeth allow the surgeon to get a better grip on larger tissue bundles

**Needle Holders**

 I. Type of forceps used to hold curved needles and aid in tying sutures
 II. Surgical preference determines the type of needle holder used
 III. Mayo-Hegar (Figure 22-8) and Olsen-Hegar needle holders are commonly used in veterinary surgery
  A. Olsen-Hegar needle holders also have a scissors to cut sutures without using a separate scissor

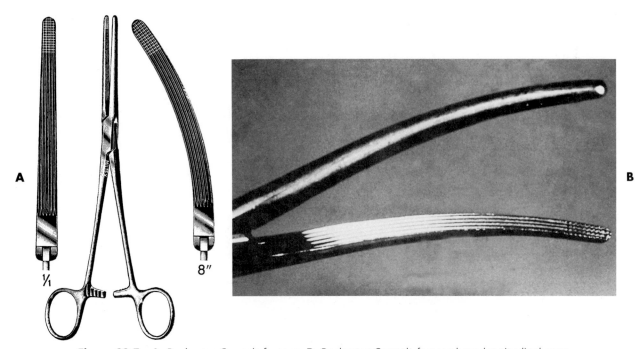

**Figure 22-6**    Halsted mosquito forceps, curved. (Courtesy The Ohio State University. From Tracy DL: *Small animal surgical nursing,* ed 3, St Louis, 2000, Mosby.)

**Figure 22-7    A,** Rochester-Carmalt forceps. **B,** Rochester-Carmalt forceps have longitudinal serrations and cross-hatched pattern at tips of each jaw. (Courtesy Miltex and The Ohio State University. From Tracy DL: *Small animal surgical nursing,* ed 3, St Louis, 2000, Mosby.)

B. The Mayo-Hegar instrument can be used only as a needle holder (no scissors)
C. Crisscross grooves assist in grasping the needle
IV. Mathieu needle holders do not have rings for the fingers; they open and close by finger pressure

## Retractors

I. Senn rake retractors are double ended and useful for skin and superficial muscle retraction
  A. One end has a three-pronged point (sharp or blunt) that curves
  B. The end looks somewhat like a rake
II. Meyerding, Hohmann, and U.S. Army retractors are hand held for larger muscle masses (Figure 22-9)
  A. U.S. Army retractors come in a set of two
  B. A U.S. Army retractor has one end shaped like a paddle so the wound edges can be opened easily
III. Malleable retractors are made of a soft metal that can be bent to accommodate hard-to-retract areas
IV. Self-retaining retractors have a locking mechanism
  A. Gelpi retractors have a single tip that extends outward to retract muscles; they are commonly used during orthopedic procedures and neurosurgery
  B. Weitlander retractors are similar to Gelpi retractors but have multiple prongs at the tips; they are also commonly used during orthopedic procedures and neurosurgery

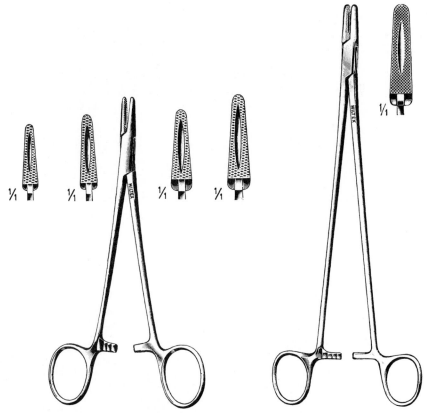

**Figure 22-8** Mayo-Hegar needle holder. (Courtesy Miltex. From Tracy DL: *Small animal surgical nursing,* ed 3, St Louis, 2000, Mosby.)

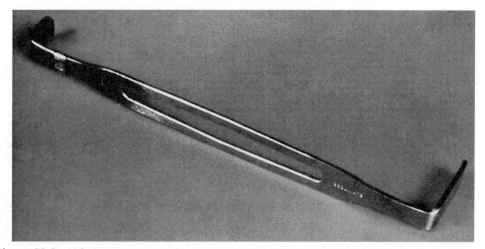

**Figure 22-9** U.S. Army retractor. (Courtesy The Ohio State University. From Tracy DL: *Small animal surgical nursing,* ed 3, St Louis, 2000, Mosby.)

C. Balfour retractors are useful in abdominal surgery to hold the abdomen open; several sizes are available

D. Finochetto retractors are used during thoracic surgery

V. The ovariohysterectomy hook or spay hook is a type of retractor (Figure 22-10)

A. The Snook spay hook has a broad, flat handle and a flat, curved tip

B. The Covault spay hook has an octagonal handle and a buttoned tip

## Common Orthopedic Instruments

I. Kern and Richards forceps have strong gripping teeth; some have a ratchet to manipulate bone fractures to reduction

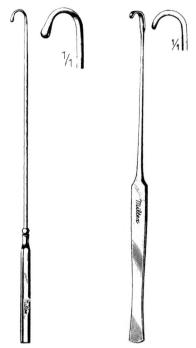

**Figure 22-10** Spay hook. (Courtesy Miltex. From Tracy DL: *Small animal surgical nursing*, ed 3, St Louis, 2000, Mosby.)

II. Verbrugge and reduction forceps can hold bone fragments in reduction while inserting fixators such as screws
III. Wire twisters look like larger needle holders
IV. Jacobs chucks are used to advance pin placement
V. Rongeurs, such as the Lempert, are used to break up and remove bone
VI. Bone-cutting forceps, such as the Liston, are used to cut bone
    A. They often have a double handle to increase power
    B. They have smooth, heavy, scissor-like jaws
VII. Osteotomes are used to cut through bone
VIII. Mallets are used to strike an osteotome or any other instrument that needs to be pounded during surgery
IX. Bone curettes have a sharp edge to remove bone
    A. Usually has a "cup" shape on one end
    B. Commonly used to scrape out osteochondritis dissecans (OCD) lesions
X. Bone rasps are used to smooth rough edges on bone
XI. Periosteal elevators, such as the Freer and Langbeck elevators, are used to remove muscle from bone by releasing the periosteum
XII. Intramedullary pins are used to stabilize fractures

## Miscellaneous Instruments

I. Suction tips
    A. Poole tips work well to remove abdominal fluid without being plugged by omentum
    B. Frazier-Ferguson tips allow variable suction strength for removing blood
    C. Yankauer tips are best for removing fluid other than blood
II. A Bard-Parker scalpel handle is used with a detachable blade
    A. Use a needle holder to attach and remove the blade
    B. A No. 3 handle and a No. 10, 11, 12, or 15 blade are most commonly used in small animal surgery
        1. No. 10 is the basic blade and is commonly used for incising skin
        2. No. 11 blade is used to sever ligaments
        3. No. 12 blade is used to lance abscesses
        4. No. 15 blade is used for precise, small or curved incisions
    C. A No. 4 handle and a No. 20 blade are most commonly used for large animal procedures
III. Groove directors are sometimes used to assist in making an incision

## Needles and Suture Material

I. Surgical needles are available in several sizes and forms
    A. Can be straight, curved, half curved, or half circle
        1. Curved needles are most commonly used
        2. Curved needles are described by their circle size (e.g., ½-inch, ⅜-inch circle)
        3. Half curved needles are straight except for a curved tip
    B. Needle points are cutting or tapered (noncutting)
        1. Type of cutting point can be reverse, triangular, or side cutting for skin, cartilage, or tendons
        2. Taper point needles are round or oval with reverse cutting points for tissues that may tear easily
    C. Needles can be eyeless (swaged) with suture already connected to the needle, or have an eye (round, square) to place suture through
        1. Needles swaged on to the suture are less traumatic because needle size is relative to suture size
        2. A separate needle and suture can cause tissue damage if used improperly
            a. Needle and suture should be similar in size
            b. Thread suture through curved needles from the inside without tension
II. Commonly used absorbable suture material
    A. Surgical gut is the most common nonsynthetic material
        1. Commonly referred to as catgut
        2. Made from the submucosal layer of sheep intestine
        3. Broken down by phagocytosis

B. Examples of synthetic suture material
  1. Polyglycolic acid (Dexon; Davis and Geck): synthetic polyester from hydroxyacetic acid
  2. Polyglactin acid (Vicryl, Ethicon): copolymer of lactic and glycolic acids
  3. Polydioxanone (P.D.S., Ethicon) and polyglyconate (Maxon, Davis and Geck): synthetic polyester
  4. Monofilament material provides less tissue drag when sutures are placed
  5. In general, absorbable suture retains its strength for several weeks

III. Nonabsorbable suture material can also be natural or synthetic
  A. Examples of natural fibers for suture material
    1. Silk is considered nonabsorbable even though its tensile strength is usually lost after 6 months
      a. Commonly braided or twisted into multifilament strands
      b. Most commonly used for cardiovascular surgery
      c. Can act as a wick, allowing migration of contamination
    2. Cottons and linens have been used for suture material
    3. Stainless steel suture is used in veterinary surgery but can be difficult to work with because of its decreased flexibility
  B. Examples of synthetic nonabsorbable suture material
    1. Polypropylene (Prolene, Ethicon): synthetic plastic
    2. Polyamide/nylon (Ethilon, Ethicon): polymerized plastic
    3. Polymerized caprolactrum (Vetafil, B. Braun, Melsungen AG): coated synthetic fiber commonly used for skin closure
  C. In general, nonabsorbable suture retains its tensile strength for 60 days or more

IV. United States Pharmacopeia (USP) sizing is generally used when asking for suture material
  A. Example: 4-0 (pronounced "4 ought"), 3-0, 2-0, 0, 1, 2 . . .
  B. As the number increases to the right after 0, the diameter of the suture becomes thicker; thus the size increases (e.g., size 3 suture is larger than size 2 suture)
  C. As the number increases to the left of 0, the diameter of the suture is thinner; thus the size decreases (e.g., size 2-0 is larger than size 3-0)
  D. Wire suture is also sized by gauge
    1. Size varies from 18 to 40 gauge
    2. The lower the gauge number, the thicker the diameter of the wire suture

V. Suture material and needle size used are based on many factors determined by the surgeon

## INSTRUMENT CARE AND PACK PREPARATION ■

Stainless steel instruments are in general expensive and of high quality. If maintained well, stainless steel instruments will last a lifetime.

### Instrument Care

I. Instruments should be kept moist or washed immediately after use to prevent residue from drying, which can cause staining, pitting, and corrosion
II. Clean instruments in distilled water and approved cleaning agents
  A. Tap water should be avoided because it can leave mineral deposits on the instruments during the sterilization process
  B. Cleaning agents should have a neutral pH between 9.2 and 11 to prevent spotting and corrosion
    1. Commercial instrument cleaners are available
  C. Instrument-cleaning brushes are helpful in removing debris from boxlocks, ratchets, and teeth
III. Use an ultrasonic cleaner to clean instruments, because it is 16 times more effective than manual cleaning
  A. Instruments should be placed in cleaner with boxlocks and ratchets open
  B. Do not overpack the cleaner with instruments
  C. To prevent electrolytic corrosion, do not mix different metals in the same cycle
  D. Run the cycle for approximately 10 minutes
IV. Place instruments in a surgical milk solution
  A. The surgical milk solution is an excellent lubricant and rust inhibitor
  B. In general, surgical milk must be used on all instruments cleaned by ultrasound, because all traces of lubricants are lost in cleaning
  C. After immersion in instrument milk, the instruments should be put on a clean paper or cloth towel to drain
  D. Surgical milk should be fresh so that it has no bacterial growth
  E. Some prefer to use an instrument milk spray
V. Additional use of a surgical lubricant on the instrument's moving parts can help to ensure a better working condition
VI. Instruments should be examined before being packed for resterilization
  A. Check that all surfaces are clean and free of foreign material
  B. Make certain that boxlocks work smoothly and are not loose
  C. Instrument tips should close tightly and evenly, especially tips on all forceps and needle holders
  D. Scissors should be sharp along the entire edge of the blade

## Preparing Instrument Packs and Linens

I. Reusable linens, such as gowns, drapes, and skin towels, should be laundered in a separate washer and dryer with minimal detergent
   A. An extra rinse cycle should be used to ensure that no detergent residue is left
   B. Leftover detergent residue can transfer via steam to surgical instruments during the sterilization process
II. The packing of instruments and linens should be consistent and allow the greatest amount of steam sterilization
   A. Use of pans or trays with perforations to hold instruments can allow better steam penetration and drying
   B. Leave boxlocks and ratchets in the open position or locked no more than one click
   C. Place heavier instruments on the bottom of the packs, and place items that are used first, such as towel clamps, on top
   D. Fold linens by the accordion style method (fan fold)
      1. Surgical gowns should be laundered and untorn
         a. Wrap inside out with all ties folded inside neatly and sleeves on top of the gown
         b. Gown pack can also include a towel for drying hands after a surgical scrub
      2. Laparotomy sheets, drapes, and skin towels should be laundered and lint free
         a. Wrap using the accordion pleat method and then fold into three sections
         b. Some surgeons prefer to have one corner of the drape folded over for easier grasping of the drape
   E. Packs must fit the size of the autoclave and allow ample room for steam movement and penetration
      1. Size should not exceed 30 × 30 × 50 cm
      2. Weight should not exceed 5.5 kg
      3. Density should not exceed 115.3 kg/m$^3$
      4. Space between packs should be 2.5 to 7.5 cm
III. The wrapping of instrument packs and linens should be consistent for proper sterile handling technique when opened
   A. Place a minimum of two appropriate-sized wrapping materials in front of you in a diamond shape
   B. Place the instrument pack or linen in the center of the first or inner wrapper
   C. Tightly pull linens with each fold
   D. Begin with the corner nearest you and fold over the top of the pack
   E. Take a small part of that corner and fold it back toward you to leave a tab

F. Do the same with one of the side corners, then the opposite side
G. The side farthest from you should always be folded over last
H. Tuck this last corner inside the two sides, leaving a tab that can be pulled to open
I. Repeat the same folding technique with the second or outer wrapper
J. Instruments should not be loose inside pack; everything should be tight and secure
IV. Indicator tape should be used on the outside of every pack and linen
   A. Tape keeps the packs sealed tighter and prevents corners from unfolding
   B. Useful for labeling information
      1. Contents of item (e.g., large gowns, general packs)
      2. Date item was sterilized and anticipated expiration date
      3. Initials of the technician who prepared and sterilized the pack
V. Sterilization pouches made of paper and/or plastic are useful for sterilizing individual items
   A. Pouches can be sealed by heat or by rolling the ends three times and securing with indicator tape
   B. Make sure you tab one end of the tape for easier opening
   C. Sterilize in an upright position to allow the best steam sterilization and drying
VI. Types of sterilization monitors
   A. More than one sterilization monitor should be used to ensure optimum sterility of the pack
   B. Indicator tape indicates only that an item has been exposed to steam or ethylene oxide
      1. Lines on the tape will change color to black
      2. Color change does not indicate that temperature has been met and maintained for a certain period of time
      3. Indicator tape on the outside of the pack means only that the outside of the pack has been exposed to steam
   C. Chemical indicator strips change color when exposed to steam or ethylene oxide for a specific period of time
      1. Place indicator in the center of the pack in the least accessible place for steam: between folds of drapes or gown. Do not place the indicator directly on instruments
      2. Must remember to check the strip as soon as pack is open
   D. A Bowie-Dick test is performed with a prepurchased dense pack with indicator tape in the center
      1. Place test pack in the most inaccessible location in the autoclave
      2. Verifies steam penetration

E. Biological indicators are excellent monitors of sterility
   1. Tests for the most heat-resistant bacteria
   2. However, it does not give an immediate answer
F. Visually check your autoclave to ensure that adequate time, temperature, and pressure have been achieved for proper sterilization

VII. Length of time steamed autoclaved items remain sterile can be extended by the type of wrapping material and where they are stored
   A. Textile wrapping material can be bulky to use and must be laundered and in good condition
      1. Cotton muslin should be double layered, and two wraps should be used for pack preparation
      2. Higher thread-count cottons can use two single-layered wraps
      3. If kept in open shelving, the items can remain sterile for 3 weeks
   B. Disposable paper wraps can be crepe or non-crepe material that can be cut to the desired size
      1. Crepe paper is easier to work with and more durable
      2. Crepe paper is more expensive
      3. Single-wrapped two-way crepe paper can remain sterile for 3 weeks with open shelving
   C. You can double the sterilization shelf life by keeping items in a clean, closed cabinet
   D. For infrequently used items, wrap and store in sterilization pouches to extend the shelf-life to 1 year in a closed cabinet
   E. Ethylene oxide sterilization can also prolong the shelf-life of sterile items

## PATIENT PREPARATION

The goal of patient preparation is to achieve asepsis or a preparation site free of germs that could cause disease or decay.

I. Patient preparation should be performed outside of the operating room
II. Before clipping, the bladder may need to be emptied, either by walking the patient outside or manually expressing the bladder
   A. Caution may be warranted when expressing a patient's bladder, and the surgeon should be consulted before performing the procedure
   B. An empty bladder can increase the space in the abdominal cavity and prevents the animal from eliminating on the surgery table while under anesthesia
III. Surgical hair removal should be completed with electric clippers and a No. 40 blade
   A. Blades should be clean and well lubricated and have no missing teeth that may tear the skin
   B. Coolants prevent clipper blades from overheating
IV. Start clipping at the proposed incision in the direction of the hair growth, then against the direction of hair growth to minimize irritation from the clippers
   A. Thick-coated animals sometimes require clipping with the direction of hair first, perhaps using a No. 10 blade initially
   B. Try not to allow clipped areas to touch unclipped areas
   C. In general, clip more hair rather than too little hair (2 to 4 cm in each direction from incision site)
   D. By consulting with the surgeon and the patient file, determine the proper site and the size of the site before clipping
   E. Water-soluble lubricant should be placed in open wounds before clipping to prevent further contamination from loose hair
V. Technicians should be familiar with common general surgical clips and animal placements for surgery
   A. Most laparotomies, such as the ovariohysterectomy and splenectomy, have a standard preparation site
      1. Animals are placed in dorsal recumbency
      2. Hair is removed cranially to the xiphoid process and caudally to the pubis
      3. Hair is removed laterally
         a. For cats, approximately one clipper blade width past the nipple line
         b. For large dogs, at least 4 inches (10 cm) of hair on either side of the midline should be removed
   B. Canine castrations require hair removal from the scrotum and prepuce extending into the inguinal area
      1. Some surgeons prefer that the tip of the prepuce remain unshaven to reduce irritation
      2. Some surgeons prefer the prepuce to be flushed with Nolvasan before surgery or being clamped off
      3. Use caution while shaving the scrotum to avoid clipper burn
   C. Feline castrations require less hair removal and can be done by plucking the hair from the testes and around the scrotum
   D. Puppy dewclaw removal and tail docking as well as feline declawing do not require hair removal before surgical scrub
   E. For perineal urethrostomies, rectal fistulas, and anal sac surgeries, the animal is placed in ventral recumbency with its hind legs hanging over the edge of the table. The tail is tied or clipped to the top or side of the body

1. Some surgical tables can be tilted upward for the surgeon's comfort
2. Hair removal should be outward from the rectum and extended up the base of the tail and down both legs

F. Orthopedic surgeries require a larger surgical area prepared to enable the surgeon to manipulate the limb (e.g., lateral and medial hind limb for a femoral intramedullary pinning)

VI. After clipping, a dust buster or central vacuum is useful to remove all loose hair from the surgery site and the surrounding area of the preparation table

VII. If performing a limb surgery, the unclipped area of hair on the foot should be wrapped
   A. Plastic wrap or examination gloves secured with tape work well
   B. Wrapping the foot after the hair is clipped prevents loose hair from sticking to the tape
      1. Hanging leg preparation can be used for shoulder and hip surgeries
         a. Operated limb is suspended by tape/rope for the surgical scrub
         b. After prep is finished, paw is wrapped with a sterile towel for easy handling by the surgeon

VIII. Recommended scrub solutions are chlorhexidine or povidone-iodophor products

IX. Surgical scrub procedure
   A. Required equipment: gloves, gauze, sponge forceps, and scrub bowl
   B. Begin at the incision and work outward in a circular motion
   C. Never return to the incision area without getting a new gauze square
   D. Produce a good lather but do not scrub too hard
   E. Scrubbing process should be completed a minimum of three times
      1. Gauze squares should appear clean after the final scrub
      2. Ask yourself if the skin is aseptic for surgery before continuing to the next step
   F. A procedure of alternating each scrub with sterile saline or isopropyl alcohol is helpful (because of its evaporative effect, be careful using isopropyl alcohol on small patients who may be prone to having increased difficulty maintaining body temperature)
   G. Final preparation should be completed so that the area of the incision is the most aseptic
      1. Apply chlorhexidine or povidone-iodine as an antiseptic
      2. There are at least three methods to accomplish the final aseptic application

   a. Method 1: using a nonsterile gauze square with antiseptic, make the first stroke medially down the incision line. Each subsequent stroke of antiseptic is to the right or left of the incision site, ending at the outermost border
   b. Method 2: begin the same way used in method 1, complete one side, and use a new sponge soaked with antiseptic to complete the opposite side in the same manner
      (1) The objective is that no stroke of antiseptic is repeated, thereby maintaining asepsis by moving any organisms away from the site
   c. Method 3: at many practices, antiseptic spray is used as the final prep in the operating room
   d. Be careful not to overapply final paint (prep), because the prep solution could seep through to the drape

X. Once surgical preparation is completed, carefully move the patient (by gurney if available) into the operating room, trying not to contaminate the surgical scrub

XI. The patient should be tied to the table in the appropriate position
   A. The knot should be a half hitch on the limb to facilitate easy release in case of an emergency
      1. Apply ties with two contact points per limb to reduce pressure problems
      2. Do not secure too tightly; this may cause muscle problems

XII. Once patient is positioned and necessary monitoring equipment is in place, a final surgical preparation is performed
   A. Reapply antiseptic using one of the methods given
   B. Repeat entire preparation if contamination occurs

## DRAPING

After the animal is secured on the table and the final skin preparation is complete, the patient is ready to be draped.

I. Drapes maintain a sterile field
II. Draping is performed by a gowned and gloved surgical assistant or team member
III. Draping begins with the placement of field drapes (also called quarter drapes)
   A. Field drapes are placed on the unprepared portion of the animal
   B. These drapes are placed one at a time at the very periphery of the prepared area
   C. After the drapes are in place, they should not be readjusted toward the incision site
      1. Readjustment carries contaminants onto the prepared skin

D. Towel clamps are placed to secure the four corners of the drapes
   1. Towel clamps secure the drapes to the skin and surround the incision site
E. Finally, a large drape or laparotomy sheet is placed over the animal with the center or fenestration over the surgical site
   1. Final drape provides a continuous sterile field

## SURGEON AND STERILE ASSISTANT SURGICAL SCRUB

I. Purpose: remove dirt, grease, and decrease bacterial flora from the hands and arms
II. Before scrubbing, set out sterile scrub brush and any packs and surgical equipment that may be needed. Put on cap and mask, remove jewelry, and ensure that nails are fingertip length and that fingernails are free of nail polish
   A. There are many variations of a surgical scrub. All variations are based on timed or stroke methods of scrubbing the surface of the hands and arms. For the purposes of this text, a stroke method will be used as an example
      1. Turn on water, checking for comfortable water temperature; thoroughly wash both hands and arms; clean nails
      2. Begin with a sterile scrub brush or prepackaged soap/brushes; wet the brush and/or apply antiseptic soap to it
      3. Artificial nails harbor bacteria and should not be permitted
      4. Scrub finger nails and tips of fingers; 30 strokes
      5. Begin with one hand, scrubbing fingertips, divide each finger into four planes, using 20 strokes. Proceed in a methodical fashion from the baby finger to the thumb, scrubbing each plane of each finger 20 times
      6. Progress to the palm and then the back of the hand and lateral hand; 20 strokes
      7. Move to wrist area, scrubbing all four planes; 20 strokes
      8. Scrub the remaining portion of the arm, ending 2 inches (5 cm) proximal to the elbow; 20 strokes
      9. During the scrubbing process, keep hands upright with fingertips above elbows at all times to move bacteria away from hands
      10. Rinse the brush, apply more antiseptic to the brush, and begin the same procedure on the opposite hand and arm
      11. After right and left arms have been scrubbed, rinse hands and arms from the fingertips to the elbows, continuing to hold hands upward
      12. Drying of hands and arms: hold sterile towel away from the body. Using one side of the sterile towel, dry one hand first, followed by the arm. Use the other side of the towel for the opposite hand and arm
III. Gowning and gloving should be completed immediately after drying hands
   A. Gowning
      1. Hold gown by inside shoulder seams; carefully pick the gown up and away from the counter
      2. The gown will unfold open
      3. Slide one arm into the sleeve and then the opposite arm into the remaining sleeve
      4. Allow unsterile personnel to tie the gown
   B. Gloves should fit snugly but not so tightly as to cut off circulation of the hands
   C. There are two standard methods of gloving: open and closed
      1. Open gloving
         a. With left hand, grasp inside cuff of the right glove; pull glove over the right hand and cuff of the gown
         b. The left glove can now be handled with the gloved right hand by placing the fingertips on the inside of the folded back cuff of the glove and pulling it on the left hand and over the cuff of the gown
      2. Closed gloving (minimizes contamination)
         a. With fingertips of the right hand covered by the cuff of the gown, pick up the glove and place it on the covered left hand with fingertips of the glove facing the shoulder
         b. The thumb of the glove is on top of the left thumb
         c. Pull the glove over the cuff and push the hand into it while pushing out of the gown cuff
         d. The same procedure is used for the right hand glove
         e. After both gloves are in place, the gloves can be repositioned for comfort
      3. After gloving is completed the hands should be held above the waist and in front of the body

## OPERATING ROOM CONDUCT

All operating rooms have the same strict rules that must be followed. Knowing and understanding aseptic technique will help any technician adapt to any operating room.

I. Aseptic conditions must be applied to the surgical suite and the patient
   A. Patients and surgery staff prep in another room
   B. Only surgery-related equipment belongs in the operating room
   C. Always clean from ceiling to floor. Every item in the operating room must be removed and cleaned regularly with disinfectants

D. Pay particular attention to flat surfaces where dust can accumulate

E. Make sure surgery lights are clean and dust free before they are adjusted over a surgical site

F. Clean daily before surgeries begin and between cases

II. Proper surgical attire is a must

A. Scrubs are specially designed for operating rooms
   1. Street clothes should never be worn
   2. Smocks should be worn over scrubs while clipping hair and when outside the surgical area

B. Surgical head attire should be a bouffant cap or a hooded cap
   1. No hair should be exposed
   2. Hooded caps cover both the head and neck and are useful for those with facial hair

C. Surgical masks are either molded or flat
   1. Molded masks have a metal nose band to assist with fit but provide less facial coverage and can allow air to escape
   2. Flat-style masks have pleats and a metal nose band to provide a more custom fit and decrease the chance of allowing air to escape

D. Foot covers or surgery shoes must be worn

III. Talking in the operating room should be minimal

A. Talking can distract a surgeon's concentration

B. Saliva weakens the filtration of the surgical mask

C. If you have to cough, turn head away from site and cough into mask

IV. Movement within the operating room should be limited, because the increased air movement can increase the risk of contamination

A. Prepare any equipment that may be used before the surgery begins

B. An organized surgery suite layout will prevent movement in the room to retrieve needed equipment and material

C. The surgery suite should be located in an isolated area of the hospital with decreased traffic volume

V. An imaginary line should be drawn around the sterile field of the surgeon, operating table, and instrument tray

A. When passing sterile equipment, do not cross that line but stand near it

B. Stand to the right or to the left, so the surgeon does not have to his or her back to the patient

C. If you are an unsterile assistant and you need to pass the surgeon or surgical assistant, do so back to back

D. Hold a sterilized packaged item away from your body when opening

E. When opening items wrapped as described earlier
   1. Open the side farthest away from you using the tab
   2. Proceed to do one side and then the other without allowing your arms to pass over the top of the item
   3. Then pull the last tab (one closest to your body) toward you, exposing the item or second sterile wrap
   4. Only outer pack wrappers should be opened by unsterile personnel before surgery: keeping the inner wrap closed ensures sterility of the contents

F. How to open items in sterilization pouches
   1. Determine which end is marked to be opened
   2. Hold both hands in fists with thumbs on top of your index finger
   3. Grab each side of the pouch, holding it between your thumb and index finger
   4. Separate the seal by rolling your fists outward as if peeling a banana
   5. Lower part of your fist can apply pressure to the item in the pouch to prevent it from sliding out

G. Always allow the surgeon to approach you to retrieve a sterile item or place the item in a sterile manner on the pack

VI. Surgical gowns should be considered sterile only on the front side, above the waist to the shoulder, and down the arms

A. Keep hands clasped in front, close to the body, and above the waist or above the surgery table

B. If trading places, pass back to back with hands folded; never turn your back toward the patient

VII. A sterile surgical assistant can perform the following functions

A. Receive sterile equipment
   1. Lift items up and out
   2. Do not reach over a patient or sterile field

B. Keep the surgical table organized and instruments clean

C. Anticipate and pass needed equipment and instruments
   1. Hand in the correct position for immediate use
   2. Tap the surgeon's palm with the instrument to ensure proper contact

D. Maintain hemostasis for the surgeon
   1. Place suction tip near tissue, not directly on the tissue
   2. Dab area with gauze square; do not wipe

3. Keep an accurate count of the gauze squares used and discarded
   E. Provide retraction of muscles and tissues with minimal trauma and good surgical exposure
   F. Cut suture material after suture placement
VIII. If a sterile item touches an unsterile item, it immediately becomes unsterile and is discarded
   A. Any item that is dropped, punctured, or wet is unsterile
   B. The patient's skin is aseptic, not sterile; avoid contact
   C. If in doubt, it is not sterile

## ACKNOWLEDGMENT ■■■■■

The editors and author recognize and appreciate the original work by Melanie K. Gramling, on which this chapter is based.

# Glossary

**asepsis** In surgery, refers to the destruction of organisms before they enter the patient's body

**fenestration** To perforate or make an opening into

**fistula** Any abnormal passage within body tissue; generally a passage leading from two internal organs or an internal organ to the body surface

**intramedullary** Within the marrow cavity of a bone

**laparotomy** An incision into the abdominal wall; exploratory laparotomy often used to physically examine the abdominal organs (also referred to as celiotomy)

**ligating** Application of a ligature or material, such as wire or suture material, to tie off blood vessels to prevent bleeding or constrict tissue

**OCD** Osteochondritis dissecans. Inflammation of the bone and cartilage that causes a piece of articulating cartilage to split off

**ovariohysterectomy** Surgical excision of the ovaries and uterus; commonly called a spay

**pedicle** Stem or stemlike structure

**perineal** Situated on the perineum

**perineum** External region between the vulva and the anus in the female or between the scrotum and anus in the male

**ratchet** Step-locking device on surgical instruments. The ratchet consists of a notched bar on each handle of an instrument; the notches are facing and overriding when the handles are closed and locked

**reduction** Correction of a hernia, luxation, or fracture

**serrations** Having a sawlike edge or border

**splenectomy** Excision of the spleen

**swaged-on** Type of suture material that is fused to the end of the needle

**transverse** Extending from side to side or at right angles to the long axis

**urethrostomy** Creation of a permanent hole for the urethra in the perineum

**viscera** Internal organs enclosed within a cavity

# Review Questions

**1** Type of scissors with long handles used for cutting delicate tissue are
   a. Littauer
   b. Metzenbaum
   c. Mayo
   d. Lister

**2** Forceps that are 20 cm (9 inches) with longitudinal grooves are
   a. Rochester-Pean
   b. Rochester-Carmalt
   c. Kelly
   d. Crile

**3** A needle holder combined with a scissors is called
   a. Mathieu
   b. Rochester-Pean
   c. Mayo-Hegar
   d. Olsen-Hegar

**4** Self-retaining tissue forceps with multiple fine intermeshing teeth at the tips are called
   a. Allis
   b. Babcock
   c. Adson
   d. Brown-Adson

**5** Which of the following is not a type of needle point?
   a. Reverse cutting
   b. Taper
   c. Side cutting
   d. Swaged

**6** An example of a nonsynthetic absorbable suture material is
   a. Surgical gut
   b. P.D.S.
   c. Silk
   d. Nylon

**7** What is the scientific name for Vetafil?
   a. Polyglycolic acid
   b. Polypropylene
   c. Caprolactrum
   d. Polydioxanone

**8** What type of detergent should be used to clean instruments?
   a. Slightly acid pH
   b. Neutral pH
   c. Slightly alkaline pH
   d. Does not matter

**9** The minimum number of surgical scrubs that should be completed on a surgical site is
   a. One
   b. Two
   c. Three
   d. Four

**10** Which of the following is a recommended antiseptic for patient preparation?
   a. Chlorhexidine
   b. Hydrogen peroxide
   c. Roccal
   d. Dish detergent

## BIBLIOGRAPHY

Berg J: Sterilization. In Slatter DJ, editor: *Textbook of small animal surgery*, vol 1, ed 2, Philadelphia, 1993, Saunders.

Boothe HW: Suture material, tissue adhesives, staplers and ligating clips. In Slatter DJ, editor: *Textbook of small animal surgery*, vol 1, ed 2, Philadelphia, 1993, Saunders.

Bubenik LJ: Small animal surgical nursing. In McCurnin DM, Bassert JM, editors: *Clinical textbook for veterinary technicians*, ed 6, St Louis, 2006, Saunders.

Busch SJ: *Small animal surgical nursing,* St Louis, 2006, Mosby.

Davidson JR, Burba DJ: Surgical instruments and aseptic technique. In McCurnin DM, Bassert JM, editors: *Clinical textbook for veterinary technicians,* ed 6, St Louis, 2006, Saunders.

Fahie MA: Thoracic and abdominal surgery: the technician's role, *Vet Tech* 18:565, 1997.

Fries CL: Assessment and preparation of the surgical patient. In Slatter DJ, editor: *Textbook of small animal surgery*, vol 1, ed 2, Philadelphia, 1993, Saunders.

Hobson HP: Surgical facilities and equipment. In Slatter DJ, editor: *Textbook of small animal surgery*, vol 1, ed 2, Philadelphia, 1993, Saunders.

Khachatoorian L, Brady M: Aseptic surgical technique, *Vet Tech* 18:115, 1997.

Knecht CD et al: Operating room conduct. In Pederson D, editor: *Fundamental techniques in veterinary surgery*, ed 3, Philadelphia, 1987, Saunders.

Knecht CD et al: Selected small animal surgical procedures. In Pederson D, editor: *Fundamental techniques in veterinary surgery*, ed 3, Philadelphia, 1987, Saunders.

Knecht CD et al: Surgical instrumentation. In Pederson D, editor: *Fundamental techniques in veterinary surgery,* ed 3, Philadelphia, 1987, Saunders.

Knecht CD et al: Suture material. In Pederson D, editor: *Fundamental techniques in veterinary surgery,* ed 3, Philadelphia, 1987, Saunders.

Lauer SL: Surgical assistance and suture material. In McCurnin DM, Bassert JM, editors: *Clinical textbook for veterinary technicians,* ed 6, St Louis, 2006, Saunders.

McCurnin DM, Jones RL: Principle of surgical asepsis. In Slatter DJ, editor: *Textbook of small animal surgery,* vol 1, ed 2, Philadelphia, 1993, Saunders.

Miltex Instrument Co, Inc: *Miltex surgical instruments,* Lake Success, NY, 1986, The Company.

Nieves MA, Merkley DF, Wagner SD: Surgical instruments. In Slatter DJ, editor: *Textbook of small animal surgery*, vol 1, ed 2, Philadelphia, 1993, Saunders.

Schultz R: The ten commandments of surgical instrument care, *Vet Tech* 19:696, 1998.

Sirois M: Principles of surgical nursing. In Sirois M, editor: *Principles and practice of veterinary technology*, ed 2, St Louis, 2004, Mosby.

Songsathagen T: *Veterinary instruments and equipment*, St Louis, 2006, Mosby.

Wagner SD: Preparation of the surgical team. In Slatter DJ, editor: *Textbook of small animal surgery,* vol 1, ed 2, Philadelphia, 1993, Saunders.

## CHAPTER 23

# Small Animal Nursing

*Monica M. Tighe*

## OUTLINE

Physical Examination
  Introduction
  General Appearance
  Examination by System
Drug Administration
  Introduction
  Oral Route
  Parenteral Route
  Topical Route
Fluid Therapy
  Introduction
  Normal Fluid Balance
  Abnormal Fluid Losses
  Signs of Dehydration
  Estimating Degree of Dehydration
  Calculation of Fluid Replacement
    Volume
  Contraindications for Fluid
    Therapy
  Routes of Fluid Administration
  Types of Fluid
Venipuncture
Blood Collection and Transfusion
  Canine Blood Collection
  Feline Blood Collection
  Administration and Reactions
  Shelf-Life
  Indications for Use of Blood
    Component Therapy
Electrocardiography
  Definition
  Supplies
  Procedure
  Normal Electrocardiographic
    Interpretation
  Abnormal Rhythms
Orogastric Intubation
  Indications

Equipment
Procedure
Precautions
Nasogastric Intubation
  Definition
  Indications
  Equipment
  Procedure
  Precautions
Canine Male Urinary
  Catheterization
  Indications
  Equipment
  Procedure
  Precautions
Canine Female Urinary
  Catheterization
  Indications
  Equipment
  Procedure
  Precautions
Cystocentesis
  Indications
  Equipment
  Procedure
  Precautions
Manual Compression of the
  Urinary Bladder
  Indications
  Procedure
  Precautions
Auricular Treatment
  Indications
  Equipment
  Procedure
  Possible Etiologies of Otitis
    Externa
Anal Sac Expression

Definition
Indications
Procedure
Precautions
Enemas
  Definition
  Indications
  Procedure
  Precautions
Ophthalmology
  Anatomy
  Tears
  Formation of the Aqueous Humor
  Medical Terminology
  Conditions of the Eye
  Therapeutic Techniques
Dermatology
  Anatomy
  Dermatology Terminology
  Types of Shampoo
  Common Dermatological
    Conditions
Wound Management
  Wound Contamination vs.
    Infection
  Wound Healing
  Types of Wound Healing
  Wound Treatment
Bandaging
  Types of Bandages
  Head and Neck
  Thorax
  Abdomen
  Limbs
  Paw
  Tail
  Specialized Bandaging
    Techniques

Casting Materials
Aftercare of Bandages, Slings,
   and Casts
Oncology
   Definition

Classification
Diagnostics
Therapy
Euthanasia and Pet Bereavement
   Euthanasia Discussion

Methods of Euthanasia
Human Pet Bond and the Grief
   Process
The Grief Process
Necropsy

## LEARNING OUTCOMES

After reading this chapter you should be able to:

1. Explain how to perform a basic physical examination.
2. Define the importance of fluid therapy, and why and how patient requirements may change.
3. Explain and identify the signs and degrees of dehydration.
4. Describe the various routes of fluid administration and why a specific route may be used.
5. Describe various routes of drug administration.
6. Define contraindications of certain routes of drug administration.
7. Describe venipuncture procedure in the canine or feline patient.
8. Describe the collection and transfusion of blood in the canine and the feline patient.
9. Define electrocardiography.
10. Describe the equipment needed and procedure for producing an electrocardiogram.
11. Describe various abnormal electrocardiographic tracings and their etiologies.
12. Describe the precautions and procedure for inserting an orogastric tube.
13. Describe the indications, equipment, procedure, and precautions involved in male dog catheterization.
14. Describe the indications, equipment, procedure, and precautions involved in female dog catheterization.
15. Describe the indications, equipment, procedure, and precautions involved in performing a cystocentesis.
16. Describe the indications, procedure, and precautions involved in performing manual compression of the urinary bladder.
17. Describe the indications, equipment, procedure, and precautions involved in auricular treatment.
18. Describe the indications, equipment, procedure, and precautions involved in anal sac expression.
19. Describe the indications, equipment, procedure, and precautions involved in enema administration.
20. Describe the anatomy of the eye, including the aqueous humor and the structures involved in tear formation.
21. Define various medical terminology related to the eye.
22. Define common conditions of the eye and common therapeutic techniques.
23. Describe how to examine the skin and differentiate between a primary and secondary lesion.
24. Define the medical terminology relating to the skin.
25. Define the most common etiologies of dermatological conditions and their possible treatments.
26. Define the difference between a contaminated and an infected wound.
27. Differentiate and describe the four phases of wound healing.
28. Describe the different types of wound healing.
29. Define the treatment protocol for wound management.
30. Describe various types of bandages.
31. Define the indications and complications in bandaging various areas in small animals.
32. Define the classification method of tumors.
33. Describe the possible therapies that are available for cancer treatment.
34. Describe euthanasia and the grief process.
35. Describe a necropsy, including required equipment, procedure, and sampling.

As a paraprofessional, the veterinary technician assists the veterinarian by performing many diagnostic and technical procedures. This chapter outlines many basic clinical techniques.

## PHYSICAL EXAMINATION

### Introduction

I. Under the supervision of a veterinarian, veterinary technicians may conduct physical examinations
   A. To assess a patient's anesthetic risk and prepare an anesthetic plan
   B. To obtain a status or progress report for monitoring an animal's recovery
   C. To verify medical record entries
   D. To evaluate abnormalities or conditions that should be brought to the attention of the veterinarian

II. A physical examination is the first step in assessing a patient and may indicate possible health problems

III. All body systems should be checked

IV. A routine should be followed to ensure that each area is thoroughly examined

    A. Example: evaluating from the nose to tail, or system by system

## General Appearance

I. Note the animal's general appearance, gait, behavior, temperament, and attitude

II. The environment of the animal should be noted

    A. Vomiting/diarrhea, urination, defecation in the cage

III. An accurate weight, temperature, pulse, and respiratory rate should be recorded

## Examination by System

The detection of physical problems is usually due to observing the animal and palpating, smelling, and listening. The description of what is detected is also important. Size, color, rate, and appearance should be included in the record. For the following systems, various clinical signs should be noted on the patient's file.

I. Skin and coat

    A. Examine the skin and coat

        1. Shiny or dull

        2. Skin turgor

            a. Normal skin pliability depends on hydration of the tissues

            b. To assess turgor: tent the skin at the thoracolumbar junction

            c. Avoid cervical area because of the extra skin in this area

            d. If the skin returns rapidly to its initial position, it is normal

            e. If the skin remains tented or returns slowly to normal resting position, it is a sign of dehydration

            f. Mild, moderate, and severe dehydration are graded at 6% to 8%, 10% to 12%, and 12% to 15%, respectively. See fluid therapy section for more information

        3. Alopecia or dryness

        4. Lesions or obvious parasites, such as fleas, lice, mites, or ticks

    B. Palpate the entire animal; note any lumps, swelling, or painful reactions to palpation

II. Eyes, ears, and nares

    A. Examine the eyes and note the following

        1. Reflexes and response to visual stimuli

        2. Discharge from the eyes

            a. Clear or purulent

        3. Corneal changes

        4. Color of conjunctiva

    B. Manipulate the ear and note the following

        1. Response to auditory stimuli

        2. Debris in the ear canal or unusual or excessive odor

        3. If the animal is shaking or tilting its head to one side

    C. Nares

        1. Discharge: color and consistency

        2. Sneezing and patency

III. Gastrointestinal

    A. Examine mouth, teeth, and gums

        1. Signs of periodontal disease and halitosis

        2. Fractured, missing, or discolored teeth

        3. Verify age in young animals

        4. Check tonsils for enlargement

        5. Excessive salivation or difficulty swallowing

        6. Signs of malocclusion

    B. Note color of mucous membrane

        1. Mucous membranes should be a pale pink color

            a. Abnormal colors are blue-purple (cyanotic), yellow (jaundice), pale pink, bright red, or muddy brown

    C. Capillary refill time (CRT)

        1. Press on gums and note when the color returns

        2. If color returns in less than 1 second, CRT is normal

        3. If color returns in greater than 1 second, CRT is increased and abnormal

    D. Palpate the abdomen gently

        1. Check symmetry from side to side

        2. Check for distention

        3. Note signs of discomfort during palpation

        4. Assess the bladder size

        5. Lymph node abnormalities

    E. Examine the anal area for any abnormalities

        1. Color

        2. Anal gland abscesses, discharge, or inflammation

IV. Respiratory

    A. Auscultate the chest

        1. Using a stethoscope, auscultate the thorax dorsally and laterally

        2. Listen for abnormal sounds, such as crackles, wheezes, stridor, and rales

        3. Be aware of referral sounds from the upper airway

            a. Listen to the trachea to rule out this source

        4. Be aware of a decrease or lack of breath sounds

    B. Note pattern, rate, depth, and effort of breathing

        1. Hyperventilation or hypoventilation

        2. Panting or shallow breathing

        3. Open mouth breathing or panting in cats is especially abnormal

        4. Watch for dyspnea

V. Musculoskeletal
   A. Observe the animal's gait
   B. Note obvious signs of joint swelling or displacement of joints
      1. Lameness, dysplasia, or pain
   C. Flex the limbs
      1. Painful reactions
      2. Range of motion
VI. Cardiovascular
   A. Palpate femoral and dorsal pedal pulses
      1. Strength and rate of pulses
   B. Auscultate the heart and check pulses at the same time
      1. Note irregularities between pulse rate and heart rate, which can indicate pulse deficits
VII. Reproductive and urinary
   A. Examine external genitalia
      1. Redness or irritation
      2. Abnormal discharge, growths
      3. Symmetry of testicles
VIII. Lymphatic
   A. Lymph nodes may or may not be palpable
      1. Lymph nodes should not be painful when palpated
      2. Note signs of enlargement
   B. Major lymph nodes and locations
      1. Submandibular: located cranial to the angle of the mandible
      2. Prescapular: cranial to the shoulder joint
      3. Axillary: where the forelimb meets the body
      4. Popliteal: dorsal stifle
      5. Inguinal: in the inguinal area near the femoral artery and vein, where the hind limb meets the body
IX. Neurological
   A. Bright and alert
   B. Check pupil size
      1. Response to light
      2. Pupils are of equal size
      3. Nystagmus
   C. Look for signs of ataxia or weakness
   D. Check tail response and/or if there is anal tone
   E. Response in all four limbs to painful stimuli
   F. Levels of consciousness
   G. Knuckling when walking

# DRUG ADMINISTRATION

## Introduction

I. Drugs are administered in several ways
II. The route depends on type of medication and health status of the animal
III. Most common routes: oral, parenteral, and topical
IV. Whichever method is used, it is important to verify correct drug, patient, dosage, time, and route

## Oral Route

I. Oral medications are contraindicated in the following situations
   A. If patient is vomiting
   B. There are injuries to the oral cavity or esophagus
   C. Patient has decreased swallowing reflex
   D. Any disease process is present that prohibits oral intake, such as pancreatitis
II. Medication can be a liquid, semisolid, tablet, or capsule
III. Liquid is administered via syringe in the cheek pouch
IV. Tablets or capsules are administered by
   A. Holding the patient's mouth open with one hand
   B. Placing the pill at the base of the tongue with the opposite hand
   C. Closing the mouth
   D. Observing the animal swallow

## Parenteral Route

I. Includes all medications that are injected
II. These drugs are not absorbed through the gastrointestinal tract
III. Commonly includes three routes
   A. Subcutaneous (SQ or SC)
   B. Intramuscular (IM)
   C. Intravenous (IV)
IV. Occasionally, drugs may also be administered
   A. Intradermally (ID)
   B. Intraperitoneally (IP)
   C. Intracardiac (IC)
   D. Intratracheal (IT) (this route is used for emergency drug administration)
   E. Intramedullary or intraosseous (IO)
   F. Intranasal (IN)
   G. Intraarterial (IA)
V. Subcutaneous injections
   A. Solutions are injected under the skin using a 22- to 25-gauge needle
      1. Vaccines are most commonly administered via this route
         a. Because of the possibility of vaccine-induced tumors, the intrascapular region in cats should be avoided
   B. Usually where excess skin is available
      1. Dorsally from the neck to the hips
   C. Bulk fluids may also be administered subcutaneously
      1. From 50 to 100 mL of isotonic body temperature fluids may be administered per site
      2. The preferred sites are dorsal left and right thoracic region and dorsal left and right lumbar region

VI. Intramuscular injections
  A. Injections into the lumbar muscles or biceps femoris muscle using a 22- to 25-gauge needle
  B. Small volumes of up to approximately 2 mL are recommended
  C. Multiple sites may be necessary
VII. Intravenous injections
  A. Via a needle or catheter inserted into a blood vessel
  B. Most common sites: cephalic, femoral, saphenous, and jugular veins
    1. Sublingual for emergency drugs
  C. Alcohol is applied to the site before venipuncture to disinfect and part the fur
  D. A restrainer or a tourniquet is used to apply proximal pressure to vein
  E. By drawing blood into the syringe before injecting, correct placement may be ensured before administering medication
    1. Best to enter at a distal point on the limb
  F. Fastest route of absorption and large volumes can be rapidly administered
  G. Fewer problems if solutions are caustic, irritating, or hypertonic
  H. IV catheters can also be inserted for long-term administration of medications or fluids
VIII. Intraosseous route
  A. Needles are placed directly into the bone cavity for administration of fluids, drugs, or blood products
  B. This method is most commonly used for neonatal and smaller animals and animals with circulatory problems
  C. Sites of administration
    1. Femur, humerus, tibia, and sometimes the ilial wing or ischium
  D. A 15- to 18-gauge bone marrow needle is commonly used
    1. In small neonatal animals, an 18- to 22-gauge hypodermic needle may also be used
  E. Sterile technique must be used to prepare the skin for needle placement

## Topical Route

I. Medications applied directly to the skin
II. Can be applied directly on top of lesions
III. The area must be clipped and clean before applying medication
IV. Directions must be followed carefully
  A. Absorption rate is variable and depends on the amount applied and how quickly it is absorbed
V. Wearing gloves as a precaution is sometimes advisable for certain medications

# FLUID THERAPY
## Introduction

I. Fluid therapy is one of the most common procedures performed in veterinary medicine
II. It is used as supportive therapy in sick and injured patients

## Normal Fluid Balance

I. The body is made up of approximately 60% water
II. This is divided into intracellular and extracellular fluids
III. The body maintains fluid balance on a constant basis
IV. Fluids are gained via
  A. Oral intake
  B. Metabolism in the body
V. Fluids are lost by
  A. Respiration
  B. Excretion
  C. Minor routes, such as sweating and milk production

## Abnormal Fluid Losses

I. Vomiting and diarrhea
II. Increased respiration (panting) in dogs
III. Disease with accompanying polyuria
IV. Any chronic or acute injury or disease that causes fluid loss
V. Any disease state or injury that prevents or decreases the oral intake of fluids

## Signs of Dehydration

I. Indicators of dehydration can be found during physical examination
  A. Evaluating weight
  B. Skin turgor
  C. Moistness of mucous membranes
  D. Heart rate
  E. CRT

## Estimating Degree of Dehydration

I. 5% dehydration
  A. Not detectable
II. 5% to 6% dehydration
  A. Slight loss in skin turgor
III. 8% dehydration
  A. Definite increase in skin turgor
  B. Slight increase in CRT
  C. Possibly dry mucous membranes
IV. 10% to 12% dehydration
  A. Skin turgor remains
  B. Sunken eyes
  C. Increased CRT
  D. Dry mucous membranes

E. Increased heart and respiratory rates

F. Cold extremities

G. Possible signs of shock

   1. Signs include rapid thready pulse, tachycardia, and tachypnea

V. 12% to 15% dehydration

A. Shock and its clinical signs

B. Very depressed patient

C. Imminent death

VI. Other indicators of dehydration

A. Packed cell volume (PCV) and total plasma protein (TPP)

   1. PCV and TPP increase with all types of fluid loss, except in cases of severe hemorrhaging, when both will decrease

B. Urine specific gravity

   1. Can be greatly increased (>1.045)

C. Decreased urine production

   1. Normal production is 1 to 2 mL/kg/hr

## Calculation of Fluid Replacement Volume

I. Emergency fluid therapy

A. For hypovolemic, shocky, or severely dehydrated patients, fluids should be administered at 60 to 90 mL/kg/hr

II. Replacement fluids

A. Replacement fluids can be given over 12 to 24 hours

B. Daily fluid requirement = replacement + maintenance + ongoing losses

   1. Replacement requirement = % dehydration × body weight (kg) × 10

      a. Examples of replacement fluids include Normosol-R or lactated Ringer's solution (LRS)

   2. Maintenance requirement = 40 to 60 mL/kg/day

   3. Ongoing losses can be estimated by the daily volume of fluids lost as urine, diarrhea, vomit, or drainage from a wound over a 24 hour period

III. Maintenance fluids at the rate of 40 to 60 mL/kg/day

A. Examples of maintenance solutions include Normosol-M or normal saline with KCl

B. When the patient needs only to be on maintenance fluids, saline with KCl should be used

   1. Replacement fluids do not have the required amount of KCl

   2. Cardiac patients should not be given normal saline because the increase in sodium could have adverse effects

## Contraindications for Fluid Therapy

I. Patients may have existing conditions that may contraindicate the rapid replacement of fluid

II. Conditions that carry a risk of pulmonary edema from fluid shifting into the lungs necessitate the need for caution and frequent monitoring

III. Some conditions that are contraindications for rapid fluid therapy are

A. Pulmonary contusions

B. Existing pulmonary edema

C. Brain injury

D. Congestive heart failure

IV. Signs of overhydration

A. Restlessness

B. Increased respiratory rate

C. Increased lung sounds (crackles and wheezes)

D. Increased blood pressure

E. Chemosis (edema of ocular conjunctiva)

F. Pitting edema

V. Subsequent body weights, urine production, and urine specific gravity should be monitored regularly

VI. Fluid rates should be adjusted according to patient response and veterinarian orders

## Routes of Fluid Administration

I. Oral

A. Contraindicated if animal is vomiting and/or has a disease such as pancreatitis

B. Can be given by syringe

C. Can be given by feeding tube

   1. Nasoesophageal or gastric tube directly into the stomach or intestinal tract

II. Subcutaneous

A. Useful for mild dehydration

B. Fluids must be isotonic; therefore cannot contain dextrose

C. Contraindicated with patients in shock or with more severe cases of dehydration

   1. In these cases, peripheral circulation is very poor and very little absorption will take place

D. Absorption can take up to 6 to 8 hours

E. Approximate guidelines: 50 to 100 mL of body temperature fluids at each site

F. Administration can be by large-gauge needle and syringe, or needle attached to an administration set and IV bag

G. Can be administered anywhere there is excess skin

   1. Dorsally, between the scapulas

   2. Dorsal flank area

III. Intravenous

A. Preferred method for correction of moderate to severe dehydration and patients in shock

B. Commonly administered via catheter through cephalic, saphenous, or jugular veins

IV. Intramedullary

A. Useful in small or young patients where quick venous access is not possible

B. Fluids administered directly into the bone marrow cavity, for rapid absorption

C. Injected through the head of the femur or humerus

D. Strict aseptic technique must be used, and local anesthetic may be needed because this procedure can be painful

## Types of Fluid

I. Crystalloids
   A. Isotonic electrolyte solutions
   B. Most commonly used
   C. Examples
      1. LRS
      2. 0.9% saline or normal saline, also called physiological saline
II. Colloids
   A. Solutions containing protein or starch molecules
   B. Stay in vascular space and expand volume
   C. Useful in patients with cerebral or pulmonary edema, and hypoproteinemia
   D. Examples
      1. Plasma
      2. Pentastarch

## VENIPUNCTURE

I. Purposes
   A. For clinical pathology tests, such as complete blood cell count (CBC) or serum chemistry tests
   B. To administer medications or fluids
II. Equipment and supplies
   A. Cotton balls soaked with 70% alcohol (isopropyl)
   B. 3- or 12-mL syringe or Vacutainer holder
   C. 20- to 22-gauge needle
   D. Blood collection tubes, with or without anticoagulant (EDTA)
      1. Blood collection tube selection will depend on which laboratory tests are requested by the veterinarian
III. Restraint and handling
   A. Jugular vein
      1. Animal should be in sternal recumbency on table
      2. The restrainer should grasp the animal's front legs with one hand and the animal's head with the other hand, extending the neck to expose the jugular vein
         a. It may be easier to facilitate venipuncture if the patient is positioned hanging over the edge of the table with legs below the table surface
      3. Cephalic vein
         a. The animal should be in sternal recumbency on an examination table

b. The restrainer should extend the animal's front leg by placing the fingers of one hand behind the animal's elbow
      c. To compress the vein
         (1) Use a tourniquet tightened cranial to elbow; or
         (2) The restrainer can use the thumb or first two fingers to roll and compress or "hold off the vein"
   B. Lateral saphenous vein
      1. The animal should be in lateral recumbency
      2. The restrainer can extend the stifle and compress the vein by grasping the animal's distal thigh or proximal tibia
   C. Femoral vein (feline patients)
      1. Place animal in lateral recumbency
         a. Cats may prefer sitting on a table with hind leg extended
      2. The restrainer can place one hand on the medial side of the upper thigh to compress the vein
IV. Procedure
   A. Prepare venipuncture site
      1. Clip the site with a No. 40 blade
      2. Check that the needle, syringe, and Vacutainer sizes are appropriate for collection
         a. Also check for needle burs and sterility
         b. Bevel of needle should be upward toward the venipuncturist
            (1) This is so that the needle facilitates flow of the incoming blood and is not occluded by the vein
      3. Swab the area with alcohol
      4. Have restrainer hold off vein
      5. Insert the needle bevel up, approximately three fourths of its length into the vein
         a. It is preferred to bury the needle in veins of most medium to large sized dogs so that if there is movement or a change in the position of the animal, the needle will remain in the vein
         b. For smaller animals, approximately half of the needle should be inserted
      6. Pull back on the plunger and check for a small amount of blood in the hub of the needle
      7. Using a gentle force, continue to pull back on the plunger of the syringe until the syringe is full or the required amount of blood is collected
         a. The restrainer should continue to hold off until the required amount of blood is collected or until the venipuncturist says that compression can be ended
      8. After the blood is collected, the restrainer should be directed to stop the compression of

the vein and the venipuncturist can then remove the needle

    a. It is best to have the restrainer at this point apply light pressure over the venipuncture site for hemostasis

  9. The blood is then placed in a Vacutainer using sterile technique

    a. The top can be removed from the Vacutainer and the blood can be gently squirted into the Vacutainer

    b. The Vacutainer can be punctured using the needle and the blood can be injected into the Vacutainer (the Vacutainer should have a vacuum, and therefore the blood will automatically be suctioned into the Vacutainer)

    c. If the venipuncturist used a Vacutainer, it should be completely filled for the sample to be viable

  10. At this time the Vacutainer should be gently rocked for all of the blood to be mixed with EDTA (lavender top Vacutainer) or left in a rack for the blood to clot (red top Vacutainer)

  11. The Vacutainer should be labeled with the name of the patient, date, and the initials of the venipuncturist

V. Administration of drugs

  A. The procedure for the administration of drugs is the same as for a collection except that after the venipuncturist is positive that the needle is in the lumen of the vein (blood in hub of needle), the restrainer must remove the compression of the vein to facilitate the induction of the drug

## BLOOD COLLECTION AND TRANSFUSION ▬▬
## Canine Blood Collection

I. Dogs have at least 19 identified canine blood groups

  A. They are designated by the acronym DEA (dog erythrocyte antigen) and a number

    1. For example, DEA 1.1, DEA 1.2, DEA 3

    2. DEA 1.1 + is the most common canine blood type

      a. Dogs with this blood type are considered to be universal recipients

    3. DEA 1.1 or 1.2 − are considered to be the universal donors

  B. After the first transfusion, dogs should be crossmatched because they can become sensitive to the type of blood they received

II. Canine donor requirements

  A. Any breed or sex may be used

  B. A dog with a good temperament and easily accessible veins is a prime candidate

  C. Blood typing should be performed on each donor

    1. Blood typing can be performed by using a commercially prepared blood typing card

    2. Typing cards are only available for DEA 1.1

  D. Ideally, donors should be neutered and weigh more than 25 kg (55 lb)

  E. Donors can be between 1 and 8 years old

  F. Donors should be tested every 6 months for parasites, including

    1. Heartworm (and maintained on a preventive medication)

    2. Intestinal parasites

  G. Donors should be fully vaccinated

    1. Blood should not be donated for 11 to 12 days postvaccination because of vaccine effects on platelets and endothelial functions

  H. Donors must be in excellent health with yearly normal blood chemistry, CBC, and urinalysis

    1. Donors' PCV should be at least 40%

    2. Donors should also be tested for von Willebrand factor and normal platelets

  I. Donors must be free of the following infectious diseases

    1. Blood parasites: *Babesia canis*, *Haemobartonella canis*

    2. Rickettsial diseases: *Ehrlichia canis*, *Ehrlichia platys*, *Borrelia burgdorferi*, and *Rickettsia rickettsii*

  J. Donors should be fasted before donation to decrease lipemic samples of blood

  K. Donors should never have received a blood transfusion

  L. 450 mL can be collected from a dog once every 4 to 5 weeks

III. Supplies

  A. Sedation requirement depends on the animal

    1. Do not use acepromazine maleate because it causes hypotension

    2. The sedative of choice is oxymorphone given approximately 15 to 20 minutes before blood collection

  B. A blood collection bag with anticoagulant added

  C. Clippers and surgical scrub solutions for preparation of the veins

  D. All supplies for IV fluid administration should also be available

  E. Scale to measure the blood

    1. The total weight of the blood (470 g) plus the weight of the collection bag and anticoagulant (117 g) should be 587 g

IV. Procedure

  A. Sedate animal

  B. Place animal in lateral recumbency with neck extended

  C. Clip a wide area around the jugular vein to be used for collection

D. Clip and prep the skin over the cephalic vein for an IV catheter for fluid replacement after blood collection

E. Place cephalic catheter

F. Prepare jugular vein for blood collection

G. Restrainer should be prepared to hold off the jugular vein in preparation for the blood collection

H. Insert 16-gauge needle attached to the blood collection bag into the jugular vein in a cranial direction
   1. Blood bags are manufactured with the needle and tubing attached

I. As blood enters the collection bag, move the bag slightly to mix the anticoagulant with the blood

J. 450 mL of blood constitutes one entire blood collection

K. Use the scale to measure the volume of blood in the collection bag so that it is not overfilled or underfilled
   1. Overfilling or underfilling the blood collection bag results in an improper ratio of anticoagulant to blood volume

L. After completion of blood collection, apply pressure to the jugular vein for 2 minutes to minimize hematoma formation

M. The amount of blood collected from a canine donor should not exceed 10 to 20 mL/kg
   1. Most facilities bleed a donor no more than once per month

N. Multiply the volume of blood collected from the patient by three to determine the volume of replacement IV fluids

O. Clearly label the collection bag with the donor's name, collection and expiration dates, and the donor's PCV, TP (total protein), and blood type

P. The donor should be observed for 1 hour after donation; mucous membrane color, pulse, and CRT should be monitored

## Feline Blood Collection

I. Feline donors are not routinely typed before blood collection

A. The AB system of blood typing is used for cats
   1. There are three recognized blood types: A, B, and AB
      a. The most common blood type is A
         (1) Most cats in North America are blood type A
      b. Nearly all domestic shorthair and longhair cats have type A
      c. Many purebred cats have type B blood

B. Since cats have naturally occurring alloantibodies against the blood-type antigen they lack, there is no universal feline blood donor
   1. Type A cats should receive type A blood, type B cats should receive type B blood. Type AB cat can receive either type A or type B blood with no clinical reactions
   2. Cats can have severe reactions to the first transfusion due to the inheritance of preformed antibodies to the opposite blood group
   3. Cats should always have their blood typed and crossmatched before the first and subsequent transfusions

II. Donor requirements

A. Less than 8 years of age

B. A lean body weight of no less than 4.5 kg (10 lb)

C. Donor must be neutered

D. A good-natured indoor cat makes donation smoother and less stressful

E. The donor should be fully vaccinated
   1. Modified live vaccine may affect platelet and endothelial function, and therefore blood should not be donated for 11 to 12 days postvaccination

F. Excellent health must be maintained by monitoring serum biochemistry, CBC, urinalysis, and fecal tests on a yearly basis
   1. The donor's PCV should be approximately 35%

G. All donors must be negative for feline leukemia, feline infectious peritonitis, feline immunodeficiency virus, and *Haemobartonella felis*

H. A donor may provide 60 mL of blood no more than once every 4 to 5 weeks

III. Supplies

A. Sedation

B. Clippers and surgical scrub solutions

C. Appropriate size catheter and butterfly (19 gauge)

D. Anticoagulant

E. IV fluids

IV. Procedure

A. The area is aseptically prepared and a catheter is placed in the cephalic vein for fluid therapy

B. Animal is sedated "to effect"

C. Monitor vital signs: pulse, respiration, and blood pressure throughout the procedure

D. Administration of replacement fluids can begin approximately halfway through the donation

E. Clip and aseptically prepare the skin over the jugular vein

F. Place cat in lateral recumbency with neck extended, or place cat in sternal recumbency with neck extended and legs over the edge of the table

G. Insert 19-gauge butterfly into the jugular vein

H. Connect the butterfly to a 60-mL syringe containing 8.5 mL of anticoagulant

I. Always try to minimize movement of the needle in the jugular vein

J. Mix anticoagulant and blood often throughout the donation

K. Blood collection from cats is a slow process; patience is a must

L. Collection is complete when the syringe reaches a volume of 60 mL

M. Remove butterfly and apply pressure to the vein to minimize hematoma formation

N. Multiply the volume of blood collected from the patient by three to determine the volume of replacement IV fluids (180 mL)

O. Clearly label the syringe with the donor's name, PCV, TP, volume, and date of collection

## Administration and Reactions

I. Patient history should be checked for previous transfusions

A. Before the transfusion all vital signs are observed and recorded

II. All blood products should be administered at room temperature using an in-line filter to remove debris and clots

III. Flush IV lines with only sodium chloride solutions during transfusions of blood products

A. Flushing IV lines with any other fluid or solution may cause red blood cells to clump, swell, or cause subsequent hemolysis

IV. For platelet administration, administration sets should not contain latex, because platelets will adhere to it

V. Initial administration should be slow (0.25 mL/kg) for the first 15 to 20 minutes

VI. If there are no signs of a transfusion reaction, the transfusion can be continued at the rate of 5 to 10 mL/kg/hr to a maximum of 22 mL/kg/dog

VII. Transfusion reactions can be either immunological or nonimmunological

A. Immunological

1. Acute immunological transfusion reaction signs include hypotension, vomiting, salivation, muscle tremors, and tachycardia

2. At 7 to 10 days posttransfusion, the recipient's body will destroy red blood cells

3. Delayed hemolytic reactions sometimes follow multiple transfusions

a. A key indicator of delayed reaction is an unexpected drop in PCV 2 to 21 days posttransfusion

b. Reactions may also be due to blood element incompatibilities

B. Nonimmunological signs are due to vascular overload

1. Signs include respiratory disease and vomiting

VIII. For further information see Chapters 2 and 3

## Shelf-Life

I. Blood in heparin or sodium citrate

A. Must be used within 48 hours because of the lack of red blood cell (RBC) preservative

1. Chemical changes could result in rapid removal of RBCs from the recipient's circulation

II. Blood with acid citrate dextrose (ACD) or citrate phosphate dextrose (CPD)

A. Blood should be stored at 1° to 6° C (33° to 36° F)

B. Can last up to 14 to 21 days in preservative when refrigerated

C. Blood stored with CPD-1 (added RBC preservative adenosine) can be stored for 35 to 45 days

III. Packed red cells without preservative

A. 21 days refrigerated (reconstitute with 1:1 saline)

B. Cannot be frozen

IV. Fresh or frozen plasma (FFP)

A. FFP is stored at −4° F to −22° F (−20° C to −30° C) for up to 1 year

B. Plasma should be thawed to 98.6° F (37° C) in a warm water bath for approximately 30 to 60 minutes before administration

V. Platelet-rich plasma

A. Should be used within 48 hours, kept at room temperature, and protected from light

## Indications for Use of Blood Component Therapy

I. Fresh whole blood (should be transfused within 4 to 6 hours)

A. Used for hemorrhagic shock, anemia, excessive surgical hemorrhage, bleeding disorders (due to thrombocytopenia or clotting factor deficiencies), non–immune-mediated hemolytic anemia, and in some circumstances, immune-mediated hemolytic anemia

II. Packed RBCs

A. Fluid balance and osmotic pressure are maintained with crystalloid given with packed cells

B. Used for hemolytic anemias and nonregenerative anemias

C. The preservative ADSOL will maintain cells without having to reconstitute them

1. Approximately 200 mL packed RBCs in 100 mL of ADSOL

2. Always add ADSOL to the packed RBCs

a. If packed RBCs are added to the ADSOL, the cells may be damaged in the process

III. An alternative to packed RBCs is Oxyglobin solution (bovine hemoglobin)

A. There is no need for blood typing or crossmatching

B. Transfusion reactions are not generally seen in the canine patient
   1. Cats may show signs of pulmonary edema
   2. Bovine plasma is a colloid solution and can cause volume overload if administered to patients with renal or heart failure
   3. Overload can also occur if given rapidly or in large amounts
   4. Discoloration of serum, urine, and mucous membranes is often seen after bovine hemoglobin administration
C. Oxyglobin can be stored for up to 3 years

IV. Plasma
A. Used for volume expansion (shock and burn patients), hypoproteinemia, pancreatitis, sepsis, and liver toxicities

V. Platelet-concentrated or platelet-rich plasma
A. Mainly used for thrombocytopenia cases

## ELECTROCARDIOGRAPHY
### Definition

I. Recording of the electrical activity on the surface of the body generated by the heart
II. Electrocardiograph: a machine that makes a recording of the bioelectrical signals on the surface of the body that arise from within the heart
   A. Electrocardiogram (ECG or EKG): a recording of the heart's bioelectrical signals on heat-sensitive paper or on a monitor
III. An ECG represents amplitude (amount of electrical activity) and duration (length of time) of electrical activity
IV. Each contraction of the heart is preceded by an electrical wave front that stimulates the heart muscle to contract (systole) and then relax (diastole) in preparation for the next heartbeat
   A. Depolarization: contraction of the myocardium
   B. Repolarization: relaxation of cells after depolarization

V. The continuous wave of electricity through the heart is organized, rhythmic, and repetitive
   A. The sinoatrial node, or pacemaker of the heart, is the point of origin of electrical activity
   B. The cells of the heart are electrically linked; therefore the depolarization spreads quickly from the sinoatrial node to the atria in a caudal direction toward the ventricles, finally reaching the atrioventricular (AV) node
   C. Electrical activity moves slowly from the AV node and into the proximal portions of the ventricular conduction system known as the bundle of His
   D. From the bundle of His, the depolarization moves to the interventricular septum. This is depolarized in a left-to-right direction
   E. The current then moves along the left and right bundle branches to the apex of the heart, where the Purkinje fibers direct the wave of depolarization through the ventricles in a cranial direction

VI. The parts of an ECG are associated with the waves of electrical activity that spread through the heart. The parts are labeled P, QRS, and T (Figure 23-1)
   A. P wave: ECG representation of the depolarization of right and left atria
   B. PR interval: ECG representation of the beginning of atrial depolarization into ventricular depolarization
      1. This interval is mainly a result of slow conduction through the atrioventricular node
      2. This interval is only the measurement of time
   C. QRS complex: ECG expression of ventricular depolarization
   D. T wave: ECG expression of repolarization of the ventricular myocardium
   E. Atrial repolarization is not seen on an ECG because it is hidden by ventricular depolarization or the QRS complex

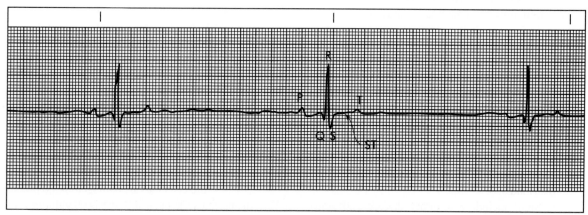

**Figure 23-1** Normal lead II complex. (Courtesy Loncke D, Rivait P, Tighe M: *Clinical procedures handbook,* Windsor, Ontario, 2006, St Clair College of Applied Arts and Technology, Veterinary Technician Program.)

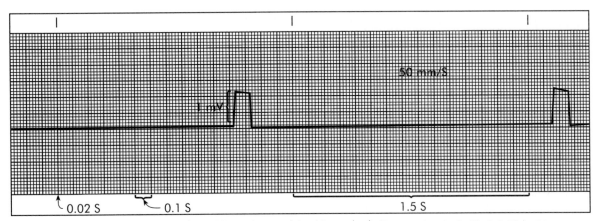

**Figure 23-2** Time intervals at 50 mm/sec and 1 mV standard. (Courtesy Loncke D, Rivait P, Tighe M: *Clinical procedures handbook*, Windsor, Ontario, 2006, St Clair College of Applied Arts and Technology, Veterinary Technician Program.)

## Supplies

I. Protective padding, blanket, or mat for steel tables (stainless steel conducts electricity)

II. Alcohol or conducting gel or paste for increased skin contact

  A. Note: alcohol should not be used in an emergency situation if defibrillation is a possibility

III. ECG machines that are manufactured for human use may need to be modified

  A. Change the snap end to an alligator clip

    1. Alligator clips should be filed or bent slightly to prevent pinching and bruising

  B. For continuous monitoring, pads or wire may be used

    1. Clip fur so that pad may be applied directly to the skin

## Procedure

I. Ideally the animal should be in right lateral recumbency during the recording of an ECG

  A. For large animals, standing position is acceptable and should be noted on the recording

  B. Cats sometimes prefer crouching on the table

II. Using manual restraint, the animal should be placed on a mat or blanket with limbs separated by paper towels or a blanket to reduce contact

III. Using alcohol or electrode gel to increase contact at the site, attach the five electrodes by alligator clips to the skin at the following locations

  A. Proximal left and right olecranons

  B. Proximal left and right stifles

  C. Chest lead: dorsal thorax near the seventh thoracic vertebra

    1. The chest lead is not universally used; however, it may provide additional data to diagnose right and left cardiac enlargement

IV. A three-lead ECG can be used

  A. The leads are labeled RA (right front), LA (left front), and LL (left hind)

V. Ideally the animal should be drug free and without stress; however, sedation can be provided to a fractious animal

  A. If sedation is needed to perform the ECG, the drug and dosage (in mg) should be recorded on the ECG, because it could affect the ECG

VI. Monitor the patient's color and respiration throughout the procedure, because many patients have compromised cardiac output and may have problems when in lateral recumbency or under stress

VII. ECG machine calibration and recording

  A. A "standard" (mV) should be recorded at the speed of 25 mm/sec on the strip before the ECG

    1. The mV standard is the measurement of the sensitivity of the machine (Figure 23-2)

  B. The paper speed should also be recorded

    1. The paper speed should be changed to 50 mm/sec for tracings

    2. A rhythm strip is run at 25 mm/sec

  C. A complete ECG consists of about 30 cm (12 inches) of each lead

    1. In general, six leads are recorded: I, II, III, aVR, aVL, and aVF

    2. A rhythm strip consisting of 30 cm or 12 inches of lead II at 25 mm/sec

  D. After completing all lead tracings, the following information should be recorded on the tracing

    1. Date of ECG

    2. Patient name, client name, and species

    3. Other relevant information

      a. Recumbency

      b. Drugs used with dose(s) in mg

    4. Name of technician

  E. The tracing may then be mounted for filing

## Normal Electrocardiographic Interpretation

I. A normal heartbeat should include P, Q, R, S, and T segments
  A. There is a P wave for every QRS complex
  B. The PR interval is relatively constant
  C. The P wave has a positive deflection (above the baseline) in lead II
  D. The T segment can have a positive or a negative deflection
II. A sinus rhythm is the normal cardiac rhythm in domestic animals
III. After completion of an ECG, the veterinarian/technician can measure the complexes and compare the measurement with normal values for each species
IV. The veterinarian/technician can also calculate the heart rate by counting the complexes in a 3-second period
  A. Most ECG paper has markings for duration of time on the top of the grid

## Abnormal Rhythms

I. Sinus arrhythmia
  A. An irregular ventricular rhythm that is sinoatrial in origin
  B. On the ECG the QRS-to-QRS interval varies, and there is a P wave for every QRS complex
  C. Most cases of sinus arrhythmia are phasic and associated with respiration
    1. The rate increases with inspiration and decreases with expiration
    2. The sinus arrhythmia of respiratory origin is due to the influence of vagal tone
    3. Individuals with respiratory disease tend to have augmented sinus arrhythmia
  D. Most sinus arrhythmias are associated with slow rates
  E. Sinus arrhythmia is normal in the dog
II. Sinus bradycardia
  A. Ventricular rate is decreased
    1. In dogs weighing less than 20 kg (45 lb): a heart rate of less than 70 beats per minute
    2. In dogs larger than 20 kg (45 lb): a heart rate of less than 60 beats per minute
    3. In cats: approximately 100 beats per minute or less
  B. Profound bradycardia will cause weakness, hypotension, and syncope
  C. Etiology of sinus bradycardia
    1. Enhanced parasympathetic tone due to
      a. Increased inspiratory effort as a result of respiratory disease
      b. Gastric irritation
      c. Increased cerebrospinal fluid pressure, hypothyroidism, hypothermia, hyperkalemia, hypoglycemia, and drug therapy

III. Sinus tachycardia
  A. Sinus rhythm with an increased ventricular rate
  B. A heart rate of 180 beats per minute or greater in dogs that are less than 20 kg (45 lb)
  C. A heart rate of 160 beats per minute or greater in dogs that are more than 20 kg (45 lb)
  D. Puppies with heart rate greater than 220 beats per minute
  E. Cats with heart rate greater than 240 beats per minute
  F. Etiology of sinus tachycardia
    1. Pain
    2. Fever
    3. Anemia
    4. Reduced cardiac output
    5. Hyperthyroidism
    6. Excitement
IV. Atrial flutter
  A. Atrial flutter appears as a regular, sawtooth formation between the QRS complexes
  B. Occurs when the ventricular rate differs from the atrial rate
  C. Atrial flutter is the precursor to atrial fibrillation
V. Atrial fibrillation
  A. No P waves are evident, and the baseline is irregular because many erratic impulses are passing through the atrial myocardium
  B. The ventricular depolarization rate is also irregular and rapid
VI. Premature ventricular contractions or complexes (PVCs)
  A. Premature beats
  B. The ventricle discharges before the arrival of the next anticipated impulse from the sinoatrial node
  C. PVCs can occur at any rate but pose a greater danger when occurring with a sustained heart rate that is tachycardic
  D. The P wave is often not seen on the ECG tracing
  E. A wide distorted QRS complex is also evident
  F. The beat preceding the PVC and the beat following the PVC are equal to the time of two normal beats
  G. Etiology of premature ventricular contraction
    1. Associated with the following
      a. Ventricular concentric hypertrophy or eccentric hypertrophy
      b. Hypoxemic states, such as anemia, gastric dilation/volvulus, and heart failure
      c. Acidosis
      d. Drugs such as digitalis, barbiturates, and antiarrhythmic agents
      e. Hypokalemia

H. Possible consequences of PVCs
   1. May initiate repetitive ventricular firing in the form of ventricular tachycardia or fibrillation
   2. Cardiac output may fall if sufficient premature beats are present
   3. PVCs should be treated if the patient shows signs due to dysrhythmia
VII. Atrial premature contraction
  A. The PR interval may be short, normal, or long, depending on the area of origin of the premature beat
   1. The origin could include the sinoatrial node or ectopic locations in the atria
  B. The atrial premature contraction may or may not be conducted to the ventricles
   1. If the beat is not conducted to the ventricles and reaches the AV node before repolarization, premature P waves without QRS complexes will appear on the ECG
   2. If depolarization is conducted through the ventricles, the QRS complex will appear normal
VIII. Ventricular tachycardia
  A. A series of four or more PVCs in sequence
IX. Ventricular fibrillation
  A. The mechanical pumping of the heart is not evident on the ECG
  B. The ECG has a bizarre baseline with prominent undulations
  C. There are no recognizable P or QRS complexes
  D. Unless controlled immediately, ventricular fibrillation will result in cardiac arrest
X. First degree AV block
  A. The PR interval is longer than normal
  B. This type of heart block is a result of a minor conduction defect
XI. Second degree AV block
  A. Some atrial pulses are not conducted through the AV node and therefore do not cause depolarization of the ventricles
  B. There are two types
   1. Type I (Mobitz type I or Wenckebach AV block): progressive lengthening of the PR interval on successive beats and then P waves occurring without QRS complexes
    a. P waves occurring without QRS complexes are called dropped beats
   2. Type II: a constant PR interval that is usually of normal duration with random dropped beats
XII. Third degree AV block
  A. Also known as a complete heart block; the most severe heart block
  B. No relationship between P waves and QRS complexes; the atria and ventricles each beat independently

XIII. Asystole
  A. Cardiac arrest
   1. The ECG tracing will appear as a flat line

## OROGASTRIC INTUBATION

### Indications

I. To remove stomach contents
II. To administer food/nutrients for orphaned or neonatal animals
III. To perform gastric lavage
IV. To administer medication or radiographic contrast material (barium)

### Equipment

I. Stomach tube
  A. 12 French (F) to 18 F infant feeding tube for puppies and kittens
  B. 18 F foal stomach tube for dogs weighing more than 10 kg (22.2 lb)
  C. Foal stomach tube for large dogs
II. Speculum
  A. Canine speculum
  B. Roll of 2-inch (2-cm) wide adhesive tape can be used
III. Adhesive tape for marking the tube
IV. Lubricant
V. Syringe containing sterile saline
VI. Syringe or funnel for administering drugs or other materials

### Procedure

I. Most animals will tolerate this procedure without tranquilization; however, light tranquilization may be required
  A. Note that the use of atropine as part of a tranquilizer will slow the motility of the intestines and should not be administered before a barium study
  B. If an animal is anesthetized during this procedure, a cuffed tight-fitting endotracheal tube should be used
   1. A tight-fitting endotracheal tube will prevent aspiration of the administered material
II. Premeasure the stomach tube
  A. The animal can be either standing or in sternal recumbency
  B. Using the tube, estimate approximately the location of the stomach (or last rib) by holding the tube next to the animal
   1. Mark the measurement on the tube at the oral end with adhesive tape
III. Lubricate the tube
IV. Insert the speculum into the mouth and have the restrainer hold the animal's jaws shut on the speculum

V. Pass the lubricated tube into the speculum and then advance to the premarked point on tube
  A. If the tube cannot be passed to the premarked point
    1. The tube is in the trachea
    2. There is an obstruction in the esophagus
    3. There is a volvulus, which is preventing the tube from passing
VI. Check the placement of the tube before administration of fluids or other material
  A. Note: if an animal is heavily sedated, check the tube placement by more than one method
    1. Palpate the neck area to check for two hard tubes: the trachea's cartilagenous rings and the stomach tube in the esophagus
    2. Blow into the tube and listen for gurgling either on the outside of the body or within the tube
    3. Inject 5 mL of sterile saline into the tube while holding the tube toward the ceiling; if the animal does not cough, the tube is in the esophagus
    4. Smell the end of the tube for gastric odors
  B. If there is any evidence that the tube is in the trachea, such as coughing, remove the tube and reinsert it
VII. Administer materials
VIII. After administration of material, flush the tube with 6 mL of water
IX. Before removing the tube, seal the end with a thumb and then remove or kink the tube
  A. This will help to prevent the leakage of the administered material and water while removing the tube
    1. The animal could aspirate the material if leakage occurs
X. Write in the patient record when and where the procedure was performed and whether any medication was administered

## Precautions

I. Administration of material into the respiratory tract, causing aspiration pneumonia
II. Esophageal trauma
III. Gastric irritation
IV. Gastric perforation

## NASOGASTRIC INTUBATION
### Definition

I. Placement of a tube through the external nares, the nasal cavity, pharynx, and esophagus and into the stomach

### Indications

I. Used for liquid nutritional support and water administration for an extended period
  A. For anorexic animals or animals too stressed to force feed

II. To administer medication or radiographic contrast medium

### Equipment

I. Nasogastric feeding tube, infant feeding tube, red rubber tube, or polyurethane tube
  A. The tube must be soft and flexible
    1. Animals less than 5 kg (12 lb) require a 5 F feeding tube
    2. Animals 5 to 15 kg (12 to 33 lb) require an 8 F feeding tube
II. Topical ophthalmic anesthetic
III. Lubricating jelly
IV. Syringe with 1 mL of sterile saline
V. Bandaging material if feeding tube is going to be used for an extended period
  A. Gauze squares and adhesive tape or elastic adhesive tape
VI. Injection cap
VII. Medication or liquid to administer

### Procedure

I. Patient should be awake
II. Premeasure the tube by placing it on the side of the patient with the tip at the thirteenth rib and the end of the tube at the nares
  A. Mark the tube with a permanent marker for future reference
III. Instill 4 to 5 drops of topical anesthetic into one nostril
  A. The patient may sneeze
  B. Hold the patient's head toward the ceiling
IV. Wait 2 to 3 minutes and apply a few more drops of topical anesthetic to the same nostril
V. Apply a small amount of lubricating jelly to the tip of the nasogastric tube
VI. Hold the head with one hand and insert the tube into the anesthetized nostril
VII. Advance the tube approximately 20 to 25 cm (10 inches)
  A. Gently rotate the tube until it is in place
VIII. Check the placement of the tube by instilling 1 mL of sterile saline into the tube
  A. If the animal coughs, the tube is in the trachea
  B. If the tube is in the trachea, remove the tube and start the procedure again
IX. If the tube is to remain in place for an extended time, bandage the tube in place on one side of the patient's neck
  A. Cachexic or debilitated cats will usually tolerate a tube for an extended period
  B. The tube can remain in place for approximately 1 week or until the animal tolerates force feeding or is eating on its own

X. The end of the tube should be covered with a cap to prevent the aspiration of air into the patient's stomach

XI. Aspirate the tube before each feeding and instill 1 mL of sterile saline into the tube to check for coughing

    A. There should be negative pressure on the tube if the tube is in the stomach

XII. Before removing the tube, seal the end with a finger or thumb to prevent leakage into the pharynx when the tube is removed

XIII. Write in the patient record the location and time of the procedure and any medications that were administered

## Precautions

I. Possible administration of materials into the respiratory tract, causing aspiration pneumonia

II. Esophageal trauma

III. Gastric irritation

IV. The procedure can be stressful to some patients

V. Contraindicated in patients with nasal tumors, esophageal disorders, or no gag reflex

VI. Possible epistaxis (nosebleed) when the tube is first inserted

VII. The tube can become obstructed by medications or nutritional supplements

## CANINE MALE URINARY CATHETERIZATION ■

### Indications

I. To collect a sterile sample of urine for analysis and culture

II. To measure urine output and drainage of urine from the urinary bladder

III. To relieve a urethral obstruction

IV. To administer medication or radiographic contrast medium into the bladder or perform pneumocystography

### Equipment

I. Mild soap

II. Sterile polyethylene, vinyl, or rubber urethral catheter

    A. These can be purchased in a variety of sizes: 3.5F, 5F, 8F, and 10F

        1. Smaller and more flexible catheters cause less trauma to the urethra

    B. Sterile lubricant

    C. Sterile syringe(s) or sterile container to collect urine

    D. Disposable gloves

### Procedure

I. The patient may be in lateral recumbency or standing

II. Wearing gloves, clip the area free of long hairs and cleanse the prepuce with a mild soap

III. Select an appropriate size of sterile catheter for the patient

    A. Dogs less than 12 kg: 3.5 or 5 F catheter

    B. Dogs greater than 12 kg: 8 F catheter

    C. Dogs greater than 35 kg: 10 or 12 F catheter

    D. Foley catheter, which has inflatable tip for long-term use

IV. Estimate the length of the catheter that will be needed to enter the urinary bladder by measuring the catheter against the dog in the approximate position of the penis and bladder

V. A restrainer can lift the dog's upper leg away from the body

VI. Open the package containing the catheter in a sterile manner

VII. Advance the catheter out of its sterile sleeve and lubricate the end of the catheter with sterile lubricant; the restrainer can then hold the catheter, which is still in the sterile sleeve

VIII. With one hand, retract the dog's prepuce so that approximately 1 to 2 inches (5 cm) of glans penis is exposed

    A. The glans penis may be cleansed again at this time

IX. With the other hand, insert the lubricated catheter into the urethral orifice, advancing slowly into the bladder

    A. Slight resistance or stoppage may be felt as the catheter passes the area of the ischial arch

    B. If this does occur, direct the penis toward the cranial end of the animal and slightly lift the penis off the body

X. Attach a syringe to the end of the catheter; extract urine by pulling back on the plunger

    A. If there is no urine entering the catheter, advance the catheter further into the bladder

XI. After the sample is obtained, label the syringe or container with name, date, time, type of sample (sterile or catheterized), and technician's initials

XII. An acceptable alternative is to remove the entire catheter from the package while wearing sterile gloves

    A. If this method is chosen, sterile technique must be used

### Precautions

I. Urinary tract infections due to a break in sterile procedure

II. Trauma to the urethra or urinary bladder by rough handling or using incorrect catheter size

## CANINE FEMALE URINARY CATHETERIZATION ■

### Indications

I. The same as for the male dog

### Equipment

I. The same as for male dog with the addition of a vaginal speculum, sterile gloves, small amount of viscous Xylocaine or 0.5% lidocaine jelly, and possibly a steel catheter

A. A human bivalve nasal speculum with a halogen bulb attached may be used instead of a vaginal speculum

   1. The use of an otoscope or a modified syringe casing as a speculum is also acceptable

## Procedure

I. Patient can be in sternal or lateral recumbency if anesthetized, or standing if awake

II. The restrainer should hold the tail out of the field of view

III. For visual technique

   A. Before performing the procedure, the area can be anesthetized with lidocaine jelly for the comfort of the patient

   B. Check the vulva and vaginal opening using a speculum

      1. Insert the closed speculum first, aiming dorsally and then cranially to avoid the clitoral fossa (blind sac at the ventral opening of the vulva)

   C. Insert lubricated sterile catheter by passing it through the speculum into the urethral orifice and advancing the catheter into the bladder

      1. The urethral tubercle leading to the urethral orifice is on the ventral surface of the vagina, approximately 1 to 2 cm (0.5 to 1 inch) from the clitoral fossa

         a. Often the urethral tubercle is white or red and appears to be puckered or in the form of a cross

   D. The catheter should be directed ventrally; if the catheter is moving in a dorsal direction, it will enter the cervical area of the uterus and will not pass farther than approximately 4 to 5 cm (2 inches)

   E. If no urine is entering the catheter, advance the catheter further into the bladder

   F. Collect the urine in a sterile container and label accordingly

      1. The urine can be collected in a sterile container or with a sterile syringe

IV. Touch technique

   A. Prepare the area as in the visual technique

   B. Lubricate the gloved index finger of one hand and palpate the urethral tubercle

   C. Pass the sterile lubricated catheter ventrally to the gloved finger in the vagina, and use a finger to guide the catheter down to the urethral tubercle and into the urethral orifice

V. A small amount of dilute povidone-iodine solution may be infused into the bladder before removing the catheter to prevent infection

## Precautions

I. The same as for the male dog

## CYSTOCENTESIS

### Indications

I. To puncture the urinary bladder for the purpose of obtaining an uncontaminated sample of urine for analysis or culture

II. To relieve distension of the urinary bladder when an obstruction cannot be relieved by catheterization

### Equipment

I. Large syringe (6 or 12 mL), 22-gauge needle (1 to 1.5 inch long), and isopropyl alcohol

### Procedure

I. This procedure can be performed on an awake, tranquilized, or anesthetized cat or dog

II. The animal should be in dorsal or lateral recumbency with the upper leg lifted away from the body to expose the inguinal area

   A. Cats and dogs may also be in standing position

III. Palpate the bladder in the ventral abdominal area just cranial to the pubis to assess whether there is urine in the bladder

IV. The location of the approximate puncture site can then be clipped and swabbed with isopropyl alcohol

V. Try to immobilize and hold the bladder in place with one hand; use the other hand to puncture the bladder with a sterile needle and syringe

VI. Puncture the bladder and direct the needle in a caudodorsal direction

VII. Using the syringe plunger and negative pressure, withdraw the sample of urine from the bladder

   A. Do not squeeze the bladder while performing cystocentesis

   B. If no fluid is obtained, remove the needle from the body and perform a second puncture using a different needle

VIII. Withdraw the needle and syringe quickly from the body after releasing the plunger

IX. Transfer the sample to a sterile collection container and label the container with the name of the patient, date, technician's initials, and type of sample

X. An alternate method is the "pooling" technique, which may help to locate the ideal location for cystocentesis

   A. The animal is in dorsal recumbency

   B. A small amount of alcohol is poured on the abdomen

   C. The area where the alcohol pools on the ventral midline is the ideal location for the puncture

   D. Withdraw the sample as described earlier

      1. In male dogs, the prepuce may be moved to one side to allow room for insertion of the needle

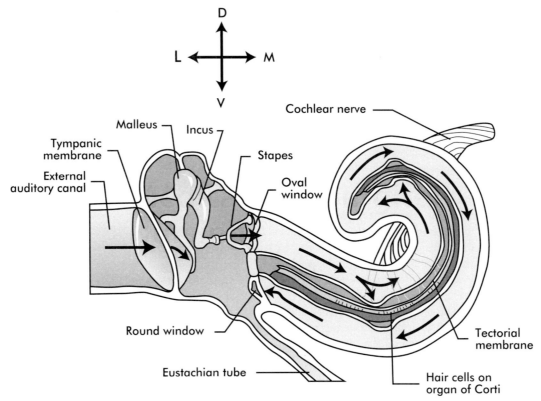

**Figure 23-3** Effect of sound waves on cochlear structures. (From Colville T, Bassert J: *Clinical anatomy and physiology for veterinary technicians*, St Louis, 2002, Mosby.)

## Precautions

I. Urine leakage and peritonitis due to a ruptured bladder
II. Contamination of urine by blood due to a bladder hemorrhage
III. Contamination of the bladder with fecal material is possible if accidental intestinal penetration occurs
IV. Cystocentesis is contraindicated in patients with a suspected pyometra, bladder neoplasms, and bleeding disorders

## MANUAL COMPRESSION OF THE URINARY BLADDER
### Indications

I. Urine collected by manual compression is unsatisfactory for urine culture but can be used to examine solute concentration, physical properties, and chemical constituents

### Procedure

I. Locate the bladder
   A. Begin palpating the abdomen starting at the last rib and move caudally; or
   B. Begin palpating the abdomen slightly cranial to the rear legs
      1. Begin dorsally and move ventrally

II. After palpating and immobilizing the bladder, exert moderate, gentle, steady pressure over the bladder
III. Direct the expressed urine into a container for analysis

## Precautions

I. Do not apply excessive force on the bladder, especially in cases of urethral blockage, because the bladder might rupture

## AURICULAR TREATMENT (Figure 23-3)
### Indications

I. Sampling of the external ear canal for yeast, bacteria, or parasites
II. The removal of cerumen, matted hair, foreign objects, and debris
III. The treatment of otitis externa
IV. Preparation of the site for surgical procedures

### Equipment

I. Bulb syringe, syringe, Auriflush unit
II. Cleansing solution and waste bowls
   1. Ceruminolytic agents, mild soap
III. Sterile cotton-tipped applicators, microscope slides, transport media tube for sampling
IV. Hemostats or forceps for hair removal
V. Otoscope with appropriate sized speculum

VI. Medication

VII. Cotton, applicator sticks for cleaning

VIII. Gloves

## Procedure

I. This procedure can be performed on awake patients; however, if the patient has a painful ear infection, the patient may need to be anesthetized or heavily tranquilized before the procedure

II. Examine the ear with an otoscope

   A. Check for redness, ulceration, odor, exudates, and parasites

   B. Check for an intact tympanic membrane

     1. If the tympanic membrane is not intact, only saline should be used to gently cleanse the ear (see Figure 23-3)

     2. The tympanic membrane (ear drum) appears in the lower external ear canal as a pearly white tissue

III. Take samples for microbiology examination first and then samples for cytology using either sterile cotton-tipped applicator sticks or transport media tube

IV. Remove hair for ease of cleansing

   A. Pluck bunches of hair with fingers or use hemostats

     1. If using hemostats, twist the handle and pull gently on the hair. It should be easy to remove

V. If the eardrum is intact, begin using a ceruminolytic agent by dropper or syringe

VI. Gently massage the external ear canal

VII. Allow waste solution to flow into a waste bowl or into a sink

VIII. Continue to add fluid, massage and empty the ear canal

IX. Use pieces of cotton to remove the loose debris

   A. Cotton-tipped applicator sticks may be used carefully to remove the debris; however, they should be used only on the outermost areas of the ear canal and not deeply inside toward the ear drum

X. Repeat this procedure as needed until ear is clean

XI. Continue to examine the ear with an otoscope

XII. Rinse ear with warm saline or tap water as the final step

XIII. Clean the folds of the pinna, making sure it is free of debris

XIV. Dry ear canal as much as possible

XV. When the ear is dry, instill prescribed medication

   A. The medication should be massaged into the ear canal for good contact

## Possible Etiologies of Otitis Externa

I. Parasites: *Otodectes cynotis*

II. Bacteria: *Staphylococcus* spp., *Streptococcus* spp., *Pasteurella* spp., *Pseudomonas* spp.

III. Fungus: *Candida albicans, Malassezia pachydermatis*

IV. Foreign bodies: grass awns, dirt

V. Tumors: squamous cell carcinoma

## ANAL SAC EXPRESSION

### Definition

I. The anal sacs are located on either side of an animal's anus at approximately the 4 and 8 o'clock positions

II. The anal sacs are filled with malodorous secretions and should normally be expressed when the animal defecates

III. This procedure is commonly performed on dogs, rarely on cats

### Indications

I. To decrease irritation to the animal caused by distention or inflammation

II. To instill medication into diseased anal sacs

III. Removal of material from anal sacs

### Procedure

I. The dog may have to be muzzled and/or securely restrained

II. There are two methods for anal sac expression

   A. External

     1. Using rolled cotton over the dog's anus, apply pressure in a medial and slightly dorsal direction of the external anus

     2. This method does not guarantee full expression of anal sacs

   B. Internal

     1. Insert a gloved, well-lubricated index finger into the anus

     2. With cotton covering the sac, gently squeeze together index finger and thumb to milk contents of the anal sac toward the medial anus

     3. After examining the contents of secretions, roll the glove over the cotton, remove from the hand, and discard

       a. Normal anal sac material should contain granular, brown, malodorous material

### Precautions

I. Rupture of abscessed anal sac

II. Perforation of rectum

## ENEMAS

### Definition

I. An enema is the infusion of fluid into the lower intestinal tract through the anus

II. Enemas are used to remove fecal material from the colon

## Indications

I. To prepare for radiographs with or without contrast medium involvement
II. To irrigate the colon of a patient who has been poisoned
III. To relieve constipation

## Procedure

I. Sedation or anesthesia may be needed in cases of severe blockage or fractious animals
II. An abdominal radiograph should be completed to rule out perforation or presence of foreign body
III. Use an enema container with a rounded, soft, pliable piece of connected tubing
IV. Place the animal in sternal or lateral recumbency, preferably on a tub table
V. Put on examination gloves
VI. Place the enema preparation into the enema container
   A. Examples of enema preparations
     1. Mild soap and water
     2. Saline for irrigation
     3. Commercial enema preparation
   B. Hyperphosphate enema solutions should not be used in cats or small dogs
     1. These solutions may cause acute collapse associated with hypocalcemia
VII. Lubricate the end of the flexible tubing
VIII. Insert the tip of the enema tubing to the colorectal junction
IX. Place the enema container above the animal so that the flow of solution into the animal is aided by gravity
X. More than one enema may be required to adequately evacuate the animal's bowels
XI. Do not continue to administer enemas if there is no sign of fecal material
XII. Do not proceed with enema if there is evidence of abdominal pain that could be associated with intestinal perforation or obstruction

## Precautions

I. Rupture of the colon
II. Leakage of enema fluid into peritoneal cavity through already ruptured intestinal tract
III. Hemorrhage in cases of ulcerative colitis
   A. Enemas are contraindicated in cases of ulcerative colitis because they may increase bleeding

## OPHTHALMOLOGY (Table 23-1)
### Anatomy (Figure 23-4)

I. Knowing the anatomical features of the eye is important in ophthalmology
II. Such structures as the conjunctiva, lens, ciliary body, cornea, sclera, choroids, retina, vitreous humor, aqueous humor, iris, and pupil all contribute to the animal's ability to see objects clearly (see Chapter 1)

III. Feline and canine eyes are different
   A. Feline differences
     1. Tapetum lucidum
       a. Iridescent epithelium of the choroid of the feline eye
       b. This epithelium causes their eyes to shine in the dark
     2. Pupil shape is oval rather than round
     3. Cats do not have true eyelashes; their hair grows to the edge of the eye

## Tears

I. Formation of tears (Figure 23-5)
   A. Lacrimal glands produce moisture (tears), and the tears empty into a conjunctival sac and flush over the eye
   B. Tears leave the eye by moving into the lacrimal puncta at the medial canthus
   C. Tears then move through the lacrimal sac, which drains into the nasolacrimal duct
   D. The nasolacrimal duct empties the tears into the nose or the tears are swallowed
II. Functions of tears
   A. Wash out foreign bodies
   B. Lubricate and moisten cornea
   C. Tears are necessary for the proper refraction of light on the cornea

## Formation of the Aqueous Humor

I. Maintains intraocular pressure and is one of the most important structures in the eye
II. Comes from the ciliary processes
III. Remains in constant amount
IV. Leaves eye via the intrascleral plexus
V. Carries waste products of the lens and corneal metabolism
VI. If the aqueous humor increases in pressure it could lead to glaucoma

## Medical Terminology

I. Proptosis: forward displacement or bulging of the eye
II. Epiphora: overflow of tears
III. Conjunctivitis: inflammation of the conjunctiva or tissue lining the eyelid
IV. Miotic: drug that makes pupils decrease in size (e.g., pilocarpine)
V. Mydriatic: drug that make pupils increase in size (e.g., 1% tropicamide or 2.5% phenylephrine)
VI. Medial canthus: area of the eye closest to the nose, at the junction of the eyelids
VII. Lateral canthus: area of the eye closest to the ears, at the junction of the eyelids
VIII. Ophthalmic drops: aqueous solution that lasts a short time on the eye

**Table 23-1** Conditions of the eye

| Condition and etiology | Description | Signs | Treatments | Common breeds affected |
|---|---|---|---|---|
| Ophthalmia neonatorum (congenital) | Infection of eye in newborn animals | Acute purulent discharge, swollen eyes | Flushing of eye and oral antibiotics | Newborn animals |
| Microphthalmia (inherited defect) | Failure of eye to reach its normal size | Eyeball decreased in size in all diameters | None | Pekingese, Poodle, Minature Schnauzer, Collie, Chihuahua, and Canary |
| Entropion (inherited) | Turning inward of eyelid, usually the lower lid | Eyelashes scratch the cornea causing ulceration | Surgical removal or eye tuck | Chow Chow, Shar-Pei |
| Ectropion (inherited) | Outward turning of eyelid, exposing conjunctiva | Dryness of eye | Surgery or eye tuck | Bloodhounds, American Eskimo, American Cocker Spaniel, Basset Hound, and Saint Bernard |
| Hypertrophy/eversion of the third eyelid, or "cherry eye" (inherited, conformation of eye) | Glandular tissue projects beyond the haw (membrane nictitans) and possibly lacrimal gland | Excessive tearing, mucoid discharge, corneal erosion, and possible rupture of the anterior chamber and iris prolapse | | Spaniels, Boston Terrier, Pug, and Beagle |
| Distichiasis (autosomal recessive trait) | Second row of eyelashes usually incomplete on upper or lower eyelid | Sometimes ectropion too; ulcerations of the cornea | Plucking or epilation of the extra eyelashes, cryosurgery | English Bulldog, Cocker Spaniel, Bull Terrier, and Poodle |
| Trichiasis (trauma, inherited) | Ingrowing hairs. Eyelashes assume an abnormal deviation | Scratches of cornea | Removal of problem hairs as for distichiasis | Poodle |
| Hordeolum/stye *Staphylococcus* spp. (bacterial infection) | Inflammation of the hair follicle or sebaceous gland | Usually involving the gland or eyelid; erythematous, swollen, cystlike lesion | Antibiotics | Any breed |
| Strabismus types: Convergent: medial movement Divergent: outward movement (inherited or congenital) | Squinting or crossing of the eyes; malfunction of the muscle that moves the eye | Congenital or acquired because of injury, cellulitis, or sinusitis | None | Congenital in the Pekingese, Pug, Boston Terrier, or Chihuahua |
| Keratoconjunctivitis sicca or "dry eye" (inherited or drug induced) | Decrease in tear production and corneal film | Conjunctivitis; sticky, stringy discharge; red, dull eyes; dry nostrils | Diagnosis by Schirmer tear test; treat with 0.2% cyclosporine ointment | Bulldogs, West Highland White Terriers, Lhasa Apso |
| Uveitis (*Brucella* spp., adenovirus, neoplasm, trauma, or keratitis) | Inflammation of the middle vascular layer of the eye; includes iris, ciliary body, choroids, and uvea | Conjunctiva and lids swollen, corneal edema, miotic pupil, swollen and discolored iris | Steroids, nonsteroidal antiinflammatory drugs (NSAIDs), mydriatics, and atropine | No specific breed |
| Pannus (autoimmune disease) | Chronic superficial keratitis | Cornea red and irritated, discharge, and itchy eyes | Lifelong steroids | German Shepherds |

**Table 23-1** Conditions of the eye—cont'd

| Condition and etiology | Description | Signs | Treatments | Common breeds affected |
|---|---|---|---|---|
| Keratitis or corneal ulcer (scratches or abrasion due to bacterial, viral infections, or trauma) | Corneal inflammation or ulcer | Can be very deep or superficial; red, swollen conjunctiva; scratching; blepharospasm; discharge | No steroids; antibiotics, atropine only if pupil is miotic; soft contact lens acting as a bandage or barrier to further infection; conjunctival flap for two days, depending on how deep the ulcer is in the eye tissue | No specific breed |
| Glaucoma (inherited or secondary infection) (acute or chronic) | Increase of intraocular pressure due to decreased draining of the aqueous humor from anterior chamber | Large swollen eyeball, painful | Mannitol, antiglaucoma medications, pilocarpine (primary glaucoma cases only), possible enucleation | Bassett Hound, American and English Cocker Spaniel, Siberian Husky, Poodles |
| Dermoid cyst (congenital) | Embryological defect; piece of skin or tissue that carries hair root has attached to the cornea and/or conjunctiva | Hair growing on cornea after newborn's eyes have opened | Surgery | No specific breed |
| Cataract (inherited) | Opacity of the lens of the eye | Cloudy/gray lens; blindness | Surgical removal of lens | Any breed |
| Nuclear sclerosis (inherited) | Normal aging of eye | Cloudy/gray eye | No treatment required; animal still has vision | Any breed |
| Progressive retinal atrophy (autosomal recessive gene, sometimes secondary to cataracts) | Degeneration of rods and cones | Starts with poor night vision; sluggish reaction of pupils to light; progresses to blindness | Vitamin A in early stages to slow down progression | English Cocker Spaniel, Poodle, Collie, and Sheltie; very common and can affect many breeds |
| Anterior uveitis (feline infectious peritonitis, feline leukemia virus, feline immunodeficiency virus, toxoplasmosis or leptospirosis) | Inflammation of the uvea, including iris and ciliary body | Blepharospasm, epiphora, swollen lids, corneal edema, miotic pupil, discoloration of the iris | Steroids, NSAIDs, antibiotics, atropine | |

IX. Ophthalmic ointments: thicker solutions that last longer than drops on the eye

X. Artificial tears: generally a solution made of methylcellulose, which lubricates the eye

## Therapeutic Techniques

I. Restraint techniques
   A. To retract the third eyelid while restraining patient
      1. Feline: shake head slightly
      2. Canine: shake head or tip head up and down
   B. Be careful to perform minimal restraint around head area
      1. If pressure is applied to the external jugular vein it may change the results of eye pressure tests
   C. Use one hand to control the muzzle by wrapping fingers around mandible and maxilla or top of muzzle

II. Examination
   A. Evaluate head symmetry
   B. Check for drooping eyelids and discharge
   C. Check pupillary light reflex by quickly shining a strong light near the eye
      1. It is possible to have pupillary light reflex and be blind
   D. Check to see if patient will follow hand or object
      1. For feline patients drop a cotton ball a few feet above their heads from behind them.

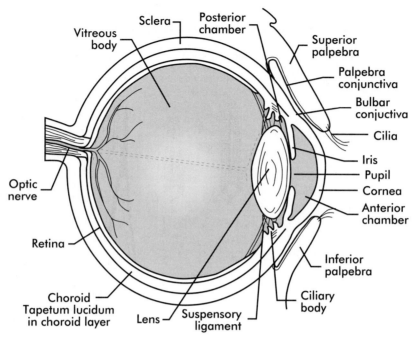

**Figure 23-4**   Cross-section of the eye. (From Colville T, Bassert J: *Clinical anatomy and physiology for veterinary technicians*, St Louis, 2002, Mosby.)

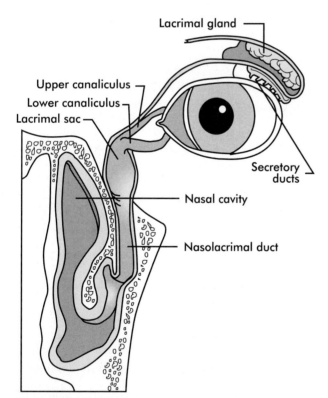

**Figure 23-5**   Lacrimal apparatus. (From Colville T, Bassert J: *Clinical anatomy and physiology for veterinary technicians*, St Louis, 2002, Mosby.)

This will ensure that the cat is following the object and not reacting to air flow movement

III. Ophthalmoscopy
   A. Examining the eye using an opthalmoscope
IV. Schirmer's tear test
   A. Used to diagnosis keratoconjunctivitis sicca (KCS) and to access the amount of tear production in each eye
   B. Patient should not be given any drugs 1 to 2 hours before test
   C. Wipe excess mucus from eye with dry swab
   D. Topical ophthalmic anesthetic can be used to anesthetize the cornea
   E. Open prepared packaged sterile strips
   F. Using sterile technique, fold strip at a 90-degree angle and insert notched end under lower eyelid
   G. Hold strip in eye for 1 minute and measure moisture on strip using the scale on package
      1. <10 mm moisture=KCS, feline
      2. <15 mm moisture=KCS, canine
      3. 18 to 25 mm is the normal amount of moisture
V. Corneal staining
   A. Performed to determine the presence or location of cornea ulcers or to check the patency of the nasolacrimal duct
   B. Moisten sterile fluorescein strip with ophthalmic irrigating solution or artifical tears solution
   C. Lift the upper eyelid
   D. Place the moistened strip under the eyelid on sclera of eye for 1 to 2 seconds

E. Remove strip

F. Flush the eye with ophthalmic irrigating solution

G. Examine the cornea in a partially dark room with either an opthalmoscope or a Wood's lamp, checking for bright green dye in ulcerated area

H. Observe the external nare of the tested eye for green dye

1. If fluorescein dye is present, it indicates patency of the nasolacrimal duct

I. Continue to flush until the eye is free of stain

VI. Rose-Bengal stain can also be used to stain devitalized epithelial tissue and to diagnose KCS

VII. Tonometry

A. Measures intraocular pressure for glaucoma

B. Anesthetize cornea using topical anesthetic

C. Tilt animal's snout upward toward ceiling and retract lower eyelid with finger of one hand

D. Place tonometer vertically, resting on cornea of the eye

1. There are several types of tonometers

a. Schiøtz; manual

b. Tono-Pen; digital read out and hand held

2. Use the average of three readings for each eye

3. There should be a difference of no more than 1 unit between the three readings

E. The same person should perform this procedure for all visits to ensure consistent and accurate readings

F. A normal reading is 15 to 25 mm Hg

VIII. Gonioscopy

A. Using an ophthalmoscope and magnification lens to examine the iris angle and anterior chamber

B. Examination for glaucoma and neoplasm

C. A very specialized procedure

IX. Lacrimal flushing

A. Anesthetize animal or apply topical anesthetic

B. Equipment required: cannulas (21 to 22 gauge) with 6 mL of sterile saline, gauze square, and strong overhead lighting

C. Find the lacrimal punctum near the medial canthus of the eye (usually it is pigmented)

D. Place the cannula in the lower punctum, positioning the cannula toward the nose and inject sterile saline

E. Place one finger over the upper punctum and allow saline to exit via the nasolacrimal duct through the nostril

F. Repeat this same procedure in the upper lid punctum while holding off the lower lid's punctum

G. Flush the puncta of both eyes

X. Surgical Preparation

A. Instill ointment in the eye to prevent hair from entering eye

1. Exception: for perforating injuries do not use ointments

a. Ointments can recede into anterior chamber of the eye and create serious problems

B. Clip the hair around the eye only; may remove eyelashes

C. Chlorhexidine gluconate or a mild solution of betadine (1 part betadine: 20 parts of saline) can be used to cleanse the area

1. Do not use alcohol or pHisoHex, because they are toxic to corneal epithelium

## DERMATOLOGY

### Anatomy

See Chapter 1 and Figure 23-6.

### Examination of the Skin

I. Examination should be performed in a well illuminated area

II. A magnifying lens should be used to examine skin lesions

III. Part the hair or clip fur to see underlying lesions

IV. Check the entire coat

V. Examine the mouth, sides of mouth, and foot pads for hidden lesions

### Primary Lesions

I. Primary lesions arise from normal skin

II. Primary lesions exhibit the initial pathological changes

III. These lesions should be used for skin biopsy and histological tests

### Secondary Lesions

I. These lesions develop from preexisting skin lesions (primary lesions)

II. They always arise from previous pathological changes rather than from normal skin

### Dermatology Terminology (Table 23-2)
### Types of Shampoo

There are many commercial brands of shampoo used for a variety of conditions. Table 23-3 lists in general the most common dermatological conditions and the most common shampoos used to treat those conditions.

### Common Dermatological Conditions

I. Bacterial

A. Pyodermas and abscesses are the most common bacterial infection

1. *Staphylococcus* spp. are the most common organisms found on canine skin

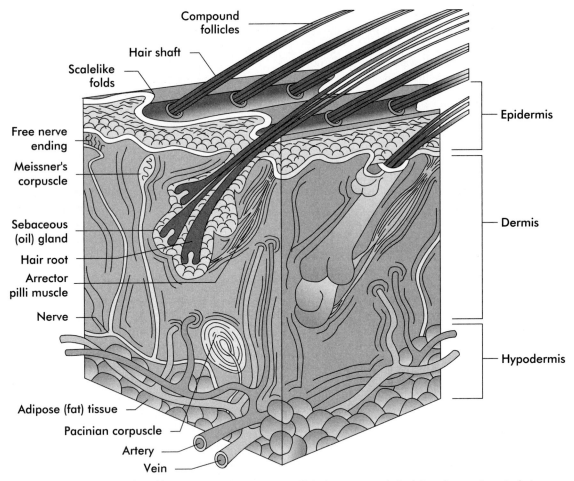

**Figure 23-6** Canine skin. (From Colville T, Bassert J: *Clinical anatomy and physiology for veterinary technicians*, St Louis, 2002, Mosby.)

B. Most bacterial infections are secondary to another disease (e.g., parasitism, allergies, endocrine disorders, immunological diseases)
C. Signs include yellow pustules; erythematous lesions; ulcerations; dry, crusted areas with alopecia; lesions are often round
D. Diagnosis
   1. Culture and sensitivity
   2. Sterile swab sample and gram stain
   3. Fine needle aspiration of pus from lesion
E. Treatment after diagnosis includes
   1. Clipping the area and washing with antibacterial soap or shampoo
      a. Careful, thorough drying
      b. Application of antibacterial ointments
   2. Oral antibiotics may also be prescribed with nutritional supplements
II. Fungal (ringworm)
   A. Etiology is generally two genera of fungi: *Microsporum canis* and *Trichophyton* spp.
   B. Ringworm is more common in young canines
   C. Fungi live in hair and nails

D. Signs include circular patches of alopecia, the center of which may be dry and crusty
   1. The head and legs of the patient are the most commonly infected
E. Diagnosis
   1. The appearance of the lesions and patient history
   2. Wood's lamp test (ultraviolet, shortwave) can be used to diagnose *Microsporum* spp. only
   3. Most reliable test is to culture the fungi found on infected areas
      a. Fungassay R (Pittman-Moore) is a special culture media used for fungus
      b. Swab the lesion with 70% alcohol to remove secondary bacteria
      c. Take hair and skin debris using sterile forceps from an area at the margin of the suspected lesion and imbed them into the small bottle of media
      d. Label the bottle with the patient's name, date, and location of lesion

**Table 23-2** Dermatology terminology

| Lesion | Description |
|---|---|
| **PRIMARY LESION TERMINOLOGY** | |
| Macule | Erythematous, not raised or depressed, visual change in skin, <1 cm |
| Papule | Erythematous, circular, elevation of skin, <0.5 cm |
| Nodule | Small node, solid elevation, extends into deep layers of skin, >1 cm |
| Tumor | Swelling or mass of varying size |
| Pustule | Small circumscribed pus-filled elevation of skin |
| Vesicle/bulla | Vesicle: small blister filled with clear fluid, <0.5 cm |
| | Bulla: large blister filled with fluid, >0.5 cm |
| Wheal | Hives; raised, flat topped, redder or paler than surrounding skin, usually accompanied by itching |
| Plaque | Flat-topped, solid elevation with alopecia and erythema |
| **SECONDARY LESION TERMINOLOGY** | |
| Scale | Dandruff; accumulation of loose epidermis |
| Epidermal collarette | Circular or semicircular accumulation of scale on skin surface |
| Erosion/excoriations | Superficial defect caused by partial loss of epidermis |
| Ulcer | Defect of skin or mucous membranes due to loss of epidermis and dermis |
| Crusts or scabs | Formed from dried exudates on the surface of a skin lesion |
| Hyperpigmentation/ hypopigmentation | More/less than normal color in skin |
| Lichenification | Thickening or hardening of the skin |
| Scar | Hard plaque of dense fibrous tissue |
| Hyperkeratosis | Extreme increase in the thickness of the corneum of the skin |
| Fissure | Deep defect (usually in a foot pad); a cracklike sore |
| Comedo | Blackhead; plug of keratin and dried sebum in a hair follicle |
| Cyst | A closed sac or pouch containing fluid or semisolid material |
| Hyperhidrosis | Excessive sweating |
| Alopecia | Loss of hair |
| Erythema | Redness of skin |
| Hot spot/acute moist dermatitis | Bacterial skin disease |

e. Place the bottle in a dark area at room temperature and check for growth daily

f. The cap should be slightly loose to allow for aerobic conditions

g. A positive sample consists of fluffy, white fungi and a change in color of the media from orange to red

F. Treatment
1. Clip the hair around the lesion, and apply a fungicidal shampoo to entire animal
2. Fungicidal ointment can also be applied to the infected area
3. Griseofulvin or ketoconazole orally may also be prescribed
4. Treatment with oral antifungals and application of ointments must be continued for several weeks to be effective

G. Zoonoses
1. Ringworm is zoonotic to humans and especially small children
2. If ringworm is suspected, the animal should be treated immediately and children should be kept away from the animal until the infection is under control

III. Allergic skin diseases
A. Etiology is usually due to a hypersensitive reaction to allergy-causing substances. These substances are known as allergens or antigens
B. Small animals can develop allergies at any age
C. Allergens include flea bites, food, mold, pollen, grass, certain soaps or shampoos, insect bites (bees, wasps, yellow jackets)
D. Signs include pruritus; red, moist patches (called hot spots); pus; and dried crusts
E. Location of lesions
1. Flea allergies are most common dorsally near base of tail
2. Dog's face and front legs are more often affected by pollen and food allergies
3. Contact allergies are seen mostly in areas of skin with the least coverage of hair, such as the armpits, chin, elbows, hocks, foot pads, and genitals
4. Dogs allergic to flea collars will show irritation around the neck area, where the collar contacts the skin
F. Diagnosis
1. History
2. Positive response to treatment
3. Intradermal skin testing or serum allergy testing
4. Biopsy
G. Treatment
1. Drugs: antihistamines, corticosteroids to decrease the pruritus

**Table 23-3** Common shampoos

| | Sulfur | Salicylic | Coal/tar | Benzoyl peroxide 2.5% | Chlorhexidine | Povidone/iodine 1% |
|---|---|---|---|---|---|---|
| Seborrhea sicca | ✓ | ✓ | | | | |
| Seborrhea oleosa | ✓ | ✓ | ✓ | ✓ | | |
| Keratolytic | ✓ | ✓ | | | | |
| Keratoplastic | ✓ | ✓ | ✓ | | | |
| Antipruritic | ✓ | | | | ✓ | |
| Antifungal | ✓ | | | | ✓ | ✓ |
| Antiparasitic | ✓ | | | | | |
| Antibacterial | ✓ | | | ✓ | ✓ | ✓ |
| **Use** | Flushes follicles | Allergic contact dermatitis and calluses | Not for use on cats; allergic contact dermatitis | Hot spots Skin fold dermatitis Deep pyodermas May bleach fabrics | Hot spots Superficial folliculitis Not inhibited by organic debris, such as dirt, scales, or crusts | Short residual May cause contact dermatitis and skin irritation Staining |

2. Avoidance of the allergen
   a. This may be the least practical treatment
3. Immunotherapy
   a. Gradual exposure of the allergen in increasing doses
   b. This should be considered only for long-term patients
   c. This can be used for patients that are intolerant of glucocorticosteroid side effects

IV. Parasites
   A. Examples
      1. Fleas are the most common parasite
         a. Itching, alopecia, crusting of the skin, flea dirt
         b. Flea dirt will turn red when exposed to water
      2. Sarcoptic mange: itchy areas most commonly around the ears, front legs, chest, and abdomen
      3. Demodectic mange: nonitching areas around the face and front legs with red and scaly ringwormlike lesions
      4. Ear mites (*Otodectes* spp.) cause scratching and red irritated ears
      5. Walking dandruff (*Cheyletiella* spp.): small, white insects found on hair
      6. Ticks
   B. Diagnosis
      1. History of contact
      2. Appearance
      3. Skin scraping
         a. A sterile blunt scalpel blade with a small amount of mineral oil is used to harvest hair and debris from several lesions

   b. If demodectic mange is suspected, pinch a fold of skin and scrape the fold until there is a slight oozing of blood
      (1) Because *Demodex* are burrowing mites, pinching a fold of skin brings the mite to the surface
   c. If *Sarcoptes* is suspected, the entire lesion should be scraped
      (1) For *Sarcoptes* at least 8 to 10 lesions should be tested to diagnose the infestation
   d. The harvested sample should be examined under a microscope immediately after sampling is completed
      4. Cellophane tape sampling
         a. A piece of clear tape is used to collect the parasite
         b. The tape containing the sample is applied to a microscope slide for microscopic examination
   C. Treatment
      1. Clip the entire hair coat for ease of treatment
      2. Medicated shampoo may be used for several weeks
         a. If using shampoo, follow directions and leave shampoo on animal for prescribed length of time
      3. Dips, shampoos, dermal applications, or oral flea medications are also commonly used
V. Hormonal
   A. Hormonal skin conditions are difficult to diagnose

B. Etiologies include hypersecretion or hyposecretion of hormones from the thyroid, adrenal, or pituitary gland
   1. Ovaries or testicles may also cause a change in skin condition
C. Signs
   1. Changes to the skin and hair coat on the lateral sides of the body
      a. The skin is often dark in color and thicker than normal
D. Diagnosis
   1. Blood tests
VI. Genetic
   A. Canine seborrheic complex
   B. A defect in the keratinization of the skin that is associated with increased scale formation, increased or decreased greasiness of the skin, and secondary inflammation
      1. Seborrhea sicca: dry skin with diffuse scaling and accumulation of white to gray scales, alopecia, erythema, and inflammation
         a. Dry, dull hair coat
         b. Common in Irish Setters, German Shepherds, Dachshunds, and Doberman Pinschers
      2. Seborrhea oleosa: excessive greasiness of skin with diffuse scaling, alopecia, erythema, and inflammation
         a. Brownish flakes adhere to skin
         b. Coat has a distinct odor and is greasy to touch
         c. Often associated with otitis externa
         d. Cocker Spaniels, Shar-Peis, West Highland White Terriers, and Basset Hounds are predisposed to this skin condition
   C. Diagnosis
      1. History and physical examination
      2. Systematic elimination of possible underlying etiologies
         a. Skin scraping, biopsy, nutritional changes, bacterial cultures, blood chemistry panels, hormone analysis
   D. Treatment
      1. Medicated shampoos daily and then every 2 weeks
      2. Possibly corticosteroids to relieve pruritus and erythema
         a. Antibiotics to control secondary infections
         b. Dietary supplements to increase fatty acids
         c. Vitamin A supplements to decrease flaking and scaling of the skin

## WOUND MANAGEMENT
### Wound Contamination vs. Infection

I. All wounds are contaminated; however, a contaminated wound elicits no immune response from the host body

A. A surgical wound is considered contaminated by microbes on the tissue and surrounding area
II. Infection is the term used for a wound where microorganisms are invading tissue and therefore eliciting an immune response from the host body
   A. A wound is considered infected if the patient is presented for treatment more than 12 hours postinjury
      1. Signs of infection can include edema, pus, fever, neutrophilia, pain, color change, exudates, and odor
III. A contaminated wound can become infected from the addition of foreign material in the wound, necrotic tissue, or excessive bleeding

### Wound Healing

I. The four phases of wound healing are the inflammatory phase, the debridement phase, the repair phase, and the maturation phase
   A. Inflammatory phase: begins directly after the injury
      1. Vasoconstriction is followed by vasodilation to control hemorrhage and then produce a clot
      2. The blood clot will dry and form a scab, which allows healing to begin
   B. Debridement phase: begins approximately 6 hours postinjury
      1. Neutrophils and monocytes travel to the site to remove foreign material, bacteria, and necrotic tissue
      2. An exudate is formed from fluid and white blood cells
   C. Repair phase: begins 3 to 5 days postinjury and depends on the debridement stage and the removal of foreign material in the wound
      1. The debridement and inflammatory phases, or the first 3 to 5 days postinjury, can also be called the lag phase
         a. The lag phase is characterized by minimal wound strength
      2. At this point, fibroblasts produce collagen that, after maturation, will become scar tissue and strengthen the wound
      3. Granulation tissue starts to appear after formation of new capillaries, fibroblasts, and fibrous tissue
         a. Granulation tissue appears under the scab as red, fleshy material
      4. Epithelialization, or the formation of new epithelial tissue, on the wound surface becomes visible 4 to 5 days postinjury
         a. Epithelial cells at the edge of the wound divide and migrate across the granulation tissue
         b. The new tissue is only one cell thick; however, over time it thickens through the formation of more cell layers

5. Wound contraction, reducing the size of the wound, occurs 5 to 9 days postinjury

D. Maturation phase: the final phase, this is the longest phase
   1. During this phase, wound strength increases to its maximum level because of remodeling of the collagen fibers and fibrous tissue
      a. Cross-linking increases and improves wound strength
   2. The scar gradually disappears because of the increased number of capillaries in the fibrous tissue
   3. This phase may continue for many years

E. Wound healing is a series of overlapping events; more than one phase may be occurring at one time

## Types of Wound Healing

I. Primary or first-intention healing
   A. Characterized by noncomplicated healing
      1. Examples: small lacerations, minor wounds, and clean wounds
      2. In the case of fractures, using pins or plates

II. Second-intention healing
   A. Wounds that are left open and allowed to heal from the internal to external areas
      1. Examples: larger wounds, infected wounds
      2. Healing of fractures through the normal formation of a callus

III. Third-intention healing
   A. Initial second-intention healing (open wound) followed by surgical repair
      1. Examples: severely contaminated wounds, very large wounds

## Wound Treatment

I. First aid
   A. Protection of the wound is important either by bandaging or by applying a makeshift splint

II. Wound evaluation
   A. Control of hemorrhaging should be the first priority, followed by an evaluation of the wound for possible contamination and infection
   B. The injury should then be assessed by obtaining a history and checking the location and size of the wound

III. Clipping, scrubbing, and wound lavage
   A. All wounds should be clipped before treatment
      1. A sterile lubricant can be put into any open wounds to avoid further contamination of the site by loose hair
      2. Ophthalmic ointment may be applied in the eye before clipping and cleaning for protection of the cornea and globe
   B. The outer edges of the wound can then be gently scrubbed using a detergent/antimicrobial surgical scrub

1. Povidine-iodine or chlorhexidine agent is recommended

C. Wound lavage is most effective when at least 7 pounds per square inch (psi) of pressure are used
   1. Equipment
      a. A 35- to 60-mL syringe with an 18-gauge needle attached
      b. Waterpik at low pressure
      c. Spray bottle
      d. Lavage solutions include
         (1) Isotonic saline, LRS, or plain Ringer's solution
         (2) Hydrogen peroxide
            (a) Its foaming effect can damage tissues
            (b) Is not antimicrobial, just sporicidal
            (c) Should be used only for first-time irrigation of dirty wounds
            (d) Should not be used under pressure because of foaming
         (3) Chlorhexidine diacetate solution (0.05%)
            (a) Broad-spectrum antimicrobial
            (b) Microbial effect is immediate with a lasting residual effect
            (c) Not inactivated by organic material
         (4) Povidone-iodine solution (1% to 2%)
            (a) Broad-spectrum antimicrobial
            (b) Antimicrobial effect lasts approximately 4 to 6 hours
            (c) It is inactivated by blood, exudates, and organic material
            (d) The detergent form is not recommended for wounds, because it causes irritation and potentiation of wound infections

IV. Debridement
   A. Debridement is the removal of necrotic tissue
   B. Necrotic tissue must be removed for new tissue to migrate over the wound
      1. Necrotic tissue is also considered a growth medium for bacteria, so its removal reduces the chances of infection
   C. Debridement is considered complete when the wound is free of necrotic tissue
      1. The wound is then considered a "clean wound"
   D. Mechanical debridement includes the use of surgical instruments, dry-to-dry bandages, wet-to-dry bandages, and irrigation
   E. Nonmechanical debridement is generally the addition of enzymatic agents or chemicals to the wound

1. Both mechanical and nonmechanical methods may be used to treat a wound
F. The procedure should be performed aseptically
V. Drainage
   A. Drains are implanted in a wound to help relieve the buildup of air or fluid
      1. The drain will reduce the possible formation of seromas, hematomas, tissue pockets, or dead space
   B. Drains are usually indicated
      1. For treatment of an abscess
      2. When foreign material in a wound cannot be removed
      3. When contamination is probable
      4. When necrotic tissue cannot be excised
      5. For prevention of the creation of dead space and to remove fluid or air after a surgical procedure
   C. Penrose drains are used most commonly
      1. They are composed of soft, latex rubber
      2. Fluid flows through the lumen of the drain and around the drain
      3. Penrose drains should not be left in place for longer than 3 to 5 days

## BANDAGING

### Types of Bandages

I. Bandages have up to three layers: primary, secondary, and tertiary
   A. Primary layer is next to the wound
   B. Secondary layer is present to absorb exudates and provide padding
   C. Tertiary layer is the outer layer, which is used for support
II. Primary layer material
   A. Adherent bandages are used to remove necrotic tissue and wound exudates when they are taken off
      1. These bandages (usually sterile gauze) are used in the very early stages of wound healing
         a. Dry-to-dry dressings are used when loose necrotic tissue is evident
            (1) Dry sterile gauze is placed over the wound with an absorbent wrap holding it in place
            (2) Bandage removal may be painful because dead tissue is adhered to the bandage
         b. Wet-to-dry dressings are used for wounds with dried or semidry exudates
            (1) The bandage is applied wet, and it absorbs the material from the wound
            (2) The exudate then adheres to the bandage and is removed when the bandage is removed

            (3) Saline or chlorhexidine can be used to moisten the bandage
         c. Wet-to-wet dressings are used on wounds with large amounts of exudates and transudates
            (1) Wet dressings tend to absorb fluid easily
            (2) Wet dressings can be used to heat the wound, which will enhance capillary action and therefore increase the drainage of the wound
            (3) These bandages are removed wet and therefore cause less pain on bandage removal
            (4) The negative aspect of this type of bandage is that there is little wound debridement because of the decreased adhesion to necrotic tissue
   B. Nonadherent primary layer
      1. Used when granulation tissue is starting to form
      2. Commonly used to minimize tissue injury during bandage changes
      3. There are many commercial products on the market
III. Secondary layer provides extra absorbency to draw fluids away from the wound and adds padding for support
   A. Generally, gauze bandaging is used, such as Kling (Johnson & Johnson)
IV. Tertiary layer holds the primary and secondary layers in place
   A. Generally made up of adhesive tapes, elastic bandages, Vetrap (3M) and a conforming stretch gauze (Conform; Kendall)

### Head and Neck

I. Reasons for bandaging
   A. Postocular surgery
   B. Repair of an aural hematoma
   C. Ear surgery
   D. To secure a jugular catheter or pharyngostomy tube
II. Precautions
   A. The bandage should be frequently checked postoperatively because edema, which could be life threatening, may occur
   B. Respiration and mucous membrane color must be monitored closely
      1. The bandage should be loose enough to enable two fingers to fit under the bandage
      2. If there are any changes in respiration, the bandage should be loosened or changed immediately
   C. If the animal tries to remove the bandage, an Elizabethan collar can be used for restraint

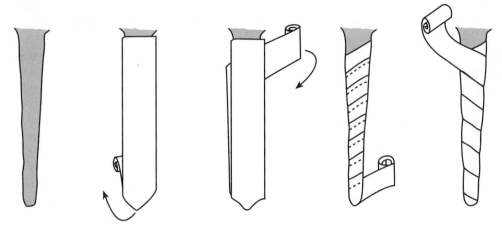

**Figure 23-7**   Tail bandage. (From Lane DR, Cooper B: *Veterinary nursing, formerly Jones' animal nursing,* ed 5, Woburn, Mass, 1998, Butterworth-Heinemann.)

## Thorax

I.  Reasons for bandaging
  A.  To secure chest drains
  B.  To protect large thoracic wounds
  C.  Spinal surgery
II. Precautions
  A.  If respiration becomes impaired, the bandage should be removed or cut to loosen it immediately

## Abdomen

I.  Reasons for bandaging
  A.  To secure a gastrostomy tube
  B.  After a radical mastectomy
  C.  For extensive wounds or dissection of the abdominal region
II. Precautions
  A.  Be careful not to incorporate the prepuce when applying the bandage to male dogs, because this can interfere with urination
  B.  The bandage should also be kept clean and dry from urine and feces

## Limbs

I.  Reasons for bandaging
  A.  Immobilization of fractures
  B.  Wound protection
  C.  Stabilization for fluid therapy
II. Most common type: Robert Jones pressure bandage
  A.  A Robert Jones bandage can be used to temporarily stabilize fractures before surgical repair
  B.  This bandage consists of several layers of rolled cotton compressed tightly with elastic gauze and elastic tape
  C.  The underlying layers of cotton prevent constriction of the limb

III. Precautions
  A.  Never bandage only the upper portion of a limb; the entire limb should be bandaged
  B.  This allows for even distribution of pressure along the limb and maintains venous return from the paw
  C.  The toes should be checked routinely for swelling, coldness, and pallor of the nail beds (where possible)
    1.  If any of these changes occur, the bandage should be loosened or changed, because these signs may indicate poor venous return
  D.  The bandage should be loose enough to allow two fingers to slip under the bandage at all times
  E.  Keep the bandage clean and dry when walking the animal
    1.  A small bag, an examination glove, or an empty fluid bag can be taped onto the distal end of the limb and then removed after exercising

## Paw

I.  Reasons for bandaging
  A.  Declawing of cats
  B.  Dewclaw removal in dogs
  C.  Repair of lacerations
II. Precautions
  A.  The accessory pad should be included when bandaging the paw
  B.  A piece of cotton under the pad, as well as between the digits (canine only) helps to prevent irritation or chafing

## Tail (Figure 23-7)

I.  Reasons for bandaging
  A.  Partial tail amputation
  B.  Protection of wounds
  C.  Tumor removal

## Specialized Bandaging Techniques

I. Ehmer sling to support the hind limb after reduction of hip luxation
II. Velpeau sling (Figure 23-8) to support the shoulder joint after surgery
III. Hobbles can be applied to hind limbs to prevent excessive abduction

## Casting Materials

I. Fiberglass cast
   A. Lightweight and strong
   B. Fast-setting cast
II. Plaster of Paris
   A. Gauze roll impregnated with calcium sulfate dihydrate

## Aftercare of Bandages, Slings, and Casts

I. Close monitoring is essential
   A. Note evidence of odor, edema, discharge, or skin irritation
   B. Note warmth, color, and swelling of toes
II. Prevent the animal from chewing or licking the bandage
   A. Discipline
   B. Sedation
   C. Elizabethan collar
   D. Covering the bandage with a T-shirt or sock
   E. Foul-tasting substances that can be applied to the dressing
III. When outdoors, protect the bandage from dirt and moisture by covering it with a plastic bag
IV. Exercise should be limited

## ONCOLOGY

The cause of tumors is not known; however, genetic factors, carcinogens, radiation, trauma, foreign material, or infectious agents may play a role in the development of some types of neoplasia.

## Definition

I. Oncology is the study of cancer
II. Cancer is defined as any malignant, cellular tumor
   A. Other terms used to describe cancer include neoplasia, neoplasm, growth, tumor, and malignancy
III. *Carcinogenic* means capable of producing cancer
IV. Benign or malignant
   A. A benign neoplasm is localized, does not infiltrate another area, and can be easily excised because it is encapsulated
     1. The harm in the neoplasm is generally due to the space the tumor is occupying
     2. *Benign* in Latin means "innocent"
   B. A malignant neoplasm can metastasize and infiltrate other tissues

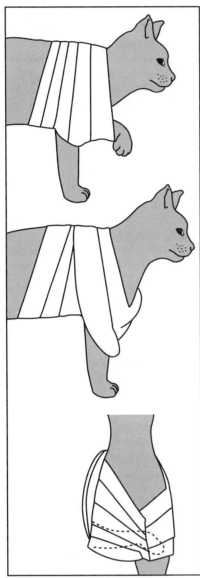

**Figure 23-8** Making a Velpeau sling. (From Lane DR, Cooper B: *Veterinary nursing, formerly Jones' animal nursing,* ed 5, Woburn, Mass, 1998, Butterworth-Heinemann.)

   D. For long-haired cats or dogs with severe diarrhea, to keep the tail as clean as possible
II. Precautions
   A. Sedation may be needed if bleeding persists from excessive tail wagging or from hitting the remaining portion of tail on a hard surface after amputation
     1. In cases of amputation, a hard tubular object fastened to the base of the tail protecting the site is often helpful
       a. Objects such as an empty cardboard roll or human finger splint can be useful
       b. Analgesics may be required for pain

**Table 23-4** Examples of common neoplasms

| Location | Malignant or benign |
|---|---|
| **MAST CELL** | |
| Skin | Both |
| **OSTEOSARCOMA** | |
| Bone | Malignant |
| **HEMANGIOSARCOMA** | |
| Blood vessels | Malignant |
| **MALIGNANT MELANOMA** | |
| Arising from the melanocytes of the skin, eye, or oral cavity | Pigs and cattle benign; all other species usually malignant |
| **SQUAMOUS CELL CARCINOMA** | |
| Conjunctiva, mouth, stomach, vulva, penis, and skin | Malignant |
| **LYMPHOSARCOMA** | |
| Lymph tissue | Malignant |
| **LEUKEMIA** | |
| Blood-forming organs | Malignant |
| **MAMMARY ADENOCARCINOMA** | |
| Mammary tissue; generally glandular tissue | Malignant |
| **FIBROSARCOMA** | |
| Fibrous tissue | Malignant |

1. Metastasis is the process in which cancer cells spread from the primary location to a secondary area, such as lymph nodes, lungs, or other viscera
   a. The secondary location is not directly connected to the primary location
2. Tumors are often classified as primary and secondary to denote which type of neoplasm was identified first

## Classification

I. Tumors are classified by their origin and whether they are malignant or benign
   A. Example: carcinomas are malignant and arise from epithelial tissues, such as skin, mucous membranes, and glandular tissue, and organs, such as liver and kidneys

B. Example: sarcomas are also malignant tumors and arise from mesenchymal tissues, such as connective tissue, cartilage, or bone

II. Tumors are also classified by their tissue of origin
   A. The prefix of a name generally indicates the specific area of origin; the suffix indicates whether it is benign or malignant (Table 23-4)
   B. The suffix -oma generally indicates a benign tumor
      1. Example: fibroma is a benign tumor of fibrous tissue
   C. The suffixes -sarcoma and -carcinoma indicate malignancy
      1. Example: chondrosarcoma is a malignant tumor of cartilage
   D. Exceptions to this rule are melanoma, which can be benign or malignant. Insulinoma and thymoma are malignant tumors

## Diagnostics

I. Early warning signs
   A. Bleeding or discharge
   B. Difficulty eating or swallowing; loss of appetite or weight
   C. Dyspnea, dysuria, abnormal stool, or problems defecating
   D. Loss of stamina, lameness, stiffness, decreased exercise
   E. Abnormal swelling, sores that do not heal, or a bad odor
II. Evaluation
   A. Obtain a patient history from the owner
      1. The history should include the duration of the problem, observations, clinical signs, previous medical problems, husbandry, and vaccination history
   B. A complete physical examination should be performed
      1. After a physical examination, which includes palpation of all lymph nodes, all masses should be checked and measured and a detailed record should be completed
   C. A CBC, serum chemistry profile, urinalysis, thoracic radiograph, abdominal radiograph, and possibly abdominal ultrasound should also be included in the evaluation of the patient
   D. Cytology
      1. To determine the cell morphology of a tumor, cytology may be performed
         a. The most common method of sample collection is fine needle aspiration biopsy
            (1) The neoplasm is cleansed with alcohol
            (2) A 22-gauge needle attached to a 6-mL syringe is inserted into the center of the neoplasm

(3) Using suction, a sample of the tumor is obtained

(4) The sample is then squirted onto a slide, air dried, and fixed with Wright's stain, new methylene blue, or a Diff-Quik or similar stain

(5) If the sample is to be shipped in a commercial laboratory pack, the slides are packed in a plastic container to protect them

(6) The history of the patient and size, location, and duration of the neoplasm should be included with the slides

E. Histopathology is the definitive method of diagnosis

1. Entire masses or large sections of a tumor may be submitted for testing

2. Biopsy techniques include

a. Needle core biopsy: a small incision is made in the mass, and the specialized needle is inserted to obtain a small sample

(1) The TruCut biopsy needle is commonly used for this procedure

b. Incisional biopsy: removal of a small wedge of tissue

c. Excisional biopsy: the entire tumor is removed and margins of surrounding tissue are included to check for cancer cells

## Therapy

I. Surgery: removal of the entire tumor

A. Surgery is most commonly used to treat localized neoplastic disease

B. If a tumor is malignant, the surgeon should remove approximately 2 to 3 cm (1 to 2 inches) of normal tissue along the margin of the tumor if possible

C. Surgery could alter organ function, change the appearance of the patient, and cause hemorrhaging

II. Cryosurgery: use of liquid nitrogen or $N_2O$ (cold) to freeze cancerous tissue

A. This method is generally used for small lesions on the external epithelium

III. Chemotherapy: the treatment of cancer with cytotoxic agents

A. Generally used for systemic or metastatic cancer and is not usually a cure

1. Often chemotherapy is used to produce remission in the patient; this method does not always eradicate cancer cells

B. Can be used after surgical excision of a malignant tumor to prevent further metastasis

C. Also used for tumors that cannot be surgically removed and to improve the quality of the patient's life

D. Can be used with other methods, such as surgery, radiation, or hyperthermia

E. Chemotherapy is often used to decrease the size of a neoplasm and to decrease the patient's pain

F. Technique

1. A combination of chemotherapeutic drugs is used most often

a. Ideally the combined drugs should have different toxicities, work through different mechanisms, and have different efficacies

2. Examples of chemotherapeutic drugs

a. Hormones, antineoplastic antibiotics, antimetabolites, alkylating agents, plant alkaloids

G. Complications

1. Most cytotoxic agents kill neoplastic cells and rapidly dividing noncancerous cells

a. Examples: bone marrow cells, intestinal cells

2. There are many side effects from chemotherapeutic agents

a. The most common are alopecia, cardiotoxicity, vomiting, diarrhea, pancreatitis, hepatosis, neutropenia, thrombocytopenia, anemia, neurotoxicity, and renal toxicity

3. Technical staff who administer the drugs can also experience side effects

a. Protective equipment should be used for safety

(1) Disposable latex gloves, long-sleeved coat or surgical gown with tight-fitting cuffs, and safety eyewear are necessities

b. Biomedical waste should be placed in a sealable plastic bag and held for biomedical waste pickup

(1) Biomedical waste includes syringes, IV administration sets, gauze, and gloves

(2) Cytotoxic waste includes urine, feces, vomitus, and other body fluids

(a) Waste from animals that have received cytotoxic drugs within the previous 48 hours is the most harmful

(b) Patient waste may be disposed of through the sewage system

IV. Radiotherapy: the use of ionizing radiation

A. The cell is killed by the disruption of its DNA

B. Radiation can be used with another therapy, such as surgery or chemotherapy

C. Radiation may be used to treat localized or regional neoplasia or as a palliative therapy in patients with terminal disease

D. Radiation is administered in frequent small doses to minimize the toxic effects and maximize the therapeutic effects

V. Hyperthermia: using a cautery unit to burn small epithelial tumors
   A. This method causes necrosis and vascular thrombosis of the area
   B. Hyperthermia is sometimes used with chemotherapy or radiation therapy

## EUTHANASIA AND PET BEREAVEMENT

Euthanasia is one of the most difficult decisions of a pet owner. Often veterinarians and veterinary technicians play an important role in the owner's decision making process by providing factual information as well as insight into ethical and personal dilemmas regarding euthanasia.

### Euthanasia Discussion

I. Where should euthanasia take place?
   A. At the client's home
   B. Most commonly at the veterinary practice
      1. The owner and other family members should be present
   C. A staff member should explain to the family about the process
      1. This should include how euthanasia is performed, the time frame, and what the animal will feel
   D. Arrangements should be made for the disposal of the body before the procedure

II. To make the experience of euthanasia the least traumatic, the staff should ensure the following
   A. Make certain that all forms and payment have been completed before the euthanasia
   B. Clients are not kept waiting in the client reception area
   C. That all staff are aware of the euthanasia and act with appropriate decorum
   D. Anyone handling the patient is aware of the procedure and uses the patient's correct name
   E. Before the procedure, confirm the client's decision and always give them a chance to change their mind
   F. Ask the client if they would like to be with the pet or wait until after the procedure to say goodbye

III. The cause and circumstances related to the death of a patient are numerous
   A. Medical conditions, acute or chronic
   B. Violent deaths (e.g., hit by car)
   C. Anesthetic deaths
      1. In these cases, it recommended that a necropsy by an external expert be performed to confirm the cause of death

D. Euthanasia of healthy pets is the most upsetting for veterinary staff and clients. The decision by a client to euthanize a pet could be due to behavioral problems, a family crisis, housing regulations, or financial problems, among other reasons

### Methods of Euthanasia

The method chosen should provide a quick, painless death with minimal stress and anxiety. When choosing the method, the veterinary team should consider the possibility of a necropsy following death.

I. Small animals
   A. Enclosed chamber or induction mask
      1. Chamber is filled with carbon dioxide
      2. This method could be also be used to induce anesthesia with halothane or isoflurane followed by a barbiturate injection
   B. Intravenous injection
      1. The use of barbiturates is the most rapid and reliable
         a. The cephalic vein is most commonly use
         b. Pentobarbital (Beuthanasia-D or Euthansol)
   C. Intraperitoneal injection
      1. Used only in very small animals (<7 kg) provided the chemical agent is nonirritating
   D. Intracardiac injection
      1. This method is used only if the patient is heavily sedated (anesthetized or comatose)

II. Large animals
   A. Physical methods
      1. In the past, captive bolt, gunshot, cervical dislocation, electrocution, exsanguinations, stunning, and pithing have been used
      2. Today euthanasia is performed by injection

### Human-Pet Bond and the Grief Process

I. The Kübler-Ross five stages of grief are
   A. Denial
      1. The client chooses to misunderstand or "not hear" a poor prognosis
      2. Often when confronted with a poor prognosis, the client will misunderstand and react with some confusion
   B. Bargaining
      1. Bargaining can include converting to homeopathic remedies, praying, negotiating with God, inquiring about a miracle cure, requesting a second opinion, or purchasing a new pet
      2. Staff members should always express empathy and answer all questions honestly
   C. Anger
      1. Anger may be specific or nonspecific and directed toward the animal or staff of the practice

2. Anger can also be expressed as guilt (anger turned inward)
3. Guilt is the hardest stage to work through and until it is realized the grief process does not continue
4. Tolerance, patience and reassurance usually helps a client deal with this stage

D. Depression
   1. This stage has also been called grief
   2. Intense grief symptoms include overwhelming sadness, appetite changes, low energy levels, withdrawing from others, inability to work, sleep irregularities, and the inability to concentrate

E. Resolution or acceptance
   1. This includes a feeling that everything is going to be okay
   2. The pet is not forgotten but rather, the pet holds a special place in the life of the client
   3. Attachments to new pets are common at this stage
   4. Children reach this stage of acceptance more quickly than adults

### The Grief Process

I. This process in not linear and can fluctuate between the five stages
   A. This process (also called stages or tasks) can take months to complete
   B. Factors that may complicate or change the grief process include
      1. Feelings of guilt about the death of the pet
      2. Loss could have been prevented or a previous pet died from the same cause
      3. Lack of explanation about the death of the pet
      4. Not being able to say goodbye to pet
      5. Multiple personal losses in the same time frame
   C. Early recognition of complications may help the client progress more easily through the grief process
   D. Advising the client to seek professional help is the best way to assist the client with the process

### NECROPSY

I. Equipment
   A. Scalpel handle, blades, sharp scissors, rat-tooth thumb forceps, a large knife, sharpening stones, a chisel, mallet, an electric saw, and pruning shears
   B. In addition the technician might need a pencil, formalin cups, measuring cups, ruler, camera, slides, stains, blood tubes, 10% neutral buffered formalin

C. Protective clothing may also be required, which includes two pairs of gloves, mask, safety goggles, overalls, plastic boots, and apron
D. A rack over a tub or a tub table is the most convenient to use with a good light source and good air ventilation

II. Before the necropsy
   A. Confirm it is the correct animal
   B. Confirm clinical history and determine the possible causes of death
   C. Label appropriate vials or collection tubes with animal's name, date, and technician's name. A necropsy record book might also need to be maintained for cross-referencing records
   D. Before removing any organs, examine all viscera in situ

III. Necropsy procedure
   A. If broken bones or gunshot wounds are a possible cause of death, a radiograph should be taken to identify sites
   B. Note the overall body condition including, skin, hair coat, mucous membrane color, discharges, staining of coat, position of body and sex
   C. Animal should be in left lateral recumbency. Make a midline incision cutting through the skin from the mandibular symphysis, around external genital organs to the pubis
   D. Cut the pectoral muscles of the accessible right front leg so that the leg can be reflected dorsally without support
   E. Repeat the same technique with the right hind leg while disarticulating or separating the coxofemoral joint at the round ligament
   F. From the ventral midline incision, reflect the skin dorsally from the right side of the animal
   G. Reflect the skin back from the face and neck to expose the prescapular and mandibular lymph nodes
   H. Make a vertical cut in the abdominal area (usually dorsal to ventral) parallel to the last rib
      1. Make a midline incision
   I. Note all findings, including
      1. Fluid: color, consistency, location
      2. Hemorrhage, jaundice, or edema
      3. Joints: joint fluid color and smoothness of joint surface
      4. Thoracic organs: note placement, color, condition, any fluid that is evident
         a. Lungs: color, palpate for firmness, crepitation, abnormal masses, and weight
         b. Heart: examine the pericardium, check vessels for size, shape, symmetry, color, and abnormal hemorrhage
         c. Heart: trace the flow of blood; check for hemorrhage, enlargement, and changes in valves; examine and cut open the

major vessels leading to and from the heart

5. Abdominal organs (liver, spleen, kidneys, urinary bladder)
   a. Check color, size, firmness, texture, and outer edges of lobes
   b. Gall bladder: squeeze and check for free-flowing bile into the duodenum
   c. Reproductive organs
      (1) Female: oviduct, ovaries, vaginal area
      (2) Male: testicles, scrotum, prostate
   d. Intestinal tract
      (1) Examine the serosa of the intestinal tract for discoloration, parasites, neoplasm, foreign bodies
      (2) Pancreas: examine for size, tumors or hemorrhaging
6. Glands: size, shape, location, and color

J. Histopathology samples
   1. 10% buffered formalin is the most commonly used fixative
   2. Tissue should be no more than 1 cm thick
   3. There should be approximately 10 times more formalin solution than tissue volume

## ACKNOWLEDGMENT

The editors recognize and appreciate the original contributions of Julie Ball-Karn and Kathy Taylor, on which this chapter is based.

# Glossary

**abduct** To draw away from the median plane

**alkylating agent** Compound that is used as a chemotherapeutic agent

**alloantibodies** An antibody produced by one individual that reacts with the alloantigens of another individual; usually occurs during a blood transfusion

**alopecia** Absence of hair from skin in areas in which it is normally present

**anaphylaxis** Manifestation of immediate hypersensitivity in which exposure of a sensitized individual to a specific antigen or protein results in life-threatening respiratory distress, usually followed by vascular collapse and shock

**antimetabolite** Substance that interferes with the use of an essential metabolite

**antineoplastic** Drug that inhibits the proliferation and maturation of malignant cells

**anuria** Complete suppression of urinary secretion from the kidneys

**aqueous humor** The fluid portion of the eye in the posterior and anterior chambers that maintains intraocular pressure

**aseptic** In a sterile manner

**aspirate** To apply suction and withdraw fluid

**ataxia** Lack of muscle coordination

**auscultate** To listen to thoracic and abdominal sounds

**canthus** The junction of the eyelids

**capillary refill time (CRT)** After applying pressure to the gum line to blanch the tissue, it is the time it takes for color to return to the area, normally 1 to 2 seconds

**cautery unit** Used in surgery to burn tissue with an electrical current

**cerumen** Ear wax

**cerumenolytic** A substance that breaks down ear wax

**chondrosarcoma** Malignant tumor of cartilage cells or their precursors

**colloid** An intravenous solution containing starch or protein molecules

**conjunctiva** Delicate membrane lining the eyelids and surrounding the eyeball

**crackles** A sharp sound heard on auscultation; usually a sign of emphysema

**crepitation** Dry cracking sound or sensation

**crystalloid** Isotonic electrolyte solution

**cytotoxic** Toxic to cells

**debridement** Removal of necrotic or devitalized tissue

**depolarization** Process of neutralizing polarity. *Depolarization phase of the cardiac cycle* means the resting phase

**distention** Abnormal swelling or size

**dressing** Bandage; material that covers a wound

**dry-to-dry bandage** Primary layer of an adherent bandage that is used on open wounds to remove necrotic tissue

**edema** Abnormally large amounts of fluid in the intercellular tissue spaces of the body

**Elizabethan collar** Special collar used in small animals to prevent self-mutilation

**epithelialization** Growth of epithelium to heal a wound

**erythema** Redness of the skin

**extracellular** Outside a cell or cells

**exudate** Fluid containing protein and cells that is excreted from the body on tissue surfaces

**F (French)** Unit used to describe the circumference of a tube. Each gauge unit is about 0.33 mm diameter

**fibroblast** Immature fiber-producing cell of connective tissue

**fibroma** Tumor of fibrous tissue, usually benign

**folliculitis** Inflammation of the hair follicle

**gait** Manner or style of walking

**gastrostomy** The creation of an opening into the stomach

**granulation** Formation of small masses of tissue during the healing process of wounds

**hemangiosarcoma** Malignant tumor of the blood vessels

**hemorrhagic shock** Hypovolemic shock resulting from hemorrhage

**hepatosis** Disorder of the liver

**hypoproteinemia** Abnormal decrease in the amount of protein in the blood, sometimes resulting in edema and fluid accumulation in serous cavities

**hypotensive** Abnormally low blood pressure

**hypovolemic** Abnormally decreased volume of circulating fluid (plasma) in the body

**hypovolemic shock** Shock resulting from insufficient blood volume for the maintenance of adequate cardiac output, blood pressure, and tissue perfusion

**intracellular** Situated or occurring within a cell or cells

**intradermal** In the dermis layer of the skin

**intramedullary** Within the marrow cavity of the bone

**intraperitoneal** Within the peritoneal cavity

**isotonic** A solution that has equal tonicity to another solution with which it is compared

**keratolytic** An agent that loosens or separates the keratin of the skin

**keratoplastic** An agent that promotes the production of keratin

**lavage** Irrigation or washing of an organ or wound

**malocclusion** Absence of proper alignment of teeth when the jaws are closed

**malodorous** Bad odor

**mesenchymal** Embryonic connective tissue such as muscle

**metastatic** Disease that is transferred from one organ to an unrelated organ

**Mobitz type 1 block** Variation of second degree heart block

**myocardium** Middle and thickest layer of the heart wall; composed of cardiac muscle

**nystagmus** Involuntary, rapid, horizontal or vertical movement of the eyeball

**oncology** Study of cancer

**oncotic pressure** Osmotic pressure due to presence of colloids in a solution; it is the force that tends to counterbalance the capillary blood pressure

**ophthalmoscope** An instrument used to examine the interior of the eye

**orogastric** Pertaining to the mouth and stomach

**osteosarcoma** Malignant tumor of bone cells

**otoscope** An instrument used to inspect the ear

**palliative** Affording relief

**palpation** Process of lightly pressing on the surface of the body to determine consistency of the parts beneath

**pancreatitis** Inflammation of the pancreas

**parenteral** Not through the gastrointestinal tract but via another route, such as intravenous

**peripheral** Outward structure or surface, as in the limbs of the body

**polyuria** Production of a large volume of urine over a specific period of time

**pneumocystography** A radiograph of the urinary bladder after injection of air or gas

**premature ventricular contraction (PVC)** Premature heartbeats where the QRS complex usually has wide and bizarre complexes

**pruritus** Itching

**purulent** Containing or forming pus

**pyrexic** Abnormal elevation of body temperature

**rales** Abnormal respiratory sound heard on auscultation. Rales are classified by their point of origin and whether the sound is dry or moist with fluid involvement

**repolarization** After depolarization, the reestablishment of polarity across a cell membrane

**sarcoma** Type of tumor that is highly malignant

**seborrhea oleosa** Moist, oily, scales and crusts on the skin

**seborrhea sicca** Dry, scaly crusts on the skin

**sinus arrhythmia** Variation in the heart rate that is normal in the dog

**stridor** Harsh, shrill respiratory sound usually heard on inspiration that is due to a laryngeal obstruction

**tachycardia** Increased heart rate

**tapetum lucidum** Iridescent reflecting layer of the choroid of the eye. This tissue layer gives the eye the property of shining in the dark

**tonometry** The measurement of tension or pressure using a tonometer

**turgor** Normal consistency of tissue or how quickly it returns to normal after being slightly pulled

**urticaria** Vascular reaction, usually transient, involving the upper dermis and representing localized edema caused by dilatation and increased permeability of the capillaries; marked by the development of wheals

**volvulus** Torsion or twisting of a loop of intestine causing obstruction

**Wenckebach AV block** Repetitive sequence seen in a partial heart block. The PR interval becomes progressively longer until ventricular response occurs

**wet-to-dry bandage** Wet dressing that is used on wounds to extract exudates

**wheeze** Whistling respiratory sound

**Wood's lamp** Used to diagnose fungal infections of the skin. A shortwave ultraviolet light

# Review Questions

**1** For the condition seborrhea sicca, which shampoos would be the most beneficial for the patient?

a. Sulfur and salicylic acid

b. Sulfur, salicylic acid, coal/tar, or 4% benzoyl peroxide

c. 2.5% benzoyl peroxide and coal/tar

d. Coal/tar, chlorhexidine, sulfur, or 4% benzoyl peroxide

**2** What is a thymoma?

a. A benign tumor on the hypothalmus

b. A malignant tumor near the thyroid cartilage

c. A malignant tumor of the thymus

d. A benign tumor of the tongue

**3** Referred sounds are generally

a. From the diaphragm

b. From the trachea

c. From the lung lobes

d. Digestion noises

**4** Kübler-Ross defined the five progressive stages of grief as

a. Bargaining, denial, depression, anger, and resolution

b. Denial, bargaining, anger, depression, and resolution or acceptance

c. Depression, anger, denial, bargaining, and resolution or acceptance

d. Bargaining, depression, denial, anger, and resolution

**5** A parenteral drug is administered

a. Topically

b. Orally

c. Not via the gastrointestinal tract

d. Intramuscularly only

**6** What is a sign of overhydration?

a. Decreased respiratory rate

b. Decreased capillary refill time

c. Increased respiratory rate

d. Increased salivation

**7** Which fluid would be considered a colloid?
   a. Ringer's lactate
   b. 5% Dextrose
   c. Plasma
   d. Saline

**8** Subcutaneous fluids are contraindicated when
   a. There is evidence of mild dehydration
   b. The patient needs dextrose
   c. The patient is very small
   d. There is evidence of chronic heart failure

**9** _____ is/are recommended before performing an enema
   a. Abdominal radiographs
   b. Abdominal palpation
   c. Intravenous fluids
   d. Large amounts of laxative

**10** A canine blood donor should weigh no less than
   a. 20 kg
   b. 25 kg
   c. 15 kg
   d. 10 kg

## BIBLIOGRAPHY

Cohan M: Euthanasia and pet bereavement, *Vet Tech* 26:706, 2005.

Crow SE, Walshaw SO: *Manual of clinical procedures in the dog, cat, and rabbit*, ed 2, Ames, Iowa, 1997, Blackwell.

DiBartola SP: *Fluid, electrolyte and acid-base disorders in small animal practice*, ed 3, St Louis, 2006, Saunders.

*Dorland's illustrated medical dictionary*, ed 30, Philadelphia, 2003, Saunders.

Dracup K: *Meltzer's intensive coronary care: a manual for nurses*, ed 5, Englewood Cliffs, NJ, 1995, Prentice-Hall.

Edwards NJ: *ECG manual for the veterinary technician*, St Louis, 1993, Saunders.

Hansen K: Canine and feline transfusion medicine, *Vet Tech* 27:410, 2006.

Heinbecker V: Small animal blood banking, Ontario Association of Veterinary Technicians Conference, Toronto, Ontario, February 15-17, 2001.

Kirk RW, Bistner SI, editors: *Handbook of veterinary procedures and emergency treatment*, ed 8, St Louis, 2006, Saunders.

Lane DR, Cooper B: *Veterinary nursing*, ed 3, Oxford, England, 2003, Butterworth-Heinemann.

Loncke D, Rivait P, Tighe M: *Clinical procedures handbook*, Windsor, Ontario, 2006, St Clair College of Applied Arts and Technology, Veterinary Technician Program.

Mathews KA: *Fluid and electrolyte maintenance and replacement, veterinary emergency and critical care manual*, ed 2, Guelph, Ontario, 2006, Lifelearn.

McCurnin D, Bassert J, editors: *Clinical textbook for veterinary technicians*, ed 6, St Louis, 2006, Saunders.

Sirois M, editor: *Principles and practice of veterinary technology*, ed 2, St Louis, 2004, Mosby.

## CHAPTER 24

# Equine Nursing and Surgery

*Susan Cornwell*    *Kim Healey*

## OUTLINE

Physical Examination and Normal
 Values
Dental Formula and Care
  Dental Formula
  Dental Care
Routes of Administration
Vaccinations
Gastrointestinal Ailments

Common Clinical Signs
Rule Outs of Gastrointestinal
 Ailments
Neuromuscular Disorders
Common Clinical Signs
Rule Outs of Neuromuscular
 Disorders
Respiratory Diseases

Common Clinical Signs
Rule Outs of Respiratory Diseases
Blood Disorder
Foot Ailments
Lameness
Equine Surgery
Bandaging

## LEARNING OUTCOMES

After reading this chapter you should be able to:

1. Recognize normal values for adult horses.
2. Understand medication treatment routes.
3. Have an understanding of disease, illnesses, and the technician's role in the animal's care.
4. Be familiar with important preoperative and postoperative care.
5. Be familiar with common vaccines.
6. Be familiar with bandaging techniques.

As veterinary technicians, we play a large role in the day-to-day care of animals. Veterinarians rely on our instincts, knowledge, and observational skills to assist and/or alert them to the progression (or deterioration) of the animal's state of health.

## PHYSICAL EXAMINATION AND NORMAL VALUES

  I. Temperature: 37° to 38.5° C (98.6° to 101.3° F)
 II. Pulse: 28 to 45 beats per minute
    A. Auscultate heart with stethoscope
       1. Heart sounds

   a. Four heart sounds may be heard, but often only two or three
   b. Normal sequence of sounds in cardiac cycle is S4, S1, S2, S3
   c. Loudest and most obvious sounds are S1 and S2
      (1) S1 is the first sound and is due to ventricular contraction
      (2) S2 is the second sound and is due to closure of semilunar valves
      (3) S3 is very faint and caused by blood rushing into the ventricles
      (4) Rarely audible S4 is caused by atrial contraction
    2. Cardiac rhythm
       a. A variety of rhythms are normal
       b. Note heart rate, rhythm, intensity, extra sounds, absence of normal sounds
       c. Abnormal rhythms
          (1) Arrhythmias: absence of rhythm
          (2) Dysrhythmia: disturbance of rhythm
          (3) Tachycardia: dysrhythmia associated with heart rates greater than 50 beats per minute
          (4) Bradycardia: dysrhythmia associated with heart rates lower than 20 beats per minute
             (a) Can occur due to hypocalcemia

d. Atrioventricular (AV) block
   (1) May occur regularly or irregularly
   (2) First degree, second degree, or third degree (complete heart block)
   (3) During second degree block, there is no S1 or S2 and no arterial pulse
   (4) Second degree heart block may be present in horses that are not fit
       (a) Not always indicative of heart disease
3. Heart murmurs
   a. Turbulent flow causes vibrations that are audible during normally quiet periods of the cardiac cycle
B. Electrocardiographic (ECG) monitor
   1. A portable ECG monitor is used on the horse while it is standing quietly
   2. Used for a definitive diagnosis of arrhythmias/dysrhythmias
C. Facial artery
   1. Located on medial aspect of mandible
   2. Palpate artery to assess blood pressure during anesthesia
   3. Use to determine if manual palpation of pulse matches the ECG
D. Coccygeal artery
   1. Located in groove on dorsal aspect of tail
   2. Use for blood pressure with a Doppler pressure monitor

III. Respiration: 8 to 20 breaths per minute
A. Observe by watching horse flanks and nostrils
B. Use stethoscope to listen to abnormal respiratory sounds
   1. Place on trachea
   2. Place on left and right lung fields
C. Horse must be relaxed in a quiet environment for assessment
D. Rhythm is important
   1. Normal horse
      a. Inspiration and expiration are followed by a pause
   2. Abnormal or excited horse
      a. Inspiration will be slightly longer than expiration
E. Signs of respiratory problems
   1. Coughing or other abnormal respiratory sounds during rest or exercise
   2. Nasal discharge
   3. Epistaxis
      a. The presence of blood in upper airway or nose as a result of
         (1) Guttural pouch infections
         (2) Exercise-induced pulmonary hemorrhage (EIPH)

4. Hyperpnea
   a. Increased rate and depth of respiration
5. Dyspnea
   a. Labored breathing causing distress
F. Pharynx and trachea examined with endoscopy
IV. Mucous membrane should be a healthypink color
V. Capillary refill time: 1 to 2 seconds
VI. Gastrointestinal motility (borborygmus)
A. Bubbling
B. Gurgling
C. Rumbling (not unlike the sound of distant thunder)
D. Cecum is heard on the right side and no sound is cause for concern
E. Recording of gut sounds
   1. By upper and lower quadrants on the left and right side
   2. 0 is absence of sound
   3. + (one plus) is hypomotile, ++ (two plus) is normal, and +++ (three plus) is hypermotile
VII. Digital pulses: none to slight
VIII. Fecal output
A. Color varies with diet
B. Should be well-formed moist balls that break easily when they hit the ground
C. Frequency: approximately 8 to 10 times daily
IX. Urine
A. Colorless to yellow
B. Can be thick or turbid from high content of mucus and calcium carbonate crystals

## DENTAL FORMULA AND CARE ▬▬▬
### Dental Formula

I. Foal has 24 temporary teeth
II. Adult has 40 to 42 permanent teeth
A. For a stallion, the dental formula is $2 \times (I\ 3/3,\ C\ 1/1,\ P\ 3/3,\ M,\ 3/3)$
B. Mares usually do not have canine teeth
C. Equine canine teeth are also called tushes

### Dental Care

I. Wolf teeth or first premolar (P1) are located in the upper jaw
A. If wolf teeth do not fall out on their own, the veterinarian will have to extract them because they can interfere with the bit
II. Anatomically the horse's upper jaw is wider than the lower jaw
A. When a horse eats, it grinds food in a side-to-side motion
B. This creates sharp edges on the buccal surface of the upper teeth and on the lingual surface of the lower teeth

C. Rasping down these sharp edges is called floating the teeth
D. A veterinarian should check the horse's teeth at least annually to determine whether teeth need floating
  1. Signs that an animal's teeth need floating include
    a. Halitosis
    b. Lacerations of oral cavity
    c. Difficulty eating (tend to drop feed)
    d. Head tilt (especially when a bit is placed in their mouth)
    e. Undigested food in feces

## ROUTES OF ADMINISTRATION

I. Oral route
  A. Powders
  B. Pastes (e.g., phenylbutazone, anthelmintics)
  C. Boluses
  D. Pills
  E. Liquids
  F. All of the above may be added to food (some after being dissolved in water) or dosed using a syringe
II. Nasogastric tube
  A. Tube is passed into the esophagus, usually by a veterinarian because of the risk of accidentally placing the tube in trachea
  B. Common route for administering Strongid (often double dosed), mineral oil, and antigas medicine as well as refluxing the stomach contents when assessing colic
  C. Nasogastric tube may be seen or felt on the left side of the neck when being passed by placing pressure above and below the tube, at the jugular groove and blowing air into the tube
III. Intravenous (IV) injection
  A. Always swab injection site with alcohol before injecting
    1. Makes vein more pronounced and disinfects skin
  B. Common sites
    1. Jugular vein is most common
    2. For small volumes the thoracic, cephalic, or saphenous veins can be used if jugular vein not accessible
  C. Use to produce rapid onset of drug action
  D. Use to administer large volumes of fluids
  E. Use for blood collection
  F. Before injecting, ensure placement in vein by getting blood flow back from needle (catheter) or aspirated in syringe
  G. Catheter placement
    1. Commonly sewn or glued in place, then secured with tape and Elastoplast

    2. Placement will depend on surgical recumbency (commonly on the nonrecumbent side)
    3. Short-term placement (several hours): Angiocath
    4. Long-term placement (several days): Mila and Arrow catheters with butterfly extensions
  H. Normal needle gauges range from 14 gauge (catheters) to 16 to 21 gauge (jugulars) to 25 or 27 gauge (some local anesthetic agents)
  I. Important to know properties of drugs before administering
  J. Only a few drugs are administered IV
  K. Incorrect route of administration could destroy the vein or cause anaphylactic reaction
  L. Administer some drugs, such as calcium, slowly so that heart rate is not adversely affected
  M. Administer some drugs as a bolus for effect (e.g., glycopyrrolate during anesthesia to regulate heart rate)
  N. Perivascular administration of some drugs can irreparably damage tissue
  O. Phenylbutazone ("bute") is the most common drug administered to horses and the most damaging to the vein perivascularly
IV. Intramuscular (IM) administration
  A. Swab injection site with alcohol to disinfect and make skin veins visible so they can be avoided
  B. Common sites
    1. Neck (Viborg's triangle, below nuchal ligament and above cervical vertebrae proximal to shoulder)
    2. Semitendinosus muscle
    3. Gluteus muscle
    4. Pectoralis descendens muscle (chest)
  C. Avoid injecting close to joints, blood vessels, or large fat deposits
  D. IM route used to prolong drug action
  E. Only safe route of administration for certain drugs
    1. To ensure that the needle is not in a blood vessel, draw back on syringe plunger to check that no blood is pulled into the syringe before injecting
    2. Procaine penicillin will cause an adverse reaction if administered into the bloodstream
    3. Mild reactions may take a few minutes to present themselves, whereas severe reactions occur immediately
    4. Reactions include restlessness, head tossing, snorting, rolling of the eyes, violent thrashing, and dropping to the ground
      a. Treat with dexamethasone (a corticosteroid) and flunixin meglumine (Banamine) (a nonsteroidal antiinflammatory drug [NSAID])

b. Treatment should be administered IV, but one may not get close enough to inject into the vein if the animal's reaction is too violent

5. A horse that has had an allergic reaction to a drug should never be given that drug again

V. Subcutaneous (SC) administration
A. Swab skin with alcohol as for IM injection
B. Administer drug by pinching a loose fold of skin and placing needle tip into space
C. Normally injected into neck
D. Will normally leave bump because of the close attachment of skin to underlying muscle
E. Always draw back on plunger to ensure that no blood is in syringe before injecting

VI. Intranasal route
A. Catheter is placed in the medial ventral nasal cavity for administration of drugs
   1. Vaccination against strangles *(Streptococcus equi)*
   2. Vaccination for the influenza virus
   3. Laryngeal/pharyngeal washes
B. The advantage to this route is direct application of the drug to the primary area of concern

VII. Inhalation route
A. Nebulizers and AeroMasks used to deliver microdroplets of a drug
   1. Mask is loosely fitted over muzzle
B. Aerosol inhalants

VIII. Topical route
A. Substances applied to skin, eyes, mucous membranes, and hooves
B. Eye creams and ointments must be placed onto the eye or into conjunctival sacs
   1. Multiple applications of liquids may require a special eye lavage system placed into the eyelid and braided through the mane

## VACCINATIONS (Table 24-1)

I. Vaccinations routinely given IM aseptically
II. Intranasal vaccine available for strangles and influenza
III. Vaccines are made from a killed virus (KV) or modified live virus (MLV), bacteria, or toxin (antigen)
IV. Routine vaccines depend on geographical area, prevalence of a disease in a specific area, and the animal's risk of exposure
V. In Ontario, Canada, horses are routinely vaccinated for
A. Rabies
B. Tetanus
C. Rhinopneumonitis (EHV-4/1)
D. West Nile virus
VI. Horses traveling outside Canada are routinely vaccinated for
A. Encephalomyelitis, Eastern and Western strains

B. Strangles (periodic outbreaks in many areas)
C. Potomac horse fever (equine *Neorickettsia risticii*)

VII. In the United States
A. Depending on the area, most horses are vaccinated for Eastern and Western encephalomyelitis, tetanus, and influenza annually
B. Rhinopneumonitis is recommended if there are yearlings
C. Strangles vaccine is common in many areas, with intranasal administration becoming more popular because of reactions at the IM injection site
D. Rabies vaccination is recommended in most areas
E. Administration of both West Nile virus and Potomac horse fever vaccine is being recommended as part of the vaccination protocol, in both high- and low-risk areas

VIII. Side effects of vaccinations
A. At 24 to 48 hours after injection
   1. Generalized muscle pain
   2. Mild lethargy
   3. Mild appetite loss
   4. Mild fever
   5. If symptoms persist longer, other causes should be examined
B. Irritation, swelling, or abscess at injection site
C. Anaphylactic reaction, although rare
   1. Treat with epinephrine

IX. Primary immunization
X. Important to read directions for each brand of vaccine
XI. Protocols for vaccination are described in Table 24-1
A. For further information, see the description under the particular vaccinations

## GASTROINTESTINAL AILMENTS

The management of all ailments and diseases is at the discretion of a veterinarian.

### Common Clinical Signs

I. Restlessness, anxiety, or agitation
II. Pawing, pacing/stall walking
III. Flank watching and possible biting at flank
IV. Kicking at abdomen
V. Sweating
VI. Getting up and down in stall
VII. Rolling
VIII. Grinding teeth
IX. Distended abdomen
X. Increased heart rate and respiration rate
XI. Mucous membranes can be pale, bright or brick red, or cyanotic

**Table 24-1** Equine vaccinations

| Foal | Brood mare (BM) or healthy horse (HH) | Wounds | Notes |
|------|---------------------------------------|--------|-------|
| **TETANUS (TOXOID)** | | | |
| At 3 mo, then 4 wk later Antibody titers usually occur 2 wk after second initial dose Then given annually | *BM:* 4-6 wk before foaling | If booster given more than 6 mo earlier Before surgery being performed | May be given as an individual vaccine or combined with another vaccine by certain manufacturers<br>If vaccination history is unknown or vaccine not previously given, treat with the tetanus anti-toxin vaccine<br>Administer separately and make sure that the injection sites are not close to each other on the horse |
| **TETANUS ANTITOXIN** | | | |
| Shortly after birth if mare unvaccinated | | Minimum dose of 1500 IU within 24 hr of exposure to tetanus toxin | Administer SQ, IV, or intraperitoneally<br>Given to treat cases of tetanus<br>Massive initial doses are better than repeated smaller doses to effect a cure<br>If wound present, increase dose relative to time of exposure to 30,000-100,000 IU |
| **RABIES** | | | |
| 3 mo of age and older | *HH:* Annual booster | | Inject a 2-mL dose IM<br>Revaccinate annually |
| **RHINOPNEUMONITIS: EHV-1, EHV-4 (EQUINE HERPESVIRUS)** | | | |
| 3 mo of age, 3-4 wk later, then 6 mo later | *BM:* At fifth, seventh, and ninth mo of gestation<br>*HH:* Primary vaccination at 6-9 mo, second dose 2-4 or 4-6 wk later, then annually | High-risk horses: every 3 mo | Both modified live and inactivated vaccine available<br>Vaccines are specifically labeled for respiration or abortion<br>Vaccines do not claim any protective properties for the neurological syndrome caused by this virus |
| **INFLUENZA** | | | |
| After 6 mo (maternal antibodies from the vaccinated mare may interfere with the vaccine for up to 6 mo of age)<br>Or<br>At 1 mo of age if mare unvacci-nated | *HH:* Primary dose of IM vaccine 9 mo and older, with second dose 2-4 or 3-6 wk later, then booster 6 mo later, then annually<br>In a high-risk area a third dose may be given within that 6-mo period<br>*Older horses:* Every 9-12 mo if in a low-risk, closed environment<br>*Show horses:* Do not vaccinate within 7-10 days of a show because of possible side effects | Booster with vaccine containing tetanus | Vaccination rarely prevents infection<br>Can reduce severity of disease and decrease its spread only<br>Side effects include fever, depression, muscle stiff-ness, reaction at injection site<br>Blood serum tests will show antibody titer levels<br>A modified live intranasal vaccine is available in the United States and Canada (Flu Avert I.N.) that has a rapid immune response at the pri-mary infection site<br>Administer 1-mL dose into nostril<br>Recommended administration twice a year, and more often in areas of high risk of exposure<br>The modified live virus intranasal route should be the first choice of administration, especially in nonpregnant mares |
| **EQUINE ENCEPHALOMYELITIS: EASTERN (EEE), WESTERN (WEE), AND VENEZUELAN (VEE)** | | | |
| 3 mo<br>Or<br>6 mo if adequate colostrum received | *BM:* 4-6 wk before foaling<br>*HH:* primary immunity, with second dose at 3-4 or 4-8 wk, then annually (titers last 6-8 mo)<br>Vaccinate if there is an outbreak | If during first 2 mo or if booster given more than 12 mo ago, administer minimum 1500 IU tetanus antitoxin | Vaccinate against EEE and WEE in Canada and the United States<br>Vaccinate against VEE in states that border Mexico<br>In cool climates, administer the vaccine in the spring when increased exposure to other horses and mosquitoes more likely<br>In warm climates, biannual vaccination is recommended |

*Continued*

**Table 24-1** Equine vaccinations—cont'd

| Foal | Brood mare (BM) or healthy horse (HH) | Wounds | Notes |
|---|---|---|---|
| **Streptococcus equi (STRANGLES)** | | | |
| Before 4 mo old | *BM:* 4-6 wk before foaling (Strepguard) | If during first 2 mo or if booster given more than 12 mo ago, administer minimum 1500 IU tetanus antitoxin | Vaccine available as whole-cell bacteria and M-protein extract for IM injection<br>Vaccination usually limited to horses at risk because of muscle soreness and incomplete protection<br>Available as modified live vaccine in intranasal form (Pinnacle I.N.)<br>Two doses 2-3 wk apart, then annual boosters<br>IM route: two or three doses 2-4 wk apart then annually<br>Not recommended for infected animals |
| **Neorickettsia risticii (POTOMAC HORSE FEVER)** | | | |
| In high-risk areas, at 4 mo for 3 doses 1 mo apart<br>In low-risk areas, treat as for healthy horses | *HH:* 3 mo of age and older, then 3-4 wk later, then at 4-mo intervals<br>*Gestating mares:* 4-6 wk before foaling | | Has been documented all across the United States and specific regions of Ontario<br>Vaccinating is generally limited to areas of high prevalence, at 4-mo intervals due to the short duration of activity |
| **WEST NILE VIRUS** | | | |
| *Nonvaccinated mare in high-risk area:* 6-8 wk of age, 3 doses 3-4 wk apart<br>*Nonvaccinated mare in low-risk area:* 3-5 mo of age, 3 doses 3-4 wk apart<br>*Vaccinated mare in high-risk area:* Give as for Nonvaccinated Mare in Low-Risk Area (3-5 mo) with 2 or 3 repeat doses<br>*Vaccinated mare in low-risk area:* 5-7 mo old, give 2 doses 3-4 wk apart<br>*Foals:* Animals a few days old have been vaccinated with no adverse effects | Administer 1 mL IM followed by second dose in 3-6 wk<br>Revaccinate annually | | Is a killed virus<br>Horses may develop immunoglobulin G (IgG) and/or IgM antibodies to the West Nile virus that would affect their ability to be exported |

XII. Toxic line (red or blue) on gums just above teeth may be present

XIII. Increased capillary refill time (CRT)

XIV. Gastrointestinal motility may be hypermotile, hypomotile, or absent

XV. Digital pulses bounding with increased heat in hoof wall

XVI. Fecal output can be absent, small number of hard, dry balls, or cow patty form to diarrhea

XVII. Sawhorse stance (standing stretched out) or dog sitting

XVIII. Decreased appetite

XIX. Reflux, via nasogastric tube, is often present (can be absent or up to 15 L [3.5 gal] in an average-size horse)

## Rule Outs of Gastrointestinal Ailments

I. Colic
   A. Refers to abdominal pain
      1. Most commonly seen ailment
   B. Gastrointestinal causes include
      1. Excessive gas
      2. Spasmodic colic
      3. Ileus (cessation of peristalsis)
      4. Parasitic infestation
      5. Volvulus (torsion of small or large intestine)
      6. Intussusception (telescoping of adjoining bowl [ileum to cecum])
      7. Impaction
      8. Obstruction
      9. Displacement
      10. Inguinal hernia
      11. Ulcer
   C. Signs vary with the severity of the colic and disposition of the horse
   D. Not all of these clinical signs will be seen in each case
   E. Management of colic consists of
      1. Fluid therapy
      2. Antiinflammatory drugs
      3. Mineral oil
      4. Antiflatulence medication
      5. Monitoring
      6. Antiulcer medications
   F. Monitoring includes
      1. Vital signs
      2. Gut sounds (motility)
      3. Fecal output
      4. Hydration status (packed cell volume [PCV] and total protein [TP])
      5. Obtaining nasogastric reflux (recording of how much)
      6. Walking
      7. Gradual introduction of food to the animal

G. In cases where surgery has been performed or toxemia occurred, digital pulses are also extremely important to monitor, because laminitis is always a concern

II. Colitis
   A. Acute inflammatory process of the large colon and cecum
   B. In most cases of acute colitis, a cause is unknown
   C. Possibilities include
      1. Dietary change
      2. Carbohydrate overload (eating too much grain)
      3. *Salmonella* spp.
      4. *Clostridium perfringens*
      5. *Clostridium difficile*
      6. Potomac horse fever
      7. Antibiotic therapy
      8. Overuse of NSAIDs
   D. Clinically, horses present with
      1. Inappetance
      2. Dull/depressed
      3. Abdominal pain
      4. Gastric motility can be either hypermotile (increased) or hypomotile (decreased)
      5. Increased heart and respiration rates
      6. Mucous membranes can be brick/dark red, muddy, or cyanotic
      7. CRT is increased (3 to 4 seconds)
      8. Diarrhea (varying from cow patty to profuse watery diarrhea)
      9. Dehydration
      10. Hypoproteinemia
      11. Electrolyte imbalances (hyponatremia, hypokalemia, hypocalcemia)
      12. Metabolic acidosis (severe cases)
      13. In severe cases, shock due to endotoxemia
   E. Management of colitis
      1. Fluid therapy with a balanced electrolyte solution (e.g., lactated Ringer's solution [LRS])
      2. If needed, addition of potassium chloride and calcium to LRS
      3. If needed, sodium bicarbonate to correct metabolic acidosis
      4. Plasma transfusion if total protein low (<4.0 g/dL)
      5. Antiinflammatory drugs
   F. Monitoring
      1. Vital signs
      2. PCV and TP
      3. Blood gas and electrolytes
      4. Digital pulses and heat (signs of laminitis) in hooves
   G. Usually free choice grass hay is offered, but grain is withheld

H. Horses with diarrhea are kept isolated because of the possibility of salmonella infection
I. When a horse is receiving IV fluids, it is vital that the indwelling catheter be monitored for
   1. Heat
   2. Swelling
   3. Pain
J. This is very important, because horses with colitis are prone to developing thrombosis of the jugular vein

III. Salmonellosis
   A. A very serious problem due to zoonotic potential and high incidence of contagion to other horses
      1. Horses may naturally carry salmonella as part of their intestinal flora
   B. Causes include
      1. Stressful situations, such as transport in a trailer
      2. Sudden changes in feeding
      3. Antibiotic use
      4. Sickness
      5. Surgery
      6. Immunosuppression
      7. Nosocomial origin
   C. Clinically, horses present with
      1. Signs similar to those of colitis
      2. Acute, profuse, watery, foul-smelling diarrhea
      3. Pyrexia
      4. Anorexia
      5. Often neutropenia
   D. Management is extremely important
      1. The horse should be isolated
      2. Handling the animal should be kept to one person to prevent the possibility of cross-contamination
      3. Anyone handling the horse should be wearing a gown, gloves, and protective boot covers
      4. When leaving the isolated animal, hands should be thoroughly washed and boots should be dipped in a foot bath containing a bactericidal solution
      5. Fluid therapy with a balanced electrolyte solution is very important, because hydration status is the number one concern
      6. Plasma transfusion may be required if hypoproteinemia is present
   E. Monitor vital signs, as with any other case of diarrhea
   F. Horse is fed free choice hay; grain is withheld

IV. Intestinal clostridial infections
   A. An acute inflammatory process of the bowel
   B. *Clostridium difficile* is the most common form
   C. Clinically, horses present with
      1. Signs similar to those of colitis
      2. Often no initial diarrhea
      3. Severe abdominal pain
      4. Increased gut motility (hypermotility)
      5. Diarrhea within a matter of hours
   D. Management is the same as for colitis and salmonellosis
   E. The antibiotic metronidazole, given orally, may be effective in some cases

V. Potomac horse fever (PHF) (monocytic ehrlichiosis)
   A. *Neorickettsia risticii* (formerly known as *Ehrlichia risticii*) is the cause of PHF
   B. This rickettsia-like organism is thought to be transmitted by aquatic insects
   C. Predominantly in northeastern United States, but outbreaks now seen throughout the United States; the peak time for PHF is June through August
   D. Horses can be tested for PHF with an enzyme-linked immunosorbent assay (ELISA) and an indirect immunofluorescent antibody (IFA) test. A polymerase chain reaction (PCR) test on blood and feces can also be used
   E. Clinically, horses present with signs similar to other bacterial infections after a 9- to 12-day incubation period
      1. Depression
      2. Anorexia
      3. Pyrexia
      4. Decreased gut sounds
      5. Some horses exhibit abdominal pain and diarrhea
   F. Infected pregnant mares may abort late in gestation
   G. Management of PHF
      1. Oxytetracycline
      2. Aggressive fluid therapy with a balanced electrolyte solution
   H. As with cases of salmonella and colitis, the same monitoring and strict isolation procedures are applied
   I. Laminitis is a major concern with PHF and should be monitored closely
   J. Vaccines available for PHF are very effective
      1. Vaccinated horses may become infected and show slightly milder symptoms of the disease
   K. Antibiotic and NSAID therapy
      1. Overuse of antibiotics and NSAIDs can cause diarrhea
      2. Clinically, horses present with
         a. Loss of appetite
         b. Depression

c. Some abdominal pain

d. Protein loss due to ulceration of the bowel or stomach

3. Antibiotics can cause diarrhea as a side effect (some are higher risk)

4. Management

a. Fluid therapy, such as LRS and plasma

b. Monitoring patient's vital signs

5. Antibiotics and NSAIDs should be discontinued

6. Gastroscopy can be performed to determine ulcerations

7. Treatment with antiulcer medication can then be initiated if needed

VI. Anterior enteritis

A. The cause is idiopathic; however, *Clostridium* spp. have been implicated

B. There is severe inflammation of the upper portion of the small intestine

C. Clinically, horses present with

1. Severe colic

2. Increased heart and respiration rates

3. Possible pyrexia

4. Gastric reflux obtained when a nasogastric tube is placed

D. Signs are often the same as with an obstruction of the bowel

E. Diagnosis is made by the veterinarian performing a rectal examination

F. In the case of anterior enteritis, colic signs decrease when nasogastric reflux is obtained. With an obstruction, colic signs usually do not decrease. The horse will then become depressed

G. Management

1. Passage of a nasogastric tube and frequent siphoning to empty fluid buildup in the stomach

2. Fluid therapy is important to replace fluid loss from the nasogastric reflux

H. Monitoring is the same as with colic, although particular attention is paid to temperature, mucous membranes, CRT, and digital pulses, because toxemia is a concern

VII. Hyperkalemic periodic paralysis (HYPP)

A. This disease originated with a genetic mutation that has been traced back to a quarter horse sire

B. Clinically, horses present with any of the following

1. Muscle fasciculations

2. Coliclike episodes

3. Sweating

4. Respiratory distress

5. Prolapsed third eye lid

6. Loose feces

7. Ataxia

C. A DNA blood test has been developed and can determine

1. If a horse is homozygous for the genetic mutation

2. A heterozygous carrier

3. A normal horse

D. If the test is positive, breeding should be discouraged and owners should be made aware that it can be dangerous to ride these horses

E. Management of HYPP consists of

1. A low potassium diet

2. Grass or oat hay (no alfalfa hay)

3. Plenty of fresh water

4. Minimizing stress in these affected horses is beneficial

## NEUROMUSCULAR DISORDERS
### Common Clinical Signs

I. Ataxia

II. Depression

III. Circling

IV. Head tilt

V. Head pressing

VI. Nystagmus

VII. Facial paralysis, drooling

VIII. Incoordination, limb knuckling, and toe dragging

IX. Muscle wasting

X. Prolapsed third eyelid

XI. Seizures

XII. Altered behavior

### Rule Outs of Neuromuscular Disorders

I. Tetanus (lockjaw)

A. Caused by the bacterium *Clostridium tetani*

B. *C. tetani* is found in the soil and infects horses through puncture wounds

C. The bacteria produce neurotoxins, which affect the horse's nervous system

D. Clinically, horses present with

1. Muscle stiffness (sawhorse stance)

2. Decreased feed and water intake

3. Sensitivity to light and sound

4. Muscle fasciculations

E. Management of tetanus should begin with the infected horse receiving high doses of tetanus antitoxin

1. This is given because the antitoxin will bind to any circulating tetanus toxins

F. Wound treatment

1. Cleaning

2. Draining

3. Local infiltration of penicillin to the site of the wound

G. Systemically, the horse should be given IV penicillin

H. The horse should be kept in a dark, quiet stall

I. IV fluids may be needed, especially if the horse is dysphagic

J. Vaccination of horses annually with tetanus toxoid to help stimulate the immune system is a preventive measure

II. Rabies

A. Caused by the rhabdovirus, which attacks the central nervous system

B. This virus most commonly is passed by a bite from an infected animal

C. Because the virus is found in large quantities in saliva, domestic animals, including humans, can become infected through open wounds and across mucous membranes

D. Clinically, horses present with signs listed previously under Common Clinical Signs, as well as the following

1. Extreme aggression (in some cases)
2. Dysphagia
3. Hydrophobia
4. Self-inflicted wounds

E. Clinical signs are always progressive and can be quite variable

F. Management of rabies

1. The suspected horse must be quarantined
2. Anyone handling the horse should wear protective clothing and gloves because of rabies zoonotic potential

G. Unfortunately, if rabies is highly suspected, the horse must be euthanized because of the threat to human life and because there is no cure

H. A definitive diagnosis can be made only at postmortem

I. An annual rabies vaccine should be given as a preventive measure

III. Equine protozoal myeloencephalitis (EPM)

A. Affects the central nervous system

B. The protozoa *Sarcocystis neurona* is the causative agent

1. The protozoa encysts in the muscle of birds
2. Opossums eat the infected birds
3. Opossum's feces contaminate the horse's feed and water supply

C. Symptoms depend on location of lesion

D. Locations of lesions from the protozoa

1. Brain stem
2. Spinal cord
3. Peripheral nerves

E. Clinically, horses may present with any of the following

1. Ataxia
2. Facial paralysis

3. Head tilt
4. Depression
5. Blindness
6. Dysphagia
7. Circling
8. Hind end weakness and ataxia
9. Gluteal, tongue, and masticatory muscle wasting
10. Incontinence
11. In some cases, recumbency

F. EPM is diagnosed by performing a cerebrospinal fluid (CSF) tap

G. The spinal fluid is then analyzed for

1. Antibodies to *Sarcocystis neurona*
2. Protozoal DNA

H. Management of EPM consists of long-term antibiotic and antiprotozoal therapy, which usually includes trimethoprim-sulfadiazine and pyrimethamine

1. Other approved antiprotozoal medications are: ponazuril (Marquis) and nitazoxanide (Navigator)

I. Unfortunately, affected animals often do not recover completely and posttherapeutic relapses are common

IV. Equine herpesvirus 1 (EHV-1)

A. This strain affects the nervous system

1. It is transmitted via direct contact or aerosols
2. Clinically, horses with EHV-1 can
   a. Be uncoordinated
   b. Be incontinent
   c. Be ataxic in hind limbs
   d. Have loss of tail tone
   e. In extreme cases, hind limb paralysis leads to dog-sitting posture or recumbency

B. Abortion can occur in pregnant mares

1. Vaccinate with Pneumabort-K +1b during months 5, 7, and 9 of pregnancy

C. If affected late in gestation, abortion may not occur; however, foals are infected in utero and may be born dead or die shortly after birth

D. Management of EHV-1 depends on the severity of the disease, and treatment includes

1. Antibiotics
2. Antiinflammatory drugs
3. Corticosteroids

E. Vaccination of horses is a preventive measure and may not be effective against neurological diseases, but is reasonably effective against abortions

F. Once infected, the virus is carried in a dormant state for the rest of the animal's life and symptoms can be reactivated by stress

V. Equine encephalomyelitides (sleeping sickness)
   A. Three strains of this alphavirus
      1. Eastern (EEE)
      2. Western (WEE)
      3. Venezuelan (VEE)
   B. Most common to Canada and the United States: eastern (EEE) and western (WEE) strains
   C. Transmitted by mosquitoes, outbreaks tend to occur late in the summer
   D. 1 to 3 week incubation period
   E. Is communicable to humans (zoonotic)
   F. Clinically, horses present with the following initial signs
      1. Pyrexia
      2. Anorexia
      3. Depression
      4. Increased heart rate
   G. Nervous signs develop later and are mostly due to EEE
      1. Anxiousness, excitement, and restlessness
      2. Exaggerated response to touch
      3. Head pressing, circling in the stall
      4. Seizures
      5. Paralysis
      6. Incoordination
      7. Loss of consciousness
   H. Death is common
   I. Management
      1. Antiinflammatory drugs
      2. Fluid therapy
      3. Corticosteroids
      4. Anticonvulsants
      5. Emphasis on supportive nursing care
   J. Vaccination of horses against this disease is an effective preventive measure
   K. Control disease by identifying and destroying or segregating affected individuals
VI. West Nile virus (meningomyeloencephalitis)
   A. This flavivirus first appeared late in 1999 in the United States
   B. The virus is transmitted by mosquitoes
      1. Mosquitoes get the virus from infected birds
      2. Horses and humans are dead end hosts
   C. Outbreaks tend to occur late summer and in the fall
   D. Especially at risk are the very young, elderly, and sick
   E. Horses do not necessarily die from this virus; some recover fully
   F. Deaths have been reported
   G. Clinically, horses can present with some or all of the following
      1. Pyrexia
      2. Front end or hind end weakness
      3. Toe dragging
      4. Ataxia
      5. Head and neck tremors
      6. Sensitivity to touch
      7. Aggression
      8. Circling
      9. Depression
      10. Listlessness
      11. Seizures
      12. Coma
   H. Management
      1. Antiinflammatory drugs
      2. Short-acting corticosteroids
      3. Fluids (LRS)
      4. May use dimethyl sulfoxide (DMSO) in fluids
      5. Vaccinations in spring and fall
      6. Control mosquito population

## RESPIRATORY DISEASES

### Common Clinical Signs

I. Coughing
II. Clear runny nasal discharge
III. Secondary bacterial infection causes purulent (puslike) discharge
IV. Depression
V. Anorexia
VI. Dyspnea, tachypnea
VII. Pyrexia

### Rule Outs of Respiratory Diseases

I. Strangles
   A. A very contagious upper respiratory tract disease
      1. Caused by the bacterium *Streptococcus equi*
   B. It is spread by the infected animal's secretions or by fomites
   C. Another bacterium that creates similar clinical signs but is not contagious is *S. zooepidemicus*
   D. Horses develop swelling of the lymph nodes
      1. Under the mandible
      2. In the guttural pouches
      3. In the throat area
   E. These abscesses can be quite painful and eventually rupture
   F. Management
      1. Infected horse isolated to prevent cross-contamination
      2. Abscesses hot packed (to speed maturation) or lanced to encourage proper drainage
      3. Fluids and feed slurries given if the horse is dysphagic
      4. Horse kept warm with plenty of fresh water available
      5. Possible use of antipyretics and antibiotics
      6. Anything that comes into contact with the infected horse should be well disinfected or burned if possible

7. Currently available vaccines may lessen the severity of the disease but will not prevent an infection
8. Intranasal vaccine now the route of choice

II. Equine herpesvirus (EHV-4) (viral rhinopneumonitis)
   A. This virus is prevalent worldwide
   B. As with EHV-1 (see Neuromuscular Disorders), this virus is also spread via direct contact or aerosols
      1. This strain of virus attacks the upper respiratory tract
   C. As well as the previously listed clinical signs of respiratory diseases, horses will have
      1. Increased lung sounds
      2. Possible swelling of the lymph nodes
   D. Management
      1. Isolate the infected animal to prevent cross-contamination
      2. Keep the horse warm in a well-ventilated stall
      3. Have plenty of fresh water available
      4. Avoid stressful situations (e.g., transport in a trailer)
      5. Exercise for brief periods to keep blood and lymph circulating
   E. A vaccine is available; although its ability to prevent the disease is questionable, it does seem to lessen its severity

III. Equine influenza (flu)
   A. An extremely contagious virus that attacks the upper respiratory tract
   B. Two subtypes: influenza A/equine/1 and influenza A/equine/2
   C. Present worldwide except for Australia and New Zealand
   D. Affects horses, donkeys, mules, and zebras
   E. Usually affects animals between 1 and 3 years of age
   F. It is spread very quickly in areas of extensive horse populations, such as
      1. Horse shows
      2. Race tracks
      3. Barns where horses are constantly moving in and out
   G. Infection is more frequent in winter and spring because of low temperatures and humidity, but can occur all year
   H. Like the other respiratory viruses, the influenza virus also is spread by direct contact and by aerosols
   I. Clinical signs may include
      1. Lethargy/depression
      2. Pyrexia
      3. Severe dry cough
      4. Increased lung sounds (in some cases)
      5. Watery nasal discharge
      6. Loss of appetite
      7. Constipation
      8. Some muscle soreness
   J. Management is the same as for EHV-4
   K. Some vaccines are reasonably effective, especially intranasal vaccines

## BLOOD DISORDER

I. Equine infectious anemia (EIA)
   A. Also known as swamp fever
   B. The virus is found in
      1. Blood
      2. Semen
      3. Tissues
   C. It is transmitted by
      1. Arthropods (most commonly biting flies)
      2. Blood transfusions
      3. Dirty needles
   D. Clinically, horses will be
      1. Pyretic
      2. Depressed
      3. Anorexic and show weight loss
      4. Anemic
   E. Coggins test is used to diagnose EIA
      1. A blood sample is taken and the serum is analyzed for antibodies
      2. This test is required for
         a. Any horse that is traveling between countries
         b. Racehorses
         c. Show horses
         d. Horses that are being sold
   F. There is no cure or prevention for this disease
   G. Infected horses will always be carriers of this virus but may be asymptomatic
   H. Euthanasia depends on
      1. State regulations
      2. Provincial regulations
      3. Federal regulations
   I. If horse is not euthanized, it must be isolated for the rest of its life

## FOOT AILMENTS

I. Laminitis (founder)
   A. Inflammation of the sensitive laminae of the feet
      1. Most commonly occurs in the front feet, but can occur in the hind feet
   B. Caused by
      1. Grain overload
      2. Ingestion of large amounts of cold water (water founder)
      3. Endotoxemia
      4. Concussion (road founder)
      5. Hormonal influences

6. Previous viral respiratory diseases
7. Previous administration of drugs
8. Overeating lush pastures, particularly in the spring

C. Clinically, horses will
1. Be reluctant to move
2. Be anxious (in extreme cases)
3. Toe point
4. Rock back on the heal to relieve the pressure on the toe
5. Be pyrexic
6. Be depressed
7. Be off feed
8. Have increased heat in the hoof wall and bounding digital pulses as a result of increased blood flow
9. Be sensitive to hoof testers

D. In extreme cases the coffin bone rotates and can come through the sole of the foot

E. Radiographs are used to determine degree of rotation

F. Management
1. Antiinflammatory drugs
2. Isoxsuprine hydrochloride (vasodilator)
3. Nitroglycerin applied to the medial and lateral digital arteries (vasodilator)
4. Acepromazine
5. Fluids (LRS)
6. Grass hay free choice, no grain
7. Corrective hoof trimming
8. Cold hosing and icing feet may also be done; however, this treatment is controversial
9. Foot pads

II. Navicular syndrome
A. Degeneration of the navicular bone
B. Exact cause unknown
C. Clinically, horses may
1. Stumble
2. Have a shortened stride
3. Be intermittently lame
D. When pressure is applied over the sole of the foot with hoof testers, a horse with navicular disease will react by pulling the foot away in response to pain
E. To further diagnose navicular syndrome, the following is performed
1. Flexion tests
2. Nerve blocking
3. Radiographs
4. MRI can be useful in some cases
F. Management
1. Antiinflammatory drugs
2. Vasodilator (isoxsuprine hydrochloride)
3. Corrective foot trimming and shoeing
4. Last resort: surgically performing a neurectomy

# LAMENESS

I. Etiology
A. Wounds/trauma
B. Bone changes
1. Congenital (e.g., osteochondritis dissecans)
2. Chip fragments in joints resulting from excessive force
C. Soft tissue damage
1. Tendon injuries
2. Suspensory ligament injuries
3. Tendon sheath and joint capsule tears
D. Neurological (e.g., EPM)
E. Circulatory disorders (e.g., laminitis)

II. Detailed medical history important
A. Duration of lameness
B. Chronic versus acute
C. Working or stall rested while lame
D. Warms out of lameness
E. Stumbling
F. Previous medication
G. Alteration in the presentation of lameness while on medication

III. Methods of diagnosing lameness
A. Visual examination
1. At rest, walk, and trot
B. Flexion testing to assess joint specific lameness
C. Palpation of tendons and suspensory ligaments to assess soft tissue lameness
D. Local anesthetics
1. Carbocaine-V 2% injected into soft tissue or intraarticularly
2. Alcohol or antiseptic scrub applied before blocking the area
3. Intraarticular blocks are evaluated after 30 minutes
4. Nonarticular blocks are evaluated after 5 to 15 minutes
5. Ensure that horse is properly restrained before veterinarian injects the anesthetic
6. Horse not sedated for this procedure to accurately diagnose an effect
7. Horse is assessed at walk and trot before and after blocking, preferably with the same person handling the horse
8. For an excited horse that is difficult to handle, acepromazine may be injected intravenously without masking the lameness
E. Radiographic examination (ionizing radiation or CR [computed radiography] and DR [digital radiography])
1. Proper holding of the plate is essential, but radiation safety is to be considered
2. Plate held parallel to the leg, with the leg positioned squarely under the horse

3. Lead aprons with thyroid protectors and lead gloves must be worn
4. Dosimeters measure radiation exposure levels
5. Views include
   a. Lateral
   b. Oblique: medial and lateral
   c. Anterior-posterior
      (1) Often referred to as dorsal to palmar for front limb and dorsal to plantar for hind limb
         (a) Views distal to and including the carpus
      (2) Proximal to the carpus or tarsus, views often named cranial to caudal
   d. Flexed for fetlock and carpus
   e. Skyline of the carpus and stifle
   f. Extra views are taken of the feet with the horse standing on a cassette covered by a strong Plexiglas shield
6. Portable units used to x-ray feet, fetlocks, carpus, and hocks
7. Larger stationary units with higher mAs and kVp used for shoulder, stifle, cervical spine, and head
8. For pelvic radiographs, horse may need to be anesthetized and have radiographs taken in dorsal recumbency, but can also be done with the horse standing and very well sedated

F. Ultrasound diagnosis
   1. Tendons: superficial and deep digital flexor tendons
   2. Ligaments: check ligament, main suspensory, and medial and lateral branches of the suspensory

G. Nuclear scintigraphy
   1. A radioactive isotope, technetium, is injected IV into the horse; 2 hours later the body is scanned for "hot spots," or areas of uptake
   2. Soft tissue of the lower limbs is scanned 2 to 20 minutes from injection
   3. The horse is radioactive for 24 to 36 hours, and contact is restricted to feeding and watering
   4. Hind end scans involve withholding water the morning of the scan so the bladder does not obscure the pelvis views
   5. Salix parental, a diuretic, is injected to help minimize bladder size
   6. Common uses
      a. Lameness that does not block out
      b. Suspected stress fractures that do not always show on radiography
         (1) Tibial stress fracture
         (2) Condylar fracture
         (3) Pelvis
         (4) Carpus and hock

c. Suspected suspensory ligament and tendon injuries

H. Extracorporeal shock wave therapy (ESWT)
   1. Ultrasound-guided shock wave therapy
   2. Speeds up healing time by increasing blood flow to the area
   3. Used on ligaments, shin saucer fractures, bucked shins, and some bone fractures
   4. Beginning to be used on navicular
   5. Has not been successful in treating tendons

I. Magnetic resonance imaging (MRI)
   1. Highly specialized diagnostic tool using a high-powered magnet
   2. Used when a specific area of pain has been localized but a diagnosis is not obtainable by traditional methods mentioned previously
   3. Creates a more detailed anatomical image and shows physiological changes in tissue composition, unlike more traditional methods
   4. Areas examined, under general anesthesia, are limited to the feet, lower leg including the carpus and hock, head, neck, and whole bodies of foals
   5. The patient should be bathed to keep dirt out of the tube and away from the magnet
   6. Horse shoes must be removed and radiographs taken to ensure that all nail fragments are removed

IV. Common lameness
   A. Laminitis
   B. Navicular
   C. Fractured splint bones
   D. Bucked shins
   E. Cortical stress fractures of shins (saucer fractures)
   F. Chip fractures in joints
   G. Condylar or P1 (first pastern bone) fractures
   H. Hoof abscesses
   I. Bowed tendons
   J. Torn suspensory ligament

## EQUINE SURGERY

I. Presurgical preparations
   A. Take horse off feed 12 hours before surgery. Water can remain
   B. TPR (temperature, pulse, and respiration) is performed
   C. Groom horse to rid excess dirt and dander; pull shoes or tape for recovery
   D. Clip and aseptically prep jugular vein; place an IV catheter
   E. Placement may depend on recumbency
   F. Throat operations require placement lower than normal
   G. PCV and TP, blood gas analysis, and electrolyte analysis if available

H. Rinse out horse's mouth before induction
I. After horse is induced, the veterinarian will
1. Direct positioning of the horse on the surgery table
2. Indicate the area that needs to be clipped and prepped
J. Horse's feet should be covered with gloves or plastic (e.g., rectal sleeves) to prevent contamination to the surgery suite

II. Positioning of horse
A. The following surgeries are performed in dorsal recumbency
1. All abdominal surgeries (e.g., colic, exploratory, cesarean section, umbilical, and inguinal hernia repair) and laryngeal ventriculectomy
2. Castrations
a. Cryptorchid (bilateral or unilateral)
b. Routine castrations
3. Arthroscopies
a. Hock
b. Stifle
c. Carpus: surgeon preference
4. Neurectomy: surgeon preference
B. When positioning a horse in dorsal recumbency, particular attention must be paid to
1. The padding underneath the shoulder and gluteal muscles
2. If padding is not sufficient, myositis can develop
C. The following operations are performed in lateral recumbency
1. Eye surgery
2. Tooth extractions
3. Mandible fracture repair (wiring)
4. Laryngotomy
5. Laryngoplasty
6. Arthroscopies
a. Carpus
b. Fetlocks
c. Shoulders
7. Periosteal strips
8. Splint fracture removal
9. Neurectomy: if more than one branch
10. Condyle fracture repair
D. When positioning a horse in lateral recumbency
1. Avoid putting pressure on the down elbow
2. The down foreleg should be pulled forward to enhance circulation and protect against radial nerve paralysis
3. The contralateral limbs should be supported with pads or leg supports, to keep the weight off the down legs
4. The head should have padding between the halter and the face when dropping and recovering

5. The head should be well padded while the horse is recumbent to protect the facial nerve from paralysis
6. Halter is removed during surgery
E. The following can be performed when a sedated horse is standing
1. Extraction of wolf teeth (first premolar)
2. Rectovaginal tears using an epidural
3. Caslick's procedure (suturing a small portion of mare's vulva to prevent air entering the vagina, commonly known as wind sucking)
4. Perianal lacerations using an epidural
5. Uncomplicated ovariectomies
6. Tendon splitting
7. Castration
8. Neurectomy, of a single branch

III. Preparation of surgical site
A. After surgical site is clipped and vacuumed, caps and masks should be worn
B. Arthroscopic surgeries may have the instrument portal sites shaved with a razor
C. Prepping
1. Clean area with a bacteriostatic agent, such as chlorhexidine or an iodine-based soap
2. Minimum 7-minute scrub
3. After site is clean, apply alcohol to defat the skin
a. Do not use alcohol as a final prep for eye surgeries or castrations
4. Move horse inside the surgical suite, where a final germicidal prep solution of tincture of Savlon or iodine is used
D. Prepping for eye surgeries
1. Clip hair around eye, including eyelashes. Prevent hair from getting into eyes
2. If the eye is being enucleated (removed), the eyelids are sutured closed
3. Bacteriostatic agents should be avoided, because they irritate the sensitive tissue around the eye and can damage the eyeball
4. A very dilute solution of povidone-iodine and saline can be used to clean skin around the eye
5. When flushing out the eye, saline is often used

IV. In surgery
A. Be aware of sterility zones
B. Assist veterinarians with their gowns and draping of horse
C. Assist with intraoperative radiographs for fracture repair surgeries
D. May assist anesthetist with blood pressure readings, depending on type of monitoring equipment
E. Values to be aware of
1. Blood pressure

a. Systolic blood pressure should be above 80 mm Hg

b. Dobutamine used to increase blood pressure; side effect is to lower heart rate

V. Recovery

A. Recover in same recumbency as during surgery

B. Padding is placed between the halter and the face and a recovery helmet is worn

C. Legs are wrapped for protection

D. Endotracheal (ET) tube is tied in place

E. When in dorsal recumbency for surgery
  1. Left lateral recumbency is preferred to right recumbency

F. Assisted recovery: ET tube is pulled when horse swallows

G. Unassisted recovery: ET tube is pulled once horse is standing

VI. Postoperative care

A. After the horse recovers and is stable, it can be moved back to its stall

B. Horse should be kept warm and quiet

C. Feeding regimen is clinic specific and determined by the type of surgery

D. Monitoring horse's feces is very important, because ileus is a risk with general anesthetic

E. Horse's vital signs, including gastrointestinal motility, are monitored twice daily

F. After horse passes feces, soft food such as a small bran mash can be introduced. A few hours later, a small amount of hay can be fed

G. If horse passes more feces and vital signs are normal, horse's regular feeding schedule can be slowly introduced, beginning with gradually increasing amount of hay fed

H. If horse does not pass any feces, a veterinarian will perform a rectal examination to determine if horse is impacted

I. If impacted
  1. A nasogastric tube is passed, and mineral oil and warm water is introduced into the stomach to help break down the impaction
  2. Food is withheld from the horse
  3. Horse may be placed on intravenous fluids (LRS) until horse is passing feces
  4. Frequent hand walking (if surgery allows)
  5. Monitor vital signs
  6. Particular attention is paid to gastrointestinal motility (gut sounds)
  7. Horse is monitored four times daily until impaction has passed

J. In cases of arthroscopic surgery
  1. Bandage is monitored for fluid discharge
  2. Leg is monitored for unusual heat, swelling, or pain

  3. Usually 24 hours after the surgery, hand walking for 5 minutes is introduced

K. In cases of fracture repair
  1. The cast is monitored for softness caused by discharge leaking from the fracture site
  2. Note unusual smell or unusual swelling above the cast
  3. On recovery, the cast may be replaced by a firm standing bandage with lots of support
    a. This will depend on the severity of the fracture

## BANDAGING

I. Much damage can be done with a poor bandage

II. Principles of bandaging

A. Smooth and wrinkle free with no bunching of material

B. Adequate thickness of wrap under the bandage is necessary

C. If too loose and it slips, it may constrict the back of the tendon and cause bowed tendons

D. If too tight, it can constrict blood supply to the wound or area distal to the bandage, or cause bowed tendons

E. Usually three layers to a bandage
  1. Primary bandage or the layer right next to the skin
  2. Secondary layer mainly used for absorption of fluid
  3. Tertiary or outer layer that protects the bandage

III. Bandage uses

A. Wound protection

B. Fracture support

C. Protection during shipping

D. Protection when dropping for surgery

E. Riding

F. Keeping foot medications in place

IV. Types of wounds and wound bandages

A. Open wounds
  1. Adherent dressing as first layer
  2. Acts to debride wound when removed
  3. As wound closes and granulation bed fills in, switch to a nonadherent dressing as the primary layer

B. Closed wounds
  1. Medicated gauze, usually until first bandage change, depending on whether discharge present
  2. Next layer is absorbent padding, evenly and smoothly applied to the area being bandaged and secured with a conforming bandage
  3. Depending on area being bandaged, the tertiary layer is Elastoplast, Vetrap, or a cotton and bandage

V. Postoperative bandages
  A. As for closed wounds
  B. When bandaging the carpus and hock
    1. A figure-eight pattern with Elastoplast adhering to the hair above and below
    2. Keep the accessory carpal bone and point of the hock uncovered to avoid pressure sores
    3. A small incision is cut into the bandage over the tendon to prevent a bandage bow
    4. A standing bandage may be placed below the carpus or hock to keep it from slipping
VI. Cast
  A. Medicated gauze and absorbent layer held in place with conform bandage
  B. A sterile, nonpervious stockinette covers the leg from the toe to above the length of the cast
  C. Vetcast plaster roll is saturated in warm water and wrapped horizontally and vertically for strength
  D. For short-term casts, "Gigli" wire is placed between the nonpervious stockinette and the cast for removal once the horse is standing
  E. For long-term casts, felt is wrapped at the top of the cast to prevent rubbing
  F. Long-term casts are removed with a cast-cutting saw or cast spreaders
  G. Horses vary in tolerance and reaction to a cast and must be monitored daily
  H. Duration of time in a cast depends on the severity of the fracture
VII. Foot bandage
  A. Used to keep medication or poultice in place
  B. Animal Lintex is a manufactured bandage poultice
  C. Often left on overnight, but are replaced daily
  D. Puncture wounds and abscesses are most common reasons for a foot bandage

## ACKNOWLEDGMENT

The editors and authors recognize and appreciate the original contribution of Colleen Hill.

# Glossary

**anorexia** Lack of appetite for food

**arthroscopy** Method of looking inside a joint through the aid of a fiberoptic scope

**ataxia** Muscle incoordination or irregular muscle action

**bandage bows** Caused by applying a bandage too tightly, creating an acute pressure injury to the tendons that may cause the area to swell once the bandage is removed, giving a "bowed" appearance

**borborygmus** Bubbling and gurgling sounds from gas moving through the gastrointestinal tract

**dysphagia** Difficulty swallowing

**dyspnea** Difficulty breathing

**endotoxemia** Endotoxins present in the blood

**fasciculations** Involuntary muscle contractions

**fecal impaction** Hardened feces in the rectum

**floating** Filing down of points of teeth

**guttural pouch** Air-filled sacs, found only in the horse, that are an extension of the eustachian tubes, closed by cartilage flaps on the side of the pharyngeal wall

**halitosis** Offensive breath odor

**hydrophobia** Fear of water; may be present in patients with rabies

**ileus** Cessation of intestinal motility, which leads to impactions/obstructions

**in utero** In the uterus

**laminitis** Inflammation of the sensitive laminae of the foot

**laryngoplasty** Surgical procedure that ties back the arytenoid cartilage that is partially or completely paralyzed because of damage by the recurrent laryngeal nerve

**laryngotomy** Incision of the larynx

**myositis** Inflammation of the muscle that results when blood flow is interrupted. This results with uneven or inadequate padding. Muscles can become damaged, and it is an extremely painful condition

**nasogastric** Long tube placed through horse's nose into the stomach

**neurectomy** Cutting the palmar digital nerves at back of the pastern to desensitize the foot to pain

**nystagmus** Involuntary rapid eye movement seen during anesthesia; may be a sign of anesthetic depth and a reaction to pain

**periosteal strips** Surgical procedure to correct angular limb deformity in foals by incising and lifting the periosteum to accelerate growth on one side of the bone

**purulent** Containing or forming pus

**pyrexia** Presence of fever

**tachypnea** Very rapid respiration

**thrombosis** Presence of a fibrin clot in vessels

**thrombus** Fibrin blood clot that remains where it is formed; can affect blood flow if it obstructs the vessels

**tushes** Canine teeth

**vasodilator** Agent that causes dilatation of the blood vessels

**volvulus** Torsion of a loop of intestine, causing obstruction

**wolf teeth** Small tooth that may be present in front of each first molar

# Review Questions

1 Which of these are zoonotic?
  a. *Neorickettsia risticii* and *Clostridium* spp.
  b. *Sarcocystis neurona* and *Streptococcus equi*
  c. *Salmonella* spp. and rabies
  d. *Escherichia coli* and *Klebsiella* spp.
2 Common signs of neuromuscular disease include
  a. Restlessness, anxiousness, or agitation
  b. Anorexia, pyrexia, or depression
  c. Grinding teeth and sweating
  d. Muscle wasting, head pressing, or ataxia

**3** The etiological agent for strangles is
  a. *Streptococcus equi*
  b. *Streptococcus zooepidemicus*
  c. *Clostridium* spp.
  d. *Sarcocystis neurona*

**4** Coggins is the test for
  a. Equine infectious anemia
  b. Equine protozoal myeloencephalitis
  c. Potomac horse fever
  d. Hyperkalemic periodic paralysis

**5** What is very important when positioning a horse in dorsal recumbency for surgery?
  a. Pulling the front legs cranially
  b. Position of the head
  c. Exposure of jugular vein for intravenous access
  d. Sufficient padding for shoulders and gluteal muscles

**6** Equine herpesvirus 1 (EHV-1) primarily affects the
  a. Reproductive system
  b. Nervous system
  c. Gastrointestinal tract
  d. Musculoskeletal system

**7** Myositis is a result of
  a. Improper padding
  b. Improper prepping
  c. Horse not taken off feed before surgery
  d. Feeding horse too soon after surgery

**8** A cessation of gastrointestinal motility is referred to as
  a. Peristalsis
  b. Ileus
  c. Volvulus
  d. Intussusception

**9** With a casted leg it is important
  a. Not to move them
  b. To watch for signs of colic
  c. To monitor for fluid discharge and unusual smell or swelling
  d. To hand walk slowly for 5 minutes

**10** A Caslick procedure prevents
  a. The passing of feces
  b. Air from entering the mare's vagina
  c. Rectovaginal tears
  d. Behavioral problems

## BIBLIOGRAPHY

Anderson DM, editor: *Dorland's pocket medical dictionary,* ed 24, Philadelphia, 1988, Saunders.

Brown CM, Bertone J: *The 5-minute veterinary consult equine,* Ames, Iowa, 2002, Blackwell.

Church SL: *West Nile virus vaccine released,* November 1, 2001, http:// www.thehorse.com/ViewArticle.aspx?ID=2827& nID=6&n=West%20Nile%20Virus%20(WNV)&case=2. Accessed July 26, 2007.

*Compendium of veterinary products,* ed 7, Hensall, Ontario, 2001, Adrian J. Bayley.

Costa LRR, Talley L, Moore RM: Equine medical and surgical nursing. In McCurnin DM, Hayes MH, Knightbridge R: *Veterinary notes for horse owners,* ed 18, New York, 2002, Simon and Schuster.

Franczek R: *West Nile firsthand,* September 12, 2001, https:// www.thehorse.com/viewarticle.aspx?ID=80. Accessed July 26, 2007.

Fraser CM et al, editors: *The Merck veterinary manual,* ed 8, Rahway, NJ, 1995, Merck & Co, Inc.

Graetz KS: *EPM Special Report,* http://www.thehorse.com. Accessed August 24, 2007.

Graetz KS: *Viewpoint: are you ready for West Nile?* http://www. thehorse.com. Accessed August 24, 2007.

Hayes MH: *Veterinary notes for horse owners,* ed 17, New York, 1987, Acro.

Horse Health: *Extreme weather conditions spark Potomac horse fever epidemic throughout U.S.,* September 2006, http://www.horsetackreview.com/article-display/861.html. Accessed July 26, 2007.

Knecht CD et al: *Fundamental techniques in veterinary surgery,* ed 3, Philadelphia, 1987, Saunders.

Line S, Kahn CM, editors: *The Merck veterinary manual,* ed 8, Hoboken, NJ, 2005, John Wiley.

McCurnin DM, Bassert JM, editors: *Clinical textbook for veterinary technicians,* ed 6, St Louis, 2006, Saunders.

Reed SM, Bayly WM, Sellon D: *Equine internal medicine,* ed 2, St Louis, 2004, Saunders.

Riegel RJ, Hakola SE: *Illustrated atlas of clinical equine anatomy and common disorders of the horse,* vol 1, Marysville, Ohio, 1996, Equistar Publications.

Rose RJ, Hodgson DR: *Manual of equine practice,* ed 2, St Louis, 2000, Saunders.

Siegal M, editor: *Book of horses: a complete medical reference guide for horses and foals,* New York, 1996, HarperCollins.

Smith BP, editor: *Large animal internal medicine,* ed 3, St Louis, 2002, Mosby.

Speirs VC: *Clinical examination of horses,* St Louis, 1997, Saunders.

Stashak TS: *A practical guide to lameness in horses,* Ames, Iowa, 1996, Blackwell.

## CHAPTER 25

# Ruminant, South American Camelid, and Pig Nursing, Surgery, and Anesthesia

*Shirley Sandoval*

## OUTLINE

Ruminant, South American Camelid,
  and Pig Nursing
  Physical Examination
  Administering Medication and
    Sample Collection
  Venipuncture
  Injections
  Milk Sampling

Diseases of Ruminants, South
  American Camelids, and Pigs
  Metabolic
  Alimentary
  Reproductive
  Respiratory
  Other Diseases

Ruminant, South American Camelid,
  and Pig Anesthesia
  Local and Regional Anesthesia
    (Analgesia)
  General Anesthesia
Ruminant, South American Camelid,
  and Pig Surgery

## LEARNING OUTCOMES

After reading this chapter you should be able to:

1. Know techniques for administering medications and collecting samples in agricultural animals.
2. Describe some of the common diseases of cattle, small ruminants, South American camelids, and pigs.
3. Recognize some of the preventable (by vaccination) diseases of agricultural animals.
4. Describe some of the common surgical procedures of agricultural animals.
5. Describe some of the species-dependent differences in surgical procedures.
6. Understand the difference between local and regional anesthesia.
7. Describe the various methods of regional anesthesia in agricultural animals.
8. Describe the considerations for each species with respect to anesthesia in agricultural animals.
9. Describe monitoring techniques for general anesthesia in agricultural animals.

Technicians in large animal practice must be familiar with common diagnostic and therapeutic techniques, various diseases, available biologicals, surgical procedures, and anesthetic principles for all domestic species. For more in-depth information, refer to the many excellent references that are available.

### RUMINANT, SOUTH AMERICAN CAMELID, AND PIG NURSING

#### Physical Examination

I. Observations
  A. Use all senses when performing a physical examination
  B. Before entering a stall or pen, helpful information can be obtained by observation
    1. Note the animal's eyes, its stance and carriage, body condition, urine and manure output, and food and water intake
    2. Describe what is normal for each type of animal. For instance, if you are used to observing beef animals, a dairy cow may look underconditioned, but her weight may be optimal for her

II. Physical examination
   A. The physical examination should be consistent in all patients
   B. Proceed from nose to tail, listening to heart, lungs, and abdomen on both sides of the animal
   C. Take note of swellings, abrasions, discharges, etc.
   D. Temperature, pulse, and respiration (TPR) should fall within normal ranges (see Appendix E)
   E. Rumen or C-1 contractions should be noted by listening with a stethoscope at the left paralumbar fossa
      1. Normal rumen motility is 2 to 4 contractions per minute; normal C-1 motility is 3 to 5 contractions per minute
   F. Palpate over the ribs, vertebral column, and pelvis of fiber animals. What may appear to be a well-muscled to overweight animal may actually be a malnourished, emaciated animal hidden under the fiber

## Administering Medication and Sample Collection

I. Oral dosing
   A. Balling gun
      1. Boluses, capsules, and magnets can be administered using this device, which may be made of plastic or metal
      2. Ruminants should be secured and the head well restrained
         a. Hold the animal around the bridge of the nose, place your fingers in the interdental space, and apply pressure to the hard palate
         b. This will force the animal to open its mouth so you can introduce the balling gun at the interdental space
         c. Position it so the medication will be deposited at the base of the tongue
         d. The head should be stabilized and held horizontally
      3. In pigs, a bar speculum can be introduced into the animal's mouth to hold the jaws open so that the balling gun can be used to deposit boluses or capsules at the base of the tongue
   B. Stomach tube
      1. For delivering large amounts of liquid medication, oral fluids, or anthelmintics or for transfaunation
         a. This technique is also used to retrieve a rumen fluid sample to examine for protozoa and measure pH
      2. Frick speculum
         a. Hollow, stainless steel tube that is used in cattle; it is inserted similarly to the balling gun

(1) It is used as a guide when introducing a stomach tube to prevent the tube from being damaged
         b. In sheep, goats, and camelids, a tape roll or appropriately sized, smooth-ended syringe case can be used
      3. Measure the distance from the nose to the rumen at approximately the thirteenth rib and insert the tube through the speculum up to the mark
         a. You may detect the odor of rumen or C-1 gas to let you know you are in the correct place; or have someone listen over the rumen or C-1 at the paralumbar fossa with a stethoscope as you blow air into the tube
            (1) A gurgling sound will be heard
         b. After you verify correct placement, the liquid can be administered
         c. Always kink off the tube or occlude the end before removing it to prevent the animal from aspirating any of the contents
      4. Rumen or C-1 fluid sampling
         a. Pass the tube as just mentioned, and siphon fluid out of the rumen or C-1 by attaching a dose syringe to the end of the stomach tube
            (1) Alternatively, while the tube is in the rumen or C-1, move the tube quickly in and out a few times, about 8 to 10 inches, and occlude the end before removing the tube
            (2) This process may have to be repeated to obtain an adequate sample
         b. Pour your sample into a clean specimen container from the fluted end of the stomach tube
            (1) Passing your sample through the end of the tube that is contaminated with saliva will change the pH of your sample
   C. Drench
      1. Small amounts of liquid medication can be given via drench
      2. A dose-syringe or unbreakable bottle is placed in the interdental space (ruminants) or at the commissure of the mouth (pigs)
         a. The head is tilted slightly so the nose is level with the eye
         b. The liquid should be given at a slow rate to allow the animal to swallow

## Venipuncture

I. Cattle
   A. Jugular vein is for sampling and administering large volumes of fluids
      1. Head is restrained in a head catch and drawn upward to the opposite side

2. Injection site is cleansed with 70% alcohol and occluded
3. A 16- or 18-gauge, 3.75- to 7.5-cm (1½- to 3-inch) needle is used and pushed with one sharp motion through the skin at a 45- to 90-degree angle
   a. The larger bore and longer needle length are used for administration of fluids
B. Tail vein (ventral coccygeal) is for sampling and injecting small volumes
   1. Confine animal to an area to prevent sideways movement and bend the tail directly forward at the base
   2. Cleanse with 70% alcohol
   3. Use an 18- to 20-gauge, 2.5- to 3.75-cm (1- to 1½-inch) needle inserted at a 90-degree angle on the midline between the hemal arches of the fourth to seventh coccygeal vertebrae
C. Milk vein (subcutaneous abdominal) forms hematomas easily and is under pressure. Use caution
   1. Occlusion is not necessary before entering with a 14-gauge, 5- to 7.5-cm (2- to 3-inch) needle
   2. Digital pressure applied for several minutes is necessary but a hematoma may still form
II. Sheep, goat, and South American camelid (SAC)
A. Jugular vein is almost always used
   1. Direct an 18- or 20-gauge, 2.5- to 3.5-cm (1- to 1½-inch) needle into the jugular furrow at about a 30- to 45-degree angle
   2. Use of cephalic and femoral veins is uncommon
III. Pigs
A. Cranial vena cava for a large volume (right side preferred because the phrenic nerve and thoracic duct are found near the left external jugular vein)
   1. An 18- or 20-gauge, 7.5- to 10-cm (3- to 4-inch) needle is used for adult pigs
   2. The jugular fossa near the manubrium sterni, a bony projection just lateral to the ventral midline and cranial to the forelegs, is used as a guideline
   3. The needle is inserted perpendicular to the plane of the neck and toward the left shoulder
B. Caudal auricular (ear) for small volumes
   1. An 18- to 22-gauge, 2.5- to 3.75-cm (1- to 1½-inch) needle is usually used with slight negative pressure maintained on the syringe
C. A 19- or 21-gauge butterfly is commonly used for intravenous administration
IV. Camelids
A. Jugular vein is almost always used

1. Direct an 18- or 20-gauge, 2.5- to 3.75-cm (1- to 1½-inch) needle into the jugular furrow at a 30- to 45-degree angle
B. The jugular furrow lies medial to the ventral transverse processes of the cervical vertebra
C. Recommended to use C-2, C-5, or C-6 as landmarks for venipuncture

**Injections**

I. Intramuscular
A. Where possible, this route should be avoided in meat-producing animals. If the drug must be administered via this route, it should be placed cranial to the shoulder in the muscles of the neck, because the blemished tissues can be easily trimmed and discarded if necessary. Current studies have shown that some antibiotics have a more favorable bioavailability of therapeutic levels when they are administered in this area
B. Cattle
   1. The location is in the lateral cervical muscles
   2. Needle commonly used for adults is 16, 18, or 20 gauge, 3.75 to 5 cm (1½ to 2 inch) with 15 to 20 mL maximum volume of medication per site
   3. Smaller gauge used for calves and up to 10 or 15 mL, depending on the size of the calf
   4. When giving intramuscular injections to cattle, it is customary to place the needle before attaching the syringe
      a. A couple of slaps with the flat part of the fist before inserting the needle tends to desensitize the area and allows the animal to steady itself before the needle is inserted
C. Sheep and goats
   1. Give in the lateral cervical muscles
      a. Use 18- to 20-gauge, 3.75-cm (1½-inch) needle for adults and 20- to 22-gauge needle for young animals
      b. Depending on the size of the animal, the average volume for adults is 5 to 10 mL with a maximum of 15 mL
D. Pigs
   1. Dorsolateral neck muscles are best for pigs
   2. For adult pigs, use 18- to 20-gauge, 3.75-cm (1½-inch) needle
   3. Depending on the size of the pig(let), a maximum of 1 to 15 mL should be given
E. SACs (not intended for the food chain)
   1. Semimembranosus or semitendinosus muscle
   2. Quadriceps muscle if cushed
   3. Triceps muscle
   4. 20-gauge, 2.5-cm (1-inch) needle
   5. Adult 5 to 10 mL maximum depending upon the size of the animal and the muscle being injected

II. Subcutaneous
   A. As concerns for meat quality assurance increase, this route is becoming increasingly popular with agricultural animal producers for pharmaceutical administration. There has also been a marked increase in the variety of pharmaceuticals approved for subcutaneous administration in food-producing animals
   B. Cattle
      1. Site of administration is cranial to the shoulder and the lateral neck
      2. Use a 16- to 18-gauge, 3.75 cm (1½-inch) needle
         a. Volume depends on the personal preference of the veterinarian; however, a good guideline is up to 250 mL/site in adults and up to 50 mL/site in calves
   C. Small ruminants
      1. Site of administration is cranial to the shoulder and lateral neck area
      2. Use an 18- to 20-gauge, 2.5-cm (1-inch) needle
      3. Inject 5 mL maximum/site
   D. Pigs
      1. Site of administration is the lateral side of the neck, close to the base of the ear
      2. Use a 16- to 18-gauge, 2.5- to 3.75-cm (1- to 1½-inch) needle
      3. Depending on the size to the pig(let), 1 to 3 mL/site maximum
   E. Camelids
      1. Site of administration is the axillary region where the fiber is thin
      2. 22- to 20-gauge, 2.5-cm (1-inch) needle
      3. 5 to 10 mL/site maximum depending upon the size of the animal being treated
III. Intraperitoneal
   A. Cattle
      1. Use a 14- to 16-gauge, 3.75- to 5-cm (1½- to 2-inch) needle
      2. Antibiotics usually given in conjunction with rehydration fluids
      3. Injection site is the right flank, midway between the last rib and the tuber coxae
         a. Go at least 10 cm (4 inches) below the lateral processes of the vertebrae to prevent retroperitoneal or perirenal injection
   B. Small ruminants (neonates)
      1. Use an 18- to 20-gauge, 2.5-cm (1-inch) needle
      2. Hold the neonate by the forelimbs
      3. Place the needle approximately 1 cm (½ inch) to the left of the umbilicus, aspirate to ensure proper needle placement (not in a vein or bowel), administer medication/fluids

   C. Pigs
      1. Use a 16- to 18-gauge, 1.25- to 2.5-cm (½- to 1-inch) needle in neonates, and a 16- to 18-gauge, 7.5-cm (3-inch) needle in adults
      2. Hold the piglet by the rear legs
      3. Place the needle between the midline and the flank, aspirate to ensure proper needle placement, and administer medication/fluids
      4. Administration in adult pigs can be performed with pig in a standing position
IV. Intradermal
   A. Used primarily for tuberculin testing
   B. Cattle
      1. Use a 22-gauge, 2.5-cm (1-inch) needle
      2. Tuberculin testing requires 0.1 mL of tuberculin to be injected into the dermis of the caudal tail fold
   C. Sheep and goats
      1. Use a 25-gauge, 1.5-cm (⅝ -inch) needle
      2. Tuberculin testing requires 0.1 mL of tuberculin to be injected into the dermis of the caudal tail fold
   D. Camelids
      1. Use a 25-gauge, 1.5-cm (⅝ -inch) needle
      2. Tuberculin testing requires 0.1 mL of tuberculin to be injected into the dermis of the axillary region

## Milk Sampling

 I. An important aspect of dairy herd health is early detection and treatment of mastitis. Because of rising laboratory costs, milk sampling (for culture) is often done on a herd basis
II. Quarters are sampled into one tube and individual quarter sampling is done on only those animals that test positive on the herd testing
   A. Sampling should be done before routine milking or at least 6 hours after milking
      1. Each teat should be washed, wiped with an alcohol swab, and allowed to dry
      2. Clean in the order of far to near
      3. The first part of the stream should be discarded into a strip cup, and a midstream sample is taken horizontally and directed into the sample vial, which is held horizontally out from under the near side of the animal
      4. Sampling is done from the nearest side first
   B. Determination of subclinical mastitis and a rough estimate of somatic cell count can be done using an on-site procedure called the California Mastitis Test (CMT)
      1. The test kit consists of a paddle with four shallow cups and a reagent containing a pH indicator

2. A small amount of milk is mixed with an equal amount of CMT reagent
3. The paddle is gently rotated, and an interpretation is made based on the amount of precipitation
4. The amount of precipitate formed is given a 0 to 4 rating

## DISEASES OF RUMINANTS, SOUTH AMERICAN CAMELIDS, AND PIGS ▬▬▬
### Metabolic

I. Hypocalcemic parturient paresis (milk fever)
  A. Incidence
    1. The incidence of milk fever in cattle increases in high-performing animals at 5 to 9 years of age
    2. Greater in Channel Island breeds (Jersey)
    3. Usually occurs at 48 to 72 hours postpartum
    4. Milk fever in sheep is most common in late pregnancy but can occur in early lactation
    5. The condition is rare in sows but may occur within a few hours of farrowing
    6. Calcium levels are reported to be fairly stable in periparturient SACs
  B. Serum calcium level is decreased; serum magnesium level may be increased (flaccid paralysis) or decreased (tetany)
    1. Low serum phosphorus level may be a contributing factor
  C. Clinical signs initially include muscle tremors, weakness, and staggering gait
    1. Classic signs include sternal recumbency, head turned into flank, anorexia, dry muzzle, atonic rumen, increased heart rate (with decreased intensity of heart sound), mydriasis, myositis, and nerve damage if animal is down too long
    2. If left untreated, depression of the circulatory system and bloat as a result of lateral recumbency will be fatal
  D. Characteristically, treatment with intravenous calcium borogluconate gives a quick positive response
    1. Careful attention must be paid to the heart during infusion, because calcium salts affect the heart muscle
    2. Animals should be fed a ration high in phosphorus and low in calcium during the later stages of pregnancy
II. Ketosis (acetonemia in cattle; pregnancy toxemia in ewes)
  A. Can occur in the period from just after calving until peak lactation in the cow (2 to 6 weeks after calving)

B. Generally occurs in the last trimester of pregnancy in ewes
C. Because of increased demand for glucose for milk production in high-producing cows and the demands of the developing fetus (or fetuses), the dam has a negative energy balance
  1. Body fat is mobilized to provide energy
  2. Ketone bodies are produced in excess of tissue needs and clinical ketosis results
D. Ketosis may be secondary to any underlying disease that causes inappetence
E. There is a characteristic acetone odor to the breath, milk, and urine
F. Two forms of the disease may manifest: the wasting and the nervous forms
  1. Wasting form is more common
    a. The cow may begin by being off grain alone, then silage, but may continue to eat hay
    b. Weight loss exceeds what one might expect from loss of appetite alone
    c. Milk production declines
  2. Nervous form presents acutely with head pressing, delirium, teeth grinding, and staggering
    a. In ewes and does, signs of the disease are more like the nervous form, and ketones may be detected on the breath
G. Treatment
  1. Intravenous infusion of glucose (dextrose) is usually successful in cows, although it often needs to be repeated
  2. Oral doses of propylene glycol and hormonal therapy may be useful
  3. The same treatment in ewes is less satisfactory
  4. Lambs may have to be removed by cesarean section to save the ewe
  5. Most incidences of ketosis can be prevented by adhering to a careful management and ration plan
III. White muscle disease (nutritional myodegeneration)
  A. Vitamin E and selenium deficiency is seen in young, rapidly growing calves, lambs, kids, and cria
  B. Most commonly, these animals are from dams that were on selenium-deficient diets during their pregnancy
  C. It manifests in two forms: cardiac and skeletal
    1. The cardiac form presents with severe debilitation or sudden death
    2. Clinical signs include depression, respiratory distress, pulmonary edema, foaming at the mouth, and weakness

3. The skeletal form presents with weakness or muscle stiffness; the animal may be recumbent. Muscle groups in the limbs may become hard and painful to palpation

4. For prevention of this disease, give injection of vitamin E and selenium

## Alimentary

I. Displaced abomasum
   A. Left displaced abomasum (LDA)
      1. Occurs when the abomasum is displaced from its normal position on the abdominal floor to the left side of the abdomen, between the rumen and the abdominal wall
   B. Occurs most commonly in large-frame, high-producing, mature dairy cows immediately after calving
      1. Clinical signs are decreased appetite, lower milk production, decreased rumen motility, intermittent diarrhea, secondary ketosis, and the presence of a ping in the left flank caused by the entrapment of gas
      2. Surgical correction is performed using a left paralumbar (abomasopexy or omentopexy), right paralumbar (omentoabomasopexy or omentopexy), or ventral paramedian (abomasopexy-open or abomasopexy-toggle) approach

II. Right displaced abomasum (RDA)
   A. Occurs within a few weeks of calving and may be complicated by right-sided torsion of the abomasum (RDA)
   B. Less common than LDA but clinical signs are similar
      1. Abomasal torsion will present with acute, severe abdominal pain and acute signs of toxicity; death may occur without a timely correction
      2. Surgical correction is made using right flank (omentoabomasopexy or omentopexy) or ventral paramedian (abomasopexy-open) laparotomy
   C. There is an increased incidence of displaced abomasum in cows fed a high-grain diet (zero grazing) in conjunction with confined housing

III. Vagus indigestion
   A. Vagus indigestion is a common disease in cattle but uncommon in sheep
      1. Characterized by anorexia, decreased movement of ingesta through the stomachs, and distention
   B. Most common cause is hardware disease (traumatic reticuloperitonitis)
      1. Hardware disease usually results from perforation of the reticulum and sometimes the rumen by an ingested foreign object
      2. Clinical signs are a sudden decrease in milk production, anorexia, "hunching," and groaning
      3. Often the cow will grunt if pressure is applied over the xiphoid ("grunt test")
      4. Rumen becomes atonic, fecal output is decreased, and ketosis often occurs
      5. Treatment includes antibiotics and placing a magnet into the reticulum
      6. If unsuccessful, a rumenotomy may be performed
      7. Because dairy cattle are most often affected, most cases can be prevented by the administration of a bar magnet to all heifers at 6 months of age and careful adherence to debris-free forage
   C. Actinobacillosis of the rumen also can cause vagal indigestion in cattle
   D. In sheep the cause may be peritonitis due to sarcosporidia

IV. Ruminal tympany (bloat)
   A. Bloat is an acute overdistention of the rumen in the form of free gas or froth mixed with ingesta
      1. Frothy bloat occurs in cattle on legume pasture and on high-grain diets
         a. The froth produced prevents the escape of normal gases during eructation
      2. Gas bloat is caused by a physical obstruction of the gases and a failure of eructation
   B. If the bloat is not life threatening, the passage of a large-bore tube into the rumen to allow the escape of gas may be sufficient
   C. If the bloat is severe, the distention causes compression of the diaphragm and the animal is unable to breathe
      1. An emergency rumenotomy may be necessary to save the animal
      2. The left paralumbar fossa can be incised using a sharp knife or a trocar and cannula
      3. Antifermentative and antifrothing agents are usually administered
      4. Frothy bloat can be controlled to some degree by careful pasture and feed management

V. Rumen acidosis (grain overload)
   A. Grain overload is an accumulation of excessive quantities of highly fermentative carbohydrates that produce lactic acid in the rumen
      1. As lactic acid increases, rumen pH may drop below 5.0 and metabolic acidosis occurs
      2. Cattle, goats, and sheep are affected
      3. Usually occurs from accidental access to large quantities of grain
      4. Clinical signs include severe toxemia, weakness, dehydration, fluid-filled static rumen, incoordination, and recumbency, leading to death

B. Principles of treatment include decreasing fermentation and acid production in the rumen using antimicrobials, neutralizing metabolic acidosis, and rehydrating the animal using intravenous fluids with sodium bicarbonate

C. C-1 acidosis occurs in SACs

VI. Neonatal diarrhea

A. An important disease of farm animals; it has multiple infectious and noninfectious causes

1. Stresses such as cold weather, changes in diet or housing, weaning, and failure of passive transfer of gamma globulins from colostrum predispose the neonate to infection

2. Absorption of immunoglobulin G occurs optimally in calves within the first 6 to 8 hours of life, but may occur up to 24 hours

   a. Goats up to 24 hours
   b. Lambs, maximally to 15 hours, but up to 24 to 48 hours
   c. Piglets up to 12 to 24 hours
   d. Cria up to 24 hours

3. Dietary diarrhea also can be due to ingestion of increased quantities of milk or inferior milk replacers

B. Diarrhea is characterized by profuse, watery, yellow feces; dehydration; metabolic acidosis; shock; and death

C. Successful treatment of diarrhea depends on cause and duration

1. Replacing fluid and electrolytes lost and correcting metabolic acidosis should be the main objectives

D. Infectious causes of neonatal diarrhea can be controlled with a vaccination regimen and provision of good-quality colostrum

E. Cattle

1. *Escherichia coli* diarrhea
   a. Clinical signs include dehydration, acidosis, weakness, and death
   b. Treatable if caught early
   c. Vaccine available

F. Sheep and goats

1. Rotavirus
   a. Causes mild diarrhea
   b. Recovery usually in a few days
   c. Mortality rate increases when animal is also infected with *E. coli*

G. Pigs

1. Swine dysentery (*Treponema hyodysenteriae*)
   a. Causes depression, weakness, anorexia, hemorrhagic diarrhea, and sometimes death
   b. Can be treated, but may return after initial treatment is discontinued

   c. Effective vaccines are not available, but there is current research for the development of biological protection for this disease

2. Transmissible gastroenteritis (TGE) (porcine rotavirus)
   a. Common viral disease in pigs
   b. High morbidity and mortality rates in piglets younger than 10 days
   c. Clinical signs include diarrhea, vomiting, anorexia, dehydration, and death
   d. Vaccination available

## Reproductive

I. Cattle

A. Mastitis

1. An inflammation of the mammary gland that can occur in all species, although it assumes economic importance only in species used for milk production

2. A large proportion of cases are subclinical and can be detected only by screening tests based on the leukocyte count

3. Clinical mastitis is characterized by heat, pain, and swelling of the gland, and marked changes in the milk, such as discoloration and clots

4. A few of the major bacteria involved are *Staphylococcus aureus, Streptococcus agalactiae,* and some of the coliform bacteria

5. Treatment must include removal of infection from the quarter and returning the milk to its normal composition

6. Several treatments are available and depend on the severity of infection
   a. Includes frequent milking out of the infected quarter (stripping), udder infusions, systemic antibiotics, and perhaps drying off of the infected quarter (i.e., not milking it)

7. Prevention of mastitis through a prophylactic routine of regular screening, proper milking technique, maintenance of milking equipment, and early recognition and treatment of subclinical cases is the best course

B. Vibriosis (*Campylobacter fetus* ssp. *venerealis*)

1. A zoonotic disease
2. Causes infertility and a prolonged diestrous period
3. Periodic abortion
4. Vaccine available

C. Brucellosis (*Brucella abortus*)

1. A zoonotic disease
2. Cows
   a. Causes mid- to late-term abortions (5+ months)
   b. Subsequent pregnancies may be term or end with abortions

    c. Metritis (uterine inflammation)

    d. Retained placenta

    e. Bacterin available for calfhood vaccination

  3. Bulls

    a. Orchitis (inflammation of the testis)

    b. Epididymitis (inflammation of the epididymis)

    c. Infertility

D. Leptospirosis *(Leptospira pomona)*

  1. A zoonotic disease

  2. Clinical signs in adult cattle include fever, anorexia, agalactia, abortion, and mastitis

  3. Clinical signs in calves include septicemia, pyrexia, anorexia, depression, hemolytic anemia, and dyspnea

  4. Bacterin available

E. Listeriosis *(Listeria monocytogenes)*

  1. Zoonotic

  2. Most commonly found in ruminants

  3. Clinical signs in adults include abortion in the last trimester, ophthalmitis (inflammation of the eyeball), and uveitis (inflammation of the uvea)

  4. Bacterin available

F. Neosporosis *(Neospora caninum)*

  1. Protozoal infection

  2 Abortion at 3 to 8 months of gestation

  3. Perinatal death

  4. Encephalomyelitis in congenitally infected calves

G. Infectious bovine rhinotracheitis (IBR)

  1. Bovine herpesvirus 1

  2. Abortion, mummification, stillbirth, or weak calves when infected in the last trimester

  3. Vaccination available

H. Trichonomiasis *(Trichomonas fetus)*

  1. Protozoal infection

  2. Sexually transmitted disease

  3. Abortion or fetal reabsorption

  4. Infertility in cows

II. Sheep

  A. Vibriosis *(Vibrio fetus)* *(Campylobacter fetus* ssp. *fetus)*

    1. A zoonotic disease

    2. Clinical signs include abortion, which occurs in the last 6 weeks of gestation

    3. Also may see stillbirths and weak lambs

    4. Ewes usually survive, but the viability of the ewe decreases with complications, such as retention of fetuses, peritonitis, and metritis

  B. Brucellosis *(Brucella ovis)*

    1. Ewes (clinical signs include abortion, stillbirths, and weak lambs)

    2. Rams (infertility due to poor-quality semen and epididymitis)

C. Listeriosis *(Listeria monocytogenes)*

  1. Also known as circling disease, it is classified into three forms: neurologic disease, abortion, and septicemia

  2. The most common form in sheep is neurologic disease. *L. monocytogenes* are gram-positive, nonsporing coccobacilli

  3. Clinical signs include nasal discharge, conjunctivitis, depression, disorientation, circling, and facial paralysis

  4. Pregnant ewes develop placentitis and abort during the third trimester of gestation, usually exhibiting no other clinical signs

  5. Septicemia in lambs is characterized by depression, anorexia, pyrexia, and diarrhea. They may die in 24 hours

  6. In adults, depression, diarrhea, and slight elevation in temperature (39° to 41.5° C) (102.2° to 106.7° F)

D. Enzootic abortion in ewes (EAE) *(Chlamydophila abortus)*

  1. A major cause of abortion in sheep and goats, EAE is characterized by abortions in the last trimester

    a. Also stillbirths and placentitis

  2. The infectious organism is present in the fluids, tissues, and fetuses at the time of parturition

  3. The main transmission of the disease is via ingestion; therefore removal of the infected tissue is important to prevent spread of the disease

  4. Pregnant women should not handle these tissues or the infected animals

E. Q fever *(Coxiella burnetii)*

  1. A zoonotic disease

  2. Causative agent: rickettsia

  3. Placentitis, stillbirth, or abortion in late gestation

  4. Organism in high concentrations in the placenta and fetal fluids, also in raw milk

  5. Transmitted by inhalation or ingestion

III. Porcine

  A. Leptospirosis *(Leptospira pomona)*

    1. A zoonotic disease

    2. Stillbirths or abortion in the last 2 to 4 weeks of gestation

    3. Term piglets may be dead or weak and die shortly after birth

    4. In its acute form, it may also cause septicemia in piglets

IV. SAC

  A. Listeriosis *(Listeria monocytogenes)*

    1. Causes abortion

    2. Encephalitis, neurological signs, and recumbency

3. Leptospirosis
4. Zoonotic
5. Can cause abortion
6. Symptoms similar to those of cattle or sheep
B. Chlamydiosis
   1. Zoonotic disease
   2. See enzootic abortion in sheep

## Respiratory

I. Cattle
  A. Bovine respiratory disease complex
     1. Infectious bovine rhinotracheitis (IBR) (viral), also known as "red nose"
        a. Caused by bovine herpesvirus 1
        b. It affects cattle of all ages, but predominantly young feedlot cattle
        c. Clinical signs include upper respiratory disease, second-degree pneumonia, enteric disease (<3-week-old calves), abortion, encephalitis, and infectious pustular vulvovaginitis (IPV)
     2. Bovine viral diarrhea virus (BVDV)
        a. Caused by a pestivirus
        b. May present with bovine viral diarrhea (BVD), which includes these clinical signs: gastroenteritis, diarrhea, respiratory disease, oral lesions, and abortion
           (1) Affects cattle 6 to 24 months old
        c. May present with mucosal disease (MD), which includes these clinical signs: oral erosions, lameness, cachexia, and diarrhea
           (1) MD affects all ages but mostly young feedlot cattle
           (2) Transplacental infection of MD will have clinical signs that include calves born with curly hair coat, weak calf syndrome, and persistently infected animals
     3. Parainfluenza III (PI3) (viral)
        a. Caused by a paramyxovirus
        b. Affects all ages of cattle
        c. Clinical signs include coughing, fever, nasal discharge, and second-degree pneumonia
     4. Bovine respiratory syncytial virus (BRSV)
        a. Caused by a paramyxovirus
        b. It is most common in 6- to 8-month-old cattle
        c. Clinical signs include cough, nasal discharge, anorexia, and fever
        d. BRSV pneumonia causes dyspnea, polypnea, mouth breathing, and interstitial emphysema
     5. *Haemophilus somnus*
        a. Affects 6- to 8-month-old feedlot calves

        b. Calves are often unresponsive to treatment
        c. Clinical signs include bronchopneumonia, central nervous system disease—depression, ataxia, paralysis, recumbency, septic arthritis, myocarditis
     6. *Pasteurella haemolytica* (shipping fever)
        a. Affects young animals stressed by weaning or transport
        b. Clinical signs include acute toxemic bronchopneumonia, dyspnea, increased lung sounds, cough, and pleuritis

II. Sheep
  A. Bluetongue (viral)
     1. Transmitted by a midge vector of the *Culicoides* spp.
     2. Bluetongue is most commonly found in sheep; less common in cattle and goats
     3. A seasonal disease, it presents in the late summer and fall
     4. Initial clinical signs include a transient fever with a temperature of 41° C+ (106° F+), facial edema (including lips, muzzle, and ears), hyperemic mucous membranes, cyanotic tongue, excessive salivation, and nasal discharge
        a. This is followed by crusty lesions of the nose and muzzle, and lesions in the oral cavity, such as petechial hemorrhage, erosions, and ulcerations
        b. This progresses to lameness, cardiomyopathy, and commonly bronchopneumonia
        c. This infection can also cause the sloughing of hooves, wool break, diarrhea, and death

III. Pigs
  A. Porcine reproductive and respiratory syndrome (PRRS, or mystery swine disease)
     1. A disease in North America, making its appearance in the 1980s
     2. Characterized by reproductive failure and increased mortality rates in farrowing and nursery room pigs
     3. Reproductive problems include return to estrus, abortion, and delivery of mummified, stillborn, or poorly viable piglets
     4. Increased mortality in piglets is associated with a "thumping" respiration with severe interstitial pneumonia and several secondary infectious diseases, such as diarrhea and septicemia
     5. PRRS appears to be spread by movement of pigs between farms and by airborne dispersion over distances of less than 3 km (1.8 miles)
     6. Recent development of a vaccine has proved encouraging
  B. Atrophic rhinitis *(Bordetella bronchiseptica, Pasteurella multocida)*

1. Atrophic rhinitis is an upper respiratory disease of young pigs
2. The nonprogressive form does not include infection from toxogenic *Pasteurella multocida*
3. A less severe disease that is slight to severe, with no transient turbinate atrophy and no clinical signs
   a. The progressive form of this disease includes infection with *P. multocida,* which causes sneezing, nasal discharge, shortening or distortion of the nose, and epistaxis
4. Acute cases affect piglets from 3 to 9 weeks of age
   a. Severe nasal and maxillary distortion can result in occlusion of the nasal passages and inability to masticate, resulting in reduced growth rates

C. *Actinobacillus pleuropneumoniae*
1. This disease has a sudden onset
   a. Discovery of dead pigs without previous illness, severe respiratory distress, and a temperature of 41° C (105.8° F) is common
2. Anorexia, weakness, labored breathing with frothy discharge from mouth and nose
3. Can cause abortion in sows

## Other Diseases

I. Cattle
A. Anthrax *(Bacillus anthracis)*
1. A zoonotic disease
2. Causes peracute and acute disease
   a. Peracute disease causes sudden death
   b. Acute disease characterized by staggers, convulsions, and death
B. Anaplasmosis *(Anaplasma marginale)*
1. A rickettsial organism
   a. Transmitted from animal to animal mainly via insect vectors
   b. Also transmitted to animals by arthropod vectors, mainly ticks
2. Calves usually get a subacute form
   a. Clinical signs include bouts of anorexia and intermittent fever and may end in death; survivors are emaciated with compromised fertility
3. Adults manifest the subacute, acute, and peracute forms of the disease
   a. Subacute is as described for calves
   b. Acute disease causes anemia, weakness, pale mucous membranes, and abortion. These animals may become aggressive and attack caretakers before death
   c. Animals with peracute cases usually die within 24 hours. They initially present with fever, anemia, and respiratory distress

4. Vaccination available
   a. The killed vaccine is not preventative but decreases the severity of the disease
   b. Immunity is considered short in duration, at least 5 months
   c. Vaccination of breeding cows may predispose calves to neonatal isoerythrolysis

II. Ovine
A. Contagious foot rot
1. *Bacteroides nodosus* acts synergistically with *Fusobacterium necrophorum* as the causative agents
   a. *B. nodosus* is a gram-negative, anaerobic rod
   b. *F. necrophorum* is a gram-negative, anaerobic coccobacillary rod
   c. Clinical signs include varying degrees of lameness in one or more feet, walking on the knees, or recumbency
      (1) The interdigital skin becomes inflamed, and there is slight undermining of the sole
      (2) Removal of the loose hoof emits a distinct foul odor
   d. Treatment includes trimming the feet close, exposing the anaerobic bacteria to air, and copper sulfate foot baths or topical 10% formalin
   e. Bacterin available
2. Contagious ecthyma, soremouth, orf (viral)
   a. A zoonotic disease of sheep and goats
   b. Affects all ages but is most common in young animals
   c. Animals present with crusty lesions on the lips, nose, and gums
   d. Older animals usually present with lesions on the udder, external genitalia, coronary band, eyelids, and conjunctiva
   e. Recovery is dependent on complications that may arise from the initial insult
      (1) Complications include second-degree bacterial infection, mastitis, screwworm infestation, pneumonia, anorexia, and death
   f. Bacterin available

III. Porcine
A. Erysipelas *(Erysipelothrix rhusiopathiae)*
1. A zoonotic disease
2. This bacterial infection of pigs can manifest in an acute or a chronic form
   a. The acute form presents with fever, anorexia, and diamond-shaped skin lesions
   b. The chronic form manifests as arthritis or vegetative endocarditis

c. Incidence is decreased in swine rearing operations where the animals are housed off soil
   (1) Most commonly affects unvaccinated pigs at 3 months to adulthood
   (2) In specific pathogen-free herds, the first signs of disease may be abortion storms and septicemic death in suckling pigs

B. Meningitis *(Streptococcus suis)*
   1. A zoonotic disease
   2. This bacterial infection occurs in pigs younger than 12 weeks
   3. Initial clinical signs include fever, anorexia, depression, stiff gait, blindness, muscular tremors, and ataxia
      a. Followed by recumbency, paddling, and death
   4. A more acute disease presents with sudden death

C. Pseudorabies (Aujeszky's disease [viral])
   1. Caused by suid herpesvirus 1
   2. It is transmitted via oronasal contact with infected pigs
   3. The nervous system is the primary site of infection
   4. Clinical signs include fever, depression, vomiting, hind limb ataxia, muscle tremors, paddling, recumbency, coughing, sneezing, and death within 12 hours in young pigs
   5. In adult pigs, the disease can cause abortion, stillbirths, and mummified fetuses
   6. Vaccination available

IV. SACs
   A. There are no current biologicals approved for use in the SAC

## RUMINANT, SOUTH AMERICAN CAMELID, AND PIG ANESTHESIA

### Local and Regional Anesthesia (Analgesia)

I. Local and regional anesthetics are commonly used in large animal practice because they are often safer and more convenient than general anesthetics
   A. Local anesthesia is the desensitization of the tissues of the surgical site by the infiltration of an anesthetic agent. Regional anesthesia is desensitization of the surgical site by blocking the nerves to the region

II. Cattle: regional anesthesia in cattle is commonly used for standing laparotomy. The following techniques (or a variation) are frequently performed. In every case, the animal is adequately restrained, the area is clipped and prepped, and attention is paid to aseptic technique
   A. Inverted L block
      1. Nerves supplying the paralumbar fossa travel in a ventrocaudal direction from the spine
      2. Local anesthetic is infiltrated in a horizontal line just ventral to the transverse processes of the lumbar vertebrae and a vertical line just caudal to the last rib
         a. In this way the nerves supplying the incision site are blocked
      3. A variation of this technique is used for regional analgesia for a ventral midline approach
   B. Paralumbar block (Cornell block)
      1. Local anesthetic is injected below the lateral edges of the transverse processes of the first four lumbar vertebrae
         a. The needle is placed horizontally below each process and directed toward the midline
         b. Twenty to 25 mL of local anesthetic is injected at each site, using an 18-gauge, 3½-inch needle
      2. In this way the branches of T13, L1, and L2 (and L3), which supply the surgical site, are blocked
   C. Paravertebral block
      1. The nerves are blocked as they come off the spinal column (T13, L1, L2, and L3)
         a. At a position about 4 cm (1½ inch) off the midline, using a long (4 to 6 inch) needle, local anesthetic is injected at the caudal edges of L1, L2, and L3
      2. Muscle relaxation and desensitization of the skin and deeper tissues will result if the block is successful
   D. Epidural block
      1. Indications for use
         a. To stop straining for obstetrical manipulations
         b. To facilitate the reduction of rectal and vaginal prolapses
         c. Perineal or udder surgery
         d. To stop straining during laparotomy and cesarean delivery
         e. Urethrostomies
      2. It is achieved by injecting a small quantity of anesthetic agent in the epidural space between the first and second coccygeal vertebrae (cranial epidural) or the sacrococcygeal junction (caudal epidural)
         a. The area blocked includes the anus, vulva, perineum, and caudal aspects of the thighs
      3. If a larger quantity of local anesthetic is used (high epidural), it may provide 2 to 4 hours of analgesia for laparotomy, limb surgery, teat surgery, etc.
      4. The animal will not remain standing in the latter case

E. Cornual nerve block: used to provide anesthesia for dehorning
1. The cornual nerve runs along the frontal crest from the lateral canthus of the eye to the horn
2. The head must be firmly secured, and the area clipped and prepped
3. Five to 10 mL of local anesthetic is injected about halfway along the nerve at the lateral border of the frontal crest

F. Peterson eye block; for eye enucleation
1. First a skin bleb is made at the point where the supraorbital process meets the zygomatic arch
   a. A 14-gauge, 2.5-cm (1-inch) needle is inserted in the bleb as a cannula
   b. An 18-gauge, 12.5-cm (5-inch) needle is inserted through the cannula and directed past the rostral border of the coronoid process to the pterygopalatine fossa. Approximately 8.75 to 10 cm (3½ to 4 inches) in depth
   c. Deposit 15 mL of 2% lidocaine at this site
2. Second, local anesthetic is injected subcutaneously lateral to the zygomatic arch
   a. This technique will desensitize the globe and surrounding tissues of the eye for enucleation

G. Retrobulbar (four point) block: local anesthetic is injected into the dorsal and ventral eyelids and at the medial and lateral canthi
1. Then approximately 30 to 40 mL of local anesthetic is directed to the nerves at the apex of the orbit with a curved needle
2. Both block techniques can be used for enucleation or extirpation of the eye

H. Ring block
1. Local anesthetic agent is deposited subcutaneously and deep into the tissues completely around the surgical site, as in teat surgery, dehorning, claw amputation, etc.

I. Vascular infusion for anesthesia of the distal limb
1. Used for digit amputation, hoof/sole surgery, corn removal, and laceration repair
2. Place a tourniquet at mid metatarsal or metacarpal region
3. Clip and prep injection site; identify a surface vein
4. Using a 19- to 20-gauge, 2.5-cm (1-inch) needle or butterfly catheter, insert the needle intravenously. Aspirate to ensure proper placement
5. Infuse 10 to 30 mL of 2% lidocaine slowly
6. Remove the needle and apply pressure to the insertion site to prevent leakage and hematoma
7. Remove tourniquet at the end of the procedure

III. Sheep and goats
A. Regional anesthesia, such as paravertebral and epidural blocks, can be used in camelids, sheep, and goats
B. Goats have a low pain threshold and require sedation
C. Cornual and infratrochlear nerve blocks are used for dehorning goats
1. The corneal nerve is blocked at the caudal ridge of the supraorbital process, 1 to 1.5 cm deep, with 2 to 3 mL of 2% lidocaine (in adults)
   a. The infratrochlear nerve is blocked by inserting a needle 0.5 cm through the skin at the dorsomedial margin of the orbit
   b. The nerve may be palpated in some animals
2. A total dose of 10 mg/kg (0.5 mL of 2% solution/kg) must not be exceeded because of the toxicity potential

IV. Pig
A. The most commonly used regional anesthetic techniques in tranquilized pigs are infiltration, lumbosacral epidural injection, and intratesticular injection
B. Lumbosacral epidural is used for cesarean section, claw amputation, prolapsed rectum repair, scrotal and inguinal hernia repair, and testectomy
C. A surgical prep is performed at the injection site
D. Depending on the size of the pig, a 16- to 18-gauge, 3- to 6-inch needle is inserted into the lumbosacral space
E. The pigs should be recovered in a quiet area, away from other pigs, until they are fully awake and aware of their surroundings

## General Anesthesia

I. Cattle
A. Bloat and regurgitation of rumen contents, respiratory depression, apnea, and poor oxygenation are problems associated with general anesthesia in cattle
1. Feed should be withheld from cattle before general anesthesia
2. Withhold roughage for 48 hours, grain and concentrates for 24 hours, and water for 12 hours
3. Withhold feed for 2 to 4 hours in preruminant calves
B. Tranquilizers are not usually administered as a preanesthetic, because they do not work well to calm fractious cattle and violent recoveries are not a problem in cattle
C. An intravenous catheter should be placed in the jugular vein
1. Use 14-gauge, 5½-inch needle

D. Anesthesia can be induced with a number of drugs, including but not limited to the following
  1. Thiamylal sodium
  2. Thiopental sodium
    a. Induction is not as prolonged as with thiamylal sodium and may cause transient apnea
  3. Guaifenesin with 2 g of a thiobarbiturate
  4. Ketamine and xylazine intramuscularly
  5. A mixture of 5% guaifenesin containing 1 mg/mL ketamine and 0.1 mg/mL xylazine
  6. Masking with isoflurane or halothane
E. In a recumbent cow, bloat and aspiration of regurgitated rumen contents are concerns
  1. If possible, position so that the animal is in right lateral recumbency, which keeps up the rumen
    a. Elevate the neck so head is downward. Position so upper front and hind limbs are parallel to the table surface, pull lower forelimb forward to help prevent radial nerve paralysis
  2. Position in sternal recumbency as soon as possible
  3. The cuff should remain inflated during extubation
F. An endotracheal tube with inflated cuff should be placed even if inhalants are not used. Also use a stomach tube for the escape of rumen gases
  1. On induction, a mouth speculum is inserted to aid in the introduction of the endotracheal tube
G. The surgical table should be covered with protective padding to prevent postanesthetic complications due to nerve paralysis
H. Halothane or isoflurane is usually used when inhalation anesthesia is chosen
  1. At surgical plane, the cattle will have slow regular breathing, a slight palpebral reflex, and anal reflex
  2. The pupil is centered between the upper and lower lids
  3. The eye is rotated ventrally and the pupil is rotated medially below the lower lid when the animal is in a light plane of anesthesia
  4. Oxygen should be continued 5 to 10 minutes after anesthetic delivery
  5. The cuff should remain inflated during extubation
  6. A stomach tube should be available to decompress the rumen in the event of bloat
 I. The technician should monitor heart rate, pulse strength, muscle relaxation, respiratory rate, mucous membranes, capillary refill time, and blood pressure

II. Sheep and goats
  A. Injectable anesthesia regimens and the use of halothane or isoflurane for general anesthesia are similar to those outlined for cattle
  B. Intravenous catheter placement: 16- to 14-gauge, 3- to 5½-inch catheters in adults; and 18- to 14-gauge, 2- to 3-inch catheters in young animals
  C. Withhold feed for 24 hours and water for 12 hours in adults
    1. Withhold feed for 2 to 4 hours in preruminant animals
  D. Small ruminants should be intubated to prevent aspiration from regurgitation
  E. Oxygen should be continued 5 to 10 minutes after anesthetic delivery
  F. The cuff should remain inflated during extubation
  G. A stomach tube should be available to decompress the rumen in the event of bloat
  H. Eye position as a measurement of anesthetic depth is not as accurate in small ruminants as in cattle
III. Pig
  A. Some concerns when anesthetizing pig
    1. A higher incidence of malignant hyperthermia
    2. Fewer accessible superficial veins and arteries
    3. Tracheal intubation is difficult in adult pigs
      a. Oral cavity is small
      b. Larynx is long and mobile
      c. Laryngeal spasm is common
      d. Pharyngeal diverticulum
    4. Withhold food 8 to 12 hours; do not withhold water
  B. Induction can be achieved using
    1. Thiamylal or thiopental sodium
      a. These can be used alone for short procedures
    2. Ketamine can be used with thiobarbiturates or inhalants, such as halothane or isoflurane
    3. A mixture of guaifenesin (5% solution), ketamine (1 mg/mL), and xylazine (1 mg/mL) can be used in adult pigs
    4. Halothane or isoflurane by face mask
    5. Droperidol and fentanyl (Innovar-Vet) intramuscularly
    6. Stresnil (Azaperone)
  C. Eye reflexes and position are unreliable for monitoring pigs
  D. Heart rate, respiratory rate, muscle relaxation, and pulse strength (if possible) should be monitored
  E. As with ruminants, continue oxygen 5 to 10 minutes after inhalation and position the animal in sternal recumbency as soon as possible
  F. Unless there is evidence of regurgitation, extubate with the cuff deflated
    1. Keep the animal away from other pigs until well recovered

IV. SACs

    A. Injectable anesthesia regimens and the use of halothane or isoflurane for general anesthesia are similar to those outlined for cattle

    B. Intravenous catheter placement: 16- to 14-gauge, 3- to 5½-inch catheters in adults; and 18- to 16-gauge, 2- to 3-inch catheters in young animals

    C. Withhold feed for 24 to 48 hours and water for 12 hours in adults

       1. Withhold feed for 2 hours in cria

    D. Intubate as with small ruminants

    E. Monitoring is as with small ruminants

    F. Keep nose lower than the pole to prevent aspiration of regurgitation

    G. Maintain on oxygen 5 to 10 minutes postanesthetic delivery

    H. The cuff should remain inflated during extubation

## RUMINANT, SOUTH AMERICAN CAMELID, AND PIG SURGERY

I. Laparotomy (cattle)

    A. A laparotomy for diagnostic purposes or for surgical intervention of a condition such as LDA or RDA or for cesarean section or rumenotomy is routinely performed with the animal standing in a chute or stocks using local anesthetic

    B. The incision is made in the paralumbar fossa, and the area to be prepped includes a wide margin surrounding the incision site

    C. The hair is clipped, any gross debris is removed, and a surgical prep is performed over the entire clipped area

    D. The tail should be tied to the animal's hind leg or attached by rope to her halter, to keep her from swinging it into the incision

       1. Never tie a cow's tail to a post or rail, because she can easily amputate her tail

    E. Sutures should be removed 2 to 3 weeks after surgery

    F. On occasion the surgeon may elect to perform a paramedian or ventral midline celiotomy for an RDA or a cesarean section

       1. The cow is cast with ropes and placed in dorsal recumbency

II. Digit amputation (cattle)

    A. The cow is placed in lateral recumbency with the affected claw up

    B. The claw and interdigital space are thoroughly cleaned of manure and debris

    C. The area is clipped from mid metacarpus to the hoof and prepped in a routine manner

    D. Anesthesia is achieved with a ring block or intravenous local using rubber tubing as a tourniquet distal to the carpus or hock

    E. Obstetrical or Gigli wire is used to amputate the claw

    F. After surgery, the foot is bandaged for 2 to 3 weeks (unless complicated by infection); the bandage may need to be changed frequently

III. Teat laceration repair (cattle and goat)

    A. This surgery may be performed with the animal standing or in dorsal recumbency

    B. A ring block is used on the affected teat, and a complete surgical prep is performed

       1. Rubber tubing used as a tourniquet will control bleeding and milk leakage

       2. A teat prosthesis may be inserted at the time of repair

    C. Postoperatively, the insert will allow the affected teat to drain while the other quarters are being milked

    D. Hand milking should not be done because it may interfere with the suture line

    E. Sutures are removed in about 2 weeks

    F. Similar surgical technique is used on the doe

IV. Eye enucleation (cattle)

    A. The cow will have to be restrained in a chute while a halter secures its head to one side

    B. Regional anesthesia is done with a Peterson eye block or a four-point retrobulbar block

    C. Usually the eyelids are sewn together; then the area is clipped and surgically prepped

    D. Typically, the prep is complicated by necrotic and contaminated tissue

    E. Postoperative care will include antibiotics and perhaps a wound spray on the surgical site

V. Castration

    A. Cattle

       1. Calves are usually castrated from 1 to 4 weeks of age

       2. No anesthesia or surgical prep is generally used, for financial reasons

       3. For open castration, an incision is made in the scrotum and an emasculator is used to sever and crush the spermatic cord

       4. Calves should be vaccinated for clostridial infections before or at the time of castration (Table 25-1)

       5. An emasculatome is used for closed castration

         a. This device crushes and severs the spermatic cord without having to incise the skin of the scrotum

       6. Calves are sometimes castrated using an elastrator, or elastic band, around the testicles

         a. This procedure is preferably performed within the first few weeks of life; however, it can be successfully performed in older animals

**Table 25-1** Clostridial diseases with biologicals

| System/Etiology | Signs | Other comments |
|---|---|---|
| | ***Clostridium chauvoei* (BLACKLEG)** | |
| | ***Cattle*** | |
| Clostridial myositis | Severe lameness; depression; anorexia; temperature of 41° C (106° F); increased pulse of 100-120 beats/min; and acute edema, hot and painful, that becomes cold and painless with emphysema as the disease progresses | Death occurs in 12-36 hr |
| | ***Sheep and Goats*** | |
| Clostridial myositis | Clinical signs include lameness, high fever, anorexia, depression, and death | Occurs when young rams are housed together, butt heads, and create wounds for the organisms to enter the body |
| | ***Clostridium septicum, Clostridium sordellii* (MALIGNANT EDEMA)** | |
| | ***Cattle*** | |
| Gas gangrene | Lesion with painful swelling, with or without emphysema, temperature of 41°-42° C (106°-107° F), depressed, weak, muscle tremor, lame, or stiff | Death occurs in 24-48 hr |
| | ***Sheep*** | |
| | May occur after lambing, shearing, or castration/tail docking "Swelled head" | Organisms are transmitted from the soil to the animals through open cuts, wounds, surgical incisions, and the umbilicus |
| | ***Clostridium novyi* TYPE B (BLACK DISEASE)** | |
| | ***Cattle*** | |
| Infectious necrotic hepatitis | Initiated by damage to the liver; causes severe depression and an initial fever followed by subnormal temperatures, rumen atony, and abdominal pain, which may last 1-2 days; animals tend to separate from the rest of the herd | |
| | ***Sheep and Goats*** | |
| Initiated by damage to the liver | Causes severe depression and an initial fever followed by subnormal temperatures | Clinical signs are not usually observed because death is rapid. Animals usually die during the night |
| | ***Clostridium haemolyticum* (BACILLARY HEMOGLOBINURIA)** | |
| | ***Cattle and Sheep*** | |
| Initiated by damage to the liver | Clinical signs include fever, rumen atony, anorexia, abdominal pain, toxemia, arched posture, and dark-red urine ("red water") | Death occurs in 12-96 hr |
| | ***Clostridium perfringens* TYPE D (PULPY KIDNEY)** | |
| | ***Cattle*** | |
| | *Peracute disease:* Animals found dead <br> *Acute disease:* Animals exhibit bellowing, mania, convulsions, and death in 1-2 hr <br> *Subacute disease:* Animals appear quiet and docile, show adipsia, and may appear blind <br> Signs may last 2-3 days <br> Quick, complete recovery | Affects calves 1-4 mo old <br> Occurs in the summer and fall in endemic areas where fields may be irrigated |

*Continued*

**Table 25-1**   Clostridial diseases with biologicals—cont'd

| System/Etiology | Signs | Other comments |
|---|---|---|
| | *Sheep* | |
| | Lambs with peracute disease present with sudden death<br>Lambs with acute disease (<2 hr) present with depression, clonic convulsions, diarrhea, opisthotonus, and death<br>Adults may live up to 24 hr, lag behind, and show staggers, knuckling, and a rapid, shallow respiration | |
| | *Goats* | |
| | Peracute disease presents with fever, abdominal pain, dysentery, and convulsions<br>Goats with acute disease present with abdominal pain and diarrhea | Death occurs in 4-36 hr<br>Goats with acute disease may recover in 2-4 days or die |
| | *Enteric Disease in Piglets* | |
| | Peracute, acute, subacute, or chronic disease<br>Peracute and acute disease each show varying degrees of hemorrhagic diarrhea and death within 2 days<br>Subacute disease produces diarrhea, which can last 7 days and produces a dehydrated piglet, resulting in death in 5-7 days<br>Chronic infections result in diarrhea, with chronic ill thrift and sometimes death | |
| | *Clostridium perfringens* **(HEMORRHAGIC ENTEROTOXEMIA)**<br>*Cattle* | |
| Gastrointestinal (GI) system; mainly affects calves up to 10 days of age | Includes diarrhea, acute abdominal pain, and nervous signs | May result in sudden death or a slow recovery in 10-14 days |
| | *Sheep* | |
| GI system; affects lambs at 1-4 days of age<br>Adult sheep | Peracute form of the disease causes sudden death<br>Acute form of the disease causes diarrhea, anorexia, and severe abdominal pain<br>"Struck": sudden death | Death occurs in 24 hr |
| | *Clostridium tetani* **(TETANUS)**<br>*Cattle* | |
| Toxins affect central nervous system | Bloat, prolapse of the third eyelid, muscle stiffness, muscle spasm, increased response to sound and tactile stimuli, and muscular rigidity ("sawhorse" stance) | |
| | *Sheep* | |
| | Clinical signs include prolapse of the third eyelid, erect ears, muscle stiffness, muscle spasms, an increased response to sound and tactile stimuli, and muscular rigidity (sawhorse stance), followed by convulsions, respiratory arrest, and death | After shearing or tail docking<br>Can give antitoxin when processing animals |

B. Small ruminants
   1. Lambs (if used for wool) are castrated within the first 1 to 2 weeks of life using an elastrator, and are tail-docked at the same time, also using an elastic or rubber band
   2. Sometimes an open or closed method of castration is used, as described previously for calves
   3. Lambs destined for meat are usually only tail docked and are often not castrated because they reach market weight before sexual maturity
   4. Kids are castrated within the first 1 to 3 weeks of life using methods described previously
   5. Other procedures performed at this time include vaccination against clostridial infection and injection of vitamin E and selenium
C. Pig
   1. Pigs are usually castrated at 1 to 2 weeks of age using an open technique
   2. Other procedures performed before or at this time are iron dextran injection to prevent anemia, tail docking to prevent cannibalism in confined housing, and clipping of milk or needle teeth (canines and third incisors) to prevent injury to the sow
   3. Frequently, inguinal hernias are discovered in the piglet at the time of castration
      a. The skin of the inguinal area should be prepped with an antiseptic solution before repair
      b. Piglets should be placed in a clean, warm pen until recovered
D. SACs
   1. Castration
   2. 2 years old
   3. May be performed standing with sedation and local anesthesia
   4. Tail should be wrapped and scrotum prepped with an antiseptic solution
   5. The scrotum is incised and the spermatic cord is stripped
   6. The cord is then transfixed and the spermatic cord is severed
   7. The scrotum is left open for drainage
VI. Dehorning
   A. Calves: dehorning in cattle is done to prevent injury from fighting
      1. It is preferable to disbud calves at 1 to 2 weeks of age using an electric dehorner
         a. Caustic pastes should be avoided
      2. If the horn buds are 1 to 2 cm (½ to 1 inch) long, a gouge-type dehorner (Barnes) can be used

   3. Mature horns can be removed with a Keystone dehorner, a hardback saw, or a wire saw
   4. Local analgesia for dehorning can be achieved with a cornual nerve block or ring block
   5. Considerations are control of pain and hemorrhage and protection against fly strike in the dehorn wound
B. Goats
   1. Goats should be dehorned using an electric dehorner as soon as the horn buds are palpable
   2. Goats are very susceptible to pain and can die of shock and fright, so analgesia is often provided
   3. Brain tissue is superficial in young goats and may be damaged if the iron is left on too long

## ACKNOWLEDGMENT

The editors and author recognize and appreciate the original contributions of Sandy Agla, on which this chapter is based.

# Glossary

**abomasopexy** Abomasum is fixed to the abdominal wall using a permanent suture. The technique is used to correct a displacement of the abomasum

**abomasopexy-toggle** Via a dorsal approach, the abomasum is attached to the ventral body wall with a toggle suture (bar suture). Used when open surgical intervention is too costly, compared with the animal's value, and the animal is being salvaged for meat

**adipsia** Absence of thirst, or the lack of desire to drink

**atonic** Lacking in tone

**balling gun** Instrument used for the administration of boluses to cattle, horses, sheep, and goats

**bolus** A large, ready to be swallowed mass of medication. Formed into an oblong tablet or gel

**C-1** The first of three compartments of the camelid stomach

**cachexia** Emaciated, malnourished

**capsule** Usually administered with a balling gun

**celiotomy** Incision into the abdominal cavity

**clonic convulsions** Seizures characterized by alternation of relaxation with jerking and flexing of muscles

**commissure of the mouth** Angled area at the most lateral portion of the mouth where the upper and lower lips meet

**cria** A young South American camelid

**cushed** The posture of a camelid when it is laying down in sternal recumbency

**drench** To give liquid medications by mouth

**emasculatome** Instrument for bloodless castration in cattle and sheep. It crushes the spermatic cord without incising the scrotum

**emasculator** Instrument used to cut and crush the spermatic cord in an open castration

**endemic** Present in an animal community at all times

**enucleation** Surgical removal of the globe of the eye

**epistaxis** Nasal bleeding

**eructation** Expelling of gas from the rumen via the oral cavity; part of the normal digestive process in ruminants

**extirpation** Surgical removal of everything within the orbit of the eye, including globe, muscles, adipose tissue, and lacrimal gland

**flaccid paralysis** Loss of voluntary movement and decreased tone of limb muscles

**fly strike** Infestation of fly larvae in the cutaneous tissues. Usually in wool or hair contaminated with feces or urine; also in skin wounds. Also called cutaneous myiasis

**grunt test** In cattle, the test is performed to detect reticuloperitonitis. It can be accomplished by a withers pinch or placing a board under the cow at the sternum, just behind the elbow. A positive test will elicit a grunt

**mydriasis** Dilation of the pupil

**myositis** Voluntary muscle inflammation

**omentoabomasopexy** Right paralumbar approach in which the abomasum is sutured in place through the ventral body wall separate from but in addition to a basic omentopexy

**omentopexy** Omentum is anchored to the abdominal wall similar to an abomasopexy, usually in the case of right-sided torsion of the abomasum

**opisthotonus** Involuntary posture in which the head and tail are bent upward and flexed over the back while the abdomen is bowed downward. It is an indicator of medulla, pons, and midbrain disease

**paralumbar fossa** Area in the flank bordered dorsally by the spinous processes of the lumbar vertebrae, cranially by the last rib, and caudally by the tuber coxae. It provides a flank approach to the abdomen for laparotomy

**paramedian** Off midline

**peracute** Duration of a few hours; very acute

**petechial hemorrhage** Small (pinpoint) round, red spots. They are not raised; may be intradermal or submucosal

**pole** The top or point of the head

**prophylactic** Prevention of disease by treatment or vaccination

**ring block** Injection of a local anesthetic in a circle around the circumference of a teat, or a lower limb, to facilitate closure of lacerations or to help in the diagnosis of lameness

**rumenotomy** Surgical procedure for evacuation of the rumen. A left flank approach is used. A rumenotomy is indicated under the following conditions: removal of metallic foreign bodies (traumatic reticuloperitonitis), rumen overload, obstructing foreign bodies, and rumen impaction

**somatic cells** Cells of the body other than germ cells

**speculum (Frick)** Instrument used to facilitate the passage of an orogastric tube by protecting the tube from damage by the animal's teeth

**subacute** Duration of disease process that is between acute and chronic. Considered to be about 1 week

**subclinical** Disease process that is not detectable by physical examination, or very mild case of disease process

**tetany** Condition in which localized spasmodic contraction of the muscle takes place. It results from a decreased level of blood calcium

**transfaunation** Reconstitution of the rumen flora through the use of cud transfer

**uvea** Structure made up of the iris, ciliary body, and choroids

**zero grazing** Animal husbandry technique in which animals are raised in confinement, on a dry lot, such as dairy cattle. Their daily feed rations are harvested plant material, concentrates, and/or grains

# Review Questions

**1** An infectious cause of abortion in ruminants
 a. *Brucella* spp.
 b. *Leptospira*
 c. *Listeria*
 d. All of the above

**2** Starting at the esophagus and going to the duodenum, the order of the ruminant's compartments is
 a. Reticulum, rumen, omasum, abomasum
 b. Abomasum, omasum, reticulum, rumen
 c. Rumen, reticulum, omasum, abomasum
 d. Omasum, abomasum, rumen, reticulum

**3** To auscultate the rumen or C-1, place the stethoscope over the
 a. Right paralumbar fossa
 b. Left paralumbar fossa
 c. Animal's left side just below the point of the elbow
 d. Animal's right side just below the point of the elbow

**4** Intradermal injections are primarily used for
 a. Antibiotic administration
 b. Vaccinations
 c. Tuberculosis testing
 d. Anesthetic administration

**5** Periparturient hypocalcemia is not common in
 a. Cattle
 b. Sheep
 c. Goats
 d. South American camelids

**6** A common clinical sign in LDA is
 a. Toxemia
 b. Ping heard with auscultation
 c. Hunching
 d. Head pressing

**7** Extubation postanesthesia in ruminant/pseudoruminant requires one to position
 a. The nose above the animal's poll
 b. The ET tube cuff to be inflated
 c. The ET tube cuff to be deflated
 d. None of the above

**8** Blackleg is a disease of ruminants caused by
 a. *Pasteurella haemolytica*
 b. *E. coli*
 c. Anthrax
 d. *Clostridium chauvoei*

**9** Which of the following veins should be used with caution when taking a blood sample from a cow?
 a. Jugular
 b. Lateral thoracic
 c. Milk
 d. Coccygeal

**10** Which of the following is not a zoonotic disease?
 a. Leptospirosis
 b. Brucellosis
 c. Anthrax
 d. Actinomyces

## BIBLIOGRAPHY

Fowler M: *Medicine and surgery of South American camelids*, ed 2, Ames, 1998, Iowa State Press.

Gill MS: Food animal medical and surgical nursing. In McCurnin DM, Bassert JM, editors: *Clinical textbook for veterinary technicians*, ed 6, St Louis, 2006, Saunders.

Line S, Kahn CM, editors: *The Merck veterinary manual*, ed 8, Hoboken, NJ, 2005, John Wiley.

Muir WW III et al: *Handbook of veterinary anesthesia*, ed 3, St Louis, 2001, Mosby.

Noordsy JL: *Food animal surgery*, ed 3, Trenton, NJ, 1994, Veterinary Learning Systems.

Pugh DG: *Sheep and goat medicine*, St Louis, 2002, Saunders.

Radostits OM et al: *Veterinary medicine: a textbook of the diseases of cattle, sheep, pigs, goats and horses*, ed 10, London, 2007, Saunders.

Reibold TW, Geiser DR, Goble DO: *Large animal anesthesia: principles and techniques*, Ames, 1995, Iowa State University Press.

Sirois M, editor: *Principles and practice of veterinary technology*, ed 2, St Louis, 2004, Mosby.

## CHAPTER 26

# Veterinary Dentistry

*Barbara Donaldson*

## OUTLINE

Anatomy of the Tooth
Dentition
Tooth Surface Terminology
Tooth Roots Using Triadan System
Tooth Function
Numbering Teeth

Dental Instruments
Complete Oral Hygiene Procedure
Safety and Infection Control
Dental Radiography
Home Care
Occlusion

Oral Lesions
Further Dental Problems
Periodontal Disease
Resorptive Lesions
Lymphocytic/Plasmacytic Stomatitis
Lagomorphs and Rodents

## LEARNING OUTCOMES

### After reading this chapter you should be able to:

1. Recognize normal and abnormal dental structures, conditions, and lesions.
2. Identify teeth by means of the Anatomical and Triadan Numbering Systems.
3. Use dental terminology to accurately chart dental morphology.
4. Recognize and correctly use, care for, and sharpen dental hand instruments.
5. List the steps to perform a complete oral hygiene procedure.
6. Describe the causes and stages of gingivitis and periodontitis.
7. Perform dental radiography.
8. Recommend a dental home care program.

It is estimated that 85% of all dogs and cats over the age of 2 years have periodontal disease. Periodontal disease is a progressive condition that affects the supporting tissues of the teeth. Bacterial plaque is the initial cause of periodontitis; it can lead to tooth loss and infections of the heart, liver, and kidney. Proper dental consideration is a vital part of the veterinary care necessary to ensure a healthy and happy pet.

## ANATOMY OF THE TOOTH

I. Tooth structure (Figure 26-1)
  A. Enamel
    1. Outer covering of the crown composed of crystals of hydroxyapatite arranged in prisms
    2. Formed by ameloblasts during tooth development. Production stops once the tooth erupts
    3. Is acellular and considered nonliving; is a relatively thin layer
       a. Cats, <0.1 to 0.3 mm thick; dogs, <0.1 to 0.6 mm thick
    4. Acts as an effective barrier to bacteria
    5. Has no sensory capacity, elasticity, or flexibility and is relatively nonporous and impervious
    6. In hypsodont teeth (long crown) of herbivores such as horses, the enamel is also invaginated into longitudinal grooves and infundibula (cups) of the teeth
  B. Dentin
    1. Makes up the bulk of the tooth
    2. Formed by odontoblasts in a tubular fashion, running from the pulp toward the enamel
    3. As hard as bone but much softer than enamel
    4. Composed of roughly 72% mineral, 18% organic matter (mostly collagen), and 10% water by weight
    5. Sensitive to heat, cold, touch, and variations in osmotic pressure. All stimuli are felt as pain
    6. Considered to be living tissue

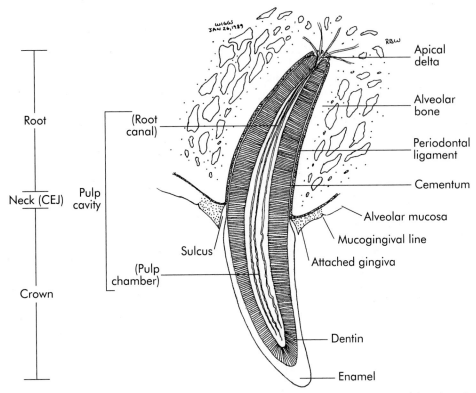

**Figure 26-1** Anatomy of a tooth and supporting structures. *CEJ*, Cementoenamel junction. (From Pratt PW: *Principles and practice of veterinary technology*, St Louis, 2001, Mosby.)

7. Collagen gives it flexibility
8. Primary dentin is formed before and during tooth eruption
9. Secondary dentin is formed continuously, causing a gradual reduction in the size of the pulp chamber
10. Tertiary dentin is formed in areas exposed to injury or irritation and is darker in color with no nerve fibers

C. Pulp
   1. Occupies the interior cavity
   2. In the crown it is called the pulp chamber, and in the root it is called the root canal
   3. Rich with blood vessels, nerves, and lymphatics
   4. Composed of odontoblasts, fibroblasts, and other cells
   5. Enters the tooth through many tiny openings in the root apex and is known as the apical delta
   6. Registers pain and quickly becomes contaminated, inflamed, and necrotic if exposed

D. Cementoenamel junction (CEJ)
   1. Junction between crown and root

II. Tooth-supporting structure; also called the periodontium. It is a collection of supporting structures surrounding the teeth

A. Cementum
   1. A type of bone that covers the root of the tooth
   2. Attached to the gingiva by the periodontal ligament fibers
   3. Inorganic content: 45% to 50% hydroxyapatite
   4. Organic content: mainly collagen fibers and Sharpey's fibers
   5. Constantly undergoing resorption and repair
   6. Is cellular at the root apex with some capacity for repair
      a. Is acellular near the crown
   7. Loss of cementum by subgingival slab fractures or by root planing will prevent gingival and ligament reattachment to the root surfaces, resulting in a permanently deep periodontal pocket

B. Periodontal ligament
   1. Holds the tooth in the alveolus (socket) by attaching the tooth to the alveolar bone
   2. Composed of collagen with some elastic fibers, blood vessels, nerves, and lymphatics
   3. Main components are the principal fibers, which are embedded in cementum and alveolar bone; termed Sharpey's fibers
   4. Absorbs shock of impact, transmitting occlusal forces to alveolar bone

5. Protects vessels and nerves in the periodontal space
6. Contains sensory nerve endings, which register pain and tactile pressure
7. Supplies nutrients to alveolar bone and cementum via arterioles and drainage via venules and lymphatics

C. Alveolar bone
   1. Surrounds and supports the teeth
   2. Constantly remodeling internally, yet remains constant throughout adult life as deposition and resorption occur
   3. Sharpey's fibers are embedded deeply into alveolar bone
   4. Lamina dura is the wall of the alveolar tooth socket that is radiographically seen as a thin white line.

D. Gingiva
   1. Soft tissue providing epithelial attachment
   2. First line of defense
   3. Divided into three regions: marginal gingiva, attached gingiva, and interdental gingiva
   4. Gingival sulcus
      a. Space between the gingiva and the tooth
      b. Normal depth in dogs is 1 to 3 mm; in cats, 0.5 to 1 mm
   5. Sulcular fluid
      a. Secreted from the gingival connective tissue, passes through sulcar epithelium
      b. Flushes the sulcus
      c. Rich in immunoglobulins and other substances with antimicrobial properties
   6. Normal aging of the periodontium
      a. Periodontal ligament shows an increase in the number of elastic fibers and a decrease in the vascularity, mitotic activity, fibroplasia, collagen fibers, and mucopolysaccharides
      b. Cementum becomes thicker
      c. The density of the alveolar bone increases with a reduction of the definition of the lamina dura and slight regression of the alveolar crest
      d. Decrease in the healing ability of the alveolar bone with increased porosity

## DENTITION

I. Mammals are diphyodonts, which means that they have two sets of teeth

| | Deciduous | Permanent | Permanent incisors | Permanent canines | Permanent premolars | Permanent molars |
|---|---|---|---|---|---|---|
| Dogs | 28 | 42 | 6/6 | 2/2 | 8/8 | 4/6 |
| Cats | 26 | 30 | 6/6 | 2/2 | 6/4* | 2/2 |
| Horses | 24 | Mare, 30-36 Male, 40-42 | 6/6 | 2/2† | 6/6 | 6/6 |
| Swine | 32 | 44 | 6/6 | 2/2 | 8/8 | 6/6 |
| Ruminants (e.g., sheep, cattle) | 20 | 32 | 0/8 | 0/0 | 6/6 | 6/6 |
| Hamsters, gerbils, rodents | | 16 | 2/2 | 0/0 | 0/0 | 6/6 |
| Guinea pigs | | 20 | 2/2 | 0/0 | 2/2 | 6/6 |
| Rabbits | | 28 | 4/2 | 0/0 | 6/4 | 6/6 |

Formulae indicated for the full jaw.
*Anatomists conclude that the first upper premolars and the lower first and second premolars are missing.
†Mares often do not have canine teeth.

## TOOTH SURFACE TERMINOLOGY

I. Crown: above the gum line
II. Root: below the gum line
III. Buccal: surface toward the cheek
IV. Lingual: surface toward the tongue
V. Labial: surface toward the lips
VI. Palatal: surface toward the soft palate
VII. Mesial: surface toward the rostral end or front of the mouth
   A. Incisor is the edge closest to the midline
VIII. Distal: surface toward the back of the tooth
IX. Rostral: surface facing the nose of the animal
X. Occlusal: chewing surface
XI. Furcation: the space between two roots where they meet the crown

## TOOTH ROOTS USING TRIADAN SYSTEM

| DOG | 1 | 1 | 1 | 1 | 1 | 2 | | 2 | 3 | 3 | | 3 | X |
|---|---|---|---|---|---|---|---|---|---|---|---|---|---|
| CAT | 1 | 1 | 1 | 1 | X | 1 (2 fused)* | | 2 | 3 | 1 (2 fused)* | | X | X |
| Right maxilla | 201 | 202 | 203 | 204 | 205 | 206 | | 207 | 208 | 209 | | 210 | 211 |
| Tooth | I | I | I | C | P | P | | P | P | M | | M | M |
| Right mandible | 301 | 302 | 303 | 304 | 305 | 306 | | 307 | 308 | 309 | | 310 | 311 |
| CAT | 1 | 1 | 1 | 1 | X | X | | 2 | 2 | 2 | | X | X |
| DOG | 1 | 1 | 1 | 1 | 1 | 2 | | 2 | 2 | 2 | | 2 | 1 |

*Usually has one root or two fused roots with a single crown.

## TOOTH FUNCTION

I. Incisors: cutting, nibbling
II. Canines: holding, tearing
III. Premolars: cutting, shearing, holding
IV. Molars: grinding
V. Carnassial teeth: largest cutting teeth
    A. Dogs: upper fourth premolars and lower first molars
    B. Cats: upper fourth premolars and lower molars

## NUMBERING TEETH

I. Anatomical system
    A. Uppercase letters: permanent teeth
    B. Lowercase letters: deciduous teeth (primary)
    C. Superscript right: upper right teeth
    D. Subscript right: lower right teeth
    E. Examples
       1. $I_2$: second permanent incisor, lower right
       2. $^1c$: primary canine, upper left
       3. $Sp^1$: supernumerary first primary premolar, upper right
II. Triadan system
    A. Uses quadrants with three-digit numbers
    B. First number indicates the quadrant in which the tooth is found and the type of tooth
    C. Permanent teeth begin with the numbers 1, 2, 3, and 4
    D. Deciduous (primary) teeth begin with the numbers 5, 6, 7, and 8

| **Upper right quadrant** | **Upper left quadrant** |
|---|---|
| 1 if permanent tooth<br>5 if deciduous tooth | 2 if permanent tooth<br>6 if deciduous tooth |
| **Lower right quadrant** | **Lower left quadrant** |
| 4 if permanent tooth<br>8 if deciduous tooth | 3 if permanent tooth<br>7 if deciduous tooth |

    E. The second and third numbers refer to the specific tooth in each quadrant, always beginning from the midline of the mouth

    F. Examples
       1. 103: upper right third permanent incisor
       2. 308: lower left last permanent premolar
    G. Cats are missing teeth 105, 205, 305, 306, 405, 406
    H. Cats

| (101-103) | 104 | (106-108) | 109 | Upper right |
|---|---|---|---|---|
| I | C | P | M | |
| (401-403) | 404 | (407-408) | 409 | Lower right |

    I. Dogs

| (101-103) | 104 | (105-108) | (109-110) | Upper right |
|---|---|---|---|---|
| I | C | P | M | |
| (401-403) | 404 | (405-408) | (409-411) | Lower right |

    J. Rule of 5 and 9
       1. First premolar will always end in a 5
       2. First molar will always end in a 9

## DENTAL INSTRUMENTS

I. Hand instruments
    A. Three parts: handle, shank, and working end
    B. Instruments are held in a modified pen grasp
    C. Use a finger rest for more stability
    D. Sickle scaler
       1. Curved or straight
       2. Is triangular and tapers to a sharp pointed tip with two parallel sharp sides
       3. Used for removing supragingival calculus and for removing calculus from pits, fissures, and interproximal areas
       4. Comes in a variety of sizes
       5. Always pull away from the gum line
    E. Curettes
       1. Have a U-shaped toe with one sharp side
       2. Used for subgingival calculus removal and root planing

3. Place the cutting edge against the tooth. The handle is held parallel to the tooth root. Pull the instrument away from the root in a series of overlapping strokes to remove the calculus until the tooth root is glassy smooth

4. Come in a variety of sizes and shapes. Two curettes used routinely are
   a. Gracey curette has the face tipped 20 to 30 degrees from the perpendicular and is area specific. Lower numbers are for incisors and canine, higher numbers are for caudal teeth
   b. Universal curette has the face perpendicular to the shank and can be used in all areas

F. Periodontal probe
   1. Has no sharp sides
   2. Used to measure the depth of the gingival sulcus
   3. Measured in millimeters with a light touch
   4. Insert the probe between the gingiva and tooth root surface, parallel to the long axis of the tooth. Walk the probe along the circumference of each tooth in at least four locations. Chart any abnormal sulcus depths
   5. Notched or color coded bands in millimeters
   6. Also comes as a Sensor Probe. The probe closes its gap once 20 grams of pressure has been reached, the pressure recommended to use to avoid trauma to the gingiva

G. Shepherd's hook or explorer
   1. Has a sharp tip only. Use a light touch to avoid gingival trauma
   2. Used to detect subgingival calculus and tooth mobility
   3. Used to detect feline external odontoclastic resorptive lesions (RLs)
   4. Used to detect cavities and broken teeth
   5. Finer tips allow greater tactile sensitivity

H. Dental elevators
   1. Serve as a wedge placed between the root and the bone to stretch and break the periodontal ligament
   2. Come in all sizes to service large and tiny spaces
   3. Must be sharp and fit the contour of the root
   4. Winged elevators are intended to wrap around the cylindrical roots
   5. Require regular sharpening
   6. Root tip picks are available for very tiny teeth and for retrieving retained root tips

I. Periosteal elevators
   1. Used to elevate and reflect gingival, mucogingival, and palatal flaps

2. Must be sharp so that they will cut rather than tear

J. Extraction forceps
   1. Come in all sizes and shapes
   2. Available with or without spring-loaded handles
   3. Have straight or angled tips
   4. Used for extractions and the removal of heavy calculus

II. Mechanical scalers
A. Ultrasonic scalers convert sound waves into mechanical vibration
   1. Magnetostrictive: tip vibrates in an elliptical motion, 18,000 to 29,000 cycles per second
      a. Use the back or sides of the distal one-sixteenth inch lightly
      b. Two types available
         (1) Flat metal strip, such as the Cavitron
         (2) Newest type is ferroceramic rod
   2. Piezoelectric: tip vibrates linearly
      a. Converts alternating current into 40,000 cycles per second through a piezoelectric crystal in the hand piece
      b. A linear tip motion is created without producing heat
      c. Vibration not evenly distributed
      d. Tip moves farther in one direction than the other
      e. Use most active side on calculus

B. Sonic: tip vibrates in an elliptical motion, up to 18,000 cycles per second
   1. Less heat buildup in these units; some units are more efficient than others
   2. Can be used subgingivally with caution

C. Mechanical scalers used for gross calculus
   1. Proper tips must be used
   2. Used lightly on the teeth to avoid heat buildup and pitting of the enamel with possible pulpal damage
   3. Maximum of 5 seconds per tooth (it depends on the unit)
   4. The scaler tip will wear with time; as it becomes shorter, its resonance frequency changes and it becomes less efficient
      a. Tips should be replaced periodically
   5. Use a lot of water to cool teeth
      a. Distilled or filtered water will prevent a mineral buildup in the tubing of the dental unit
      b. If you use a water bottle, rinse it with disinfectant, such as 0.12% chlorhexidine solution, and let the bottle air dry at the end of the day
   6. Roto-Pro burs
      a. Spin at 300,000 to 400,000 rpm

b. Used to remove tartar and calculus

c. Can easily damage the enamel, dentin, and soft tissue

7. Air-driven units

a. Basic units come with low-speed hand piece, high-speed hand piece, and a three-way air/water syringe

b. More elaborate units have piezoelectric scaler or outlet for sonic scaler, suction, fiberoptic illumination, extra electrical outlets, electrosurgical outlets, and a variety of other options

c. Air is provided by compressors or compressed gas in bulk tanks

d. Converts air into mechanical vibration

e. Compressors are either oil cooled or oil free

(1) Very quiet oil-cooled compressors are available

(2) Oil-free dental compressors tend to be noisier and more expensive

8. Unit maintenance

a. The oil level of the oil-cooled compressors must be checked weekly to ensure that the level of oil is adequate

b. The oil should be changed every 6 months

c. Prophy heads that are not self-lubricating and hand pieces should be oiled weekly and disinfected/autoclaved after each use, depending on the hand piece

d. Clean biofilm from water lines and tubing with a noncorrosive dental unit product

e. Filtration units are available to treat and purify dental water

f. Use surface barrier sleeves on parts of the dental unit that cannot be autoclaved, such as the air/water syringe, hand pieces, drills, and curing lights

III. Sharpening hand instruments

A. Sharpen after each use before sterilization

B. Use an acrylic stick to test for sharpness

C. If light reflects from the cutting edge, the instrument is dull

D. Sharpening stones vary from coarse to fine

1. Ruby stone: coarse; water lubricant

2. Arkansas stone: fine; oil lubricant

3. India stone: fine or medium; oil lubricant

4. Carborundum stone: coarse; water lubricant

5. Ceramic stone: fine or medium; water or dry lubricant

E. Sharpening guides are available from D-Sharp Dental Instruments at www.dsharp.ca

1. Consists of three lines: a center perpendicular line, and one line on either side at a 110-degree angle from the center line

2. Come as pads of disposable guides

3. For scalers and universal curettes, align the terminal shank with the vertical central line and align the stone with either of the 110-degree lines depending on the edge that is being sharpened. Using short strokes move the stone back and forth from toe to heel. Finish with a down stroke

4. For Gracey curettes, align the terminal shank with one of the 110-degree lines and align the stone with the other 110-degree line. Proceed as previously mentioned

F. Sharpening stones

1. Lubricate with water or oil, depending on the stone type

2. Available as rectangular, square, wedge, or cone shape

3. 1000 grade is a coarse grit; 4000 is a fine grit for smoother surfaces

4. Disk-honing machines are available to quickly sharpen with precision

## COMPLETE ORAL HYGIENE PROCEDURE

I. Examine the patient, beginning with the history followed by a complete physical exam

A. Look for symmetry of the head and face

B. Look for nasal or ocular discharges or swellings

C. Following anesthesia, examine lips, mouth, tongue, palates, oropharyngeal area, tonsils, floor of the mouth, and occlusion

D. For human and animal safety, chlorhexidine rinse can be used to decrease bacterial load prior to oral examination

E. Examine teeth and gums. Include dental radiographs

F. Measure the gingival sulcus all the way around each tooth

1. May be measured after cleaning

2. Normal sulcus depth for dogs, 1 to 3 mm; for cats, less than 1 mm

G. Record clinical findings on the procedure chart

H. Scale the teeth above and below the gum line

1. Use proper method and equipment as discussed previously

2. Use a finger rest to ensure fine control of the instruments

a. Standard position is with a modified pen grip

b. Place the instrument between the thumb and index finger

c. Extend the middle finger onto the terminal end of the shank and rest the third finger on an adjacent surface

d. Always pull away from the gingiva

3. Remove gross calculus with calculus removal forceps or dental extractors
   a. Avoid damaging the gingival tissue, enamel, and cementum
4. Remove supragingival calculus and plaque with a mechanical power scaler
   a. Use a light stroke with adequate water spray
   b. Use the side of the tip and begin at the edge of the calculus
   c. Use the air syringe to dry the tooth surface to reveal remaining calculus, which will appear dull and chalky against the shiny enamel
   d. Can also use a disclosing solution to reveal remaining plaque and calculus (may stain hair and clothing)
5. Remove subgingival plaque, calculus, and necrotic cementum with hand curettes
   a. Follow the contour of the tooth at a 70- to 80-degree angle. Pull away from the gingival margin
   b. Root planing may be necessary on the root surfaces
      (1) Use curettes
      (2) Closed root planing is often sufficient for shallow depths less than 5 mm
      (3) Deeper pockets will require a gingival flap for access (open root planing)
      (4) Overzealous root planing will remove cementum, which will prevent gingival and ligament reattachment
   c. Subgingival curettage is important to remove infected soft tissue from periodontal pockets
      (1) Use a curette
      (2) May require a specific periodontal incision
I. Polish to remove plaque and stain
1. Keep prophy cup moving to avoid heating the tooth, maximum 5 seconds per tooth
2. Use plenty of paste
3. Wet teeth with water to cool them
4. Use a light touch but sufficient pressure to flare the cup
5. Polish the enamel in the sulcus
6. Use a medium or fine paste
7. Set the polisher below 3000 rpm
8. Wet the teeth periodically to cool them
9. Use a soft prophy cup to minimize the pressure necessary to flare the cup
J. Flush the gingival sulcus to remove all paste and loose debris

1. Use an air/water syringe or a 20- to 60-mL syringe attached to a small intravenous catheter
2. If there is no attachment loss, use a solution of 0.12% chlorhexidine
3. Use only saline if there is attachment loss. Chlorhexidine and fluoride will interfere with reattachment
K. Wipe and air dry the teeth if using fluoride
L. Can use a disclosing solution to reveal any remaining plaque (solution may stain hair or clothing)
M. Dry teeth, apply fluoride, and leave on 1 to 4 minutes (optional). There has been no confirmed benefit of using fluoride on veterinary dental patients
1. Wipe off; water deactivates fluoride
2. Serves as an antibacterial agent
3. Desensitizes the teeth
4. Strengthens the enamel
5. Fluoride is found in some brands of prophy paste
N. Charting
1. Each hospital should select a dental charting system
2. The chart becomes part of the patient's medical file
3. Charts should depict each tooth and tooth surface
4. Charts should allow space to record calculus, caries, fractures, gingivitis index, gingivitis recession, periodontal index, mobility index, malocclusions, RLs, and oral lesions
5. Dates when dental procedures were performed, what was done, treatment, and prognosis should also be recorded
6. Accurate charting will allow for an accurate assessment at future dental appointments
O. Animal positioning
1. The animal is usually in lateral recumbency, with the head positioned downward
2. Always turn the animal sternally to avoid gastric torsion
3. To minimize the number of times required to turn the animal, include the labial surfaces, followed by the opposite palatal and lingual surfaces
   a. Then turn the animal and complete the scaling/polishing on the remaining labial, palatal, and lingual surfaces
   b. Work is completed first on one half of the mouth, the animal is turned, and then work is completed on the second half of the mouth

## SAFETY AND INFECTION CONTROL ▬▬▬

I. In animals, dentistry involves oral and environmental bacteria. Sterilization and bacterial control are essential to protect cross-contamination of patients and personnel
  A. Use sterile and well-maintained instruments and equipment
    1. At the end of every procedure, wash, rinse, and wipe off gross debris
    2. Use ultrasonic instrument bath with a detergent solution, with the lid on
    3. Use surgical milk for hinged and sharp instruments
    4. Sharpen instruments before sterilization
    5. Most dental instruments can be sterilized in an autoclave
    6. To reduce the length of time to achieve sterilization, package in autoclave film or envelopes
    7. Can also use autoclavable instrument trays
    8. For equipment that is not autoclavable, use disposable, plastic infection barriers such as tray sleeves
    9. Most air driven hand pieces can be autoclaved
    10. Disposable items, such as prophy cups, should be disposed after each use. They cannot be adequately decontaminated
    11. Note: read the manufacturer's recommendations for sterilization procedures
    12. Keep the lid on bulk pots of prophy paste to avoid airborne contamination. Use small amounts as required
    13. Empty the water from the water bottle at the end of each day, and rinse it at least twice weekly with disinfectant
    14. Can use 0.1% to 0.2% chlorhexidine mixed with the water to give a 0.12% solution (60 mL 2% chlorhexidine in 1 L water). Chlorhexidine bonds to the teeth, so it must be polished off before applying restoratives or fluoride
    15. Flush all lines with disinfectant, rinse with distilled water, and air dry the lines
    16. Handpieces should be washed and lubricated regularly
  B. Use an appropriately sized mouth gag to avoid problems in the temporomandibular joints. Ensure that the teeth contact rubber/plastic inserts and not metal. Mouth props are also available and are autoclavable
  C. Use a cuffed endotracheal tube
  D. Place gauze sponges in the back of the throat as a protection against excessive water and debris. Replace them when they become wet and ensure that all gauze squares are accounted for
  E. Keep the patient's head downward
  F. Cover the patient's eyes
  G. Roll the patient with the sternum under, especially in large breed dogs
  H. Maintain the patient's body temperature to prevent hypothermia. The oral cavity is highly vascular. Cooling takes place quickly

II. Human safety
  A. Wear a surgical mask, glasses, and gloves to protect against oral bacteria. Anything within 4 feet of a scaler will be contaminated
  B. May help to spray the patient's mouth with 0.12% chlorhexidine to reduce the bacterial load
  C. Work comfortably while seated on a stool with a backrest at a proper height, and follow proper ergonomic procedures to minimize fatigue and muscle strain
  D. The patient's mouth should be at elbow height so the hands can be level with the elbow
  E. Hands and elbows should be well below shoulder level to maintain relaxed shoulders and to avoid neck fatigue
  F. Avoid hunching the back and twisting the neck. Vary finger movements
  G. Support the working hand on a surface in the same quadrant you are working in
  H. Use adequate light source, such as one worn on the head
  I. Do strengthening exercises
  J. The most common injury for dental workers is carpal tunnel syndrome

## DENTAL RADIOGRAPHY ▬▬▬

I. Purpose
  A. Ascertain condition of teeth and gingival sulcus
  B. Identify cavities and RLs
  C. Identify retained roots
  D. Identify bone and root system of the teeth
  E. Help evaluate intraoral neoplasia
  F. Identify number of teeth in the mouth
  G. Identify periapical abscesses

II. Recommendations
  A. Obtain routine dental radiographs in young animals to identify the permanent dentition
  B. In the treatment of periodontal disease, obtain radiographs every 12 to 24 months
  C. Use radiographs before extractions to determine condition of the roots and number of teeth and roots involved. Follow up with a radiograph to document that there are no retained roots or fragments
  D. Perform radiography during endodontic procedures to confirm the procedure

E. Obtain radiographs as follow-up to root canal procedure to check the file depth

F. Radiograph chipped teeth with pulp exposure to determine how much dentin is protecting the pulp

G. Radiograph fractured teeth with pulp exposure to assess the periapical disease

H. Radiograph every tooth in patients with a history of RLs

III. Equipment

A. Intraoral film for detail

1. Comes in a variety of sizes; common sizes used in dogs and cats are 0, 2, and 4
   a. Size 0 works well in cats
   b. Size 2 works well in dogs and cats
   c. Size 4 is necessary in dogs to radiograph the incisors and canines
      (1) Called occlusal film
   d. Size 2 is the least expensive because it is the size used routinely in human dentistry and therefore is produced in quantity
2. Available in D (Ultra-speed), E (Ektaspeed), and F (Insight) speeds
   a. Insight is a fast film with good image clarity but costs more

B. Chairside darkroom will free up the main dark room

1. Rapid processing solutions
2. Purchase dental film clips
3. Can use regular bulk tanks
4. Automatic processors are available

C. Dental x-ray machine with a lead-lined cone will achieve greater detail and versatility

1. Digital dental x-ray machines are available

D. Protective shielding, film-holding devices, finger-ring dosimeter badges

IV. Positioning

A. Routine dental survey of six films

V. Techniques

A. If possible, use

1. Twelve-inch source image distance (SID) for dental films and 30 inches for standard screens
2. Nonscreen film, which gives high detail
3. Small focal spot
4. Collimate as much as possible

B. Parallel technique (Figure 26-2)

1. For mandibular molars and premolars
2. Place the dental film parallel to the end of the x-ray tube and the long axis of the tooth
3. The central ray will be perpendicular to the teeth and the film
4. Place folded gauze between the top edge of the film and the occlusal surfaces of the teeth to securely push the film down into the bottom of the mouth

C. Bisecting angle (Figure 26-3)

1. Place the film inside the animal's mouth behind the affected tooth
2. Direct the central ray perpendicular to the line that bisects the angle formed by the film and the long axis of the tooth
3. This technique will reduce the artifact of foreshortening or elongation
   a. Foreshortening makes the tooth appear shorter than it is
      (1) Occurs when the x-ray beam is more perpendicular to the film
   b. Elongation makes the tooth appear much longer
      (1) Occurs when the x-ray beam is more perpendicular to the tooth axis
4. Can be used for intraoral and extraoral films
5. Can apply the tube shift technique to better visualize such structures as the three roots of the upper fourth premolar
   a. The lateral view will superimpose the two mesial roots
   b. Use the SLOB rule to separate the two mesial roots

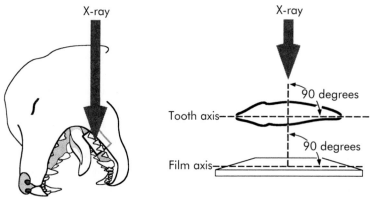

**Figure 26-2** Parallel position technique for dental radiographs of the mandibular premolar teeth. (From Harvey CE, Emily PE: *Small animal dentistry*, St Louis, 2001, Mosby.)

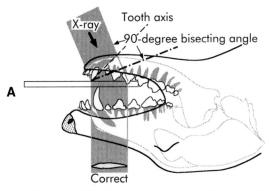
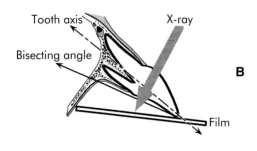

**Figure 26-3** Bisecting angle technique for dental radiographs. **A,** Lower canine tooth. **B,** Carnassial tooth. (From Harvey CE, Emily PE: *Small animal dentistry*, St Louis, 2001, Mosby.)

(1) Acronym means *s*ame, *l*ingual; *o*pposite, *b*uccal

c. Objects (e.g., roots) that are lingual to a reference point will appear to shift in the same direction in which the tube head has been moved

d. Objects that seem to move in the opposite direction to the tube head will be on the buccal side

e. Move the tube head back toward the ear so that the beam is directed obliquely from distal to mesial. The palatal root will appear to move back toward the ear. The buccal root will appear to move toward the nose

f. The root that seems to shift in the same direction as the tube head is on the palatal side, and the root that moves in the opposite direction is on the buccal side

| Quadrant and teeth | No. of films | Technique | Position |
|---|---|---|---|
| Mandibular canines and incisors | 1 | Bisecting angle | Dorsal or lateral |
| Mandibular premolars and molars | 2 | Parallel lateral oblique | Dorsal |
| Maxillary canines | 1 each | Bisecting angle | Lateral or rostro-caudal oblique |
| Maxillary incisors | 1 | Bisecting angle | Sternal or lateral |
| Maxillary premolars and molars | 2 | Bisecting angle | Sternal or lateral |
| | | | Rostrocaudal or caudo-rostral oblique |

## HOME CARE

I. Goal: to control plaque and tartar buildup. Should begin following a recent and thorough oral exam. Home care can cause pain if dental problems exist

  A. Genetics plays a major role in determining dental disease. Not all pets require home care due to natural resistance

  B. Other factors include diet, chewing habits, health status, and shape of mouth

  C. Daily brushing with a soft bristle brush using veterinary products. The mechanical action of the brushing is the most significant factor

II. May involve use of antibacterial and fluoride products

III. Feed hard food and other products that do not stick to the teeth. Feeding large pieces of raw vegetable or cooked fibrous meat at least twice weekly will remove some plaque

IV. Use chew toys to provide an abrasive action, to strengthen the periodontal ligaments, and to increase crevicular flushing

  A. Use toys that are softer than the teeth to avoid fractures and chronic trauma

  B. Do not feed dried hooves, which may cause slab fractures

  C. Nylon chew bones can cause slab fractures

  D. Nylon rope toys should be avoided, because they can cause gingival trauma when the fine nylon threads slice the gingiva

  E. Dense rubber toys are safer and work the jaw bones well

  F. Rawhide strips reduce plaque and calculus and are unlikely to cause fractures

    1. They absorb saliva, become mushy, and are squished between the teeth to remove debris

    2. If swallowed in small pieces, they are digestible

V. Chemical plaque control agents reduce or retard plaque but do not stop it from forming

VI. The Veterinary Oral Health Council (VOHC) issues their registered seal on products that meet their standards for effectiveness in retarding plaque and tartar when used as directed
   A. Recognized world wide
   B. Publishes a list of acceptable products at www. vohc.org

## OCCLUSION

I. Normal occlusion
   A. Scissor bite
   B. The upper incisors close just in front of the lower incisors
   C. The lower canines lie between the upper incisors and canines without touching either
   D. The lower first premolars are the most rostral, with the upper arcade fitting into the spaces between the lower premolars and forming a zigzag pattern
   E. The upper fourth premolars overlap the lower first molars, forming the carnassial teeth in dogs
   F. In cats the upper third and fourth premolars tightly overlap the lower fourth premolars, as well as the first molars. The upper fourth premolars and lower molars are the feline carnassial teeth
   G. Well proportioned skull width and maxillary length is referred to as mesaticephalic
II. Malocclusions
   A. Class I malocclusion
      1. Maxillary and mandible correctly proportioned, but one or more teeth are misaligned
      2. Known as neutroclusion
      3. Examples of Class I malocclusion
         a. Anterior crossbite
            (1) One or more of the maxillary incisors displaced so they are lingual to mandibular incisors
         b. Posterior crossbite
            (1) Mandible is wider than the maxilla in the area of the premolars
            (2) One or more of the premolar or molar teeth is displaced
            (3) Occurs occasionally in boxers and long nosed breeds
         c. Base narrow canines
            (1) The mandibular canines are lingually displaced
            (2) Can cause trauma to palatal tissue
      4. All three Class I malocclusions can be part of Class II and III malocclusions
   B. Class II malocclusion
      1. Referred to as distoclusion
      2. Teeth in mandible are distal to maxillary equivalents

3. Can be an abnormally short mandible or abnormally long maxilla
4. Has been referred to as brachygnathism, overshot jaw, or parrot mouth
   a. Often not possible to identify which jaw is abnormal
   b. *Brachygnathic* means the mandible is shorter than the maxilla
5. More likely to occur in dolichocephalic breeds with narrow skull and long maxilla (Collies)
   C. Class III malocclusion
      1. Referred to as mesioclusion
      2. Mandibular teeth occlude mesial to maxillary equivalent
      3. Can be due to abnormally short maxilla or long mandible
      4. Has been referred to as prognathism or undershot jaw
      5. Often not possible to identify which jaw is abnormal
      6. Prognathic means the mandible is longer than maxilla
      7. Normal for brachycephalic breeds
         a. These breeds have wide skulls with a short maxilla
      8. Often associated with anterior crossbite
   D. Other malocclusion abnormalities
      1. Level bite
         a. End-to-end bite of the incisors
         b. Genetically a degree of prognathism
      2. Wry mouth
         a. Genetically affects only one quadrant of the mandible or maxilla
         b. One segment of the jaw is disproportionately sized relative to the other half
      3. Oligodontia
         a. Fewer teeth than normal
      4. Anodontia
         a. Missing teeth
      5. Polydontia
         a. More teeth than normal
      6. Abnormal dental interlock
         a. Deciduous teeth that erupt in an abnormal pattern
         b. The upper deciduous canine teeth are pushed rostral to the lower canine teeth, which prevents the forward growth of the mandible
         c. Occurs in Class II malocclusion and base-narrow malocclusion by impeding growth of the mandible
      7. Retained deciduous teeth
         a. Permanent teeth erupt lingually to the deciduous teeth (except the upper canine teeth)
         b. Common in toy breed dogs

## ORAL LESIONS ▬▬▬▬▬▬▬

I. Malignant tumors
  A. Melanoma
    1. Most common in dogs; rare in cats; poor prognosis
    2. Spreads early to regional lymph nodes, bone, or lungs
  B. Squamous cell carcinoma
    1. Second most common tumor in dogs; most common in cats
    2. Spreads slowly, invades bone
    3. May affect lips but more commonly affects tissues within the oral cavity
  C. Fibrosarcoma
    1. Third most common tumor in dogs
    2. Metastasizes slowly but is aggressively invasive, requiring wide surgical resection
    3. Guarded prognosis
  D. Osteosarcoma
    1. May affect bones of mandible or maxilla
    2. Oral osteosarcoma spreads slower than the appendicular version, so it is more responsive to surgery
II. Nonmalignant tumors
  A. Epulis (an oral mass)
    1. Requires biopsy to differentiate
    2. Classified as peripheral odontogenic fibromas or peripheral acanthomatous ameloblastoma
      a. Peripheral odontogenic fibroma is benign, not very locally invasive, rough surfaced, and protrudes from the gingiva
        (1) Grows from the periodontal ligament
        (2) Also known as fibromatous epulis
      b. Peripheral acanthomatous ameloblastoma is benign, with a rough surface of an even yellow-pink color, more locally invasive, requiring aggressive surgical resection. Arises from periodontal tissue subgingivally
    3. Involves the periodontal ligament
    4. Can be locally invasive to bone
III. Gingival hyperplasia
  A. Thickening of gingiva as a result of chronic inflammation
  B. Most commonly seen in Boxers. Also in Huskies and Collies. Also affects large breeds, such as Wolfhounds and Saint Bernards
  C. Gingiva grows to engulf crowns. Traps food, hair, debris, and bacteria
IV. Stomatitis
  A. Inflammation of soft tissue of the oral cavity
  B. Can be caused by foreign bodies or chemical or electrical burns, or can be immune related

V. Contact ulcers
  A. Lesions caused when a tooth makes contact with the mucosa
VI. Eosinophilic ulcers
  A. Rodent ulcers that occur on the lip of cats; benign

## FURTHER DENTAL PROBLEMS ▬▬▬▬▬

I. Gemini
  A. One root with two crowns
II. Fusion
  A. Two tooth buds grow together to form one larger tooth
III. Enamel hypoplasia
  A. Known as distemper teeth, where sections of enamel are reduced or missing
IV. Misdirected teeth
  A. Teeth that erupt in an abnormal direction
V. Retained deciduous
  A. Retained primary teeth
VI. Tetracycline staining
  A. Yellow stain due to the administration of tetracycline to a pregnant dog or to young pups
VII. Impaction
  A. The inability of the tooth to erupt through the gum
VIII. Abscessed teeth
  A. Advanced periodontal disease may result in root abscesses
  B. Most commonly seen abscessed tooth in dogs is the upper fourth premolar
IX. Oronasal fistula
  A. Caused by an abscess of the maxillary canine; can show clinical signs of nasal discharge and/or swelling over the root
X. Caries
  A. True coronal caries not a common problem in carnivores compared with humans
  B. If present, caries are often multiple advanced lesions affecting several teeth
  C. Upper first and second molars and lower first molar are most commonly affected
  D. Classified by location as pit and fissure, smooth surface, or root surface
XI. Worn teeth
  A. Exhibit a brown center but does not allow access by an explorer
  B. Odontoblasts are stimulated to produce tertiary dentin, which will protect the tooth if the rate of wear is gradual
XII. Trauma
  A. Caused by chewing hard objects or by blows to the head
  B. Crown fracture with pulp exposure
    1. Will always become inflamed causing irreversible pulpitis

2. Patient feels stabbing pain until the pulp dies
3. Pulp chamber will fill with necrotic soft tissue and bacteria, causing chronic periapical periodontitis, which is very painful
4. Requires endodontic treatment or extraction

C. Chip fracture
   1. Exposes dentin, but still has a thick layer protecting the pulp
   2. Can cause sensitivity
   3. May require coating with a dentin bonding agent or no treatment, depending on the thickness of the dentin layer

## PERIODONTAL DISEASE

I. Causes of periodontal disease
   A. Lack of daily dental care, genetics, and physical factors
   B. Accumulation of plaque, which is composed of bacteria, saliva, epithelial cells, leukocytes, macrophages, and water
   C. Formation of calculus, which is mineralized plaque
      1. Plaque can form within 6 hours
      2. Plaque can mineralize within 24 to 48 hours to form a brown or yellow calculus around the teeth
      3. Plaque is a biofilm of bacteria, saliva, and debris. It is a glycoprotein component of saliva, known as the acquired pellicle, that attaches to the tooth surface
      4. The pellicle takes only 20 minutes to form. Bacteria attaches to the pellicle. The bacteria then absorbs calcium from saliva and calcifies into calculus
      5. Bacterial endotoxins are released that damage the gingival tissue and cause the animal's immune system to react
   D. Systemic factors, such as hormonal changes, play a secondary role by exaggerating the tissue response
   E. 80% of dogs and cats demonstrate some degree of periodontal disease by 4 years of age

II. Gingivitis
   A. Inflammation of the gingiva caused by plaque
   B. If treated properly, gingivitis is entirely reversible
   C. If not treated it will advance to periodontal disease
   D. Nonmotile, aerobic, gram-positive rods and cocci predominate
   E. Gingivitis index: designates the degree of inflammation
      1. GI0: normal, healthy gingiva; shrimp colored; normal gingival sulcus depth; no odor
      2. GI1: marginal gingivitis, mild inflammation, slight edema, no bleeding on probing, no increase in gingival sulcus depth
      3. GI2: moderate gingivitis, increased hyperemia, edema, bleeds on gentle probing, normal sulcar depth
      4. GI3: advanced gingivitis, inflammation, edema, hyperemia, tendency to bleed spontaneously, may have attachment loss

III. Periodontitis
   A. Inflammation of the supporting structures of the teeth, the periodontal ligament, alveolar bone, and cementum
   B. Further progression and destruction of the periodontium caused by bacteria in plaque
   C. Progressive, usually nonregenerative and incurable. If treated properly can be managed
   D. Bacterial flora changes to motile, anaerobic, gram-negative rods and filamentous organisms that produce endotoxins and exotoxins; very resistant to antibiotics and chemical oral rinses
      1. BPAB (black pigmenting anaerobic bacteria) found in periodontal pockets of dogs and cats
         a. Known as *Porphyromonas gulae, P. denticanis*, and *P. salivosa*
         b. Pfizer manufactures a monovalent companion animal periodontal disease vaccine against BPAB
   E. Periodontal index: amount of periodontal attachment loss as a percentage of the periodontal support that has been destroyed by the disease
      1. Measured with a periodontal probe in millimeters from the CEJ to apex of the defect
      2. PI0: healthy gingiva, deeper structures, no clinical disease
      3. PI1: gingivitis only with no attachment loss
      4. PI2: less than 25% attachment loss
      5. PI3: 25% to 50% attachment loss
      6. PI4: greater than 50% attachment loss
   F. Mobility index helps to assess the prognosis for a tooth
      1. M0: no tooth mobility
      2. M1: slight mobility, less than 1 mm laterally with no apical mobility
      3. M2: moderate tooth mobility, 1 to 2 mm laterally, no apical mobility
      4. M3: both lateral and apical mobility, requires extraction
   G. Gingival recession is estimated by measuring from the CEJ to the current free gingival margin and then adding 1 to 2 millimeters to account for the normal free gingival margin coronal to the CEJ
   H. Furcation index records the degree of exposure of the furcation of a multirooted tooth
      1. F1 furcation can be probed, but there is no evidence of bone loss

   2. F2 furcation allows a probe to detect it. There is reduced bone density

   3. F3 furcation allows a probe to penetrate all the way through because of bone loss

   4. F4 furcation is entirely visible

IV. Classification of gingival disease

  A. Gingivitis index

   1. As above

  B. Periodontal index

   1. Criteria described above

   2. As the disease advances, pockets become deeper, pus forms, and the tooth becomes mobile

   3. Gram-positive aerobic cocci and rods change to anaerobic gram-negative rods

V. Treatment

  A. Depends on disease classification and discretion of the veterinarian

   1. Thoroughly scale and polish the teeth and take radiographs

   2. Root planing and gingival curettage

   3. Antibiotics and chemical plaque control agents

   4. Possible gingival surgery

   5. Possible tooth extraction and wound closure

   6. Home care

   7. Dry food

   8. Chew toys

   9. Reevaluate every 3 to 12 months

## RESORPTIVE LESIONS

I. Also called feline cervical neck lesions, neck lesions, enamel erosions, and feline odontoclastic RLs

II. Etiology involves many facets, including

  A. Nutritional hyperparathyroidism leading to resorption of calcium

   1. Has since been proven groundless

  B. Chronic calicivirus has not been a consistent finding

  C. Viral infection at the time of tooth development

  D. Chronic hair balls

  E. Low-pH diets causing a chronic acidic environment

   1. No evidence to support this

   2. Genetics: higher incidence in Persians, Abyssinians, Siamese, Russian blue, Scottish fold, and Oriental shorthairs

  F. Hypervitaminosis D

   1. Many canned cat foods contain excess vitamin D. Studies have indicated that excess vitamin D causes changes similar to RLs

III. Periodontal disease is the most consistent factor associated with neck lesions

IV. Usually starts at CEJ

V. Not the result of bacterial digestion of teeth, such as in human caries

VI. Lesions are filled with granulation tissue high in odontoclasts that actively resorb dentin and enamel

VII. Lesions spread in all directions

  A. Once it reaches the pulp, it spreads quickly

  B. The crown may look normal, but the tooth may have very little or no root left

VIII. Neck lesions create excruciating pain

IX. Advanced lesions require extraction

X. Teeth with resorptive lesions require extraction

XI. Graded from class I to V (the most advanced)

XII. Two distinct types of RLs

  A. Type I lesions are less common and typically start at the CEJ

  B. Type II lesions arise at any location on the root and are associated with extensive root resorption, loss of periodontal ligament, and ankylosis

## LYMPHOCYTIC/PLASMACYTIC STOMATITIS

I. Seen commonly in cats; very painful

II. Very inflamed gums, often with minor calculus accumulation

III. Many cats have underlying disease that interferes with cat's local immunity in the gingiva

IV. Cats should be screened for diseases, such as feline leukemia virus (FeLV), feline immunodeficiency virus (FIV), and feline infectious peritonitis (FIP)

  A. Can be associated with disorders of the circulation, such as diabetes mellitus and immune disorders

V. Complete intolerance to dental plaque

VI. Higher incidence in highly bred cats, such as Siamese, Himalayans, and Abyssinians

VII. Thoroughly clean teeth, treat with antibiotics and oral antiseptics, brush daily with antibacterial solution, maintain hard diet, and recheck monthly

VIII. If the condition recurs, extract all premolars, molars, and retained roots

  A. Clean canines and incisors

  B. If problem still recurs, remove the remaining teeth

## LAGOMORPHS AND RODENTS

I. Most problems are related to anatomical peculiarities of their dentition and poor husbandry

II. Two basic types of teeth

  A. Brachyodont

   1. Short crown to root ratio with a true root

   2. No potential for further tooth growth once matured

B. Hypsodont
1. Long crown, short root
2. Either radicular or aradicular
3. Radicular hypsodont grows for most of the animal's life until the root apex closes late in life
4. Horses and ruminants have radicular hypsodont teeth
5. Aradicular hypsodont never forms a true root and grows continuously
6. Rabbits, guinea pigs, and chinchillas have aradicular hypsodont teeth
7. Incisors of all rodents are aradicular hypsodont, whereas the cheek teeth can be either radicular or aradicular, depending on the species

III. Lagomorphs (rabbits) do not have canine teeth
IV. Rabbits do not gnaw like rodents (unless a cheek tooth poses a problem)
V. Tooth overgrowth is the most common dental problem and is usually caused by feeding a nonabrasive diet in lagomorphs or by lack of gnawing material in rodents
VI. In guinea pigs, cheek tooth overgrowth is associated with vitamin C deficiency. Overgrowth has also been linked to excessive selenium
VII. Nail clippers should not be used to shorten overgrown incisors because they shatter the teeth, which causes a fracture to extend subgingivally. Burs, rasps, and files can be used
VIII. Tooth trimming should be performed under anesthesia to allow a good examination of the cheek teeth
IX. Gingivitis in the front of the mouth is caused by rough edges on watering devices and food bowls
X. Periodontal disease is generally found in the cheek teeth
XI. Tooth caries are generally found in the cheek teeth of rodents with brachyodont teeth
XII. Caries and root resorption have been described in chinchillas

# Glossary

**acanthomatous** Pertaining to a benign tumor of the gingiva

**alveolar bone** Cancellous bone adjacent to tooth roots

**alveolus** Socket within bone in which a tooth is normally located

**ameloblast** Enamel-producing cells

**ameloblastoma** A tumor of the jaw arising from enamel-forming cells, ameloblasts

**ankylosis** Fusion of cementum and alveolar bone and obliteration of the periodontal ligament

**anodontia** Absence of teeth

**apex** Bottom of the root

**apical** Toward the apex

**attached gingiva** Gingiva from the free gingival groove to the mucogingival line

**brachygnathism** The maxilla is too long in relation to the mandible—overshot jaw

**buccal** Tooth surface nearest the cheek

**calculus** Mineralized plaque

**canine tooth** Large single-rooted tooth used to grasp and tear

**caries** Cavities

**carnassial tooth** Upper fourth premolar and lower first molar used to shear

**caudorostral oblique** Tube head of x-ray machine is at the back of the head and aimed toward the nose at about 45-degree angle from the lateral position

**cementoblasts** Cells that form cementum

**cementoenamel junction (CEJ)** Where the enamel meets the cementum

**cementum** Bony tissue covering the dentin of the root

**collagen** Produced by fibroblasts; found in gingiva and cementum

**coronal** Toward the crown

**crevicular fluid** Secreted from the gingiva

**crown** Portion of the tooth covered by enamel

**cusp** Tip of the crown

**deciduous teeth** Baby or primary teeth

**dental quadrant** Half of an arch when divided by the midline

**dentin** Bulk of the tooth covered by cementum in the root and enamel in the crown

**diphyodonts** Two sets of teeth as possessed by mammals: deciduous and permanent teeth

**distal** Away from the midline

**enamel** Hydroxyapatite covering of the crown

**endodontic** Pertains to tissue within a tooth. Endodontics is the study and the treatment of the tissue within the tooth and the periapical tissues. Also known as root canal therapy

**epulis** Fibrous tumor of the gum

**erosion** Loss of tooth structure by chemical means not involving bacteria

**exodontia** Extraction of the teeth

**fibroma** A fibrous, encapsulated, connective tissue tumor, irregular in shape and slow growing

**fibroplasia** Development of fibrous tissue

**free gingiva** Portion of gingiva not attached to the tooth

**free gingival margin** Free edge of the gingiva on the tooth

**furcation** Space between two roots where they join the crown

**gingiva** Connective tissue surrounding the teeth

**gingival hyperplasia** Proliferation of the gingiva

**gingival sulcus** Space between the free gingiva and the tooth

**hydroxyapatite** Inorganic crystals found in enamel and cementum

**hyperemia** Excess bleeding

**incisal** Biting surface of the anterior teeth

**interdental** Area between the proximal surfaces of adjacent teeth in the same arch

**labial** Surface of the incisors nearest the lips

**lamina dura** Wall of alveolar tooth socket that is radiographically seen as a thin white line

**lingual** Surface of the mandibular teeth nearest the tongue

**malocclusion** Deviation from the normal bite

**mandible** Bone of the lower jaw

**maxilla** Bone of the upper jaw

**mesial** Toward the midline of the dental arch; can also be the surface or edge of the tooth closest to the rostral end (front of the mouth)

**mesocephalic** Another term for mesaticephalic, which is a well-proportioned skull width and maxillary length

**molar** Large multicusped tooth used for grinding

**mucogingival line** Line where the gingiva meets the alveolar mucosa

**neck** Cementoenamel junction

**occlusal** Chewing surface of the posterior teeth

**odontoblasts** Cell in the pulp that produces dentin

**oligodontia** Fewer teeth than normal

**oronasal fistula** Abnormal opening between the nasal and oral cavities

**orthodontics** Refers to the correction and prevention of malocclusions of the teeth

**palatal** Surface of the maxillary teeth nearest the palate

**palate** Structure separating the oral and nasal cavities

**pellicle** Amorphous coating of salivary proteins and glycoproteins attached to exposed tooth surfaces

**periapical abscess** Abscess at the apex of the tooth

**periodontal ligament** Network of fibers connecting the tooth to the bone

**periodontium** Supporting structures of the teeth

**plaque** Thin film covering the teeth; composed of bacteria, saliva, food, and epithelial cells

**premolars** Teeth between the canines and the molars used for shearing

**primary teeth** First teeth to erupt

**prognathism** The mandible is too long relative to the maxilla—undershot jaw

**proximal** Surface of the tooth adjacent to another tooth

**pulp** Soft tissue inside the tooth; composed of blood vessels, nerves, lymphatics, and connective tissue

**pulpitis** Inflammation of the pulp; may be caused by thermal, chemical, infective, or traumatic insults

**radicular** Pertaining to the tissues on or around a tooth root

**resorption** Loss of substance by a physiological or pathological process

**restorative dentistry** Use of caps or prosthetic crowns on the teeth

**root** Part of the tooth covered by cementum

**root canal** Part of the tooth containing the pulp

**root planing** Scaling of the tooth root

**rostral** Toward the nose of the animal

**rostrocaudal oblique** Tube head is at the nose and aimed towards the back of the head at about a 45-degree angle from the lateral position

**saliva** Secretions from the salivary glands, containing enzymes

**Sharpey's fibers** Terminal portions of collagen fibers of the periodontal ligament

**stomatitis** Inflammation of the soft tissues of the mouth

**subgingival curettage** Removal of plaque and calculus from the gingiva below the gum line

**temporomandibular joint (TMJ)** A joint composed of the condylar process of the vertical ramus of the mandible and the mandibular fossa of the temporal bone of the skull

**tertiary dentin** Formed as a result of injury or irritation to the pulp; reparative dentin

# Review Questions

**1** The normal depth of the gingival sulcus in a dog is
   a. 0.5 to 1 mm
   b. 1 to 2 mm
   c. 1 to 3 mm
   d. 4 to 6 mm

**2** The most common oral malignant tumor in cats is
   a. Melanoma
   b. Fibrosarcoma
   c. Squamous cell carcinoma
   d. Osteosarcoma

**3** The teeth that are radiographed using standard parallel technique are the
   a. Maxillary incisors
   b. Mandibular canines
   c. Maxillary premolars
   d. Mandibular molars

**4** The third premolar in the upper left quadrant is
   a. 203
   b. 207
   c. 107
   d. 307

**5** The recommended speed (rpm) for the polisher is
   a. 1000
   b. 3000
   c. 5000
   d. 300,000

**6** Sharpey's fibers connect the
   a. Gingiva to the cementum
   b. Tooth to the alveolar bone
   c. Cementum to the enamel
   d. Dentin to the enamel

**7** A new theory regarding the cause of resorptive lesions in cats is the prevalence of
   a. Hypervitaminosis D
   b. Hyperparathyroidism
   c. Calicivirus
   d. A low pH diet

**8** Type II resorptive lesions arise
   a. At the CEJ
   b. At any location on the root
   c. On the crown
   d. In the pits of the molars

**9** The lubricant to use on an Arkansas stone is
   a. Water
   b. Oil
   c. Silicone
   d. None required

**10** Bacterial contamination from a power dental scaler will reach distances of
   a. 4 feet
   b. 5 feet
   c. 6 feet
   d. 8 feet

## BIBLIOGRAPHY

Bellows J: *Home study course*, Venice, Fla, 1995, American Society of Veterinary Dental Technicians.

Burns S: *It's about time: longer life for dental instruments*, Chicago, 1995, Hu-Friedy.

Emily P, Penman S: *Handbook of small animal dentistry*, Toronto, 1993, Pergamon Press.

Gorrel C, Derbyshire S: *Veterinary dentistry for the nurse and technician*, Edinburgh, 2005, Butterworth-Heinemann.

Hale F: *Understanding veterinary dentistry*, Guelph, Ontario, 2004, Author.

Harvey CE: *Small animal dentistry*, St Louis, 1993, Mosby.

Holmstrom S: *Veterinary dentistry for the technician and office staff*, Philadelphia, 2000, Saunders.

Miller B, Harvey C: Sharpening of dental instruments, *Vet Tech* 15:29, 1994.

Piasentin W: Techniques of veterinary dental radiography, *Vet Tech* 17:419, 1996.

## CHAPTER 27

# Emergency Medicine

*Sally R. Powell   Elisa A. Petrollini*

## OUTLINE

Cardiopulmonary Cerebral
  Resuscitation
Triage
Systemic Approach to Triage
  Respiratory System
  Cardiovascular System
  Central Nervous System

Renal System
  Life-Threatening Wounds
Monitoring Status of Emergency
  Patients
  Respiratory System
  Cardiovascular System
  Central Nervous System

Renal System
Endocrine and Metabolic
  Emergencies
Gastrointestinal Emergencies
Reproductive System Emergencies
Toxic Substance Emergencies
Ocular Emergencies

## LEARNING OUTCOMES

After reading this chapter you should be able to:

1. Describe triage and the guidelines for executing triage.
2. Describe how to monitor respiratory, cardiovascular, renal, and neurological status of the emergency patient.
3. Describe the clinical signs, treatment, and monitoring of patients with respiratory, cardiovascular, central nervous system, renal, and reproductive system emergencies.
4. Describe emergencies caused by the ingestion of toxic substances by defining the clinical signs and treatment.
5. Describe cardiopulmonary cerebral resuscitation (CPCR).
6. List equipment and supplies that may be needed to perform first aid and CPCR.

Clinical evaluation of the emergency patient should initially focus on four major organ systems: respiratory, cardiovascular, central nervous, and renal. It is essential for the veterinary technician to understand how to rapidly evaluate each system to provide emergency care and monitor the critically ill patient. This chapter describes cardiopulmonary cerebral resuscitation (CPCR) and first aid and discusses guidelines for triage (initial evaluation). It also outlines in chart form the common disease processes that affect the four major organ systems, including clinical signs, initial treatment, and parameters that should be monitored.

## CARDIOPULMONARY CEREBRAL RESUSCITATION

CPCR can be performed only by a team, and therefore the first step should always be to alert the veterinarian and other technicians of an emergency situation involving cardiac arrest.

I. A common memory cue for the steps to perform CPCR is ABCD

    A Airway      C Cardiac

    B Breathing   D Drugs

  A. Airway

    1. Establish and secure a patent airway

      a. Endotracheal intubation

      b. Tracheostomy if unable to intubate

  B. Breathing

    1. Resuscitation bag connected to oxygen supply or anesthesia machine, 30 to 60 breaths per minute

      a. Maximum of 20 cm of $H_2O$ pressure for dog (if using anesthesia machine)

b. Maximum of 15 cm of $H_2O$ pressure for cat (if using anesthesia machine)
2. Mouth to endotracheal tube if there is no oxygen supply
3. Mouth to muzzle if needed
C. Cardiac/Circulation
1. Continuous electrocardiographic monitoring
2. Chest compressions (external cardiac massage)
   a. Animal should be in right lateral recumbency; exceptions are cats and large, round-chested dogs
      (1) Cats should be in dorsal recumbency
      (2) Large, round-chested dogs should be in right lateral or dorsal recumbency
   b. Count four to six rib spaces or use point of the elbow to locate the heart
   c. Using two hands in large dogs, press down on the chest with heal of the lower hand
      (1) For cats and small dogs, squeezing the chest between the index finger and thumb is adequate
      (2) Compress the chest for 1 second and release for 1 second
      (3) A ventilation rate of 1 ventilation to 1 chest compression is recommended
3. Volume replacement
   a. Isotonic crystalloids
   b. Blood components
   c. Synthetic colloids
D. Drugs
1. Intravenous access
2. Intravenous drugs
   a. Atropine sulfate: increases heart rate
   b. Epinephrine: increases heart rate and force of contraction
   c. Lidocaine: used in occasional arrest situations as an antiarrhythmic
   d. Sodium bicarbonate: used in occasional arrest situations to correct metabolic acidosis
3. Intratracheal drugs
   a. When venous access cannot be obtained immediately, the following drugs should be administered via endotracheal tube
      (1) Using a syringe, inject the drug down the tube and forcefully blow air through the tube
      (2) Epinephrine
      (3) Atropine
4. Intracardiac drugs
   a. To be used only as a last resort: this route is not recommended
   b. Use lower dose of drug, place needle in the area where the heart would be

anatomically, aspirate and check for blood, and administer drug
   c. Epinephrine
   d. Isoproterenol
II. Hints for successful CPCR
A. An arrest station or special area to conduct CPCR is ideal; however, many practices have crash carts so that all necessary supplies are readily available
B. Necessary supplies include
1. Oxygen
   a. S-bag or anesthesia machine
2. Crash cart or emergency kit
   a. Endotracheal tubes
   b. Laryngoscope
   c. Intravenous catheters, fluids, administration sets, tape, syringes, needles, tourniquet
      (1) Venous cutdown supplies: scalpel blades, catheter introducers, suture material
   d. Drugs; do not predraw drugs into syringes. Many drugs are sensitive to light and plastic. Have syringes and drug labels available in arrest drugs drawer
   e. Chart of dose rates for all drugs in the kit
   f. Clippers
   g. Electrocardiographic monitor
   h. Defibrillator
   i. Suction and suction tips

## TRIAGE

I. Definitions
A. An emergency can be described as any situation that arises suddenly and unexpectedly, resulting in a sudden need for action
B. Triage is the initial assessment of the emergency patient
1. Triage is performed immediately on presentation and should take less than 5 minutes
2. Triage is the evaluation of the four major organ systems (cardiovascular, respiratory, neurological, and renal systems) while simultaneously obtaining a capsule history
   a. Acquiring the history can be the most difficult step
   b. Conversation should be limited to salient points only, avoiding irrelevant details
   c. The history should include the primary complaint, duration of the problem, and any current drug therapy
II. After triage the patient is categorized as stable or unstable, allowing appropriate prioritization of care
A. A stable patient is not in a life-threatening condition
B. An unstable or an emergent patient is in life-threatening circumstances and requires quick judgment and prompt action

III. There are several classification systems for triage; however, every case is unique and classifications do not cover every scenario
IV. If a patient is critical, a primary survey should be performed by a veterinarian with the assistance of a veterinary technician

## SYSTEMIC APPROACH TO TRIAGE

### Respiratory System

I. Airway: determine patency of airway
  A. Normal (patent/clear breath sounds)
  B. Upper airway noise (stridor/stertor)
  C. Distress with inspiration associated with stridor
II. Breathing
  A. Assess respiratory rate
    1. Normal: cat, 24 to 42 respirations per minute; dog, 10 to 30 respirations per minute
    2. Tachypnea: increased respiratory rate
    3. Apnea: no respirations
    4. Cheyne-Stokes: tachypnea interspersed with apnea
  B. Assess respiratory effort
    1. Normal: there should be no effort
    2. Labored inspiration
    3. Labored expiration
    4. Labored inspiration and expiration
    5. Paradoxical respiration: chest wall and abdominal wall do not move synchronously
  C. Postural adaptations of dyspnea
    1. Normal: patient should not be posturing to breathe
    2. Orthopnea
      a. Stand rather than sit
      b. Abduct elbows
    3. Abdominal movement
    4. Extended neck, open mouth, head lifted

### Cardiovascular System

I. Mucous membrane color
  A. Pink: normal
  B. Muddy or gray: poor perfusion
  C. Pale or white: anemia or poor perfusion
  D. Brick red (hyperemic): septic shock (not to be confused with severe gingivitis)
  E. Dark blue (cyanosis): hypoxia
  F. Yellow (jaundice): hepatic dysfunction, hemolysis, or biliary obstruction
  G. Brown: methemoglobinemia (most commonly seen with acetaminophen toxicity)
II. Capillary refill time (CRT)
  A. Normal: 1 to 2 seconds
  B. Prolonged: greater than 2 seconds; indicates poor perfusion
  C. Rapid: less than one second; indicates hyperdynamic state or hemoconcentration

III. Normal pulse rate
  A. Dog: 70 to 160 beats per minute (beats/min)
    1. Less than 70 beats/min: bradycardia
    2. Greater than 160 beats/min: tachycardia
  B. Cat: 150 to 210 beats/min
    1. Less than 150 beats/min: bradycardia
    2. Greater than 210 beats/min: tachycardia
IV. Pulse quality
  A. Normal: strong and synchronous with heart rate
  B. Weak: indicates poor perfusion
  C. Snappy: anemia (tall and thin pulse quality)
  D. Bounding: sepsis, hyperdynamic state

### Central Nervous System

The following should be assessed on triage. Their severity will determine the stability of the patient.
I. Gait
  A. Ataxia/weakness
  B. Loss of motor function
II. Muscular twitching
  A. Hypocalcemia (i.e., eclampsia)
  B. Pyrethrin toxicity
III. Head trauma
IV. Nystagmus: rapid eye movement
V. Head tilt
VI. Level of consciousness
  A. Alert
  B. Depressed
    1. Quiet, unwilling to perform normally; responds to environmental stimuli
  C. Delirium/dementia: responds abnormally to environmental stimuli
  D. Stuporous: unresponsive to environmental stimuli; responds to painful stimuli
  E. Comatose: no response to environmental and painful stimuli

### Renal System

On triage, the renal system is assessed with abdominal palpation when urinary blockage is suspected. Other emergencies affecting the renal system are identified while assessing the patient's cardiovascular status.
I. Acute renal failure
II. Chronic end-stage renal failure
III. Disruption of the urinary tract
  A. Ruptured ureter
  B. Ruptured bladder
  C. Ruptured urethra
IV. Urinary obstruction

### Life-Threatening Wounds

I. Open or penetrating chest wounds
II. Wounds to upper airway
III. Open or penetrating abdominal wounds
IV. Wounds affecting major blood vessels

## MONITORING STATUS OF EMERGENCY PATIENTS

Frequent and perceptive evaluation of physical examination parameters is the fundamental basis of emergency and critical care monitoring. The four major organ systems should be closely monitored at all times. The status of the emergent patient can rapidly change; therefore it is essential that the emergency technician be capable of noticing slight changes in the patient's physical parameters. If changes occur in the patient's status, the veterinarian should be notified immediately. The following sections will not discuss normal parameters; only abnormal parameters will be addressed.

### Respiratory System

Patients in respiratory distress are often very unstable; minimizing stress to the animal is extremely important. Physical examination, diagnostics, and treatments are performed in stages to allow the patient to rest and breathe in an oxygen-enriched environment. It may be necessary to rule out primary heart disease before sedation in some cases.

Patient monitoring should include respiratory status, cardiovascular status, renal status, and temperature (Table 27-1).

I. Postural adaptations of dyspnea
  A. Orthopnea
    1. Patient would rather stand than sit or lie sternally
    2. Abducted elbows
II. Respiratory rate
  A. Tachypnea: increased respiratory rate
  B. Apnea: no respiratory rate
  C. Cheyne-Stokes: tachypnea interspersed with apnea
III. Respiratory effort
  A. Labored inspiration
    1. Upper airway disorders
      a. Collapsing trachea
      b. Laryngeal paralysis
      c. Foreign body
      d. Soft tissue swelling
      e. Brachycephalic occlusive syndrome
  B. Labored expiration
    1. Feline asthma
  C. Labored inspiration and expiration
    1. Parenchymal disorders
      a. Pneumonia
      b. Contusions
      c. Pulmonary edema
      d. Neoplasia
  D. Short inspiration and expiration
    1. Pneumothorax
    2. Pleural effusion
    3. Diaphragmatic rupture

  E. Paradoxical respiration: chest wall and abdominal wall do not move synchronously
IV. Auscultation of lungs
  A. Dull lung sounds ventrally
    1. Indicates a pneumothorax
  B. Dull lung sounds dorsally
    1. Indicates a pleural effusion
  C. Harsh lung sounds
    1. Indicates parenchymal disorders
      a. Pneumonia
      b. Pulmonary contusions
      c. Pulmonary edema
      d. Neoplasia
  D. Rales
    1. Parenchymal disorders
      a. Cardiogenic
        (1) Right-sided heart failure
      b. Noncardiogenic
        (1) Fluid overload
        (2) Strangulation
        (3) Electrocution
V. Oxygenation status
  A. Arterial blood gas is more invasive and more accurate
    1. It requires placement of an arterial line (most commonly placed in the metatarsal artery) or obtaining sample via a blood gas syringe
    2. $Pao_2$ (partial pressure of oxygen in the arterial blood) less than 80 mm Hg: may require oxygen supplementation or mechanical ventilation
    3. $Paco_2$ (partial pressure of carbon dioxide in the arterial blood) greater than 45 mm Hg: may require mechanical ventilation
  B. $Sao_2$ (percentage of available hemoglobin that is saturated with oxygen) reading
    1. Less invasive and potentially less accurate
    2. Readings can be falsely high or low because of equipment failure, heart arrhythmias, human error, motion, and patient's pigmentation
    3. Requires a pulse oximeter
    4. Less then 92% indicates hypoxia

### Cardiovascular System

Emergencies affecting the cardiovascular system result from failure of the heart to pump blood throughout the body or from an inappropriately low blood volume. The mainstay of therapy for hypovolemic, septic, neurogenic, and anaphylactic shock is aggressive volume replacement. In contrast, volume replacement can be fatal in the patient with heart failure; therefore it is essential to differentiate between these conditions. Monitoring devices, such as those for direct and indirect blood pressure, are necessary; however, physical examination parameters are most important.

Patient monitoring should include respiratory status, cardiovascular status, neurological status, renal status, and temperature. Serial evaluations of an emergency blood screen are an integral part of patient monitoring (Table 27-2).

I. Mucous membrane color
II. Capillary refill time
III. Pulse rate
IV. Pulse quality
V. Blood pressure reading
    A. Direct arterial pressure readings
    B. Indirect pressure readings by
        1. Oscillometric pressure monitor
        2. Doppler blood flow monitor
VI. Electrocardiography

## Central Nervous System

Emergencies of the central nervous system (CNS) may affect the brain and/or the spinal cord. It is important to rule out hypoglycemia as a cause of seizures in patients presenting with continuous seizure activity. Behavior, pupillary reflexes, pupil size, and eye movement are used to evaluate the brain. The spinal cord is assessed by noting conscious proprioception, voluntary motor function, and superficial and deep pain (Table 27-3).

The causes of seizures include congenital/hereditary factors; inflammatory disease processes; viral, bacterial, fungal, protozoal, or rickettsial organisms; metabolic or nutritional deficiencies; trauma; a central vascular system breakdown; neoplasia; epilepsy; and toxicity.

I. Level of consciousness
    A. Alert: normal
    B. Depressed: quiet, unwilling to perform normally; responds to environmental stimuli
    C. Delirium/dementia: responds abnormally to environmental stimuli
    D. Stuporous: unresponsive to environmental stimuli; responds to painful stimuli
    E. Comatose: no response to environmental and painful stimuli
II. Pupillary reflexes
    A. Blink
    B. Menace
    C. Pupillary light response
        1. Direct
        2. Consensual
III. Pupil size
    A. Miosis: pinpoint
    B. Anisocoria: asymmetrical or unequal
    C. Mydriasis: dilated
IV. Eye movement/position
    A. Nystagmus
        1. Horizontal eye movement
        2. Vertical eye movement
    B. Strabismus: abnormal eye position

V. Evaluate spinal cord compression by
    A. Conscious proprioception
    B. Voluntary motor function
    C. Superficial pain
    D. Deep pain

## Renal System

The causes of renal system emergencies include acute and chronic renal failure, urethral obstructions, ruptured ureter/bladder, and urethral tears. Patients with renal disease should be monitored by measuring urine production, serum, creatinine, blood urea nitrogen (BUN), electrolytes (sodium, potassium, phosphorus, calcium), and acid-base parameters on a pretreatment basis and throughout the patient's treatment. Patient monitoring should include respiratory status, cardiovascular status, neurological status, temperature, and serial emergency blood screen readings (Table 27-4).

I. Urination
    A. Monitor urination
    B. Measure urine output
        1. Indwelling urinary catheter with closed collection system
        2. Normal values are 1 to 2 mL/kg/hr
    C. Central venous pressure: evaluates ability of the right ventricle to handle fluid therapy
        1. An early indicator of fluid overload
        2. Used when aggressive fluid therapy is indicated to treat renal failure
II. Temperature
    A. Hypothermia because of poor perfusion, anesthesia, exposure to cold
    B. Hyperthermia because of infection, sepsis, heat prostration, malignant hyperthermia, seizures, upper airway obstruction
III. Fluid losses should be assessed and recorded
    A. Vomiting
    B. Diarrhea
    C. Blood loss
    D. Effusions
    E. Edema
    F. Respiratory losses: excessive panting
IV. Emergency blood screen
    A. Packed cell volume/total solids
    B. Blood urea nitrogen and glucose analysis
    C. Electrolyte analysis
        1. Sodium
        2. Potassium
        3. Chloride
        4. Calcium
        5. Magnesium
    D. Acid-base analysis
        1. pH
        2. $Po_2$
        3. $Pco_2$
        4. $HCO_3^-$

## ENDOCRINE AND METABOLIC EMERGENCIES ▬

The treatment for a patient with an endocrine and/or metabolic emergency includes correcting dehydration, electrolyte abnormalities, and metabolic abnormalities and providing appropriate drug therapy. Metabolic disorders are always associated with a primary disease process.

Patient monitoring should include respiratory status, cardiovascular status, renal status, temperature, and serial emergency blood screen analysis (Table 27-5).

## GASTROINTESTINAL EMERGENCIES ▬

Patient monitoring should include respiratory status, cardiovascular status, renal status, and serial emergency blood screen readings. For gastric dilation, serial measurement of abdominal girth may be performed. A patient with severe vomiting and diarrhea can be classified as emergent because of the cardiovascular effects of fluid loss (Table 27-6).

## REPRODUCTIVE SYSTEM EMERGENCIES ▬

Patient monitoring should include respiratory status, cardiovascular status, renal status, and temperature. Note vomiting/diarrhea, serial database readings, and serial emergency blood screen analysis. The female patient should also be closely observed for active contractions, vaginal discharge, and delivery. Reproductive emergencies affecting the male often require prompt surgical intervention (Table 27-7).

## TOXIC SUBSTANCE EMERGENCIES ▬

Because of the wide variety of effects caused by toxins, it can be difficult to recognize an intoxicated patient without a detailed history. A local poison control center can often give treatment options to the veterinarian. There are a variety of plants that may potentially be toxic to animals. If plant toxicity is suspect, refer to a plant toxicity reference or contact poison control. Patient monitoring should include respiratory status, cardiovascular status (electrocardiogram), renal status, vomiting/diarrhea, coagulopathy, and neurological status. See Table 27-8 for the most common toxins.

## OCULAR EMERGENCIES ▬

Ocular emergencies can be caused by trauma, primary medical problems, penetrating foreign objects, or increased intraocular pressure. It is essential that the eye(s) be rechecked frequently so progress can be monitored. More complicated ophthalmic emergencies require the expertise of an ophthalmologist. Misdiagnosis and improper treatment can lead to the loss of vision (Table 27-9).

**Table 27-1** Respiratory emergencies

| Clinical signs | Treatment |
|---|---|
| **COLLAPSING TRACHEA (most commonly seen in small breed dogs)** ||
| Loud goose honk cough with expiration, ± postural indications of dyspnea, ± hyperthermia | Supply oxygen, calm with sedation when necessary (rule out primary heart disease before sedation), ± surgical intervention |
| **LARYNGEAL PARALYSIS (most commonly seen in large breed dogs)** ||
| Noisy breathing, distress with inspiration, postural adaptations of dyspnea | Supply oxygen, calm with sedation, endotracheal intubation, ± surgical intervention, ± tracheostomy |
| **FOREIGN BODY** ||
| Noisy breathing, distress with inspiration, acute onset of gagging with severe respiratory distress, postural adaptations of dyspnea, ± hyperthermia | Supply oxygen, remove obstruction |
| **SOFT TISSUE SWELLING: ALLERGIC REACTION** ||
| Facial swelling, ± generalized urticaria (hives) ± noisy breathing, ± distress with inspiration, ± postural indications of dyspnea | Dexamethasone sodium phosphate (antiinflammatory agent), diphenhydramine HCl (inhibits histamine release) |
| **SOFT TISSUE SWELLING: TUMOR** ||
| Noisy breathing, distress with inspiration, postural adaptations of dyspnea, ± hyperthermia | Supply oxygen, calm with sedation, ± intubation, ± tracheostomy, ± surgical intervention |

**Table 27-1** Respiratory emergencies—cont'd

| Clinical signs | Treatment |
|---|---|
| **BRACHYCEPHALIC OCCLUSIVE SYNDROME (elongated soft palate, stenotic nares, hypoplastic trachea, everted laryngeal saccule)** ||
| Upper airway stertor, distress with inspiration, postural adaptations of dyspnea, ± hyperthermia | Supply oxygen, calm with sedation, ± intubation, ± surgical intervention, ± tracheostomy |
| **SMALL AIRWAY DISEASE: FELINE ASTHMA** ||
| Dyspnea (prolonged expiration), postural indications of dyspnea, expiratory wheeze | Supply oxygen, bronchodilator, corticosteroids |
| **PNEUMONIA** ||
| Tachypnea, dyspnea (inspiration and expiration), postural indications of dyspnea, ± pyrexia, ± cyanosis, lung auscultation (harsh sounds), ± rales | Supply oxygen (100% initially), 40% oxygen is suggested for long-term therapy (100% oxygen for more than 12 hr can result in pulmonary oxygen toxicity), appropriate antibiotic therapy, nebulize, coupage, ± positive pressure ventilation |
| **CONTUSIONS** ||
| Tachypnea, dyspnea, postural indications of dyspnea, evidence of recent trauma, ± shock, ± cyanosis, ± hemoptysis, lung auscultation (harsh lung sounds), ± rales | Supply oxygen, ± fluid therapy, ± positive pressure ventilation |
| **PULMONARY EDEMA** ||
| Tachypnea, dyspnea, postural adaptations of dyspnea, ± cyanosis, ± burns in mouth (suggestive of electric shock), ongoing fluid therapy (suggestive of fluid overload), harsh lung sounds, ± rales, ± heart murmur | Supply oxygen, diuretics, ± positive pressure ventilation |
| **PULMONARY NEOPLASIA** ||
| Tachypnea, dyspnea, ± cyanosis, harsh lung sounds, ± rales | Supply oxygen, ± positive pressure ventilation |
| **PNEUMOTHORAX** ||
| Tachypnea, dyspnea, (rapid and short inspirations and expirations), ± cyanosis, postural indications of dyspnea, decreased/muffled lung sounds dorsally, evidence of recent trauma | Supply oxygen, evacuate air (thoracocentesis), ± chest tube (placed when negative pressure is not achieved or when it is necessary to tap chest repeatedly) |
| **PLEURAL EFFUSION (hemothorax, pyothorax, chylothorax, and serous effusion)** ||
| Tachypnea, dyspnea, postural adaptations of dyspnea, ± cyanosis, decreased muffled lung sounds ventrally | Supply oxygen, evacuate fluid (chest tap), ± chest tube |
| **DIAPHRAGMATIC RUPTURE** ||
| Tachypnea, dyspnea (paradoxical abdominal movement), postural adaptations of dyspnea, ± cyanosis, ± evidence of trauma, ± auscultation of borborygmus in thorax, decreased/muffled lung sounds, cardiac displacement | Supply oxygen, surgical correction |

**Table 27-2** Cardiovascular emergencies

| Clinical signs | Treatment |
|---|---|
| **HYPOVOLEMIC SHOCK** | |
| Pale, gray, or muddy mucous membrane color; prolonged capillary refill time; rapid pulse rate, weak pulse quality; ± evidence of acute blood loss; ± evidence of fluid loss (vomiting, diarrhea); ± evidence of fluid sequestration | Shock fluid therapy (isotonic crystalloid, hypertonic crystalloids, blood products, artificial colloid), ± oxygen supplementation |
| **SEPTIC, NEUROGENIC, OR ANAPHYLACTIC SHOCK** | |
| Brick red mucous membrane color, hyperdynamic, rapid capillary refill time (less than 1 sec), tachycardia, bounding pulse quality, ± hyperthermia, ± hypoglycemia | Shock fluid therapy, ± blood culture (for septic shock), ± antibiotics for septic shock, ± corticosteroids for anaphylactic shock, ± diphenhydramine for anaphylactic shock |
| **CARDIOGENIC SHOCK: CONGESTIVE HEART FAILURE, PERICARDIAL TAMPONADE** | |
| Pale or muddy mucous membrane color, prolonged capillary refill time, rapid pulse rate, weak pulse quality, ± tachypnea/dyspnea, ± postural indications of dyspnea, ± cyanosis, ± evidence of trauma | *Congestive heart failure:* oxygen supplementation, diuretics, inotropes, vasodilators, ± fluid therapy (very conservative, minimize stress levels) *Cardiac tamponade:* oxygen supplementation, pericardiocentesis, ± fluid therapy (very conservative, minimize stress levels) |

**Table 27-3** Central nervous system emergencies

| Clinical signs | Monitoring | Treatment |
|---|---|---|
| **EPILEPSY** | | |
| Hyperthermia, hyperdynamic state, ± nystagmus/strabismus, ± pupillary changes (miosis, mydriasis, anisocoria) | Respiratory status (potential for aspiration during seizure); cardiovascular status; neurological status (mental status: alert and responsive; depressed, stupor, coma, and pupillary light response); renal status, body temperature | Diazepam (good anticonvulsant activity, must give to effect), phenobarbital, pentobarbital (heavy anesthesia) |
| **HEAD TRAUMA** | | |
| Depression, ± stupor, ± coma, ± convulsions, ± pupillary changes (miosis, mydriasis, anisocoria), ± nystagmus/strabismus, ± blood in aural canal, ± hyphema, ± scleral hemorrhage, ± skull/facial fractures | Respiratory status (trauma to the brain stem can cause altered ventilatory status, important to keep carbon dioxide levels normal to low, increased carbon dioxide will cause increased intracranial pressure), cardiovascular status, neurological status, renal status | Corticosteroids, ± mannitol (osmotic agent, can decrease intracranial pressure through its osmotic effects), elevate head (place patient on flat board and elevate board to approximately 30 degrees in attempt to decrease intracranial pressure), ± ventilation (to decrease carbon dioxide levels) |
| **ACUTE PARESIS/PARALYSIS** | | |
| Loss of conscious proprioception, loss of voluntary motor function, loss of superficial pain, loss of deep pain | Respiratory status (patients with tetraparesis can experience loss of function to intercostal muscles), cardiovascular status, neurological status (conscious proprioception, voluntary motor activity, superficial pain, deep pain), renal status (upper motor neuron: hypertonic sphincter), (lower motor neuron: bladder hypotonia) | Conservative (commonly used when voluntary motor function is still present), corticosteroids, strict cage rest, surgical intervention (myelogram, laminectomy) |

**Table 27-4**  Renal system emergencies

| Clinical signs | Treatment |
|---|---|
| **ACUTE RENAL FAILURE** ||
| Vomiting, diarrhea, dehydration, ± evidence of exposure to toxins (e.g., ethylene glycol or gentamicin) | Pretreatment, emergency blood screen and creatinine and phosphorus, fluid therapy (isotonic crystalloid solutions, measure urine output, diuretics after rehydration), ± peritoneal dialysis, gastrointestinal protectants |
| **CHRONIC END-STAGE RENAL FAILURE** ||
| Weight loss, vomiting, anorexia, dehydration, anemia, lethargy | Fluid therapy, electrolyte replacement (e.g., potassium), ± blood transfusion, measure urine output |
| **FELINE URETHRAL OBSTRUCTION** ||
| Dysuria, ± hematuria, vomiting, vocalizing, painful abdomen, distended bladder on abdominal palpation, ± hyperkalemia, ± hypocalcemia | Fluid therapy, electrocardiogram, treat arrhythmias with calcium gluconate, emergency blood screen, treat hyperkalemia because it can cause life-threatening arrhythmias |
| **URETER/BLADDER RUPTURE** ||
| Vomiting, diarrhea, ± hematuria, ± evidence of trauma, ± abdominal effusion, ± red blood cells in urine, abdominal pain, ± hypovolemic shock, ± decreased urine output | Radiographs, urinary catheter, ± excretory urogram, ± retrograde urethrography/cystography, surgical intervention, ± abdominocentesis |
| **URETHRAL TEARS** ||
| ± Vomiting, ± dysuria/hematuria, ± anuria, ± abdominal effusion, ± subcutaneous edema of hind limbs and ventral abdomen ± hypovolemic shock, ± hyperkalemia | ± Urinary catheter, ± surgical intervention, ± abdominocentesis |

**Table 27-5**  Endocrine and metabolic emergencies

| Clinical signs | Treatment |
|---|---|
| **ADDISONIAN CRISIS (hypoadrenocorticism)** | |
| Hyponatremia, hyperkalemia (causing bradycardia), ± hypovolemic shock, hypoglycemia, hypercalcemia, vomiting, diarrhea, polyuria/polydipsia (PU/PD) | Fluid therapy: normal saline, glucocorticoid (dexamethasone most commonly used) will not interfere with adrenocorticotropic hormone stimulation test; correct acidosis (if severe, give sodium bicarbonate, supply oxygen) |
| **DIABETIC KETOACIDOSIS** | |
| PU/PD, vomiting, diarrhea, dehydration, ± hypovolemic shock, hyperglycemia, glucosuria, ketonuria, acidemia, tachypnea | IV fluid therapy, insulin therapy, ± KCl replacement, ± phosphorus replacement |
| **HYPERGLYCEMIA** | |
| Vary depending on underlying disease process | When diabetes is suspected, insulin therapy will be initiated |
| **HYPOGLYCEMIA** | |
| Depressed, weakness, ataxia, stupor, blindness, seizure activity, coma | Supplement with dextrose; a dextrose bolus must be diluted 1:4 with a crystalloid to prevent phlebitis |
| **HYPERCALCEMIA** | |
| Vary depending on cause of hypercalcemia | Hypercalcemia is a medical emergency because of its effects on the kidney; fluid therapy with 0.9% NaCl for rehydration and increased calcium excretion; find underlying cause of increased calcium |
| **HYPOCALCEMIA** | |
| Increased neuromuscular excitability (muscular twitching), generalized muscle tremors, seizures, hyperthermia | Calcium supplementation, must be given slowly with continuous electrocardiogram (ECG) monitoring; if arrhythmias or bradycardia occur, calcium administration should be discontinued |
| **HYPERNATREMIA** | |
| Dehydration, neurological signs | Slowly correct dehydration and gradually lower sodium levels |
| **HYPONATREMIA** | |
| Protracted vomiting and diarrhea, lethargy, coma | Electrolyte replacement, correction of dehydration |
| **HYPERKALEMIA** | |
| ECG: increased amplitude of T wave with decreased amplitude of R wave and prolonged PR interval, then bradycardia with widening of QRS complex are eventually seen; cardiac arrest | Restore potassium balance; fluid therapy, administration of intravenous regular insulin followed by dextrose administration is used to lower potassium levels; ongoing fluid therapy with dextrose supplementation; administer calcium gluconate to protect myocardium and reverse arrhythmias |
| **HYPOKALEMIA** | |
| Severe muscle weakness, ventroflexion of neck, stilted forelimb gait | Potassium supplementation via intravenous fluid administration; if giving shock bolus of fluid, do not use fluids that have been supplemented with potassium |

**Table 27-6**  Gastrointestinal (GI) emergencies

| Clinical signs | Treatment |
|---|---|
| **GASTRIC DILATION AND/OR VOLVULUS** ||
| Abdominal distention; nonproductive retching; pale, muddy, or gray mucous membrane color; prolonged capillary refill time; tachycardia; weak pulse; ± tachypnea; dyspnea | Fluid therapy (rapid IV bolus), decompression (trocharization or gastric intubation/lavage), corticosteroids, abdominal radiographs (right lateral most important), surgical intervention if torsion |
| **GI OBSTRUCTION (foreign body, intussusception, tumor)** ||
| Vomiting; diarrhea; red, pale, gray, or muddy mucous membrane color; fast or prolonged capillary refill time; abdominal pain; tachycardia; weak pulse quality; dehydration; tachypnea; dyspnea | Fluid therapy, ± endoscopy, ± surgical intervention, abdominal radiographs, ± upper GI study, ± abdominal ultrasound |
| **PERITONITIS (GI perforation, ruptured prostatic abscess)** ||
| Hyperemic; brick-red mucous membrane, rapid capillary refill time, tachycardia, bounding pulse quality, hyperthermia, ± hypoglycemia, abdominal pain | Fluid therapy, appropriate antibiotics, abdominocentesis (obtain sample for cytology), ± diagnostic peritoneal lavage, surgical intervention |
| **PARVOVIRUS INFECTION** ||
| Vomiting; diarrhea; pale, gray, or muddy mucous membrane color; prolonged capillary refill time; tachycardia; weak pulse quality; dehydration; ± hypoglycemia; ± hypokalemia; ± leukopenia | Fluid therapy, antibiotics to prevent secondary bacterial infection, correct hypoglycemia, correct hypokalemia, ± antiemetics, abdominal palpation to rule out intussusception |
| **LIVER FAILURE** ||
| Vomiting; ± hematemesis; diarrhea; ± melena; polyuria/polydipsia; ± dementia; ± seizures; ± jaundice; ± anemia; ± coagulopathy; hypoalbuminemia; hypoglycemia; hyperbilirubinemia; hypocholesterolemia; low blood urea nitrogen | Fluid therapy, GI protectants, ± lactulose, vitamin $K_1$, ± antibiotics, ± fresh frozen plasma |
| **HEMORRHAGIC GASTROENTERITIS** ||
| Hematochezia, vomiting, dehydration, lethargy, anorexia | Fluid therapy, ± colloid replacement, GI protectants |
| **PANCREATITIS** ||
| Vomiting, diarrhea, lethargy, anorexia, painful abdomen, pyrexia | Fluid therapy, ± colloid therapy, ± antibiotic therapy, ± pain medication |

**Table 27-7** Emergencies of the reproductive system

| Clinical signs | Treatment |
|---|---|
| **PYOMETRA** ||
| Polyuria/polydipsia, recent estrus, vomiting, ±hyperthermia, ±vaginal discharge (depends on whether the cervix is open or closed), ±abdominal distention | Fluid therapy (isotonic crystalloid), antibiotic therapy, surgical intervention |
| **ECLAMPSIA** ||
| Muscle tremors, evidence of whelping and lactation usually 2-3 wk before, brick-red mucous membranes (hyperemic), tachycardia, bounding pulse quality, hyperthermia, hypocalcemia | Calcium gluconate (slow IV bolus), fluid therapy (when hyperthermia, isotonic crystalloid solution), oral calcium throughout lactation, electrocardiogram while administering calcium gluconate; if bradycardia, arrhythmia, or vomiting occurs, stop treatment |
| **DYSTOCIA** ||
| Active contractions for more than 30 min, more than 2 hr between deliveries, green discharge with no delivery of fetus | Rule out obstructive dystocia (digital examination, abdominal radiographs), oxytocin, ±calcium gluconate, ±glucose, ±surgical intervention |

**Table 27-8** Emergencies caused by toxic substances

| Clinical signs | Treatment |
|---|---|
| **ACETAMINOPHEN (Tylenol) TOXICOSIS** ||
| 1-2 hr postingestion (salivation, vomiting, tachypnea, brown or cyanotic mucous membrane color, dark or chocolate-colored blood, edema of face) | Induce emesis if less than 1 hr postingestion (not performed if showing signs of tachypnea), acetylcysteine, ascorbic acid, fluid therapy (isotonic crystalloid), supply oxygen |
| **ANTICOAGULANT RODENTICIDE TOXICITY** ||
| No clinical signs: ingested recently, dyspnea, hematuria, hematemesis, epistaxis, melena, hemothorax | Induce emesis (if recently ingested, activated charcoal, vitamin $K_1$), prothrombin time analysis 2 days postingestion, then prothrombin time analysis 2 days after vitamin $K_1$ finished, fresh whole blood or fresh frozen plasma if coagulopathy is present |
| **CHOCOLATE TOXICOSIS (methylxanthine) (active ingredient theobromine) ($LD_{50}$: 100 mg/kg)** ||
| Vomiting, diarrhea, hyperactivity, muscle tremors, tachycardia, arrhythmia, hypertension, ±seizures | Induce emesis, ±gastric lavage, activated charcoal, cathartics, fluid therapy (isotonic crystalloid), ±oxygen supplementation |
| **ETHYLENE GLYCOL TOXICITY ($LD_{50}$: dog, 4-6 mL/kg; cat, 1.5 mL/kg)** ||
| Vomiting, polyuria/polydipsia, tachypnea, tachycardia, azotemia, increased serum osmolality, metabolic acidosis, hypocalcemia, oliguria, ataxia, seizures, stupor, coma | Gastric lavage, cathartics, fluid therapy (isotonic crystalloid), ethanol (7%), peritoneal dialysis, ±methylpyrazole test for ethylene glycol within 12 hr of ingestion; if patient is exhibiting seizure activity, obtain blood for ethylene glycol test before administration of diazepam (propylene glycol in diazepam can make ethylene glycol test falsely positive) |
| **LEAD POISONING** ||
| Vomiting, diarrhea, lethargy, abdominal pain, ataxia, blindness, seizures, evidence of nucleated red blood cell on blood smear with no evidence of anemia | Remove lead from gastrointestinal (GI) tract, enema, emetic, surgical intervention, remove lead from tissues and blood, calcium EDTA, penicillin, control seizures |

**Table 27-8**   Emergencies caused by toxic substances—cont'd

| Clinical signs | Treatment |
|---|---|
| **NONSTEROIDAL ANTIINFLAMMATORY DRUGS** ||
| Vomiting, diarrhea, GI bleeding (hematemesis, melena) | Fluid therapy (isotonic crystalloid, isotonic colloid, blood products, artificial colloid), GI protectants (sucralfate, cimetidine HCl) |
| **ORGANOPHOSPHATE TOXICITY** ||
| Acronym: DUMBELS = *d*iarrhea, *u*rination, *m*iosis, *b*radycardia, *e*mesis, *l*acrimation, *s*alivation; dyspnea, fasciculation, vomiting, diarrhea, seizures | Remove toxin (bathe with soap and water), atropine sulfate, diphenhydramine, ± pralidoxime (2-PAM), fluid therapy (isotonic crystalloid), control fasciculation/convulsions (diazepam or pentobarbital) |
| **PYRETHRINS** ||
| Central nervous system signs, severe muscular twitching, ± hypothermia ± hyperthermia, ± dyspnea | Bathe patient immediately, initially administer diazepam IV to effect, methocarbimal IV p.r.n. to effect (do not exceed 330 mg/kg/day), ± fluid therapy |
| **PHILODENDRON/DUMB CANE (insoluble calcium oxalate)** ||
| Pain and burning of throat, oral mucosa, and lips. Mucosal edema and dyspnea can occur if severe | Will resolve without treatment |
| **MARIJUANA (tetrahydrocannabinol)** ||
| Depression, ataxia, animal appears anxious, abnormal vocalization, ± vomiting | Induce vomiting, ± gastric lavage, activated charcoal, place animal in a quiet environment |
| **EASTER AND TIGER LILIES (unknown poison)** ||
| Anorexia, vomiting, renal failure | Treat for acute renal failure (see Table 27-4) |
| **RHODODENDRON AZALEA (andromedotoxins)** ||
| Salivation, diarrhea, vomiting, muscle weakness, bradycardia, hypotension, coma, and convulsions | Induce vomiting, ± gastric lavage, activated charcoal, electrocardiogram, fluid therapy, treat bradycardia |

**Table 27-9**   Ocular emergencies

| Clinical signs | Treatment |
|---|---|
| **GLAUCOMA** ||
| Enlarged eyeball, dilated pupil, negative menace response, absent papillary light response, corneal edema, and pain<br>Diagnosis is determined by measuring intraocular pressure (IOP). IOP is measured by the use of a Schiøtz or electronic tonometer | Treat with drugs, such as mannitol and pilocarpine, that will reduce IOP by drawing fluid out of the vitreous chamber |
| **CORNEAL FOREIGN BODIES AND LACERATIONS** ||
| Blepharospasm, ocular discharge, photophobia as a result of pain | *Corneal foreign body:* gentle irrigation with sterile saline to dislodge foreign object, ± surgical intervention<br>*Laceration:* surgical intervention, topical antibiotics and atropine sulfate, oral antibiotics |
| **HYPHEMA** ||
| Hemorrhage in anterior chamber | Treat underlying cause (trauma, infection ± uveitis, neoplasia ± uveitis, coagulopathy) |

*Continued*

**Table 27-9**  Ocular emergencies—cont'd

| Clinical signs | Treatment |
|---|---|
| **UVEITIS** | |
| Painful, red, inflamed iris; blepharospasm; miotic pupil; prolapsed nictitans; decreased IOP; ± hypopyon; ± hyphema | Topical atropine; if secondary glaucoma is present, use adrenaline (epinephrine), topical corticosteroids |
| **PROPTOSIS** | |
| Proptosis of eye | First note severity of proptosis: ± enucleation, ± replacement of eye |
| **CORNEAL ULCERS** | |
| Blepharospasm, ocular discharge, photophobia as a result of pain | *Superficial ulcers:* topical antibiotics, ± atropine sulfate<br>*Indolent ulcers (Boxer ulcers):* debride edges of ulcer, keratectomy, topical antibiotics<br>*Deep ulcer:* avoid excessive restraint, which may lead to perforation; topical antibiotics; topical atropine sulfate; patients with melting or infected ulcers need topical anticollagenase (autologous serum administered every hour for the first day of treatment); ± Elizabethan collar to prevent patient scratching of eye |
| **DESCEMETOCELE** | |
| Descemet's membrane penetrated through ulcer, looks transparent; cornea is in danger of penetration | Surgical intervention, topical antibiotics |

# Glossary

**abducted**  Drawn away from an axis or a median plane

**acidemia**  Abnormal acidity of the blood

**acidosis**  State characterized by actual or relative decrease of alkali in body fluids in relation to acid content

**ACTH**  Adrenocorticotropic hormone

**anaphylactic**  Serious reaction (shock) brought about by hypersensitivity to an allergen, such as a drug or protein (anaphylaxis)

**anisocoria**  Unequal or asymmetrical pupil size

**anticollagenase**  Drug that is used to prevent the body from breaking down collagen

**anuria**  No urine production

**apnea**  No respirations

**ataxia**  Incoordination of limb movement

**auscultation**  Listening for sounds produced within the body

**autologous**  Of the self

**azotemia**  Retention of renal excretory products

**blepharospasm**  Spasm of the eyelid

**borborygmi**  Rumbling or gurgling noises produced by movement of gas in the gastrointestinal tract

**cardiac tamponade**  Reduction of venous return to the heart because of increased volume of fluid in the pericardium

**cathartics**  Agent that increases gastrointestinal flow

**chylothorax**  Accumulation of milky chylous fluid in the pleural space, usually on the left side

**coagulopathy**  Any disorder of blood coagulation

**colloid**  Solution containing large molecules that cannot pass out of blood vessels

**coma**  State of unconsciousness with no response to external stimuli

**coupage**  Striking the thoracic area to aid in the removal of secretions

**crystalloid**  Solution containing small molecules that can pass out of blood vessels

**cyanosis**  Bluish discoloration of skin and mucous membranes

**cystography**  Radiography of the urinary bladder using a contrast medium

**descemetocele**  Herniation of Descemet's membrane, usually through a corneal ulcer

**Descemet's membrane**  Posterior portion of the cornea; a membrane

**diuretic**  Agent that promotes excretion of urine

**Doppler monitor**  Device that uses ultrasound for measuring blood flow

**dyspnea**  Difficulty breathing

**dysuria**  Difficult urination

**ecchymosis**  Large area of nonelevated bruising in the skin or mucous membranes

**edema**  Accumulation of an excessive amount of watery fluid in cells, tissues, or serous cavities

**effusion**  Escape of fluid from blood vessels or lymphatics into tissues or cavities

**encephalitis**  Inflammation of the brain

**epistaxis**  Nasal hemorrhage; nosebleed

**fasciculation**  Localized involuntary muscular contraction

**hematemesis**  Vomiting blood

**hematochezia** Blood in feces

**hematuria** Blood in urine

**hemoptysis** Coughing blood

**hemothorax** Blood in the pleural cavity

**hydrocephalus** Condition marked by an excessive accumulation of fluid in the brain

**hyperdynamic** Excessive muscular activity

**hyperkalemia** Abnormally high potassium levels

**hypernatremia** Increased sodium in the blood

**hyperthermia** Increased body temperature

**hyphema** Blood in the anterior chamber of the eye

**hyponatremia** Deficiency of sodium in the blood

**hypoplasty** Underdevelopment of an organ or tissue

**hypopyon** Pus in the anterior chamber of the eye

**hypothermia** Decreased body temperature

**hypoxia** Decrease in oxygen

**indwelling (urinary catheter)** Catheter that is designed to stay in the urethra to drain urine from the bladder

**intussusception** Infolding of one segment of the intestine into another

**IOP** Intraocular pressure

**isotonic** Of similar osmolality to normal plasma

**lactulose** A synthetic sugar used as a cathartic to enhance the excretion of ammonia in patients with liver disease

**laminectomy** Surgical excision of the dorsal arch of a vertebra

**lavage** Washing out or irrigating the intestinal tract or stomach

**LD$_{50}$** Dose that will kill 50% of the tested population

**menace reflex or menace response** Reflex assessed by stabbing a finger toward an eye. Positive response is closing of the eyelids; absence of response could indicate paralysis of the eyelids or serious depression of consciousness

**methemoglobinemia** Presence of methemoglobin in the circulating blood

**miosis** Contraction of the pupil

**mydriasis** Dilation of the pupil

**myelogram** Graphic representation of cells found in a bone marrow sample

**nebulization** Treatment by a spray

**neoplasia** Pathological process that results in the formation and growth of a tumor

**neurogenic** Originating in the nervous system

**nystagmus** Rhythmic involuntary movement of the eyeballs in a vertical, horizontal, or rotary direction

**occlusive** State of being closed; an obstruction or a closing

**oliguria** Reduced daily output of urine

**orthopnea** Discomfort in breathing aggravated by lying flat: minimizing chest wall compression by standing or sternal recumbency with elbows abducted

**osmolality** Concentration of a solution in terms of osmoles or solutes per kilogram of solvent

**paralysis** Loss of power of voluntary movement in a muscle

**paraphimosis** Inability to retract the penis

**parenchyma** Distinguishing or specific cells of a gland or organ, contained in and supported by the connective tissue framework

**paresis** Incomplete voluntary movement

**perfusion** Passage of fluid through the vessels of an organ

**pericardiocentesis** Passage into the pericardium with a needle or hollow instrument for the purpose of removing fluid

**periodontitis** Inflammation of the area surrounding a tooth or the periodontium

**pleura** Serous membrane enveloping the lungs and lining the walls of the pleural cavity

**pneumothorax** Presence of air or gas in the pleural cavity

**postural** Pertaining to position or posture

**prolapsed nictitans** Prolapsed third eyelid. When the eye is depressed within the socket because of dehydration or emaciation and the third eyelid is moved across the eye

**proprioceptive** Capable of receiving stimuli originating in muscles, tendons, and other internal tissues

**protectant** Agent that promotes defense immunity against a harmful substance

**PU/PD** Polyuria/polydipsia

**pyothorax** Empyema (pus) in the pleural cavity

**pyrexia** Fever

**rales** Crackling sounds heard on lung auscultation

**septic** Pertaining to sepsis; the presence of toxins in the blood or other tissues

**sequestration** Abnormal separation of a part or a whole portion by a disease process

**serous** Relating to, containing or producing, or a substance having a watery consistency

**shock** Stage in which the body is unable to adequately deliver oxygen to tissues

**status epilepticus** Repeated seizure or a seizure prolonged for at least 30 minutes

**stenotic** Abnormal narrowing or constriction

**stertor** Snoring; a noisy inspiration sometimes because of obstruction of the larynx or upper airway

**strabismus** Change in the visual axis; examples: wandering eye, walleye, cross-eye, squint

**stridor** High-pitched, noisy respiration sometimes caused by obstruction of the larynx or upper airway

**stupor** State of impaired consciousness with response to noxious stimuli

**tachypnea** Rapid respirations

**tetraparesis** Muscular weakness affecting all four extremities

**thoracocentesis** Passage into the pleural cavity with a needle or hollow instrument for the purpose of removing fluid or air

**tonometer** Instrument for measuring intraocular tension or pressure

**torsion** Act of twisting

**urogram** Radiography of any part of the urinary tract

**urticaria** Vascular reaction of the skin that is a response to direct exposure to a chemical or an immunological response; wheals or hives

**ventroflexion** Flexion of the cervical spine with movement of the head towards the ventral surface

# Review Questions

1 What are the four major organ systems that are immediately evaluated in an emergency situation?
   a. Renal, gastrointestinal, cardiovascular, respiratory
   b. Endocrine, central nervous, gastrointestinal, renal
   c. Musculoskeletal, gastrointestinal, endocrine, renal
   d. Respiratory, cardiovascular, renal, central nervous

**2** What are the postural adaptations for dyspnea?
  a. Coughing, tachypnea, extended neck, upper airway noise
  b. Lay rather than sit, labored expiration, abdominal movement
  c. Stand rather than sit, abducted elbows, abdominal movement, extended neck
  d. Dyspnea, stertor, extended neck, abdominal movement

**3** Forty percent oxygen is suggested for long-term therapy; 100% oxygen for more than _____ can result in pulmonary oxygen toxicity
  a. 6 hours
  b. 8 hours
  c. 12 hours
  d. 24 hours

**4** What disease process requires nebulization as a treatment?
  a. Contusions
  b. Pulmonary edema
  c. Laryngeal paralysis
  d. Parenchymal lung problems

**5** A capillary refill time of greater than 2 seconds is indicative of
  a. Hyperdynamic state
  b. Liver problems
  c. Cerebral edema
  d. Poor perfusion

**6** Emergency situations treated with vitamin $K_1$ include
  a. Liver and anticoagulant rodenticide toxicity
  b. Chocolate toxicity and NSAID toxicity
  c. Acute paresis and acute renal failure
  d. Ethylene glycol and lead toxicities

**7** Initial treatment for a patient in respiratory distress is
  a. Electrocardiogram
  b. Chest radiographs
  c. Diuretics
  d. Oxygen supplementation

**8** Dull lung sounds ventrally on auscultation indicate
  a. Pneumonia
  b. Pleural effusion
  c. Pulmonary edema
  d. Pneumothorax

**9** The clinical signs of anaphylactic shock are
  a. Brick-red mucous membranes, CRT of 1 second, and tachycardia
  b. Pale mucous membranes, CRT of 1 second, and bradycardia
  c. Muddy colored mucous membranes, prolonged CRT, and weak pulse
  d. Pale mucous membranes, CRT of 1 second, and tachycardia

**10** Clinical signs for eclampsia are caused by
  a. Hypoglycemia
  b. Hyperkalemia
  c. Hypocalcemia
  d. Hypernatremia

## BIBLIOGRAPHY

Battaglia A: *Small animal emergency and critical care for veterinary technicians*, ed 2, St Louis, 2007, Saunders.

Hensyl WR, editor: *Stedman's medical dictionary*, ed 27, Baltimore, 2000, Lippincott Williams & Wilkins.

King L, Hammond R, editors: *Manual of canine and feline emergency and critical care*, Shurdington, Cheltenham, United Kingdom, 1999, British Small Animal Veterinary Association.

Kirby R et al, editors: *The veterinary clinics of North America: small animal medicine, vol 24(6), Emergency medicine*, Philadelphia, 1994, Saunders.

Kirk RW et al: *Current veterinary therapy*, ed 13, Philadelphia, 2000, Saunders.

Mathews KA: *Veterinary emergency and critical care manual*, ed 2, Guelph, Ontario, 2006, Lifelearn Publication.

Murtaugh RJ et al: *Veterinary emergency and critical care medicine*, St Louis, 1992, Mosby.

Plunkett SJ: *Emergency procedures for the small animal veterinarian*, Philadelphia, 2001, Saunders.

## CHAPTER 28

# Zoonoses

*Kisha L. White-Farrar*

## OUTLINE

Bacterial Zoonoses
Rickettsial Zoonoses
Viral Zoonoses

Parasitic Zoonoses
Mycotic Zoonoses

Prion/Transmissible Spongiform
Encephalopathy Zoonoses

## LEARNING OUTCOMES

After reading this chapter you should be able to:

1. Define bacterial, rickettsial, viral, parasitic, mycotic, and other miscellaneous zoonotic diseases.
2. Recognize etiology, symptoms (human and animal), transmission, diagnosis, treatment, prevention, and control of various zoonotic diseases.

**Z**oonoses are infections or parasitic diseases that can be transmitted between humans and animals. It is beyond the scope of this chapter to address all of the known zoonoses, but descriptions of many important or commonly encountered diseases are presented. Any ill or infected animal represents a potential source of zoonotic infection, but with the use of proper precautions the chances of disease transmission can be greatly reduced. People who are immunocompromised (e.g., the very young, the aged, those on chemotherapeutic regimens), have had their spleen removed, or are immunodeficient should avoid contact with sick animals, because most pathogenic organisms can "set up shop" in atypical host species if an individual has greatly lowered (or absent) body defenses.

The practice of epidemiology analyzes factors that influence the incidence, distribution, and control of infectious disease. By understanding how to recognize the symptoms, transmission, diagnosis, treatment, and control of transmittable diseases, the incidence of serious illness in humans and animals can be reduced (Tables 28-1 to 28-6).

**Table 28-1** Bacterial zoonoses

| Etiology | Symptoms—human | Symptoms—animal | Transmission | Diagnosis | Treatment | Prevention control |
|---|---|---|---|---|---|---|
| **AVIAN CHLAMYDIOSIS (psittacosis, parrot fever, ornithosis)** | | | | | | |
| *Chlamydia psittaci*; susceptible species: primary reservoirs are birds (common in psittacines, pigeons, sea/shore birds, poultry, waterfowl) | Severity ranges from mild, flulike illness to death; may include flulike symptoms, pneumonitis, pneumonia, myocarditis, encephalitis, thrombophlebitis | Acute or latent carriers (intermittently shedding infective organisms); stress induces disease/shedding; may include depression, anorexia, ocular/nasal discharge, dyspnea, diarrhea (green) | Fecal-oral route; inhalation/ingestion of infected aerosolized fecal matter | Cloacal/fecal culture and isolation, serological testing (collected 2 wk apart) | Antibiotic (AB) therapy | Quarantine/detection/treatment of infected animals, protective clothing, dampen cage floor before cleaning (to reduce aerosolization) |
| **Bacillus anthracis** | | | | | | |
| *Bacillus anthracis*; susceptible species; all mammals, most birds | Three clinical presentations: cutaneous, intestinal, pulmonary; disseminated septicemia and/or meningitis may occur; disseminated septicemia is rapidly fatal if untreated | Three clinical presentations: peracute, acute, subacute/chronic | Direct contact with infected animal or animal products; insect vectors and contaminated water possible | Culture/isolation, microscopic identification | Human: AB therapy; Animal: AB therapy (effective early in disease) | Vaccines available for humans and animals; disinfection/sterilization of animal products; do not perform necropsy on suspected cases; incinerate or bury deeply and cover carcass with quicklime |
| **BRUCELLOSIS (Bang's disease, undulant fever)** | | | | | | |
| *Brucella* spp.; susceptible species: most mammals; common in cattle, dog | Clinical presentation, from latent to chronic, may include flulike symptoms, fatigue, weight loss, depression, meningitis, encephalitis, endocarditis; common in vocationally high-risk persons | Varied, may include abortion, retained placenta, mastitis, fistulous withers, arthritis, orchitis, lymphadenopathy, sterility | Direct contact with infected animals or animal products; humans are always accidental hosts | Culture/isolation, serum agglutination, ELISA, CF (most reliable) | AB therapy | Test/slaughter, vaccinate cows and calves, protective clothing, good sanitation/hygiene, proper food handling |

| | Clinical signs (humans) | Clinical signs (animals) | Transmission | Diagnosis | Treatment | Prevention |
|---|---|---|---|---|---|---|
| **CAMPYLOBACTERIOSIS (vibriosis)** | | | | | | |
| Campylobacter spp.; susceptible species: most species, common in birds | May include: abdominal pain, acute (possibly bloody) diarrhea for 3-5 days; spontaneous recovery is common, without AB therapy; latent carriers may result | May include: 3-7 days of watery, mucoid, or bloody diarrhea; anorexia; abortions; spontaneous recovery with or without AB therapy; may become latent carriers | Fecal-oral contact, contaminated water, infected food products (animal and vegetable) | Culture/isolation, cytological examination of feces | AB therapy—does not shorten clinical course of disease, but eliminates carrier state | Primarily good sanitation/hygiene |
| **Capnocytophaga canimorsus INFECTIONS** | | | | | | |
| Capnocytophaga canimorsus; susceptible species: primarily dog and cat | Can be asymptomatic or self-limiting, but may present as nonspecific febrile illness that frequently progresses to a severe septicemia; DIC, cellulitis, endocarditis, renal failure and gangrene may occur | No signs in animals; C. canimorsus may be a commensal organism in dog and cat | Directly, or indirectly transmitted by domestic dogs through bites or scratches; domestic cats have also been indicated in transmission | Clinical presentation/ appropriate history, culture/ isolation, serology, cytological identification | AB therapy (usually penicillin) | Prevention of bites and scratches, thorough cleaning/irrigation of all bites, immediate medical attention if fever or cellulitis develops |
| **CAT SCRATCH DISEASE (cat scratch fever)** | | | | | | |
| Multiple bacterial species have been implicated; examples: Afipia felis, Bartonella henselae, Pasteurella multocida; susceptible species: primarily cat | Primarily in children <12 yr; may include identifiable primary inoculatory lesion, regional lymphadenopathy, flu-like symptoms, anorexia, osteolytic lesions, oculoglandular syndrome | Cats display few if any clinical signs; endocarditis, usually self-limiting with no recurrence in recovered patients | Directly or indirectly transmitted by domestic cats (bacilli may be normal oral flora, transmitted to claws during grooming), usually transmitted through bite/scratch. Most commonly from male, intact cats (<1 yr), with fleas, not declawed, and indoor/outdoor access | Clinical presentation/appropriate history, primary inoculatory lesion, positive Hangar-Rose skin test, culture/ isolation | Usually self-resolving but may require AB therapy | Declaw young cats; owners should not allow cats to lick their (owners') open wounds; good sanitation/hygiene; handle cats gently to prevent bites/scratches |

*Continued*

**Table 28-1** Bacterial zoonoses—cont'd

| Etiology | Symptoms—human | Symptoms—animal | Transmission | Diagnosis | Treatment | Prevention control |
|---|---|---|---|---|---|---|
| | | | **ERYSIPELOTHRIX INFECTION** | | | |
| *Erysipelothrix rhusiopathiae*; susceptible species: pig, wild and domestic fowl | Cutaneous infection known as erysipeloid on fingers and hands; raised lesions accompanied by severe pain and swelling | Acute, subacute or chronic; septicemia; raised, reddish purple, rhomboidal lesions (diamond skin disease) Chronic; may cause arthritis, endocarditis, and death | Occupational exposure via scratches, abrasions, or puncture wounds | Culture/isolation | AB therapy | Good sanitation/hygiene |
| | | | **LEPTOSPIROSIS (Weil's disease, Fort Bragg fever)** | | | |
| *Leptospira* spp.; susceptible species: wide variety mammals/ reptiles, but rodents are a primary reservoir | Incubation 1-2 wk, duration 1-7 days; may include flulike symptoms, jaundice, anuria, rash, conjunctivitis, liver/kidney failure, death | Three clinical presentations: acute hemorrhagic, subacute, subclinical; acute/subacute may include high fever, septicemia, anorexia, depression, icterus, hemolytic anemia, endotoxemia, abortion, mastitis, infertility | Contact with infective urine, contaminated water/soil, direct contact with infected animals | Culture/isolation (blood, urine), microagglutination and macroagglutination, ELISA | AB therapy: treatment or prophylactic | Protective clothing, rodent control, good sanitation/hygiene, avoid contaminated water sources, vaccination (moderately effective) |
| | | | **LISTEROSIS** | | | |
| *Listeria* spp.; susceptible species: many mammals, fowl, fish (common in ruminants) | Several clinical presentations: depends on route of infection; may include dermal lesions, enteritis, septicemia, encephalitis, abortion/ stillbirth, birth of infected neonates | May include diarrhea, flulike symptoms, excessive salivation, mastitis, monocytosis, septicemia, purulent/necrotic lesions of visceral organs/lymph nodes, abortion/ stillbirth, encephalitis | Exposure to infected animal/ bird products, contaminated silage/vegetables | Culture/isolation | AB therapy | Good sanitation/hygiene, protective clothing |

| | | | | | | |
|---|---|---|---|---|---|---|
| **PLAGUE** | | | | | | |
| *Yersinia* spp.; susceptible species: chief reservoirs are rodents, birds, lagomorphs; also common in carnivores | Three main clinical presentations: bubonic (acute), septicemic, pneumonic; may include acute fever, painful lymphadenitis, anorexia, flulike symptoms, dyspnea, fatigue | May include: fever, lymphadenitis/abscess formation; some species may show high mortality rates | Flea bites, direct contact with infected animals, inhalation of aerosolized contaminants | Culture/isolation, IFA, serological testing | AB therapy | Rodent/flea control, protective clothing, good sanitation/hygiene |
| **COXIELLOSIS (Q fever)** | | | | | | |
| *Coxiella burnetii*; susceptible species: cattle, sheep, goat; many other mammals can be carriers | Acute febrile disease, respiratory involvement, flulike symptoms, pneumonia, meningoencephalitis and cardiac involvement; most cases are mild and self-limiting; if left untreated, causes fatal endocarditis | Asymptomatic, although sometimes causes abortion | Inhalation of aerosol spores from infected birth fluid and ruminant placentae; wool or hides; unpasteurized milk from infected animals can lead to human infection | Serological testing | AB therapy | Avoid contact with infected animals |
| **SALMONELLOSIS (enteric fever)** | | | | | | |
| *Salmonella* spp.; susceptible species: almost all species (especially prevalent in reptiles) | Incubation: 6-72 hr; primarily presents as acute gastroenteritis; may also include focal infections, chronic rheumatoid conditions, colitis, autoimmune disorders, chronic enteric hyperplastic/inflammatory conditions; shedding of infected organisms occurs for days to weeks | Four clinical presentations: subclinical, acute enteritis, subacute enteritis, chronic enteritis  Acute: may include high fever, explosive diarrhea (possibly bloody), depression, death within 48 hr  Chronic: may include mild symptoms, low-moderate fever, soft feces/mild diarrhea, abortion | Primarily fecal-oral route; commonly found in beef and poultry products; unthrifty appearance; stress can induce shedding of infective organisms | Clinical presentation/ appropriate history, culture/ isolation | AB therapy | Good sanitation/hygiene; proper cooking/handling of beef/poultry products; do not bathe animals or wash cage items in kitchen or bathroom sink |

*Continued*

**Table 28-1** Bacterial zoonoses—cont'd

| Etiology | Symptoms—human | Symptoms—animal | Transmission | Diagnosis | Treatment | Prevention control |
|---|---|---|---|---|---|---|
| | | | **TUBERCULOSIS (TB)** | | | |
| *Mycobacteria* spp.; susceptible species: most species | Two clinical presentations: acute, chronic Acute: may include acute miliary TB meningitis, secondary infections Chronic: may include pulmonary/bone/joint lesions, meningitis, genitourinary infections, cervical lymphadenitis | May include lymphadenopathy, lesions/granulomas of organs, anorexia, weakness, weight loss, coughing/dyspnea, pleural pneumonia, death; latent carrier state is common | Primarily fecal-oral route; ingestion of contaminated food products; contact with infected tissues/animal products | Reaction to interdermal tuberculin test(s), culture/isolation | Human: anti-TB drug therapy/prophylaxis (for known exposure) | Intradermal tuberculin testing (animals and vocationally high-risk persons), animal test/cull programs, proper preparation/handling of food |
| | | | **TULAREMIA (rabbit fever)** | | | |
| *Francisella tularensis*; susceptible species: many species of vertebrates/invertebrates | Incubation 2-3 days; several clinical presentations, depending on route of infection: ulceroglandular, typhoidal, oculoglandular, glandular, tularemic pneumonia | Usually manifests as septicemia (may show high mortality rates), heavy tick infestation may be concurrent | Blood/tissue of infected animals, fluids/feces of infected ticks, bites from infected ticks | Culture/isolation, FA testing, serology (later in disease) | AB therapy | Protective clothing, tick control, sanitation/hygiene |

**Table 28-2** Rickettsial zoonoses

| Etiology | Symptoms—human | Symptoms—animal | Transmission | Diagnosis | Treatment | Prevention control |
|---|---|---|---|---|---|---|
| | | | **EHRLICHIOSIS** | | | |
| *Ehrlichia* spp.; susceptible species: primarily canids | May include acute fever, flulike symptoms, leukopenia | Three clinical presentations: acute, subacute, chronic; thrombocytopenia, elevated hepatic enzyme activity (especially aspartate amino-transferase, alanine amino-transferase) May include fever, anorexia, depression, lymphadenopathy, thrombocytopenia, "fading puppy syndrome" | Primarily bite from an infected tick, also oral (splashed, infective urine), placental transmission | Clinical presentation/ appropriate history, IFA, isolation from tissues | Antibiotic (AB) therapy | Use of protective clothing, tick repellents, preven-tion of prolonged tick attachment, environmental tick treatment, treat-ment of pets for ticks, vaccine available |
| | | | **LYME BORRELIOSIS (Lyme disease)** | | | |
| *Borrelia burgdorferi*; susceptible species: variety of wild/domestic animals | Three stages First stage: "bull's eye" red lesion (usually at site of tick bite), maculopapular/ petechial/vesicular rashes, flulike symptoms Second stage: duration 3 days– 6 wk, meningitis, encephalitis, cardiac complications, musculoskeletal pain Third stage (months to years later): central nervous system (CNS) involvement, arthritis, chronic dermatological complications | May include: fever, arthralgia, arthritis, lameness, CNS involve-ment, encephalitis, abortion | Primarily bite from an infected tick, also oral (splashed, infective urine), placental transmission | Clinical presenta-tion/history of tick exposure, culture/ isolation, IFA and ELISA available but false positive/ negative results have been reported | AB therapy | Use of protective clothing, tick repellents, preven-tion of prolonged tick attachment, environmental tick treatment, treat-ment of pets for ticks, vaccine available |

*Continued*

**Table 28-2** Rickettsial zoonoses—cont'd

| Etiology | Symptoms—human | Symptoms—animal | Transmission | Diagnosis | Treatment | Prevention control |
|---|---|---|---|---|---|---|
| **ROCKY MOUNTAIN SPOTTED FEVER** | | | | | | |
| *Rickettsia* spp.; susceptible species: variety of wild/domestic animals | May include abdominal pain, flulike symptoms, rash on palms/soles, CNS abnormalities, hepatomegaly, jaundice, myocarditis, meningo-encephalitis, DIC | Similar to human course of disease | Primarily bite from an infected tick, also oral (splashed, infective urine), placental transmission | Clinical presentation/appropriate history, CF and micro-IFA (false positive is rare but false negative occurs) | AB therapy | Use of protective clothing, tick repellents, prevention of prolonged tick attachment, environmental tick treatment, treatment of pets for ticks, vaccine available |

**Table 28-3** Viral zoonoses

| Etiology | Symptoms—human | Symptoms—animal | Transmission | Diagnosis | Treatment | Prevention control |
|---|---|---|---|---|---|---|
| **ARBOVIRAL ENCEPHALITIS (sleeping sickness)** | | | | | | |
| Family Arboviridae; examples: eastern equine encephalomyelitis, western equine encephalomyelitis, Venezuelan equine encephalomyelitis, St. Louis encephalitis; susceptible species: many bird/wild animals (primarily rodent) reservoirs, common in equines | Usually biphasic First phase may include headache/high fever, which may abate before disease progresses Second phase (encephalitic): cervical stiffness, nausea/vomiting, disorientation, frequent progression to coma/convulsions | Symptoms vary but may include fever, depression, impaired vision, irregular gait, wandering, incoordination, slowed reflexes, facial/general paralysis, death | Viral reservoir is maintained by mosquito vectors | Culture/isolation, serological testing | Antibiotic (AB) therapy and antiviral therapy in humans | Avoid bite of mosquitoes; use protective screening/clothing; liberal use of insect repellent; use of vaccines |

**AVIAN INFLUENZA (bird flu): INFLUENZA A, SUBTYPE H5N1**

| | | | | | |
|---|---|---|---|---|---|
| Family Orthomyxoviridae; susceptible species: all birds, especially wild waterfowl, migrating species, and poultry; mammals include exotic felids, swine, hoofstock, whales, seals | Fever, malaise, bone pain, blood stained sputum, diarrhea, shortness of breath, elevated alanine aminotransferase, decreased lymphocyte count, coagulopathy, rapidly progressive pneumonia, severe adult respiratory distress syndrome with multiorgan failure, death (approaching 70%+ human mortality)  Wide spectrum of symptoms, ranging from asymptomatic/mild illness to a highly pathogenic avian influenza (highly contagious, severe and rapidly fatal, with mortality approaching 100%) with coughing, sneezing, excessive lacrimation, cyanosis of unfeathered skin, cranial edema, ruffled feathers, diarrhea, nervous system disorders, sudden death (often with no clinical signs) | Close human contact with domestic poultry 3-7 days before illness; possible limited aerosol transmission human-to-human (primarily patient to healthcare workers); exposure to wild, infected birds' respiratory secretion/saliva/feces; spread among domestic poultry farms via contaminated birds or inanimate vectors; virus can survive several months in feces, 4-30 days in water, and indefinitely in frozen material | RT-PCR; viral culture from nasopharyngeal aspirates, monoclonal AB-based immunofluorescent assay; serology of paired samples (days 1-3 and days 10-14) showing a $\geq 4\times$ AB increase | In humans: neuraminidase inhibitors (oseltamivir and zanamivir) as treatment and prophylaxis | Due to natural reservoir species, not able to eradicate virus; continuous surveillance of flu strains in humans and birds; appropriate personal protective equipment; use of human flu vaccine in vocationally high-risk persons (to decrease the possibility of H5N1/human flu hybrid virus mutation); avoid contact with poultry; good personal hygiene; with human patients/samples: minimize aerosol/droplet formation, use of airborne isolation rooms; disinfection: heat sterilization, alcohol, 5% bleach, formalin, iodine compounds; during an outbreak: rapid destruction of the entire domestic poultry population, proper disposal of carcasses, rigorous disinfection of farms, mandated quarantine, testing before importation, restrict movement of live poultry, removal of all ducks, geese, and quail from retail markets, monthly market "clean days" (empty and disinfect all bird areas simultaneously) |

*Continued*

**Table 28-3** Viral zoonoses—cont'd

| Etiology | Symptoms—animal | Symptoms—human | Transmission | Diagnosis | Treatment | Prevention control |
|---|---|---|---|---|---|---|
| | | | **HERPES B VIRAL INFECTION** | | | |
| *Herpesvirus simiae*; susceptible species: primarily macaque species (principally rhesus) | Chiefly gingivostomatitis with buccal mucosal lesions; asymptomatic infection is believed to be common | Causes an ascending encephalitis that is usually fatal; those who survive often have severe, permanent neurological damage; symptoms usually occur within 30 days of exposure; may include vesicular skin lesions, localized neurological symptoms, regional lymphadenopathy, fever, headaches, ataxia, encephalitis, death—usually 2-3 days after onset of clinical signs | Primarily by exposure to infected monkey saliva/tissues | Culture/isolation, serological testing | Thoroughly clean/disinfect all primate bite/scratch wounds; immediately report any rash/itching/ numbness at wound site; evidence suggests that early administration of acyclovir may aid recovery | Thoroughly clean/disinfect all bites/scratches; use protective clothing, liberal use of chemical/ mechanical restraint |
| | | | **NEWCASTLE DISEASE** | | | |
| An RNA virus, paramyxovirus; especially susceptible species: primarily poultry, also wild birds | Respiratory: gasping, coughing Central nervous system: drooping wings, twisted neck, paralysis, depression, anorexia Viscerotropic: acute watery, green diarrhea, facial edema, tracheal exudate, necrosis of intestinal mucosa, high mortality rate associated with this type | Conjunctivitis, swelling of subconjunctival tissues; occasionally systemic with flu-like symptoms, lymphadenitis of the lymph nodes in front of the ear | Virus can be aerosolized or passed in feces; improper handling/use of vaccine | Viral isolation from tracheal exudate, lung or spleen; serological testing | Usually self-resolving in humans | Good hygiene, vaccinate flocks with a live lentogenic vaccine; use care when handling live vaccine, use mask/eye protection, avoid creating aerosols when cleaning or when handling vaccine |

## POXVIRAL DISEASE (contagious ecthyma, bovine papular stomatitis, pseudopox)

| | | | | | | |
|---|---|---|---|---|---|---|
| Family Poxviridae | Usually progressive, localized skin lesions, may progress to cellular proliferation/necrosis | Same course as human | Direct contact (usually through dermal abrasion) | Clinical presentation/appropriate history, culture/isolation, CF, IFA | AB therapy for secondary bacterial infection | Use of protective clothing, use of vaccines |

## RABIES (hydrophobia, "mad" dog disease)

| | | | | | | |
|---|---|---|---|---|---|---|
| Rhabdovirus; susceptible species: all mammals (common in skunk, bat, dog, cat, horse) | Incubation 9 days–2+ yr, clinical course usually 2-8 days; may include anxiety, hyperesthesia, hyperactivity, aerobia, increased salivation, laryngopharyngeal muscular spasms, convulsions, coma, and ultimately death | Two stages. First stage: duration 1-6 days, may include behavioral changes (unusual friendliness/aggression), excitability, altered vocalizations. Second stage: duration 1-4 days, progressive paralysis and death | Primarily contamination of a wound (bite, abrasion) by infected saliva; ingestion/mucosal contact with infected saliva | Clinical presentation/appropriate history, IFA (optimal recovery from hippocampus, brain stem, cerebellum) | Practice prophylactic treatment | Immunization of applicable species, preexposure prophylaxis for vocationally high-risk persons |

## WEST NILE VIRUS

| | | | | | | |
|---|---|---|---|---|---|---|
| A flavivirus; susceptible species: wild birds, especially crows, jays, geese, birds of prey, domestic equids, also domestic dog and cat, bears, crocodiles, alligators, bats | Most are asymptomatic; acute illness, fever, dysphagia/anorexia, convulsions, paralysis, and death | Many are asymptomatic; acute illness, fever, headaches, fever, headaches, and myalgia, often with roseolar/macopapular rash and regional lymphadenitis; severe encephalic infection may show high fever, cervical stiffness, disorientation, convulsions, paralysis, coma, or death (3%-15%) | Viral reservoirs maintained by mosquito vectors, primarily Culex spp. In wild bird populations, ticks have been found infected with virus, but their role in disease maintenance and transmission is uncertain | Culture/isolation, serological testing, MAC-ELISA, histopathology, PCR (tissues) | There is no specific therapy, intensive supportive therapy, AB therapy to prevent secondary infection, good nursing care | Avoid mosquito bites, use protective screening/clothing, liberal use of insect repellant, wear gloves when handling/cleaning game birds, cook wild game thoroughly, conditional vaccine for domestic equine use, human vaccine, human blood product screening |

**Table 28-4** Parasitic zoonoses

| Etiology | Symptoms—human | Symptoms—animal | Transmission | Diagnosis | Treatment | Prevention control |
|---|---|---|---|---|---|---|
| **ANCYLOSTOMIASIS (hookworm disease) (cutaneous larval migrans)** | | | | | | |
| Many species of hookworms may infect man and animals; susceptible species: most species | May include bloody diarrhea, anemia (which may lead to tachycardia, heart failure, hypoproteinemia, ascites), cutaneous infection, dermatitis, generalized edema, regional lymphadenitis, pneumonitis, corneal opacities | May include anemia, dark/tarry stools, dehydration, emaciation; fatalities are common in young animals | Fecal-oral route, cutaneous penetration by larvae | Ova on fecal flotation, clinical presentation/ appropriate history | Anthelmintic therapy | Good sanitation/ hygiene; treat infected animals; cover sandboxes; use protective clothing |
| **CRYPTOSPORIDIOSIS** | | | | | | |
| Cryptosporidium parvum (coccidian protozoan parasite); susceptible species: cattle, cat, and other domestic animals | Profuse, watery diarrhea with abdominal cramps, symptoms may recur, but is often self-limiting; resolution usually occurs within 30 days, but can be fatal | Often subclinical in adult animals, newborns/juveniles usually demonstrate profuse diarrhea | Primarily fecal-oral route | Detection of oocysts from feces, histopathology, ELISA, and an immunofluorescence test | No specific therapy; supportive therapy and nursing care | Good sanitation and hygiene, thorough disinfection procedures |
| **SARCOPTIC MANGE (scabies)** | | | | | | |
| Sarcoptes scabei mite; susceptible species: many species | Intensely pruritic dermal lesions, may develop alopecia/skin crusting/skin thickening, peripheral lymphadenopathy | Same as human | Direct contact with infested animal | Visualization of mites/ ova from skin scraping | Anthelmintic therapy | Treat infected animals, protective clothing, regular washing/changing of animal bedding, prophylactic ivermectin |
| **TAPEWORM INFECTION (low pathogenicity): MULTIPLE SPECIES** | | | | | | |
| Dipylidium spp., Taenia spp., Hymenolepis spp.; susceptible species: most species | Common in very young children, symptoms usually mild; may include abdominal discomfort, diarrhea, pruritus, anemia, weight loss | Migrating proglottids may cause anal irritation; may include weight loss, unthrifty appearance | Ingesting infected fleas or proglottids/ova | Primarily by presence of proglottids on feces/perianally (rarely observed on fecal flotation) | Anthelmintic therapy | Flea control; treat infected animals; good sanitation/ hygiene |

**TAPEWORM INFECTION (high pathogenicity)**

| Agent / Susceptible species | Clinical signs | Transmission | Diagnosis | Treatment | Prevention |
|---|---|---|---|---|---|
| *Echinococcus* spp.; susceptible species: many species (common in dog, cat, rodents) Predator-prey cycle: predator species are the definitive hosts, prey species are intermediate hosts, human is (accidental) intermediate host | Alveolar hydatid disease; progressive onset of symptoms may include epigastric pain, malaise, progressive jaundice, hepatomegaly, hepatic cysts | See Tapeworm Infection (Low Pathogenicity) | Because of small size of proglottids, very difficult to detect on or in feces, indistinguishable ova (from other cestodes) | Animals: anthelmintic therapy Humans: surgical excision of cysts | See Tapeworm Infection (Low Pathogenicity) |

**TOXOCARIASIS (visceral larval migrans [VLM], ocular larval migrans [OLM])**

| Agent / Susceptible species | Clinical signs | Transmission | Diagnosis | Treatment | Prevention |
|---|---|---|---|---|---|
| *Toxocara* spp.; susceptible species: most species | VLM: larval migration through somatic tissues; may include fever, hepatomegaly, bronchiolitis, asthma, pneumonitis, central nervous system <br> Usually inapparent in adults (larval encystation in tissues); in young may include diarrhea, dehydration, intestinal distention/obstruction, exaggerated immunological response OLM: larva enter into orbit of the eye, usually no other signs | Fecal-oral (2-wk incubation period) | Ova found on fecal flotation, clinical presentation, appropriate history, ELISA | Anthelmintic therapy | Good sanitation/hygiene, treat infected animals |

**TOXOPLASMOSIS**

| Agent / Susceptible species | Clinical signs | Transmission | Diagnosis | Treatment | Prevention |
|---|---|---|---|---|---|
| *Toxoplasma gondii*; susceptible species: most species, but cat is definitive and intermediate host | Most adults show subclinical symptoms, but may include flulike symptoms, transient cervical lymphadenopathy, myocarditis, splenomegaly, hepatomegaly, encephalitis, retinochoroiditis; congenital infections may manifest a subclinical or clinical presentation of variable severity; fatalities do occur | Fecal-oral, ingestion of improperly cooked meats; congenital-transplacental transmission | Leukocytosis, eosinophilia, observation/isolation of tachyzoites from blood/tissues, Sabin-Feldman dye test, IFA, CF, ELISA, oocyst identification from fecal flotation (requires sporulation) | Anticoccidial anthelmintic therapy | Proper handling/preparation of food, keep pet cats indoors (reduce hunting opportunities), clean litter box regularly (ova require 3+ days incubation before infective), good sanitation/hygiene, gloves when cleaning litter box/gardening, cover sandboxes |

*Continued*

**Table 28-5** Mycotic zoonoses

| Etiology | Symptoms—human | Symptoms—animal | Transmission | Diagnosis | Treatment | Prevention control |
|---|---|---|---|---|---|---|
| | | **DERMATOPHYTOSIS (ringworm, dermatomycosis)** | | | | |
| Most common: *Microsporum* spp., *Trichophyton* spp.; susceptible species: most common in young mammals | Incubation 1-2 wk; superficial infections of skin/hair/nails; acute inflammatory reaction; lesions usually papulosquamous with circular/reddened borders (but may be dry/alopecic or moist/eczematous lesions) | Lesions are usually circular/crusty, with or without redness/ alopecia | Direct contact with an infected animal (or its hair, skin, leashes/brushes), equipment, or contaminated soil | Dermatophyte/ mycological culture/ isolation, ultraviolet fluorescence (Wood's lamp), biopsy/cytology | Topical/oral antifungal therapy, vaccine (limited use) | Protective clothing, good sanitation/ hygiene, treat infected animals |
| | | **SYSTEMIC MYCOSES** | | | | |
| Most common: *Histoplasma* spp., *Coccidioides* spp., *Blastomyces* spp., *Cryptococcus* spp.; susceptible species: most species | Usually begin as pulmonary infection with fever/myalgia/ congestion; may progress into chronic/ granulomatous pneu- monia or disseminate to other organs; may develop into subacute or chronic meningoen- cephalitis | Similar to course of disease in human | Usually aerosolized organisms (fecal/ infective soil) | Culture/isolation, ELISA | Antifungal therapy | Protective clothing (when handling infected animals or cleaning their pens/supplies) |

**Table 28-6** Prion/Transmissible Spongiform Encephalopathy Zoonosis

| Etiology | Symptoms—human | Symptoms—animal | Transmission | Diagnosis | Treatment | Prevention control |
|---|---|---|---|---|---|---|
| **BOVINE SPONGIFORM ENCEPHALOPATHY (mad cow disease/Creuzfeldt-Jakob disease)** | | | | | | |
| Prion infection; susceptible species: cattle, sheep, goats, deer, exotic hoofstock | Incubation varies from months to decades; once symptoms develop, disorder is usually fatal within 1 yr; rapidly progressive dementia/cognitive imbalance, psychiatric/behavioral abnormalities, coordination deficits, myoclonus, distinct triphasic and polyphasic electrocardiogram readings; noninflammatory pathological process of the central nervous system | Similar to course of disease in humans, plus hypersensitivity, nervousness, high-stepping gait, anorexia/weight loss, pruritus, excessive licking, ataxia; other transmissible spongiform encephalopathies: scrapie in sheep and goats, exotic encephalopathy, chronic wasting disease in mule deer and elk, feline/bovine encephalopathy | In animals: consumption of prion infected/contaminated rendered foodstuffs/tissues; transplacental; evidence of genetic susceptibility In humans: consumption of prion infected meat (primarily beef); direct inoculation; implantation or transplantation of infected materials/tissue | No reliable lab tests, only histological exam of brain tissue (florid amyloid plaque formation, presence of spongiform lesions) | No specific therapy available for prion disease at this time; all cases are fatal | Feed bans of animal tissue to food animals; selective DNA guides breeding programs; test/slaughter cattle; use of disposable surgical instruments; prions exhibit unusual resistance to conventional and physical decontamination methods; successful disinfection protocols include: 1 N NaOH, steam sterilization at 100°-121° C (212°-250° F) with exposure to formalin/formic acid solution, 0.09 N NaOH for 2 hr with steam sterilization at 121° C (250° F) for 1 hr |

## Glossary

**acute** An abrupt, brief onset of serious or severe symptoms that are rapidly progressive and need urgent care

**anthelmintic** Chemical agent that destroys, kills, or expels parasites

**CF** Complement fixation (test)

**chronic** Symptoms with virtually no change, of indefinite duration, generally lasting 3 months or more

**clinical** Showing signs

**commensal** Two nonparasitic organisms that live together; one benefits from the association whereas the other is neither benefited nor harmed

**DIC** Disseminated intravascular coagulation

**dysphagia** Difficulty swallowing

**ELISA** Enzyme-linked immunosorbent assay (test)

**epidemiology** Scientific study of the factors that influence the incidence, distribution, and control of infectious diseases

**FA** Fluorescent antibody assay (test)

**flulike symptoms** Usually sudden onset of fever, shivering, headache, myalgia, and malaise

**IFA** Indirect fluorescent antibody assay (test)

**latent carrier** State where disease-causing organisms are present but clinical disease symptoms are not manifested

**lentogenic vaccine** Only marginally virulent

**miliary TB** Disseminated tuberculosis, usually manifested by small, millet seed–sized nodules

**myalgia** Muscle pain

**mycotic** Relating to fungi or vegetating microorganisms

**myoclonus** Involuntary twitching/jerking of the limbs

**peracute** Very acute onset of severe, violent symptoms of a short duration

**petechial** Minute, pinpoint hemorrhaging

**prion** A unique class of pathogens that are associated with the genetic mutation of a host cellular protein; a proteinaceous infectious agent

**proglottids** Cestode segments that contain fertile, infective oocytes

**pruritic** Itchy

**reservoir** Alternative host or a pathogenic agent

**roseolar rash** Red rash that develops primarily on the neck and trunk

**RT-PCR** Reverse transcriptase–polymerase chain reaction

**spongiform** Having or developing vacuoles/holes

**subacute** Rather recent onset or somewhat rapid change of symptoms; between acute and chronic in duration

**subclinical** Without clinical manifestations; the early signs or stages of a mild form of a disease

**typhoidal** Symptoms marked by sustained high fever, severe headache, and a rash

**undulant** To fluctuate in wavelike patterns

**vector** Carrier, usually an arthropod, that transfers an infective agent from one host to another

**VLM** Visceral larval migrans

## Review Questions

1 Most infectious organisms have certain species that are preferred hosts. Which statement is most true about infectious organisms?
   a. They will always invade any animal, regardless of the immune status of that individual
   b. They will never invade outside their preferred host species
   c. They may invade outside their normally preferred hosts if an individual is sufficiently immunocompromised
   d. If an individual is immunocompromised, an infectious organism will always invade the preferred host

2 The rhabdovirus that causes hydrophobia is not capable of infecting a/an _____ patient
   a. Canine
   b. Equine
   c. Avian
   d. Feline

3 Antibiotic therapy would be indicated for a patient who has
   a. Visceral larval migrans
   b. Rabies
   c. Salmonellosis
   d. Toxoplasmosis

4 Echinococcal
   a. Proglottids are identical to the *Taenia* spp. proglottids
   b. Ova are indistinguishable from those of other species of cestodes
   c. Human infestations are treated with anthelmintic therapy
   d. Infection in humans is considered benign

5 Ringworm infection
   a. Is caused by a small parasite
   b. Affects only cats
   c. Commonly occurs in healthy adult animals
   d. Is treated with a regimen of antifungal agents (topical and/or oral)

6 Cat scratch disease can be prevented in part by
   a. Allowing a cat to lick open wounds, thus raising antibody levels
   b. Administering a vaccine to cats
   c. Administering a vaccine to humans
   d. Declawing young cats and handling them gently

7 Salmonellosis
   a. Is transmitted by flea bites
   b. Can be prevented with yearly vaccination
   c. Is not commonly shed by latent carriers
   d. Can be transmitted in food products such as chicken or eggs

8 In humans, the first stage of Lyme disease can be diagnosed by the presence of a characteristic lesion. The lesion is similar to a/an
   a. Bull's eye
   b. Mosquito bite
   c. Red rash
   d. Area of petechiae

**9** Psittacosis can be contracted only from _____ species
  a. Bovine
  b. Avian
  c. Ovine
  d. Equine

**10** A preventive flea program is an important factor in controlling _____ infestations
  a. *Toxascaris*
  b. Toxoplasmosis
  c. *Sarcoptes* spp.
  d. *Taenia* spp.

## BIBLIOGRAPHY

Apisarnthanarak A et al: *Atypical avian influenza (H5N1),* Emerg Infect Dis 10:1321, 2004.

August JR: *Zoonosis updates,* ed 2, Schaumberg, Ill, 1995, American Veterinary Medical Association.

Benenson AS: Cryptococcosis. In Benenson AS, editor: *Control of communicable diseases manual,* Washington, DC, 1995, American Public Health Association.

Bonagura J, editor: *Kirk's current veterinary therapy, XIII: small animal practice,* Philadelphia, 1999, Saunders.

Bowman DD: *Georgis' parasitology for veterinarians,* ed 8, St Louis, 2003, Saunders.

Brown P et al: Bovine spongiform encephalopathy and variant Creutzfeldt-Jakob disease: background, evolution and current concerns, *Emerg Infect Dis* 7:6, 2001.

Clark WH, Dawkins B, Audin JH: *Zoonosis updates,* Schaumberg, Ill, 1990, American Veterinary Medical Association.

Colville JL, Berryhill DL: *Handbook of zoonoses: identification and prevention,* St Louis, 2007, Mosby.

Fowler ME, Miller RE, editors: *Zoo and wild animal medicine,* ed 5, St Louis, 2003, Saunders.

Groves MG, Harrington KS: Zoonoses and public health. In McCurnin DM, Bassert JM, editors: *Clinical textbook for veterinary technicians,* ed 6, St Louis, 2006, Saunders.

Hendrix CM, Sirois M, editors: *Laboratory procedures for veterinary technicians,* ed 5, St Louis, 2007, Mosby.

Howard JL, Smith R, editors: *Current veterinary therapy: food animal practice,* ed 4, Philadelphia, 1998, Saunders.

Hugh-Jones ME, Hubbert WT, Hagstad HV: Newcastle disease. In *Zoonosis: recognition, control and prevention,* Ames, 1995, Iowa State University Press.

Kirk RW, editor: *Kirk's veterinary therapy, small animal practice,* ed 7, Philadelphia, 1995, Saunders.

Morris D: Dealing with avian influenza and other viral infections. *The Sports Journal: The Sport Supplement,* http://www.thesportjournal.org/sport-supplement/vol14no3/05_morris.asp. Accessed July 9, 2007.

Rakel RE, Bope ET, editors: *Conn's current therapy, 2001: latest approved methods of treatment for the practicing physician,* Philadelphia, 2001, Saunders.

Robinson NE, editor: *Current veterinary therapy in equine medicine,* ed 5, St Louis, 2003, Saunders.

Rutala WA, Weber DJ: Creutzfeldt-Jakob disease: recommendations for disinfection and sterilization, *Clin Infect Dis* 32:1348, 2001.

Sampathkumar P: West Nile virus: epidemiology, clinical presentation, diagnosis and prevention, *Mayo Clin Proc* 78:1137, 2003.

Sasaki DM, Katz AR, Middleton CR: *Capnocytophaga* and related infections. In Beran GW, Steele JH, editors: *Handbook of zoonoses,* ed 2, Boca Raton, Fla, 1994, CRC Press.

Sejvar JJ et al: Neurologic manifestations and outcome of West Nile virus infection, *JAMA* 290:511, 2003.

Trampuz A et al: Concise review for clinicians—H5N1 outbreak, *Mayo Clin Proc* 79:523, 2004.

# PART VI

# Practice Management
# and Self-Management

# Personal, Practice, and Professional Management Skills and Ethics

*Monica Dixon Perry*     *Sheila R. Grosdidier*     *Marg Brown*

## OUTLINE

Practice Management Communication
  Overview
  Verbal Communication
  Nonverbal Communication
  Listening
Special Communication Situations
  Client Communication
  Co-Worker Communication
  Written Communication
  Electronic Communication
Practice Management
  Organization Management
  Business Management
  OSHA and WHMIS

Personal Management
  Time Management
  Goals
  Decision Making
  Stress Management
  Coping with Burnout
  Negotiating Conflict Resolution
Career Management
  Personal Finance
  Job Search
  Interview
Marketing
  Internal Marketing
  External Marketing

Professionalism
  Education
Ethics
  History of Ethics
  Personal Ethics
  Professional Ethics
  Professional Association Ethics
Veterinary Technology as a Profession
Professional Organizations
Accomplishments of Veterinary
  Technology
Registration, Licensing, and
  Certification
Summary

## LEARNING OUTCOMES

After reading this chapter you should be able to:

1. Outline the elements of communication, including verbal, written, and electronic.
2. Describe techniques that can increase client communication and communication in the workplace.
3. Define basic management and business principles for hospital managers and employees.
4. List personal management techniques.
5. List career management techniques and personal growth strategies.
6. Describe internal and external marketing strategies.
7. Define *ethics*.
8. Differentiate between professional and personal ethics.
9. Describe why there is a need for professional ethics.
10. List the components of a code of ethics.
11. Identify a personal code of ethics in a mission statement.
12. Describe the ethics of NAVTA and the CAAHTT.
13. Define the purpose of a professional association.
14. Describe and understand the role of a veterinary technician.
15. Describe the role of the veterinary state boards in veterinary technology.

The work environment for many veterinary technicians has changed over the past decade. Now veterinary technicians must not only be skilled in the medical and technical aspects of veterinary medicine but also take responsibility for many of the business decisions that occur in the workplace. For this reason, communication skills, management skills, and marketing have become important tools for the veterinary technician. These skills are also important for personal career planning and professional advancement.

## PRACTICE MANAGEMENT COMMUNICATION ▬
### Overview

Communication is the process individuals or organizations use to create meaning with others.
I. Components of communication
   A. Sender: the sender develops a message or thought that will be conveyed
      1. The message will determine the channel
   B. Receiver: individual who receives the sender's message
   C. Message: thoughts or ideas expressed by the sender
   D. Feedback: response by the receiver as perceived by the sender
      1. Feedback enables the sender to determine how much of the message was accurately understood and interpreted by the receiver
   E. Channels: mechanisms for communication based on the five senses of sight, sound, smell, touch, and taste, including verbal, written, and electronic channels
   F. Interference: any interruption (external or internal) that enters the communication loop
      1. Interruptions can include physical noise, receiver interpretation, incorrect grammar, electronic failure, and body language
   G. Listening: a crucial element of verbal communication
II. Flow of communication
   A. Communication within an organization travels in at least three directions: downward, upward, and horizontal
      1. Downward: information from figures of authority to subordinates, providing instructions related to the task at hand
      2. Upward: information from subordinates to authority figures
      3. Horizontal: communication that takes place among individuals with the same status

### Verbal Communication

Verbal communication is involved in many types of conversations that take place on a daily basis. Effective communication also includes nonverbal elements.

### Nonverbal Communication

I. Definition: The unspoken elements that replace, reinforce, or contradict verbal communication; they include visual, temporal, vocal, and spatial
II. Visual cues include posture, facial expressions, eye contact, and hand gestures, among others
   A. Posture communicates mood of the sender
      1. Upright posture can imply confidence
      2. Slouched posture can indicate insecurity, sadness

   B. Facial expressions are good indicators of how messages are received
   C. Direct eye contact between sender and receiver indicates an open communication channel
      1. Indirect eye contact can imply uneasiness in or a closure of the communication process
   D. Hand gestures such as a handshake or a touch on the arm add meaning to communication
III. Temporal cues are in relation to time of day
   A. Receiving a message the first thing after arriving at work indicates urgency
   B. A message sent at the end of the day with a "see me at your convenience tomorrow" does not indicate the same level of urgency
   C. Timely response indicates a commitment to the message and sender
   D. A failure to respond indicates a lack of interest
IV. Vocal cues are voice qualities that qualify verbal messages. Some vocal cues are pitch, rate, and volume
   A. Voice pitch ranges from low to high
      1. Monotone can imply disinterest in the topic
      2. Varied range or pitch implies enthusiasm and commitment to the topic
      3. A voice pitch inconsistent with the message may indicate incongruence
   B. Rate of speech
      1. Normal speech is 125 to 150 words per minute
      2. Both rapid and slow speech may lose the receiver
   C. Volume of voice
      1. Lack of volume can indicate tension, insecurity, lack of commitment to message
         a. An intentionally low volume can better illustrate a point by forcing the receiver(s) to listen more intently
      2. A volume that is too high can indicate enthusiasm and excitement but also tension and insecurity
V. Spatial cues refer to the use of space often determined by culture, which significantly affects communication
   A. Personal space is the area around oneself, known as the comfort zone
      1. Intrusion into the receiver's personal space can create interference in the message being sent
      2. If a person is leaning away from you as you are speaking, you are probably inside his or her personal space
      3. It is best to be on the same level or plane as the person to whom you are speaking (e.g., both standing, both sitting)
      4. The generally recognized area of personal space is approximately 46 cm to 1.2 m (18 inches to 4 feet)

B. Office space often dictates a professional tone of a communication
   1. If the sender is separated from the receiver by a desk, there is an implied message of an authority/subordinate relationship
   2. This set-up should be reserved for formal conversations, reprimands, and negotiations
   3. Informal conversations are best held in a neutral setting within the office, such as around a small work table or sitting in chairs next to one another

## Listening

Effective communication requires listening capabilities of the sender and the receiver.

I. The listening process requires total concentration on the message being sent

II. Active listening implies that you are aware of both the speaker's words and feelings on a subject. Being attentive to both gives the listener an advantage in truly understanding the message. There are basic principles to active listening
   A. Using words and expressions to encourage the speaker to share information with you freely (being sincere is the key to making the speaker feel he or she can share with you)
   B. Repeating the speaker's message will give him or her confidence that you understand what was said and will encourage him or her to share more
      1. Often referred to as paraphrasing
   C. Perform periodic checks of the message by asking short questions that will clarify a point
   D. Make sure you capture the feelings that are presented along with the message; to make sure you understand, question the speaker by asking, for example, "You are excited about this opportunity?"

III. Barriers to effective listening can be avoided by
   A. Concentrating on the message being sent with a clear, undivided mind
   B. Avoiding judgment of the message sender. Do not let personal and emotional opinions distort the message
   C. Understanding
      1. The mind can process information faster than the words can be spoken
         a. To effectively listen, do not get ahead of the message being sent
   D. Presenting a communication from a supervisor in a way that encourages feedback from subordinates

IV. Better listening requires practice of the following
   A. Do not interrupt the sender while the message is being delivered
   B. Ask for clarification of the message if necessary
   C. Ignore distractions in the environment
   D. Respond to the message; provide feedback

E. Observe the sender's body language to uncover other meanings in the message
F. Do not place personal opinions or preconceived opinions into the message

## SPECIAL COMMUNICATION SITUATIONS ▬▬▬
## Client Communication

Clients are the most important people in any practice. Effective communication is essential. Communication with clients takes place in different ways, such as client education, information gathering, grief counseling, emergency situations, telephone conversations, and dealing with angry/hostile clients.

I. Client education is a vital component of the veterinary technician's role in the hospital
   A. Technicians communicate with the client by describing routine procedures performed on pets using terminology understood by the client
   B. To assist in this communication the technician often develops visual tools, including diagrams, charts, specimens, and newsletters
   C. Special explanations for children can be developed to assist them in understanding procedures performed on their pets
   D. Technicians may be responsible for obtaining information from clients
      1. If detailed answers are required, use open-ended questions
         a. Begin with "What?" "When?" "Where?" "Who?" and "How?"
      2. Ask leading questions only if a yes or no answer is desired
         a. Include "Did it ...?" or "Was it ...?"
         b. Avoid asking leading questions, because a client may feel the need to answer yes or no, even if unsure of the answer
      3. Use active listening techniques

II. Grief counseling is an important communication tool used to help clients deal with grief and emotional pain resulting from the loss of a pet
   A. Listening skills are an essential component of grief counseling
   B. Elizabeth Kübler-Ross, MD, was the first to identify the stages in the grieving process
   C. The six stages of grief a client may experience at various times (not necessarily in order)
      1. Denial—usually the first stage the body goes through to prepare for emotional trauma. During this stage, the client refuses to deal with the pet's condition
         a. The client needs support, understanding, and permission to grieve
         b. Communicate clearly and listen actively, rephrase if necessary and avoid medical jargon

c. Remain nonjudgmental; give client time to move out of the denial stage at his or her own pace

d. Allow client to feel a sense of closure such as viewing the body or saying goodbye

2. Bargaining—often an irrational attempt to reverse or control a situation and may include negotiation with a higher being for the health/life of the pet

a. This phase is not seen as often in pet loss as in the loss of a human

b. It is important to not become defensive and to patiently answer any questions or concerns

3. Anger—often follows denial. The veterinary technician or the veterinarian may be the target of that anger

a. The client may place the blame for the death of the pet on the ones who were entrusted with its medical care

b. It is particularly important not to become defensive or to mirror the anger

c. Give the client permission to vent anger

d. Listen actively by mirroring, maintaining eye contact, using empathetic statements

4. Guilt—often accompanies this stage, so relieve it by assuring the client that the best decision was made

a. Guilt inhibits progress toward resolution

b. Dealing with the guilt is key in moving on

5. Depression—sadness that follows after anger subsides

a. This phase begins and ends at different times for each client

b. Allow clients to express feelings and follow up after the death of the pet

c. Listen actively and empathetically; a touch on the forearm or shoulder may convey compassion

d. Validate normalcy of the client's feelings

e. This may be a good time to encourage memorialization of the pet, such as planting a tree or starting a scrapbook

6. Resolution—when the pet owner accepts the fate of the pet

a. Memories become a comfort rather than a source of sorrow

b. It is during this phase that clients may consider getting another pet

III. Emergency situations require quick assessment and response to patient needs

A. The first key to successfully handling an emergency is to be familiar with the hospital's policies for such situations

1. Know the protocols that the hospital follows

2. Be familiar with the standard recommendations to the clients that the veterinarians prefer that you use

3. You must be prepared technically to be able to "take charge"

B. Assessing the needs of the animal and/or client is the first step once an actual emergency has taken place. This assessment requires that appropriate instructions be given to the client for management of the emergency

1. To determine if you understand the situation, summarize and repeat the client's situation

2. Once you have given directions, ask the client to repeat the instructions back to you and ask if he or she has any questions

C. Clients under stress may not have appropriate listening capabilities, so communications must be short, concise, and without an emotional tone of voice

IV. Telephone conversations with clients are an important means of communication

V. Telephone etiquette includes

A. Use of professional greetings, name of the business, and name of the person answering the telephone

B. The ability to assess the caller's needs (e.g., an emergency)

C. Appropriate voice tones

D. Following rules associated with length of time to keep a client on hold

E. Answering the telephone before a predetermined number of rings, usually a maximum of three

F. Appropriate use of voice mail systems

G. Protocol for taking and returning messages

VI. Communication with angry/hostile clients requires recognizing the potentially hostile situation before it escalates. Considerations include

A. A proper place for conversation with an angry client

B. Disassociation of the problem from the person so that solutions might be more easily seen

C. One of the best ways to diffuse a hostile situation is to use active listening skills

1. Appearing to agree may diffuse the problem

D. Never argue with a dissatisfied client because the client is always right, even when wrong

E. Use conflict resolution techniques. The steps include

1. Recognize and define each piece of the problem

2. Generate ideas to develop a resolution plan

3. Make and implement a decision where everyone wins

4. Evaluate the outcome

F. If the client seems unreasonable, ask the veterinarian to handle the problem as quickly as possible

G. People on drugs or alcohol could become violent and uncontrollable, so be careful

  1. Law enforcement officials may have to be called if substances are used in excess

VII. There are many veterinary grief counseling hotlines and veterinary schools and colleges with grief counseling programs. Other referral sources include the Delta Society

## Co-Worker Communication

Communication with co-workers is the key to success of the team. Positive idea exchange, the act of providing and receiving constructive criticism, is essential.

I. Types of co-worker communication

  A. Supervisor and employee

  B. Employee and supervisor

  C. Employee and employee

II. Mechanisms of positive idea exchange

  A. Communication on work-related issues should focus on identifying the issue with the end result of identifying a solution

    1. The work environment should be conducive and support exchange of information and ideas

  B. Staff meetings provide an open forum for exchange of ideas and should be scheduled regularly

  C. Goals of the practice provide all staff members with a clear understanding of the direction in which the organization is heading

  D. New techniques learned at continuing education meetings or seminars should be shared

  E. Clearly worded manuals containing written policies and protocols, including job responsibilities, should be available

III. Conflict resolution: handling of conflict through appropriate channels within the workplace is essential for their resolution. The following are further pertinent elements of conflict resolution

  A. Face-to-face conversation about a problem allows all parties an opportunity to air opinions

  B. A mediated session can be held where a neutral party is identified and serves as an intermediary to observe, listen, and keep the discussion focused on issues, not individuals

  C. A written grievance can be filed, following steps accepted by the hospital

  D. Staff meetings can be a good source for conflict resolution, because all variables surrounding a conflict can be discussed openly

  E. Conflict can result in positive change in the work environment in the form of constructive criticism or critique of current protocols, techniques

  F. Conflict should be resolved immediately

    1. Waiting provides an opportunity for conflict to build into a larger problem

    2. Immediate handling allows clear memory of the situation by those involved

    3. Waiting too long to address a conflict gives the "injured party" a sense that the problem is not important

## Written Communication

I. Definition: communication through messages delivered in written form. Good writing skills are essential for the veterinary technician

II. The technician will have to communicate in writing with co-workers and other professionals in the form of letters, memos, and reports

III. The technician will communicate with clients and the general public via client information handouts, written take-home directions, hospital newsletters, public education information in newspapers, etc.

IV. Main components of business communications

  A. Audience should be identified and materials tailored to educational/knowledge level

  B. Correct grammar and punctuation are a must

  C. Pitfalls to avoid

    1. Wordiness

    2. Slang terms or expressions

    3. Long words and medical terminology not familiar to the reader

    4. Vague expressions: be concise and direct

    5. Condescending statements

    6. Sexist language

    7. Negative expressions

  D. All written communication should be printed on good-quality paper with attention to appearance of the final document

    1. Typographical errors must be eliminated by repeated proofreading

## Electronic Communication

Also known as telecommunications, electronic communication is a means to transmit voice, data, and images from one location to another through the use of a host of electronic equipment. Computers have become vital in most veterinary practices for the management of information and communication.

I. Patient records, data, financial management, inventory of medical supplies, and communication with colleagues are now performed with computers

II. Software packages specifically designed for veterinary hospitals allow word processing, database management, ordering, and inventory control

III. Electronic communication, such as e-mail, has become popular because of its speed and ease of use

A. Messages are posted in the receiver's electronic mailbox in a fraction of the time of conventional methods

B. E-mail should not take the place of talking about a problem and listening to co-workers about concerns

C. Tips for being a responsible e-mail user
  1. Keep the message short and concise
  2. Always show respect for the person to whom you are sending the message
  3. Refrain from using derogatory terms and inappropriate language
  4. Use appropriate spelling and grammar
  5. Identify the purpose and receiver of the e-mail and draft the message accordingly
  6. Use humor sparingly

D. E-mail provides a written record of your thoughts and ideas
  1. This is a written record so it is important to not state anything in an e-mail that you will later regret

IV. The Internet has revolutionized the way information is disseminated. This has affected veterinary medicine by connecting a once fragmented community. The latest political and scientific information is now as close as your nearest computer

A. Latest information on veterinary related subjects is provided

B. Online discussion or chats also provide continuing education opportunities and the opportunity to network with colleagues thousands of miles away

C. Many places of employment have their own Web pages and podcasts that clients access

V. Telephone systems with multiple features allow better communication with the client

A. On-hold message feature: allows client on hold to listen to messages developed by the veterinary hospital describing available services or facilities

B. Call waiting feature: signals when another call is coming in and can ensure a quicker response to a client's inquiry

C. Conference call option: allows multiple individuals to be included simultaneously in a conversation

D. Cellular telephones: send messages by using radio transmitters. These telephones allow greater mobility and portability for individuals
  1. Can be used to keep communication lines open between the hospital and individuals traveling to clients by vehicle
  2. Also allow access to computer on-line networks for consultations, drug formulas, and new information regarding medical issues in combination with portable computers while in the field

## PRACTICE MANAGEMENT
### Organization Management

Veterinary practice management is the analyzing, planning, evaluating, advising, organizing, supervising, directing, and implementing of policies and procedures for all aspects of a veterinary practice. It also includes the funds and resource management, which includes overseeing the health care team, inventory, and the practice's performance so that the mission and goals of the veterinary practice can be achieved.

I. In veterinary medicine, practice management continues to evolve and is a constant and integral part of a practice's business platform

A. The size of a practice is irrelevant because all practices regardless of size need an active management structure

B. Managing a practice is the driving force for a practice's success

C. Clients search for a progressive, professional, and accommodating facility to not only meet their expectations, but exceed them

D. Veterinary medicine continues to be an industry that is client and patient driven
  1. Constant demands to provide quality medicine to the patients while simultaneously providing superior customer service to their advocates, the clients
    a. A well-managed practice anticipates what is required before clients even know what their needs may be
    b. Pets are usually regarded as family members
      (1) When this relationship is completely understood, the level of commitment and obligation placed on management becomes clear

E. Embracing the idea and acknowledging that practice management is the backbone and the brain center for a practice is essential
  1. Important to keep a solid planning program in place by staying current with the changes in the industry
  2. Must be creative and innovative to assist in the practice's success
  3. A new practice initially has much vision and many goals, but a seasoned practice must maintain this level of enthusiasm and interest

II. Members of a management team are expected to possess the following three key elements: leadership, vision, and communication skills

A. Successful management will support a practice's future growth and development

B. A visionary will focus on the future and have insight into the practice's direction

C. In addition, the day to day operations of a veterinary practice demand excellent leadership and communication skills
  1. How can you lead if you are a ineffective communicator?
  2. What value is an effective communicator if he or she lacks strong leadership and mentoring skills?
D. These skills are so interdependent that if one is absent, the direction of a practice can be greatly compromised
E. Personal discipline and focus are needed to strategically and successfully enhance these skills

III. Within a veterinary hospital, managerial tasks may be delegated to a practice manager, who may be a veterinary technician. The practice manager is involved with four functions
A. Planning: thinking through and making decisions about goals and actions in advance so that objectives can be defined and procedures established
  1. Planning and analyzing the practice are imperative pieces for the continued growth and development of a practice
    a. Planning in a veterinary practice involves the establishment of goals, policies, and procedures
    b. Proper and strategic planning continually facilitates and supports a practice's focus, direction, and ability to obtain its business, patient care, and customer service goals
    c. Clearly identifying and analyzing the vision and direction of a practice relies on sound, concise, and thorough communication between the practice owner(s) and its management team
  2. For a practice to remain successful, constant planning, analyzing, and vision are required and become a fundamental part of the practice's lifeline and existence
    a. The primary reason that clients select a practice is that they hope it will provide quality care for their pets
  3. Each facility should have a mission statement that all employees know and implement
  4. Goals should be established
  5. Policies and procedures becomes essential to support the practice's objectives
    a. Key elements for consistency, continuity, success and unification
    b. They support and help sustain the practice's vision, mission, and philosophy
  6. Policy manual
    a. Provides a written record of organization policies, including those that govern organization-wide actions and those that cover the actions of individuals
    b. Organization-wide activities include history, the organization's purposes and goals, mission statement, policies on community affairs, etc.
    c. Individual activities, or what the employee needs to know
    d. Policies on personnel guidelines, job descriptions of all team members, scheduling, absenteeism, tardiness, injury on the job, impairment on the job, etc.
  7. Procedures manual
    a. Outlines protocols for various procedures performed within an organization, such as surgery, laboratory, or radiology protocols and safety procedures
    b. Helps ensure that all employees adhere to the standards of the organization
    c. Written clearly and provides suggestions on the efficient completion of tasks
    d. Highlights government rules and regulations and quality control measures
    e. Sometimes referred to as SOP (standard operating procedure)
B. Organization: the next step after planning, so that human and material resources of a practice will achieve goals of the organization
  1. Critical to the practice's structure and foundation
  2. Organization commands conformity, which will provide structure and stability within a practice

IV. Lack of stability compromises the quality of care and services provided to a client and also increases the likelihood of a decreased perception of value for both clients and the health care team
A. Leadership: directing and influencing the practice's employees to carry out the organization's objectives
  1. Developing communication and leadership skills is very important and necessary in practice management
  2. The health care team and owner(s) seek daily guidance and direction from the brain center of the practice
  3. Important for management to take speaking and debating courses, read communication enrichment books, attend seminars of leadership
  4. Various skills are important
    a. Supervisory skills: involve the ability to direct a co-worker or subordinate's work to meet goals of the organization
    b. An effective supervisor motivates, provides constructive criticism, and evaluates performance

c. Delegation: formally assigning responsibility for completion of a task to a subordinate
   (1) For delegation to be effective the following rules apply
      (a) Carefully consider who should be given the assignment and which tasks can and should be delegated
      (b) Provide all pertinent information about the responsibility at the time of delegation
      (c) Provide a system for feedback
D. Control: monitoring and evaluating performance
   1. Managing staff or the health care team requires a strong sense of organization and structure
      a. Most problems arise within a veterinary practice because of lack of or inappropriate communication, which often results from inappropriate training procedures
      b. Training and the implementation of phase training programs into the practice is essential
         (1) Phase training programs map out training for the team members, providing structure and guidance, so that the trainer and trainee know what to focus on daily
         (2) The checklist of responsibilities is outlined
            (a) All parties know what is to be expected
            (b) Can be signed off once the training has been completed
   2. The understanding of certain management principles will facilitate efficiency and harmony among the employees. These include, but are not limited to, the following concepts
      a. Teamwork: the result of all members of an organization understanding their roles and working together to accomplish the goals of an organization
         (1) Teamwork is an essential component of the organizational structure
         (2) Each position should have specified tasks based on education and legal limits of the practice
         (3) More efficiency will result if the task is given to the lowest paid qualified worker
   3. Personnel management is important
      a. The ability to properly recruit, hire, and train the health care team is one of the biggest tests for practice management

## Business Management

I. Definition: practices required for the successful financial operation of a facility
II. Time is often a limiting factor, but without proper business policies there would be no practice
III. Properly managing the funds and resources of a practice ensures that the practice remains profitable and runs efficiently
   A. Several factors are important when managing the funds of a practice
      1. Financial management requires a solid accounting background and ability to forecast, budget, and analyze the trends within the practice as well as in the industry
         a. There are daily, monthly, quarterly, and annual obligations placed on members to manage the financial status of a practice
            (1) Monthly analysis should be completed to establish trends, make comparisons of past months and past years, note immediate changes, and review fees, inventory comparisons, and credit policies
         b. Assessing and interpreting data generated from the practice's veterinary software provides a plethora of information for management
         c. The information and reports that can be obtained allow the analysis of number invoices generated within the practice, which provides a basis to determine the number of veterinarians needed to support the volume of the practice
         d. Guidelines have been established by the American Animal Hospital Association (AAHA) and other veterinary organizations to assist veterinary professionals with assessing their practice's financial position
   B. In financial management, practice management is responsible for managing the practice's accounts receivable, accounts payable, and bookkeeping practices
      1. The ability to interpret, analyze, and evaluate all of the data related to the practice's available funds and resources must be monitored or overseen daily
      2. Practice management is expected to give ownership feedback on the financial standing of the practice as well as provide financial guidance for future goals and planning for the practice
      3. In conjunction with the hospital's bookkeeper, if that is not the practice manager, management works with the practice's accountant

4. The financial team works collectively to ensure and safeguard the financial well-being of the practice
5. Having a strong and unified financial team allows management to budget and plan for two of the primary expenditures management can control—inventory and payroll
    a. Although a practice is faced with many more expenses, these are two areas that if not properly monitored and supervised can become extremely costly to a practice and compromise its profitability

IV. Inventory control
  A. Two goals
    1. Have items on hand when needed
    2. Minimize expense of keeping supplies in stock
  B. Turnover rate should be six to eight times per year depending on the product
    1. Calculated by: yearly inventory expense ÷ average cost of inventory on hand
    2. Inventory turned over close to once a month so items used up before the bills are due
    3. Turnover rate can be calculated on the 80:20 rule, whereby 20% of items stocked account for 75% to 85% of the expenditures
  C. Elements of a good inventory system include
    a. Good record keeping that includes a reorder log, purchase order records, individual inventory records, inventory master list, and vendor files
    b. Effective use of inventory control cards or computer control
    c. Appropriate arrangement and storage of inventory
    d. Effective monitoring of inventory levels and expiration dates
    e. Smart purchasing policies, including knowledge of products

V. Accounts payable should be paid close to the due date to maximize use of capital
  A. Arrange for discounts for prompt payment
  B. Do not allow accounts to proceed beyond due date (credit rating may drop)

VI. Other various aspects of business include
  A. Records
    1. Involved in all aspects of hospital operation
    2. Many formats available, but whatever format is used, there must not be complete obliteration or erasure
    3. Handwritten records must be legible, accurate, and written in permanent ink
        a. Any errors should be crossed out with a single line, corrections made, dated, and initialed by the person making the entry
    4. Some records and consent forms may require client's signature
        a. A minor cannot legally enter into a contract
    5. Ownership
        a. The veterinary practice, not the client, owns the records
        b. Original records are a legal document and must be retained by the practice
        c. Any release of information is at the discretion of the veterinarian or practice
        d. A request for transfer should be made in writing; best to mail prepared records directly to referring or new veterinarian
    6. Information contained in all medical records is confidential and should not be discussed with outside parties without client's written permission
        a. Exception is the reporting of certain contagious and zoonotic diseases
    7. Statute of limitations requires that records be legally retained for a certain length of time, usually 5 to 7 years (depending on the state or province) from the date of last visit or discharge
    8. Many record filing systems are available; most medical records are arranged alphabetically by the owner's last name
    9. Any lost records should be explained to the client and a new record begun immediately
    10. Medical records include
        a. Log books: contain entries of services provided and include controlled drugs (required by law), radiography, surgery, euthanasia, laboratory, and necropsy logs
        b. Animal records: must be individualized and contain certain information such as signalment (owner's name, address, and telephone number; patient's name, sex, species, age, breed, and color), as well as date seen, chief complaint, history, clinical signs, diagnosis, prognosis, authorization records, radiographic data, laboratory reports, and vaccination and surgical records
        c. Financial information may be included in medical records, but separate billing is becoming more common practice
    11. Basic formats include
        a. Chronological or conventional method: events are entered as they occur
        b. Problem-oriented method includes separating out the problems, database, comprehensive history and physical examination, and progress notes
        c. Progress notes are divided into SOAP

(1) S = subjective data
(2) O = objective data
(3) A = assessment
(4) P = procedure for diagnosis and treatment
  d. Vaccination and spaying/neutering certificates need to be accurate
  e. Authorization or consent forms are not legal requirements, but they protect the veterinarian and ensure that the client understands all treatments and procedures
    (1) Includes treatment, surgery, fee estimate, euthanasia, and necropsy
    (2) Should be part of permanent record
    (3) Euthanasia authorization essential
  f. Medication labels must be complete and accurate
B. Credit and collection policies
  1. Policies should be written and strictly adhered to
  2. A written estimate should always be used
  3. Accounts receivable should be kept to a minimum
C. Consider use of a computer if the practice does not already have one
  1. Much of the hospital operation can be provided by the computer, including inventory control, medical records management, client communication and information analysis, vaccination reminders, and accounting
  2. Many well-designed programs are available
  3. Research particular needs so that the proper system can be purchased
D. A fax (facsimile) is an efficient, rapid mode of communication
  1. Strict confidentiality must be maintained

## OSHA and WHMIS

I. OSHA stands for the Occupational Safety and Health Administration
  A. OSHA is the federal agency that is responsible for enforcing the safety practices of businesses throughout the United States
  B. The Occupational Safety and Health Act (OSH Act) implemented in 1971 and falls under the Department of Labor
  C. OSHA's mission is to prevent work-related injuries, illnesses, and deaths
    1. Top priority for OSHA's inspectors are reports of imminent dangers—accidents about to happen
    2. Second are fatalities or accidents serious enough to send three or more workers to the hospital
    3. The third priority is employee complaints
    4. Referrals from other government agencies are fourth

5. Fifth are targeted inspections, such as the site-specific targeting program, which focuses on employers that report high injury and illness rates, and special emphasis programs for hazardous work, such as trenching, or equipment, such as mechanical power presses
6. Follow-up inspections are the final priority
  D. Implementing a firm OSHA program takes few basic steps
    1. It is recommended to form a committee that includes a committee leader
    2. To be designated as the OSHA Safety Officer
    3. To be required to research, investigate, and communicate with the other committees all of the requirements mandated by law
    4. Within the practice's OSHA program, the practice should include a minimum of new employee training and annual training for the entire health care team
    5. In addition, ongoing training should be done as needed to ensure the safety of the team and facility
II. The Workplace Hazardous Materials Information System (WHMIS) is Canada's national hazard communication standard
  A. The key elements of the system are cautionary labeling of containers of WHMIS controlled products, the provision of material safety data sheets (MSDSs), and worker education and training programs
  B. WHMIS is implemented through coordinated federal, provincial and territorial legislation
  C. Supplier labeling and MSDS requirements are set out under the federal Hazardous Products Act and associated Controlled Products Regulations
  D. All of the provincial, territorial, and federal agencies responsible for occupational safety and health have established WHMIS employer requirements within their respective jurisdictions
    1. These requirements obligate employers to ensure that controlled products used, stored, handled, or disposed of in the workplace are properly labeled
    2. MSDSs are to be made available to workers
    3. Workers must receive education and training to ensure the safe storage, handling, use and disposal of controlled products in the workplace
III. Incorporating a sound and solid OSHA and WHMIS program is a legal requirement for veterinary practices and is not optional

## PERSONAL MANAGEMENT

I. Definition: skills and techniques required of each individual member of an organization to make the team function most efficiently

II. Personal management skills allow the veterinary technician to manage within the team to the benefit of the team. Components of personal management are time management, goal setting, decision making, stress management, coping with burnout, and negotiating

## Time Management

I. Effectively using available time during the workday maximizes productivity for the employee and helps alleviate stress
   A. Time is a unique resource in that it cannot be accumulated and each person has the same amount
   B. Time management is a personal process and must fit into one's lifestyle and circumstances
   C. The following suggestions can be applied to almost everyone to help manage time and reduce stress
      1. Make a daily "to do" list
      2. Develop daily, weekly, and yearly lists of goals
      3. Learn to say no; gain control of what takes up your time
      4. Establish priorities
      5. Use technology to increase efficiency: computer, calculator, and new laboratory equipment
      6. Never handle a piece of paper more than twice
      7. Learn to skim what you read
      8. Keep procrastination to a minimum
      9. Work at meeting deadlines
      10. Exercise at least 20 minutes per day to help you focus

## Goals

I. Life offers a series of choices and decisions that need to be made
II. Establishing goals allows an individual to have a choice in the course of action required to accomplish a certain task and help lead in this direction
III. Set effective goals
   A. Identify possible needs in such areas as career, personal life, financial concerns, physical fitness, community involvement, and leisure time
   B. Set a goal for each identified need by describing the result
   C. Prioritize
   D. Define objectives required to achieve the goal (steps to be done to achieve the goal)
   E. Select activity to complete each objective
   F. Indicate time frame for implementation
   G. Evaluate and monitor accomplishments
IV. As much as possible, make sure the objectives set for achieving the goals are measurable, clear, realistic, and stated as required results

V. Greater success will be achieved if one
   A. Prioritizes
   B. Draws up written plans to help achieve goals
   C. Breaks goals into smaller sequential steps that can be achieved one at a time
   D. Begins now

## Decision Making

I. The process of identifying and selecting a course of action for a specific problem or situation
II. Indecision or making no choice paralyzes the ability of an organization or an individual to move forward
III. Key components to making a decision are similar to problem-solving techniques and include
   A. Listing options
   B. Evaluating options (thinking it over)
   C. Factoring in personal feelings
   D. Evaluating how the decision will affect priorities already set
   E. Making the decision and discarding other options
   F. Committing to the decision (mentally not looking back)
   G. Doing everything possible to make the decision work

## Stress Management

I. Stress is the feeling of tension and pressure that results when a demand cannot be readily dealt with or if there is a perceived or real threat
II. Stress is response to a force that upsets one's equilibrium
   A. Strain is the adverse effects of stress on an individual's mind, body, and actions
III. Stressor: a force that brings about stress
IV. The body's physiological and chemical changes resulting from the fight-or-flight response include an increase in heart rate, blood pressure, blood glucose, and blood clotting
V. Short-term physiological changes and prolonged stress can lead to annoying and life-threatening conditions and a weakening of the immune system
VI. Due to lack of control, job pressures create stress for many people
VII. Not all stress is bad; some stress leads to achieving goals and meeting or exceeding personal potential
   A. Referred to as eustress
   B. Stress management is individual and varies from highly specific techniques to a change in lifestyle
      1. Identify stress signals
      2. As much as possible, eliminate or modify stressors
      3. Improve work habits

4. Physical exercise reduces tension and keeps one in good condition and more resistant to fatigue
5. Stress can be managed through mental relaxation techniques, including relaxation response, biofeedback training, muscle monitoring, and concentration techniques

## Coping with Burnout

I. Burnout is closely related to stress and is defined as a state of exhaustion (physical, mental, and emotional) caused by involvement in situations that are demanding
II. Burnout is a set of behaviors that result from strain
III. Persons suffering from burnout exhibit many symptoms—some physical, some emotional
IV. Employer role: reduce the amount of burnout
   A. Jobs should be clearly defined and provide the employee with a sense of purpose and opportunities for growth
V. Employee role: find significance in something other than work
   A. Develop new interests that provide satisfaction outside the workplace
   B. Time management and goal setting might also be effective
VI. Counseling and support are needed for recovery from burnout

## Negotiating Conflict Resolution

I. Differences of opinion or situations of conflict frequently arise
II. A win-win solution is a key to being a valuable team member
III. To prepare for negotiation
   A. Always separate the person from the problem
   B. Focus on the interest at hand, not the position taken
   C. Identify options for a viable solution
   D. Discuss options after clearly weighing all possible solutions

## CAREER MANAGEMENT ▬▬▬▬

I. Make career decisions that move one closer to self-fulfillment
II. Key components to finding the right job opportunity include personal finance, job search, and interview

## Personal Finance

I. Step 1 in career planning is to determine the type of income that will be required to meet financial obligations
   A. Prepare a budget that will allow you to view your obligations and make correct important career decisions

1. Budget is defined as a statement of resources allocated for specific activities over a certain period of time
2. All income, which includes salary, return on investments, and interest income, is projected and should be listed
3. List all expected expenses
   a. Housing, utilities, telephone, property tax, all types of insurance, automobile expenses (including loan payments, gas, and maintenance), other outstanding loan payments (including credit cards), food, household repairs, clothing, entertainment, travel, and miscellaneous expenses
4. The goal is to have more income than expenses
   a. If there are more expenses, one of the categories will have to be adjusted
   b. It is wise to only accept jobs that will allow you to meet current financial obligations

## Job Search

I. Career choices and options for veterinary technicians are not limited to practice settings
   A. Opportunities also exist in biomedical research, specialty practice, education, universities, industry, zoos, animal husbandry related areas, military service, and humane societies
   B. Research each of the areas that interest you and note pros and cons
   C. A career choice is not necessarily a long-term decision, because changing career paths is not uncommon
II. Seek job notices in placement services, classified advertisements, and through networking
   A. Résumé, cover letter, references
     1. Résumé
      a. Summarizes your background, qualifications, and accomplishments
      b. Key components of a résumé
       (1) Personal identification, including name, address, and telephone number where you can be reached
       (2) Career objective defines what type of job you are seeking
       (3) State clearly what you hope to achieve in your professional career
       (4) Traditionally, work history is in reverse chronological order
       (5) Accomplishments highlight pertinent achievements at each job
       (6) Traditionally, education is also in reverse chronological order
       (7) Personal interests are optional
       (8) May be best to include job-related activities only

(9) The traditional chronological résumé, functional résumé, or a combined format can be used

2. Cover letter
   a. Usually read before the résumé, its goal is to get you to the interview stage
   b. Key components
      (1) The letter should be one page in length with approximately three paragraphs
      (2) First paragraph: introduces yourself and identifies the position for which you are applying
      (3) Second paragraph: lists accomplishments that would be beneficial for the business
      (4) Third paragraph: serves as a closing and indicates your next step, which is usually a telephone call in a few days
   c. Rules governing cover letter and résumé
      (1) Always use premium paper and matching envelopes
      (2) Check very carefully for typographical errors, including spelling and punctuation
      (3) Make sure the appropriate person at the prospective place of employment is addressed
      (4) Keep copies of all documents you send out and a list to whom they were sent
      (5) Do not include photographs or mention your race, color, creed, or political affiliation
      (6) Proofread all materials several times and have some one else proofread them as well
      (7) If sent via e-mail, ensure proper formatting

3. References
   a. Provided by former employers, college instructors, and clients (check with an individual before using them as a reference)
   b. Provide prospective employers with a telephone number where a reference can be contacted
   c. If a written reference is required, provide references with the correct address and background information

## Interview

I. Provides a personal opportunity to impress a potential employer
II. Research your potential employer
   A. Obtain a detailed job description
   B. Determine the background on the business, including type of practice and number of owners
   C. Contact employees of the business and/or company representatives
   D. Gather information from the Chamber of Commerce or a local newspaper on the community in which the business is located
   E. Make a list of questions you have about the job
   F. Estimate the wages you will need to earn (as indicated by your budget) to take the job
   G. Prepare a list of potential questions the interviewer may ask and format your responses
III. During the interview your objective is to gather information as well as provide the potential employer with knowledge about you
   A. In less than 10 seconds you will make a first impression on the interviewer, and in less than 4 minutes the interviewer will acquire a lasting impression of you
   B. Personal appearance for the interview is very important
      1. Your appearance should convey a clean, conservative, and professional person
   C. Be punctual
   D. Relax
   E. Listen to and answer questions carefully
   F. Ask questions you have about the potential employment
   G. Stress your strengths as well as what you can offer
   H. Encourage the employer to make you an offer. A decision can be made later on whether to accept or not
IV. Certain questions do not have to be answered during an interview. These involve marital status, child care, plans for having a family, arrest record, and age
   A. These are questions that can be construed as prejudicial
V. Be prepared to negotiate salary and benefit packages
   A. Best to have offer presented in writing
   B. Consider the entire package, not just salary
      1. A lower salary with health insurance, life insurance, and paid vacation may be better
   C. Benefits are a vital portion of any job offer and add to value of the job. Benefits that may be offered include, but are not limited to
      1. Health insurance/dental insurance
      2. Life insurance
      3. Bonuses
      4. Discounted pet care and uniforms
      5. Paid vacation
      6. Paid sick days
      7. Expenses for continuing education, including registration, time off, travel, lodging, and per diem expenses
      8. Professional association dues

VI. It is important to personally thank each person who was involved in your interview process at the conclusion of the interview
  A. The thank you may also be sent in writing 24 hours after the interview is complete
VII. Wait at least 1 day before accepting any offer to allow time to compare all propositions

## MARKETING

I. Definition: communication to others about goods or services that are offered
  A. In veterinary medicine, marketing is the process of educating the client/public on services that can be provided for quality care
  B. Marketing consists of all activities employed to promote goods and services
  C. Veterinary technicians have an important role in these activities
  D. Marketing in a veterinary hospital can be divided into two distinctly different areas: internal marketing and external marketing

### Internal Marketing

Internal marketing is the process of marketing veterinary services to clients and potential clients. The following are areas of the veterinary hospital suited to internal marketing.

I. Outward appearances: the initial visual image that a client/potential client sees when approaching and entering the veterinary hospital
  A. Exterior of building, parking lot, and grounds should all be well kept
  B. First impressions of the inside of the building and waiting room are important, including cleanliness and freedom from odor
  C. Consider equipment, including availability of modern equipment and computers
  D. Professional appearing staff, clean uniforms, name tags
  E. A sense of order
II. A caring attitude should be displayed by *all* staff members at all times
  A. The staff should be positive and enthusiastic and not display anger or dissatisfaction with their jobs
III. Client needs must be evaluated in any marketing plan, consider
  A. Location of the practice
    1. Clients in rural areas will require different services than those in a strictly urban environment
      a. Goods and services should be provided accordingly
  B. The time commitment made by your client in coming to your practice. Do not minimize
    1. Today's consumer should be greeted with fast, courteous service

  C. Conveying the importance of clients and their pets will make them more eager to return to your practice for future veterinary care
  D. Client needs can be evaluated by focus groups, questionnaires, and listening to complaints
IV. Marketing tangible products to the client can be done most effectively by identifying a need of a client and/or pet and finding a product within the hospital to fill it
  A. The veterinary technician must be knowledgeable about the products being sold to clients
  B. Improper information about a product can be hazardous to the pet and to the confidence the client has in the practice
  C. The veterinary/client/patient relationship must be considered when dispensing products
    1. This relationship means the client's animal has had contact with the veterinarian within a specified period of time
  D. Over-the-counter products versus professional products should be handled accordingly
V. Tangible items that can be used to market goods or services include
  A. Client reminders—a simple postcard reminder to the client of routine vaccinations and dental and heartworm checks can go a long way to keeping clients coming back year after year. This is also seen as an extension of the caring veterinary hospital
  B. Commercial handouts—many companies provide materials that are available to describe their product and its benefits to the client and pet when used
    1. These materials provide excellent marketing of goods without expense of preparation
  C. Practice newsletters and health bulletins keep the client in contact with the practice throughout the year
    1. They can provide valuable information on seasonal needs of pets, special promotions being run by the practice, and updates on new or common diseases
    2. All newsletters must clearly indicate the hospital, be printed in a professional appropriate manner, and be free of typographical errors
  D. Sympathy communication—a very personal and caring message is sent (through a card or letter from the practice staff) when client's grief at the loss of a pet is recognized
  E. Sales point displays—often corporations will provide displays for their products for use in the clinic's waiting area
    1. Display products in a visually appealing manner
    2. Use such displays only for marketable products

F. Animal care talks—the practice that provides puppy and kitten talks, behavior classes, etc., has opened another avenue for marketing its goods and services and for showing care

VI. Intangible items such as services cannot be overlooked even though results are not often visually beneficial. Preventive health care programs fall into this category and may or may not be equated with veterinary care

## External Marketing

External marketing activities are aimed at expanding current client activity within the practice and increasing the exposure of goods and services to those who are currently not clients.

I. External marketing usually involves advertising and can be done in some of the following ways
   A. External visual signs promoting the practice include use of hospital signs and distribution of business cards for the veterinarian and the veterinary technician
   B. Media routes for advertising services include telephone directories, newspaper articles or advertisements, and radio and television commercials
   C. Direct mail provides information to a targeted audience via the postal service
      1. Primarily to acquaint nonclients with services

II. Community activities can be seen as gestures of good will and can be accomplished by talking to community groups about good quality pet care, by promoting the veterinary technology profession, and by participating in community service, such as volunteering to judge children's animal projects at a local fair
   A. The veterinarian and the veterinary technician should volunteer their expertise to the community
   B. The veterinary technician also has an obligation to provide information about his or her career to the general public, co-workers, and peers as a means of promoting the profession and their own career

## PROFESSIONALISM ▬▬▬▬

Professionalism includes demeanor, appearance at work and in the community, and ethics.

I. The perception of the entire profession can be affected

II. Key components of professionalism
   A. Demeanor: outward behavior or conduct should always reflect positively on you, your employer, and the profession
      1. A professional will always project a proper image to those around them

III. Dress: clothing, hairstyle, jewelry, etc., worn during the workday and in the community reflect a person's level of professionalism
   A. Workplace: clothing should be appropriate for the job

1. Uniforms with a name tag identifying you as a veterinary technician are appropriate for a practice setting
   a. The uniforms should be changed if soiled
2. Business casual clothing is most appropriate for continuing education seminars, workshops, or presentations
   a. T-shirts, jeans, and shorts are generally not acceptable and do not portray a sense of professionalism

IV. Speech: words used to communicate with the public, clients, co-workers, and even patients reflect a level of professionalism
   A. Avoid personal problems, gossip, health, controversial social issues, politics, religion, sex, and slang phrases
   B. Maintaining confidentiality is essential when dealing with business matters. Office situations, clients, and their pets should not be discussed socially or in the presence of the general public
   C. Jokes and terminology that may be offensive to those of a certain sex, physical appearance, or ethnic origin should be avoided

## Education

The veterinary technician has an obligation to remain current with technical information that pertains to the job. This involves a commitment to continuing education and lifelong learning and may even require higher-level education for advancement.

I. Continuing education comes in various forms, including advanced, review, and new information
   A. Registration requirements in certain areas demand proof of attendance
   B. Lifelong learning shows a commitment to growth

II. Advanced degrees
   A. Most veterinary technicians' education consists of a 2-year program in the field of veterinary technology
   B. As career plans change and job opportunities become available, a bachelors or masters degree may become important
   C. Investigate all options for degrees, including those offered through computer access and special programs set up for the employed adult learner

## ETHICS ▬▬▬▬
### History of Ethics

I. The word "ethics" comes from the Greek word *ethos,* which means "character"
   A. Philosophers such as Socrates, Plato, and Aristotle espoused moral ethics, based on a man's experience and education
      1. Socrates initiated the need for definitions of courage, justice, law, and government before we could be called good citizens

2. The social ethics or values of current times have diversified with geography and social history, including traditions and the church

3. These morals are the principles that govern our views of right and wrong

## Personal Ethics

I. Personal ethics are the values and beliefs that we use each day to decide how we will interact with team members, clients, and patients. The best way to connect with our values and create a set of ethics is the creation of a mission statement
   A. To create a personal mission statement, think about the answers to these questions
      1. What would you like to have achieved by the end of your life?
      2. You are in a room with your family and friends; one by one those people come up to you and give you a gift, what would you like that gift to be?
      3. What do you find the most meaningful about your life?
      4. Who are the people you most admire and why?
      5. How can you make a difference in the world?
      6. What would you like to be remembered for?
      7. Make a list of the 10 strengths that you possess; what do you do well?
      8. Ask friends and family what they like best about you
   B. Creating a mission statement takes time and reflection and will change over time
   C. Share your mission statement with friends and family to get their ideas and feedback, to refine it
   D. The end result can be in any form: a verse, poem, letter, or just a few words
      1. An example of a mission statement: Live simply. Love generously. Care deeply. Speak kindly
   E. Personal ethics provides a power in purpose, the sense that there is meaning to life
II. Create a personal mantra to use in setting an ethics standard when working with clients
   A. Think of the three words you would like to have a client used to describe you
      1. What would you like them to think of you and your interaction with them and their pet?
   B. When you have identified those three words, say them to yourself before speaking with a client or working with a patient, it will enhance your conscious and subconscious demonstration of those words in your actions
   C. An example mantra might be "professional, knowledgeable, compassionate"

III. Use your set of values and ethics to define who you are in the practice and how you will decide what is important on a daily basis. It is also valuable in determining how to proceed in difficult situations when an answer is not readily apparent
   A. As an example, consider what you might do in this situation, based upon your ethics
      1. Example A: Sharon, someone you have worked with for the last 2 years has a habit of being chronically late for work. Lately, the supervisor has counseled her that her chronic problem with being on time could result in her termination if it doesn't improve immediately. You have always enjoyed working with Sharon and consider her a friend, not just a co-worker. Sharon calls you and asks if you would clock her in on the computer because she overslept or she will be 15 minutes late and most likely lose her job. The clinic policy clearly states that clocking someone else into the practice is expressly forbidden. Sharon says she is afraid she will lose her job if you don't help her out this one time and no one will know. What would you do? What personal ethics do you find are in conflict with this situation?
      2. Example B: Mrs. Jones has been coming to the practice for over 15 years with Benji, her mixed breed dog. Benji's health has been declining over time and Mrs. Jones has brought the dog into the practice to determine if it may be time to have him euthanized. The doctor agrees that it is time to consider having him euthanized, but you can see the conflict in deciding in Mrs. Jones' face. When the doctor steps out of the exam room, she asks you what you would do. Would you agree with what the doctor says even though you don't believe in euthanasia? What would you say? Is there a correct answer?
      3. Personal ethics and seeking a practice that shares common values increases job satisfaction and decreases stress in the workplace
         a. When there is a dramatic difference in ethics between team members, there is likely to be significant conflict in the practice and often contributes to burnout in the technician profession

## Professional Ethics

Ethics are rules established by organizations to set guidelines for and influence behavior and actions of the group.
   I. As legal agents for veterinary employers, technicians must "accept [their] obligations to practice [their] profession conscientiously and with sensitivity, adhering

to the profession's Code of Ethics" (from the North American Veterinary Technician Association [NAVTA])

II. Veterinarians are held liable for the actions of veterinary technicians

III. In Ontario, the Ontario Association of Veterinary Technicians governs legislation that makes RVTs accountable for their own actions

IV. Veterinary technicians are under supervision and control of a veterinarian and must never engage in practices reserved for the veterinarian
   A. These include diagnosing, prognosing, performing surgery, and prescribing medication
   B. Technicians must never complain about veterinarians or other employees to or in the presence of a client

V. As professionals the actions of technicians must be based on the best interests of patients and clients

VI. The veterinary technician code of ethics
   A. Communicates the profession's ideals to the public and members of the profession
   B. Is a general guide for professional ethical conduct
   C. Provides disciplinary procedures to members who are not operating at an acceptable level of conduct

VII. There are a number of reasons why a profession should have a code of ethics
   A. There are ethical expectations from employers, clients, and co-workers
   B. Members of a profession perform a special function in society
      1. That function involves special education, situations, and decisions that not all people face
      2. In most societies, it is assumed that the people in a profession understand the ethical issues that they come in contact with and can therefore construct their own rules, standards, and bylaws
   C. A code of ethics establishes a framework of professional behavior and responsibilities
      1. It promotes high standards of practice and provides a benchmark for individual evaluation
   D. Professional ethics is the middle ground between moral ethics, which each person holds as an individual, and the social ethics, which are expected by society as a whole
      1. With autonomy it is important that members of the profession maintain records and regulate themselves in a way that meets with the understanding of society
      2. This is especially important with the social concern regarding the treatment of animals
   E. The establishment of a code of ethics for a profession can also mark the maturity of the profession
      1. The development of the ethics includes having a large number of people think through their mission and obligations as a group and as individuals with respect to society
   F. A code of ethics will often have two components
      1. The ideals of the organization
      2. The rules or principles that the members of the organization or profession are expected to follow
   G. Ethics can also be outlined as a statement of values, a policy, or a mission statement
      1. The mission statement for the National Association of Veterinary Technicians of America (NAVTA) is "Connecting veterinary technicians to one another and the profession to the world"
      2. The mission statement of the Canadian Association of Animal Health Technologists and Technicians (CAAHTT) is "Dedicated to fulfilling the goal of professional recognition nationally and internationally through communication, direction, and support of the provincial AHT/VT associations"
   H. Once the professional ethics have been approved and documented, it is important to have a way to present this information and ensure that it is made public both internally and externally
      1. It is also important that the code of ethics values be included in the organization's policies and be reviewed and revised as required by the organization
      2. It is important to define a method to enforce the code of ethics and to describe the possible results of noncompliance

## Professional Association Ethics

I. In the preamble to the Code of Ethics of NAVTA, it is stated that "Veterinary Technology includes the promotion and maintenance of good health in animals, the control of diseased and injured animals, and the control of diseases transmissible from animals to man"
   A. Although a code of ethics can help with professional identity and form a foundation for an organization, there are still many other purposes and characteristics of a professional organization (Box 29-1)
      1. NAVTA has stated that the association's purpose is to represent and promote the profession of veterinary technology; provide direction, education, support, and coordination for its members; and work with other allied professional organizations for the competent care and humane treatment of animals

---

**Box 29-1** NAVTA Code of Ethics

**NATIONAL ASSOCIATION OF VETERINARY TECHNICIANS IN AMERICA (NAVTA) CODE OF ETHICS**
Veterinary technicians shall
- Aid society and animals through providing excellent care and services for animals
- Prevent and relieve the suffering of animals
- Promote public health by assisting with the control of zoonotic diseases and informing the public about these diseases
- Assume accountability for individual professional actions and judgments
- Protect confidential information provided by clients
- Safeguard the public and the profession against individuals deficient in professional competence or ethics
- Assist with efforts to ensure conditions of employment consistent with the excellent care of animals
- Remain competent in veterinary technology through a commitment to lifelong learning
- Collaborate with members of the veterinary medical profession in an effort to ensure quality health care services for all animals

From NAVTA 2001 Resource Guide.

---

2. The objectives of the CAAHTT are similar to those of NAVTA with the addition of promoting greater communication nationally and internationally, through direction and support of the provincial AHT/VT associations
3. Professional associations can begin to govern their members through the ethics and purpose of the association

## VETERINARY TECHNOLOGY AS A PROFESSION

I. Definition of a profession: A vocation or occupation requiring advanced education and training, and involving intellectual skills
II. Definition of a professional: according to Webster's Third New International Dictionary, a professional is "a calling requiring specialized knowledge and often long and intensive preparation including instruction in skills and methods as well as in the scientific, historical or scholarly principles underlying such skills and methods, maintaining by force of organization or concerted opinion high standards of achievement and conduct and committing its members to continued study and to a kind of work which has for its prime purpose the rendering of a public service"
  A. This definition is based on both the description of the professional role and what is required to achieve the status of the profession
  B. As a description of the role, the Ontario Association of Veterinary Technicians (OAVT) has stated that "Veterinary Technicians are specifically trained professionals who work as an integral part of the

veterinary medical team, to provide humane quality animal health care"
  C. NAVTA further defines this role: "The Veterinary Technician/Technologist is educated to be the veterinarian's nurse, laboratory technician, radiography technician, anesthetist, surgical nurse and client educator." With this must also come the requirements to fulfill the role. In both statements, the words *trained* and *educated* lead the definition
  D. In the United States, a veterinary technician is a graduate of a 2-year, American Veterinary Medical Association (AVMA)–accredited program from a community college, college, or university
  E. A veterinary technologist is a graduate from an AVMA-accredited bachelor's degree program
  F. Almost every state requires a veterinary technician/technologist to pass a credentialing examination
    1. The examination is a means to ensure the public that veterinary technicians have entry-level knowledge of the duties they are asked to perform in a veterinary clinic or hospital

## PROFESSIONAL ORGANIZATIONS

Professional organizations for veterinary technicians provide members with the opportunity for career advancement by supporting groups who work to advance the entire profession.
I. During their careers, technicians have obligations to their profession and professional organization, as well as to themselves
II. National/international organizations
  A. Organizations that deal with issues affecting a broad range of topics, including public image of the veterinary technician, laws and legislation governing the profession, and effective use of the veterinary technician within the veterinary health care team
  B. These organizations actively interact with other organizations, looking for ways that a collaborative effort might benefit the entire health care team
    1. Career building and professionalism are important goals of these associations
III. State/provincial/local organizations
  A. Provide members with information pertinent to the profession on a local level
  B. Become actively involved in laws pertinent to their specific location, providing information to residents of their area, and updating members on local issues

## ACCOMPLISHMENTS OF VETERINARY TECHNOLOGY

I. The first formal academic program was started in the United States in 1961 and in Canada in 1967
II. Animal Technician was the official title chosen to recognize graduates of an accredited program in 1967

---

**Box 29-2** Objects of the CAAHTT

**THE CANADIAN ASSOCIATION OF ANIMAL HEALTH TECHNOLOGISTS AND TECHNICIANS**
The objects of the Corporation are to
- Establish and maintain a national standard of membership
- Promote and assist in continuing education for AHT/VTs
- Promote greater communication nationwide
- Promote the profession of AHT/VT within the animal health community and to the general public
- Be a resource regarding national and international issues

---

III. The name was changed to Veterinary Technician in 1989 to recognize graduates of AVMA-recognized colleges
IV. The first credentialing examination: the Veterinary Technician National Examination (VTNE) was administered by PES (Professional Examination Service) in 1978. The examination process was the responsibility of a committee of the American Veterinary Medical Association (AVMA) until 1995, when PES signed on with the American Association of Veterinary State Boards (AAVSB)
V. Continuing education programs for technicians have been available since the 1970s
VI. Publications specific to technicians have been in print since the 1980s
VII. The NAVTA Executive Board adopted a resolution in June 1993 declaring the third week in October as National Veterinary Technician Week (NVTW)
   A. The CAAHTT has also declared the third week of October as NVTW and continues to pursue an official proclamation
VIII. In April 1970, a nucleus of Animal Health Technology graduates formed the Canadian Association of Animal Health Technicians
IX. To incorporate their objects into a strong national body, representatives of seven provincial associations founded the CAAHTT in July 1989 (Box 29-2)
   A. In 1993 the CAAHTT adopted reciprocity for the VTNE, through PES
X. In 1991 at Michigan State University, the North American Veterinary Technician Association was formed
XI. In January 2002, NAVTA changed their name to the National Association of Veterinary Technicians in America to delineate their focus

## REGISTRATION, LICENSING, AND CERTIFICATION

I. In the United States, once a veterinary technician has passed the VTNE, he or she is then eligible to use one of the following designations

A. Licensed Veterinary Technician
B. Certified Veterinary Technician
C. Registered Veterinary Technician
D. The three designations, or licenses, are granted by a state agency or board
   1. Each state has its own Veterinary Practice Act or rules of practice
   2. Veterinary state boards write these rules and regulations
   3. These regulations can include education, continuing education, and specific duties
   4. Most states require a continuing education component to maintain credentialing
II. In Canada, animal health technician and veterinary technician/technologist are titles given to graduates of postsecondary programs, as approved by their provincial associations
   A. To use the designation of *registered* with the graduate program title, the candidate must pass the VTNE, as well as meet any other requirements designated by the governing provincial association
   B. One of these requirements may be a mandatory continuing education component to maintain registered status
   C. The VTNE is used by all Canadian provinces to designate registered status, which allows for reciprocity across Canada

## SUMMARY

I. There has been much growth and accomplishment in the field of veterinary technology
II. It started with common goals, mission statements, and the development of a code of ethics to provide a solid foundation for the profession and to continue the establishment of specialty organizations within the profession
III. There are still many areas in which the profession can expand, including continuity within the profession from state to state and internationally, improvements to self-regulation, and a clear definition of the role of veterinary technicians in practice
IV. Through participation in provincial or state professional organizations, maintaining a high quality of education, pursuing an ongoing firm belief in the goals and ethics of the profession, and continuing to improve relationships between associations and related professions, many more accomplishments will be possible in the future

## ACKNOWLEDGMENT

The editors acknowledge and appreciate the original contribution of Carlene A. Decker, A. Patrick Navarre, and Julie Ovington, whose work has been incorporated into this chapter.

# Glossary

**accounts payable** Money owed by one business to another

**accounts receivable** Money owed to a business, usually owed by the clients

**burnout** State of emotional, mental, and physical exhaustion in response to prolonged stress

**business management** Practices required for the successful financial operation of a facility

**call-waiting feature** A telephone feature that signals when another call is coming in and can ensure a quicker response to a client's inquiry

**career development** Planned approach to achieving growth and satisfaction in work experiences

**chronological résumé** Job résumé that presents education, work experience, interests, and accomplishments in reverse chronological order

**communication** Sending, receiving, and interpreting messages

**conference call option** A telephone feature that allows multiple individuals to be included simultaneously in a conversation

**conflict** Situation in which there is disagreement, incompatibility, or mutual exclusiveness

**control** A function of practice manager to monitor and evaluate performance

**counseling** Formal discussion method, usually with a professional, in which an individual is encouraged to overcome a problem or improve his or her potential

**delegation** Formally assigning responsibility for completion of a given task to a subordinate

**ethics** Rules established by an organization to influence actions and behaviors of the group, not enforced in a court of law

**electronic communication** Also known as telecommunications, a means to transmit voice, data, and images from one location to another through the use of electronic equipment

**eustress** Positive or good stress that rejuvenates, excites, or stimulates an individual

**fight-or-flight response** Body's physiological and chemical response to stressors in which the individual attempts to avoid or cope with the situation

**functional résumé** One that organizes skills and accomplishments into the functions or tasks required for the position sought

**leadership** Directing and influencing the practice's employees to carry out the organization's objectives

**nonverbal communication** The unspoken elements that replace, reinforce, or contradict verbal communication; they include visual, temporal, vocal, and spatial

**on-hold message feature** A telephone feature that allows client, while on hold, to listen to messages developed by the veterinary hospital describing services or facilities that are available

**organization** A function of a practice manager to help achieve human and material resource goals of the organization

**organizational management** Working with and through people to accomplish organizational goals

**personal management** Skills and techniques required of each member of an organization to make the team function most efficiently

**phase training programs** A component of training personnel that maps out training by providing structure and guidance so that on a daily basis, the trainer and trainee know what their training focus is

**planning** A function of practice management that involves thinking through and making decisions about goals and actions in advance so that objectives can be defined and procedures established

**policy manual** A manual that provides a written record of organization policies and includes policies that govern organization-wide actions and those that cover the actions of individuals

**profession** A vocation or occupation requiring advanced education and training, and involving intellectual skills

**professional** Engaged in or worthy of the high standards of a profession

**relaxation response** Lowered metabolism, heart rate, respiration, and blood pressure

**signalment** Data on records that include owner's name, address, and telephone; patient's name, sex, species, age, breed, and color; and date seen. Technically it is a detailed physical description for purposes of identification

**SOP** Standard operating procedure, or another term for "procedures manual" that outlines protocols for various procedures performed within an organization, such as surgery, laboratory or radiology protocols, and safety procedures

**stress** Body's response to stressors that threaten to disturb homeostasis

**stressor** Anything that causes stress

**supervisory skills** Involve the ability to direct a co-worker or subordinate's work to meet goals of the organization

**teamwork** The result of all members of an organization understanding their roles and working together to accomplish the goals of an organization

**veterinary practice management** The analyzing, planning, evaluating, advising, organizing, supervising, directing and implementation of policies and procedures for all aspects of a veterinary practice as well as the funds and resource management

**win-win conflict resolution** A method of resolving conflict whereby both sides gain something of value

**written communication** Communication through messages delivered in written form

# Review Questions

1 Feedback is from the receiver and allows the sender to
   a. Interpret the message
   b. Interpret the interference
   c. Understand how much of the message is comprehended
   d. Understand the receiver's message
2 Body language does not include
   a. A handshake
   b. Direct eye contact
   c. Slouched posture or upright posture
   d. A kind word in a low voice

**3** "Good" communication techniques include all of the following skills except
  a. Concentrating on the message
  b. Processing the information too rapidly
  c. Providing feedback
  d. Avoiding judgment of the message sender

**4** The six stages of grief a client may experience are
  a. Denial, bargaining, anger, depression, blame, and celebration
  b. Denial, bargaining, anger, guilt, depression, and resolution
  c. Anger, violence, sadness, bargaining, grief, and depression
  d. Anger, sadness, grief, resolution, celebration, and guilt

**5** Which of the following actions diminishes a successful resolution of a problem with a staff member?
  a. A staff meeting
  b. Waiting 2 months before talking about the problem
  c. Allowing all parties to express opinions
  d. A written grievance filed with the manager

**6** All of the following techniques may be used to increase a veterinary technician's time management abilities except
  a. Making a daily list of jobs to do
  b. Establishing priorities
  c. Learning to say no to your employer
  d. Procrastinating less and meeting deadlines more

**7** The best personal reference for a potential position in a large progressive veterinary practice is
  a. Your childhood neighbor
  b. Your family physician
  c. Your college instructor
  d. A former client, whom you have not seen in 2 years

**8** An example of a tangible internal marketing tool is
  a. An advertisement in the telephone directory
  b. An announcement of a new practice in the area
  c. A sympathy card to a client who recently lost a pet
  d. A visit to the local primary school

**9** A message sent in a loud voice indicates
  a. Tension
  b. Insecurity
  c. Enthusiasm
  d. All of the above

**10** The area of personal space or "comfort zone"
  a. Depends on personal preference
  b. Is approximately 4 to 6 m (13 to 19 ft)
  c. Is approximately 46 cm to 1.2 m (18 inches to 4 ft)
  d. Depends on gender of the individual

## BIBLIOGRAPHY

Bassert JM: An introduction to the profession of veterinary technology. In McCurnin DM, Bassert JM, editors: *Clinical textbook for veterinary technicians*, ed 6, St Louis, 2006, Saunders.

Brock SL: *Better business writing*, Los Altos, Calif, 1988, Crisp Publications.

Brounstein M: *Communicating effectively for dummies*, New York, 2001, Hungry Minds.

Dessler G: *Personnel/human resource management*, ed 8, Englewood Cliffs, NJ, 2000, Prentice-Hall.

Dubrin A: *Human relations for career and personal success*, ed 4, Englewood Cliffs, NJ, 1995, Prentice-Hall.

Haynes ME: *Personal time management*, Los Altos, Calif, 1987, Crisp Publications.

Lipitz BA: Ethical, legal, and safety issues in veterinary medicine. In Sirois M, editor: *Principles and practice of veterinary technology*, ed 2, St Louis, 2004, Mosby.

MacDonald C: www.ethicsweb.ca. Accessed July 9, 2007.

Perreault WD: *Basic marketing*, ed 13, Boston, 2000, Irwin.

Quible ZK: *Administrative office management*, ed 7, Englewood Cliffs, NJ, 2000, Prentice-Hall.

Rollin BE: Veterinary ethics, social ethics and animal welfare, Colorado State University, 1999, OAVT Conference Proceedings.

Rose RJ: Overview of veterinary technology. In Sirois M, editor: *Principles and practice of veterinary technology*, ed 2, St Louis, 2004, Mosby.

Rosenberg MA: *Companion animal loss and pet owner grief*, ed 2, Lehigh Valley, Pa, 1993, Alpo Pet Foods.

Tannenbaum J: *Veterinary ethics: animal welfare, client relations, competition and collegiality*, ed 2, St Louis, 1995, Mosby.

# Abbreviations and Symbols

**A**

Å  Angstrom; anode; anterior

**a**  Ampere; anterior; area; artery

**A₂**  Aortic second sound

**a̅a̅**  Of each

**AAHA**  American Animal Hospital Association

**AALAS**  American Association for Laboratory Animal Science

**AAVSB**  American Association of Veterinary State Boards

**ab**  Antibody

**ABO**  Three basic human blood groups

**AC**  Alternating current; adrenal cortex

**a.c.**  Before meals *(ante cibum)*

**ACE**  Adrenocortical extract

**ACh**  Acetylcholine

**ACH**  Adrenocortical hormone

**ACTH**  Adrenocorticotropic hormone

**ACTTSA**  Association Canadienne des Techniciens et Technologistes en Santé Animale

**AD**  Right ear

**ad lib**  As much as desired *(ad libitum)*

**ADH**  Antidiuretic hormone

**A/G; A-G ratio**  Albumin-globulin ratio

**Ag**  Silver

**ag**  Antigen

**AHT**  Animal Health Technician

**AIDS**  Acquired immune deficiency syndrome

**AKC**  American Kennel Club

**AL**  Left ear

**Al**  Aluminum

**ALAT**  Assistant Laboratory Animal Technician

**Alb**  Albumin

**ALT**  Alanine aminotransferase (formerly SGPT)

**AMA**  American Medical Association

**AMI**  Acute myocardial infarction

**amp**  Ampere

**ana**  So much of each, or **a̅a̅**

**anat**  Anatomy or anatomical

**ANS**  Autonomic nervous system

**A-P; AP; A/P**  Anteroposterior

**A.P.**  Anterior pituitary gland

**APHIS**  Animal and Plant Health Inspection Service

**Aq**  Water *(aqua)*

**ARD**  Acute respiratory disease

**As**  Arsenic

**ASD**  Atrial septal defect

**AST**  Aspartate aminotransferase (formerly SGOT)

**AU**  Both (left and right) ears

**Au**  Gold

**A-V; AV; A/V**  Arteriovenous; atrioventricular

**Av**  Average *(avoirdupois)*

**AVECCT**  Academy of Veterinary Emergency Critical Care Technicians

**AVMA**  American Veterinary Medical Association

**AVTA**  Academy of Veterinary Technician Anesthetists

**ax**  Axis

**B**

**B**  Boron; bacillus

**Ba**  Barium

**Bact**  Bacterium

**BBB**  Blood-brain barrier

**BE**  Barium enema

**Be**  Beryllium

**BER**  Basal energy requirement

**Bi**  Bismuth

**bid; b.i.d.**  Twice a day *(bis in die)*

**BM**  Bowel movement

**BMR**  Basal metabolic rate

**BP**  Blood pressure

**bp**  Boiling point

**BPH**  Benign prostatic hypertrophy

**BSA**  Body surface area

**BSP**  Bromsulphalein

**BUN**  Blood urea nitrogen

**BVD**  Bovine virus diarrhea

**BW**  Body weight

**C**

**C**  Carbon; centigrade; Celsius

**c̄**  With

**Ca**  Calcium; cancer; cathode

**CAAHTT**  Canadian Association of Animal Health Technologists and Technicians

**CaCO₃**  Calcium carbonate

**Cal**  Large calorie

**cal**  Small calorie

**CALAS**  Canadian Association for Laboratory Animal Science

**CBC; cbc**  Complete blood count

**cc**  Cubic centimeter

**CCl₄**  Carbon tetrachloride

**CD**  Canine distemper

**CDC**  Centers for Disease Control and Prevention

**cf**  Compare or bring together

**CFT**  Complement-fixation test

**cg; cgm**  Centigram

**CHCl₃**  Chloroform

**CH₃COOH** Acetic acid
**CHD** Canine hip dysplasia
**ChE** Cholinesterase
**CHF** Congestive heart failure
**C₂H₅OH** Ethyl alcohol
**C₅H₄N₄O₃** Uric acid
**CH₂O** Formaldehyde
**CH₃OH** Methyl alcohol
**CKC** Canadian Kennel Club
**Cl** Chlorine
**cm** Centimeter
**CMT** California Mastitis Test
**CNS** Central nervous system
**CO** Carbon monoxide
**CO₂** Carbon dioxide
**Co** Cobalt
**CPC** Clinicopathologic conference
**CRF** Chronic renal failure
**CRT** Capillary refill time
**C&S** Culture and sensitivity
**CSF** Cerebrospinal fluid
**CT; CAT** Computed (axial) tomography
**Cu** Copper
**CuSO₄** Copper sulfate
**CVA** Cerebrovascular accident
**CVMA** Canadian Veterinary Medical Association
**CVP** Central venous pressure
**CVT** Certified Veterinary Technician
**CVTS** Committee on Veterinary Technician Specialties

**D**

**D** Dose; vitamin D; right (dextro)
**DC** Direct current
**DCA** Deoxycorticosterone acetate
**DEA** Drug Enforcement Administration; dog erythrocyte antigen
**Deg** Degeneration; degree
**DES** Diethylstilbestrol
**dg** Decigram
**diff** Differential blood count
**dil** Dilute
**dimone** Half
**DJD** Degenerative joint disease
**DLH** Domestic longhair (cat)
**DNA** Deoxyribonucleic acid
**DOA** Dead on arrival
**D/S** Dextrose in saline
**DSH** Domestic shorthair (cat)
**DVM** Doctor of Veterinary Medicine
**Dₓ** Diagnosis

**E**

**E** Eye
**ECC** Emergency and critical care
**ECG** Electrocardiogram; electrocardiograph
**ED** Effective dose
**ED₅₀** Median effective dose
**EDTA** Ethylenediaminetetraacetic acid
**EEG** Electroencephalogram; electroencephalograph
**EENT** Eye, ear, nose, and throat
**EFA** Essential fatty acid

**EIA** Equine infectious anemia; enzyme immunoassay
**EKG** Electrocardiogram; electrocardiograph
**ELISA** Enzyme-linked immunosorbent assay
**EMB** Eosin-methylene blue
**EMC** Encephalomyocarditis
**EMG** Electromyogram
**EMS** Emergency medical services
**ENT** Ear, nose, and throat
**ER** Emergency room (hospital); external resistance
**ESR** Erythrocyte sedimentation rate
**ext** Extract

**F**

**F** Fahrenheit; formula
**FA** Fatty acid
**FANA** Fluorescent antinuclear antibody test
**F&R** Force and rhythm (pulse)
**FB** Foreign body
**FBS** Fasting blood sugar
**FD** Fatal dose
**FDA** Food and Drug Administration
**Fe** Iron
**FeCl₃** Ferric chloride
**FeLV** Feline leukemia virus
**FFD** Film focal distance
**FIP** Feline infectious peritonitis
**FIV** Feline immunodeficiency virus
**Fl** Fluid
**fld** Fluid
**fl oz; fl. oz.** Fluid ounce
**FLUTD** Feline lower urinary tract disease
**FPV** Feline panleukopenia virus
**FR** Flocculation reaction
**FSH** Follicle-stimulating hormone
**ft** Foot
**FUO** Fever of undetermined origin
**FUS** Feline urological syndrome
**Fx** Fracture

**G**

**g** Gram
**gal** Gallon
**Galv** Galvanic
**GB** Gallbladder
**GBS** Gallbladder series
**GDV** Gastric dilatation volvulus
**GFR** Glomerular filtration rate
**GH** Growth hormone
**GI** Gastrointestinal
**GLPs** Good laboratory practices
**Gm; gm** Gram
**GnRH** Gonadotrophin-releasing hormone
**GP** General practitioner; general paresis
**gr** Grain(s)
**GSW** Gunshot wound
**gt** Drop (gutta)
**GTT** Glucose tolerance test
**gtt** Drops (guttae)
**GU** Genitourinary
**Gyn** Gynecology

**H**

**h**  Hour
**H**  Hydrogen
**H⁺**  Hydrogen ion
**H$_x$**  History
**H&E**  Hematoxylin and eosin (stain)
**Hb; Hgb**  Hemoglobin
**HBC**  Hit by car
**H$_3$BO$_3$**  Boric acid
**HC**  Health certificate
**HCG**  Human chorionic gonadotropin
**HCl**  Hydrochloric acid
**HCN**  Hydrocyanic acid
**H$_2$CO$_3$**  Carbonic acid
**HCT; Hct**  Hematocrit
**HDL**  High-density lipoprotein
**H of A**  Health of Animals
**He**  Helium
**Hg**  Mercury
**HNO$_3$**  Nitric acid
**H$_2$O**  Water
**H$_2$O$_2$**  Hydrogen peroxide
**HR**  Heart rate
**hs**  At bedtime *(hora somni)*
**H$_2$SO$_4$**  Sulfuric acid

**I**

**I**  Iodine
**¹³¹I**  Radioactive isotope of iodine (atomic weight 131)
**¹³²I**  Radioactive isotope of iodine (atomic weight 132)
**IB**  Inclusion body
**IBR**  Infectious bovine rhinotracheitis
**IC**  Intracardiac
**ICF**  Intracellular fluid
**ICH**  Infectious canine hepatitis
**ICS; IS**  Intercostal space
**ICSH**  Interstitial cell-stimulating hormone
**ICU**  Intensive care unit
**id**  The same *(idem)*
**ID**  Intradermal
**IM**  Intramuscular
**IOP**  Intraocular pressure
**IP**  Intraperitoneal
**IT; i.t.**  Intratracheal
**IU**  Immunizing unit; international unit
**IV**  Intravenous
**IVP**  Intravenous pyelogram
**IVT**  Intravenous transfusion
**IVU**  Intravenous urogram/urography

**K**

**K**  Potassium
**k**  Constant
**K$_9$**  Canine
**Ka**  Cathode or kathode
**KBr**  Potassium bromide
**kc**  Kilocycle
**kcal**  Kilocalorie
**KCl**  Potassium chloride

**keV**  Kiloelectron volt
**kg**  Kilogram
**KI**  Potassium iodide
**km**  Kilometer
**KOH**  Potassium hydroxide
**kV**  Kilovolt
**kW**  Kilowatt

**L**

**L**  Left; liter; length; lumbar; lethal
**LAT**  Laboratory Animal Technician
**LATG**  Laboratory Animal Technologist
**lb**  Pound *(libra)*
**LCM**  Left costal margin
**LD**  Lethal dose
**LD$_{50}$**  Median lethal dose
**LDA**  Left displaced abomasum
**LDL**  Low-density lipoprotein
**LE**  Lupus erythematosus
**LFD**  Least fatal dose of a toxin
**LH**  Luteinizing hormone
**Li**  Lithium
**lig**  Ligament
**Liq**  Liquor
**LN**  Lymph node
**LPF**  Leukocytosis-promoting factor
**LRS**  Lactated Ringer's solution
**LTH**  Luteotrophic hormone
**LV**  Left ventricle
**LVT**  Licensed Veterinary Technician

**M**

**M**  Muscle; thousand
**m**  Meter; milli; thousand
**μCi**  Microcurie
**mcg; μg**  Microgram
**MCH**  Mean corpuscular hemoglobin
**MCHC**  Mean corpuscular hemoglobin concentration
**mCi; mc**  Millicurie
**mcm; μm**  Micron
**MCV**  Mean corpuscular volume
**MCT**  Mast cell tumor
**MED**  Minimal effective dose
**mEq**  Milliequivalent
**mEq/L**  Milliequivalent per liter
**ME ratio**  Myeloid-erythroid ratio
**Mg**  Magnesium
**mg**  Milligram
**MI**  Myocardial infarction; mitral insufficiency
**MID**  Minimum infective dose
**MIP**  Mare's immunological pregnancy test
**ML**  Midline
**mL; ml**  Milliliter
**MLD**  Median or minimum lethal dose
**MLV**  Modified live virus
**MM**  Mucous membrane
**mm**  Millimeter; muscles
**mm Hg**  Millimeters of mercury
**Mn**  Manganese
**mN**  Millinormal

**mol/liter**  Mole per liter
**MRI**  Magnetic resonance imaging
**MS**  Mitral stenosis; morphine sulfate
**MT**  Medical technologist
**mu**  Mouse unit

**N**

**N**  Nitrogen
**n**  Normal
**Na**  Sodium
**NaBr**  Sodium bromide
**NaCl**  Sodium chloride
**Na$_2$C$_2$O$_4$**  Sodium oxalate
**Na$_2$CO$_3$**  Sodium carbonate
**NaF**  Sodium fluoride
**NaHCO$_3$**  Sodium bicarbonate
**Na$_2$HPO$_4$**  Sodium phosphate
**NaI**  Sodium iodide
**NaNO$_3$**  Sodium nitrate
**Na$_2$O$_2$**  Sodium peroxide
**NaOH**  Sodium hydroxide
**Na$_2$SO$_4$**  Sodium sulfate
**NAVTA**  National Association of Veterinary Technicians in America
**NAVTTC**  North American Veterinary Technician Testing Committee
**NCC**  Nucleated cell count
**Ne**  Neon
**NH$_3$**  Ammonia
**Ni**  Nickel
**NMR**  Nuclear magnetic resonance
**non rep**  Do not repeat
**NPL**  Nonpalpable lesion
**NPN**  Nonprotein nitrogen
**NPO; n.p.o.**  Nothing by mouth *(non per os)*
**NR**  Not remarkable
**NRBC**  Nucleated red blood cell
**NS**  Normal saline
**NSF**  No significant findings
**NSR**  Normal sinus rhythm
**NTP**  Normal temperature and pressure
**NVL**  No visible lesions

**O**

**O**  Oxygen; oculus
**O$_2$**  Oxygen
**O$_3$**  Ozone
**OAVT**  Ontario Association of Veterinary Technicians
**OBGYN**  Obstetrics and gynecology
**OCD**  Osteochondritis dissecans
**OD**  Right eye *(oculus dexter);* optical density; overdose
**OFA**  Orthopedic Foundation for Animals
**OHE**  Ovariohysterectomy
**Ol**  Oil *(oleum)*
**OR**  Operating room
**OS**  Left eye *(oculus sinister)*
**Os**  Osmium
**OSA**  Osteosarcoma
**OSHA**  Occupational Safety and Health Administration

**OU**  Both eyes
**oz**  Ounce

**P**

**P**  Phosphorus; pulse; pupil
**P$_2$**  Pulmonic second sound
**P-A; P/A; PA**  Posteroanterior
**P&A**  Percussion and auscultation
**PAB; PABA**  Para-aminobenzoic acid
**PAC**  Premature atrial contraction
**PAS; PASA**  Para-aminosalicylic acid
**Pb**  Lead
**PBI**  Protein-bound iodine
**p.c.**  After meals *(post cibum)*
**PCV**  Packed cell volume
**PDA**  Patent ductus arteriosus
**PDR**  *Physician's Desk Reference;* passive defense reflex
**PE**  Physical examination; pulmonary edema
**PEG**  Pneumoencephalography
**per os**  Orally
**PET**  Positron emission tomography
**PFF**  Protein-free filtrate
**PG**  Prostaglandin
**PGA**  Pteroylglutamic acid (folic acid)
**pH**  A measure of alkalinity/acidity of a solution based on hydrogen ion concentration
**Pharm; Phar.**  Pharmacy
**PI**  Parainfluenza virus
**PM**  Postmortem; evening
**PMN**  Polymorphonuclear neutrophil
**PMSG**  Pregnant mare serum gonadotrophin
**PN**  Percussion note
**PNS**  Parsympathetic nervous system
**PO; p.o.**  Orally *(per os);* postoperatively
**POVMR**  Problem-oriented veterinary medical records
**PPB**  Parts per billion
**PPD**  Purified protein derivative (TB test)
**PPM**  Parts per million
**PPV**  Porcine parvovirus
**PRN; prn**  As required *(pro re nata)*
**pro time**  Prothrombin time
**PRRS**  Porcine reproductive and respiratory syndrome
**PS**  Pulmonic stenosis
**PSP**  Phenolsulfonphthalein
**Pt**  Platinum; patient
**PT**  Pint
**PTA**  Plasma thromboplastin antecedent
**PTC**  Plasma thromboplastin component
**PTH**  Parathyroid hormone
**Pu**  Plutonium
**PVC**  Premature ventricular contraction or complex
**PZI**  Protamine zinc insulin

**Q**

**q**  Every
**QBC**  Quantitative buffy coat
**qd**  Every day *(quaque die)*
**qh**  Every hour *(quaque hora)*
**qid; q.i.d.**  Four times daily *(quater in die)*
**ql**  As much as desired *(quantum libet)*

**qns** Quantity not sufficient
**qod** Every other day
**q.p.** As much as desired *(quantum placeat)*
**qs** Sufficient quantity
**qt** Quart
**qv** As much as you please *(quantum vis)*

**R**

**R** Respiration; right; *Rickettsia*; roentgen
**R$_x$** Take
**Ra** Radium
**RAD** Radiograph
**rad** Unit of measurement of the absorbed dose of ionizing radiation
**RAI** Radioactive iodine
**RAIU** Radioactive iodine uptake
**RBC; rbc** Red blood cell; red blood count
**RDA** Right displaced abomasum
**RE** Right eye; reticuloendothelial tissue or cell
**Re** Rhenium
**Rect** Rectified
**Rep.** Let it be repeated *(repetatur)*
**RES** Reticuloendothelial system
**Rh** Symbol of rhesus factor; rhodium
**RHF** Right heart failure
**Rn** Radon
**RNA** Ribonucleic acid
**R/O** Rule out
**RPM; rpm** Revolutions per minute
**RT** Radiation therapy
**RVT** Registered Veterinary Technician

**S**

**S** Sulfur
**S.** Sacral
**s̄** Without *(sine)*
**S-A; S/A; SA** Sinoatrial
**SD** Skin dose
**Se** Selenium
**Sed rate; SR** Sedimentation rate
**SGOT** Serum glutamic oxaloacetic transaminase (see AST)
**SGPT** Serum glutamic pyruvic transaminase (see ALT)
**Si** Silicon
**Sig** Label; prescription
**SMEDI** Stillbirths, mummified, embryonic death infertility
**Sn** Tin
**SNS** Sympathetic nervous system
**SOAP** Subjective objective assessment plan
**Sol** Solution
**sp** Species
**Sp** Spirit
**sp. gr.; SG** Specific gravity
**SPCA** Society for the Prevention of Cruelty to Animals
**Sr** Strontium
**SR** Suture removal
**s̄s̄** One half *(semis)*
**Staph** *Staphylococcus*
**Stat** Immediately *(statum)*
**STD** Sexually transmitted disease
**STH** Somatotropic hormone

**Strep** *Streptococcus*
**SVBT** Society of Veterinary Behavior Technicians
**S$_x$** Sign or symptom; surgery
**Sym** Symmetrical

**T**

**T** Temperature; thoracic
**t** Temporal
**T$_3$** Triiodothyronine
**T$_4$** Thyroxine
**tab** Tablet
**TAT** Tetanus antitoxin
**TB** Tuberculin; tuberculosis; tubercle bacillus
**TBW** Total body water
**TDN** Total digestible nutrient
**Te** Tetanus
**TGC** Time gain compensation
**TGE** Transmissible gastroenteritis
**Th** Thorium
**tid; t.i.d.** Three times daily *(ter in die)*
**T-L** Thoracolumbar vertebrae
**Tl** Thallium
**TLC** Tender loving care
**TP** Total protein
**TPP** Total plasma protein
**TPR** Temperature, pulse, and respiration
**tr** Tincture
**TS** Test solution
**TSH** Thyroid-stimulating hormone
**TSI** Triple sugar iron
**TT** Tetanus toxoid
**T$_x$** Treatment

**U**

**U** Uranium; unit
**UA** Urinalysis
**ung** Ointment *(unguentum)*
**UO** Urinary obstruction
**URI** Upper respiratory infection
**US** Ultrasonic
**USDA** United States Department of Agriculture
**USP** U.S. Pharmacopeia
**Ut. dict.** As directed *(ut dictum)*
**UTI** Urinary tract infection

**V**

**v** Vein
**V** Vanadium; vision
**V** Volt; vein
**VC** Vital capacity
**VEE** Venezuelan equine encephalomyelitis
**VHD** Valvular heart disease
**VLDL** Very low-density lipoprotein
**VMD** Veterinary Medical Doctor
**VS** Volumetric solution; vital signs
**VSD** Ventricular septal defect
**VTA** Veterinary Technician Anesthetist
**VTNE** Veterinary Technician National Examination
**VTS** Veterinary Technician Specialty
**VW** Vessel wall

## W

**w**  Watt
**WBC; wbc**  White blood cell; white blood count
**WEE**  Western equine encephalomyelitis
**WL**  Wavelength
**WNL**  Within normal limits
**Wt; wt**  Weight

## X

**X-ray**  Roentgen ray
**XRT**  Radiation therapy

## Z

**z**  Symbol for atomic number
**Zn**  Zinc

## Symbols

> greater than
< less than
♀ Female
♂ Male

# The Metric System and Equivalents

The basis of measurement in science is the Système International d'Unités (SI), in which the main units are the meter, the gram, and the liter. Although the English system is still used in the United States, the metric system is the preferred system because of its logic and accuracy.

## SI ABBREVIATIONS

The rules for writing metric units are (1) use lowercase letters for abbreviations, except for the symbol for liter (L) or if the units are named after a person; (2) symbols are never pluralized; and (3) decimals are used instead of fractions.

| | |
|---|---|
| centimeter | cm |
| deciliter | dL |
| decaliter | dkL |
| gram | g |
| hectoliter | hL |
| kilogram | kg |
| kilometer | km |
| liter | L |
| meter | m |
| microgram | mcg or mg |
| milliliter | mL |
| millimeter | mm |

## Units of Length

Given are metric linear decimal scale and English (U.S.) equivalents.

| | | | | |
|---|---|---|---|---|
| 10 millimeters | = 1 centimeter | | = | 0.3937 inch |
| 10 centimeters | = 1 decimeter | | = | 3.937 inches |
| 10 decimeters | = 1 meter | | = | 39.37 inches (3.2808 feet) |
| 10 meters | = 1 decameter | | = | 10.936 yards |
| 10 decameters | = 1 hectometer | | = | 19.884 rods |
| 10 hectometers | = 1 kilometer | | = | 0.62137 mile |
| 10 kilometers | = 1 myriameter | | = | 6.2137 miles |
| 1 inch | = 2.54 centimeters | or | 25.4 millimeters | |
| 1 foot | = 3.048 decimeters | or | 304.8 millimeters | |
| 1 yard | = 0.9144 meter | or | 914.40 millimeters | |
| 1 rod | = 0.5029 decameter | | | |
| 1 mile | = 1.6093 kilometers | | | |

## Units of Weight

Given are metric weights and English (U.S.) equivalents.

| | | | | |
|---|---|---|---|---|
| 1 milligram | = | 0.001 gram | = | 0.015 grain |
| 1 centigram | = | 0.01 gram | = | 0.154 grain |
| 1 decigram | = | 0.10 gram | = | 1.543 grains |
| 1 gram | = | 1 gram | = | 0.035 ounce |
| 1 dekagram | = | 10 grams | = | 0.353 ounce |
| 1 hectogram | = | 100 grams | = | 3.527 ounces |
| 1 kilogram | = | 1000 grams | = | 2.205 pounds |
| 1 grain | = | 0.0648 gram | | |
| 1 ounce | = | 28.349 grams | | |
| 1 pound | = | 0.453 kilogram | | |
| To convert kg to lb: | | lb = kg × 2.204 | | |
| To convert lb to kg: | | kg = lb ÷ 2.204 | | |

## Units of Volume

Given as metric liquid measure capacity and English (U.S.) equivalents.

| | | | | |
|---|---|---|---|---|
| 1 milliliter (cc) | | | = | 16.23 minims or 0.0338 fluid ounce |
| 1 liter | | | = | 33.8148 fluid ounces or 2.1134 pints or 1.0567 quarts or 0.2642 gallon |
| 1 teaspoon | | | = | 5 mL |
| 1 tablespoon | | | = | 15 mL |
| 1 fluid ounce | | | = | 29.573 mL |
| 1 pint | = | 16 ounces | = | 473.166 mL or 0.473 L |
| 1 quart | = | 2 pints | = | 946.332 mL or 0.946 L |
| 1 gallon | = | 4 quarts | = | 3.785 L |

## Temperature Equivalents

To convert Fahrenheit to Celsius: $°C = °F - 32 \times \frac{5}{9}$

To convert Celsius to Fahrenheit: $°F = °C \times \frac{5}{9} + 32$

## Other Equivalents

Freezing point: 0° C or 32° F at 1 atmosphere pressure

Boiling point: 100° C or 212° F at 1 atmosphere pressure

# Medical Terminology

For further information, consult excellent veterinary terminology texts that are available.

## PREFIXES

**a-, ab-, abs-** From; away; departing from the normal

**ad-** Addition to; toward; nearness

**amb-, ambi-** Both; ambidextrous; having the ability to work effectively with either hand

**amphi-** On both sides

**ampho-** Both

**an-** Negative; without or not

**ana-** Upper; away from

**andro-** Signifying man

**angi-** Vessel

**aniso-** Unequal

**ant-, anti-** Against

**ante-, antero-** Front; before

**auto-** Self

**bi-** Two

**bili-** Pertaining to bile

**brady-** Slow

**brom-, bromo-** A stench

**broncho-** Relating to the bronchi

**cac-** Bad; ill

**cardi-, cardio-** Relating to the heart

**cata-** Down or downward

**centi-** Hundred

**cervico-** Relating to the neck

**circa-** About

**circum-** Around

**co-** With or together

**con-, com-** Together with

**contra-** Opposite; against

**de-** Down from

**deci-** One tenth

**demi-** Half

**di-** Twice

**dia-** Through, apart, across, or between

**dialy-** To separate

**dis-** Reversal; separation; duplication

**dys-** Bad; difficult; disordered

**en-** In

**end-, endo-, ento-** Inward; within

**ep-, epi-** On; in addition to

**eu-** Normal; good; well; easy

**ex-** Out; away from

**exo-** Without; outside of

**extra-** Outside of; in addition to

**fibro-** Relating to fibers

**hecto-** Hundred

**hemi-** Half

**hemo-** Relating to the blood

**heter-, hetero-** Meaning other; relationship to another

**homeo-** Denoting likeness or resemblance

**homo-** Denoting sameness

**hyper-** Above; excessive; beyond

**hypo-** Below; less than

**ideo-** Pertaining to mental images

**idio-** Denoting relationship to one's self or to something separate and distinct

**in-** Not; in; inside; within; also intensive action

**infra-** Below

**inter-** In the midst; between

**intra-** Within

**intro-** In or into

**iso-** Equal or alike

**juxta-** Of close proximity

**karyo-** Relating to a cell's nucleus

**kilo-** One thousand

**kypho-** Humped

**laryngo-** Pertaining to the larynx

**mal-** Illness, disease

**medi-** Middle

**micro-** Small

**milli-** One thousandth

**multi-** Many

**my-, myo-** Relating to muscle

**myc-, mycet-** Denoting a fungus

**nano-** Dwarf; small size

**necro-** Denoting death

**neo-** New

**noci-** Harm, injury

**omni-** All

**pan-** All, entire

**para-** Pair; beside

**per-** Through; by means of

**peri-** Around; about; near

**poly-** Many

**post-** Behind or after

**pre-** Before

**pro-** Before; in front of

**pseudo-** False

**quadri-** Four
**re-** Back; again (contrary)
**retro-** Backward
**semi-** Half
**steato-** Fatty
**sub-** Under; near
**sym-, syn-** With; along; joined together
**tachy-** Swift
**trans-** Across; over
**tri-** Three
**un-** Not; reversal
**uni-** One

## SUFFIXES

**-able, -ible, -ble** The power to be
**-ad** Toward; in the direction of
**-aemia, -emia** Pertaining to blood
**-age** Put in motion; to do
**-agra** Denoting a seizure; severe pain
**-algia** Denoting pain
**-ase** Forms the name of an enzyme
**-blast** Designates a cell or a structure
**-cele** Denoting a swelling
**-centesis** Denoting a puncture
**-ectasia** Expansion; dilatation; distention
**-ectomy** A cutting out
**-emia** Condition of the blood
**-esthesia** Denoting sensation
**-gog, -gogue** To make flow
**-gram** A tracing; a mark
**-graph** A writing; a record
**-iasis** Denoting a condition or pathological state
**-id** Denoting shape or resemblance
**-ism** State; process; condition
**-ite** Of the nature of
**-itis** Denoting inflammation
**-logia, -logy** Denoting discourse, science, or study of
**-lysis** Dissolution
**-malacia** Softening
**-megaly** Enlargement
**-oid** Denoting form or resemblance
**-oma** Denoting a tumor
**-osis** Denoting any morbid process
**-ostomosis, -ostomy, -stomy** Denoting an outlet; to furnish with an opening or mouth
**-paresis** Slight or incomplete paralysis
**-pathy** Morbid condition or disease
**-penia** Deficiency
**-pexy** Surgical fixation
**-plasty** Denoting molding or shaping
**-plegia** Paralysis
**-prandial** Meal
**-ptosis** Drooping
**-rhagia, -rrhagia** Denoting a discharge; usually a bleeding
**-rhaphy, -rrhaphy** Meaning suturing or stitching
**-rhea, -rrhea** Meaning a flow or discharge
**-rrhexis** Rupture of a blood vessel
**-scopy** Generally, an instrument for viewing
**-tomy** Denoting a cutting operation

**-tripsy** Crushing
**-trophy** Denoting a relationship to nourishment

## ROOTS AND COMBINING FORMS

**aer, aer/o** Denoting air or gas
**alge, algesi, alg/o** Relating to pain
**all/o** Other; differing from the normal
**ankyl/o** Bent; crooked; in the form of loop
**anomal/o** Denoting irregularity
**arth/ro** Relating to a joint or joints
**brevi** Short
**cac, cac/o** Bad, diseased
**celi/o** Denoting the abdomen
**centr/o** Center
**cheil, cheil/o** Denoting the lip
**chol, chole, cholo** Relating to bile
**chondr, chondri** Relating to cartilage
**chrom, chrom/o** Relating to color
**cole, cole/o** Denoting a sheath
**colp, colp/o** Relating to the vagina
**crani/o** Relating to the cranium of the skull
**crym/o, cry/o** Denoting cold
**crypt** To hide; a pit
**cyan/o** Dark blue
**cycl/o** Pertaining to a cycle
**cyst/o** Relating to a sac or cyst
**cyt/o** Denoting a cell
**dacr/yo** Pertaining to the lacrimal glands
**dactyl/o** Relating to digits
**dent, dent/o** Relating to teeth
**derma, dermat** Relating to the skin
**desm/o** Relating to a bond or ligament
**dextr/o** Right
**dipl/o** Double; twofold
**dorsi, dors/o** Referring to the back
**duoden/o** Relating to the duodenum
**electr/o** Relating to electricity
**encephal/o** Denoting the brain
**enter/o** Relating to the intestines
**episi/o** Relating to the vulva
**erythr/o** Red; erythrocyte
**es/o** Inward
**esthesi/o** Relating to feeling or sensation
**facient** That which makes or causes
**faci/o** Relating to the face
**gangli, gangli/o** Relating to a ganglion
**gaster, gastr, gastr/o** Pertaining to the stomach
**gen/o** Relating to reproduction
**gene, genesis, genetic, genic** Denoting production; origin
**ger/o, geront/o** Denoting old age
**gigant/o** Huge
**gingiv/o** Relating to the gingiva or gum
**gloss, gloss/o** Relating to the tongue
**gluc/o** Denoting sweetness
**glyc/o** Relating to sugar
**gon** Denoting a seed
**graph/o** Denoting writing
**hapt, hapte, hapt/o** Relating to touch or a seizure
**hel/o** Relating to a nail or a callus

**hepat, hepatic/o, hepat/o** Pertaining to the liver
**hist, histi/o, hist/o** Relating to tissue
**hol/o** Relating to the whole
**hyal, hyal/o** Transparent
**hydr, hydr/o** Denoting water
**hygr/o** Denoting moisture
**hyl, hyle, hyl/o** Denoting matter or material
**ileo** Relating to the ileum
**ipsi** Meaning self
**irid/o** Relating to a colored circle
**iso** Equal
**jejun/o** Referring to the jejunum
**kerat/o** Relating to the cornea
**kin/o** Denoting movement
**labi/o** Pertaining to the lips
**lact/o** Relating to milk
**lapar/o** Pertaining to the loin or flank
**later/o** Pertaining to the side
**leid/o, lei/o** Smooth
**leuk, leuko** Denoting deficiency of color
**lip, lip/o** Pertaining to fat
**lith/o** Denoting a calculus
**macr, macr/o** Large; long
**mast, mastr/o** Relating to the breast
**meg, mega** Great; large
**melan/o** Black; melanin
**meli** Sweet
**mening/o** Denoting membranes; covering the brain and spinal cord
**micr, micr/o** Small in size or extent
**mon/o** One
**morph/o** Relating to form
**myel/o** Pertaining to the spinal cord or bone marrow
**myring/o** Denoting tympani or the eardrum
**myx, myx/o** Pertaining to mucus
**narc/o** Denoting stupor
**nas/o** Relating to the nose
**nephr, nephr/o** Denoting the kidney
**norm/o** Normal or usual
**ocul/o** Denoting the eye
**odyn/o** Denoting pain
**ole/o** Denoting oil
**onc/o** Denoting a swelling or mass
**onych/o** Relating to the nails
**oo** Denoting an egg
**ophthal, ophthalm/o** Pertaining to the eye
**opisth, opisth/o** Backward
**optic/o** Relating to the eye or vision
**orchi, orch/o** Relating to the testes
**or/o** Relating to the mouth
**orth/o** Straight; right
**oscill/o** Denoting oscillation
**oste/o** Relating to the bones
**ot, ot/o** Denoting an egg
**ovari/o** Pertaining to the ovary
**palat/o** Denoting the palate
**path/o** Denoting disease
**pedia, ped/o** Denoting a child
**perine/o** A combining form for the region between the anus and either the scrotum or the vulva

**phag/o** Denoting a relationship to eating
**pharyng/o** Pertaining to the pharynx
**phleb, phleb/o** Denoting the veins
**phon, phon/o** Denoting sound
**phot, phot/o** Relating to light
**phren** Relating to the mind
**picr, picr/o** Bitter
**pil/o** Denoting hair
**plasm/o** Relating to plasma or the substance of a cell
**pnea** Respiration, breathing
**pneuma, pneumon/o, pneumot/o** Denoting air or gas
**pod, pod/o** Foot
**postero** Relating to the posterior
**proct, proct/o** Denoting the anus and rectum
**psych, psych/o** Relating to the mind
**ptyal/o** Denoting saliva
**pubio, pub/o** Denoting the pubic region
**pulm/o** Denoting the lung
**pupill/o** Denoting the pupil
**py, py/o** Denoting pus
**pyel, pyel/o** Denoting the pelvis
**pylor/o** Relating to the pylorus
**rect/o** Denoting the rectum
**rhin, rhin/o** Denoting the nose
**rrhagia** Denoting abnormal discharge
**salping/o** Denoting a tube, specifically the fallopian tube
**schiz/o** Split
**scler/o** Denoting hardness
**scot/o** Relating to darkness
**ser/o** Pertaining to serum
**sial/o** Relating to saliva or the salivary glands
**sider/o** Denoting iron
**sinistr/o** Left
**somat/o** Denoting the body
**somni** Denoting sleep
**spasm/o** Denoting a spasm
**spermat/o, sperm/o** Denoting sperm
**spher/o** Denoting a sphere; round
**sphygm/o** Denoting a pulse
**splen, splen/o** Denoting the spleen
**staphyl, staphyl/o** Resembling a bunch of grapes
**sten/o** Narrow; short
**sterc/o** Denoting feces
**steth, steth/o** Relating to the chest
**stomat/o** Denoting the mouth
**tars/o** Relating to the flat of the foot
**therm/o** Heat
**thorac/o** Relating to the chest
**thromb/o** Denoting a blood clot
**toxic/o, tox/o** Denoting poison
**trache/o** Denoting the trachea
**trichi, trich/o** Denoting hair
**ur, ur/o, uron/o** Relating to urine
**varic/o** Denoting a twisting or swelling
**vas/o** Denoting a vessel
**ven/o** Denoting a vein
**ventri, ventr/o** Denoting the abdomen
**vertebr/o** Relating to the vertebra
**vesic/o** Denoting the bladder
**viscer/o** Denoting the organs of the body

**vivi** Denoting alive
**xanth/o** Denoting yellow
**xer/o** Denoting dryness

## TERMINOLOGY FREQUENTLY USED TO DESIGNATE BODY PARTS OR ORGANS

**abdomen** Abdomin/o, celi/o, lapar/o
**anus** Anal, an/o
**arm** Brachial, brachi/o
**belly** Ventr/o
**blood** Heme, hemat, sanguin/o
**body** Soma, somata
**brain** Encephal/o, cerebrum
**breast** Mamm/o, mastos
**cartilage** Chondr/o
**cell** Cyto
**cheek** Buccal
**chest** Thoracic, thorax
**ear** Auricle, ot/o
**eye** Ocular, ocul/o, ophthalm/o
**fingers, toes** Dactyl/o
**foot** Pedal, ped, pod
**gallbladder** Chole, chol
**gland** Aden/o
**gum** Ul, gingiva
**hair** Trichos, capillus, pilo
**head** Cephalic, cephal/o
**heart** Cardium, cardiac, cardi/o
**intestines** Cecum, colon, duodenum, ileum, jejunum
**jaw** Gnath/o
**joint** Arthron, articulus
**kidney** Renal, nephric, nephr/o
**ligament** Syndesm/o
**lip** Cheil, labia
**liver** Hepatic, hepat/o
**lungs** Pulmonary, pulmonic, pneum/o

**membrane** Meninx, meningos
**mind** Psych/o, ment/o
**mouth** Oral, os, stoma, stomat
**muscle** Myo, muscul/o
**neck** Cervix, cervical, cervico
**nerve** Neuron, nervus
**nose** Nasus, rhinos
**peritoneum** Peritone/o
**penis** Penile
**pulse** Sphygm/o
**pupil** Core/o
**rectum** Rectal, rect/o proct/o
**saliva** Sial/o, pty, ptyal
**shoulder blade** Scapul/o
**skin** Derma, integumentum, cutis
**spinal chord** Myelos, chord/o
**spleen** Splen/o
**stomach** Gastric, gastr/o
**tear** Dacry/o, lacrim
**teeth** Odont/o, dent/o
**testicle** Orchi/o, orchi, orchid/o, testis
**thigh** Femur, femoris
**tissue** Histos
**tongue** Lingua, gloss/o
**tooth** Odontus, dentis
**ureter** Ureter/o
**urethra** Ureter/o
**urinary bladder** Cysti, cyst/o
**uterus** Hyster/o, metra
**vagina** Vulv/o, vaginal
**vessel** Angi/o, vascul/o, hemang/io
**viscera** Splanchn/o, viscer/o
**vein** Phlebos, venus
**vulva** Episi/o
**womb** Hystera, uter/o, metra
**wrist bones** Carp/o

# Species Names

| Common name | Scientific name (generic) | Male/female terminology | Neutered male | Act of parturition | Young called |
|---|---|---|---|---|---|
| Cat | *Felis catus* (feline) | Tom/queen | | Queening | Kitten |
| Cattle | *Bos taurus* *Bos indicus* (bovine) | Bull/cow | Steer | Calving | Calf |
| Chicken | *Gallus gallus* | Rooster/hen | Capon | Laying/hatching | Chick |
| Chinchilla | *Chinchilla brevicaudata* | Male/female | | Parturition | |
| Dog | *Canis familiaris* (canine) | Dog/bitch | | Whelping | Puppy |
| Ferret | *Mustela putorius furo* | Hob/jill | Male: gib Female: sprite | Kindling | Kit |
| Gerbil (jird) | *Meriones unguiculatus* | Male/female | | Parturition | Pup |
| Goat | *Capra hircus* (caprine) | Buck/doe | Wether | Kidding | Kid |
| Guinea pig (cavy) | *Cavia porcellus* | Boar/sow | | Farrowing | Pup/piglet |
| Hamster | *Mesocricetus auratus* | Male/female | | Parturition | Pup |
| Horse | *Equus caballus* (equine) | Stallion/mare | Gelding | Foaling | Foal (either sex) Colt (male) Filly (female) |
| Llama | *Lama glama* | Bull/cow | Gelding | | Cria |
| Mouse | *Mus musculus* | Male/female | | Parturition | Pup |
| Pig | *Sus scrofa* (porcine) | Boar/sow | Barrow | Farrowing | Piglet, pig |
| Rabbit | *Oryctolagus cuniculus* | Buck/doe | Lapin | Kindling | Bunny, nestling |
| Rat | *Rattus norvegicus* | Male/female | | Parturition | Pup, nestling |
| Sheep | *Ovis aries* (ovine) | Ram/ewe | Wether | Lambing | Lamb |

Modified from McBride DF: *Learning veterinary terminology,* St Louis, 1996, Mosby.

# Normal Values

| Species | Temperature | | Heart rate (beats/min)* | Respiratory rate (min)* | Onset of puberty (mo) | Gestation (days) | Length of estrous cycle | Length of estrus‡ |
| | °F | °C | | | | | | |
|---|---|---|---|---|---|---|---|---|
| Alpaca | 99.5-102 | 37.5-38.9 | 60-90 | 10-30 | 12-13 | 335-365 | 12-14 days† | |
| Bovine | 100.4-102.2 | 38-39 | 40-80 | 12-36 | 9-10 | 285 | 21 days | 18-24 hr |
| Canine | 99.5-102.2 | 37.5-39 | 70-160 | 10-30 | 6-8 | 63-65 | 7-8 mo | 5-9 days |
| Caprine | 101.3-104.9 | 38.5-40.5 | 40-60 | 12-20 | 3-7 | 149 | 21 days | 40 hr |
| Equine | 98.6-101.3 | 37-38.5 | 28-50 | 8-20 | 12-18 | 336 | 22 days | 6 days |
| Feline | 100.4-102.2 | 38-39 | 150-210 | 24-42 | 5-9 | 63-65 | 6 mo | 4 days |
| Llama | 99.5-102 | 37.5-38.9 | 60-90 | 10-30 | 12-13 | 342-359 | 12-14 days† | |
| Ovine | 100.4-104 | 38-40 | 60-120 | 12-72 | 6-7 | 148 | 17 days | 10-30 hr |
| Porcine | 100.4-104 | 38-40 | 58-100 | 8-18 | 5-7 | 114 | 21 days | 48-55 hr |

*These values are estimated for mature animals. In general, immature animals have slightly higher ranges for respiration and heart rate.
†These species are induced ovulators, and the length of estrus applies only if they are mated, ovulate, and fail to become pregnant.
‡Alpacas and llamas are induced ovulators and will be continuously receptive to the male with brief periods of nonreceptivity of 2-3 days between follicular waves.

# Additional Veterinary Technician Resources

Due to the changing nature of websites, one or more of the following URLs may be obsolete at the time of printing.

A plethora of information can be found on the following websites, including such information as state/provincial veterinary and technician associations, state/provincial representatives, international associations, registration of technicians, and countless other links.

| | |
|---|---|
| http://www.navta.net | NAVTA—National Association of Veterinary Technicians in America |
| http://www.caahtt-acttsa.ca/ | CAAHTT/ACTTSA—Canadian Association of Animal Health Technologists and Technicians |
| | Association Canadienne Des Techniciens Et Technologistes En Santé Animale |
| http://www.vetweb.co.uk/sites/ivna/ | IVNTA—International Veterinary Nurses and Technicians Association |
| http://www.aavsb.org | American Association of State Boards |
| | List licensing requirements for veterinary technicians |
| http://www.avma.org/ | American Veterinary Medical Association |
| http://www.avte.net | Association of Veterinary Technician Educators |
| http://canadianveterinarians.net/ | Canadian Veterinary Medical Association |
| http://www.oavt.org/ | Ontario Association of Veterinary Technicians |

# Comprehensive Test with Answer Key

This comprehensive examination is meant as a study aid only and thus covers 10 questions from each chapter. The number in parenthesis represents the chapter in which the answer can be found.

**1** Which of the following is a function of bile? *(1)*
   a. Activation of pancreatic sucrase
   b. Emulsification of fat
   c. Decreasing intestinal motility
   d. Causing contraction of the gallbladder

**2** Which of the following chemical constituents in urine is the result of fatty acid catabolism? *(2)*
   a. Acetone
   b. Bilirubin
   c. Glucose
   d. Hemoglobin

**3** A common neoplasm of cats is *(3)*
   a. Pyelonephritis
   b. Feline infectious peritonitis
   c. Mastitis
   d. Renal lymphosarcoma

**4** The term *mange* means *(4)*
   a. Hair loss
   b. Infestation by mites
   c. Infestation by lice
   d. Rough hair coat

**5** Salmonella *(5)*
   a. Can infect the gastrointestinal tract of humans, mammals, birds, and reptiles
   b. Is a gram-positive rod
   c. Normally inhabits the respiratory tract
   d. Are lactose fermenters on MacConkey agar

**6** All of the following are commonly measured in a liver profile *except (6)*
   a. Total bilirubin
   b. Urea
   c. Total protein
   d. AP

**7** Viruses may possess one of four different genomic constructs. *(7)*
   a. True
   b. False

**8** Clients should be educated as to the possible adverse reactions an animal may have to a vaccination. *(8)*
   a. True
   b. False

**9** To restrain a cat it is important to *(9)*
   a. Immediately apply the maximum restraint possible
   b. Make friends first and then apply the maximum restraint
   c. Make friends first and then apply least restrictive restraint
   d. Immediately apply the least restrictive restraint

**10** An appropriate chemical disinfectant for stainless steel tables is *(10)*
   a. Bleach
   b. Alcohol
   c. Iodine solution
   d. Peroxide

**11** The purpose of an aluminum filter in an x-ray machine is to *(11)*
   a. Limit the size of the x-ray beam
   b. Focus the x-ray beam to the focal spot
   c. Remove the long wavelength x-rays from the x-ray beam
   d. Increase the number of short wavelength x-rays in the beam

**12** At which area does the ultrasound beam reach its narrowest point? *(12)*
   a. Focal point
   b. Near field
   c. Far field
   d. Reverberation point

**13** The breakage of two chromosomes, resulting in repair in an abnormal arrangement is called *(13)*
   a. Deletion
   b. Anomalies
   c. Duplication
   d. Translocation

**14** Which of the following statements regarding puppy classes is false? *(14)*
   a. Puppies will learn canine language through puppy class
   b. All puppies should be neutered in a puppy class
   c. Owners will learn how to prevent the most common behavior problems
   d. Veterinarians should encourage their clients to participate in a puppy class

**15** Average moisture (water) content of canned food is *(15)*
   a. 25% to 40%
   b. 72% to 82%
   c. 40% to 60%
   d. 10% to 12%

16 The trace mineral that is an essential part of vitamin B$_{12}$ is *(16)*
   a. Copper
   b. Zinc
   c. Cobalt
   d. Molybdenum

17 In an animal colony, how can you be assured that you are maintaining disease-free animals? *(17)*
   a. Absence of clinical signs
   b. Use of sentinel animals
   c. By purchasing only SPF and VAF animals
   d. By housing animals within a barrier facility

18 Suitable sites for blood collection in birds are *(18)*
   a. Jugular, cephalic, and saphenous
   b. Jugular, brachioulnar, and medial tibiotarsal
   c. Jugular, cephalic, and femoral
   d. Jugular, brachioulnar, and toenail

19 Which of the following is an indication to include an anticholinergic in preanesthetic medication? *(19)*
   a. To produce analgesia
   b. To produce sedation
   c. To prevent bradycardia
   d. To treat tachypnea

20 Many drugs used in chemotherapy can cause severe side effects. Side effects may include *(20)*
   a. Liver and kidney toxicities, low blood cell counts, vomiting and diarrhea
   b. Hemorrhage, seizures, gastroenteritis, hair loss
   c. Allergic reaction, anorexia, cardiac and nervous system toxicities
   d. All of the above

21 A patient must be given 1 L of fluids and a vitamin mixture (50 mg/mL) at the rate of 75 mg/kg. The patient weighs 35 kg. The IV line has to run for 5 hours with an administration set calibrated at 15 drops/mL. The drip rate is calculated at *(21)*
   a. 9 drops/min
   b. 0.9 drop/sec
   c. 8 drops/sec
   d. 49 drops/min

22 An ultrasonic cleaner is how many times more effective than manual cleaning of the instruments? *(22)*
   a. 3
   b. 10
   c. 16
   d. 25

23 The most common vein used for blood donation is the *(23)*
   a. Jugular
   b. Cephalic
   c. Saphenous
   d. Femoral

24 When positioning a horse in lateral recumbency for surgery, it is important to pull the *(24)*
   a. Upper foreleg forward to enhance circulation
   b. Upper hind leg forward to enhance circulation
   c. Down foreleg forward to enhance circulation
   d. Down hind leg forward to enhance circulation

25 When performing orogastric intubation in ruminants, which of the following is false? *(25)*
   a. Measure the tube length to the last rib
   b. Occlude the tube before removal
   c. Rumen gas may be detected on correct placement
   d. Visual observation of esophageal tube placement may be made on the right side of the neck

26 The percentage of dogs and cats over the age of 2 years with some form of periodontal disease has been estimated to be *(26)*
   a. 50%
   b. 65%
   c. 75%
   d. 85%

27 Which of the following signs is common in acetaminophen toxicity? *(27)*
   a. Icterus
   b. Hemolysis
   c. Methemoglobinemia
   d. Hematuria

28 A nocturnal animal foraging for food at 11:00 in the morning may be infected with *(28)*
   a. Rabies
   b. Anthrax
   c. Tularemia
   d. *Capnocytophaga canimorus*

29 Which of the following is not true of good e-mail policy? *(29)*
   a. Message should be short and concise
   b. You should never e-mail a co-worker when you are very angry
   c. E-mail is a great way to share jokes and humorous stories
   d. E-mail should not take the place of conversation

30 Which of the following cells would most likely have the largest number of mitochondria? *(1)*
   a. Osteocytes
   b. Smooth muscle cells
   c. Skeletal muscle cells
   d. Adipocytes

31 Iron deficiency is a common cause of which of the following erythrocyte findings? *(2)*
   a. Polychromasia
   b. Hypochromasia
   c. Macrocytosis
   d. Basophilic stippling

32 Infections with *Histoplasma* or *Balantidium* organisms are commonly identified using *(3)*
   a. Fine needle aspiration
   b. Intestinal biopsy
   c. Rectal mucosal scraping
   d. Fecal smear

33 The Baermann technique is used for the recovery of *(4)*
   a. Lungworm larvae
   b. Microfilariae
   c. Mites
   d. Cryptosporidia oocysts

34 *Candida albicans* is a yeast that *(5)*
   a. Can grow on some bacteriological media and can cause opportunistic infections
   b. Is found only in the gastrointestinal tract
   c. Does not produce germ tubes
   d. Is encapsulated

35 The test of choice for assessing whether animals have exocrine pancreatic insufficiency is *(6)*
   a. Serum lipase
   b. Serum amylase
   c. Serum trypsin
   d. TLI

36 Samples for virology testing may include which of the following? *(7)*
   a. Frozen postmortem tissues
   b. EDTA plasma samples
   c. Frozen serum samples
   d. All of the above

37 To provide maximal immunity to the neonate, all vaccines should be given *(8)*
   a. Just before parturition
   b. According to the vaccine protocol
   c. Immediately after parturition
   d. Before the dam becomes pregnant

38 White around the eyes, sharp movements of the head and ears, trembling lips, and boisterous behavior indicate a dog is *(9)*
   a. Nervous/frightened
   b. Happy
   c. Normal acting
   d. Hostile

39 Which of the following disinfectants is toxic to cats? *(10)*
   a. Alcohols
   b. Quaternary ammonium compounds
   c. Phenols
   d. Aldehydes

40 The degree of overall blackness on a radiograph is termed *(11)*
   a. Density
   b. Contrast
   c. Radiolucent
   d. Radiopaque

41 The purpose of the time-gain compensation is to *(12)*
   a. Make tissues look alike
   b. Decrease contrast of the image
   c. Increase speed of the returning image
   d. Adjust brightness of the image

42 Colostrum is *(13)*
   a. Formed in the ovary after ovulation and produces progesterone
   b. The act of artificial insemination
   c. The period of ovulation
   d. The immunoglobulin-rich milk secreted from the mammary gland shortly after parturition

43 When using drug therapy to modify pet behavior, what should be done to obtain the maximum results? *(14)*
   a. Monitor the side effects
   b. Keep the animal in a calm and noise-free environment
   c. Combine drug therapy with a behavior modification program
   d. Combine drug therapy with an extensive physical exercise program

44 What is the best feeding method for puppies that are growing? *(15)*
   a. Free choice
   b. Food-restricted meal feeding
   c. Time-restricted feeding
   d. Food- and time-restricted feeding

45 Ruminants use nonprotein nitrogen (NPN) through *(16)*
   a. Microbial fermentation in the rumen
   b. Digestion in the omasum
   c. Digestion in the abomasum
   d. Direct absorption into the blood stream

46 What is a HEPA filter? *(17)*
   a. High energy particle absorber
   b. High efficiency particle absorber
   c. High efficiency particulate air
   d. High energy particulate air

47 In lizards and turtles, IM injections are best given in the *(18)*
   a. Rear leg
   b. Lumbar muscles
   c. Front leg
   d. Renal portal system

48 Which opioid preanesthetic agent has a higher incidence of producing vomiting and should be avoided with cases such as gastrointestinal obstruction or diaphragmatic hernia? *(19)*
   a. Butorphanol
   b. Morphine
   c. Meperidine
   d. Oxymorphone

49 Antitoxin and antiserum vaccines *(20)*
   a. Stimulate the body to create antibodies
   b. Last at least 1 year
   c. Create passive immunity
   d. Should not be given to pregnant animals

50 An animal is given 26 mg of a drug. The dose rate is 1 mL/15 kg. The concentration of the drug is 10 mg/mL. How much does this animal weigh? *(21)*
   a. 2.6 kg
   b. 3.9 kg
   c. 26 kg
   d. 39 kg

51 Which is not a type of sterilization monitor? *(22)*
   a. Indicator tape
   b. Chemical indicator strips
   c. Biological indicators
   d. David Bowie test

52 A constricting bandage is not likely to cause *(23)*
   a. Difficulty breathing
   b. Swelling or edema
   c. Coldness of the extremity
   d. Normal color of the body part

**53** Twelve hours before surgery, the horse must *(24)*
  a. Be taken off feed
  b. Have water withheld
  c. Have the surgical site clipped
  d. Have the mouth rinsed out with water

**54** By visual inspection, malnutrition or emaciation in cattle may be difficult to detect in *(25)*
  a. Older animals
  b. Young animals
  c. Fully haired animals
  d. Freshly shorn animals

**55** The normal bite of a dog is best described as *(26)*
  a. An anterior crossbite
  b. A scissor bite
  c. A level bite
  d. A posterior bite

**56** Which of the following statements is true regarding ethylene glycol toxicity? *(27)*
  a. The ethylene glycol test can be performed days after ingestion
  b. Seizure activity is not commonly related to ethylene glycol toxicity
  c. Ethylene glycol toxicity causes liver failure
  d. A blood sample to test for ethylene glycol should be obtained before administering diazepam in patients with seizure activity

**57** Which steps should be taken to prevent human infection with *Toxoplasma gondii*? *(28)*
  a. Eating rare meat
  b. Allowing pet cats the opportunity to hunt and eat prey
  c. Leaving the cover off children's sandboxes
  d. Cleaning the litter box every 1 to 2 days

**58** Active listening *(29)*
  a. Means that you interrupt the speaker to interject your thoughts
  b. Involves speaking in a loud voice with many hand gestures
  c. Implies that you are aware of the speaker's words and feelings
  d. Encourages everyone in the room to participate in the conversation

**59** The vertebral column of the cat would be represented by *(1)*
  a. C7 T13 L7 S3 Cd 21-23
  b. C7 T18 L6 S5 Cd 16-18
  c. C7 T12 L5 S5 Cd 4-5
  d. C5 T13 L8 S3 Cd 20-23

**60** Which term describes cells as having spiny projections around the margin and is often the result of slow drying of the blood film? *(2)*
  a. Target cells
  b. Acanthocyte
  c. Schistocyte
  d. Crenation

**61** The presence of cells with prominent dark black granules indicates *(3)*
  a. Purulent inflammation
  b. Mast cell tumor
  c. Mesothelioma
  d. Melanoma

**62** Which of the following is not a zoonotic parasite? *(4)*
  a. *Cryptosporidium*
  b. *Toxocara canis*
  c. *Gasterophilus* spp.
  d. *Ixodes* spp.

**63** *Mycobacterium* spp. are bacteria that are *(5)*
  a. Often the cause of diarrhea in many animals
  b. Gram-negative rods
  c. Easy to grow on usual bacteriological media
  d. Acid-fast negative

**64** Which of the following is considered to be a very specific test for all forms of liver disease in most species? *(6)*
  a. AST
  b. ALT
  c. Bile acids
  d. AP

**65** The best animals to sample for virology testing are those that are showing the severest clinical signs. *(7)*
  a. True
  b. False

**66** In which of the following species can IgG antibody cross the placental barrier? *(8)*
  a. Horse
  b. Cattle
  c. Cat
  d. Pig

**67** Which dog would be most likely to show aggressive behavior? *(9)*
  a. Large dog like a Newfoundland
  b. A medium-size dog like a Beagle
  c. A small dog like a Chihuahua
  d. All dogs can be equally aggressive

**68** The use of _____ on a contaminated open wound may result in the formation of a coagulum. *(10)*
  a. Peroxide
  b. Alcohol
  c. Iodine
  d. Quaternary ammonium compound

**69** An example of positive contrast media that may be injected intravascularly is *(11)*
  a. Nonsoluble barium
  b. Water-soluble barium
  c. Water-soluble iodine
  d. Both b and c

**70** The transducer needs crystals that can transform electrical energy into sound, etc. The effect exhibited by these crystals is *(12)*
  a. Electromagnetic
  b. Impedance
  c. Piezoelectric
  d. Attenuation

**71** In what breed does maintenance of pregnancy depend on luteal progesterone? *(13)*
  a. Sheep
  b. Pig
  c. Goat
  d. Cat

**72** Which is the least effective procedure to prevent barking? *(14)*
   a. Counterconditioning
   b. Cage training
   c. Obedience training
   d. Muzzling the dog

**73** Puppies should be weighed and body condition score monitored every_____ to ensure proper growth. *(15)*
   a. Week
   b. 2 weeks
   c. Month
   d. 2 months

**74** Which of the following is the major site for roughage fermentation in the horse? *(16)*
   a. Stomach
   b. Small intestine
   c. Cecum
   d. Rectum

**75** If restrained improperly, which of the following animals will have "fur slip"? *(17)*
   a. Chinchilla
   b. Degu
   c. Rabbit
   d. Mouse

**76** The clinical signs of lead toxicity in a bird include *(18)*
   a. Lethargy, depression, green diarrhea, and paresis
   b. Bradycardia, pale mucous membranes, and high blood pressure
   c. Tachycardia, hyperemic membranes, and high blood pressure
   d. Hypoventilation, muddy mucous membranes, and low blood pressure

**77** Which inhalation anesthetic agent has the quickest induction and recovery? *(19)*
   a. Halothane
   b. Isoflurane
   c. Methoxyflurane
   d. Pentobarbital

**78** Antiulcer drugs can work in any of the following ways *except (20)*
   a. Decreasing the pH in the stomach
   b. Neutralizing stomach acid
   c. Protecting the stomach lining
   d. Stimulating mucus production

**79** If a bucket holds 5 gallons, how much iodine must be added to make a concentration of 2 ppm? (1 gallon = 3785 mL) *(21)*
   a. 0.1 g
   b. 0.04 g
   c. 0.002 g
   d. 9.46 g

**80** Storing sterile packs in what type of cabinet will provide the longest shelf-life? *(22)*
   a. Open
   b. Closed
   c. Perforated
   d. Does not matter

**81** Anal sacs are expressed *(23)*
   a. To decrease odor caused by fecal material
   b. To increase the chances of a ruptured anal sac
   c. Due to perforation of the rectum
   d. To instill medication in diseased anal sacs

**82** Parasitic infestations in horses can cause *(24)*
   a. Colic
   b. Swamp fever
   c. West Nile virus
   d. Colitis

**83** Under general anesthesia, all of the following are used to judge the depth of anesthesia in small ruminants *except (25)*
   a. Heart rate
   b. Respiratory rate
   c. Pulse quality
   d. Eye signs

**84** Retained deciduous teeth *(26)*
   a. Present no problems for the pet
   b. Affect larger breeds more often
   c. Cause malocclusions and gingivitis
   d. Occur commonly in a wry bite

**85** Pericardiocentesis is indicated for which condition? *(27)*
   a. Pericarditis
   b. Pericardial tamponade
   c. Hemothorax
   d. Peritonitis

**86** Which of the following statements is least often true regarding brucellosis? *(28)*
   a. Carried by cattle
   b. Small animal veterinarians and staff are not at risk
   c. Can cause abortions in bovids
   d. Can lead to sterility

**87** The guilt phase of grieving *(29)*
   a. Is with a person forever; you never get over it but can move on to the other stages
   b. Is the first stage
   c. Inhibits progress toward resolution
   d. Is usually targeted at the veterinarian

**88** Which of the following is a strong protective covering of the heart? *(1)*
   a. Epicardium
   b. Myocardium
   c. Visceral pericardium
   d. Parietal pericardium

**89** Which intracellular parasite appears fairly large, paired, and teardrop shaped? *(2)*
   a. *Haemobartonella felis*
   b. *Anaplasma marginale*
   c. *Babesia canis*
   d. *Haemobartonella canis*

**90** An example of a noninflammatory, nonneoplastic lesion is *(3)*
   a. TVT
   b. Hematoma
   c. Metastasis
   d. Fibroma

**91** The common name for an ascarid is *(4)*
a. Whipworm
b. Bloodworm
c. Roundworm
d. Tapeworm

**92** Enteral bacteria are bacteria that *(5)*
a. Are normal flora of the gastrointestinal tract
b. Do not cause infections
c. Grow well on CNA agar plates
d. Are identified using the germ tube test

**93** Which of the following pairs of electrolytes have an inverse relationship in the body; that is, when the level of one increases in the body, the level of the other decreases? *(6)*
a. Calcium and phosphorus
b. Sodium and calcium
c. Potassium and chloride
d. Sodium and potassium

**94** Which of the following is true about viral samples? *(7)*
a. They should be frozen to ensure stability
b. They survive up to 3 weeks without refrigeration
c. They are inherently unstable and must be submitted as soon as possible
d. Only naked virus samples can be shipped because they are very refractory

**95** Which antibody class is produced during the secondary immune response? *(8)*
a. IgM
b. IgG
c. IgA
d. IgE

**96** Which tool is considered the main tool(s) of restraint on a horse? *(9)*
a. Halter and lead rope
b. Stanchion
c. Stocks
d. Lariat

**97** The mode of action of moist heat is *(10)*
a. Oxidation
b. Protein denaturation
c. Hydrolysis
d. Reduction

**98** To increase the radiographic detail or definition *(11)*
a. Increase the object film distance
b. Decrease the source image distance
c. Increase the source image distance
d. Increase the focal-spot size

**99** In ultrasonography, the artifact that is exhibited posterior to a bladder stone is *(12)*
a. Mirror image
b. Reverberation
c. Refraction
d. Shadowing

**100** The order of the stages of the estrous cycle is *(13)*
a. Proestrus, estrus, metestrus, anestrus
b. Proestrus, anestrus, metestrus, estrus
c. Estrus, proestrus, anestrus, metestrus
d. Estrus, anestrus, proestrus, metestrus

**101** Which statement best describes the advice you would give to the owner of a 3-month-old puppy who asks how to housetrain the dog? *(14)*
a. Set up a newspaper area in each room of the house
b. Rub the animal's nose in his feces when it eliminates in the house
c. Set a regular routine to go outside
d. The puppy cannot be trained before 4 months of age

**102** Cats are *(15)*
a. Omnivores
b. Carnivores
c. Herbivores
d. Vegetarian

**103** Pigs are not usually fed *(16)*
a. Diets high in nonprotein nitrogen
b. Protein supplements
c. Ground grains
d. Pelleted premixes

**104** What type of bedding is inappropriate for use as a contact bedding for laboratory animals? *(17)*
a. Hardwood shavings
b. Cedar chips
c. Corn cob bedding
d. Aspen chips

**105** The normal gastrointestinal flora of psittacines include *(18)*
a. Predominantly gram-positive bacteria
b. Predominantly gram-negative bacteria
c. *Klebsiella* and *Salmonella*
d. Predominantly anaerobic bacteria

**106** How do you prevent diffusion hypoxia after discontinuation of $N_2O$ use in general anesthesia? *(19)*
a. Increase the $O_2$ flow rate for at least 5 minutes
b. Provide intermittent positive pressure ventilation
c. Increase the intravenous fluid rate
d. Turn off inhalant anesthetic agent

**107** A goal of antimicrobial therapy is to *(20)*
a. Kill microorganisms in the host and restore normal flora
b. Prevent microorganisms in the host from infecting other animals
c. Kill microorganisms in the host without killing the host
d. Prevent microorganisms in the host from moving to other places in the body

**108** How much NaCl should be measured out to produce 500 mL of a 4.5% w/v solution? *(21)*
a. 225 g
b. 22.5 g
c. 1111.1 g
d. 111.1 g

**109** What size of clipper blade should be used for patient preparation? *(22)*
a. 10
b. 20
c. 30
d. 40

**110** The origin of electrical activity in the myocardium is *(23)*
   a. AV node
   b. SA node
   c. Atrium
   d. Ventricle

**111** The etiological agent for tetanus is *(24)*
   a. *Clostridium difficile*
   b. *Clostridium perfringens*
   c. *Clostridium tetani*
   d. *Ehrlichia coli*

**112** The vein most commonly used in ruminants for IV catheterization in large animals is *(25)*
   a. Cephalic
   b. Saphenous
   c. Jugular
   d. Mammary

**113** The most common oral tumor in dogs is a(n) *(26)*
   a. Melanoma
   b. Squamous cell carcinoma
   c. Fibrosarcoma
   d. Eosinophilic ulcer

**114** _____ is used for cardiac arrest and is commonly administered via the intratracheal route. *(27)*
   a. Lidocaine
   b. Atropine
   c. Epinephrine
   d. Sodium bicarbonate

**115** Intradermal skin testing is used to detect *(28)*
   a. Mycobacteria
   b. Rabies
   c. Cryptosporidium
   d. *Sarcoptes scabiei*

**116** The Internet can be used by veterinary technicians for all *except (29)*
   a. Searching for the latest information on a disease process
   b. Keeping current on the political happenings in the profession
   c. Plagiarizing assignments
   d. Sharing ideas via chat rooms

**117** Which of the following contains valves? *(1)*
   a. Arteries and veins
   b. Veins and lymphatic vessels
   c. Veins and capillaries
   d. Arteries and lymphatic vessels

**118** A large leukocyte with variable nuclear shape with diffuse chromatin, blue-gray cytoplasm, vacuoles, and possible fine pink granules is descriptive of a(n) *(2)*
   a. Lymphocyte
   b. NRBC
   c. Monocyte
   d. Basophil

**119** An epithelial cell tumor that usually exfoliates sheets of cells is also referred to as *(3)*
   a. Sarcoma
   b. Carcinoma
   c. Lipoma
   d. Hematoma

**120** The intermediate host for *Dipylidium caninum* is a(n) *(4)*
   a. Infective egg
   b. Rodent
   c. Flea
   d. Mosquito

**121** The goal of streaking for isolation is to *(5)*
   a. Cover the surface of the bacterial plate as evenly as possible
   b. Sterilize the loop used for streaking
   c. Determine if a bacterium is gram positive or gram negative
   d. Obtain bacterial colonies that are isolated from each other so they can be identified

**122** Which of the following enzymes is considered a liver-specific enzyme in dogs and cats? *(6)*
   a. Alkaline phosphatase
   b. Aspartate aminotransferase
   c. Sorbitol dehydrogenase
   d. Alanine aminotransferase

**123** Viruses are *(7)*
   a. The smallest form of life
   b. Never found outside the host
   c. Obligate intracellular parasites
   d. Always difficult to disinfect

**124** Why is a second vaccine administered to elicit a secondary immune response in a patient? *(8)*
   a. To stimulate the production of more phagocytes
   b. To stimulate the production of an increased IgM antibody titer
   c. To cause the patient to produce an acquired artificial passive immunity
   d. To result in a stronger, faster immunity by causing a secondary immune response

**125** A lead shank in a horse is used for all *except* when you need *(9)*
   a. It to lift up the horse's leg
   b. More restraint
   c. A distraction technique
   d. To discipline a horse

**126** Which of the following disinfectants has sporicidal activity? *(10)*
   a. Alcohols
   b. Aldehydes
   c. Phenols
   d. Peroxides

**127** There is about a 1-inch clear band along one of the narrow film edges of the manually processed radiograph. This occurred because the *(11)*
   a. Developer is too low
   b. Fixer is too low
   c. Field size was collimated in too far
   d. Film edge was exposed to light

**128** Ultrasound uses sound that is in what range of frequency of human hearing? *(12)*
   a. Within
   b. Below
   c. Above
   d. Equal to

**129** A masking of one allele over the genes on another is called *(13)*
   a. Polygenic
   b. Epistasis
   c. Expressivity
   d. Codominance

**130** Which of the following is not a cause of inappropriate urination in the house? *(14)*
   a. Diet change
   b. Separation anxiety
   c. Fear
   d. Medical condition

**131** The minimum time for an elimination food trial is *(15)*
   a. 4 weeks
   b. 6 weeks
   c. 4 months
   d. 6 months

**132** How many gallons of water does a lactating cow require to produce 1 gallon (3.8 L) of milk? *(16)*
   a. 1 to 2 (3.8 to 7.5 L)
   b. 3 to 5 (11.4 to 18.9 L)
   c. 8 to 10 (30.2 to 37.8 L)
   d. 12 to 15 (45.5 to 56.7 L)

**133** Newborn offspring from which of the following species are precocious, with hair, erupted teeth, and open eyes? *(17)*
   a. Guinea pig, chinchilla, and degu
   b. Guinea pig, rabbit, and hedgehog
   c. Mouse, guinea pig, and rat
   d. Gerbil, hamster, and degu

**134** The avian pectoral girdle is composed of *(18)*
   a. Clavicle, scapula, and humerus
   b. Clavicle, coracoid, and scapula
   c. Humerus, radius, and ulna
   d. Femur, tibia, and fibula

**135** To reduce the amount of rebreathing during the use of a rebreathing system, which of the following would you do? *(19)*
   a. Increase the total fresh gas flow rate
   b. Decrease the total fresh gas flow rate
   c. Increase percent of inhalant anesthetic gas
   d. Decrease percent of inhalant anesthetic gas

**136** Which class of reproductive drug can be potentially dangerous to pregnant females who come into contact with it? *(20)*
   a. Gonadotropins such as hCG
   b. Prostaglandins such as dinoprost (Lutalyse)
   c. Estrogens such as estradiol cypionate (ECP)
   d. Progestins such as megestrol acetate (Ovaban)

**137** There is a client on the telephone trying to figure out an old prescription. She reads to you the following: "Put 2 drops O.S. q.4h for 3 days then q.8h for 3 days until finished. Not for p.o. use." What does this label mean? *(21)*
   a. Put 2 drops on the mouth every 4 hours for 3 days, then every 8 hours for 3 days until finished
   b. Put 2 drops in the right eye about 4 times a day for 3 days, then about every 8 hours for 3 days until finished. Before meals
   c. Put 2 drops in the left eye about 3 times a day for 3 days, then about 4 times a day for 3 days until finished. Not for oral use
   d. Put 2 drops in left eye every 4 hours for 3 days, then every 8 hours for 3 days until finished. Not for oral use

**138** What is a standard method of gloving when preparing for surgery? *(22)*
   a. Open hand gloving
   b. Open cuffed gloving
   c. Closed gloving
   d. Closed hand gloving

**139** What is not represented on an ECG tracing? *(23)*
   a. Ventricular systole
   b. Atrial systole
   c. Ventricular repolarization
   d. Atrial repolarization

**140** Potomac horse fever is transmitted by *(24)*
   a. Mosquitoes
   b. Ticks
   c. House flies
   d. Snails

**141** All of the following are zoonotic *except (25)*
   a. Orf
   b. Blue tongue
   c. Leptospirosis
   d. Erysipelas

**142** The lesion that occurs at the neck of the tooth in cats is called a(n) *(26)*
   a. Epulis lesion
   b. Crevicular lesion
   c. Root cavity
   d. External odontoclastic resorption (EOR)

**143** What are the clinical signs of dystocia? *(27)*
   a. Active contractions for more than 30 minutes
   b. More than 2 hours between deliveries
   c. Green discharge with no delivery of fetus
   d. All of the above

**144** *Capnocytophaga canimorsus* causes which of the following in canids? *(28)*
   a. Profuse, watery diarrhea
   b. Abortions
   c. No symptoms
   d. Eating of feces

**145** A good supervisor will *(29)*
   a. Tell people what to do at the start of each day
   b. Delegate only those things that they do not want to do
   c. Motivate and provide constructive criticism
   d. Control employees' activities so the job is done correctly

**146** The four primary body tissues are *(1)*
  a. Dense, muscle, nervous, bone
  b. Epithelial, bone, muscle, areolar
  c. Nervous, cartilage, connective, reticular
  d. Muscle, nervous, epithelial, connective

**147** Staining urine sediment can be easily accomplished by using which of the following? *(2)*
  a. Papanicolaou stain
  b. Sedi-stain
  c. Gram stain
  d. Wright-Giemsa

**148** A mesenchymal cell tumor that usually exfoliates single cells may be referred to as *(3)*
  a. Sarcoma
  b. Carcinoma
  c. Lipoma
  d. Hematoma

**149** *Taenia* spp. ova are *(4)*
  a. Dark brown and nearly spherical with striations evident
  b. Different colors compared with other ova
  c. Larger than *Toxascaris leonina* ova
  d. Indistinguishable from other ova

**150** Salmonella-Shigella agar does all of the following *except* *(5)*
  a. Select pathogenic enteric bacteria
  b. Select gram-positive bacteria
  c. Differentiate on the basis of lactose fermentation
  d. Differentiate on the basis of hydrogen sulfide production

**151** The anticoagulant of choice for collecting samples for electrolyte determination is *(6)*
  a. Heparin
  b. EDTA
  c. Sodium fluoride
  d. Sodium citrate

**152** A latent infection is *(7)*
  a. One that never causes clinical signs
  b. Often dormant until the host is stressed
  c. Caused by a cancer-causing oncogenic virus
  d. One against which the animal is vaccinated

**153** Ingestion of colostrum is an example of *(8)*
  a. Acquired artificial passive immunity
  b. Acquired natural active immunity
  c. Acquired natural passive immunity
  d. Innate immunity

**154** Where is the safest place to stand when you are next to a cow? *(9)*
  a. Slightly in front and to the left of the head
  b. Slightly in front of the shoulder
  c. Next to the abdomen
  d. Slightly in front of the back leg

**155** Liquids to be autoclaved must be placed in a container at least _____ time(s) the size as the liquid volume. *(10)*
  a. One
  b. Two
  c. Three
  d. Six

**156** Which of the following will give you 20 mA? *(11)*
  a. 100 mA and $\frac{1}{10}$ second
  b. 100 mA and $\frac{1}{20}$ second
  c. 200 mA and $\frac{1}{10}$ second
  d. 300 mA and $\frac{1}{20}$ second

**157** A mechanical sector scanner consists of one or more crystals mechanically moved to produce what type of image? *(12)*
  a. Rectangular
  b. Pie-shaped
  c. Square
  d. Linear

**158** In which animal is the age of puberty directly related to body weight? *(13)*
  a. Cat
  b. Dog
  c. Cattle
  d. Goat

**159** The owner of two cats complains about feces found outside of the litter box. Which of the following is least likely to resolve the problem? *(14)*
  a. Provide a second litter box
  b. Clean the litter boxes more frequently
  c. Avoid perfumed litter substrate
  d. Confine both cats in the same room as the litter box

**160** The most common nutrient of concern in adverse food reactions is *(15)*
  a. Carbohydrate
  b. Protein
  c. Vitamins
  d. Fat

**161** A disease that is associated with a lack of usable carbohydrates during late gestation in sheep or early lactation in cattle is *(16)*
  a. Milk fever
  b. White muscle disease
  c. Rickets
  d. Ketosis

**162** Normal rabbit urine is *(17)*
  a. Clear and brown
  b. Clear and orange
  c. Cloudy and thick
  d. Blood-tinged

**163** When restraining a bird, it is important to *(18)*
  a. Not restrict movement of the sternum
  b. Cover its eyes
  c. Use large leather gloves
  d. Hold it by its wings

**164** During a surgical plane of anesthesia, where will the eye position be? *(19)*
  a. Ventral-medial
  b. Dorsal-medial
  c. Lateral
  d. Central

**165** Why is it important to know the cause of vomiting before giving an antiemetic? *(20)*
   a. Different drugs work on different emetic centers
   b. Giving an inappropriate drug could make the problem worse
   c. In some cases vomiting should be encouraged
   d. All of the above

**166** A patient needs to receive 1.2 L of lactated Ringer's solution at the drip rate of 50 drops/min using a 15 drops/mL administration set. How long will it take for the fluids to be administered? *(21)*
   a. 4 hours
   b. 3 hours
   c. 6 hours
   d. 120 minutes

**167** Which style of surgical mask allows the least amount of air to escape? *(22)*
   a. Molded
   b. Hooded
   c. Flat pleated
   d. See through

**168** What would be evident in a lightly tranquilized dog if an orogastric tube has been placed in the patient's trachea? *(23)*
   a. Dyspnea and coughing occur
   b. Popping and gurgling sounds are coming from the tube
   c. After palpation, there appears to be two tubes in the neck region
   d. Vomiting occurs

**169** Which of the following is transmitted by mosquitoes? *(24)*
   a. *Clostridium difficile* and *Salmonella* spp.
   b. *Ehrlichia risticii* and colitis
   c. Equine encephalomyelitis and West Nile virus
   d. HYPP and EPM

**170** In cattle undergoing general anesthesia, which of the following will not assist in the prevention of bloat in the patient? *(25)*
   a. An orogastric tube should be placed
   b. They should be placed in sternal recumbency for recovery
   c. Withhold feed 24 to 48 hours
   d. Deflate cuff before extubation

**171** The bulk of the tooth is composed of *(26)*
   a. Enamel
   b. Dentin
   c. Cementum
   d. Pulp

**172** How is hyperkalemia treated if a cat has a urinary obstruction? *(27)*
   a. Insulin/dextrose
   b. Calcium gluconate
   c. Lidocaine
   d. Sodium bicarbonate

**173** Leptospirosis is mainly passed through contact with *(28)*
   a. Skin of infected animal
   b. Infective urine
   c. Aerosolized discharges
   d. Fomites

**174** Greater success in achieving goals can be realized if *(29)*
   a. Priorities are set
   b. You wait to start to determine if the goal will change—you never know
   c. Give all responsibility for completing the goal to someone else who is faster
   d. Use procrastination to your advantage

**175** The receptors for hearing are part of the _____ within the _____. *(1)*
   a. Stapes/cochlea
   b. Cochlea/middle ear
   c. Organ of Corti/inner ear
   d. Organ of Corti/middle ear

**176** The presence of intact RBCs in the urine is referred to as *(2)*
   a. Oliguria
   b. Pollakiuria
   c. Azotemia
   d. Hematuria

**177** A stain used specifically for staining of nuclei, mast cells, or infectious agents is *(3)*
   a. Romanovsky
   b. Giemsa
   c. New methylene blue
   d. Gram stain

**178** *Giardia* spp. have *(4)*
   a. Undulating membrane
   b. Long flagella from the anterior end
   c. Bipolar plugs
   d. An operculum

**179** Which of the following cannot be used to sterilize a bacteriology loop? *(5)*
   a. An electric heating element
   b. An incubator
   c. A Bunsen burner
   d. An alcohol lamp

**180** Many of the electrolytes act closely with other electrolytes. Which of the following combinations of electrolytes are closely related? *(6)*
   a. Sodium, potassium, and hydrogen
   b. Calcium, phosphorous, and magnesium
   c. Sodium and bicarbonate
   d. All of the above

**181** The order of the viral replication cycle is *(7)*
   a. Attachment, penetration, uncoating, assembly, and release
   b. Attachment, penetration, assembly, uncoating, and release
   c. Attachment, assembly, and release
   d. Attachment, penetration, assembly, release, and uncoating

**182** Atopy is a genetically based condition where the patient *(8)*
   a. Does not possess IgE antibody
   b. Has an overreactive immune system
   c. Produces an excess of IgE antibody
   d. Is deficient in cell-mediated immunity

**183** What is the sheep's main means of defense? *(9)*
   a. Speed and flocking instinct
   b. Hooves and head
   c. Teeth and hooves
   d. Speed and head

**184** Which of the following disinfectants is inactivated by the presence of organic debris? *(10)*
   a. Aldehydes
   b. Chlorine
   c. Phenols
   d. Biguanides

**185** As the contrast of a radiograph decreases, you will have a *(11)*
   a. Brighter radiograph with few steps but greater differences between each step
   b. Brighter radiograph with many steps but little differences between each step
   c. Grayer radiograph with few steps but greater differences between each step
   d. Grayer radiograph with many steps but little differences between each step

**186** A structure that contains cystic and solid lesions is *(12)*
   a. Hypoechoic
   b. Anechoic
   c. Complex
   d. Sonolucent

**187** On a pedigree chart, what symbol represents unknown sex? *(13)*
   a. Half solid symbol
   b. Diamond
   c. Square
   d. Open symbol

**188** Which statement is the best advice for cat owners who do not want to declaw their cat? *(14)*
   a. Buy leather furniture instead of fabric furniture
   b. Provide an alternative scratching post
   c. Rub the furniture with mothballs
   d. Get a second cat to entertain the first one

**189** What is the most essential nutrient required for survival? *(15)*
   a. Water
   b. Protein
   c. Fat
   d. Carbohydrate

**190** A nutritional disease of equines associated with acute overconsumption of grain, lush pasture, or water is *(16)*
   a. Heaves
   b. Rickets
   c. Laminitis
   d. Water belly

**191** Which species has two pair of upper incisors (peg teeth)? *(17)*
   a. Degu
   b. Gerbil
   c. Hamster
   d. Rabbit

**192** Autotomy in exotic medicine is the *(18)*
   a. Study of the parts of the body
   b. Slow movement of a turtle
   c. Ability of a lizard to shed its tail when captured
   d. Shedding of the skin in reptiles

**193** Paradoxical breathing is characterized as which of the following? *(19)*
   a. Holding of breath on inspiration
   b. Increased respiration rate
   c. Abdomen rising and chest falling during an inspiration
   d. Increased tidal volume

**194** Chemotherapeutic drugs require specific precautions for safe handling to prevent occupational exposure because they *(20)*
   a. Can cause a miscarriage
   b. Can affect rapidly growing cells in humans
   c. Will cause an allergic reaction in humans
   d. Are toxic to the skin and mucous membranes

**195** The veterinarian gives you the following prescription to fill. "Levothyroxin sodium tablets 0.1 mg/10 pounds, SID for 4 weeks." The canine patient weighs 27 kg. The available tablet sizes are 0.1-, 0.2-, 0.3-, 0.5-, and 0.8-mg tablets. What should be written on the prescription label? *(21)*
   a. Give ¾ tablet each day for 28 days (0.8-mg tablet, quantity 21 tabs)
   b. Give 1 tablet each day for 28 days (0.2-mg tablet, quantity 28 tabs)
   c. Give 1 tablet each day for 4 weeks (0.2-mg tablet, quantity 28 tabs)
   d. Give 1 tablet twice a day for 28 days (0.1-mg tablet, quantity 28 tabs)

**196** Which of the following is not a duty of a sterile assistant? *(22)*
   a. Providing hemostasis
   b. Touching the instruments with the bare hands
   c. Providing retraction of tissues
   d. Keeping count of gauze squares

**197** A Foley catheter is inserted in *(23)*
   a. The jugular vein for extended periods of time
   b. Only the female dog for collection of urine
   c. The male dog to facilitate a sterile collection of blood
   d. A dog's urethra for long periods of catheterization

**198** In horses, there is a vaccine available for *(24)*
   a. Equine protozoal myeloencephalitis
   b. Equine infectious anemia
   c. Sleeping sickness
   d. Hyperkalemic periodic paralysis

**199** In animals entering the food chain, intramuscular injections should be given in the *(25)*
   a. Gluteal muscles
   b. Semimembranosus muscles
   c. Semitendinosus muscles
   d. Lateral cervical muscles

200 With the triadan numbering system, the lower left fourth premolar is tooth number *(26)*
a. 108
b. 208
c. 308
d. 408

201 What statement best describes paradoxical respirations? *(27)*
a. Labored inspiration
b. Cheyne-Stokes
c. Abdominal wall and chest wall do not move synchronously
d. Labored expiration

202 *Toxocara* larva (in humans) typically does not migrate through which organs? *(28)*
a. Viscera, somatic tissues
b. Eyes
c. Intestines
d. Ears

203 All of the following are true about stress, *except* that it *(29)*
a. Creates a feeling of tension and pressure
b. Is never healthy
c. Causes physical as well as mental symptoms
d. Is created by lack of control over one's life

204 Which of the following is not a function of the autonomic nervous system? *(1)*
a. Causing muscles of the foreleg to contract
b. Contracting and dilating blood vessels
c. Causing changes in heart rate
d. Causing muscles of the intestine to contract

205 Which of the following is considered the least reliable method of determining urine specific gravity? *(2)*
a. Reagent test strips
b. Refractometer
c. Urinometer
d. All are unreliable

206 A sample that contains macrophages and 65% neutrophils is classified as *(3)*
a. Purulent
b. Granulomatous
c. Suppurative
d. Pyogranulomatous

207 All of the following are true of trematodes *except* that they *(4)*
a. Are hermaphroditic
b. Have two suckers (oral and ventral)
c. Are all host specific
d. Require an intermediate host

208 *Campylobacter* spp. are bacteria that *(5)*
a. Do not grow well on usual microbiology media
b. Can be presumptively identified on a gram stain by their shape
c. Are anaerobic
d. Both a and b

209 If the exocrine function of the pancreas is abnormal, one would expect to find *(6)*
a. Chronic or acute pancreatitis
b. Hyperglycemia or hypoglycemia
c. Normal blood lipase or amylase
d. Abnormal blood or urine glucose

210 Which of the following is not a virology test that is commonly performed in veterinary clinics? *(7)*
a. FA
b. ELISA
c. EM
d. LA

211 Characteristics of killed or inactivated vaccines are that they *(8)*
a. Usually require repeated administrations to produce a healthy level of immunity
b. May cause a mild form of the disease in some patients
c. Do not store well
d. Cause abortions in pregnant patients

212 What method works best to move a pig from one place to another? *(9)*
a. Yelling and shouting
b. Get a large group of people to herd the pigs
c. Use a dog to chase the pigs
d. Use a hurdle or plastic pipe

213 Items sterilized in an ethylene oxide chamber must be ventilated for at least ___ hours to remove residual ethylene oxide. *(10)*
a. 24
b. 18
c. 12
d. 2

214 If you do not follow proper safelight procedures in the x-ray dark room, you will cause *(11)*
a. Fogging of the film
b. Underexposure of the film
c. Clearing of the film when it is developed and fixed
d. A dark border around the edges of the film

215 Lateral resolution depends on beam *(12)*
a. Bandwidth
b. Frequency
c. Wavelength
d. Width

216 Lordosis is *(13)*
a. Vocalization
b. Tail deflection
c. Crouching and rolling on the floor
d. A clear discharge from the vulva

217 For which of these behavior problems is drug therapy not a solution? *(14)*
a. Obsessive/compulsive disorder
b. Running away/escaping
c. Separation anxiety
d. Aggression

218 Ideal weight loss per week for a cat is *(15)*
a. 0.25 lb (0.11 kg)
b. 0.5 lb (0.22 kg)
c. 1.0 lb (0.45 kg)
d. 1.5 lb (0.68 kg)

219 Two animals that benefit nutritionally from consuming browse are *(16)*
a. Pig and sheep
b. Goat and llama
c. Horse and cattle
d. Horse and sheep

**220** The most common health condition to affect workers in a laboratory animal facility is *(17)*
   a. Salmonellosis
   b. Giardiasis
   c. Laboratory animal allergens
   d. Pasteurellosis

**221** The normal Ca/P ratio in a bird is *(18)*
   a. 5:1
   b. 1.5:1
   c. 1:5
   d. 10:1

**222** Which of the following is an indication of hypoventilation? *(19)*
   a. Respiratory acidosis
   b. Respiratory alkalosis
   c. Metabolic acidosis
   d. Metabolic alkalosis

**223** An otic drug may not be effective if _____ and may cause toxicity if _____. *(20)*
   a. The ear canal is dirty/the eardrum is ruptured
   b. The ear is infected/the eardrum is covered with wax
   c. The bacteria are not correctly identified/the patient has kidney or liver disease
   d. Parasites are present in the ear canal/parasites are present in the middle ear

**224** What is the dose range in mg and mL for a 13-kg dog for atropine sulfate (0.5 mg/mL) at dosage of 0.02 to 0.04 mg/kg? *(21)*
   a. 2.6 to 6.5 mg/5.2 to 13 mL
   b. 0.26 to 0.52 mg/0.052 to 0.104 mL
   c. 0.26 to 0.52 mg/0.52 to 1.04 mL
   d. 0.26 to 0.52 mg/kg/0.052 to 1.04 mL/kg

**225** What size surgical blade attaches to a No. 4 Bard Parker scalpel handle? *(22)*
   a. 20
   b. 15
   c. 11
   d. 10

**226** A squamous cell carcinoma may be located in *(23)*
   a. The nasal cavity of a white cat and is malignant
   b. Mammary tissue and is benign
   c. Axillary lymph tissue and is cancerous
   d. Fibrous tissue and is metastatic

**227** How are horses infected with equine protozoal myeloencephalitis? *(24)*
   a. Fomites
   b. Opossum feces
   c. Arthropods
   d. Aerosol

**228** Which of the following is considered a quick-release knot? *(25)*
   a. Tom fool
   b. Square knot
   c. Bowline
   d. Slipknot

**229** The surface of the incisor tooth facing the roof of the mouth is *(26)*
   a. Lingual
   b. Buccal
   c. Palatal
   d. Labial

**230** What is the antidote for organophosphate toxicity? *(27)*
   a. Vitamin $K_1$
   b. Ethanol
   c. 2-PAM (pralidoxime)
   d. Methylpyrazole

**231** Which group of animals is most likely to be a vector for human herpes B infection? *(28)*
   a. Reptiles
   b. Primates
   c. Canids
   d. Felids

**232** Internal marketing does not include:
   a. Building appearance and equipment
   b. Media routes for providing services available
   c. Staff and veterinarian knowledge
   d. Practice newsletters and health bulletins

**233** In glomerular filtration, metabolic waste from the plasma would *(1)*
   a. Pass into the distal convoluted tubule
   b. Remain in the plasma
   c. Pass into peritubular capillaries
   d. Pass into Bowman's capsule

**234** Which of the following is not a granulocyte precursor? *(2)*
   a. Prorubricyte
   b. Myeloblast
   c. Band
   d. Metamyelocyte

**235** A sample that contains few macrophages and greater than 70% neutrophils is classified as *(3)*
   a. Purulent
   b. Granulomatous
   c. Suppurative
   d. Pyogranulomatous

**236** Examples of parasites in ruminant hosts that produce GIN-type eggs are *(4)*
   a. *Cooperia, Moniezia, Ostertagia*
   b. *Cooperia, Trichuris, Haemonchus*
   c. *Cooperia, Eimeria, Ostertagia*
   d. *Cooperia, Ostertagia, Haemonchus*

**237** A lactose-fermenting bacterial colony is what color on MacConkey agar? *(5)*
   a. Black
   b. Clear
   c. Dark pink or purple
   d. White

**238** The following is true of hyperglycemia *except* that it *(6)*
   a. May be induced by stress
   b. Must be accompanied by glycosuria to confirm a diagnosis of diabetes mellitus
   c. Often accompanies pancreatitis
   d. Always leads to a diagnosis of diabetes mellitus

**239** Which of the following is true regarding the analysis of viral samples? *(7)*
   a. It is usually performed to determine a course of treatment
   b. It is always performed in a clinic
   c. The virus is most easily cultured from animals just before and just after the onset of clinical signs
   d. Previous history is not needed

**240** Once a vaccine is administered to a healthy patient, it is known that the patient is immune to the disease for which it was vaccinated. *(8)*
   a. True
   b. False

**241** A hog snare has an optimum effect of *(9)*
   a. 3 to 5 minutes
   b. 8 to 10 minutes
   c. 15 to 20 minutes
   d. 25 minutes

**242** The recommended method of quality control for autoclave sterilization in the veterinary clinic is *(10)*
   a. Bowie-Dick test
   b. Surface sampling
   c. Biological testing
   d. Thermocouple

**243** When you increase the object-film distance, you will have a *(11)*
   a. Sharper image that is smaller
   b. Sharper image that is larger
   c. Fuzzier image that is smaller
   d. Fuzzier image that is larger

**244** In ultrasonography, which organ is the most echogenic? *(12)*
   a. Bladder
   b. Liver
   c. Kidney
   d. Spleen

**245** A gene that has been altered by the addition of exogenous DNA is called a(n) *(13)*
   a. Transgenic gene
   b. Independent allele
   c. Hybrid vigor
   d. Karyotype

**246** Which of the following is not an example of olfactory communication in cats? *(14)*
   a. Urine spraying
   b. Feces in obvious locations
   c. Meowing
   d. Rubbing

**247** An ingredient panel lists ingredients in *(15)*
   a. Alphabetical order
   b. Ascending order
   c. Descending order
   d. No order

**248** Copper *(16)*
   a. Toxicity is a serious issue in cattle and sheep
   b. Is not needed for iron absorption
   c. Deficiency leads to reproductive failure
   d. Is a macromineral

**249** Ringworm, a common zoonotic disease carried by rodents, guineas pigs, rabbits, and other animals, is caused by a *(17)*
   a. Parasite
   b. Bacterium
   c. Fungus
   d. Virus

**250** A turtle's respiration is controlled by *(18)*
   a. The diaphragm
   b. The intercostal muscles
   c. Water depth during swimming
   d. Alternating body cavity pressure during locomotion and pharyngeal pumping

**251** Replacement crystalloids during anesthesia are administered at which of the following rates? *(19)*
   a. Up to 5 mL/kg/hr
   b. 5 to 10 mL/kg/hr
   c. 10 to 15 mL/kg/hr
   d. 15 to 20 mL/kg/hr

**252** Ophthalmic steroidal antiinflammatory drugs are contraindicated when *(20)*
   a. There is no corneal ulcer
   b. There is an infection in the cornea
   c. The patient is also receiving an antiviral drug
   d. The patient is also receiving a miotic drug

**253** Meloxicam at 1.5 mg/mL is prescribed for an arthritic 45-kg Irish Wolfhound. On the first day of treatment the patient should receive 0.2 mg/kg SID PO AC. The maintenance dosage is 0.1 mg/kg body weight every other day. How much meloxicam should be prescribed for a 2-week period? *(21)*
   a. 8 mL
   b. 16 mL
   c. 15 mL
   d. 24 mL

**254** What type of forceps has fine intermeshing teeth on the edges of the tips? *(22)*
   a. Brown-Adson
   b. Dressing
   c. Russian thumb
   d. Halstead mosquito

**255** Which of the following statements is false: *(23)*
   a. Chemotherapy utilizes cytotoxic agents
   b. Radiotherapy is the use of ionizing radiation
   c. Cryosurgery is the application of heat
   d. Hyperthermia causes necrosis and vascular thrombosis of an area

**256** The term *floating teeth* in reference to horses refers to *(24)*
   a. When a horse chews side to side
   b. Rasping down the sharp edges of teeth
   c. The removal of wolf teeth
   d. When a horse reacts to the bit

**257** Tail bleeding is most commonly performed in which species? *(25)*
   a. Cattle
   b. Goat
   c. Sheep
   d. Pig

258 The number of permanent teeth in cats is *(26)*
   a. 26
   b. 30
   c. 35
   d. 42

259 The most commonly occurring electrolyte imbalances associated with Addison's disease are *(27)*
   a. Hyperchloremia and hyperkalemia
   b. Hypernatremia and hypokalemia
   c. Hypokalemia and hypernatremia
   d. Hyponatremia and hyperkalemia

260 Newcastle disease causes which of the following symptoms in domestic poultry? *(28)*
   a. Watery, green diarrhea; tracheal exudate; facial edema; intestinal mucosa necrosis
   b. Gasping, coughing
   c. Twisted neck; paralysis; drooping wings; anorexia
   d. All of the above

261 When dealing with conflict, make sure you do all *except (29)*
   a. Separate the person from the problem
   b. Always walk away from the source of the conflict
   c. Identify options for possible solutions
   d. Focus on the interest, not the position

262 The part of a synovial joint that encloses the joint in a strong fibrous covering is *(1)*
   a. Synovial membrane
   b. Articular cartilage
   c. Joint capsule
   d. Synovial ligaments

263 The term for a variation in the size of erythrocytes is *(2)*
   a. Poikilocytosis
   b. Stomatocytosis
   c. Crenation
   d. Anisocytosis

264 A transudate would be expected to have a total protein concentration of *(3)*
   a. >7.5
   b. 7.5
   c. <7.5
   d. <3

265 A technician notes that during a patient's bath, the rinse water turned a red color. This could be an indication of an infestation of *(4)*
   a. *Ctenocephalides canis*
   b. *Ancylostoma caninum*
   c. *Strongylus vulgaris*
   d. *Oxyuris equi*

266 A bacterium that grows only on the TSA/blood agar plate is *(5)*
   a. An anaerobic bacteria
   b. Probably *Mycobacterium* sp.
   c. A fastidious organism
   d. All of the above

267 TLI (trypsinlike immunoreactivity) *(6)*
   a. Is highly specific for canine exocrine pancreatic insufficiency
   b. Uses EDTA anticoagulant
   c. Is completed on nonfasting animals
   d. Is used to determine if an animal has endocrine pancreatic insufficiency

268 What information is not needed when submitting virology samples for diagnosis? *(7)*
   a. The number of animals affected
   b. The clinical signs and treatment administered to date
   c. The veterinarian's tentative disease diagnosis
   d. Animal eye color

269 Which of the following is false with regard to maternal antibodies? *(8)*
   a. They are obtained by the neonates of all species via colostrum
   b. The antibodies do not prevent neonatal diarrhea
   c. They may block the effectiveness of vaccines when given too early in the neonate's life
   d. They convey short-lived immunity to the neonate

270 What does the standing part of the rope refer to? *(9)*
   a. The part of the rope that is attached to the animal
   b. The shortest part of the rope when tying a knot
   c. The part of the rope attached to an inanimate object
   d. The middle part of the rope

271 The recommended method of quality control for disinfection of the surgical suite in the veterinary clinic is *(10)*
   a. Bowie-Dick test
   b. Surface sampling
   c. Biological testing
   d. Thermocouple

272 A black mark on a radiographic film could be caused by all of the following *except* for *(11)*
   a. Debris in the intensifying screen
   b. Static electricity
   c. Light leak
   d. Linear lines due to grid cutoff

273 *Hertz* refers to *(12)*
   a. Velocity
   b. Density
   c. Cycles per second
   d. Wavelength

274 In mares, the incidence of dystocia is *(13)*
   a. <1%
   b. <3%
   c. <5%
   d. <6%

275 Which factor is least important to consider when selecting a pet? *(14)*
   a. Exercise requirement
   b. Grooming requirement
   c. Financial resources
   d. Child's preferences

276 Food allergy/intolerance in pets may manifest as *(15)*
   a. Gastrointestinal or dermatological signs
   b. Gastrointestinal or renal signs
   c. Hepatic or renal signs
   d. Cardiac or hepatic signs

277 The most critical nutritional requirement for newborns is *(16)*
   a. Water intake
   b. Carbohydrate intake
   c. Protein intake
   d. Colostrum intake

**278** You have been asked to give a dehydrated adult mouse intraperitoneal fluid therapy. What would be the absolute maximum that you could safely give? *(17)*
 a. 1 mL
 b. 2 mL
 c. 3 mL
 d. 4 mL

**279** In housing reptiles, the term *POT* refers to *(18)*
 a. Preferred outdoor tank
 b. Plastic outdoor tank
 c. Plastic oblong tank
 d. Preferred optimal temperature

**280** If the patient's total protein is 3.5 g/dL, which of the following is not considered a suitable choice for intravenous fluids during anesthesia? *(19)*
 a. Plasma
 b. Crystalloids
 c. Dextran
 d. 15 to 20 mL/kg/hr

**281** Analgesics that may be toxic to cats include *(20)*
 a. Narcotic analgesics
 b. Local anesthetics
 c. Nonsteroidal antiinflammatory drugs
 d. Steroids

**282** What volume of fluids did a patient receive if the drip rate was approximately 45 drops/min using a 20 drops/mL administration set, the IV line was in place at 800 mL, and the patient removed it at 1500 mL? *(21)*
 a. 945 mL
 b. Approximately 2 L
 c. 5.67 L
 d. 260 mL

**283** When labeling sterile packs, what information is not necessary? *(22)*
 a. Content
 b. Date of sterilization
 c. Initials of the person who prepared the pack
 d. Intended patient

**284** When performing wound lavage the most effective treatment is rinsing the wound with *(23)*
 a. Hydrogen peroxide using a Waterpik
 b. Normal saline in a 3-mL syringe using an 18-gauge needle
 c. Chlorhexidine diacetate solution in a spray bottle
 d. Povidone-iodine solution (10%) with a 60-mL syringe and an 18-gauge needle

**285** A major postoperative concern for the horse is *(24)*
 a. PCV and TP
 b. Moving the horse back to its stall as quickly as possible
 c. Proper grooming and shoe removal
 d. Ileus

**286** When performing a tuberculin test, the tuberculin is injected *(25)*
 a. Intramuscularly
 b. Subcutaneously
 c. Intradermally
 d. Intravenously

**287** The instrument used to scale the root of the tooth is a(n) *(26)*
 a. Sickle
 b. Explorer
 c. Probe
 d. Curet

**288** What does $Spo_2$ measure? *(27)*
 a. Hemoglobin saturation
 b. $Pao_2$
 c. $Paco_2$
 d. Lung sounds

**289** Hookworm disease is not likely to be transmitted to humans via *(28)*
 a. Mosquitoes
 b. Walking barefoot where animals have defecated
 c. Fecal-oral route
 d. Poor sanitation and hygiene

**290** When setting up a budget, you should *(29)*
 a. Just list household expenses
 b. List all expenses and income
 c. Include only your salary as income
 d. Make sure you have more expenses than income

**291** Ad lib is the abbreviation that means *(Appendix A)*
 a. As much as desired
 b. As needed
 c. Toward freedom
 d. After meals

**292** 5 kilograms is equal to *(Appendix B)*
 a. 5000 mg
 b. 5000 g
 c. 0.005 g
 d. 2.25 lbs

**293** The suffix for drooping or prolapse is *(Appendix C)*
 a. -poietic
 b. -plakia
 c. -phthisis
 d. -ptosis

**294** The genus and species for swine is *(Appendix D)*
 a. *Equus caballus*
 b. *Ovis aries*
 c. *Oryctolagus cuniculus*
 d. *Sus scrofa*

**295** The normal temperature and respiration rate for cats are *(Appendix E)*
 a. 105.5 ° F (41° C) and 150 to 210 breaths per minute
 b. 100.4° F (38° C) and 100 to 150 breaths per minute
 c. 100.4° F (38° C) and 150 to 200 breaths per minute
 d. 104° F (40° C) and 150 to 200 breaths per minute

**296** When you see the abbreviation Q.I.D., you should *(Appendix A)*
 a. Give the medication every 4 hours
 b. Give the medication 4 times a day
 c. Give the medication 2 times a day
 d. Give medication as desired

**297** Hypo- is the prefix that means *(Appendix C)*
 a. Decreased or less than
 b. Increased or more than
 c. The same
 d. Below

**298** The gestation and estrous cycles for ovines are *(Appendix D)*

    a. 68 and 12 days

    b. 148 and 17 days

    c. 114 and 21 days

    d. 335 and 17 days

**299** The abbreviation for *treatment* is *(Appendix A)*

    a. $D_x$

    b. $P_x$

    c. $T_x$

    d. $S_x$

**300** The prefix that means around, near, or about is *(Appendix C)*

    a. Peri-

    b. Para-

    c. Per-

    d. Pan-

| # | Ans | # | Ans | # | Ans | # | Ans | # | Ans | # | Ans |
|---|-----|---|-----|---|-----|---|-----|---|-----|---|-----|
| 1 | b | 46 | c | 91 | c | 136 | b | 181 | a | 226 | a |
| 2 | c | 47 | c | 92 | a | 137 | d | 182 | c | 227 | b |
| 3 | d | 48 | b | 93 | a | 138 | c | 183 | a | 228 | d |
| 4 | b | 49 | c | 94 | b | 139 | d | 184 | b | 229 | c |
| 5 | a | 50 | d | 95 | b | 140 | d | 185 | d | 230 | c |
| 6 | b | 51 | a | 96 | a | 141 | b | 186 | c | 231 | b |
| 7 | a | 52 | d | 97 | c | 142 | d | 187 | b | 232 | b |
| 8 | a | 53 | a | 98 | c | 143 | d | 188 | b | 233 | d |
| 9 | c | 54 | c | 99 | d | 144 | c | 189 | a | 234 | a |
| 10 | b | 55 | b | 100 | a | 145 | c | 190 | c | 235 | d |
| 11 | c | 56 | d | 101 | c | 146 | d | 191 | d | 236 | d |
| 12 | a | 57 | d | 102 | b | 147 | b | 192 | c | 237 | c |
| 13 | d | 58 | c | 103 | a | 148 | a | 193 | c | 238 | d |
| 14 | b | 59 | a | 104 | b | 149 | a | 194 | b | 239 | c |
| 15 | b | 60 | d | 105 | a | 150 | b | 195 | a | 240 | b |
| 16 | c | 61 | d | 106 | a | 151 | a | 196 | b | 241 | c |
| 17 | b | 62 | c | 107 | c | 152 | b | 197 | d | 242 | c |
| 18 | b | 63 | b | 108 | b | 153 | c | 198 | c | 243 | d |
| 19 | c | 64 | c | 109 | d | 154 | b | 199 | d | 244 | d |
| 20 | d | 65 | b | 110 | b | 155 | c | 200 | c | 245 | a |
| 21 | b | 66 | c | 111 | c | 156 | c | 201 | c | 246 | c |
| 22 | c | 67 | d | 112 | c | 157 | b | 202 | d | 247 | c |
| 23 | a | 68 | b | 113 | a | 158 | c | 203 | b | 248 | a |
| 24 | c | 69 | c | 114 | c | 159 | d | 204 | a | 249 | c |
| 25 | d | 70 | c | 115 | a | 160 | b | 205 | a | 250 | d |
| 26 | d | 71 | c | 116 | c | 161 | d | 206 | d | 251 | b |
| 27 | c | 72 | d | 117 | b | 162 | c | 207 | c | 252 | a |
| 28 | a | 73 | b | 118 | c | 163 | a | 208 | d | 253 | d |
| 29 | c | 74 | c | 119 | b | 164 | a | 209 | a | 254 | a |
| 30 | c | 75 | a | 120 | c | 165 | d | 210 | c | 255 | c |
| 31 | b | 76 | a | 121 | d | 166 | c | 211 | a | 256 | b |
| 32 | c | 77 | b | 122 | d | 167 | c | 212 | d | 257 | a |
| 33 | a | 78 | a | 123 | c | 168 | a | 213 | a | 258 | b |
| 34 | a | 79 | b | 124 | d | 169 | c | 214 | a | 259 | d |
| 35 | d | 80 | b | 125 | a | 170 | d | 215 | d | 260 | d |
| 36 | c | 81 | d | 126 | b | 171 | b | 216 | c | 261 | b |
| 37 | b | 82 | a | 127 | a | 172 | a | 217 | b | 262 | c |
| 38 | a | 83 | d | 128 | c | 173 | b | 218 | a | 263 | d |
| 39 | c | 84 | c | 129 | b | 174 | a | 219 | b | 264 | d |
| 40 | a | 85 | b | 130 | a | 175 | c | 220 | c | 265 | a |
| 41 | d | 86 | b | 131 | a | 176 | d | 221 | b | 266 | c |
| 42 | d | 87 | c | 132 | b | 177 | c | 222 | a | 267 | a |
| 43 | c | 88 | d | 133 | a | 178 | b | 223 | a | 268 | d |
| 44 | b | 89 | c | 134 | b | 179 | b | 224 | c | 269 | a |
| 45 | a | 90 | b | 135 | a | 180 | d | 225 | a | 270 | d |

| | | | | | |
|---|---|---|---|---|---|
| **271** b | **276** a | **281** c | **286** c | **291** a | **296** b |
| **272** a | **277** d | **282** a | **287** d | **292** b | **297** a |
| **273** c | **278** c | **283** d | **288** a | **293** d | **298** b |
| **274** a | **279** d | **284** c | **289** a | **294** d | **299** c |
| **275** d | **280** b | **285** d | **290** b | **295** c | **300** a |

# Answer Key to Chapter Review Questions

**Chapter 1**
1 b
2 a
3 d
4 b
5 d
6 b
7 b
8 c
9 d
10 d

**Chapter 2**
1 b
2 d
3 d
4 b
5 a
6 b
7 c
8 c
9 a
10 c

**Chapter 3**
1 c
2 b
3 a
4 d
5 c
6 a
7 b
8 c
9 b
10 a

**Chapter 4**
1 b
2 a
3 a
4 c
5 b
6 b
7 a
8 d
9 d
10 d

**Chapter 5**
1 d
2 b
3 c
4 a
5 d
6 c
7 c
8 a
9 b
10 a

**Chapter 6**
1 d
2 c
3 b
4 d
5 c
6 b
7 a
8 a
9 d
10 a

**Chapter 7**
1 c
2 c
3 a
4 d
5 a
6 b
7 d
8 c
9 d
10 a

**Chapter 8**
1 d
2 d
3 d
4 c
5 d
6 b
7 a
8 b
9 a
10 a

**Chapter 9**
1 a
2 d
3 a
4 d
5 d
6 c
7 a
8 d
9 b
10 b

**Chapter 10**
1 c
2 b
3 c
4 a
5 d
6 c
7 d
8 b
9 d
10 c

**Chapter 11**
1 c
2 b
3 d
4 b
5 c
6 c
7 a
8 b
9 d
10 a

**Chapter 12**
1 a
2 b
3 c
4 c
5 d
6 a
7 d
8 b
9 c
10 d

**Chapter 13**
1 d
2 a
3 a
4 b
5 c
6 b
7 a
8 c
9 d
10 d

**Chapter 14**
1 d
2 d
3 a
4 b
5 d
6 d
7 b
8 b
9 c
10 a

**Chapter 15**
1 b
2 c
3 d
4 a
5 c
6 d
7 c
8 b
9 c
10 d
11 c
12 b
13 a

## Chapter 16

1 d
2 c
3 c
4 a
5 a
6 c
7 c
8 a
9 b
10 b

## Chapter 17

1 b
2 a
3 c
4 a
5 b
6 a
7 b
8 c
9 b
10 c

## Chapter 18

1 b
2 c
3 b
4 a
5 a
6 b
7 b
8 b
9 d
10 d

## Chapter 19

1 b
2 c
3 a
4 d
5 d
6 c
7 c
8 a
9 b
10 c

## Chapter 20

1 c
2 b
3 a
4 a
5 c
6 a
7 c
8 c
9 d
10 b

## Chapter 21

1 a
2 b
3 c
4 d
5 a
6 d
7 a
8 a
9 c
10 c

## Chapter 22

1 b
2 b
3 d
4 a
5 d
6 a
7 c
8 b
9 c
10 a

## Chapter 23

1 a
2 c
3 b
4 b
5 c
6 c
7 c
8 b
9 a
10 b

## Chapter 24

1 c
2 d
3 a
4 a
5 d
6 b
7 a
8 b
9 c
10 b

## Chapter 25

1 b
2 c
3 b
4 b
5 a
6 b
7 c
8 d
9 c
10 a

## Chapter 26

1 c
2 c
3 d
4 b
5 c
6 b
7 a
8 b
9 b
10 a

## Chapter 27

1 d
2 c
3 c
4 d
5 d
6 a
7 d
8 b
9 a
10 c

## Chapter 28

1 c
2 c
3 c
4 b
5 d
6 d
7 d
8 a
9 b
10 d

## Chapter 29

1 c
2 d
3 b
4 b
5 b
6 c
7 c
8 c
9 d
10 c

# Index

## A

AAFCO. *See* Association of American Feed Control Officials
AAHA. *See* American Animal Hospital Association
AAVSB. *See* American Association of Veterinary State Boards
Abbreviations/symbols, 562-567
ABCD. *See* Airway Breathing Cardiac Drugs
Abdomen
  bandaging, 444
  palpation, 416
Abdominal ballottement, definition, 227
Abdominal fluid, removal/evaluation, 67
Abdominocentesis, 55
  definition, 71
Abnormal dental interlock, 500
Abomasum,15. *See also* Displaced abomasum
Abscessed areas, specimen type, 101
Absolute, definition, 51
Absolute count, definition, 51
Absorbable suture material, 405-406
Absorbed due, definition, 190-192
*Acanthocheilonema*, examination, 75
Acanthocyte, 38f
  definition, 51
Acariasis, definition, 95
Accessory sex glands, 18
ACE. *See* Angiotensin-converting enzyme
Acemannan, usage, 387
Acetaminophen toxicosis, 518t
Acetonemia. *See* Ketosis
Acetylcholine agonists, usage, 361
Acetylcholine antagonists, usage, 361
Acid-base balance, 363
Acid-base disturbances, categories, 363
Acid citrate dextrose (ACD), addition. *See* Blood
Acid-fast stain, 104
Acoustic coupling gel, usage, 199
Acoustic impedance, 195
  definition, 202
Acquired artificial active immunity, 136
Acquired artificial passive immunity, 136
Acquired deficiencies, 138
Acquired immunities, 355
  types, 136-137
Acquired natural active immunity, 136
Acquired natural passive immunity, 136
Active immunity, 355
Active processes, 4
Active transport, 4
Actual focal spot, definition, 191

Acute intraoperative blood loss, fluid replacement, 363
Acute paresis/paralysis, emergency, 514t
Acute renal failure, emergency, 515t
Adaptive immunity, 135
Addisonian crisis (hypoadrenocorticism), emergency, 516t
Additive, definition, 284
Adenocarcinoma, definition, 70
Adenoma, definition, 70
Adenomyosis, definition, 227
Adenosine triphosphate (ATP), production, 3
ADH. *See* Antidiuretic hormone
Adipocytes, definition, 70
Adjuvant, definition, 131, 141
Ad libitum, definition, 284
Adrenal cortex function tests, 121b
Adrenal gland, sonographic appearance, 200
Adrenergic blockers, 377
Adrenergics
  list, 379t
  sympathetic effects, 377
Adson tissue forceps, 401
Adsorb, definition, 131
Adult cats, nutritional requirements, 254-255
Adult dogs, nutritional requirements, 252
Aerobic, definition, 110
Aerobic gram-positive rods, 108-109
Afferent nerve processes (sensory nerve processes), 11-12
African clawed frog *(Xenopus laevis)*, 303-305
  behavioral/physiological characteristics, 303-304
  breeding considerations, 304
  dropsy/bloat, 307
  fungal infections, 305
  handling/restraint, 304
  health conditions, 305
  pain/distress, signs, 304-305
  parasitic infections,305
  red leg, 305
  research origin/uses, 303
  sampling, 304
Agar, definition, 110
Aggression. *See* Canine
  definition, 240
Agouti, definition, 227
Agranulocyte, definition, 51
Air-driven units, 495
Air filtration, usage, 166
Air sacculitis, 317
Air sacs, avian/mammalian comparison, 313
Airway Breathing Cardiac Drugs (ABCD), 507

Alanine aminotransferase (ALT), 117-118
Alanine transaminase, 117-118
Albumin
  change, 117
  levels, change. *See* Serum
Albumin-globulin ratio (A:G), 117
Alcohol lamps, usage, 99
Alcohols, usage, 168
Aldehydes, usage, 167-168
Aleutian disease (AD). *See* Ferrets
Alimentary canal, walls (division), 14
Alkaline phosphatase (AP), 118
Alkylating agents, list, 388t
Alleles, 207
  definition, 227
  duplication, 211
Allelomimetic, definition, 162
Allergens. *See* Food allergies/intolerance
  definition, 141
  list, 257
Allergic reaction, 512-513t
Allergic skin diseases, 439-440
Allis tissue forceps, 401
Alopecia. *See* Hedgehogs; Rabbit
  definition, 95
Alpha2 adrenergic agonists, 360
Alpha2 agonists, 544
Alpha2 reversal agonists, 338
Alpha-hemolysis, 105
Altered self, definition, 131
Alternative imaging technology
  glossary, 202-203
  learning outcomes, 194
  review questions, 203-204
Alveolar bone, 472
Alveolar macrophages, nucleus placement, 64
AMDUCA. *See* Animal Medicinal Drug Use Clarification Act of 1994
American Animal Hospital Association (AAHA), 548
American Association of Veterinary State Boards (AAVSB), 558
American Society of Anesthesiologists (ASA) scale, 336t
American Veterinary Medical Association (AVMA)
  accredited program, 558
  AMDUCA brochure, 368
  prescription guidelines, 396
Amidate. *See* Etomidate
Amorphous phosphates, 36
Amorphous urates, 34f, 36
Amperage, definition, 191
Amphiarthrosis, 8

Page numbers followed by *f* indicate figures; *t,* tables; *b,* boxes.

Amphibians, blood specimen, 103
Amplexus, definition, 309
Amplitude, definition, 202
Amplitude mode (A-mode), 197
    definition, 202
    peaks, usage, 197f
Amylase, 15
Amyloclastic test, definition, 124
Amyloidosis, definition, 71
An-, definition, 51
Anaerobic, definition, 110
Anal area, examination, 416
Analgesia, 359
Analgesic agents/techniques, examples,
    359
Analgesic drugs, 370-375
    list, 374-375t
Analgesic usage, reasons, 359
Analog, definition, 191
Analog-to-digital converter (ADC), 189
Anal sac expression
    definition, 432
    indications, 432
    precautions, 432
    procedure, 432
Anaphylactic shock, emergency, 514t
Anaplamosis. *See* Cattle
Anasarca, definition, 227
Anatomy, definition, 3
*Ancylostoma caninum,* 96f
Ancylostomiasis, parasitic
    zoonosis, 534t
Androgens
    anabolic steroids, usage (rarity), 390
    list, 386t
Anechoic, definition, 202
Anechoic image, 197
Anemia, 279
    acute blood loss, impact, 362
    definition, 51
Anesthesia
    environmental concerns, 353
    glossary, 365
    health hazards, 353
    hepatotoxicity, 353
    induction, 483
    learning outcomes, 334
    machine, components, 351f
    monitoring techniques, 355
    reproductive problems, 353
    review questions, 365
    stages, 358
    subplanes, 358
    techniques, vigilance, 354
Anesthetic agents. *See* Injectable anesthetic
    agents
    classification, 340
    pharmacological properties, 348t
Anesthetic drugs, 375
    list, 376-377t
    overdose, 375
Anesthetic equipment, 348
    low pressure leaks, problems, 354
    maintenance/concerns, 354-355
    monitoring, objective, 358

Anesthetic machine, 348-352
    Bain mount/system, 351
    carbon dioxide absorber, 350-351
    check valve, 348
    circle/breathing system, 350
    components, 348-352
    concerns, 354-355
    flowmeters, 349
    gas supply, 348
    oxygen flush valve, 351
    pop-off valve, 350
    pressure gauge, 348-349
    pressure manometer, 351
    pressure-reducing valve/regulator,
        349
    reservoir bag, usage, 350
    scavenging systems, 351
    unidirectional valves, 350
    vaporizers, usage, 349-350
Anesthetic protocol, selection, 335
Anesthetic risk, 335
Anestrus, 19
    cell population identification, 69
Anger, grief stage, 448, 544
Angiotensin-converting enzyme (ACE)
    inhibitors, list, 379t
Animal anatomy/physiology
    glossary, 22
    learning outcomes, 2
    review questions, 23
Animal Medicinal Drug Use Clarification
    Act of 1994 (AMDUCA), 368
Animals
    behavior. *See* Applied animal
        behavior
    consumption, usage, 270
    needs, assessment, 544
    treatment. *See* Pregnant animals
Anion, definition, 124, 171
Anisocytosis, definition, 51, 71
Anisokaryosis, 62
    definition, 71
Anisonucleoliosis, definition, 71
Ankylosis, definition, 227
Anode
    definition, 191
    types, 175
    usage, 175
Anodontia, 500
Anorexia, definition, 284
ANS. *See* Autonomic nervous system
Anterior direction, 7
Anterior enteritis
    management, 461
    rule out, 461
Anthelmintic, definition, 95
Anthrax. *See* Cattle
Antiarrhythmics
    list, 380t
    usage, 378
Antibiotic-associated enterotoxemia. *See*
    Guinea pig
Antibiotics
    bacterial resistance, 370
    list, 388t

Anticholinergics
    classification, 336
    list, 379t
    side effects, 377
Anticoagulants
    definition, 124
    list, 380t
    rodenticide toxicity, 518t
    usage, 390
Anticonvulsants, list, 376t
Antidiabetics, list, 387t
Antidiarrheals
    list, 383t
    usage, 380
Antidiuretic hormone (ADH) release, 114
Antidotes, list, 389t
Antiemetics
    list, 382t
    usage, 378-380
Antigen, definition, 141
Antigenic drift
    capability. *See* Viruses
    definition, 141
Antihistamines, list, 381t
Antiinflammatory drugs, 370-375
    list, 374-375t
Antikicker, definition, 162
Antimetabolites, list, 388t
Antimicrobial agents, mechanisms, 370
Antimicrobial drugs, 370
Antimicrobials, list, 371-373t
Antineoplastic agents, impact, 389
Antineoplastic drugs, types, 389
Antiparasitic drugs
    list, 384-385t
    usage, 383
Antiseptic, definition, 171
Antisera
    antibodies, inclusion, 387
    definition, 141
    usage, 139
Antispasmodics, list, 382t
Antitoxins, antibodies (inclusion), 387
Antitussives
    list, 381t
    usage, 378
Antiulcer drugs, list, 382t
Antiulcer medications, usage, 381-383
Anuria, 27
    definition, 51
Anus, 15
Aortic arch, branches, 13
AP. *See* Alkaline phosphatase
Apnea, definition, 17
Appendicular skeleton, 7
Appetite stimulants, list, 382t
Applicator sticks, usage, 100
Applied animal behavior, 236
Aqueous humor, 21
    formation, 433
Arachidonic acid, 244
    requirement, 317
Arboviral encephalitis, viral zoonosis, 530t
Arterial blood gas, invasiveness, 496
Arteries, 14

Arterioles, 14
Arthrocentesis, 55
 definition, 71
Arthropod, definition, 95
Articular cartilage, 8
Articulations (joints), 8-9
Artifacts. *See* Film
 definition, 191
 technical areas, 181b
Artificial immunity, 136
Artificial vagina (AV), 211, 220
 definition, 227
ASA. *See* American Society of Anesthesi-
  ologists
Ascites, definition, 227
Asepsis, definition, 171
Aseptic technique, 110
Aspartate aminotransferase (AST), 118
Aspartate transaminase, 118
Aspergillosis, 317
Aspermatogenesis, definition, 261
Aspirate, expelling, 58f
Aspiration method, 54
Aspirin, NSAID example, 375
Assembly-release, replication stage, 127
Association areas, 10-11
Association of American Feed Control Of-
  ficials (AAFCO), 259
 calorie/fat content regulation, 213
 definition, 261
 nutrient profiles, guidelines, 260
Assortative mating, 209
 definition, 227
Asystole, 427
Ataxia, definition, 261
Atelectasis, definition, 17
Atomic absorption, 120
Atopy, definition, 141
Atrial fibrillation, 426
Atrial flutter, 426
Atrial premature contraction, 427
Atrial repolarization, absence, 424
Atrioventricular (AV) block, 454
Atrophic rhinitis. *See* Pigs
Atropine, usage, 336
Attachment, replication stage, 127
Attenuated-live vaccines, 138
Attenuation, 195
 artifacts, 198
 definition, 202
Auditory, definition, 240
Aujeszky's disease. *See* Pseudorabies
Auricular treatment, 431-432
 equipment, 431-432
 procedure, 432
 purpose, 328
Autoclave
 advantages, 169
 chamber, loading, 170-171
 definition, 131
 disadvantages, 169
 function, 169
 load, preparation, 170
 operation, 170-171
 types, 169-170
 usage, 169-171

Autoimmune disorder, result, 138
Autoimmune hemolytic anemia, 138
Autoimmune reaction, definition, 141
Autolysis, definition, 131
Autonomic division, 11-12
Autonomic nervous system (ANS), drugs
  (impact), 377
Autosomal
 definition, 227
 usage, 208
Autosomal dominant, 209
Autosomal recessive, 209
AV. *See* Artificial vagina;
  Atrioventricular
Aversive, definition, 240
Aves, class, 312
Avian anesthesia/analgesia, 316
 monitoring, 316
Avian bacterial diseases, 317
Avian beak trimming, 315-316
Avian blood
 analysis, 315
 collection, 315
 specimen , 103
Avian chlamydiosis, emergency, 524t
Avian cholera, 317
Avian classification, 312
Avian clinic caging, 314
Avian diets/problems, 316
Avian ectoparasites, 318
Avian endoparasites, 318
Avian gastric yeast, 317
Avian home caging, 314
Avian housing, 314
 quarantine, 314
Avian infectious diseases, 317-318
Avian influenza, viral zoonosis, 531t
Avian intramuscular injections, performing,
  315
Avian intraosseous catheter placement, 315
Avian intravenous catheter placement, 315
Avian leukocyte count, 46
Avian medicine, 312
Avian mycobacteriosis, 317
Avian mycotic diseases, 317-318
Avian nail trimming, 315
Avian noninfectious diseases/conditions,
  316-317
Avian nursing care, 314-316
Avian nutrition, 316
Avian oral drug administration/gavage
  feeding, 316
Avian parasites, 318
Avian physical examination, 314-316
Avian predisposing factors, 316-317
Avian restraint/handling, 312
Avians, mammals, anatomical/physiological
  comparison, 312-314
Avian subcutaneous injections, usage,
  316
Avian trauma, 316
Avian viral diseases, 317
Avian wing clipping, 315
Avirulent, definition, 141
AVMA. *See* American Veterinary Medical
  Association

Axenic, definition, 309
Axial resolution, definition, 202
Axial skeleton, 7
Azaperone, usage, 337
Azotemia, definition, 124
Azoturia, 283
Azurophilic granules, definition, 51

**B**

Babcock intestinal forceps, 401
*Bacillus anthracis*, 524t
Backcross, definition, 227
Background, definition, 284
Backhaus towel clamps, 401
Backhaus towel clips, 402f
Bacterial dermatological conditions,
  364-365
Bacterial enteritis, 317
Bacterial flora, change, 502
Bacterial pneumonia. *See* Guinea pig
Bacterial toxemia, 317
Bacterial zoonosis, 524-528t
Bacteriological media, 100-101
Bacteriostat, definition, 171
Baermann technique. *See*
  External parasite identification
 definition, 95
Bailey ejaculator, 220
Bain mount/system. *See* Anesthetic machine;
  Breathing circuits
Balfour retractors, 403-404
Balling gun
 definition, 162
 usage, 472
Bandages
 aftercare, 445
 layers, 443
 types, 443-445
 uses, 468
Bandaging. *See* Equine
 principles, 468
 techniques, 445
Barbering, definition, 309
Barbiturates
 examples, 341-342
 lipid solubility, 11
 list, 376t
 protein binding, 11
 usage, 340
Bar cells, 38f
Bard-Parker scalpel handle, 405
Bargaining, grief stage, 448, 543
Barking. *See* Canine
Barrier sustained, definition, 309
Barrow, definition, 227
Basal cells, size, 69
Basophilia, definition, 51
Basophilic stippling, definition, 51
Beef cattle
 calcium, 268
 calves, creep feeding, 270
 cobalt, 268
 copper, 269
 feeding, 267
 feed sources, 267
 iodine, 268

Beef cattle *(Continued)*
  iron, 269
  life stages, 269
  minerals, 268
  nutrition, disease (relationship), 271
  nutritional requirements, 268
  phosphorus, 268
  protein, 268
  replacement/breeding animals, feeding, 270
  selenium, 269
  sodium/chloride, 268
  vitamins, 269
  water, 268
  zinc, 269
Behavioral problems, 238
Behavior modification, 240
Benign, definition, 71
Benzodiazepines
  anxiety reduction, 377
  usage, 337
Beta blockers
  list, 379t
  usage, 377
Beta decay, definition, 202
Beta-hemolysis, 105
Beta particles, definition, 202
Beta ray
  definition, 202
  radiation, 200
BHI. *See* Brain heart infusion
Bight, definition, 162
Biguanide, usage, 168
Bile, definition, 124
Bile acids, 118-119
Bile esculin (BE)
  agar, 100
  test, 104
Bile pigments, chemical component, 31
Bilirubin
  conjugated/unconjugated forms, 115-116
  crystals, 36
  false-positive results, 116
  production, 115-116
Bilirubinuria, 31
  definition, 51
Binding energy, definition, 191
Biochemical reference values, 122t
Biochemistry data, conversion factors, 123t
Biochemistry reference intervals, 122t
Biological enzymes, classification, 117
Biological indicators, 408
Biological testing, 171
Biological value, definition, 284
Biopsy, definition, 71
Birth canal. *See* Vagina
Bitch, 213
  examination, 213
Black marks. *See* X-ray film
Black pigmenting anaerobic bacteria (BPAB), 502
Bladder
  rupture, failure, 515t
  sonographic appearance, 199

Bloat, 271, 274. *See also* Ruminal tympany
Blood
  acid citrate dextrose (ACD), addition, 423
  cells, avian/mammalian comparison, 313
  chemical component, 31-32
  citrate phosphate dextrose (CPD), addition, 423
  component therapy, use (indications), 423
  gas results, interpretation, 364
  gas samples, disorders (presence), 364-365
  loss, monitoring, 362
  parasite examination, 73-75
    buffy coat method, 75-76
    commercial filter technique, 75
    modified Knott's technique, 75
  parasites, diagnostic characteristics. *See* Domestic animals
  pressure, monitoring, 356
    technique, recommendation, 360
  products, administration, 363
  profiles (hemograms), expansion, 37
  samples, serum separation, 113
  shelf-life, 423
  specimen, 103
  substitutes, impact, 390
  transfer, 37
  tubes, 113
  vessels, 14
Blood-brain barrier, 11
Blood collection
  administration/reactions, 423
  sampling, 37
  transfusion, 421-424
Bloom, definition, 284
B-mode. *See* Brightness mode
Boars, 225
  definition, 227
Body
  cellular damage, types, 186
  condition
    definition, 227
    scoring, 252b
  fluid discoloration, inflammation (impact), 56
  supporting bones, 8
  systems, 7-22
Bone curettes, 405
Bone-cutting forceps, 404-405
Bone marrow
  cells, characteristics, 66
  core biopsy, 120
  films, evaluation, 66
  lesions, collection/evaluation, 66
  smears, preparation, 66
Bone rasps, 405
Bones
  cells, types, 7-9
  classification, 7-9
  formation, 8
  function, 7-9
    classification, 8
  structure, classification, 8-9
  types, 7-9

Borborygmus, 454
*Bordetella* spp., 108
Bovine, 217-219
  breeding soundness examination, 217-218
  dystocia, causes, 219
  estrous cycle, 210-211
  estrus, signs, 218
  gestation, 218-219
  locomotor abnormalities, 217-218
  maternal dystocia, 219
  neonatal care, 219
  parturition, stages, 218-219
  pregnancy diagnosis, 218
  puberty, 217
  Q fever, 218
  reproductive abnormalities, 218
  semen characteristics, 218
  semen collection techniques, 218
  semen evaluation, 218
Bovine respiratory disease complex, 479
Bovine respiratory syncytial virus (BRSV), 479
Bovine viral diarrhea virus (BVDV), 479
Bowel, sonographic appearance, 200
Bowie Dick test, 171
  performing, 407
Bowline knot, 161f
  usage, 161
BPAB. *See* Black pigmenting anaerobic bacteria
Brachiocephalic artery. *See* Innominate artery
Brachycephalic occlusive syndrome, emergency, 513t
Brachyodont, 503
Brain, 10-12
  capillaries, endothelial cells, 11
  stem, 11
Brain heart infusion (BHI), 100
Breakaway collar, definition, 162
Breathing, triage, 493
Breathing circuits, 437
  Bain system, 353
  universal F-circuit, 352
Breathing system. *See* Anesthetic machine
  usage, 352
Breech, definition, 227
Breeding, systems/terminology, 209-210
Breeding sows/litters, management, 279
Brightness mode (B-mode), 197
  definition, 202
Broad bandwidth transducer, 196
Bronchi, 16
Bronchial samples, collection/evaluation, 64
Bronchial washes, 56
  orotracheal technique, 56
  percutaneous technique, 56
Bronchiole, 17
Bronchoalveolar lavage (BAL), orotracheal technique, 56
Bronchodilators
  impact, 378
  list, 381t
  usage, 378

Bronchoscopy, preference, 56
Broth, definition, 110
Brown-Adson tissue forceps, 401
   illustration, 402f
Browse, definition, 284
BRSV. *See* Bovine respiratory syncytial
   virus
Bruce effect, 309
Brucellosis, 220, 223
   bacterial zoonosis, 524t
   *Brucella abortus. See* Cattle
   *Brucella ovis. See* Sheep
Buck, 220
   examination, 220
Buffy coat
   definition, 51
   method. *See* Blood
Bull, 217
Bull to cow/heifer ratio, 218
Bunsen burner, usage, 99
Bupivacaine, usage, 359
Burnout, coping, 552
Business communications, components,
   545
Business formats, 549
Business management, 548
Butyrophenones, usage, 337
BVDV. *See* Bovine viral diarrhea virus

**C**

CAAHTT. *See* Canadian Association of
   Animal Health Technologists and
   Technicians
Calcinosis, definition, 261
Calcium carbonate, 36
Calcium channel blockers, list, 379t
Calcium oxalate, 36
Calcium oxalate monohydrate, 34f
Calcium oxalate urolithiasis, 36
Calculus
   formation, 502
   removal, 496
California Mastitis Test (CMT), 474-475
Calipers, definition, 191
Calves
   dehorning, 487
   indigestion, 272
Camelids. *See* South American
   camelid
   diseases, 475-481
   energy requirements, 275
   feeding, 275
   feed sources, 275
   forages, usage, 275
   intradermal injections, 474
   life stages, 276
   minerals, usage, 276
   nutrition, disease (relationship), 276
   nutritional requirements, 275
   proteins, ingestion, 275
   subcutaneous (SC) injections, 474
   venipuncture, 473
   water, usage, 275
*Campylobacter fetus* ssp. *venerealis. See*
   Cattle
Campylobacteriosis, 525t

Canadian Association of Animal Health
   Technologists and Technicians
   (CAAHTT), 557
Canadian Food and Drug Act Schedules,
   drug specification, 368
Canaliculi, 7
Cancellous bone. *See* Spongy bone
*Candida albicans*, 109
Candidiasis, 317
Canine, 213
   aggression, 238
   auditory sense, 232
   barking, 238
   behavior, 231
   behavioral development, 231
   behavioral problems, 238
   blood collection, 421-422
      procedure, 421
      supplies, 421
   breeding soundness examination, 213
   cancer, 258-259
   development stages, 232t
   donor requirements, 421
   dystocia
      causes, 215
      signs, 215
   estrous cycle, 214
   estrus, signs, 214
   eyes 433
   gestation, 214-215
   house soiling, 239
   neonatal care, 215
   olfaction, 499
   parturition, stages, 215
   postural signaling, 232
   pregnancy diagnosis, 214
   puberty, 213
   seborrheic complex, 441
   semen characteristics, 213-214
   semen collection technique, 213-214
   skin, 438f
   social development, 231-233
   vision, 232
Canine castrations, 408
Canine female urinary catheterization,
   429-430
   equipment, 429
   indications, 429-430
   precautions, 430
   procedure, 430
Canine male urinary catheterization, 429
   equipment, 429
   indications, 429
   precautions, 429
   procedure, 429
Canine skeleton, 9f
Canine thyroid stimulating hormone,
   120
Capillaries, 14
Capillary refill time (CRT)
   monitoring, 355
   observation, 416
   usage, 509
*Capnocytophaga conimorsus* infections,
   525t
Capnograph, usefulness, 361

Caprine, 220-222
   breeding soundness examination, 220
   dystocia
      causes, 221-222
      signs, 222
   estrous cycle, 220-221
   estrus, signs, 221
   gestation, 221
   neonatal care, 222
   parturition, stages, 221
   pregnancy diagnosis, 221
   puberty, 220
   Q fever, 220
   semen characteristics, 220
   semen collection techniques, 220
Caprofen, NSAID example, 375
Capsid, definition, 131
Capture pole, usage, 147
Carbohydrates
   definition, 261
   nutrients, 244
Carbonaceous, definition, 284
Carbon dioxide
   absorber. *See* Anesthetic machine
   monitor, usefulness, 361
Carcinoma, definition, 71
Cardiac cycle, 13-14
Cardiac muscles (myocardium), 10
Cardiac muscle tissue, 5-6
Cardiogenic shock, emergency, 514t
Cardiopulmonary cerebral resuscitation
   (CPCR), 507-508
   success, advice, 508
Cardiovascular drugs, 378
   list, 379-380t
Cardiovascular emergencies, 514t
Cardiovascular system, 12-14
   anesthesia monitoring techniques,
      355-357
   components, 12
   function, 12-14
   physical examination, 417
   protective layers, 12-14
   status, monitoring, 499
   structure, 12-14
   triage, 493
Career management, 552
Carnassial tooth, dental radiography
   (bisecting angle technique), 148f
Carnivore, 14
Carrier females, 208
Cartilaginous structure, 8-9
Casting
   definition, 162
   materials, 445
Casts, aftercare, 445
Casts (cylinduria), 34f, 33-36
Catalase test, 104
Catecholamines, usage, 378
Cathode
   definition, 191
   electron source, 174
Cation, definition, 124, 171
Cat restraint, 147-149
   considerations, 148
   equipment, 148-149

Cats
  back legs, securing, 149f
  behavioral characteristics, 147-148
  cat bag, advantages/disadvantages, 149
  cornering, 148
  depressed behavior, 148
  friendliness, 233
  gloves, usage, 149
  head restraint, 148f
  lower urinary tract disease, risk factors, 255b
  neck, scruffing, 149f
  nutritional requirements, 250-255. See also Adult cats; Geriatric cats
  towel wrapping, 149f
Cat scratch disease, 525t
Cattle
  acetonemia, 475
  anaplasmosis (Anaplasma marginale), 480
  anthrax (Bacillus anthracis), 480
  bite, infrequency, 154
  brucellosis (Brucella abortus), 477-478
  casting, 156
  castration, 484-487
  digit amputation, 484
  Escherichia coli diarrhea, 477
  eye enucleation, 484
  feet, restraint, 154
  flank restraint, 156
  front foot, rope usage, 155f
  general anesthesia, 482-483
  head, restraint, 153,155
  head chute, usage, 154f
  herding, 154-155
  hind feet, danger, 154
  hobbles, usage, 155
  intradermal injections, 474
  intramuscular (IM) injections, 473
  intraperitoneal injections, 474
  jugular vein, 472
  laparotomy, 484
  leptospirosis (Leptospira pomona), 478
  listeriosis (Listeria monocytogenes), 478
  mastitis, 477
  milk vein (subcutaneous abdominal), 473
  neosporosis (Neospora caninum), 478
  parainfluenza III, 479
  regional anesthesia, 481
  subcutaneous (SC) injections, 474
  tail
    annoyance, 154
    jacking, 155
    jack procedure, 156f
    restraint, 154
  tail vein (ventral coccygeal), 473
  teat laceration repair, 484
  trichonomiasis (Trichomonas fetus), 478
  venipuncture, 46
  vibriosis (Campylobacter fetus ssp. vene-realis), 477
Cattle restraint, 153-156
  behavioral characteristics, 154
  body, restraint, 153
  considerations, 148

Cattle restraint (Continued)
  danger potential, 147, 153-154
  equipment, 148-149
  usage, 154-156
Caudal direction, 7
Caudate cells, 34f
Caudocranial (CdCr), definition, 191
Caveman pets, 148, 152
  definition, 162
CCD. See Charge-coupled device
CdCr. See Caudocranial
Cecotrophs, definition, 309
Cecum, anatomy/physiology, 277
Cell-mediated immune response, 135
Cell-mediated immunity (CMI), 138
  definition, 141
Cell-mediated immunodeficiency, 138
Cell membrane, damage, 370
Cellophane tape
  method. See External parasite identification
  sampling, 420
Cells
  drinking. See Pinocytosis
  eating. See Phagocytosis
  microscopic examination, 54
  movement, 4
  populations, estrous cycle identification, 69
  size, variations, 51
  structure/physiology, 3
Cellular casts, 35
Cellular changes, 62
Cementum, 472
Centesis, 55
  definition, 71
Central haversian canal, 7
Central nervous system (CNS), 10
  anesthesia monitoring techniques, 355
  depression, absence, 360
  drugs, 376-377t
  emergencies, 514t
  glial cells, 12
  organization, 11f
  status, monitoring, 500
  triage, 493
Central vascular system, 14
Centrifugal flotation technique. See Feces
Centrioles, 4
Cephalic vein, venipuncture, 420
Cereal grains, usage, 268
Cerebellum, 11
Cerebrospinal fluid (CSF), 11-12
  evaluation, 68
  taps, 55
Cerebrum, 10
Cervical dilation failure, 221
Cervical lymphadenitis. See Guinea pig
Cervix, 19
Cestode
  definition, 95
  impact, 318
Chain leashes, 146
Chairside darkroom, usage, 498
Chapter review questions, answer key, 594-595

Charge-coupled device (CCD), definition, 191
Chelonians, nutrition/diets (problems), 321-322
Chemical agent, usage, 166-169
Chemical buffers, usage, 363
Chemical indicator strips, color change, 407
Chemicals
  -cidal activity, ranking, 167f
  usage, 166-169
Chemotactic, definition, 71
Chemotherapeutic agents, list, 388-389t
Chemotherapeutic drugs, 389-390
  DNA alteration, permanence, 389
Chemotherapy, 447
Chest
  auscultation, 416
  compressions, 508
Chew toys, usage, 499
Chinchilla (Chinchilla langier), 297-298
  behavioral/physiological characteristics, 302
  breeding considerations, 302-303
  handling/restraint, 302
  health conditions, 303
  pain/distress, signs, 295
  research origin/uses, 302
  sampling, 303
Chinese letters look, 108
Chlamydiosis, 317
Chlaymydia psittaci. See Enzootic abortion in ewes
Chlorhexidine diacetate solution, usage, 442
Chlorine, usage, 168
Chocolate toxicosis, 518t
Choke, 283
  definition, 285
Choker collars, usage, 146
Cholangiohepatitis, definition, 71
Cholecystokinin, impact, 16
Cholinergics
  parasympathetic effects, 377
  side effects, 377
Chondrosarcoma, definition, 71
Chorioallantoic membrane, definition, 227
Choroid, 21
Chromatin pattern, coarseness, 62
Chromodacyorrhea, definition, 309
Chromosomal abnormalities, 211
Chromosomes
  definition, 227
  deletion, 211
  duplication, 211
  translocation, 211
Chronic egg-laying, 316
Chronic end-stage renal failure, emergency, 515t
Chronic founder, 284
Chronic renal disease (CRD), 259
Chylous effusion, definition, 71
Chyme, pancreatic enzymes (action), 16
Ciconiiformes, carnivores, 316
-cide (-cida), definition, 171
Cidex. See Glutaraldehyde

Circle system, 350, 352. *See also* Anesthetic machine
  components, 352
Circular folds, 15
Circulating metabolites, filtration, 370
Circulation, emergency medicine, 490
Circulatory flight endurance, avian/mammal comparison, 313
Circulatory system, reptilian/mammalian system, 319
Citrate phosphate dextrose (CPD), addition. *See* Blood
Clasmatocyte, definition, 71
Claws, 21
Cleaning, definition, 171
Client-collected samples, 25
Clients
  communication, 543, 544
  education, 543
  reminders, 554
  telephone conversations, 544
Clinical chemistry
  glossary, 124
  information, 112-113
  learning outcomes, 112
  review questions, 124-125
  sample handling, 113
Clinitest tablets (Ames), usage, 114
Closed gloving, 410
Closed wounds, 468
Clostridial diseases, biologicals (usage), 485-486t
*Clostridium piliforme. See* Syrian hamster
Clove hitch, 162f
CMI. *See* Cell-mediated immunity
CMOS. *See* Complementary metal-oxide semiconductor
CMT. *See* California Mastitis Test
CNS. *See* Central nervous system
Coagulase test, 104
Coagulum, definition, 171
Coat, physical examination, 416
Coccidiosis. *See* Rabbit
  impact, 318
Coccobacillus, definition, 110
Cochlear structures, sound waves (effect), 431f
Codocyte, definition, 51
Co-dominance, 207
  definition, 227
Coggins test, usage, 464
Cognitive dysfunction, 261
Colibacillosis, definition, 227
Colic, 283
  management, 459
  rule out, 459
Colitis. *See* Diarrhea
  management, 459
  monitoring, 459
  rule out, 459-460
Collapsing trachea, emergency, 512t
Colloids, 420
Colon, anatomy/physiology, 277
Colorimetric methods, 120
Colostrum, definition, 141, 227, 285

Columbia colistin-nalidixic agar (CNA), 100
Columnar epithelium, 5
Comet tail artifacts, 198
Commensual, definition, 141
Commercial handouts, 554
Common lesions, collection/evaluation, 64-70
Communication. *See* Practice management communication; Verbal communication
  effectiveness, 543
  flow, 542
  process, 542
  special situations, 543
Compact bone (dense bone), 7
Companion animal behavior
  glossary, 240-241
  learning outcomes, 231
  review questions, 241-242
Complementary metal-oxide semiconductor (CMOS), definition, 191
Complete blood count (CBC), 36
Compounded drugs, 368
Comprehensive test, answer key (inclusion), 576-593
Compression prep method. *See* Slide preparation
Computed radiography (CR), definition, 191
Computed tomography (CT), 189
  definition, 202
  F-FDG/X-ray, 202
  usage, 201
Concentrates
  definition, 285
  usage, 268
Concentrations, expression, 395
Concentration techniques. *See* Cytology
Conflict resolution
  negotiation, 552
  techniques, usage, 544
Congenic, definition, 309
Congenital, definition, 141
Congestive heart failure, emergency, 514t
Conjunctiva, 21
  samples, evaluation, 65
Conjunctivitis, 433
Connective tissue, 5
  categories, 6t
  cell types, 5
  fiber types, 5
Consciousness, level, 509, 511
Conspecifics, definition, 240, 309
Contagious ecthyma, 480
Contagious foot rot, 480
Continence, 27
  definition, 51
Continuous-wave transducers, 195
Contrast radiography, 189
  concepts, 189
  media, 189
  patient preparation, 189
  positioning, 189
Contusions, emergency, 513t
Coprophagia, definition, 309
Cornea, 21

Corneal foreign bodies/lacerations, 519t
Corneal lesions, samples (evaluation), 65
Corneal reflex, monitoring, 355
Corneal staining, 436-437
Corneal ulcers, emergency, 520t
Cornell block. *See* Paralumbar block
Cornual nerve block, 482
Coronary circulation, 13-14
Coronaviruses. *See* Rat
Corpus luteum, definition, 227
Corticosteroids, list, 374t
*Corynebacterium* spp., 108
Coryza, 317
Cotton-tipped applicators, usage, 100
Cotyledonary placentation, definition, 227
Coulometric methods, 120
Counterconditioning, 238
  definition, 240
Covault spay hook, 404
Cover letter, usage, 553
Co-worker communication, 545
  types, 545
*Coxiella burnetii. See* Sheep
CPCR. *See* Cardiopulmonary cerebral resuscitation
CR. *See* Computed radiography
Cradle
  definition, 162
  usage. *See* Horses
Cranial direction, 7
CRD. *See* Chronic renal disease
Creatinine, production, 113
Credit/collection policies, 550
Crenated RBC (CR), 34f
Crenation, definition, 51
Crepuscular, definition, 309
Crile forceps, 402
Critical care nutrition, 257
Cross tying, definition, 162
CRT. *See* Capillary refill time
Cryosurgery, 447
*Cryptococcus neoformans*, 109
Cryptorchid, definition, 227
Cryptosporidiosis
  definition, 227
  parasitic zoonosis, 534t
*Cryptosporidium* oocysts, OVC puddle technique, 75
Crystalloid fluids, 420
Crystalloid volume, 363
Crystals, 35-36
CSF. *See* Cerebrospinal fluid
Cuboidal epithelium, 5
Culture, definition, 110
Curettes, usage, 493
Cushing's syndrome, definition, 124
Cutaneous membranes (integument/skin), 7
Cutaneous tissues, lesions (collection/evaluation), 64
Cyclohexamines
  classification, 342-343
  usage, 342
Cyclosporine, usage, 387
Cylinduria. *See* Casts
Cystic lesions, 200
  definition, 202

Cystine, 36
Cystocentesis, 25, 70, 430-431
  definition, 71
  equipment, 430
  indications, 430
  precautions, 431
  procedure, 430
Cytologic preparations, evaluation algorithm, 382t
Cytology. *See* Inflammation
  cells, examination. *See* Exfoliative cytology
  concentration techniques, 56
  evaluation/interpretation, 60
  fixation/staining techniques, 58
  glossary, 70-71
  indications, 54
  learning outcomes, 54
  review questions, 71-72
  slides, 58
    fixation, 58
    preparation, 57
  specimen collection, 54
  stains, usage, 59
  usage, 446-447
Cytoplasm, 3
  abundance, 64, 69
Cytoplasmic changes, 62
Cytosis, definition, 51
Cytoskeleton, 191

**D**

DA. *See* Displaced abomasum
Dairy cattle
  calcium, 268
  calves, feeding process, 270
  cobalt, 268
  copper, 269
  feeding, 267
  feed sources, 267
  iodine, 268
  iron, 269
  life stages, 269
  minerals, 268
  nutrition, disease (relationship), 271
  nutritional requirements, 268
  phosphorus, 268
  protein, 268
  replacement/breeding animals, feeding, 270
  selenium, 269
  sodium/chloride, 268
  vitamins, 269
  water, 268
  zinc, 269
Darkroom
  considerations, 179-180
  processing techniques, 179
  safelight, usage, 180
DDR. *See* Direct digital radiography
DE. *See* Digestible energy
Dead space, 17
Deafness, 22
Decision making, 551
Decongestants, list, 381t
Defensive aggression, 233

Deficiency, effects, 248-250t
Degenerated WBC, 34f
Degloving, definition, 309
Deglutition, definition, 285
Degu
  anesthesia/analgesia, 326
  behavioral/physiological characteristics, 325
  breeding considerations, 326
  health conditions, 326
  housing/nutrition, 325
  medicine, 325
  nursing care, 326
  origin, 325
  pain/distress, signs, 326
  restraint/handling, 326
Dehydration
  degree, estimation, 418
  signs, 418
  treatment, 362
Demodectic mange, 440
Denial, grief stage, 448
Dense bone. *See* Compact bone
Dental elevators, 147
Dental instruments, 493-495
  hand instruments, sharpening, 495
  sharpening stones, usage, 495
  unit maintenance, 495
Dental problems, 501-502
Dental procedures, horse restraint, 151
Dental radiography, 497-499
  bisecting angle, 498
    technique. *See* Carnassial tooth; Lower canine tooth
  equipment, 498
  parallel position technique. *See* Mandibular premolar teeth
  parallel technique, 498
  positioning, 498
  recommendations, 378
Dentin, 472
Dentition, 492
Denuding, definition, 309
Deoxyribonucleic acid (DNA)
  definition, 131
  mutation, 211
  transcription. *See* Double-stranded DNA
  usage, 3
Depression, grief stage, 449, 544
Dermatitis. *See* Hedgehogs; Rabbit
Dermatological conditions, 437-441
Dermatology, 437-441
  examination, 437
  primary lesions, 437
  secondary lesions, 437
  terminology, 437
    list, 439t
Dermatophytes, identification, 109
Dermatophyte test medium (DTM), 100
  color change, 103
Dermatophytosis, mycotic zoonosis, 536t
Dermis, 21
Descemetocele, emergency, 520t

Desflurane
  pharmacological effects, 346
  physical/chemical properties, 346
  usage, 346
Detail, definition, 191
Detergents, usage, 165
Detomidine, usage, 129
Dexamethasone, corticosteroids, 375
Diabetes mellitus, diagnosis, 114
Diabetic ketoacidosis, emergency, 516t
Diagnostic microbiology/mycology
  equipment, 99
  glossary, 110
  learning outcomes, 98
  purpose, 98
  review questions, 110-111
Diagnostic radiographic examinations, positioning techniques, 187
Diagnostic tests, 335
Diaphragmatic rupture, emergency, 513t
Diaphysis, 8
Diarrhea (colitis), 283
Diastema, definition, 162
Diencephalon, 11
Diestrus, 19
Diets, types, 14-16
Differential medium, definition, 110
Diffuse, definition, 203
Diffuse placenta, definition, 227
Diffusion, 4
Digestible energy (DE), definition, 285
Digestion, definition, 285
Digestive system, 14-16
  avian/mammal comparison, 312
  function, 14
  histological layers, 14
  organs, involvement, 15-16
  process, 14-16
  reptilian/mammalian system, 319
  structures, 15-16
Digestive tract tests, 121b
Digital, definition, 191
Digital radiography (DR), 189-190
  definition, 191
  overview, 189
  types, 189
Dihybrid cross, 197, 208f
  definition, 227
  offspring prediction, 208
Diluted solutions, strength (calculation), 395
Dilutions, 395
  definition, 395
Dimorphic fungi, 110
  definition, 110
Diploid, definition, 227
*Dipylidum caninum*, 96f
Direct digital radiography (DDR), 189
  definition, 191
Directional terminology, 7
Direct smear. *See* Feces
*Dirofilaria immitis*, examination, 75
Disbudding, definition, 162
Diseases, vaccine (availability), 130-131t
Disinfectant, definition, 171

Disinfection. *See* Sanitation/sterilization/dis-
    infection
    levels, 167t
Displaced abomasum (DA), 271, 476
Display. *See* Ultrasound
    format
    monitor controls, brightness/contrast, 196
Disposable paper wraps, 408
Distal, definition, 191
Distal direction, 7
Diuretics
    list, 380t
    usage, 378
Diurnal, definition, 309
DMI. *See* Dry matter intake
Doe, 220
    examination, 220
Dog restraint, 145-147
    behavioral characteristics, 145
    considerations, 145-146
    danger potential, 145
    equipment, 146-147
Dogs
    aggression/hostility, 145
    head/body, restraint, 145f
    life stage nutritional requirements, 253t
    lower urinary tract disease, risk factors,
        255b
    nervousness/fear, 145, 146
    nutritional requirements, 250-255 251-
        252. *See also* Adult dogs; Geriatric
        dogs; Young dogs
    old/young, 146
    viciousness/aggressiveness, 145
    weaning, 251
Domestic animals
    blood parasites, diagnostic characteristics,
        89t
    internal parasites, diagnostic characteris-
        tics, 78-89t
Dominance signaling, 232
Dominant gene, 227
Doppler imaging, 198
Doppler monitor, usage, 356
Doppler shift, definition, 203
Dorsal direction, 7
Dorsopalmar (DPa), definition, 191
Dorsoplantar (DPl), definition, 191
Dorsoventral (DV), definition, 191
Dosage calculations, 394-395
Dosimeter, definition, 191
Double-stranded DNA, transcription, 127
Doyen intestinal forceps, 401
DR. *See* Digital radiography
Draping, 409-410
    initiation, 409-410
Drench, usage, 472
Dressing forceps, 401
Drip rates, 396
    calculation, 396
    formula, variations, 396
Droperidol, usage, 337
Drug
    abuse, potential, 368
    approval, 368
    classes, 370

Drug *(Continued)*
    compounding, concerns, 369
    concentrations, observation, 369
    definition, 367-369
    elimination process, 369
    emergency medicine, 492
    generic name, 367
    manufacture, 368
    milligram dose, recordation, 454
    package insert, information, 368-369
    postadministration path, 369
    storage, 368
    target tissue time, 369
    withdrawal times, 368
Drug administration, 417-418
    exclusivity, 369
    five rights, 369
    introduction, 417
    oral route, 416
    parenteral route, 417
    topical route, 418
Dry, definition, 162
Dry chemistry, definition, 124
Dry heat, physical method, 169-171
Drying, efficacy, 165
Dry matter basis, definition, 261
Dry matter intake (DMI), definition,
        285
Dry sterile gauze, usage, 443
Dry-to-dry dressings, 443
Dry weight analysis, calculation, 260b
DTM. *See* Dermatophyte test medium
Ductus deferens. *See* Vas deferens
Dumb cane, toxic substances (impact),
        519t
DV. *See* Dorsoventral
Dyspnea
    definition, 17
    postural adaptations, 507, 510
Dystocia, 20
    emergencies, 518t
Dysuria, 27
    definition, 51

E
EAE. *See* Enzootic abortion in ewes
Ears
    anatomy, 21
    canals, secretions (collection), 65
    manipulation, 416
    mites, 440
    physical examination, 416
    swabs, usage, 55
Easter/tiger lilies, toxic substances (impact),
        519t
ECG. *See* Electrocardiography
Echogenic (echoic) image, 197
Echoic, definition, 203
Eclampsia, emergencies, 518t
Ectoparasites, 93-94t
EDIM. *See* Epizootic diarrhea of infant
        mice
EDTA. *See* Ethylenediaminetetraacetic
        acid
EFAs. *See* Essential fatty acids
Effective focal spot, definition, 191

Efferent nerve processes (motor nerve
        processes), 11-12
Efficacy, definition, 95
Effusions
    classification algorithm, 34f
    definition, 71
Egg-binding, 316
Ehmer sling, 445
Ehrlichiosis, bacterial zoonosis,
        529t
EHV-1. *See* Equine herpesvirus (EHV-1)
EHV-4. *See* Equine herpesvirus (EHV-4)
EIA. *See* Equine infectious anemia
Eicosapentaenoic acid (EPA), usage, 254
Electrical impulses, conduction, 6
Electric heating element, usage, 99
Electrocardiography (ECG/EKG), 14
    components, 424
    definition, 424
    interpretation, 426
    machine calibration/recordation, 425
    monitor, usage, 454
    procedure, 425
    rhythms, abnormality, 426-427
    time intervals, 425f
Electroejaculation, 211, 214
Electrolytes
    clinical chemistry, 119-120
    definition, 124
    function test, 121b
    measurement, 120
Electromagnetic radiation, 174
    definition, 191
Electron, definition, 191
Electron beam, definition, 191
Electronic communication, 444
Electrophoresis, 117
    definition, 124
ELISA. *See* Enzyme linked immunosorbent
        assay
Emergency, toxic substances (impact),
        518-519t
Emergency blood screen, 511
Emergency fluid therapy, 419
Emergency medicine
    glossary, 520-521
    learning outcomes, 507
    review questions, 521-522
Emergency patients, status (monitoring),
        510-511
Emergency situations, assessment/response
        (requirement), 544
Emetics
    impact. *See* Vomiting
    list, 383t
Enamel, 471
Enamel hypoplasia, 501
Encephalomalacia, definition, 261
End, definition, 162
Endochrondral bones, 8
Endocrine drugs
    examples, 383
    list, 386-387t
    usage, 383-385
Endocrine emergencies, 512
    list, 516t

Endocrine function tests, 121b
Endocrine glands, 20, 20t
Endocrine system, 20
   characteristics, 20
   control, 20
Endocytosis, 4
Endogenous, definition, 124
Endometrium, 19
Endoplasmic reticulum (ER), 3
Endosteum, 8
Enemas
   definition, 432
   indications, 433
   precautions, 433
   procedure, 433
Energy-producing nutrients, 244-245
Energy requirements, 245-250
   maintenance, calculations, 250t
Ensiling, definition, 285
Enteral, definition, 261
Enteral bacteria, definition 110
Enteral nutrition, 257
Enterobacteriaceae (enteric bacteria/gut
   bacteria), 107-108
Enterocolitis, definition, 227
Enterotexmia, 271, 274
Entropion, definition, 227
Entry portal. *See* Portal of entry
Enzootic abortion in ewes (EAE) (*Chlamy-
   dia psittaci*), 478
Enzyme linked immunosorbent assay
   (ELISA)
   definition, 95
   tests, 30
   usage, 76, 129
Enzymes, 117
   classification. *See* Biological enzymes
EO. *See* Ethylene oxide
Eosinopenia, definition, 51
Eosinophilia, definition, 51
Eosinophilic inflammation, 60
Eosinophils, examination, 60
Eosin stain, usage, 59
EPA. *See* Eicosapentaenoic acid
Epidermis, 21
Epididymitis, definition, 227
Epidural block, 481-482
Epilepsy, emergency, 514t
Epiphora, 433
Epiphyseal cartilage, 8
Epiphysis, 8
Epistasis, definition, 227
Epithelial cells, sediment (component),
   33
Epithelial tissue, 5
   subtypes, 5
Epitope, definition, 141
Epizootic diarrhea of infant mice (EDIM),
   290
EPM. *See* Equine protozoal myeloencepha-
   litis
Epulis, 501
   definition, 71
Equine, 215-217
   administration routes, 455-456
   bandaging, 468-469

Equine *(Continued)*
   blood disorder, 445
   breeding soundness examination,
      215-216
   cardiac rhythm, 453
   care, 454-455
   cast, 469
   dental formula, 454-455
   dystocia
      causes, 217
      signs, 217
   encephalomyelitis, vaccination,
      457t
   estrous cycle, 216
   estrus, signs, 216
   fecal output, 454
   foot ailments, 464-465
   foot bandage, 469
   gastrointestinal (GI) ailments, 456-461
      clinical signs, 456-459
      rule outs, 459-461
   gastrointestinal (GI) motility, 454
   gestation, 216-217
   inhalation route, 456
   intramuscular (IM) administration,
      455
   intranasal route, 456
   lameness, 465
   mucous membrane, 454
   neonatal care, 560
   neuromuscular disorders, 461-463
      clinical signs, 461
      rule outs, 461-463
   normal values, 453-454
   parturition, stages, 216-217
   physical examination, 453-454
   postoperative bandages, 469
   postoperative care, 468
   pregnancy diagnosis, 216
   presurgical preparations, 466-467
   puberty, 215
   pulse, 453
   respiration, 454
   respiratory diseases, 463-464
      clinical signs, 463
      rule outs, 463-464
   semen characteristics, 216
   semen collection techniques, 216
   subcutaneous (SC) administration, 456
   surgery, 466-468
      process, 467-468
      recovery, 468
   surgical site, preparation, 467
   urine, 454
   vaccinations, 456
      list, 457-458t
Equine encephalomyelitides (sleeping sickness)
   management, 463
   rule out, 463
Equine herpesvirus (EHV-1), rule out,
   462
Equine herpesvirus (EHV-4) (viral rhinopneumonitis)
   management, 464
   rule out, 464

Equine infectious anemia (EIA), 138, 464
   diagnosis, 464
Equine influenza (flu), rule out, 464
Equine nursing/surgery
   glossary, 469
   learning outcomes, 453
   review questions, 469-470
Equine protozoal myeloencephalitis
   (EPM)
   management, 462
   rule out, 462
Equine recurrent uveitis, 284
ER. *See* Endoplasmic reticulum
Eructation, definition, 285
Erysipelas (*Erysipelothrix rhusiopathiae*),
   480-481
Erysipelothrix infection, 526t
*Erysipelothrix rhusiopathiae*, 108-109
Erythema, definition, 95
Erythrocytes. *See* Red blood cells
Erythrocytophagia, definition, 71
Erythroid cells, characteristics, 66
Erythrophagocytosis, definition, 51
Erythropoiesis, definition, 51
Erythropoietin, growth hormone, 390
Esophagus, 15
   anatomy/physiology, 277
Essential fatty acids (EFAs), 244
   definition, 261
   requirement, 254
Estrogens
   list, 386t
   usage, 383
Estrous cycles, 19-20
   types, 19
Estrus (standing heat), 19
   cell population identification, 69
ESWT. *See* Extracorporeal shock wave
   therapy
Ethics, 555
   glossary, 560
   history, 555
   learning outcomes, 541
   review questions, 560
   veterinary technician code, 557
Ethylenediaminetetraacetic acid (EDTA),
   104
   anticoagulant, 37
Ethylene glycol toxicity, emergency,
   518t
Ethylene oxide (EO/EtO)
   definition, 171
   usage, 168-169
Etiological agent, definition, 141
Etodolac, NSAID example, 375
Etomidate (Amidate), usage, 343
Eukaryote (true nucleus), 3
Eukaryotic cells, composition 3
Eupnea, definition, 17
Euthanasia, 448
   discussion, 448
   grief process, 448, 449
   intracardiac injection, 448
   intraperitoneal injection, 448
   intravenous injection, 448
   methods, 448

Ewes, 222
  enzootic abortion. *See* Enzootic abortion
    in ewes
  examination, 222
  pregnancy toxemia, 475
Excess, effects, 248-250t
Excisional biopsy, 447
Excretory system, 17-18
  anatomy, 17
  filtration, 18
  hormonal influence, 18
  physiology, 18
  reabsorption, 18
  secretion, 18
Exfoliative cytology
  cells, examination, 60
  definition, 5171
Exocytosis, 4
Exotic animal medicine
  glossary, 330
  learning outcomes, 311
  review questions, 331
Expectorants, usage, 378
Expiration (exhalation), 17
Expiratory reserve volume, 17
External marketing, 555
External parasite identification, 76
  Baermann technique, 77
  cellophane tape method, 76
External respiration, 17
Extinction, 238
  definition, 240
Extracellular, definition, 4
Extracorporeal shock wave therapy (ESWT),
    usage, 466
Extreme (marked), definition, 51
Exudates
  classification, 57f
  definition, 51, 71
Eyelid press, usage. *See* Horses
Eyes
  anatomy, 21
  conditions, 434-435t
  cross-section, 436f
  immobilization, 360
  movement/position, 498
  physical examination, 416
  position, monitoring, 355

**F**

F₁F₂, definition, 227
Face-to-face conversation, 545
Facilitated diffusion, 4
Failure of passive transfer (FPT), 271, 274,
    276, 280, 283
  definition, 285
Failure to thrive (FTT), 276
False-positive test outcomes. *See* Urine
Farrowing, definition, 162
Farrowing crates, usage. *See* Pigs
Far side, definition, 162
*Fasciola hepatica*, 96f
FA test. *See* Fluorescent antibody test
Fats, nutrients, 244
Fatty casts (lipid casts), 35
Fatty liver disease, 271

FDG. *See* Fluorodeoxyglucose
Fearful signaling, 232
Feather abnormalities, 316
Fecal cultures, 103
Fecalyzer, usage, 74
Feces
  centrifugal flotation technique, 74-75
  direct smear, 74
  examination, 73-75
  flotation kits, 74
  gross examination, 73
  quantitative fecal examination, 74
  vial gravitation flotation technique, 73-74
Fecundity, definition, 309
Feeding
  costs, calculation, 259t
Feeding methods. *See* Small animal nutrition
Feedlot, definition, 285
Feedstuff, definition, 285
Feet, picking up. *See* Horses
Feline, 211-213
  auditory sense, 128
  behavior, 233
  behavioral development, 233
  behavioral problems, 239
  blood collection, 422-423
    procedure, 422-423
    supplies, 422
  body postures, 234f
  breeding soundness examination, 211
  communication, 235f
  developmental stages, 233t
  donor requirements, 422
  dystocia
    causes, 212
    signs, 212
  ears/neck/head positions, 235f
  elimination, problem, 240
  estrous cycle, 212
  estrus, signs, 212
  eyes, 278
  gestation, 212
  male, examination, 211
  natural breeding, 212
  neonatal care, 212-213
  olfaction, 234
  parturition, stages, 212
  postural signaling, 233
  pregnancy diagnosis, 212
  puberty, 211
  scratching, 240
  semen characteristics, 211-212
  semen collection techniques, 211-212
  social development, 233-236
  spraying, 239
  uroliths, mineral composition, 256t
  vision, 233
Feline immunodeficiency virus (FIV), 128
Feline leukemia virus (FeLV), 129
Feline lower urinary tract disease (FLUTD),
    211
  definition, 261
  prevention, 255
Feline restraint bag (cat bag), 149
Female anatomy, 18
Female physiology, 19

Female reproductive system, 18-20
  histological layers, 19
Femoral vein, venipuncture, 420
Fentanyl, usage, 343
Ferguson angiotribe forceps, 401
Ferrets
  Aleutian disease (AD), 329
  analgesia, 328-329
  anesthesia, 328-329
  aplastic anemia, 329-330
  behavioral/physiological characteristics,
    327
  blood collection, 328
  breeding considerations, 327-328
  fluid therapy, 328
  health conditions, 329-330
  housing/nutrition, 327
  human influenza, impact, 329
  hyperadrenocorticism (adrenal disease),
    329
  insulinoma (pancreatic beta cell
    tumors), 329
  intramuscular injections, 328
  intraosseous catheters, 328
  intravenous catheters, placement, 328
  isoflurane, usage, 328
  lymphoma, 329
  medicine, 326
  nomenclature, 326
  nursing care, 328
  origin, 326
  proliferative bowel disease, 329
  restraint/handling, 327
  viral enteritis, 329-330
Fertilization/pregnancy, 19
Fetal circulation, 14
Fetal dystocia, 212
Fetal monster, definition, 228
Fiberglass cast, 445
Fibrinogen, coagulation factors, 117
Fibroma, definition, 71
Fibrosarcoma, 446t, 501
  definition, 71, 141
Fibrous structure, 8-9
Filament, definition, 191
Filial, definition, 228
Filiform, 22
Film. *See* X-ray film
  contrast, definition, 191
  graininess, definition, 191
  latitude, definition, 191
Filter paper, usage, 100
Filtration, 4
Final host, definition, 95
Final image, 197-198
  characteristics, 197-198
Financial management, 548
Fine needle aspiration, usage, 65
Fine needle biopsy, 54
Finochetto retractors, 403-404
First degree AV block, 427
First-intention healing, 442
Fish, research usage, 305
Fish blood specimen, 103
Fistula, definition, 71
FIV. *See* Feline immunodeficiency virus

Fixation techniques. *See* Cytology
Flagellum, definition, 95
Flame photometry, 120
Flanking, definition, 162
Flank restraint. *See* Cattle
Flat bones, 8
Fleas, impact, 440
Flies, impact, 318
Flow cytometry, 50
Fluids
   abnormal losses, 418
   administration, routes, 419-420
   anesthesia monitoring, 357
   aspirates, fluid accumulation (removal/
     evaluation), 67
   calculations, 362
   characteristics, 362
   filtration, 166
   normal balance, 418
   replacement volume, calculation, 419
   samples
     characteristics, 56
     color/turbidity, 56
   therapy, 362-365, 418-420
     contraindications, 419
     monitoring, 362
   types, 420
Fluorescent antibody (FA) test, 129
Fluorodeoxyglucose (FDG), usage, 201
Flushing, definition, 228
FLUTD. *See* Feline lower urinary tract
   disease
Foals, capture/restraint, 153
Focal changes, definition, 203
Focal point, focusing, 196-197
Focal range, definition, 191
Fogging, detail, 191
Foliate papillae, 22
Follicular phase, definition, 228
Food allergies/intolerance, 257-258
Food-restricted meal feeding, 247-250
Foot rot. *See* Contagious foot rot
Foot rot, definition, 228
Forages
   classification, 267
   definition, 285
Forbs, definition, 285
Forceps, 401-402
Formaldehyde, usage, 168
Founder. *See* Laminitis
Founder, definition, 285
Four-chambered heart, avian/mammalian
   comparison, 313
FPT. *See* Failure of passive transfer
Frazier-Ferguson tips, 405
Free radicals, definition, 261
Free thyroid hormone (FT$_4$), 120
Frenulum, definition, 228
Frequency
   bandwidth, 196
   definition, 203
   wavelength, inverse proportion, 195f
Freshen, definition, 228
Fresh whole blood, transfusion, 423
Frick speculum, usage, 472
Full jaw, formulae, 492t

Functional ruminants, 267
Fungal cultures, 103
Fungal dermatological condition, 438
Fungal identification, 109-110
Fungal media, 100-101
Fungi
   identification, 109
   visibility, 64
Fungicide, definition, 171
Fungiform papillae, 22
Furcation index, 502

**G**
GA. *See* Guaranteed analysis
Gallbladder, 16
   sonographic appearance, 199
Gamma-glutamyltransferase (GGT), 118
Gamma-hemolysis, 105
Gamma ray
   definition, 203
   radiation, 200
Gantry, definition, 203
Gastric dilatation-volvulus (GDV), 363
   emergency, 517t
Gastrointestinal (GI) drugs, 378-380
   list, 382-383t
Gastrointestinal (GI) emergencies, 512
   list, 517t
Gastrointestinal (GI) obstruction, emer-
   gency, 517t
Gastrointestinal (GI) system, physical
   examination, 416
Gastrointestinal (GI) tract, walls (division),
   14
Gauze muzzle, 147
   fit, 147f
Gavage, definition, 309
GDV. *See* Gastric dilatation-volvulus
GE. *See* Gross energy
Gelding, definition, 228
Gene, definition, 228
Gene-deleted, definition, 141
General examination, horse restraint, 151
Genes, inheritance, 208
Genetics, 207
   concepts, 207
   definition, 228
   glossary, 227-229
   learning outcomes, 207
   review questions, 229-230
Genomes, 127
   definition, 131, 141, 228
Genotype, definition, 228
Gentle leaders, 146
Geometric unsharpness, definition, 191
Geriatric cats, nutritional requirements, 255
Geriatric dogs, nutritional requirements, 252
Gestation
   definition, 228
   nutritional requirements, 250-251
Gestation period, 20
GGT. *See* Gamma-glutamyltransferase
Gilt, definition, 228
Gingiva, 472
Gingival disease, classification, 503
Gingival hyperplasia, 501

Gingivitis, 502
   index, 503
Glandular epithelium, 5
Glandular tissues, lesions (collection/evalu-
   ation), 65
Glass microscope slides/coverslips,
   usage, 100
Glaucoma, emergency, 519t
Glial. *See* Neuroglial cells
Globulin
   fractions, 117
   levels, changes, 117
Glossal edema, definition, 228
Gloves, usage. *See* Cats
Gloving. *See* Closed gloving; Open gloving
   completion, 410
Glucose, chemical component, 30-31
Glucosuria, definition, 51
Glutaraldehyde (Cidex), usage, 167
Glycerol guaiacolate. *See* Guaifenesin
Glycoprotein
   definition, 261
   impact, 257-258
Glycopyrrolate, usage, 336
Glycosuria (glucosuria), 114
GN broth. *See* Gram-negative broth
Gnotobiotic, definition, 309
GnRH. *See* Gonadotropin-releasing hormone
Goat restraint, 157-158
   danger potential, 157-158
   usage, 158
Goats
   anatomy, 158
   behavioral characteristics, 158
   castration, 158
   dehorning, 158, 487
   energy, requirements, 272
   feeding, 272
   feed sources, 272
   head, usage, 157-158
   hooves, front foot (picking up), 159f
   intradermal injections, 474
   intramuscular (IM) injections, 473
   life stages, 274
   minerals, ingestion, 273
   nutrition, disease (relationship), 274
   nutritional requirements, 272
   protein, 272
   regional anesthesia, 482
   rotavirus, 477
   teat laceration repair, 484
   venipuncture, 473
   vitamins, necessity, 273
   water, usage, 272
Goiter, definition, 261
Goldberg refractometer, usage, 116
Goldi complex (Golgi apparatus), 3-4
Gonadotropin-releasing hormone (GnRH),
   definition, 228
Gonioscopy, usage, 437
Gowning, completion, 410
Grain overload. *See* Rumen acidosis
Gram-negative (GN) bacilli, visibility, 64
Gram-negative (GN) broth, 100
Gram-negative (GN) cocci, 106-107

Gram-negative (GN) coccobacilli, 108
Gram-negative (GN) identification, miniature biochemical test kits (usage), 105
Gram-negative (GN) rods, 107-108
    flowchart, 107f
Gram-negative (GN) spirochetes, 108
Gram-positive cocci, 106f
    visibility, 64
Gram-positive rods, 108-109
Gram staining, usage, 59
Gram stain test, 104
Granular casts, 35
Granulocyte, definition, 51
Granuloma, definition, 141
Granulomatous, definition, 51, 71
Granulomatous inflammation, 60
Grass tetany (hypomagnesemic tetany), 271, 274
Gravity displacement autoclave, 169
Grid. See X-ray machine
    cutoff, definition, 191
    ratio, definition, 191
Grief counseling, 543
Grief process. See Euthanasia
Groove directors, 405
Gross calculus, removal, 496
Gross energy (GE), definition, 285
Growing/finishing market hogs, management, 279
Guaifenesin (glycerol guaiacolate), usage, 343
Guaranteed analysis (GA), 260
    definition, 261
Guilt, grief stage, 544
Guinea pig (Cavia porcellus), 300-302
    anesthetic complications/considerations, 302
    antibiotic-associated enterotoxemia, 301
    bacterial pneumonia, 301
    behavioral/physiological characteristics, 300
    breeding considerations, 300
    cervical lymphadenitis, 301
    handling/restraint, 300
    health conditions, 301
    malocclusion, 301
    pain/distress, signs, 301
    research origin/uses, 300
    Salmonella, 301-302
    sampling, 300-301
    scurvy (hypovitaminosis C), 301
Gums, physical examination, 416

H

Habituation, 238
    technique, definition, 240
Hair, 21
    components, 21
    types, 21
Half hitch/loop, definition, 162
Half-life, definition, 203
Half-life decay, 200
Halogens, usage, 168
Halophilic, definition, 110

Halothane, 345
    pharmacologic effects, 345
    physical/chemical properties, 345
    usage, 483
Halsted mosquito forceps, 402
    illustration, 403f
Halter tie, 161f
    usage, 162
Halti collars, 146
Haploid, definition, 228
Harderian gland, definition, 309
Hard rope leashes, 146
Harem mating, 210
    definition, 228, 309
Harness, process, 147
Haylage, definition, 285
Hays, division, 267
H-blockers, impact, 381
hCG. See Human chorionic gonadotropin
Head
    bandaging, 443
    trauma, emergency, 514t
Headgate, definition, 162
Hearing, 21-22
    physiology, 22
Heart
    anatomy, 13f
    electricity, continuous wave, 424
    murmurs, 454
    sonographic appearance, 199
Heart rate (HR), 14
    monitoring, 355-356
Heartworm, 129
Heat labile, definition, 172
Heaves, 284
Hedgehogs
    alopecia, 324
    anesthesia/analgesia, 324
    behavioral/physiological characteristics, 323
    breeding considerations, 324
    cardiac disease, 325
    dermatitis, 324
    health conditions, 324-325
    housing/nutrition, 323
    medicine, 323
    nursing care, 324
    obesity, 325
    origin, 323
    pain/distress, signs, 324
    respiratory disease, 324
    restraint/handling, 323-324
Heel effect, definition, 191
Heifer, 217
Heinz body, 38f
Hemangiosarcoma, 446t
    definition, 71
Hematinics, usage, 389-390
Hematocrit (HCT), 37
    centrifuges, 45
Hematology, 36-51
    bibliography, 53
    glossary, 51-52
    learning outcomes, 24
    review questions, 52-53
Hematoxylin stain, usage, 59

Hematuria, 31-32
    definition, 51
Hemoglobin
    formation, support, 390
    impact, 45
Hemoglobinuria, definition, 51
Hemolysis, definition, 51, 124
Hemorrhagic gastroenteritis, emergency, 517t
Hemosiderin
    definition, 71
    presence, 67
Hemosporidia, 318
Hemostatic forceps, 402
HEPA. See High efficiency particle absorption
Heparin, usage, 68
Hepatic lipidosis, definition, 261
Hepatobiliary tissues, samples, 67
Hepatocytes, definition, 71
Hepatotoxicity. See Anesthesia
Herbivore, 14
    definition, 285
Hermaphrodite, definition, 228
Herpes B viral infection, 532t
Heterophil, definition, 51
Heterosis, definition, 228
Heterosis (hybrid vigor), 210
Heterozygous, definition, 228
Hexacanth, definition, 95
High efficiency particle absorption (HEPA)
    filter, 172
    definition, 309
High-voltage circuit. See X-ray machine
Histiocytoma, 62
    definition, 71
Histological layers. See Digestive system; Female reproductive system
Histology, definition, 405
Histomoniasis, 318
Histopathology
    definition, 71
    usage, 447
Hitches
    definition, 162
    usage, 162
HMP. See Sodium hexametaphosphate
Hobble, definition, 162
Hog snare, definition, 162
Hohmann retractors, 403
Homemade treats, usage, 254b
Homozygous, definition, 228
Hooves, 21
Hormonal influence. See Excretory system
Hormonal skin conditions, 440-441
Hormones
    list, 386-387t
    usage, 383-385
Horns, 21
Horse restraint, 149-153
    behavioral characteristics, 150
    danger potential, 149-150
    distraction techniques, 151-152
    ears, restraint, 150
    tail, restraint, 150
    usage. See Dental procedures; General examination

Horses
  approach, 150
  blindfolds, usage, 151
  capture, 150
  carbohydrates, usage, 280
  casting, 153
  chain shank, usage, 152f
  cradle, usage, 152
  cross tying, 151
  eyelid press, usage, 152
  feeding, 282-283, 280-284. *See also*
    Mature horse
  feed sources, 280
  feet, picking up, 153
  front foot, picking up, 153f
  grains, usage, 280
  leading, 150
  life stages, 281
  microminerals, 281
  minerals/vitamins, 280
  nutrition, disease (relationship),
    283
  nutritional requirements, 280
  protein, ingestion, 281
  shoulder roll, usage, 152
  stocks, usage, 151
  surgical positioning, 467
  tail tie, 153f
    usage, 152
  twitch, application, 152f
  tying, 151
  water, ingestion, 441
Hospitalized horses, feeding,
  283
Hot air oven, usage, 165
House soiling. *See* Canine
Howell-Jolly body, 38f
HR. *See* Heart rate
Human chorionic gonadotropin (hCG),
  definition, 228
Humane twitch, usage, 152
Human-pet bond, 448
Humoral immunodeficiencies, 138
Hyaline casts, 35
Hybrid, definition, 228
Hybrid vigor. *See* Heterosis
Hydrocephalus, definition, 228
Hydrogen peroxide, usage, 442
Hydrolysate, definition, 261
Hydrolysis, definition, 172, 261
Hydrophilic, definition, 172
Hyper-, definition, 51
Hyperadrenocorticism (adrenal disease). *See*
  Ferrets
Hypercalcemia
  definition, 124
  emergency, 516t
Hypercapnia, monitoring, 357
Hypercellularity, definition, 71
Hyperchloremia, definition, 124
Hyperchromasia, 45
Hyperechoic, definition, 203
Hyperglycemia, 31
  definition, 124
  emergency, 516t
  result, 114

Hyperkalemia
  definition, 124
  emergency, 516t
Hyperkalemic periodic paralysis (HYPP)
  management, 461
  rule out, 461
Hyperkeratosis, definition, 261
Hypernatremia
  definition, 124
  emergency, 516t
Hyperparathyroidism, definition, 124
Hyperphosphatemia, 120
  definition, 124
Hyperplasia (benign neoplasia), 65
  definition, 71
Hypersegmentation, definition, 71
Hypersegmented, definition, 51
Hypersensitivity, definition, 141
Hypersensitivity reactions, types, 137
Hyperthermia, 448
  monitoring, 358
Hyperthyroidism, occurrence, 385
Hypertonic, definition, 4, 52
Hypervitaminosis D, 503
Hyphema, emergencies, 519t
Hypo-, definition, 52
Hypocalcemia
  definition, 124
  emergency, 516t
Hypocalcemic parturient paresis (milk
  fever), 475
Hypochloremia, definition, 124
Hypochromasia, 45
Hypochromic, definition, 52
Hypodermis, 21
Hypodont, 504
Hypoechoci, definition, 203
Hypoglycemia
  emergency, 516t
  result, 114
Hypokalemia
  definition, 124
  emergency, 516t
Hypomagnesemic tetany. *See* Grass tetany
Hyponatremia
  definition, 124
  emergency, 516t
Hypoparathyroidism, definition, 124
Hypophosphatemia, 120
  definition, 124
Hypothermia
  impact, 360
  monitoring, 358
Hypothyroidism, occurrence, 385
Hypotonic, definition, 4, 52
Hypovolemic shock, emergency, 514t
Hypoxemia, cause, 357
Hypoxia, risk, 347
HYPP. *See* Hyperkalemic periodic
  paralysis
Hypsodontic, definition, 309

**I**

IBR. *See* Infectious bovine rhinotracheitis
Ibuprofen, NSAID example, 375
Icterus, definition, 124

IM. *See* Intramuscular
Image. *See* Final image
  brightness/contrast
    gain/power, 196
    organ brightness, 197f
    physics, 196
  production, 195
  receptors, 177-181
    screen construction, 178
  resolution, 196
Image reader device (IRD), 190
Imaging
  techniques, 200
    client preparation, 202
  technology. *See* Alternative imaging
    technology
Immune-mediated thrombocytopenia, 138
Immune system, strength, 135
Immunodeficiency, 138
  combination, 138
  definition, 141
Immunoglobulin A (IgA), 135-136
Immunoglobulin D (IgD), 136
Immunoglobulin E (IgE), 136
Immunoglobulin G (IgG), 135
  definition, 228
Immunoglobulin M (IgM), 135
Immunological agents, list, 388-389t
Immunological drugs, 385-387
Immunological transfusion reaction, 423
Immunology
  glossary, 141
  learning outcomes, 134
  review questions, 141
Immunopathological mechanisms,
  137-138
Immunoproliferative disorders, 137
  definition, 141
Immunostimulants, list, 388t
Immunosuppressants, list, 388t
Immunosuppressed, definition, 309
Impedance counter, 50
Inactivated, definition, 131
Inactivated vaccines, usage, 138
Inanition, 277
  definition, 285
Inbred, definition, 309
Inbreeding, 210
  definition, 228
  depression, 210
    definition, 228
Incision, clipping, 408
Incisional biopsy, 447
In-clinic laboratory testing. *See* Virology
Incomplete dominance, 207
  definition, 228
  lethal gene, 211
Incontinence, 27
  definition, 52
Incubator, usage, 99
Indicator tape, usage, 407
Indirect digital conversion systems
  CCD, usage, 190
  computed radiography, usage, 190
  flat panel detectors, usage, 190
Indirect digital radiography, 189

Infectious bovine rhinotracheitis (IBR), 478, 479
Infective, definition, 95
Inflammation, cytology, 60
Influenza. *See* Equine influenza
    vaccination, 457t
Ingredient, definition, 261
Ingredient panel, usage, 260
Inguinal hernia, definition, 228
Inhalant anesthetics, potency, 344
Inhalants
    classification, 344
    list, 376t
Inhalation anesthetic agents, usage, 344
Inhalation anesthetics, physical properties, 344t
Inhaled steroids, list, 381t
Inheritance
    concepts, 207
    patterns, 208
Injectable anesthetia, inhalation anesthetic
    agents (comparison), 344
Injectable anesthetic agents, usage, 340
Innate immunity, 134-135
Inner ear, 21
Innominate artery (brachiocephalic artery), 13
Inotropic drugs, list, 379t
In situ, definition, 71
Inspiration (inhalation), 17
    shortness, 510
Inspiratory reserve volume, 17
Instrument care, 406-408
    glossary, 412
    learning outcomes, 400
    review questions, 412
Instrument cleaning, 406
Instrument packs, preparation, 407-408
Insulin, endocrine drug, 383
Insulinoma (pancreatic beta cell tumors).
    *See* Ferrets
Integument
    avian/mammal comparison, 312
    reptilian/mammalian comparison, 319
Integumentary system, 21
    anatomy, 21
    function, 21
Intensifying screens, care, 178
Intercellular, definition, 4
Intermediate host, definition, 95
Intermediate inheritance, definition, 228
Intermittent positive pressure ventilation
    (IPPV), 361
Internal marketing, 554
Internal parasites. *See* Zoonotic internal
    parasites
    diagnostic characteristics. *See* Domestic
    animals
Internal respiration, 17
International Commission on Radiological
    Protection (ICRP), 186
Internet, impact, 546
Interview
    objective, 553
    process, 553
Intestinal clostridial infections, 460
Intestinal villi, 15

Intracardiac drugs, usage, 508
Intracellular, definition, 4
Intramedullary fluid administration, 419
Intramedullary pins, 405
Intramembranous bones, 8
Intramuscular (IM) administration, 455
Intramuscular (IM) drug route, 417
Intramuscular (IM) injections, 418
Intraoral film, usage, 498
Intraosseous drug route, 418
Intraruminal pH, range, 267
Intratracheal drugs, usage, 508
Intravenous (IV) access, 508
Intravenous (IV) drugs
    route, 417
    usage, 508
Intravenous (IV) fluids
    administration, 419
    usefulness, 362
Intravenous (IV) injections, 418
    usage, 455
Intussusception, definition, 95
Inventory control, 549
    turnover rate, 549
Inventory system, elements, 549
Involuntary muscle. *See* Smooth muscles
Iodine, usage, 168
Ionization, definition, 191
Ionizing radiation, 174
    hazards, 185
Ion-selective electrodes, 120
IPPV. *See* Intermittent positive pressure
    ventilation
IRD. *See* Image reader device
Iris, 21
Iris scissors, 400-401
Irregular bones, 8
Iso-, definition, 52
Isoechoic, definition, 203
Isoflurane
    anesthesia, usage, 316. *See also* Ferrets
    pharmacological effects, 346
    physical/chemical properties, 345-346
    usage, 345, 483
Isolation, streaking, 102f
Isotonic, definition, 4
Isotonic saline, usage, 442

**J**

Jacking, definition, 162
Jacobs chucks, 404-405
Jaw tone (muscle tone), monitoring, 355
Job search, management, 552
Joints. *See* Articulations
Jugular vein, venipuncture, 420

**K**

Karyolysis, definition, 71
Karyorrhexis, 68
    definition, 71
Karyotype, definition, 228
Kelly forceps, 402
Keratoconjunctivitis sicca (KCS), diagnosis, 436
Keratomalacia, definition, 261
Kern and Richards forceps, 404-405

Ketamine, usage, 342
Ketones, chemical component, 31
Ketonuria, definition, 52
Ketosis (acetonemia), 271, 274
    presence, 475
Kidneys, 17
    function
        clinical chemistry, 113-114
        test, 121b
    sonographic appearance, 199
    tissues, samples, 68
Kids, life stage, 274
Killed vaccines, usage, 138
Kilovoltage, film impact, 183
Kilovolt peak (kVp), definition, 191
Kinetoplast, definition, 95
Kirby-Bauer sensitivity, 104-105
Kittens, nutritional requirements, 254
Knots
    definition, 162
    usage, 160-162
Kübler-Ross, Elizabeth, 543
Kübler-Ross grief stages, 448-449

**L**

Labor, 20
Laboratory animal allergy (LAA), 307-308
Laboratory animals
    caging/housing, 305-307
    housing data, 306t
    medicine
        glossary, 309
        learning outcomes, 287
        review questions, 309-310
    parasites, presence, 91-92t
Lacrimal apparatus, 21
    illustration, 436f
Lacrimal flushing, 437
Lactate dehydrogenase (LDH), 118
Lactation (milk production), 20
    definition, 162
    nutritional requirements, 250-251
Lacunae, 7-9
Lagomorphs, 504
    rodents, relationship, 503-504
Lamb
    identification, 225
    life stage, 274
Lamellae, 7-9
Lameness. *See* Equine
    diagnosis, methods, 465
    etiology, 465
    nuclear scintigraphy, 466
    radiographic examination, 465-466
    ultrasound diagnosis, 466
Laminitis (founder), 284
    impact, 464-465
Laparatomies, 408
Large animal nutrition/feeding
    concepts, 263-266
    glossary, 284
    learning outcomes, 263
    process, 263
    review questions, 285
Large animals, euthanasia, 448
Large-breed puppies, feeding, 251-252

Large intestine, 15
  anatomy/physiology, 277
  function, 16
Laryngeal paralysis, emergency,
  512t
Larynx (voice box), 16
Latent, definition, 132
Latent image, definition, 191
Latent infection, definition, 309
Lateral canthus, 433
Lateral direction, 7
Lateral resolution, definition, 203
Lateral saphenous vein, venipuncture, 420
Laxatives
  list, 382t
  usage, 380
LDA. *See* Left displaced abomasum
LDH. *See* Lactate dehydrogenase
Lead II complex, 424f
Lead poisoning, emergencies, 518t
Lead shank
  definition, 162
  usage, 152
Learning theory, usage. *See* Pet behavior
Leashes, types, 146
Leather leases, usage, 146
Left displaced abomasum (LDA), 476
Left shift, definition, 52
Left subclavian artery, 13
Legumes, definition, 285
Lempert rongeur, 404-405
Lens, 21
Leptocytes, 38f
  definition, 52
Leptospirosis. *See* Cattle
  bacterial zoonosis, 526t
Lesions
  appearance, 200
  classification, 200
  collection/evaluation. *See* Common
    lesions
  sonographic appearance, 200
Lethal genes, 211
  definition, 228
Leucine, 36
Leukemia, 446t
  definition, 52
Leukemoid response (reaction), definition,
  52
Leukocytes. *See* White blood cells
Leukocytosis, definition, 52
Leukopenia, definition, 52
LH. *See* Luteinizing hormone
Lice, impact, 318
Lidocaine, usage, 359
Life stage nutritional requirements. *See*
  Dogs
Life-threatening wounds, 495-497
Light microscope, usage, 99
Limbs, bandaging, 444
Limb surgery, performing, 409
Linear array transducer, 196
Linear scanner, definition, 203
Line breeding, 210
  definition, 228
Linens, preparation, 407-408

Line smear
  concentration technique, 59f
  usage, 57
Linoleic acid, 244
Linolenic acid, 244
Lipase, 15
Lipemia, definition, 124
Lipid-soluble substances, 11
Lipoic acid, definition, 261
Lipophilic, definition, 172
Liquid specimen, 101
Listening, 543
  barriers, 543
  practice, 543
Lister bandage scissors, 401
  illustration, 402f
*Listeria monocytogenes,* 108-109
Listeriosis
  bacterial zoonosis, 526t
  *Listeria monocytogenes. See* Cattle;
    Sheep; South American camelid
Littauer suture removal scissors
Litter pan, usage, 25
Liver, 15-16
  failure, emergency, 517t
  function
    clinical chemistry, 115-119
    tests, 121b
  sonographic appearance, 199
Livestock
  body condition scoring classification, 265t
  calcium/phosphorus, usage, 265
  carbohydrates, usage, 264
  fats, ingestion, 264
  macrominerals, 265
  magnesium, relationship, 265
  minerals, usage, 264
  nutrition, basics, 263-264
  potassium, 265
  protein, ingestion, 263
  vitamins, usage, 266
  water, adequacy, 266
Lizards, nutrition/diets (problems), 322
Local anesthetics
  list, 375t
  usage, 359
Lochia, definition, 228
Lockjaw, rule out, 461-462
Locus, definition, 228
Long bones, 7-9
  parts, 8f, 8
Lordosis, definition, 228-309
Lower canine tooth, dental radiography
  (bisecting angle technique), 499
Low-voltage circuit. *See* X-ray machine
Lungs, 17
  auscultation, 496
  tissue, samples (collection/evaluation),
    65
  volume, 17
Luteal phase, definition, 228
Luteinizing hormone (LH), definition, 228
Lyme borreliosis (Lyme disease), rickettsial
  zoonosis, 529t
Lymphadenitis, 65
  definition, 71

Lymphatic system, 16
  function, 16
  physical examination, 417
  structure, 16
Lymph nodes, 16
  characteristics, 65
  lesions, collection/evaluation, 65
Lymphoblast, definition, 71
Lymphocytes, examination, 60
Lymphocytic choriomeningitis (LCM) virus.
  *See* Syrian hamster
Lymphocytic stomatitis, 503
Lymphocytosis, definition, 52
Lymphokines, examples, 135
Lymphoma. *See* Ferrets
Lymph organs, 16
Lymphosarcomas, 446t
  identification, 70
  recognition, 62-64
Lymph vessels, 16
Lyophilized, definition, 141
Lysin, definition, 132
Lysogenic cycle, definition, 132
Lysosomes, 3

**M**

MA. *See* Microalbumin
MacConkey II agar (MAC), 100
Machine housing, 175
Macro-, definition, 52
Macrocyte, definition, 52
Macrocytic, definition, 52
Macrocytosis, definition, 71
Macrophages
  appearance, 67
  attack, 135
  definition, 71
  examination, 60
Magnesium ammonium phosphate. *See*
  Struvite
Magnetic resonance imaging (MRI),
  189
  definition, 203
  usage, 202
Maintenance energy requirements (MER),
  definition, 261
Maintenance fluids, 419
Maintenance nutrient requirements (MNRs),
  definition, 285
Malabsorption, definition, 124
Malassimilation, definition, 124
Male anatomy, 18
Male physiology, 18
Male reproductive system, 18
Malignancy
  criteria, 62
  general/nuclear criteria, 63t
Malignant, definition, 71
Malignant melanoma, 446t
Malignant neoplasia, 62
Malignant tumors, 501
Malleable retractors, 403
Mallets, usage, 405
Malocclusion. *See* Guinea pig
  abnormalities, 500
  classes, 500

Malocclusion *(Continued)*
definition, 309
level bite, 500
Malpresentation, definition, 228
Mammals
blood specimen, 103
respiration, 17
Mammary adenocarcinoma, 446t
Mandibular premolar teeth, dental radiography (parallel position technique), 498f
Mange, definition, 95
Mantle, definition, 309
Mare, 215
examination, 215
Marijuana, toxic substances (impact), 519t
Marked (extreme), definition, 52
Marketing, 554
Marrow. *See* Medullary cavity
smears, preparation. *See* Bone marrow
mAs. *See* Milliampere-second
Mast cells, 446t
definition, 52, 71
examination, 60
presence, 64
recognition, 64
Mastication, definition, 285
Material Safety Data Sheet (MSDS)
availability, 368
consultation, 389
Maternal dystocia, 212
Maternal immunity, transfer, 137
Mature horse, feeding, 282
Maximum permissible dose (MPD), 186, 186t. *See also* Radiation
definition, 191
Mayo dissecting scissors, 401f
Mayo-Hegar needle holders, 402-403
illustration, 401
Mayo scissors, 400
ME. *See* Metabolizable energy
Mean corpuscular hemoglobin concentration (MCHC), 45-46
Mean corpuscular hemoglobin (MCH), 45
Mean corpuscular volume (MCV), 45
Mean platelet volume (MPV), 50
Mechanical scalers, 494
Mechanical scalers, usage, 494
Mechanical sector transducer, 196
Meconium, definition, 228
Medetomidine, usage, 338
Media. *See* Plates; Tubes
selection, 99
types, 100
Medial direction, 7
Mediated session, holding, 545
Medical canthus, 433
Medical records, usage, 549
Medical terminology, 569-572
Medical units/conversions, 394t
Medications (dispensation), veterinary technician (role), 396
Medullary cavity (marrow), 8
Megabacteria, 317
Megacalorie (Mcal), definition, 285
Megakaryocytes, characteristics, 66

Meiosis, definition, 228
Melanoma, 501
characterization, 64
definition, 71
Melena, definition, 95
Membrane-bound nucleus, 3
Membranes, 6-7
composition, 6-7
types, 6-7
Memory, definition, 141
Meninges, 11-12
Meningitis *(Streptococcus suis)*, 481
Meningomyeloencephalitis. *See* West Nile virus
Meniscus, definition, 95
MER. *See* Maintenance energy requirements
Merocrine glands, definition, 240
Mesenchymal, definition, 71
Mesenchymal cell tumors, 62
Mesoderm, definition, 71
Mesothelial, definition, 71
Mesothelial cells
appearance, 67
examination, 60
Mesothelioma, definition, 71
Meta-, definition, 52
Metabolic acidosis, 364
treatment, 364
Metabolic alkalosis, 364
treatment, 364
Metabolic bone disease. *See* Rickets
Metabolic cage, definition, 309
Metabolic emergencies, 512
list, 516t
Metabolism cage, usage, 25
Metabolizable energy (ME), definition, 285
Metacercaria, definition, 95
Metaclopramide, 377
Metal loop, usage, 100
Metastasis, definition, 71, 124
Metestrus, 19
cell population identification, 69
Methohexital, usage, 342
Methoxyflurane
pharmacologicla effects, 345
usage, 344
Methylated oxybarbiturates, usage, 341
Metric conversions, 393-394
Metric date, 394
Metric mass, 394
Metric system, 393-394
equivalents, 568
Metric temperature, 394
Metric time, 394
Metric units
abbreviation, 394t
base unit, 394t
conversion methods, 393
prefix, 394t
Metzenbaum scissors, 400-401
Meyerding retractors, 403
MH. *See* Mueller-Hinton agar
Micro-, definition, 52
Microaerophilic, definition, 110
Microalbumin (MA) test, 30
Microanatomy, definition, 4

Microbial cell, development (disruption), 370
Microbial control
action, mode, 165
chemical methods, 166-169
degrees, 165
efficacy, 165
methods, 165-166
process, 165
physical methods, 165-166
Microbial metabolic activity, disruption, 370
Microbial protein synthesis, interference, 370
Microbial resistance, levels, 164
Microbicidal, definition, 172
Microbiology, purpose. *See* Diagnostic microbiology/mycology
Microcotyledonary placentation, definition, 228
Microcyte, definition, 52
Microcytic, definition, 52
Microenvironment, definition, 309
Microorganisms
definition, 172
resistance ranking, 165f
Microscopic evaluation. *See* Urine
Microscopic grooves, removal. *See* Teeth
Microvilli, 15
Micturition, 27
definition, 52
Middle ear, 21
Milk fever (parturient paresis), 271. *See also* Hypocalcemic parturient paresis
Milliampere-second (mAs), definition, 191
Milligram dose calculation, 394
Milliliter dose calculation, 394
Minerals
clinical chemistry, 119
functions, 246-247t
function test, 121b
nutrients, 245
Miniature biochemical test kits, usage. *See* Gram-negative identification
Minnesota Urolith Center, reports, 36
Miotic, definition, 433
Miotics, usage, 387
Mirror image, impact, 198
Mites. *See* Mouse
impact, 318
Mitochondria, 3
Mitosis, definition, 228
Mitotic activity, increase, 62
Mitotic inhibitors, list, 388t
Mixed lesions, 200
definition, 203
MLV. *See* Modified-live vaccines
M-mode. *See* Motion mode
MNRs. *See* Maintenance nutrient requirements
Modified compression preparation. *See* Slide preparation
Modified Knott's technique. *See* Blood
Modified-live vaccines (MLV), 138
Modified transudates
classification, 57f
definition, 71

Moist heat, usage, 166
Monday morning sickness, 283
Monestrus, definition, 228
Mongolian gerbil *(Meriones unguiculatus)*, 295-297
  behavioral/physiological characteristics, 296
  breeding considerations, 296
  handling/restraint, 296
  health conditions, 297
  nasal dermatitis (sore nose), 297
  pain/distress, signs, 296
  research origin/uses, 295
  Salmonella, 297
  sampling, 296
  Tyzzer's disease *(Clostridium piliforme)*, 297
*Moniezia* sp., 96f
Monoclonal vaccines, 139
Monocytopenia, definition, 52
Monocytosis, definition, 52
Monogastric, definition, 309
Monogastric digestion, 277
  anatomy/physiology, 277
Monohybrid cross, 197, 208f
  definition, 228
  genotype prediction, 208
Moon blindness, 284
*Moraxella bovis,* 108
Morula, definition, 95
Motility test medium, 100-101
Motion mode (M-mode), 197
  definition, 203
  motion display, 197f
Motor control, site, 10-11
Motor nerve processes. *See* Efferent nerve processes
Mouse *(Mus musculus)*, 288-292.
  *See also* Epizootic diarrhea of infant mice
  behavioral/physiological characteristics, 288
  breeding considerations, 289
  handling/restraint, 288-289
  health conditions, 289-292
  hepatitis virus, 289-290
  injection/sampling, needle sizes/sites (recommendation), 291-292t
  mites, 290-291
  pain/distress, signs, 289
  pinworm, 290
  reproductive data, 290t
  research, origin/uses, 288
  respiratory disease, 289
  restraint technique, 289f
  sampling, 289
  Tyzzer's disease, 294-295
Mouth, 15
  anatomy/physiology, 277
  physical examination, 416
  rot. *See* Stomatitis
MPD. *See* Maximum permissible dose
MSDS. *See* Material Safety Data Sheet
Mucocele, definition, 71
Mucolytics, list, 381t

Mucosa, 14
Mucous membranes, 6-7
  color, 509, 511
  monitoring, 357
  observation, 416
Mueller-Hinton agar (MH), 100
Mueller-Hinton sensitivity test, 105
Multicellular organisms, eurkayotic cell composition, 3
Multinucleation, 62
Mummified fetus, definition, 228
Murine mycoplasmosis. *See* Rat
Muscles
  acute inflammatory disease, 283
  disease, tests, 121b
  relaxants, 361-362
    list, 374-375t
    usage, 360
  tissue, 5-6
  tone, monitoring. *See* Jaw tone
  types, 9-10
Muscularis externa, 14
Muscular system, 9-10
  function, 9-10
Musculoskeletal system
  physical examination, 417
  tissue samples, 70
Mutation, definition, 228
Muzzles. *See* Gauze muzzle
  types, 147
*Mycobacterium* spp., 108-109
Mycology, purpose. *See* Diagnostic microbiology/mycology
Mycoplasma, 109
Mycosel agar, 100
Mycotic diseases. *See* Avian mycotic diseases
Mycotic zoonosis, 536t
Mydriatic, definition, 433
Mydriatics, usage, 387
Myeloid cells
  characteristics, 66
  erythroid cells (M:E) ratio, 66
Myiasis, definition, 95
Myocardium. *See* Cardiac muscles
Myometrial contraction, definition, 228
Myopathy, definition, 261
Myositis, 283
Mystery swine disease, 479

**N**

N₂O, usage. *See* Nitrous oxide
NA. *See* Nutrient agar
Naked virus
  definition, 132
  envelope, absence, 126-127
Narcotic agonist drugs, 375
Nares
  manipulation, 416
  physical examination, 416
Nasal cavity, 16
Nasal dermatitis (sore nose). *See* Mongolian gerbil
Nasal flush, 56

Nasogastric intubation, 428
  definition, 428
  equipment, 428
  indications, 428
  precautions, 429
  procedure, 428-429
Nasogastric tube, usage, 455
National Council on Radiation Protection and Measurements (NCRP), 186
National Research Council (NRC), 259-260
  definition, 261
Natural fibers, 406
Natural immunity, 136
Navicular syndrome, 465
  management, 465
NAVTA. *See* North American Veterinary Technician Association
N:C ratio, variation, 62
Near side, definition, 162
Neck, bandaging, 443
Necropsy, 449
  equipment, 449
  procedure, 449-450
Necrosis, definition, 141
Necrotic cementum, removal, 496
Needle holders, 402-403
Needle points, 405
Needles, 405
Needle spread, preparation, 59f
Needle teeth, definition, 162
Negative punishment, 237
Negative reinforcement, 237
  definition, 240
Nematode
  definition, 95
  impact, 318
Neonatal, definition, 228
Neonatal care
  glossary, 227-229
  learning outcomes, 541
  relationship. *See* Theriogenology
  review questions, 229-230
Neonatal diarrhea, 12
Neonatal isoerythrolysis, definition, 228
Neonates
  immune system, 137
  nutritional requirements, 251
Neoplasia
  definition, 71
  occurrence, 65
Neoplasms, examples, 416
Neoplastic lesions, 60-64
Neoplastic lymphocytes, appearance, 68
Neoplastic tissue cells, 62
*Neorickettsia risticii. See* Potomac horse fever
Neosporosis. *See* Cattle
Nerve deafness, 22
Nerve processes, 11-12
Nerve stimulator, usage, 360
Nervous system, 10-12
  cells, 12
  drugs, 375-378
Nervous tissue, 6
  specialization, 6
Neubauer hemocytometer, usage, 46

Neurogenic shock, emergency, 514t
Neuroglial cells (glial), 12
Neuroleptanalgesics, usage, 339
Neurological system, physical examination, 417
Neuromuscular blocking agents, 360-361
    classification, 361
    side effects, 361
Neutropenia, definition, 52
Neutrophilia, definition, 52
Neutrophils
    comparison, 64
    examination, 60
    predominance, 67
Newcastle disease, 532t
New methylene blue (NMB)
    definition, 52
    stain, usage, 59
Nictitating membrane, 21
Nitrogenous, definition, 261
Nitrous oxide (N₂O)
    clinical use, 347
    pharmacological effects, 347
    physical/chemical effects, 346-347
    usage, 346
        precautions, 347
nlf. *See* Non–lactose fermenter
NMB. *See* New methylene blue
Nocturnal, definition, 309
Nonabsorbable suture material, 406
Nonbreeding dairy calves, feeding, 264
Non–energy-producing nutrients, 245
Nonimmunological transfusion reaction, 423
Noninfectious inflammation, result, 64
Noninfective, definition, 95
Noninflammatory nonneoplastic lesions, 64
Non–lactose fermenter (nlf), definition, 110
Nonmalignant tumors, 501
Non–plasma specific enzymes, 117-118
Nonprecision vaporizers, 350
Nonprotein nitrogen (NPN), definition, 285
Nonrebreathing system, 352
Nonscreen film, 179
Nonspecific immunity, 134-135
Nonsterile areas, specimen type, 101
Nonsteroidal antiinflammatory drugs (NSAIDs), 360
    list, 374t
    toxic substances, impact, 519t
Nonstriated muscle. *See* Smooth muscles
Nonverbal communication, 542
Normal flora, definition, 110
Normal values, 574
Normo-, definition, 52
Normochromic, definition, 52
Normocyte, definition, 52
North American Veterinary Technician Association (NAVTA), 557
    ethics code, 557
    list, 558b
Nostrils (nares), 16
Novel, definition, 261
NPN. *See* Nonprotein nitrogen
NRC. *See* National Research Council
NSAIDs. *See* Nonsteroidal antiinflammatory drugs

Nuclear changes, 62
Nuclear medicine (NM), 189
    definition, 203
    introduction, 200
Nuclear molding, 62
Nuclear scintigraphy, 200-201
    definition, 203
    usage, 466
Nucleated red blood cell, 38f
    definition, 52
    interference, 46
Nucleic acid
    core, definition, 132
    production, inhibition, 370
Nucleus, 4
Nutrient, definition, 261-285
Nutrient agar (NA) slant, 100-101
Nutrition. *See* Small animal nutrition
Nutritional adequacy, statement, 260-261
Nutritional myodegeneration. *See* White muscle disease
Nutritional therapy, necessity, 257

**O**

Obesity. *See* Hedgehogs
    management, 255
Object-film distance (OFD)
    definition, 191
    increase, 517t
Obligate intracellular bacteria, 109
Obligate intracellular parasite, definition, 132
Occlusion, 500
Occult blood, presence, 32
Occupational Health and Safety Administration (OHSA), anesthesia recommendations, 353
Occupational Safety and Health Administration (OSHA), 550
    drug handling procedures, 368
Occupational Safety and Health (OSH) Act, 550
Ocular emergencies, 512
    list, 519t
OF. *See* Oxidation fermentation
OFD. *See* Object-film distance
Offensive aggression, 233
Olfaction, definition, 241
Oligodontia, 500
Oliguria, 27
    definition, 52
Olsen-Hegar needle holders, 402-403
Omasum, 15, 267
Omnivore, 14
Omphalitis, definition, 228
Oncogenesis, definition, 132
Oncology, 445-448
    classification, 446
    definition, 445
    diagnostics, 446
    therapy, 447
Ontario Veterinary College (OVC)
    definition, 95
    puddle technique. *See Cryptosporidium* oocysts

Oocysts
    definition, 95
    OVC puddle technique. *See Cryptosporidium* oocysts
Open-air scanner, usage, 201
Open gloving, 410
Open wounds, 468
Operant conditioning, 237
    definition, 241
Operating room
    aseptic conditions, 410-411
    conduct, 410-412
    items, opening procedure, 411
    movement, limitation, 411
    sterile field, imaginary line, 411
    sterilization pouches, items (opening procedure), 411
    surgical attire, requirement, 411
    talking, minimization, 411
Operating scissors, 400
Operculum, definition, 95
Ophtalmoscopy, 436
Ophthalmic agents, formulation, 387-389
Ophthalmic drops, 433
Ophthalmology, 433
    anatomy, 433
    medical terminology, 433-435
    tears, 433
    therapeutic treatments, 435
Opioids
    administration route, 339
    analgesics, 370
        list, 374t
    classification, 338-339
    clinical effects, 339
    component, reversal, 340
    differences, 360
    perianesthetic agents, 370
    summary, 340t
    usage, 338
Opportunistic pathogen, definition, 110
Optochin susceptibility test, definition, 110
Oral cavity, lesions (collection/evaluation), 65
Oral fluid administration, 419
Oral health, 258
    diet, characteristics, 258
    hygiene procedure, 495-497
Oral lesions, 501
Orchitis, definition, 228
Organ
    appearance, 198
    brightness, 197f
    sonographic appearance, 199
Organization management, 546
Organophosphate toxicity, toxic substances (impact), 519t
Ornithosis, 317
Orogastric intubation, 427-428
    equipment, 427
    indications, 427
    precautions, 428
    procedure, 427-428
Orphaned young, life stage, 274
Orthopedic instruments, 404-405

OSHA. *See* Occupational Safety and Health Administration
Osmometry, usage, 29
Osmosis, 4
Osmotic pressure, definition, 124
Osteoarthritis, definition, 261
Osteoblast, 7
    component, 66
Osteoclast, 7
    components, 66
Osteocyte, 7
Osteogenesis (ossification), 8-9
Osteology, definition, 7-9
Osteomalacia, definition, 261
Osteomyelitis, definition, 71
Osteoporosis, definition, 261
Osteosarcoma, 446t, 501
    definition, 71
Osteotomies, 405
Otic preparations, 387-389
Otitis externa, etiologies, 432
Outbred, definition, 309
Outbreeding, 209
    definition, 228
Outer ear, 21
Ovaries, 18
Ovariohysterectomy hook, 403-404
Ovassay, usage, 74
Ovatector, usage, 74
OVC. *See* Ontario Veterinary College
Overhand knot, definition, 162
Overventilation, indication, 361
Oviduct, 18
Ovine, 222-225
    breeding soundness examination, 222-223
    brucellosis, 223
    dystocia
        causes, 224
        signs, 224
    estrous cycle, 223
    estrus, signs, 223
    forelegs, malposition, 224
    gestation, 223-224
    neonatal care, 224-225
    parturition, stages (lambing), 223-224
    pregnancy diagnosis, 223
    puberty, 222
    Q fever, 223
    semen characteristics, 223
    semen collection techniques, 223
    tail dock/castration, 225
    vitamin E/selenium supplementation, 225
Ovine diseases, 480
Ovulation, definition, 228
Ovum, strongyle type, 96f
Oxidation, action mode, 169-171
Oxidation fermentation (OF) medium, 100-101
Oxidizing agent, definition, 172
Oxybarbiturates, usage, 341
Oxygen, usage, 378
Oxygenation
    anesthesia monitoring, 357
    anesthetic equipment problems, 365
    status, 510

Oxygen flush valve. *See* Anesthetic machine
Oxyglobin, impact, 390
Oxytocin, usage, 383
*Oxyuris equi*, 96f

**P**

Packed cell volume (PCV), 36. *See also* Red blood cells
    definition, 52, 95
    dehydration indicator, 419
    improvement, total volume (necessity), 362
    level, impact, 362
Packed RBCs, usage, 423
Pack preparation, 406-408
PACS. *See* Picture archiving and communication system
Pain response, monitoring. *See* Pedal reflex
Pain treatment, reasons, 359
Palmar direction, 7
Palpebral reflex, monitoring, 355
Pan-, definition, 52
Pancreas, sonographic appearance, 200
Pancreatic beta cell tumors. *See* Ferrets
Pancreatic enzymes, delivery, 16
Pancreatic function
    clinical chemistry, 114-115
    tests, 121b
Pancreatitis, emergency, 517t
Pancytopenia, definition, 52
Papanicolaou's stains, usage, 59
Papilloma, definition, 71
Parabasal cells, appearance, 69
Parakeratosis, 280
    definition, 261-285
Paralumbar block (Cornell block), 481
Paraphimosis, definition, 309
*Parascaris equorum*, 96f
Parasites
    definition, 132
    examination. *See* Blood
    examples, 440
    host, relationship, 73
    identification. *See* External parasite identification
    presence. *See* Laboratory animals
    visibility, 64
Parasitic samples, preservation, 75
Parasitic zoonosis, 534-535t
Parasitology
    appendix, 96
    glossary, 95
    learning outcomes, 73
    review questions, 95-96
Parasympathetic nerve fibers, 12
Paratenic host, definition, 95
Parathyroid hormone (PTH), regulation, 119, 120
Paraverebral block, 481
Parenchymal disorders, 496
Parenteral, definition, 261
Parenteral nutrition, 257
Parovirus, 129. *See also* Rat
    infection, emergency, 517t
Particulate radiation, 174
Parts per million (ppm), 395-396

Parturient paresis. *See* Milk fever
Parturition (birth), 20
    definition, 228
Passive immunity, 556
Passive processes, 4
*Pasteurella* spp., 226
Pasteurellosis *(Pasteurella multocida)*, 317. *See also* Rabbit
Pathogen, definition, 172
Patients
    identification/history, 335
    preparation, 408-409
        goals, 408
    sighing/bagging, 361
Paws, bandaging, 444
Pedal reflex (pain response), monitoring, 355
Pediculosis, definition, 95
Pedigree charts, 210f
    definition, 228
    usage, 209
Pemphigus, 138
    definition, 141
Penetrance, definition, 228
Penetration-uncoating, replication stage, 127
Penia, definition, 52
Penis, 18
    composition/description, 18
Penrose drain, usage, 443
Pentobarbital, usage, 341
Pentobarbital sodium, euthanizing agent, 375
Penumbra
    definition, 191
    magnification, increase, 185f
Percutaneous, definition, 71
Performance horse, feeding, 283
Pericardial tamponade, emergency, 514t
Perinuclear, definition, 71
Periodic ophthalmia, 284
Periodontal disease, 502-503
    causes, 502
Periodontal index, 502, 503
Periodontal ligament, 472
Periodontal probe, 494
Periodontium, aging, 492
Periosteal elevators, 405, 494
Periosteum, 8
Peripheral nervous system (PNS), 11-12
    division, 11-12
    glial cells, 12
    organization, 11f
Peritonitis, emergency, 517t
Perosomus elumbis, definition, 228
Peroxisomes, 3-4
Peroxygen compounds, usage, 168
Personal ethics, 556
Personal finance, management, 543
Personal management, 550
    goals, 551
Personal management skills
    glossary, 560
    learning outcomes, 541
    review questions, 560
Personal mantra, creation, 556
Personnel management, importance, 548

PET. *See* Positron emission tomography
Pet behavior
    correction, 237
    modification, learning theory (usage), 237
    problem, 237
Peterson eye block, 482
Pet food, 259-260
    label, 259-260
    selection process, 259
Pets
    acquisition, 236
    bereavement, 448
    euthanasia, grief process, 448
    health care, 236
    intervention techniques, 293
    physiological modification, 237
    selection, 236
    signalment, 237
    socialization/training, 236
pH. *See* Urine
    diet, impact, 30
    regulation mechanisms, 363
Phagocytes, definition, 141
Phagocytosis (cell eating), 4
Phantom mare, definition, 229
Pharmaceutical calculations
    learning outcomes, 393
    review questions, 397-398
Pharmacokinetics, 369-370
Pharmacology
    definitions/terminology, 367-369
    glossary, 390-391
    learning outcomes, 367
    review questions, 391-392
Pharynx, 15, 16
Phased array sector scanner transducer, 196
Phase training programs, 548
Phenobarbital, usage, 341
Phenols, usage, 167
Phenothiazines
    anxiety reduction, 377
    usage, 337
Phenotypes
    definition, 229, 309
    prediction, 207-208
Phenylbutazone
    NSAID example, 375
    usage, 360
PHF. *See* Potomac horse fever
Philia, definition, 52
Philodendron, toxic substances (impact), 519t
Phimosis, definition, 229
Phosphor crystals, size (increase), 178f
Photon, definition, 191
Photostimulable phosphor (PSP) detector screen, usage, 190
Physical examination, 415-417
    animal appearance, observation, 416
    introduction, 415-416
    system approach, 416
    usage, 335
    veterinary technician, role, 415
Physical problems, detection, 416
Physiology, definition, 3
Pica, definition, 285

Picture archiving and communication system (PACS), definition, 191
Piezoelectric effect, 196
    definition, 203
Piglets, management, 279
Pig restraint, 158-160
    danger potential, 158
    usage, 159-160
Pigs
    *Actinobacillus pleuropneumoniae*, 480
    alimentary disease, 476-477
    anatomy/physiology, 159
    atrophic rhinitis *(Bordetella bronchiseptica, Pasteurella multocida)*, 480
    behavioral characteristics, 158-159
    castration, 487
    collection sample, 472
    diseases, 475-476, 480-481
    farrowing crates, usage, 159
    general anesthesia, 483-484
    glossary, 487-488
    herding instincts, 158
    hog panels, 159
    hog snare
        placement, 160f
        usage, 159
    holding, 160f
    intramuscular (IM) injections, 473
    learning outcomes, 471
    lifting, 160
    local/regional anesthesia/analgesia, 481-482
    medication, administration, 472
    metabolic diseases, 475-476
    movement, hurdle (usage), 159f
    observations, 471-472
    peritoneal injections, 474
    physical examination, 471-472
    recumbency, 160
    reproductive diseases, 477-479
    respiratory diseases, 479-480
    review questions, 488-499
    squeeze pens, usage, 159
    subcutaneous (SC) injections, 474
    surgery, 484-487
    swine dysentery *(Treponema hyodysenteriae)*, 477
    venipuncture, 473
Pilocarpine, 377
Piloerection, definition, 241
Pinocytosis (bulk-phase/cell drinking), 4
Pinworm. *See* Mouse
Piriform, definition, 95
Pituitary hormones, list, 386t
Pixel
    definition, 191
    placement, 195
Pizzle rot, definition, 229
Placentophagia, definition, 309
Plague, bacterial zoonosis, 527t
Plantar direction, 7
Plaque
    accumulation, 502
    formation, 502
    removal, 496
Plasma, definition, 52, 124

Plasma cells
    definition, 71
    examination, 60
    inclusions, 66
Plasmacytic stomatitis, 503
Plaster of Paris, 445
Plate, definition, 110
Platelet-concentrated plasma, 424
Platelet evaluation. *See* Thrombocyte evaluation
Plates (media), 100
Pleomorphic, definition, 71, 110
Pleural effusion, emergency, 512t
Pleuritis (pleurisy), definition, 17, 71
Pluriparous, definition, 229
Pneumatic bones, 8
Pneumonia, 317, 322
    definition, 17
    emergency, 513t
Pneumothorax
    definition, 17, 71
    emergency, 513t
    ventilation, caution, 362
Poikilocytosis, definition, 52
Poison, definition, 367
Polioencephalomalacia. *See* Thiamine-deficiency polio
Poll, definition, 162
Pollakiuria, 27
    definition, 52, 261
Polled, definition, 162
Polychromasia, definition, 52
Polychromatic beam, definition, 191
Polyclonal, definition, 141
Polydontia, 500
Polyestrous, definition, 229
Polygenic traits, definition, 229
Polyuria, 27
    definition, 52
Polyvalent vaccines, 139
Poole tips, 405
Pop-off valve. *See* Anesthetic machine
    reopening, 361
Porcine, 225-227
    breeding soundness examination, 225
    diseases, 480-481
    dystocia
        causes, 226
        signs, 226
    estrous cycle, 226
    estrus, signs, 226
    gestation, 226
    neonatal care, 227
    parturition, stages, 226
    pregnancy diagnosis, 226
    puberty, 225
    semen characteristics, 225
    semen collection techniques, 225
Porcine reproductive and respiratory syndrome (PRRS), 479
Porcine reproductive diseases, 478
Porcine rotavirus. *See* Transmissible gastroenteritis
Portal of entry, definition, 132

Positioning
  criteria/principles, 188
  techniques. *See* Diagnostic radiographic
    examinations
Positive idea change, mechanisms, 545
Positive inotropes, usage, 378
Positive punishment, 237
Positive reinforcement, definition, 241
Positron emission tomography (PET), 201
  definition, 203
  F-FDG/X-ray, 202
  PET/CT, definition, 203
  unit, 201f
Postcava, 13
Postcentrifugation, 32
Posterior direction, 7
Postmortem tissues, aseptic collection,
    128
Postprandial, definition, 52
Potable water, definition, 285
Potomac horse fever (PHF) *(Neorickettsia
    risticii)*
  rule out, 460-461
  vaccination, 458t
Poultry diet, 316
Povidone-iodine solution, usage, 442
Poxviral disease, viral zoonosis, 533t
ppm. *See* Parts per million
ppp. *See* Prepatent period
Practice management, 546
  responsibility, 548
Practice management communication, 542
  overview, 542
Practice management skills
  glossary, 560
  learning outcomes, 541
  review skills, 560
Preanesthetic agents
  classifications, 336-340
  usage, 335
Preanesthetic assessment, 335
Precava (cranial vena cava/superior vena
    cava), 13
Precentrifugation, 32
Precision vaporizers, 349-350
Precursor blood cells, 51t
Prednisone, corticosteroids, 375
Pregnant animals, treatment, 146
Prehepatic, definition, 124
Prehepatic jaundice, 115-116
Premature ventricular contraction/complex
    (PVC), 426
Premix, definition, 285
Prepatent infection, definition, 95
Prepatent period (ppp), definition, 95
Prescriptions, 396-397
  guidelines, 396
  labels, 396
Pressure manometer. *See* Anesthetic
    machine
Prevacuum autoclave, 169-170
Primary healing, 442
Primary immune responses, secondary
    immune responses (contrast), 136
Primary lesions, 437
  terminology, 439t

Primary uterine inertia, definition, 229
PR interval, 424
Prion, definition, 132
Prion/transmissible spongiform encepha-
    lopathy zoonosis, 537t
Pro-, definition, 52
Procedures manual, 547
Proestrus, 19
  cell population identification, 69
Professional association ethics, 557
Professional ethics, 556
  middle ground, 557
Professionalism, 555
  components, 555
  education, 555
Professional management skills
  glossary, 560
  learning outcomes, 541
  review questions, 560
Professional organizations, career advance-
    ment opportunity, 558
Progesterone, definition, 229
Progestins
  list, 386t
  usage, 383
Prokaryote (before nucleus), 3
Proliferative bowel disease. *See* Ferrets
Proliferative ileitis, 295
Propagation artifacts, 198
Proparacaine, usage, 387
Propofol, usage, 343
Proportion equation, 368
Proptosis, 433
  emergency, 520t
Prostaglandins
  list, 386t
  usage, 383
Prostate, sonographic appearance, 199
Protective fetal membranes, 20
Protein
  chemical component, 30
  content, 267
  definition, 261
Proteinaceous, definition, 285
Protein-containing fluid, absorption, 16
Proteins, nutrients, 244
Proteinuria, definition, 52
Protozoa
  definition, 95
  impact, 318
Proximal direction, 7
PRRS. *See* Porcine reproductive and
    respiratory syndrome
Pseudorabies (Aujeszky's disease), 481
Pseudostratified columnar epithelium, 5
Psi, definition, 132
Psittacine diet, 316
  deficiencies, 316
Psittacosis, 317
PSP. *See* Photostimulable phosphor
Psychoactive drugs, definition, 241
Puberty, definition, 229
Pulmonary circulation, 13
Pulmonary edema, emergency, 513t
Pulmonary neoplasia, emergency,
    513t

Pulsed-wave transducers, 195
Pulse rate, monitoring, 356
Punch biopsy, 55
Punnett square
  definition, 229
  usage, 207
Pupil, 21
  size, monitoring, 355
Pupillary reflexes, 511-512
Puppies, nutritional requirements, 251
Purulent, definition, 71
Purulent inflammation, 60
PVC. *See* Premature ventricular contrac-
    tion/complex
P wave, 424
Pyelonephritis, 68
Pyknosis, 68
  definition, 71
Pyodermas, 437
Pyogranulomatous, definition, 71
Pyogranulomatous inflammation, 60
Pyometra, emergencies, 518t
Pyrethrins, toxic substances (impact),
    519t

**Q**
Q fever. *See* Sheep
  bacterial zoonosis, 527t
QRS complex, 424
Quality, definition, 191
Quantitative buffy coat (QBC) analysis,
    50
Quantitative fecal examination. *See* Feces
Quantity, definition, 191
Quantum mottle, definition, 191
Quaternary ammonium compounds, usage,
    167
Queen, 211
Quick release knot, 162

**R**
Rabbit *(Oryctolagus cuniculus)*, 297-299
  behavioral/physiological characteristics,
    297-298
  breeding considerations, 298
  coccidiosis, 299
  dermatitis/alopecia, 299
  handling/restraint, 298
  health conditions, 299
  pain/distress signs, 299
  pasteurellosis *(Pasteurella multocida)*,
    299
  research origin/uses, 297
  sampling, 298-299
  transporting technique, 298f
  trichobezoars (hairballs), 299
Rabies
  management, 462
  rule out, 462
  vaccination, 457t
  viral zoonosis, 533t
Rabies pole, usage, 147
Radiation
  measurement, 186
  permissible dose, maximum, 186, 186t
  responsibilities, 185

Radiation *(Continued)*
 safety, 185-187
  practices, 187
 types, 200
 usage, 166
Radiodense (radiopaque), definition, 191
Radiograph
 beam direction, 187
 exposure, digital radiography unit (usage), 188
Radiographic contrast, 182
 definition, 191
 technical factors, impact, 184t
Radiographic density, 181
 definition, 192
 step wedge, example, 182f
Radiographic detail/definition, absence (errors), 184t
Radiographic examinations, positioning techniques. *See* Diagnostic radiographic examinations
Radiographic quality, 181
 definition, 192, 181
Radiography. *See* Contrast radiography
 definition, 192
 glossary, 190-191
 learning outcomes, 173
 review questions, 192-193
Radioimmunoassay, definition, 124
Radiology, definition, 192
Radiolucent, definition, 192
Radionuclides, 200
 definition, 203
Radiotherapy, 447
Rales, 510
Ram, 222
 examination, 222
Random breeding, 209
Raptoral species, carnivores, 316
Ration, definition, 285
Rat *(Rattus norvegicus)*, 292-294
 behavioral/physiological characteristics, 292
 breeding considerations, 293
 coronaviruses, 293
 handling/restraint, 292-293
 health conditions, 293-294
 mammary tumors, 294
 murine mycoplasmosis, 293-294
 pain/distress, signs, 293
 parovirus, 293
 research origin/uses, 292
 sampling, 293
 Sendai virus, 293
Rat-tooth thumb forceps, 401
Rayon swabs, usage, 55
RBCs. *See* Red blood cells
RDA. *See* Right displaced abomasum
Reactive lymphocytes, comparison, 68
Reagent sticks, usage, 114
Reagent strips, 29-30
 usage, 116
Reagent test strips. *See* Specific gravity
Rebreathing system, 352. *See also* Nonrebreathing system
 closed system, 352
 semiclosed system, 352

Recessive gene, definition, 229
Recombinant, definition, 132
Recombinant vaccines, 138-139
Records, usage, 549
Rectal mucosa, tissue samples, 70
Rectification, definition, 192
Rectum, 15
Red blood cells (RBCs/erythrocytes), 34f
 casts, 35
 definition, 52
 evaluation, 37-46
 examination, 60
 increase, 68
 indices, 45-46
 mean size, 45
 morphological changes/inclusions, 38f
 number, excess, 33
 PCV, 37-45
 percentages, determination, 37-45
 total numbers, 45
 variations, 381t
Red leg. *See* African clawed frog
Reduction forceps, 404-405
References, usage, 553
Reflexes, 12
 responses, 12
Refraction, impact, 198
Refractometer, usage, 28-29
Refractory, definition, 132
Regurgitation
 definition, 285
 problems, 316
Relative, definition, 52
Remnant beam, definition, 192
Renal disease, 259
Renal system
 emergencies, 515t
 pH regulation, 363
 status, monitoring, 501
 triage, 493-495
Renal tubular (RT), 34f
 irritation, 35
Renal tubular (RT) epithelial cells, 68
Replacement fluids, 419
Replacement heifer, definition, 285
Replication, 127
 stages, 127
Reproductive system. *See* Female reproductive system; Male reproductive system
 emergencies, 503, 518t
 physical examination, 417
Reptiles
 anesthesia/analgesia, 321
 bacterial diseases, 322
 blood
  analysis, 321
  collection, 320
  specimen, 103
 classification, 318-319
 clinical conditions/diseases, 322
 clinic housing, 320
 diets, problems, 321-322
 ectoparasites, 322-323
 endoparasites, 323
 housing, 320
 infectious diseases, 322

Reptiles *(Continued)*
 intramuscular injection, 321
 intraosseous catheterization, 321
 intravenous injection, 321
 leukocyte count, 46
 medicine, 318
 meds, oral administration, 321
 mycotic diseases, 322
 nursing care, 320-321
 nutrition, 321-322
 parasites, 322-323
 physical examination, 320
 protozoal diseases, 322
 restraint/handling, 320
 stomach feeding, 321
 viral diseases, 322
Reptiles/mammals, anatomical/physiological comparison, 319-320
Reptilia, class, 318
RER. *See* Rough endoplasmic reticulum
Reservoir bag, usage. *See* Anesthetic machine
Residual volume, 17
Resolution/acceptance, grief stage, 449, 544
Resorptive lesions, 503
 etiology, 503
Respiration, control, 17
Respiratory acidosis, 363
 treatment, 363
Respiratory alkalosis, 364
 treatment, 364
Respiratory drugs, 378
 list, 381t
Respiratory effort
 assessment, 509
 status, monitoring, 510
Respiratory emergencies, 512-513t
Respiratory rate, 17
 assessment, 493
 status, monitoring, 495
Respiratory system, 16-17
 avian/mammal comparison, 313
 lesions, collection/evaluation, 64
 pH regulation, 363
 physical examination, 416
 physiology, 17
 reptilian/mammalian comparison, 319
 status, monitoring, 497
 structures, 16
 terminology, 17
 triage, 493
Restraint/handling
 glossary, 162-163
 learning outcomes, 144
 review questions, 163
Résumé, usage, 552
Retained deciduous teeth, 500
Reticulocyte count, usage, 46
Reticulum, 267
 hardware compartment, 15
Retina, 21
Retractors, 403-404
Retrobulbar block, 482
Reusable linens, 407
Reverberations, impact, 198
Reversal agents, list, 389t

Reverse transcriptase RNA, definition, 132
Revolutions per minute (rpm), definition, 95
Rhabdomyolysis, 283
   definition, 285
Rhinopneumonitis, vaccination, 457t
Rhododendron azalea, toxic substances
      (impact), 519t
Rhythm, monitoring, 356
Ribonucleic acid (RNA)
   definition, 132
   transcription, 127
Ribosomes, 3
Rickets (metabolic bone disease), 271, 274,
      277, 284
Rickettsial zoonosis, 529-530t
Right displaced abomasum (RDA), 476
Right shift, definition, 52
Ring block, 482
Ring down artifacts, 198
Ringwomb, definition, 229
Ringworm, 438-439
Robert Jones pressure bandage, 444
Rochester-Carmalt forceps, 402
   illustration, 403f
   longitudinal serrations, 403f
Rochester-Ochsner forceps, 402
Rochester-Pean forceps, 402
Rocky Mountain spotted fever, 530t
Roeder towel forceps, 401
Romanowsky stains, usage, 59
Romifidine, usage, 338
Rongeurs, 404-405
Rope leashes, usage, 146
Rose-Bengal stain, usage, 437
Rotating anode, 274
Roto-Pro burs, 494-495
Roughages
   classification, 267
   definition, 285
Rough endoplasmic reticulum (RER), 3
Rouleaux, definition, 52
Round cell tumors, discreteness, 62
rpm. *See* Revolutions per minute
Rumen, 267
   acidosis, 272, 274
   fermentation vat, 15
Rumen acidosis (grain overload), 476-477
Ruminal tympany (bloat), 476
Ruminants
   alimentary disease, 476-477
   anatomy/physiology, 266
   collection sample, 472
   concentrates, usage, 267b
   digestion, 266
   diseases, 475-481
   glossary, 487-488
   intradermal injections, 474
   intramuscular (IM) injections, 473
   intraperitoneal injections, 474
   learning outcomes, 471
   local/regional anesthesia/analgesia, usage,
      481-482
   medication, administration, 472
   metabolic diseases, 475-476
   milk sampling, 474-475
   observations, 471-472

Ruminants *(Continued)*
   peritoneal injections. *See* Small ruminants
   physical examination, 471-472
   reproductive disease, 477-479
   respiratory diseases, 479-480
   review questions, 488-489
   roughage, usage, 267b
   stomach, 15
   subcutaneous (SC) injections. *See* Small
      ruminants
   surgery, 445
Russian tissue forceps, 401
Rut, definition, 162

**S**
SAC. *See* South American camelid
Saccharogenic test, definition, 124
Sagittal, definition, 203
Sales point displays, 554
Salmonella, 322. *See also* Guinea pig;
      Mongolian gerbil
*Salmonella-Shigella* (SS) agar, 100
*Salmonella* spp. *See* Syrian hamster
Salmonellosis
   bacterial zoonosis, 527t
   management, 460
   rule out, 460
Sanitation/sterilization/disinfection
   glossary, 171-172
   learning outcomes, 164
   quality control, 171
   review questions, 172
Sanitize, definition, 172
Saprophytes, identification, 109
Sarcoma, definition, 71
Sarcoptic mange, 440
   parasitic zoonosis, 534t
SC. *See* Subcutaneous
Scanning planes, 198
Scatter radiation
   definition, 192
   impact, 183
Scavenging systems. *See* Anesthetic
      machine
Schedule II drugs, regulation, 368
Schirmer's tear test, 436
Schistocyte, 38f
   definition, 52
Schistosomus reflexus, definition, 229
SCID. *See* Severely compromised immune
      deficient
Scintillating devices, definition, 192
Scissors, 400-401
Sclera, 21
Scours, definition, 285
Scraping, usage, 55
Screen film, 178
Scrubbing, preparation, 410
SCUD. *See* Septicemic cutaneous ulcer disease
Scurvy (hypovitaminosis C). *See* Guinea pig
SD. *See* Sorbitol dehydrogenase
Seasonally polyestrous, definition, 229
Seborrhea oleosa, 441
Seborrhea sicca, 441
Secondary immune responses, contrast. *See*
      Primary immune responses

Secondary lesions, 437
   terminology, 439t
Secondary radiation, definition, 192
Secondary uterine inertia, definition, 229
Second degree AV block, 427
Second-intention healing, 442
Sector scanner, definition, 203
Sedatives
   list, 376t
   usage, 336
Sedimentation rate, definition, 52
Seizures, causes, 511
Selective medium, definition, 110
Self-retaining forceps, 55
Self-retraining retractors, 403-404
Semen evaluation, 70
Sendai virus. *See* Rat
Senn Rake retractors, 403
Senses, 21
Sensory impulses, interpretation, 10-11
Sensory nerve processes. *See* Afferent nerve
      processes
Sensory organs, lesions (collection/evalua-
      tion), 65
Sensory system
   avian/mammal comparison, 312
   reptilian/mammalian comparison, 319
Sentinel, definition, 172, 309
Septicemia, 322
Septicemic cutaneous ulcer disease (SCUD),
      215
Septic shock, emergency, 514t
SER. *See* Smooth endoplasmic reticulum
Seroconversion, definition, 141
Serology, 171
Serosa, 14
Serous membranes (serosa), 7
Serum
   albumin, levels (change), 114
   ALT, increase, 118
   calcium, presence, 119-120
   chloride, abundance, 119
   cholesterol, 120-124
   conjugated bilirubin levels, increase, 116
   magnesium, 120
   phosphorus, 120
   potassium, level, 119
   quality, 113
   sodium, abundance, 119
Serum amylase, existence, 114-115
Serum glutamic-oxaloacetic transaminase
      (SGOT), 118
Serum glutamic pyruvic transminase
      (SGPT), 117
Serum lipase, existence, 115
Serum/plasma glucose, usage, 114
Serum separator tube (SST), definition,
      309
Sesamoid bones, 8
Setting up, definition, 162
Severely compromised immune deficient
      (SCID) animal, 309
Sevoflurane
   pharmacological effects, 346
   physical/chemical properties, 346
   usage, 346

Sex chromosomes, 208
definition, 229
SGOT. *See* Serum glutamic-oxaloacetic transaminase
SGPT. *See* Serum glutamic pyruvic transminase
Shampoo
list, 440t
types, 437
Shaping, 237-238
definition, 241
Sheep
anatomy/physiology, 156
behavioral characteristics, 156
bluetongue, 479
brucellosis *(Brucella ovis)*, 478
casting
final position, 157f
starting position, 157f
energy, requirements, 272
feeding, 272
feed sources, 272
intradermal injections, 474
intramuscular (IM) injections, 473
life stages, 274
listeriosis *(Listeria monocytogenes)*, 478
minerals, ingestion, 273
nutrition, disease (relationship), 274
nutritional requirements, 272
protein, 272
Q fever *(Coxiella burnetii)*, 478
regional anesthesia, 482
rotavirus, 477
venipuncture, 473
vibriosis *(Vibrio fetus)*, 478
vitamins, necessity, 273
water, usage, 272
Sheep restraint, 156-157
danger potential, 156
usage, 156-157
Sheet bend knot, 161f
usage, 160-161
Shepherd's hook/explorer, 494
Short bones, 8
Shoulder roll, usage. *See* Horses
SI. *See* Système International d'Unités
Sialocele, definition, 71
Sickle hocks, definition, 229
Sickle scaler, usage, 493
SID. *See* Source-image distance
Signalment, definition, 241
Silage
definition, 285
roughage, 303
Simple stomach, 15, 16
Sinus arrhythmia, 426
Sinus bradycardia, 426
Sinus tachycardia, 426
Skeletal divisions, 7-9
Skeletal muscles (striated muscles/voluntary tissues), 9-10
actions, 10
contraction, 10
Skeletal muscle tissue (striated muscle tissue), 5

Skeletal species, differences, 8-9
Skeletal system, 7-9
avian/mammalian comparison, 312
reptilian/mammalian comparison, 319
Skin
digestion technique, 76
layers, 21
lesions, samples, 55
physical examination, 416
scraping, 76, 440
Slant, definition, 110
Sleeping sickness. *See* Equine encephalomyelitides
Slide preparation. *See* Cytology
compression prep method, 57
modified compression preparation, 57
starfish method, 57
Sliding-filament theory, 10
Slings, aftercare, 445
Slow drying, 181b
Small airway disease, emergency, 513t
Small animal nursing
glossary, 450
learning outcomes, 415
review questions, 451
Small animal nutrition
basics, 243
feeding methods, 245-250
glossary, 261
learning outcomes, 243
review questions, 261-262
Small animals, euthanasia, 448
Small intestine, 15
anatomy/physiology, 277
enzymes, secretion, 16
Small ruminants
castration, 487
peritoneal injections, 406
subcutaneous (SC) injections, 474
Smears, preparation
fluid samples, usage, 57
solid masses, usage, 57
Smell, 22
Smooth endoplasmic reticulum (SER), 3
Smooth muscles (visceral muscle/nonstriated muscle/involuntary muscle), 10
Smooth muscle tissue, 5-6
Smudge cell, definition, 52
Snakes, nutrition/diets (problems), 321
Snook spay hook, 404
Socialization period, definition, 241
Sodium hexametaphosphate (HMP), addition, 258
Sodium polyphosphate, addition, 258
Softer masses, syringes (usage), 54
Soft tissue swelling, emergency, 512t
Solid, definition, 203
Solid lesions, 200
Solid mass imprinting, 55
Solid specimen, 101-102
Solute, definition, 4, 352
Solutions, 395
definition, 4, 395
percent strength, calculation, 5
Solvent, definition, 4
Sonolucent image, 197

Sorbitol dehydrogenase (SD), 118
Sound
beam zones, 196
frequency, 195
velocity, 195
wavelength, 195
waves, 195
Source-image distance (SID)
definition, 192
increase, 185f
South American camelid (SAC)
alimentary disease, 476-477
castration, 487
collection, sample, 472
diseases, 480-481
general anesthesia, 484
glossary, 487-488
intramuscular (IM) injections, 473
learning outcomes, 471
listeriosis *(Listeria monocytogenes)*, 478-479
local/regional anesthesia/analgesia, 481-482
medication, administration, 472
metabolic diseases, 475-476
observations, 471-472
physical examination, 471-472
reproductive diseases, 477-479
respiratory diseases, 479-480
review questions, 488-489
surgery, 484-487
venipuncture, 473
Sows, 225
Spatial cues, 550
Spay hook, 403-404
illustration, 405f
Specialized integument, 21
Species, names, 573
Specific gravity (SG). *See* Urine
reagent test strips, 29
Specific immunity, 135
Specificity, definition, 141
Specific pathogen-free (SPF), definition, 309
Specimens
collection, 54-56, 101, 128. *See also* Virology
culture, 101-103
diagnostic tests, 104
transport/shipping, 103-104
types, 103
Speed, definition, 192
Spencer suture removal scissors, 401
Spermatozoa, definition, 229
Spherocyte, definition, 52
Spinal cord, 11-12
compression, evaluation, 498
Spindle cell tumors, 62
Spleen, 16
sonographic appearance, 199
tissue samples, 70
Sponge forceps, 401
Spongy bone (cancellous bone), 7
Sporicide, definition, 172
Sporocyst, definition, 95
Sporozoite, definition, 95

Springing heifer, definition, 285
Squamous cell carcinoma, 446t, 501
Squamous epithelium, 5
Square knot, 161f
    usage, 160
Squash preparation, 58f
    modification, 58f
Squeeze chute, definition, 163
Squeeze pens, usage. *See* Pigs
SS. *See* Salmonella-Shigella
SSA. *See* Sulfosalicylic acid
SST. *See* Serum separator tube
Stability (absence), care quality (compromising), 547
Staff meetings, usefulness, 545
Staining techniques. *See* Cytology
Stains
    types, 59
    usage. *See* Cytology
Stallion, 215
    examination, 215
    feeding, 283
    libido/manner, 216
Stanchion, definition, 163
Standing part, definition, 163
*Staphylococcus* spp., 105-106
Starfish method. *See* Slide preparation
Starfish preparation, 59f
Starter pigs, 279
Starvation, 277
Stationary anode, 36
Steamed autoclave, time length, 408
Steam sterilization
    temperature/pressure chart, 169t
    usage. *See* Viruses
Steatitis, definition, 261
Steatorrhea, definition, 124
Steer, definition, 229
Stereotypical behavior, 241
Sterilant, definition, 172
Sterile areas, specimen type, 101
Sterile assistant surgical scrub, 410
Sterile surgical assistant, functions, 411
Sterilization. *See* Sanitation/sterilization/disinfection
    monitors, types, 407-408
    quality control, 171
Sterilize, definition, 172
Sterilized packs, storage times (recommendation), 170t
Sterilizing heat sources, usage, 99
Steroid inhibitors, list, 386t
Steroids, list, 386t
Stimulants, list, 381t, 382t
Stocks, definition, 163
Stomach, 15
    anatomy/physiology, 277
    sonographic appearance, 200
    tube, usage, 472
Stomatitis (mouth rot), 322, 501
Stomatocytes, 38f
Strangles *(Streptococcus equi)*
    management, 463-464
    rule out, 463-464
    vaccination, 458t
Streaking, goal, 102f

*Streptococcus* spp., 105
Stress management, 551
Striated muscles. *See* Skeletal muscles
Structure mottle, definition, 192
Struvite (magnesium ammonium phosphate/triple phosphate), 36
Stud, 213
    examination, 213
Subclinical, definition, 132
Subcutaneous (SC) drug route, 417
Subcutaneous (SC) fluid administration, 419
Subcutaneous (SC) injections, 417
    usage, 456
Subcutaneous (SC) tissues, lesions (collection/evaluation), 64
Subgingival plaque, removal, 496
Subject contrast, 182
    definition, 192
Subject densities, 183f
Submucosa, 14
Subordinate signaling, 232
Sub-unit, definition, 141
Successive approximation, 241
Suckling foals, 282
Suction tips, 405
Sulcular fluid, 492
Sulfosalicylic acid (SSA) turbidometric test, 30
Suppurative, definition, 71
Supragingival calculus, removal, 496
Supravital staining, definition, 52
Surface sampling, 171
Surgeon, surgical scrub, 410
Surgeon's knot, 161f
Surgery, definition, 447
Surgical gowns, sterility (consideration), 411
Surgical hair removal, completion, 408
Surgical instruments, 400-406
    parts, 401f
Surgical milk solution, instrument placement, 406
Surgical needles, 405
Surgical preparation
    glossary, 412
    learning outcomes, 400
    review questions, 412
Surgical scrub
    procedure, 409
    variations, 410
Suture material, 405-406
Swab specimen, 101
Swab technique, usage, 55
Sweet itch, definition, 141
Swine
    dysentery *(Treponema hyodysenteriae)*, 477
    energy requirements, 278
    feeding, 278
    feed sources, 278
    grains, preparation/feeding, 278
    life stages, 279
    minerals, 278
    nutrition, disease (relationship), 279
    nutritional requirements, 278
    protein/amino acids, 278
    vitamins, 278
    water, usage, 278

Sympathetic nerve fibers, 12
Sympathy communication, 554
Synarthrosis, 8
Synovial fluid, evaluation, 68
Synovial joints, types, 10t
Synovial structure, 9
Synthetic colloids, administration, 363
Synthetic nonabsorbable suture material, 406
Synthetic suture material, 406
Synthetic T$_3$, supplementation, 385
Synthetic T$_4$, supplementation, 385
Syrian hamster *(Mesocrietus auratus)*, 294-295
    antibiotic sensitivity, 295
    behavioral/physiological characteristics, 294
    breeding considerations, 294
    endoparasites/ectoparasites, 295
    handling/restraint, 289
    health conditions, 295
    lymphocytic choriomeningitis (LCM), 295
    pain/distress, signs, 295
    pneumonia, 295
    research, origin/uses, 294
    *Salmonella* spp., 295
    sampling, 294-295
    Tyzzer's disease *(Clostridium piliforme)*, 295
    wet tail, 303
Systematic desensitization, 241
Système International d'Unités (SI), 367
Systemic antacids, impact, 381
Systemic circulation (somatic circulation), 13-14
Systemic lupus erythematosus, 138
Systemic mycoses, 536t

T
Tablet dose calculation, 394-395
Tachypnea, result, 357
Tail, bandaging, 444
Tail deflection, definition, 229
Tail docking, definition, 229
Tail tie, usage. *See* Horses
Tangible products, marketing, 554
Tankage, definition, 285
Tapeworm infection, parasitic zoonosis, 534-535t
Taste, 22
Taurine, definition, 261
TD. *See* Transdermal
TDNs. *See* Total digestible nutrients
Tears
    formation, 433
    function, 433
Teaser bitch, 213
Technical errors. *See* X-ray film
Technique chart, development. *See* X-ray film
Teeth
    anatomical system, 493
    anatomy, 490-492
        illustration, 491f
    animal positioning, 496

Teeth *(Continued)*
  charting, 496
  chip fracture, 502
  function, 493
  hand instruments, 493
  home care, 499-500
  human safety, 497
  impaction, 501
  instruments/equipment, sterility, 497
  microscopic grooves, removal, 496
  numbering, 493
  quadrants, 499t
  roots, triadan system (usage), 509
  safety/infection control, 497
  scaling, 495
  structure, 471-472
  supporting structures, 96f
  surface terminology, 492
  trauma, 501
  types, 503
Teeth, physical examination, 416
Telephone etiquette, inclusion, 544
Telephone systems, usage, 546
Temperature, anesthesia monitoring, 357-358
Temporal cues, 542
Tension pneumothorax, indication, 362
Test cross, 209
  definition, 229
Testes, cell population identification, 69
Testicles, 18
  description, 18
Tetanus
  antitoxin, 457t
  definition, 229
  rule out, 461-462
  vaccination, 457t
Tetracaine, usage, 387
Textile wrapping material, 408
TGE. *See* Transmissible gastroenteritis
T-helper lymphocytes, 135
Themocouples, usage, 171
Therapeutic Index (TI), definition, 369
Theriogenology
  glossary, 227-229
  learning outcomes, 207
  neonatal care, relationship, 211-227
  review questions, 229-230
Thermionic emission, definition, 192
Thermoluminescent dosimeter, definition, 192
Thermoregulation, reptilian/mammalian comparison, 319
Thiamine-deficiency polio (polioencephalo-malacia), 271, 274
Thiobarbiturate, usage, 547
Thioglycollate (THIO) broth, 101
  usage, 108-109
Thiopental, usage, 341-342
Third degree AV block, 354
Third-intention healing, 442
Thoma erythrocyte-diluting pipettes, usage, 45
Thoracic fluid, removal/evaluation, 67
Thoracocentesis, 55
  definition, 71

Thorax, bandaging, 444
Three-dimensional ultrasound, 198-199
Thrombocyte (platelet) evaluation, 50
  estimates, 50
Thrombocyte (platelet) number, decrease, 50
Thrombocytopenia, 50
  definition, 52
Thrombocytosis, 50
  definition, 52
Thrombolytics, effectiveness, 390
Throw, definition, 163
Thymus, 16
Thyroidectomy, option, 385
Thyroid function, clinical chemistry, 120-124
Thyroid hormone, 120
  drugs, impact (list), 387t
Thyroid medication, endocrine drug, 385
Thyroid stimulating hormone (TSH), 385
Thyroxine ($T_4$), 120
TI. *See* Therapeutic Index
Ticks, 440
Tidal volume, 17
Tiletamine, usage, 343
Time-gain compensation, 196
Time management, 551
Time-restricted meal feeding, 245
Tissues, 4-6
  biopsy, 55
  definition, 4
  drug, impact, 369
  origin, 62-64
  scraping/impression, 65
  types, 4-5
Titer, definition, 132
T lymphocyte, definition, 132
TM. *See* Transmucosal
TMR. *See* Total mixed ration
TNCC. *See* Total nucleated cell count
Tocopherol, definition, 285
Tolerance, definition, 132, 141
Tom, 211
Tonometry, usage, 437
Tonsils, 16
Tooth-supporting structure, 472
Topical drugs, 387-388
  absorption, problems, 387
  application, 387
Total digestible nutrients (TDNs), definition, 285
Total leukocyte counts, 46
Total mixed ration (TMR), definition, 285
Total nucleated cell count (TNCC)
  basis, 57f
  determination, 56
Total plasma protein (TPP), 45
  dehydration indicator, 419
Total protein, 50
  count, basis, 57f
  determination, 56
Total serum/plasma proteins, 116-117
Total serum protein (TSP), 116
Total solids (TS) meter, usage, 28-29
Toxic neutrophils, definition, 52
Toxic substances, emergencies, 512
Toxins, impact, 316

*Toxocara canis*, 96f
Toxocariasis, parasitic zoonosis, 535t
Toxoid, definition, 141
Toxoplasmosis, parasitic zoonosis, 535t
TPP. *See* Total plasma protein
Trachea, 16
Tracheal samples, collection/evaluation, 64
Tranquilizers
  list, 376t
  usage, 336
Transabdominal ultrasound, definition, 229
Transdermal (TD) administration, 387
Transducers, 195-196
  crystals, 195
  definition, 203
  types, 196
Transfaunation, definition, 285
Transfusion reactions, 423
  signs, observation, 363
Transgenic, definition, 229
Transgenic animals, 227-229
  definition, 309
Transitional epithelium, 23
Transmissible gastroenteritis (TGE) (porcine rotavirus), 477
Transmissible ileal hyperplasia, 295
Transmucosal (TM) administration, 387
Transtracheal washes, 56
  orotracheal technique, 56
  percutaneous technique, 56
Transudates
  classification, 96f
  definition, 71
Transurethral catheterization, 25-26
Transverse, definition, 203
Trematode
  definition, 95
  impact, 318
Triadan system, 508
  usage. *See* Teeth
Triage, 508-509
  definitions, 508
  patient categorization, 508-509
  systemic approach, 509
Trichobezoars (hairballs). *See* Rabbit
  definition, 309
Trichomoniasis, 318
Trichonomiasis. *See* Cattle
*Trichuris vulpis*, 96f
Triple phosphate. *See* Struvite
Trophozoite, definition, 95
Tropicamide, usage, 387
TruCut biopsy needle, usage, 447
True nucleus. *See* Eukaryote
Trypsin, 15
Trypsinlike immunoreactivity, 115
Trypticase soy agar (TSA), 100
Trypticase soy broth (TSB), 101
TS. *See* Total solids
TSH. *See* Thyroid stimulating hormone
TSP. *See* Total serum protein
Tuberculosis (TB), bacterial zoonosis, 528t
Tubes (media), 100-101
  definition, 110
Tularemia, bacterial zoonosis, 528t

T wave, 424
Twitch, definition, 163
Twitching, 271
Tyrosine, 36
Tyzzer's disease. *See* Mongolian gerbil;
 Mouse; Syrian hamster
Tzanck preparations, 55

U
Ultrasonic cleaner, usage, 406
Ultrasonic vibration, usage, 166
Ultrasoni scalers, sound wave conversion,
 494
Ultrasound (US), 189
 axial resolution, 196
 definition, 203
 diagnosis, 466
 display, 197
 equipment controls, 196
 examination, 199
 lateral resolution, 196
 machine, 195-196
 patient preparation, 199
 physics, 194
Umbilical evisceration, definition, 229
Underventilation, indication, 361
Unidirectional valves. *See* Anesthetic
 machine
United States Pharmacopeia (USP) sizing,
 406
Universal F-circuit. *See* Breathing circuits
Unopette dilution system, 46
Urea agar slant (UREA), 101
Urea toxicity, 272
Urea (urea nitrogen), product, 113-114
Uremic, definition, 261
Ureters, 17
 failure, 515t
Urethral tears, emergency, 515t
Uric acid, 34f, 36
Urinalysis, 24
 bibliography, 53
 components, 24
 glossary, 138
 learning outcomes, 24
 physical evaluation, 27
 preservation, 26
 review questions, 52-53
 sample deterioration, variation, 26t
 sample variables, 26
 specimen collection/handling, 24-29
  collection methods, 25
 test methods, influences, 26t
Urinary bladder, 17
 manual compression, 431
  indications, 431
  precautions, 431
  procedure, 431
Urinary system, physical examination, 417
Urinary tract, cytological evaluation, 69
Urination (micturition), 18
Urine
 blood, color interpretation, 32
 chemical components, 29-32
 color, 27
 concentration tests, 114

Urine *(Continued)*
 false-positive test outcomes, 114
 formation, timing, 25
 glucose, existence, 114
 illumination, reduction, 33
 microscopic evaluation, 32-36
 nitrite level, 32
 odor, 27-28
 pH, 29-30
 RBCs, presence, 31-32
 sample preparation, 32-33
 sediment
  cells, presence, 36
  components, 33, 34f
 specific gravity (SG), 28
  evaluation, methods, 28-29
  values, 29
 specimen, 102-103
 transparency/turbidity/cloudiness, 27
 urobilinogen, 116
 volume/output, terminology, 27
Urine protein-to-creatinine (UPC) ratio, 30
Urinometer, usage, 29
Urobilinogen, formation, 32
Urogenital system
 avian/mammalian comparison, 313
 lesions, collection/evaluation, 68
 reptilian/mammalian system, 319
Urolithiasis, definition, 228
Uroliths, 36
Uroperitoneum, definition, 229
U.S. Army retractors, 403
 illustration, 401
USP. *See* United States Pharmacopeia
Uterine caruncles, definition, 229
Uterine horns (uterus), 19
Uterine inertia, 222
 definition, 229
Uterine torsion, 221
 definition, 229
Uterus, sonographic appearance, 199
Uveitis, emergency, 520t

V
Vaccinations. *See* Equine
 side effects, 456
Vaccines
 adverse reactions, 140-141
 availability, 385
 difficulties, 139
 passive immunity production, 387
 precautions, 139-140
 protocol, 137, 140t
 role, 137
 types, 138-140
 usage, 385
Vagina (birth canal), 19
Vaginal cytology, 55
 characteristics, 69-70
Vagus indigestion, 476
Vallate, 22
Values/ethics, set (usage), 556
Vaporizers. *See* Nonprecision vaporizers;
 Precision vaporizers
 usage. *See* Anesthetic machine
Variable expressivity, definition, 229

Vascular infusion, usage, 482
Vas deferens (ductus deferens), 18
 function, 18
Vasodilators
 list, 380t
 usage, 378
Vectored, definition, 141
Veins, 14
Velocity, definition, 203
Velpeau sling, 445
 making, 445f
Venereal tumor, transmission (ability),
 62
Venipuncture, 420
 drugs, administration, 421
 equipment/supplies, 420
 procedure, 420-421
 restraint/handling, 420
Ventilation, 17
 anesthesia monitoring, 357
  techniques, 361
 concerns, 361
 indication. *See* Overventilation; Underventilation
Ventral direction, 7
Ventricular fibrillation, 427
Ventricular tachycardia, 427
Venules, 14
Verbal communication, 542. *See also* Nonverbal communication
Verbrugge forceps, 404-405
Vertebral formulas, 9t
Veterinary anatomic terminology, 186f
Veterinary dentistry
 glossary, 488-489
 learning outcomes, 471
 review questions, 176
Veterinary hospital, managerial tasks,
 547
Veterinary medicine, abbreviations (usage),
 397t
Veterinary Oral Health Council (VOHC),
 seal of approval, 258
 issuance, 500
Veterinary practice management, 546
Veterinary technician
 registration/licensing/certification, 559
 resources, 571
 role. *See* Medications; Small animal
  nursing
Veterinary Technician National Examination
 (VTNE), 558
Veterinary technology
 accomplishments, 558
 profession, 558
Vial gravitation flotation technique. *See*
 Feces
Vibriosis. *See* Sheep
Viral antibody free (VAR), definition,
 309
Viral antigen, presence, 129
Viral enteritis. *See* Ferrets
Viral rhinopneumonitis, management. *See*
 Equine herpesvirus
Viral zoonosis, 530-533t
Viremia, definition, 132

Viricidal, definition, 132
Virion, definition, 132
Virology
  composition/control, 126-128
  glossary, 131-132
  learning outcomes, 126
  nomenclature, 128
  prevention, 129-131
  review questions, 132-133
  samples
    in-clinic laboratory testing, 129
    submission, 128-129
  sampling techniques, 128
  specimens, collection, 128
Virucidal, definition, 172
Viruses
  acellularity, 126
  antigenic drift, capability, 139
  components, 127
  death, steam sterilization (usage),
    127
  envelope, absence. *See* Naked virus
  infections, 128
  limitation, 127-128
  lipid membrane, 126
  obligate intracellular parasites, 126
  size, variation, 126
Visceral muscle. *See* Smooth muscles
Vision, 21
Visual cues, 542
Vitamins
  functions, 248-250t
  nutrients, 180
Vitreous humor, 21
Vocal cues, 542
Voice box. *See* Larynx
Voice commands, usage, 147
Volatile anesthetic, brain concentrations,
  344
Volume replacement, 508
Voluntary muscle. *See* Skeletal muscles
Volvulus, definition, 95
Vomiting
  emetics, impact, 378
  problems, 316
VTNE. *See* Veterinary Technician National
  Examination
Vulva, 19

**W**

Walking dandruff, 440
Wasting syndrome, 276
Water, nutrients, 245
Water belly, 274, 284, 501
Water deprivation, test, 114
Waterfowl diet, 316
Wavelength. *See* Sound
  definition, 203
  inverse proportion. *See* Frequency
Waxy casts, 35
Weanlings, 282
Wedge smear, usage, 58
Weigh-in periods, scheduling, 256
Weight loss
  program, 256
  rate, 256

West Nile virus (meningomyeloencephalitis)
  rule out, 463
  vaccination, 458t
  viral zoonosis, 533t
Wethe, definition, 229
Wet tail. *See* Syrian hamster
Wet-to-dry dressings, 443
Wet-to-wet dressings, 443
Whelping, definition, 229
White blood cells (WBCs/leukocytes), 34f
  casts, 35
  definition, 52
  differentiation, 46
  evaluation, 46-49
  morphology, 47-49t
  presence, 33
  tests, 32
White marks. *See* X-ray film
White muscle disease, 272, 274
  nutritional myodegeneration, 475-476
Whitten effect, definition, 309
WHMIS. *See* Workplace Hazardous Materials Information System
Whole blood, components, 112-113
Winking, definition, 229
Wire-cutting scissors, 400
Wire twisters, 404-405
Working horse, feeding, 283
Workplace Hazardous Materials Information
  System (WHMIS), 550
  hazard communication standard, 550
Worn teeth, 501
Wound
  bandages, 468
  contamination, infection (contrast), 441
  debridement phase, 441
  healing, 441
    types, 442
  inflammatory phase, 441
  lavage, 442
  management, 441
  maturation phase, 442
  repair phase, 441
  treatment, 442-443
  types, 468
Written communication, 545
Written grievance, filing, 545
Wry mouth, 500

**X**

*Xenopus laevis. See* African clawed frog
X-linked dominant inheritance, 209
X-linked inheritance, 208
X-linked recessive, 209
X-ray equipment, 176
X-ray film
  automatic processing, 180
  black marks, 181b
  care, 179
  density (change), technical errors
    (impact), 182t
  filing, 179
  green areas, 181b
  manual processing pointers, 180
  screen systems, 179
  technical errors/artifacts, 183

X-ray film *(Continued)*
  technique chart, development, 183
  types, 178
  usage, 217
  white marks, 181b
X-ray machine, 176-177
  collimation, 176
  electrical circuits, 176
  grid, 176
    cross section, 177f
    types, 177
  high-voltage circuit, 176
  low-voltage circuit, 176
  rectification circuit, 176
  technique selection/control panel, 176
  timer switch, 176
X-ray production, 173-174
X-rays
  definition, 174, 192
  discovery, 174
  production, 174
  tissues, interaction, 186
X-ray tube, 174-176
  anatomy, 175f
  envelope, 175
  failure, causes, 176
  rating chart, 176
Xylazine, usage, 315

**Y**

Yankauer tips, 405
Yearlings, feeding, 282
Yeast, identification, 109-110
Yellow radiograph, 181b
Young dogs, nutritional requirements,
  251-252

**Z**

Zonary placentation, definition, 229
Zoonoses, 307, 325, 439
  definition, 95
  glossary, 538
  learning outcomes, 523
  listing, 307t
  review questions, 538-539
Zoonotic, definition, 110
Zoonotic internal parasites, 90t
Zoonotic potential, 218, 220
Zygote, definition, 95